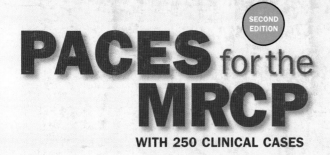

PACES for the
MRCP
WITH 250 CLINICAL CASES

SECOND
EDITION

For Elsevier
Commissioning Editor: Ellen Green/Pauline Graham
Development Editor: Helen Leng
Project Manager: Anne Dickie
Design Direction: Erik Bigland
Illustration Manager: Merlyn Harvey
Illustrator: Oxford Illustrators

PACES for the MRCP

WITH 250 CLINICAL CASES

Tim Hall MB ChB MRCP MRCGP DipMedEd

Consultant in Geriatric Medicine and Acute and
General (Internal) Medicine
Plymouth Hospitals NHS Trust, South West Peninsula Deanery,
Plymouth, UK

With forewords by

Professor Sir John Tooke DM DSc(Oxon) FRCP FMedSci

Dean, Peninsula College of Medicine and Dentistry,
Universities of Exeter and Plymouth, UK

Dr Jim Copper MA FRCP FRCP(Ed)

Honorary Consultant Physician, Plymouth Hospitals
NHS Trust, Plymouth, UK

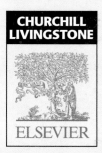

CHURCHILL
LIVINGSTONE

ELSEVIER

Edinburgh   London   New York   Oxford   Philadelphia   St Louis   Sydney   Toronto   2008

CHURCHILL
LIVINGSTONE
ELSEVIER

An imprint of Elsevier Limited

First edition 2003
Second edition 2008
  Reprinted 2009

ISBN: 978-0-443-10370-4

British Library Cataloguing in Publication Data
A catalogue record for this book is available from the British Library

Library of Congress Cataloging in Publication Data
A catalog record for this book is available from the Library of Congress

The
publisher's
policy is to use
**paper manufactured
from sustainable forests**

Printed in China

Contents

Preface   xi

Acknowledgements   xii

Forewords   xiii

Introduction

The Practical Assessment of Clinical Examination Skills (PACES)   2

PACES for the MRCP   2

References and further reading   8

Station 1
Respiratory and abdominal system

RESPIRATORY SYSTEM

Examination of the respiratory system   10

Cases

1.1   Chronic obstructive pulmonary disease   15

1.2   Consolidation   19

1.3   Dullness at the lung base   21

1.4   Pneumonia   21

1.5   Lung cancer   24

1.6   Pancoast's syndrome   28

1.7   Superior vena cava obstruction   29

1.8   Collapse/pneumonectomy/lobectomy   30

1.9   Bronchiectasis   30

1.10 Cystic fibrosis   32

1.11 Kartagener's syndrome   34

1.12 Tuberculosis   34

1.13 Idiopathic pulmonary fibrosis and diffuse parenchymal lung disease   37

1.14 Rheumatoid lung   42

1.15 Extrinsic allergic alveolitis   42

1.16 Asbestos-related lung disease and pneumoconiosis   43

1.17 Pulmonary sarcoidosis   44

1.18 Pulmonary hypertension   47

1.19 Cor pulmonale   49

1.20 Pulmonary embolism   49

1.21 Pleural effusion   54

1.22 Pleural rub   56

1.23 Pneumothorax   57

1.24 Obstructive sleep apnoea–hypopnoea syndrome   59

1.25 Lung transplant   60

ABDOMINAL SYSTEM

Examination of the abdominal system   62

Cases

1.26 Chronic liver disease   66

1.27 Jaundice   71

1.28 Ascites   73

1.29 Alcoholic liver disease   74

1.30 Viral hepatitis   75

1.31 Autoimmune hepatitis   79

1.32 Primary biliary cirrhosis   81

1.33 Genetic haemochromatosis   82

1.34 Wilson's disease   84

1.35 Hepatomegaly   85

v

Contents

1.36 Splenomegaly   86

1.37 Hepatosplenomegaly   86

1.38 Felty's syndrome   87

1.39 Abdominal mass   87

1.40 Crohn's disease   87

1.41 Ulcerative colitis   90

1.42 Enteric and urinary stomas   92

1.43 Carcinoid syndrome   93

1.44 Chronic myeloid leukaemia   95

1.45 Polycythaemia vera, myeloproliferative
      disorders and myelodysplasia   98

1.46 Chronic lymphocytic leukaemia   101

1.47 Lymphadenopathy and lymphoma   103

1.48 Polycystic kidney disease   106

1.49 Nephrotic syndrome   107

1.50 Renal transplant   107

References and further reading   110

Station 2
History-taking skills

INTRODUCTION TO HISTORY-TAKING SKILLS

Clinical reasoning   114

The traditional medical history model   114

**Incorporating the patient's perspective – ideas, concerns
and expectations**   114

**History-taking skills – the communication skills that make
history taking effective**   116

**The traditional model and communication skills – putting
these together**   119

Cases

RESPIRATORY PROBLEMS

2.1   Breathlessness   121

2.2   Asthma   125

ABDOMINAL PROBLEMS

2.3   Dyspepsia   129

2.4   Dysphagia   133

2.5   Abdominal pain   136

2.6   Altered bowel habit   139

CARDIOVASCULAR PROBLEMS

2.7   Prevention of cardiovascular disease and
      weight gain   144

2.8   Chest pain and angina   151

2.9   Acute coronary syndrome   155

2.10 Heart failure   161

2.11 Palpitations   166

2.12 Atrial fibrillation   170

2.13 Dyslipidaemia   175

2.14 Hypertension   182

NEUROLOGICAL PROBLEMS

2.15 Headache   188

2.16 Transient ischaemic attack   192

2.17 Weakness and wasting   196

2.18 Multiple sclerosis   198

2.19 Tremor   202

LOCOMOTOR PROBLEMS

2.20 Back pain and osteoporosis   205

2.21 Joint pain   211

EYE PROBLEMS

2.22 Visual loss   213

ENDOCRINE PROBLEMS

2.23 Type 1 diabetes mellitus   215

2.24 Type 2 diabetes mellitus   220

RENAL AND METABOLIC PROBLEMS

2.25 Acute renal failure   228

2.26 Chronic kidney disease and renal
      replacement therapy   233

2.27 Glomerulonephritis   239

2.28 Systemic vasculitis   244

2.29 Hypercalcaemia   248

2.30 Hyponatraemia   252

2.31 Poisoning and metabolic disturbance   256

HAEMATOLOGICAL PROBLEMS

2.32 Anaemia   260

2.33 Sickle cell disease and thalassaemia   264

2.34 Purpura   267

2.35 Haemophilia   271

2.36	Deep vein thrombosis	273
2.37	Thrombophilic tendency	276
2.38	Myeloma	279

INFECTIOUS DISEASE PROBLEMS

2.39	Human immunodeficiency virus infection	284

OTHER GENERAL MEDICAL AND ELDERLY CARE PROBLEMS

2.40	Falls and rehabilitation	291
2.41	Syncope	295
2.42	Seizures	300
2.43	Acute confusion	304
2.44	Mild cognitive impairment and dementia	307
2.45	Incontinence	314
2.46	Raised inflammatory markers	317
2.47	Polymyalgia and giant cell arteritis	325
2.48	Pyrexia and sepsis	327
2.49	Weight loss	333
2.50	Tiredness	334
	References and further reading	336

Station 3
Cardiovascular and nervous system

CARDIOVASCULAR SYSTEM

Examination of the cardiovascular system		346
Cases		
3.1	Mitral stenosis	355
3.2	Mitral regurgitation	357
3.3	Aortic stenosis	359
3.4	Aortic regurgitation	361
3.5	Tricuspid regurgitation and Ebstein's anomaly	363
3.6	Other right-sided heart murmurs	364
3.7	Mixed valve disease	365
3.8	Mitral valve prolapse	365
3.9	Prosthetic valves	367
3.10	Permanent pacemaker	368
3.11	Infective endocarditis	370
3.12	Congenital acyanotic heart disease	373
3.13	Cyanotic heart disease	375
3.14	Hypertrophic (obstructive) cardiomyopathy	375
3.15	Pericardial rub and pericardial disease	378

NERVOUS SYSTEM

Examination of the nervous system – overview		380
Examination of the cranial nerves		380
Examination of higher cortical function and specific lobes		387
Examination of speech and language		389
Examination of coordination		390
Examination of power and sensation – overview		392
Examination of the upper limbs		397
Examination of the lower limbs		402
Examination of gait		406
Cases		
3.16	Visual field defects	406
3.17	Ocular nerve lesions	407
3.18	Internuclear ophthalmoplegia	409
3.19	Nystagmus	411
3.20	Ptosis	412
3.21	Large pupil	413
3.22	Small pupil	414
3.23	Horner's syndrome	415
3.24	Cerebellopontine angle syndrome	416
3.25	Facial nerve palsy	418
3.26	Bulbar palsy	420
3.27	Anterior circulation stroke syndromes	421
3.28	Dysphasia and dysarthria	431
3.29	Pseudobulbar palsy	431
3.30	Agnosias and apraxias	432
3.31	Posterior circulation stroke syndromes	435
3.32	Parkinson's disease	438
3.33	Cerebellar disease	442
3.34	Spastic paraparesis and Brown–Séquard syndrome	443
3.35	Syringomyelia	446
3.36	Absent ankle jerks and extensor plantars	447

Contents

3.37 Motor neurone disease   449

3.38 Cervical myeloradiculopathy   451

3.39 Cauda equina syndrome   452

3.40 Carpal tunnel syndrome (median nerve lesion)   454

3.41 Ulnar nerve lesion   455

3.42 Radial nerve lesion   457

3.43 Wasting of the small (intrinsic) muscles of the hand   459

3.44 Common peroneal nerve lesion   460

3.45 Peripheral neuropathy   461

3.46 Charcot–Marie–Tooth disease and hereditary neuropathies   468

3.47 Guillain–Barré syndrome   469

3.48 Myasthenia gravis   472

3.49 Myopathy and myositis   474

3.50 Myotonic dystrophy   479

References and further reading   482

Station 4
Communication skills and ethics

INTRODUCTION TO COMMUNICATION SKILLS AND ETHICS

Communication skills   486

Ethics   487

Cases

DISCUSSING CLINICAL MANAGEMENT

4.1 Explaining a diagnosis   488

4.2 Explaining an investigation   489

4.3 Discussing treatment   492

4.4 Discussing management, prognosis and possible complications in a patient with multiple problems   494

4.5 Discussing diagnostic uncertainty   496

4.6 Discussing risk and treatment effect   497

4.7 Negotiating a management plan for a chronic disease/long-term condition   500

4.8 Encouraging concordance with treatment and prevention   502

COMMUNICATION IN SPECIAL CIRCUMSTANCES

4.9 Cross-cultural communication   505

4.10 Communicating with angry patients or relatives   506

4.11 Communicating with upset or distressed relatives   508

4.12 Discharge against medical advice   509

4.13 Delayed discharge   511

BREAKING BAD NEWS

4.14 Cancer – potentially curable   514

4.15 Cancer – probably incurable   516

4.16 Cancer – patient not fit for active treatment   518

4.17 Chronic disease   520

4.18 Discussing an acutely terminal situation with relatives   522

CONFIDENTIALITY, CONSENT AND CAPACITY

4.19 Legal points in confidentiality   524

4.20 Breaching confidentiality when a third party may be at risk   526

4.21 Breaching confidentiality in the public interest   527

4.22 Confidentiality when talking with relatives and other third parties   529

4.23 Consent for investigation or treatment   530

4.24 Consent and capacity   533

4.25 Refusal of consent   537

4.26 Deliberate self-harm   540

END OF LIFE ISSUES

4.27 Resuscitation-status decision-making – discussion with patient   543

4.28 Resuscitation-status decision-making – discussion with relative   547

4.29 Appropriateness of intensive therapy unit transfer   548

4.30 Withholding and withdrawing life-prolonging treatments – antibiotics and drugs   550

4.31 Withholding and withdrawing life-prolonging treatments – artificial hydration and nutrition   553

4.32 Percutaneous endoscopic gastrostomy feeding   556

4.33 Palliative care   558

4.34	Advance directives/decisions	561
4.35	Persistent vegetative state	563
4.36	Brainstem death	565
4.37	Discussing live organ donation	568
4.38	Requesting an autopsy (post mortem)	569

CLINICAL GOVERNANCE

4.39	Critical incident	572
4.40	Managing a complaint and the question of negligence	575
4.41	Fitness to practise – poor performance in a colleague	578
4.42	Fitness to practise – misconduct in a colleague	580
4.43	Fitness to practise – health problems in a colleague	582
4.44	Recruitment to a randomised controlled trial	584

OTHER COMMUNICATION, ETHICAL AND LEGAL SCENARIOS

4.45	Genetic testing	589
4.46	HIV testing	590
4.47	Needlestick injury	591
4.48	Medical opinion on fitness for anaesthesia	593
4.49	Fitness to drive	595
4.50	Industrial injury benefits	596
References and further reading		598

**Station 5
Skin, locomotor system, eyes, endocrine system**

SKIN

Examination of the skin		600
Cases		
5.1	Psoriasis	600
5.2	Dermatitis	605
5.3	Lichen planus	607
5.4	Blistering skin disorders	608
5.5	Facial rash	612
5.6	Scleroderma, vitiligo and autoimmune skin disease	617

5.7	Oral lesions	619
5.8	Nail lesions	620
5.9	Shin lesions	621
5.10	Neurofibromatosis	625
5.11	Tuberose sclerosis	627
5.12	Neoplastic skin lesions	628
5.13	Skin vasculitis	630
5.14	Xanthomata and xanthelasmata	631
5.15	Skin and soft tissue infection	632

LOCOMOTOR SYSTEM

Examination of the joints – overview		635
Examination of the hands and arms		635
Examination of the legs		640
Examination of the spine		642
Cases		
5.16	Rheumatoid hands and rheumatoid arthritis	643
5.17	Ankylosing spondylitis and spondyloarthropathies	652
5.18	Systemic lupus erythematosus	655
5.19	Scleroderma	659
5.20	Crystal arthropathy	662
5.21	Osteoarthritis	664
5.22	Paget's disease	666
5.23	Marfan's syndrome	668
5.24	Ehlers–Danlos syndrome	670
5.25	Osteogenesis imperfecta	671

EYES

Examination of the eyes		673
Cases		
5.26	Diabetic retinopathy	675
5.27	Hypertensive retinopathy	678
5.28	Swollen optic disc and papilloedema	679
5.29	Optic atrophy	680
5.30	Chorioretinitis	682
5.31	Retinitis pigmentosa	682

Contents

5.32 Central retinal vein occlusion   683

5.33 Central retinal artery occlusion   684

5.34 Retinal detachment and vitreous
      haemorrhage   685

5.35 Drusen and age-related macular
      degeneration (asteroids)   686

5.36 Angioid streaks   688

5.37 Myelinated nerve fibres   688

5.38 Glaucoma   689

5.39 Cataracts   690

5.40 Uveitis and red eye   691

ENDOCRINE SYSTEM

Examination of the thyroid   693

Cases

5.41 Hyperthyroidism and Graves' disease   693

5.42 Hypothyroidism   697

5.43 Goitre and neck lumps   699

5.44 Hypopituitarism   700

5.45 Acromegaly   703

5.46 Cushing's syndrome   705

5.47 Hypoadrenalism and Addison's disease   707

5.48 Hirsutism and polycystic ovarian syndrome   711

5.49 Hypogonadism and gynaecomastia   712

5.50 Pseudohypoparathyroidism   713

References and further reading   714

Appendix – 100 tips for passing PACES

Before PACES   716

On the day of PACES   716

After PACES   719

Index   721

Preface

The aim of this book is to help you pass PACES.

The real challenge was to produce a book containing all of the information that candidates might be asked, and yet be concise. Whilst candidates invariably 'just want to pass the exam', a broad grasp of relevant clinical medicine favours candidates in PACES, particularly when faced with examiners' questions. The remit of cases and examiners' questions is far reaching, and most candidates ask how to 'prepare' for PACES rather than how to 'cram' for it.

This book, therefore, remains a textbook for PACES with explanations of why things are so, rather than a series of steps or lists to be learnt by rote. The aim is to promote deeper learning, and so more ready recall of information 'in the heat of' the exam. Most candidates find that time in the exam goes fleetingly fast, but those who perform more strongly are those who have prepared widely, practised their examination skills thoroughly and envisaged lots of potential questions; the one or two questions that are then asked in each case are then answered with 'second nature' confidence. There is certainly more rather than less information needed to pass PACES in this book, but candidates who know more usually pass!

Following extensive feedback from candidates and examiners a number of new features have been introduced into this second edition. The most obvious changes are a substantial increase in the number of clinical images and illustrations, and the use of full colour throughout.

My editor, Ellen Green, and the team at Elsevier have done a remarkable job in producing a book that is very easy to navigate. There are now 50 cases in each station, and the format throughout is consistent and logical. The ease of orientation makes it a lot easier for you to skip through areas where you feel confident, and linger in areas where you feel lost.

This second edition of *PACES for the MRCP* has been fully rewritten and updated to complement a now established exam. And with the emphasis in medical schools increasingly on problem-based learning and outcome-based assessment, this book should continue to appeal to aspiring medical students seeking a case-based textbook of medicine.

PACES provides valid, reliable evidence of attainment in knowledge, clinical skills and behaviour, and passing it remains essential for career progression in the new era of specialty training; it is a mandatory requirement for achievement of the Certificate of Completion of Training and a key informer for allocation of specialist training posts. A marking scheme based on competencies and a new format for Station 5 (enabling a number of competencies to be assessed – focused history taking, focused examination and the interpretation and discussion of findings) are proposed, but the basic format of the exam, and its attainment as a necessary hurdle, seem here to stay.

Whilst it is likely that fine-tuning of the assessment process will continue in years to come, let me worry about that and update future editions accordingly. Your job is to see patients in preparation for the exam. This book is the map. The adventure is yours!

Good luck.

Tim Hall

Acknowledgements

As ever, I am indebted to an awful lot of people.

I am hugely grateful to all patients who kindly agreed to appear in this book; I am equally grateful to all consultant colleagues who agreed for their patients to participate, and I am equally grateful to the Hospital Trusts who gave their permission – Grampian Royal Hospitals Trust (Aberdeen Royal Infirmary), Plymouth Hospitals NHS Trust (Derriford Hospital), South Devon Healthcare Trust (Torbay Hospital) and Royal Devon and Exeter Foundation Trust. Particular mention should go to Keith Duguid, Head of Aberdeen's Department of Medical Illustration, Trevor McCausland at Derriford, Graham Slocombe at Royal Devon and Exeter, and Pete Worlledge at Torbay. Pete Worlledge and his secretary Jill Chalk gave an extraordinary amount of help and patience that was hugely appreciated.

I am indebted to all those colleagues who have inspired and taught me over the last few years, whose collective wisdom is distilled strongly into this text. I particularly thank Dr Jim Copper, Dr Jamie Fulton, Dr Richard Warrell, Dr Salim Mahadik, Dr Garry Kendall, Dr Peter Sleight, Dr Chris Uridge, Dr Karen Broadhurst, Dr Vaughan Pearce, Dr Martin James, Dr Mike Jeffreys, Dr Susie Harris, Dr Anthony Hemsley, Dr Jane Sword, Dr Doug MacMahon and Dr Chris Bellamy for their teaching and example.

I am very grateful also to Dr Carolyn McNeill, Dr Bethia Bradley, Dr Sophia Bratanow and Dr Yvonne Mukasa for comprehensive feedback on the first edition.

I remain, of course, grateful to all those acknowledged in the production of the first edition, paving the way to this one.

Enormous thanks to Frances Kelly (my agent), Ellen Green (formerly Commissioning Editor at Elsevier), Helen Leng (Development Editor) and the production team at Elsevier. I am grateful for permission from Elsevier to reproduce Figs 1.51, 1.52 and 3.2 from Douglas G, Nicol F, Robertson C (2005) *Macleod's Clinical Examination*, 11e, and adapt the following figures from the same book: Figs 1.2A,C, 1.3B, 1.4, 1.37, 1.38, 1.58, 3.3, 3.4, 3.21, 3.22, 3.23, 3.24, 3.28, 3.30, 3.31B, 3.32, 3.38, 3.39, 3.69, 5.37 and 5.38 and some figures in Tables 5.27 and 5.30. Further sincere thanks to Gillian Whytock and the team at Pre-press Projects; her unfailing energy, efficiency, patience and attention to detail was hugely appreciated.

Special thanks to Dr Claire Todd, Dr Paul Hancock, Ms Deborah Howland, Reverend Bill Anderson, Mr G. Oat and my family for their unique support.

Forewords

Society expects its doctors to be confident and competent in their clinical skills – and to aspire to continually better themselves in this regard. Society also expects that through appropriate examinations such skills are assured. PACES is one such examination that has been carefully crafted to provide such assurance. It is well known in educational circles that 'assessment drives learning', and thus a comprehensive treatise on PACES, such as this book represents, provides a crucial framework for the necessary skills and knowledge.

The challenge for any trainee doctor is to build on those skills and knowledge whilst involved in very significant service provision. In many ways such experiential learning is aided by the cases – the people with the illnesses and their reactions to them – who are not only rich sources of insight through their narrative but also provide the hooks upon which to hang an understanding of the biology of medicine. For this reason I commend the approach taken in PACES for the MRCP, firmly rooting the content knowledge in 250 carefully considered cases.

The MRCP remains an important milestone for trainee physicians. I recommend this book to candidates and I am confident that it will aid preparation for the assessment. I only wish that I had had access to similar material at that stage!

Professor Sir John Tooke

Medicine is not an exact science, and never will be. This is not because of any inherent variability in disease processes that prevents their rational scientific dissection, but the inherent variable factor in their host, man. That factor is the interplay between mental, physical and, arguably, spiritual facets that makes a disease episode unique to the individual affected, at once a challenge and a stimulus to the clinician.

One of the strengths of this book is that, although presenting a comprehensive account of clinical medicine in an exceptionally lucid format suitable for a wider audience than the PACES candidates for which it was originally intended, it places emphasis, in the sections on Stations 2 and 4 especially, on the interaction between clinician and patient that is at the heart of successful management of a disease process. Written with clarity, compassion and insight, these sections are a key to building trust and rapport between patient and doctor, as vital in practice as in the examination.

The above qualities also give a guide to the character of Tim Hall, whose wide experience in primary and secondary medical care contributes not only to his medical expertise but also to his evident skills in communication and education. This book is an excellent guide to success in the PACES section of the MRCP(UK) examination, in that its study will lead to a progressive enhancement of skills rather than simply acting as a reference text. Indeed, it may be used on this basis with value by students of medicine at any level, and that this is so is a tribute to the author.

Dr Jim Copper

Introduction

THE PRACTICAL ASSESSMENT OF CLINICAL EXAMINATION SKILLS (PACES)

PACES comprises a series of timed assessment stations where various competencies are tested by examiners with an objective marking scheme. Its main strength is in minimising bias, and it has been shown to have validity, reliability and relative practicality. The aims of PACES are to ensure that candidates are able to:

- Examine and detect the presence or absence of physical signs
- Interpret physical signs
- Make appropriate diagnoses
- Develop and discuss emergency, immediate and long-term management plans
- Demonstrate the clinical skills of history taking
- Communicate clinical information to colleagues, patients or their relatives
- Discuss ethical issues

Structure

There are five stations, each timed at 20 minutes (Fig. 1).

The start and finish of each station is signalled by a bell, although it is the duty of examiners to indicate the passing of time during each station. A different pair of examiners is at each station. One examiner takes the lead in conduct-

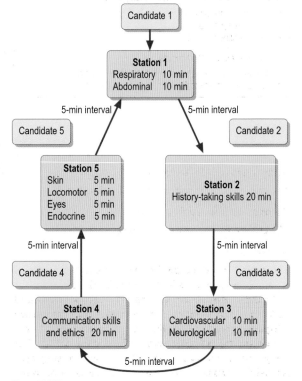

Fig. 1 PACES carousel.

Candidate 1

Station 1
Respiratory 10 min
Abdominal 10 min

5-min interval

5-min interval

Candidate 5

Candidate 2

Station 5
Skin   5 min
Locomotor   5 min
Eyes   5 min
Endocrine   5 min

Station 2
History-taking skills 20 min

5-min interval

5-min interval

Candidate 4

Candidate 3

Station 4
Communication skills
and ethics   20 min

Station 3
Cardiovascular 10 min
Neurological   10 min

5-min interval

ing the examination with the first candidate, the other examiner conducts the next, and so on. There is a five-minute seated interval between stations.

The two system stations (1 and 3)

After the five-minute interval, an examiner takes the candidate to the station and provides a written instruction for the first case. The response involves the relevant examination of the system and questions from the examiners about investigation and management of the clinical problem. Candidates should aim to complete their examination by around six minutes, and examiners may prompt at the five-minute point if that looks unlikely; this is a change from the previous situation whereby if at seven minutes the clinical examination had not been completed the examiner warned the candidate that they should finish to allow time for discussion. At 10 minutes the second examiner starts the second case at the second substation exactly as above.

Stations 2 and 4

The candidate receives a general practitioner's (GP) letter or case scenario to read during the five-minute interval. Notes may be made on paper provided. At the bell, the candidate enters the examination room. The interview with the patient/subject lasts for 14 minutes and includes history taking at Station 2 and some form of counselling or advising at Station 4. Examiners advise candidates when there are two minutes remaining (i.e. at 12 minutes). At 14 minutes the patient/subject leaves the room and the candidate is given one minute to gather his or her thoughts. The examiners may then invite the candidate to summarise the important features in the remaining five minutes. At Station 2 the examiners will ask about the implications of problems identified and strategies for management. At Station 4 the examiners are encouraged to identify ethical implications and discuss issues arising from the interview.

Station 5

After the five-minute interval one examiner takes the candidate to the station and gives written instructions for the first of the four systems. The response involves the relevant examination of the system and questions from the examiners about investigation and management of the clinical problem. The same follows for each of the four substations, and each examiner takes the lead for two of these, swapping after 10 minutes.

Examiners

There are 11 examiners for PACES, two at each station and one who oversees other matters such as the correct filling in of mark-sheets. New examiners are always paired with an experienced examiner. Each candidate is assessed by both examiners at each station; the examiners mark independently and at any one point one examiner assumes the lead role. At Stations 1 and 3 each examiner leads for one

10-minute substation then the roles are reversed for the next candidate. At Stations 2 and 4 examiners lead candidates in turn for 20 minutes. At Station 5 examiners lead the candidate for 10 minutes each during the 20 minutes and then the order is reversed for the next candidate.

Marking system – anchor statements and mark-sheets

Marking system

All marks are recorded on a four-point grading system as detailed on the PACES mark-sheets as:

- Clear pass (4 points)
- Pass (3 points)
- Fail (2 points)
- Clear fail (1 point)

Candidates are given a set of blank mark-sheets at the start of the examination (seven in total – two each for Stations 1 and 3 and one for each of the remaining stations) and hand appropriate sheets to the examiners at each station. Each mark-sheet is divided into sections to help the examiners make judgements about candidates more reliably and examiners are reminded to use only those statements relevant to the particular station. The overall mark (used in calculating the candidate's total score) is a global judgement of the candidate's performance, taking into account the sections of the form and *anchor statements*. Anchor statements are statements that assist in determining whether a candidate has achieved a clear pass, pass, fail or clear fail on a particular criterion. These are detailed on the MRCP website but the anchor statements that confer a clear pass are listed here because even although most candidates will fall below in many stations this is the standard you should aim for:

- *System of examination* – examines thoroughly and systematically
- *Language and communication skills* – talks to patient in a structured but flexible manner, using intelligible language and avoiding jargon
- *Confidence and rapport* – displays confidence, rapport and empathy
- *Clinical method* – demonstrates correct and comprehensive clinical method and skills, eliciting the correct physical signs
- *Discussion and appreciation of patient's concerns* – discusses clinical issues sensibly, spontaneously and with confidence, while able to negotiate and acknowledge areas of doubt/ignorance. Shows awareness of patient concerns
- *Clinical thinking* – clear, appropriate and professional

Clinical examination stations

The criteria for these stations are outlined in Box 1.

Box 1 Criteria for the clinical examination stations

Physical examination
- The criteria relate to the system of examination

Identification and interpretation of physical signs
- Identifies abnormal physical signs correctly
- Interprets signs correctly
- Makes correct diagnosis

Discussion
- Familiar with appropriate investigation and sequence
- Familiar with appropriate further therapy and management

   Note that for Stations 1 and 3, there are separate mark-sheets for each system but for Station 5 there is only one mark-sheet and each system is judged on the three main headings.

Box 2 Criteria for the history-taking skills station

Data gathering in the interview
- Elicits presenting complaints, documents in logical and systematic way and includes systems review
- Enquires about past medical history/family/alcohol/smoking/treatment history
- Follows leads about relevant psychosocial factors
- Appropriate verbal and non-verbal (eye contact, posture etc.) responsiveness, good balance of open and closed questions, appropriate pace

Interpretation and use of information gathered
- Checks information is correct with patient
- Able to interpret history
- Able to create a problem list

Discussion related to the case
- Able to discuss the implications of the patient's problems
- Able to discuss strategies for solving the problems

History-taking skills station

The criteria for this station are outlined in Box 2.

Communication skills and ethics station

The criteria for this station are outlined in Box 3.

Mark-sheets

The overall mark for the PACES examination is out of a possible 56 points, as illustrated in Table 1.

   An initial Royal College consensus was that a mark of 42/56 (75%) was likely to be necessary to demonstrate adequate competence in the core skills assessed at each station and thus pass the examination (equivalent to a 3 at every station or substation) but this has subsequently been revised downwards because the examination proved more difficult than at first anticipated.

Box 3 Criteria for the communication skills and ethics station

Communication skills – conduct of interview

- Introduces self to patient and explains role clearly
- Agrees purpose of the interview with the patient
- Puts the patient at ease and establishes good rapport
- Explores patient concerns, feelings and expectations – demonstrates empathy, respect and non-judgemental attitude
- Prioritises problems and redirects interview appropriately

Exploration of problem and problem negotiation

- Appropriate questioning style – generally open-ended to closed as the interview progresses
- Provides clear explanations (jargon-free) that the patient understands
- Agrees a clear course of action
- Summarises and checks the patient's understanding
- Concludes the interview appropriately

Discussion related to the case

In relation to the clinical scenario the candidate demonstrates knowledge of the relevant ethical and legal principles and appropriate attitudes in making decisions

- Knowledge of ethical principles
- Understanding of legal constraints applicable to case
- Provides adequate reasoning as appropriate to case

Documents and setting of cases for Station 2

The documents include candidate, patient and examiner information sheets. The format of these information sheets is reflected in the format of the cases in Station 2 of this textbook, the template for which is outlined later in this chapter. Below is an outline of the information that candidates and patients receive and the information that examiners receive and expect.

Candidate information

- The *role of the candidate* (e.g. you are a doctor in the medical outpatient clinic/on the ward).
- The *name and age of the patient/subject*.
- The *scenario*. This is either a scenario or a referral letter from the patient's GP. This should be addressed to the doctor in the outpatient department or admissions unit and not to a location requiring specialist knowledge such as a neurology clinic. It should pose a question (e.g. asking for advice on diagnosis, investigation, drug therapy,

Table 1 Marking scheme for the PACES examination

Station	System		Examiner 1	Examiner 2
1	Respiratory	Physical examination	/4	/4
		Identification and interpretation of physical signs		
		Discussion related to case		
	Abdominal	Physical examination	/4	/4
		Identification and interpretation of physical signs		
		Discussion related to case		
2	History-taking skills	Data gathering in the interview	/4	/4
		Interpretation and use of information gathered		
		Discussion related to case		
3	Cardiovascular	Physical examination	/4	/4
		Identification and interpretation of physical signs		
		Discussion related to case		
	Neurological	Physical examination	/4	/4
		Identification and interpretation of physical signs		
		Discussion related to case		
4	Communication skills and ethics	Communication skills – conduct of interview	/4	/4
		Exploration and problem negotiation		
		Discussion related to case		
5	Skin Locomotor Eyes Endocrine		/4	/4
Total			/28 /56	/28

complications or specialist referral) so that a task is posed for the candidate. It should be brief, not providing all of the history but sufficient information to sustain a 14-minute interview. Aspects of the social, family and past medical history may be mentioned to allow candidates to explore these in more detail. Relevant examination findings and values of investigations (with normal ranges for less common investigations) may be given. The topic should not be esoteric or obscure and the candidate should be expected to have some knowledge of it. The candidate is invited to make notes on paper provided. The description of patients by their diagnoses should be avoided ('diabetic', 'epileptic') in favour of 'patients with diabetes . . .' Abbreviations are avoided wherever possible except universally accepted abbreviations such as ECG and CXR. Trade names of drugs should be avoided. The station should be seen as an exercise in information-gathering to reach a differential diagnosis. The content and instruction should not divert the candidate to predominantly engage in a communication skills exercise.

- A reminder of the *time allowed* and that the *examiners will warn candidates when 12 minutes have elapsed.*
- A reminder that the *candidate is not required to examine* the patient.

Patient/subject information

- Whether the patient/subject is *real* or *simulated*. The patient/subject should be trained in advance whether giving his or her own or a pre-determined history, and the scenario should not be so complex that a patient or surrogate could not play the role.
- The *scenario*. The information should include presenting complaint, systems review, drug history, social history (including occupational history, home life, smoking, alcohol, recreational drugs, sexual) and family history. Patients are requested not to withhold information but not to volunteer information that has not been appropriately sought.

Examiner information

- A good candidate is expected to take a history including a detailed social history and activities of daily living, and to particularly focus on the questions posed in the referral letter.
- At the end of the consultation the candidate should have discussed solutions to the problems posed by the case and have agreed a summary with the patient.
- A good candidate would also give the patient an opportunity to ask any further questions before closure.
- Examiners are encouraged to make a rough record of the consultation as it progresses, highlighting omissions, unresolved ambiguities and additional points 'not in the script'.
- Examiners should advise candidates when two minutes remain.

- The examiner is expected to ask the candidate whether they have formed a problem list or preferred diagnosis and to answer the questions in the GP's letter. Following discussion of the answers to these questions the discussion should explore the issues raised.
- To pass, the candidate must explore the following issues or make the following diagnoses . . . (listed are as many as are required for the 'just passing' candidate).

Documents and setting of cases for Station 4

These include candidate, patient and examiner information sheets. The format of these information sheets is reflected in the format of the cases in Station 4 of this textbook, the template for which is outlined later in this chapter. Below is an outline of the information candidates and patients receive and the information examiners receive and expect.

Candidate information

- A brief definition of the *problem* (e.g. breaking bad news).
- The *role of the candidate* (e.g. you are a doctor in the medical outpatient clinic/on the ward).
- The *name and age of the patient/subject*.
- The *scenario*. The scenario should reflect everyday clinical practice and not be too obscure or complex. It should not rely on detailed knowledge of one condition, investigation, current management or prognosis. It should be sufficiently detailed to sustain a 14-minute discussion and as comprehensible as possible such that the candidate does not engage primarily in a history-taking exercise but has enough information to communicate. It should have an ethical component because it may be difficult for examiners to sustain a discussion based solely on communication skills. The topic should be a universal problem applicable to global medicine and must not require detailed knowledge of UK law. Emotionally charged topics need not be avoided if the role-player is experienced in handling these although particularly sensitive issues such as sexual history may be best avoided. The scenario should clearly define the *task* for the candidate (e.g. explaining the meaning of a diagnosis).
- A reminder of the *time allowed and that the examiners will warn candidates when 12 minutes have elapsed.*
- A reminder that the *candidate is not required to examine* the patient.

Patient/subject information

- The *name and age* and whether the patient/subject is *real* or *simulated*. A member of medical or nursing staff, or an actor (role-player) may be used.

- The *scenario*. The role of the subject should be clear (e.g. wife of a patient). The scenario should include presentation of complaint, past history, systems review, family history, drug therapy, social history, agreed emotional responses, a list of concerns or questions the subject may have and the desired outcome and negotiated conclusion.

Examiner information

- A brief definition of the problem.
- Examiners have all three briefing sheets so there is no need for the scenario to be repeated here.
- Examiners should advise candidates when two minutes remain and how long is left if they finish early.
- A reminder that a good candidate is expected to have agreed a summary and plan of action with the subject before closure but nevertheless, in discussion, the examiners will usually ask the candidate (after one minute's reflection) to summarise the problems raised.
- A reminder that the candidate should be asked to identify the ethical and legal issues raised in the case and how they would address them (detailed or local legal knowledge is not required).
- A reminder that the candidate should recognise his or her limit in dealing with a problem and know when, and from where, to seek further advice and support (e.g. from a more senior member of the team).
- A list of what the candidate should be able and would be expected to do, and the desired outcome of the scenario.

PACES FOR THE MRCP

Stations 1, 3 and 5: the clinical examination cases

The clinical examination cases should reflect everyday clinical medicine, with less emphasis these days on esoteric conditions. However, an *important difference between these cases and real practice is that these cases bypass history taking and focus on clinical examination*:

- The ability to *examine* systems
- The ability to *recognise* signs
- The ability to *interpret* those signs
- The ability to *discuss* matters arising from the case

To help you prepare for Stations 1, 3 and 5, the cases in *PACES for the MRCP* follow a consistent approach. This approach is designed to structure your knowledge and sharpen your clinical skills to directly meet the needs of the PACES examination. The approach can also be used on the wards in preparation for PACES so that you are 'primed' for using it in the examination.

Instruction

An example of the type of written instruction for candidates is given for each case within each system.

Individual cases follow the Recognition–Interpretation–Discussion (RID) format:

Recognition

You are accustomed in practice to converging upon diagnoses through history taking, examination and investigations. In PACES, examination skills are paramount in eliciting diagnoses and patients tend to have diagnoses that are readily disclosed by examination. This is not always so in practice, and in some ways PACES requires the reverse of your approach in practice.

The first thing to do in the examination case is to work out what it is that you are being asked to look at. This book describes (in a form which can be easily recited to the examiners) the *clinical signs* that help you to decide this.

You will be looking at one of two broad abnormalities:

1. *A specific diagnosis* (e.g. rheumatoid arthritis)
2. *A pattern of signs for which there may be numerous differential diagnoses* (e.g. lung consolidation, chronic liver disease, Horner's syndrome, spastic paraparesis)

Interpretation

Recognising the abnormality is your first goal. To comfortably pass you must then attempt to further interpret your initial findings. You should *know what to do next before presenting your initial findings* and *decide how you are going to present all of your findings* to the examiners.

The important extra information to gather next and a framework for presenting it all (Box 4) is organised within one or more of four subheadings.

Confirm the diagnosis

This is important, especially if there is *diagnostic ambiguity*. For example, examining the elbows in a patient with 'rheumatoid hands' for nodules or psoriatic plaques may confirm or revise your initial impression.

What to do next – consider causes or assess other systems

Considering causes may be important in cases in which you have recognised a *pattern of signs for which there could be numerous differential diagnoses*. An example is to look for or tell your examiners that you would look for signs of a Pancoast's tumour if you find Horner's syndrome.

Assessing other systems may be important in cases where you have recognised a *specific diagnosis*. For example, if you diagnose rheumatoid hands you should consider the possible extra-articular features of

---

Box 4

You will not have time to examine for all the features given under the 'Interpretation' headings in this book. Many of the features can merely be reported to examiners as ones you would look for in practice. Most important is having a framework to guide you through examining and presenting.

It may seem artificial to separate signs under the headings 'Recognition', and 'Interpretation'. For example, you may have recognised aortic stenosis and during your initial examination elicited signs of severity. The 'Interpretation' section serves merely to organise these signs in a checklist, which aids thought gathering and subsequent presentation.

Furthermore, 'Interpretation' in this book does not always mean actively examining. Time may be more wisely spent demonstrating your wide knowledge than examining. The classic signs of acromegaly may be instantly recognisable, and a good candidate may proceed to check the blood pressure but find it more productive to tell the examiners that he/she would be alert to the risks of glucose intolerance, bitemporal hemianopia, obstructive sleep apnoea and colorectal cancer than spend all of his/her time examining the visual fields.

---

rheumatoid disease. There would not be time to examine for all of them, but this book outlines those your examiners would expect you to know. You might look briefly for one or two and mention some others.

Consider severity/decompensation/complications

In many cases it is important to determine if there are signs associated with increased morbidity and mortality. An example is aortic stenosis, for which there are established signs indicating severe disease.

It may be important to look specifically for signs of decompensation, such as for signs of hepatocellular failure in chronic liver disease.

Consider function

Awareness of the possible effects of a diagnosis on your patient's functional status is very important. For example, a patient with rheumatoid arthritis may have marked difficulty with grip and a patient with chronic lung disease may be housebound.

Discussion

The key to impressing examiners is in ever striving 'to go further'. Examiners prefer candidates who spontaneously present their findings and thoughts. Examiners are less certain of candidates from whom information has to be 'dragged'.

From an examiner's perspective you do two things in each case. Firstly, you *examine* your patient. Secondly, you *present* your findings. From your perspective you are doing a lot more. While examining you are looking for signs, deciding how to further interpret your findings and thinking about how you might present them. The recognition and interpretation framework in this book should aid both your examination of patients and your presentation to examiners. By adopting this framework of *diverging* from

your initially recognised findings and reporting more information to the examiners spontaneously, you will perform well. The examiners can interrupt at any point with questions but are less likely to do so early if you appear to have a structured approach. At some stage, however, examiners will ask you questions, and your presentation will merge into a discussion.

The discussion sections of each case in this book provide, through questions and answers, revision of important areas of 'MRCP medicine' you might be expected to discuss. You are expected to have a working knowledge of the causes, underlying pathophysiology, symptoms, investigation and further management of the wide range of conditions that you could encounter in PACES.

Questions and answers tends to be a more effective way of learning information than straight text. It is very easy to skim through pages of text thinking 'I know this' without really knowing it at all! Questions, on the other hand, make you think. The answers given in this book are sometimes quite long, often covering more than the examiners would expect (especially in the short time available) but have been designed to maximise your understanding of each disease. Remember that the emphasis in PACES is on common conditions, and that you even know which system you are being examined on. Recognising common conditions may not be especially discriminating. Rather, the examiners will be testing your wider knowledge about these common conditions.

Station 2: history-taking skills

The introduction in Station 2 gives details on developing history-taking skills. The template used for the 50 cases described in this station is as follows.

Candidate information

Role

You are a doctor in the medical outpatient clinic/on the ward about to see the patient below. Please read the letter from this patient's GP. You may make notes on the paper provided. When the bell sounds, enter the examination room to begin the consultation.

Scenario

> Dear Doctor
> Re: Mr/Mrs/Ms . . .
> Details of case . . .
> Yours sincerely

Please take a history from the patient (if you wish you may continue to make notes on the paper provided). Your examiners will warn you when 12 minutes have elapsed. You have 14 minutes to take a history from the patient followed by 1 minute of reflection. There will then follow

5 minutes of discussion with the examiners. Be prepared to discuss solutions to the problems posed by the case and how you might reply to the GP's letter. You are not required to examine the patient.

Patient/subject information

Details are given.

How to approach the case

Data gathering in the interview and interpretation and use of information gathered

There follows a list of areas to cover in the interview, under the following headings:

- Presenting problems and symptom exploration
- Patient perspective
- Past medical history
- Drug and allergy history
- Family history
- Social history

These are followed by a summarising box.

SUMMARY – ASSESSMENT AND PLAN

Although you are not required to close the interview with a summary, most candidates find that it is natural to do so, that it helps to organise their thoughts and that it is a springboard for inviting questions from the examiners. The summaries included here cover initial differential diagnoses, investigations and treatments, which in any event are the points likely to arise initially in the discussion.

Discussion

A series of questions and answers relating to the case are designed to improve your knowledge of the topic and equip you to answer the examiners' questions.

Station 4: communication skills and ethics

The introduction in Station 4 gives details on developing communication skills and understanding the principles of medical ethics. The template used for the 50 cases described in this station is as follows.

Candidate information

Role

You are a doctor in the medical outpatient clinic. Please read this summary.

Scenario

Re: Mr/Mrs/Ms . . .
Details of the problem(s) to be discussed
Your task(s) is/are to . . .

Your examiners will warn you when 12 minutes have elapsed. You have 14 minutes to communicate with the patient/subject followed by 1 minute of reflection. There will then follow 5 minutes of discussion with the examiners. Do not take the history again except for details that will help in your discussion with the patient/subject. You are not required to examine the patient/subject.

Patient/subject information

Details are given.

How to approach the case

Communication skills (conduct of interview, exploration and problem negotiation) and ethics and law

There follows a list of 10 points to cover in the interview.

Discussion

A series of questions and answers relating to the case are designed to improve your knowledge of the topic and equip you to answer the examiners' questions.

References and further reading

Dacre J, Besser M, White P. MRCP (UK) Part 2 Clinical Examination (PACES): a review of the first four examination sessions (June 2001–July 2002). Clin Med 2003; 3:452–459

Royal College of Physicians (UK). PACES Examiner Booklet. London: RCP; June 2004

Royal College of Physicians (UK). PACES Examination – Clinical Mark-sheets. London: RCP

Royal College of Physicians (London) www.rcplondon.ac.uk

Royal College of Physicians (Edinburgh) www.rcpe.ac.uk

www.mrcpuk.org

Station 1
Respiratory and abdominal system

RESPIRATORY SYSTEM
Examination of the respiratory system 10
Cases
1.1 Chronic obstructive pulmonary disease 15
1.2 Consolidation 19
1.3 Dullness at the lung base 21
1.4 Pneumonia 21
1.5 Lung cancer 24
1.6 Pancoast's syndrome 28
1.7 Superior vena cava obstruction 29
1.8 Collapse/pneumonectomy/lobectomy 30
1.9 Bronchiectasis 30
1.10 Cystic fibrosis 32
1.11 Kartagener's syndrome 34
1.12 Tuberculosis 34
1.13 Idiopathic pulmonary fibrosis and diffuse parenchymal lung disease 37
1.14 Rheumatoid lung 42
1.15 Extrinsic allergic alveolitis 42
1.16 Asbestos-related lung disease and pneumoconiosis 43
1.17 Pulmonary sarcoidosis 44
1.18 Pulmonary hypertension 47
1.19 Cor pulmonale 49
1.20 Pulmonary embolism 49
1.21 Pleural effusion 54
1.22 Pleural rub 56
1.23 Pneumothorax 57
1.24 Obstructive sleep apnoea–hypopnoea syndrome 59
1.25 Lung transplant 60

ABDOMINAL SYSTEM
Examination of the abdominal system 62
Cases
1.26 Chronic liver disease 66
1.27 Jaundice 71
1.28 Ascites 73
1.29 Alcoholic liver disease 74
1.30 Viral hepatitis 75
1.31 Autoimmune hepatitis 79
1.32 Primary biliary cirrhosis 81
1.33 Genetic haemochromatosis 82
1.34 Wilson's disease 84
1.35 Hepatomegaly 85
1.36 Splenomegaly 86
1.37 Hepatosplenomegaly 86
1.38 Felty's syndrome 87
1.39 Abdominal mass 87
1.40 Crohn's disease 87
1.41 Ulcerative colitis 90
1.42 Enteric and urinary stomas 92
1.43 Carcinoid syndrome 93
1.44 Chronic myeloid leukaemia 95
1.45 Polycythaemia vera, myeloproliferative disorders and myelodysplasia 98
1.46 Chronic lymphocytic leukaemia 101
1.47 Lymphadenopathy and lymphoma 103
1.48 Polycystic kidney disease 106
1.49 Nephrotic syndrome 107
1.50 Renal transplant 107

References and further reading 110

RESPIRATORY SYSTEM

Examination of the respiratory system

Inspection

General

- Introduce yourself, ensure that the patient is sitting comfortably at 45° and then stand back. Placing your hands behind your back is a good way to show you remember the importance of inspection.
- Look around the bedside for metered dose inhalers, nebulisers or sputum pots.
- Note any cachexia.
- Count the respiratory rate (tachypnoea, defined as a respiratory rate > 20 breaths/minute (normal is 12–20 breaths/minute, albeit arbitrary), is often the first sign of respiratory or haemodynamic compromise) and note if the patient is breathless at rest.

Listen

- Listen to the breathing with unaided ears, noting any of the sounds listed in Box 1.1.

Hands

- Look for tar staining, clubbing (Case 5.8), peripheral cyanosis or wasting. Clubbing very rarely progresses to hypertrophic pulmonary osteoarthropathy, characterised by swelling and tenderness around the wrists and ankles associated with toe clubbing.
- Feel the pulse while inspecting the hands to determine if it is bounding; note any flapping tremor.

Face

- Look for central cyanosis (best seen at the tongue).
- Look for pursed lip breathing.
- Note any Horner's syndrome.

Neck

- Look at the jugular venous pulse. This is raised and pulsatile in cor pulmonale but fixed in superior vena cava obstruction, the latter characteristically causing marked venous distension in the neck and sometimes distension of veins in the hands, the underside of the tongue and upper chest wall.
- Note any phrenic nerve crush scars in the supraclavicular fossae.

Chest

- Look at the the size and shape (Box 1.2) of the chest, and note any deformities (e.g. kyphoscoliosis, pectus carinatum, pectus excavatum), thoracotomy scars, radiotherapy field markings, telangiectasia or muscle wasting.
- Look at chest wall movement (upwards in emphysema; asymmetrical in fibrosis, collapse, pleural effusion or pneumothorax).
- Note any use of accessory muscles, including abdominal or scalene muscles, or intercostal indrawing.

Palpation

Neck

- Feel the trachea to determine any mediastinal shift (using the middle finger as the exploring finger and the index and ring fingers resting on the manubriosternum either side, Fig. 1.1) and note the approximate cricoid–suprasternal notch distance, decreased in hyperinflation from the normal three-finger breadths.
- Feel for cervical, supraclavicular and axillary lymph nodes, always from behind using flat fingers and not poking with fingertips.

Chest

- Start at the front or back (you are more likely to find signs at the back) but complete all of the front or back examination before moving to the other. Remember that the lower lobes occupy most of the

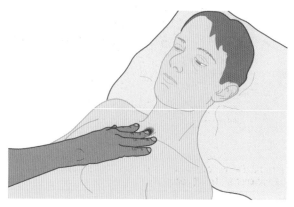

Fig. 1.1 Determining the position of the trachea.

Box 1.1 Sounds in respiratory disease you might hear before auscultation

- Expiration longer than inspiration (obstructive airways disease)
- Expiratory wheeze (obstructive airways disease)
- Inspiratory stridor (obstruction of upper airways, e.g. mediastinal mass, bronchial carcinoma)
- Clicks (bronchiectasis)
- Gurgling (airway secretions)

Box 1.2 Big or small chest?

As a simple rule, a 'big chest' (with a large anteroposterior diameter, little lateral expansion, and lifting of the rib-cage on inspiration) alerts you to COPD, while a 'small chest' alerts you to possible fibrotic lung disease.

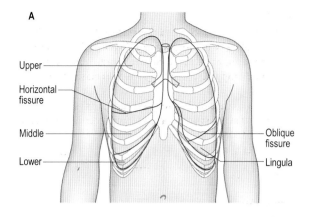

A

Upper

Horizontal
fissure

Middle

Lower

Oblique
fissure

Lingula

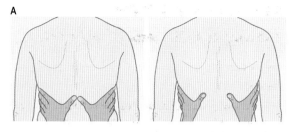

A

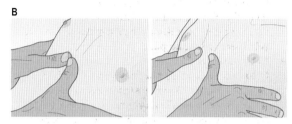

B

Fig. 1.3 Assessing chest expansion: (A) anterior, (B) posterior.

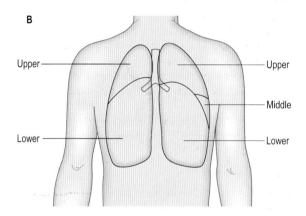

B

Upper

Lower

Upper

Middle

Lower

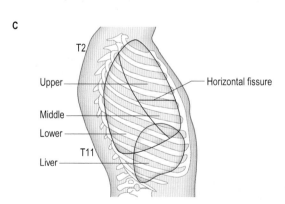

C

T2

Upper

Horizontal fissure

Middle

Lower

T11

Liver

Fig. 1.2 Surface markings of the lobes of the lungs: (A) anterior, (B) posterior, (C) lateral view.

posterior chest and the upper lobes occupy most of the anterior chest (Fig. 1.2).

- Examine chest expansion. For the inframammary area and for the back of the chest use a 'bucket handle' approach with your fingers in the intercostal spaces either side of the chest and your thumbs floating in the midline (Fig. 1.3). This allows the ribs to move outwards. For the supramammary area, where the ribs move predominantly upwards, place your hands on the chest wall with thumbs meeting.
- Tactile vocal fremitus gives the same information as vocal resonance and may be omitted.

Percussion

Percussion sites

- Percuss the supraclavicular areas, clavicles and chest on both sides (Fig. 1.4). Performing more than four or five levels of percussion is time consuming as a screen but percuss further to delineate any abnormality you find.

Percussion technique

- Compare right with left and superior with inferior (left → right at same level → right inferiorly → left at same level → left inferiorly → right at same level and so on).
- Ensure that the finger applied to the chest (left middle) is applied firmly, and aligning it with the ribs is preferable; the pad of the partly flexed percussing finger (right middle) should tap the middle phalanx of the chest finger lightly, springing away quickly after contact to avoid dampening of the note. This relaxed swinging motion should come from the wrist, not the forearm (see Fig. 1.4).
- Remember that the upper level of liver dullness is around the sixth rib in the right mid-clavicular line. Resonance below this level is a sign of hyperinflation. Cardiac dullness may also be elicited.

Auscultation

Auscultation is traditionally with the diaphragm, but the bell may not provoke as much extraneous sound from hairy chests and is able to get into the supraclavicular

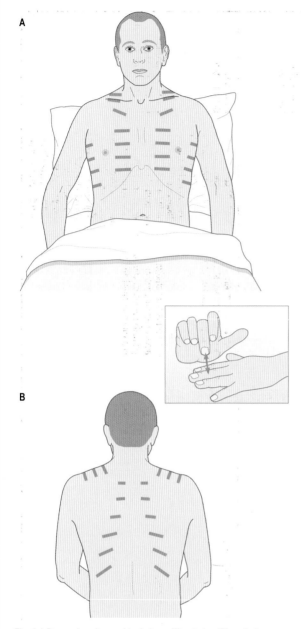

Fig. 1.4 Percussion sites and technique: (A) anterior, (B) posterior.

Vocal resonance

- Vocal resonance, like tactile vocal fremitus, represents the transmission of sound from the central airways to the chest wall. Sound transmission is enhanced through solid tissue (consolidation), provided the airways are patent, and attenuated through fluid (pleural effusion) compared with transmission through air (normal). The principles are as for bronchial breathing in consolidation and reduced breath sounds in a pleural effusion. Enhanced sound transmission in consolidation is analogous to the vibration of an earthquake that can be felt through the ground before it can be heard through the air. Attenuated sound in a pleural effusion is analogous to diving underwater, the sound of people on land suddenly muffled. 'Ninety-nine' is the conventional sound used to assess vocal resonance, but the intended nasal 'oi' is better demonstrated by 'neun-und-neunzig'.
- Whispering pectoriloquy, when whispered sounds are heard clearly, confirms consolidation because a whispered voice is clearly audible through solid lung. Aegophony is an unusual sign, in which compressed lung above a pleural effusion creates a high-pitched bleat from a conducted voice.

Additional ward tests

- Mention that you would perform ward spirometry and pulse oximetry as part of your examination.

Integration

Some patterns of important focal abnormalities are shown in Fig. 1.5.

Summary

A summary of the respiratory system examination sequence is given in the Summary Box.

SUMMARY BOX – RESPIRATORY SYSTEM EXAMINATION SEQUENCE

- From a distance look for bedside clues, look for cachexia and count the respiratory rate.
- Look at the hands for clubbing, cyanosis or wasting.
- Look at the face for pursed lip breathing or Horner's syndrome.
- Look at the jugular venous pulse.
- Look at the shape of the chest and chest wall movement and note any use of accessory muscles.
- Feel for tracheal deviation and feel for any lymphadenopathy.
- Assess chest expansion.
- Percuss for areas of dullness (consolidation, collapse, pleural effusion) or hyperresonance (hyperinflation, pneumothorax).
- Listen to breath sound quality (normal or vesicular) and intensity (reduced in consolidation, collapse, pleural effusion, hyperinflation, pneumothorax).
- Listen for added sounds (crackles, wheeze).
- Listen to vocal resonance (increased in consolidation, decreased in pleural effusion).

---

areas. The patient should breathe comfortably with the mouth open.

- Auscultate, as for percussion, the supraclavicular areas, axillae and upper, middle and lower chest for breath sounds, added sounds and vocal resonance.

Breath sounds and added sounds

These are described in Table 1.1.

Table 1.1 Breath sounds and added sounds

	Sounds		What they represent	What they sound like	When they are heard
Breath sounds	**Quality**	Normal (vesicular) breath sounds	Air turbulence in large airways filtering through lung substance to chest wall	Louder and longer in inspiration than expiration No gap between inspiratory and expiratory sounds	Normally
		Bronchial breath sounds	Air turbulence in large airways not filtered by alveoli, producing a different quality They occur in any situation where normal lung is replaced by uniformly conducting tissue, since solid lung conducts unfiltered sound to chest wall Note: Amphoric breath sounds occur over a large cavity and have exaggerated bronchial breathing quality, with lower pitch but higher resonance (likened to air passing over the top of a hollow jar)	Hollow, blowing Heard throughout expiration Inspiration and expiration more equal in duration Pause between inspiration and expiration Resemble sound when stethoscope applied to neck (but quieter)	Over an area of consolidation (very rarely over localised fibrosis, collapse or just above a pleural effusion)
	Intensity (it is preferable to describe breath sounds as normal or reduced in intensity, and not use the term 'air entry', which cannot be directly determined from breath sounds)	Normal Reduced	Breath sounds are produced in airways and not alveoli (vesicles) as once thought; intensity varies with voluntary effort Filtered sound	Loud or quiet depending on effort Quiet	Normally Consolidation Collapse Pleural effusion Hyperinflation Pneumothorax
Added sounds	**Crackles**	Early and mid-inspiratory	Sounds come from larger airways and so are similar in different areas of lung	Tend to be coarse If clear or change on coughing and occur in expiration are probably the result of airway secretions	Pneumonia Bronchiectasis
		Late inspiratory	Sounds come from smaller airways and depend on gravitational forces and so can vary over small areas	Tend to be fine Best heard at lung bases where small airways close on expiration Pulmonary fibrosis sounds like 'Velcro' (in early disease basal posterior crackles that are reduced leaning forward); positional changes occur slowly in pulmonary oedema	Pulmonary fibrosis Pulmonary oedema (occasionally coarse)

Table 1.1 Breath sounds and added sounds—cont'd

	Sounds	What they represent	What they sound like	When they are heard
Wheeze (continuous sound)	Polyphonic expiratory	Flow through narrowed airways Pitch depends more on flow rate than airway calibre	Expiratory Polyphonic	COPD Asthma
	Monophonic	Diffuse narrowing of airways		
		Usually expiratory, since airways dilate on inspiration, inspiratory wheeze tending to indicate severe obstruction		
		Narrowing of single large airway	If fixed obstruction similar in inspiration and expiration When large airway narrowing subject to pressure change, site of narrowing determines pattern; stridor is a loud monophonic wheeze prominent on inspiration (extrathoracic narrowing)	Laryngeal obstruction Tumour
	Biphasic noise	Often obstruction above the larynx – stertorous breathing	Inspiratory and expiratory noise	Tracheal obstruction Severe tonsillitis
Pleural rub		Superficial scratching or grating sound on deep inspiration (like the crackle of leaves underfoot on an autumn forest floor, or the crunching underfoot of freshly fallen snow)	Sounds 'close' to the stethoscope Does not change with coughing Can vary with time and position	Pulmonary embolism Pneumonia
		Note: A pericardial crunch is a rare sound synchronous with the heartbeat in a pneumomediastinum or small left-sided pneumothorax		

		Tracheal deviation (mediastinal shift)	Chest expansion	Percussion note ↓ duller ↑ hyper-resonant	Breath sounds ↑ louder ↓ softer	Added sounds	Vocal resonance
Consolidation	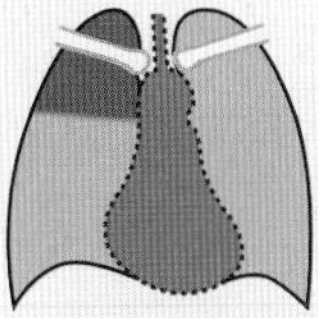	No	Normal or ↓	Normal or ↓	↑ (Bronchial – the best sign)	Coarse crackles +/– rub	↑ Whispering pectoriloquy
Lobar collapse	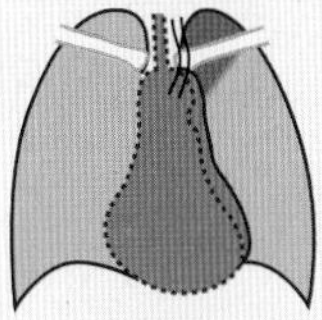	Yes (towards collapse – the best sign)	↓	↓	↓	No	↓
Pleural effusion	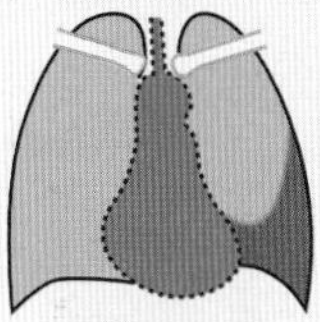	No or away from effusion	↓	↓ (Stony dull – the best sign)	↓	Occasional rub	↓
Pneumothorax	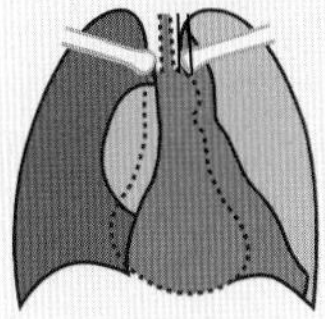	No (without tension) Yes (with tension)	Normal or ↓	↑	↓ (The best sign)	Occasional click	↓

Fig. 1.5 Patterns of important focal abnormalities.

CHRONIC OBSTRUCTIVE PULMONARY DISEASE

Instruction

This 67-year-old lady has been troubled with cough, wheeze and shortness of breath. Please examine her chest and discuss your findings.

Recognition

There may be *tar-stained fingers* (Fig. 1.6), *central cyanosis* (Box 1.3), *pursed lip breathing* and a generally *plethoric* appearance. A *bounding pulse* and *flapping tremor* suggest CO_2 retention.

Chest

There are signs of *hyperinflation* (Box 1.4, Fig. 1.7), but many patients have a degree of cachexia from chronic disease (Fig. 1.8). There may be an *expiratory*

Box 1.3 Cyanosis

Cyanosis refers to blue discolouration of skin and mucous membranes and requires a deoxygenated haemoglobin concentration of > 5 g/dL. Thus it does not occur in anaemia. Central cyanosis (blue and warm) is seen at the lips and tongue and occurs in hypoventilation (e.g. COPD, neuromuscular disease), V/Q mismatch, impaired gas transfer (e.g. pulmonary oedema) and right to left cardiac shunts. Peripheral cyanosis (pink lips, cool peripheries) is the result of local vascular effects and occurs in shock and peripheral vascular disease.

Box 1.4 Signs of hyperinflation

- Increased anteroposterior chest diameter ('barrel chest')
- Indrawing of the intercostal muscles and supraclavicular fossae
- Flattening of the subcostal angle
- A shortened cricoid-notch distance (normally greater than three finger breadths)
- Decreased chest expansion
- Attenuation of heart and liver dullness (with diminished heart sounds)
- Hyperresonance

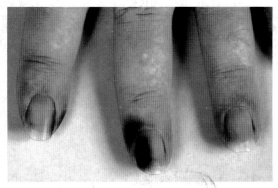

Fig. 1.6 Tar staining.

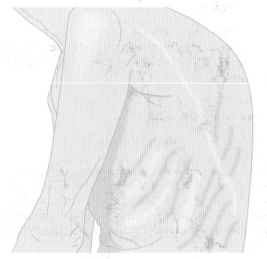

Fig. 1.7 'Barrel chest' and intercostal indrawing of chronic obstructive pulmonary disease.

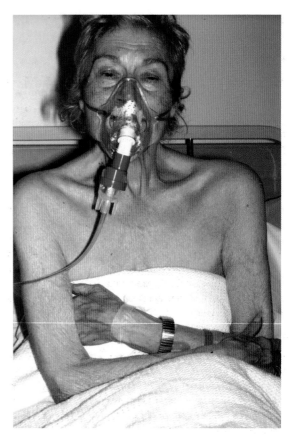

Fig. 1.8 Chronic obstructive pulmonary disease cachexia.

wheeze. Inspiratory crackles suggest superimposed infection.

Interpretation

Confirm the diagnosis

Tell the examiners you would perform spirometry.

What to do next – consider causes

Smoking is by far the commonest cause, confirmed by tar-staining; α1-antitrypsin deficiency causes lower zone emphysema.

Consider severity/decompensation/complications

Tell the examiners that you would be alert to cor pulmonale (right-sided heart failure due to pulmonary hypertension in chronic lung disease) and CO_2 retention (type 2 respiratory failure). Cachexia may imply underlying malignancy.

Box 1.5 Functional scale for breathlessness
• I only get breathless with strenuous exercise.
• I get short of breath when hurrying on the level or walking up a slight hill.
• I walk slower than people of the same age on the level because of breathlessness or have to stop for breath when walking at my own pace on the level.
• I stop for breath after walking about 100 yards or after a few minutes on the level.
• I am too breathless to leave the house or breathless when dressing or undressing.

Consider function

Tell the examiners that you would assess the scale of breathlessness (Box 1.5).

Discussion

What do you understand by the term chronic obstructive pulmonary disease (COPD)?

COPD is a chronic, progressive disease characterised by signs of airflow obstruction and obstructive lung disease on spirometry. There is minimal reversibility with bronchodilators. It affects about 5% of the population over the age of 45. The terms chronic bronchitis and emphysema are sometimes used synonymously.

Chronic bronchitis

This is defined clinically (UK Medical Research Council) as chronic, productive cough for at least three months of two consecutive years in the absence of other diseases causing sputum production. Mucus hypersecretion results from gland hypertrophy and increased goblet cell numbers. Large airways (bronchitis) and small airways (bronchiolitis) are affected in continuum.

Emphysema

This is defined pathologically as permanent enlargement of airways distal to the terminal bronchiole. There is destruction of their walls without obvious fibrosis. It may be predominantly centriacinar (destruction of alveoli at the centre of the acini, especially associated with smoking and affecting upper lobes), panacinar, paraseptal or localised around scars. Bullae are large emphysematous spaces > 1 cm in diameter.

Development of pulmonary hypertension

Chronic bronchitis and emphysema overlap and pulmonary vasculature changes – intimal and medial thickening, smooth muscle proliferation and inflammatory cell infiltration – with hypoxaemia and vasoconstriction lead to pulmonary vascular remodelling and ultimately sustained pulmonary hypertension.

What is the pathogenesis of COPD?

This is related to the inflammatory response to environmental triggers, an imbalance between proteinases and antiproteinases and an imbalance between oxidants and antioxidants.

What is one smoking pack year?

One pack year is equivalent to smoking 20 cigarettes a day for one year.

List some causes of COPD other than smoking

- α1-antitrypsin deficiency
- Environmental (short-term exposure to high-level particulate air pollution correlates with exacerbations)
- Occupational, e.g. coal workers, cadmium workers
- Genetic polymorphisms (probably determine susceptibility to environmental causes)

What is α1-antitrypsin deficiency?

α1-antitrypsin is a protease inhibitor (Pi) enzyme, synthesised in the liver during the acute-phase response, which inhibits neutrophil elastase. Low levels of the enzyme, determined by various genotypes (PiZZ the most severe with enzyme levels < 10% of those with normal M alleles), fail to protect the lung from proteolytic attack, resulting in destruction of alveolar walls, particularly in times of infection when vigorous elasteolytic activity is unopposed.

This ultimately results in basal, panlobular emphysema, accelerated in smokers, and cirrhosis. Patients typically present in the fourth or fifth decades.

How may the diagnosis of COPD be confirmed?

A post-bronchodilator FEV_1 < 80% of the predicted value with a ratio of FEV_1:FVC < 70% that is not fully reversible is consistent with COPD.

List some other tests that you might consider in assessing a patient with COPD

- Full blood picture (polycythaemia)
- Arterial blood gases (ABGs)
- Chest X-ray (hyperinflation, bullae, prominent pulmonary vessels)
- ECG (p pulmonale, right axis deviation, right bundle branch block)

How might you grade COPD severity?

The Global Initiative for Chronic Obstructive Lung Disease (GOLD) classification (Table 1.2) is prognostically informative.

What management options are there in COPD?

These are outlined in Table 1.3.

How can treatment response be assessed in stable COPD?

There is often minimal improvement in spirometry. Short-term changes in FEV_1 in response to bronchodilators or steroids are poor predictors of symptomatic benefit in moderate to severe COPD. Symptomatic improvement is more useful, e.g. reduced breathlessness, increased exercise capacity and improved sleep.

What are the indications for long-term oxygen therapy?

Long-term oxygen therapy is indicated for managing respiratory failure in stable COPD and is one of the few interventions shown to improve survival in patients with COPD. Oxygen is administered via nasal cannulae at 2–4 l/min via a concentrator for at least 15 hours a day. Patients must not smoke! Eligibility criteria are shown in Box 1.6.

How does chronic COPD progress to exacerbations with type 2 respiratory failure?

Alveolar ventilation (i.e. the volume of useful air exchanged) refers to minute ventilation (the total volume of air moving

---

Box 1.6 Indications for long-term oxygen therapy (LTOT)

- pO_2 < 7.3 kPa (55 mmHg) on air
- pO_2 7.3–8.0 kPa (55–60 mmHg) if there is pulmonary hypertension or nocturnal hypoxaemia
- FEV_1 < 1.5 litres

   ABGs should be measured when clinically stable and on two occasions at least three weeks apart (pO_2 should rise with treatment above 8 kPa without unacceptable hypercapnia).

Table 1.2 GOLD staging of chronic obstructive pulmonary disease (COPD)

Stage	At risk	I Mild	II Moderate	III Severe	IV Very severe
FEV_1 (% of predicted)	Normal spirometry (FEV_1/FVC > 70%)	≥ 80	< 80	< 50	< 30
Characteristics	Chronic symptoms + risk factors	With or without symptoms	With or without symptoms	With or without symptoms	Chronic respiratory failure or right-sided heart failure (cor pulmonale)
Stepwise treatments	Avoidance of risk factors Influenza vaccination	Add inhaled short-acting bronchodilator when needed	Add inhaled regular bronchodilator(s) Rehabilitation	Add inhaled regular glucocorticoid if repeated exacerbations	Add LTOT if chronic respiratory failure Consider surgical treatments

FEV_1, 1-second forced expiratory volume; FVC, forced vital capacity; LTOT, long-term oxygen therapy.

Table 1.3 Treatments in chronic obstructive pulmonary disease (COPD)

Problem	Treatment	Benefit	Notes
Stable COPD	Smoking cessation	The most important intervention to modify disease	
	Inhaled bronchodilator therapy	Symptom prevention or relief	Choice of β-agonist or anticholinergic determined by individual symptom response
	Long-acting bronchodilator (LABD) therapy with β-agonist such as salmeterol or formoterol, or anticholinergic (dissociates slowly from M1 and M3 receptors) reduces exacerbations and improves quality of life	Improve lung emptying in expiration and so limit hyperinflation LABDs improve symptoms and exercise capacity, reduce exacerbation rates and seem not to promote tachyphylaxis	Little evidence for nebulisers over inhaled therapy via a spacer device
	Theophyllines	Benefit uncertain	
	Inhaled corticosteroids	Do not modify natural history (evidence emerging for mortality reduction) High doses may improve FEV_1 and combined with LABD therapy may reduce exacerbations	Reasonable to recommend in patients with demonstrable FEV_1 response or moderate to severe disease (FEV_1 < 50% predicted) with recurrent exacerbations requiring antibiotics or oral corticosteroids
	Antioxidant and mucolytic drugs	Need further evaluation	
	Long-term oxygen therapy (LTOT)	Discussed below	
	Pulmonary rehabilitation (exercise, smoking cessation, nutritional assessment, education, empowering patients)	Improves exercise capacity and reduces the sensation of breathlessness and the number of hospital admissions	Depression should always be considered a cause of poor concordance
	Lung volume reduction surgery (LVRS) Bronchoscopic lung reduction (e.g. stents with one-way valves) experimental	Increases exercise capacity by reducing dynamic hyperinflation, improving diaphragmatic function and improving elastic recoil	May be useful for large bullae, especially upper lobe disease Contraindicated if FEV_1 < 20% or emphysema homogeneous
	Vaccination	Annual influenza vaccination	5- to 10-year pneumococcal vaccination uncertain
Exacerbation of COPD	Antibiotics and systemic corticosteroids (± nebulised bronchodilators)	Useful in infective exacerbations No evidence in prophylaxis	
	Non-invasive ventilation	Discussed below	

FEV_1, 1-second forced expiratory volume; FVC, forced vital capacity; LTOT, long-term oxygen therapy.

in and out of the lungs per minute, given by tidal volume × respiratory rate) minus the dead space (the proportion of minute ventilation trapped in the lungs). Dead space is increased in COPD because of expiratory airflow obstruction that is only partially compensated for by increased expiratory time, leading to hyperinflation. This ultimately leads to decreased muscle function, flattening of the diaphragm from its optimum dome shape and failure of the intercostal muscles to exert adequate upward pull. This leads to intrinsic positive end expiratory pressure (PEEP); normally, resting pressure is atmospheric but in COPD it is always greater, causing positive airway pressure, a situation demanding extra work to get air into the lungs. Tidal volume ultimately decreases and the respiratory rate must increase to compensate, creating a vicious cycle because an increased respiratory rate exacerbates gas trapping with worsening type 2 respiratory failure.

How would you manage acute respiratory failure in COPD?

Controlled oxygen therapy and supportive ventilation (non-invasive ventilation or invasive mechanical ventilation) aim to prevent tissue hypoxia and control acidosis and hypercapnia while medical therapy maximises lung function and reverses any precipitating cause.

Intravenous aminophylline is falling from favour following a Cochrane review demonstrating its failure to increase FEV_1 or shorten hospital admission, while at the same time increasing adverse effects. Oral prednisolone 30 mg is generally given for 7–14 days and then stopped. Assessment for LTOT should occur six weeks after an exacerbation.

The best marker of severity is pH; it reflects acute deterioration in alveolar hypoventilation (acute rise in pCO_2) compared with the chronic stable state. pH < 7.26 is associated with 30% mortality.

Increases in pCO_2 are associated with significant mortality but the absolute pCO_2 and pO_2 are less significant than pH; for example, a pCO_2 of 8.5 kPa associated with a bicarbonate of 35 mmol/L and a normal pH might merely reflect chronic respiratory acidosis with metabolic compensation whereas a pCO_2 of 9 kPa with a normal bicarbonate and low pH more likely reflects acute decompensation.

Some typical ABG results are shown in Table 1.4.

Oxygen therapy

Uncontrolled oxygen therapy can produce respiratory acidosis and CO_2 narcosis; the mechanism is still poorly understood. However, hypoxia is potentially life-threatening and can trigger arrhythmias. pO_2 should be maintained between 7.3 and 10 kPa (higher is dangerous and unnecessary) if the pH is normal and with adequate ventilation, aiming to stop the pH falling to < 7.26. Controlled oxygen is via a fixed percentage Venturi mask or low-flow nasal cannulae (the latter are associated with a more variable FiO_2). An oxygen saturation of 85–92% may be perfectly acceptable in COPD, although in other situations > 90% is important because the slippery slope of cellular dysfunction mirrors the tailing of the oxygen dissociation curve. ABGs are needed to check baseline pH but there-after oximetry and respiratory rate are good guides to underlying changes.

Non-invasive positive pressure ventilation (NIV)

NIV in COPD is outlined in Box 1.7.

What is cor pulmonale?

This is ventricular enlargement and failure occurring secondary to lung/chest wall/pulmonary circulatory disease. Central to cor pulmonale development is pulmonary hypertension. The 5-year mortality in patients with COPD who develop peripheral oedema is 70–100%.

CASE 1.2

CONSOLIDATION

Instruction

This patient is breathless. Please examine his respiratory system and discuss your findings.

Recognition

There may be *tachypnoea*. There may be *reduced expansion on the affected side* but the *trachea is central*. There is

Table 1.4 Typical arterial blood gas (ABG) results and action needed					
	Normal	**Unwell (non-respiratory illness)**	**Stable COPD**	**Acutely unwell COPD**	**Acutely unwell COPD**
pO_2 (kPa)	13	9	8	8	6
pCO_2 (kPa)	5	6	8	8	9.5
pH	7.4	7.2	7.4	7.3	7.25
HCO_3	26	24	34	24	18
Action needed	None	Treat underlying cause	None if patient well	Consider non-invasive ventilation	Consider non-invasive ventilation (NIV) + ITU/invasive ventilation

Box 1.7 Non-invasive ventilation (NIV) in chronic obstructive pulmonary disease (COPD)

NIV is indicated for acute exacerbations of COPD with respiratory failure. The respiratory stimulant doxapram is now seldom used.

Indications

Ideally, patients should be capable of protecting their airway, cooperative and otherwise medically stable. The following parameters are indications for such patients.

- pH < 7.35 (but most effective when pH is between 7.30 and 7.35)
- pO_2 falling despite high-flow oxygen
- pCO_2 > 8 kPa (a relative indication, pH much more important)
- respiratory rate > 23

NIV is not appropriate for those in an end-stage episode of illness but it may be the 'ceiling' of care for those in whom intubation is deemed inappropriate.

Exclusion criteria

- pH < 7.25 (NIV is not a substitute for invasive ventilation and patients appropriate for the latter should be discussed with ITU early because mortality is around 30%; in practice, however, many patients with pH < 7.25 are tried on NIV, especially if successful weaning from invasive ventilation seems unlikely)
- Unresponsive/comatose
- Pneumothorax, pneumonia or acute severe asthma (consider ITU)
- Systolic blood pressure < 90 mmHg (NIV lowers blood pressure)
- Vomiting/hypersecretory states

How NIV works

NIV is delivered via a tightly fitting face-mask with humidifier and a BIPAP box with or without oxygen. NIV overcomes auto-PEEP and reduces inspiratory effort. It is patient triggered. The patient initiates a breath and the box kicks in to raise inspiratory positive airway pressure (IPAP) to a set reading. The patient learns to 'relax' into what at first may be an uncomfortable apparatus. Expiratory positive airway pressure (EPAP) = PEEP and IPAP can be balanced with a small amount of PEEP. Oxygen can be entrained to maintain saturations between 85% and 92%. BIPAP is different to continuous PAP (CPAP), which delivers 5–10 cmH_2O throughout the breathing cycle.

IPAP, by providing positive airway pressure, assists ventilation, while EPAP recruits under-ventilated lung and improves the ventilation : perfusion ratio as well as reducing rebreathed air by eliminating exhaled air via the expiratory port.

Practical approach to using NIV

Treat in the standard way with controlled oxygen, nebulised bronchodilators and steroids (± antibiotics) with ABG analysis on admission and repeat ABG analysis at one hour whereupon pH 7.25–7.35 is the main indication for NIV. Typical starting pressures are an IPAP of 12 cmH_2O and an EPAP of 4 cmH_2O, IPAP increased in 2- to 4-cmH_2O increments up to a maximum of 20 cmH_2O but EPAP generally unaltered as higher pressures are rarely tolerated. ABG analysis repeated at four hours may guide further management:

- pH < 7.3   adjust NIV settings and consider ITU
- pH 7.30–7.35   continue NIV (80% chance of improvement)
- pH > 7.35   consider stopping NIV

Patients typically need NIV for approximately 24 hours.

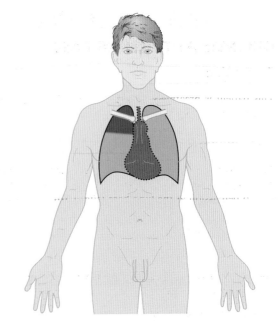

Fig. 1.9 Consolidation.

Interpretation

Confirm the diagnosis

The main differential diagnoses are pleural effusion and collapse:

- A pleural effusion produces stony dullness on percussion, reduced breath sounds and reduced vocal resonance.
- Collapse may cause the trachea to deviate towards the affected side.

What to do next – consider causes

The commonest cause is pneumonia (breathlessness, pyrexia, purulent sputum). Lung cancer with distal infection should always be considered (clubbing, cachexia).

Consider severity/decompensation/complications

Tell the examiners you would determine the CURB score (see Case 1.4, Box 1.8).

Consider function

Tell the examiners you would establish the limitations caused by breathlessness.

Discussion

What is whispering pectoriloquy?

Whispered sounds are heard clearly on auscultation, confirming consolidation because a whispered voice is clearly audible through solid lung, just as vocal resonance is increased in consolidation.

dullness to percussion over one or more lobes (Fig. 1.9). There are *bronchial breath sounds* (± *coarse crackles*) and *vocal resonance is increased* over the affected lobe(s). There may be *whispering pectoriloquy* and a *pleural friction rub*.

CASE 1.3

DULLNESS AT THE LUNG BASE

Instruction

This patient is breathless. Please examine his respiratory system and discuss your findings.

Recognition

There may be *tachypnoea*. There may be *reduced expansion on the affected side* but the *trachea is central*. There is *dullness* to percussion at the lung base (Fig. 1.10).

Interpretation

Confirm the diagnosis

The main differential diagnoses are pleural effusion, consolidation and collapse:

- A pleural effusion produces stony dullness on percussion, reduced breath sounds and reduced vocal resonance.
- Consolidation produces dullness to percussion, bronchial breath sounds, increased vocal resonance and whispering pectoriloquy.
- Collapse may cause the trachea to deviate towards the affected side.

What to do next – consider causes

Unilateral pleural effusions are often exudates (parapneumonic, lung cancer); if a pleural effusion seems likely, tell the examiners you would aspirate it (after chest X-ray) to differentiate causes. Tell the examiners that common causes of consolidation or collapse are pneumonia and lung cancer.

Consider severity/decompensation/complications

If consolidation seems likely, tell the examiners you would consider pneumonia and determine the CURB score (see Case 1.4; Box 1.8) but also wish to exclude malignancy.

Consider function

Tell the examiners you would establish the limitations caused by breathlessness.

Discussion

List some causes of dullness at the lung base

- Pleural effusion
- Consolidation
- Collapse
- Raised hemidiaphragm, e.g. hepatomegaly, phrenic nerve palsy
- Pleural thickening

CASE 1.4

PNEUMONIA

Instruction

This patient is breathless. Please examine his respiratory system and discuss your findings.

Recognition

There may be *tachypnoea*. There may be *reduced expansion on the affected side* but the *trachea is central*. There is *dullness* to percussion over one or more lobes (Fig. 1.11). There are *bronchial breath sounds* (± *coarse crackles*) and *vocal resonance is increased* over the affected lobe(s). There may be *whispering pectoriloquy* and a *pleural friction rub*.

Interpretation

Confirm the diagnosis

Pyrexia and rigors may or may not be present.

What to do next – consider causes

Streptococcus pneumoniae is the commonest pathogen in community-acquired pneumonia, even in patients with chronic obstructive pulmonary disease (COPD), followed by *Haemophilus influenzae* in older people. Other pathogens include 'atypical organisms' (especially in younger people), *Staphylococcus aureus*, *Moxarella catarrhalis* and influenza viruses A and B (especially in older people),

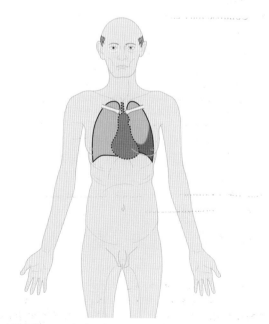

Fig. 1.10 Dullness at the lung base.

Table 1.5 CURB-65 score prognosis and management

CURB-65 score	Mortality (%)	Management
0 or 1	1.5	Home treatment likely
2	9.2	Short admission likely
≥3	22	Hospital management for severe pneumonia ITU possible if CURB-65 score > 3

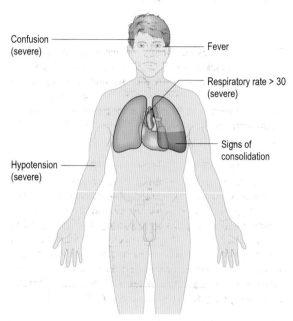

Confusion (severe)

Fever

Respiratory rate > 30 (severe)

Signs of consolidation

Hypotension (severe)

Fig. 1.11 Pneumonia.

Box 1.9 Possible complications of pneumonia

- Respiratory failure
- Pleural effusion (common)
- Empyema (less common) associated with treatment failure, persistent fevers, malaise and weight loss
- Lung abscesses (rare)
- Cavitation
- Fibrosis

Gram-negative bacteria and anaerobic bacteria (aspiration). Organisms are not isolated in up to half of cases. Streptococcal pneumonia is more common in winter. It is characterised by its abrupt onset and often causes high fever and rigors. Lobar consolidation is typical. Herpetic cold sores are common. Vaccination is recommended for high-risk patients.

Consider severity/decompensation/complications

Tell the examiners you would determine the CURB score. The six-point CURB-65 score stratifies patients into different prognostic groups suitable for different management pathways (Box 1.8, Table 1.5). Other signs of serious infection associated with a poor prognosis that do not enter the CURB score include albumin < 30 g/l, white cell count < 4 × 10⁹/l or > 20 × 10⁹/l, severe hypoxia and multilobar or bilateral disease. The CURB score is only a guide, and a low CURB score can sometimes be falsely reassuring.

Possible complications are listed in Box 1.9.

Consider function

Tell the examiners you would establish the limitations caused by breathlessness.

Discussion

What types of lower respiratory tract infection (LRTI) are there?

These include cough with sputum (acute bronchitis), acute exacerbations of COPD, community acquired pneumonia (CAP) and atypical pneumonia.

When might you treat acute bronchitis with antimicrobial therapy?

Acute bronchitis is common after upper respiratory tract infection and is usually self-limiting. Pathogens are similar to those in CAP. Antimicrobials are indicated if there is clinical deterioration or if focal chest signs develop.

When might you treat an acute exacerbation of COPD with antimicrobial therapy?

An acute exacerbation of COPD may be defined as increased cough, sputum and dyspnoea without focal signs. The pathogen is usually viral. The British Thoracic Society recommends antimicrobials if two or more of worsening dyspnoea, increased sputum purulence or increased sputum volume are present.

What is pneumonia?

Pneumonia is an inflammatory, usually infectious, disease of lung parenchyma. Most is managed in primary care. The most common symptoms are cough, sputum, dyspnoea and pleuritic pain. The most common signs are fever, tachypnoea, tachycardia and signs of consolidation. The presentation may be different in the elderly, such as confusion.

How common is community-acquired pneumonia (CAP)?

The annual incidence is six per 1000 population in the 16–59 year age group rising to 34 per 1000 population in those aged 75 and over. Hospital admission is required in 20–40% of cases and of those 5–10% need admission to ITU.

What investigations would you consider in pneumonia?

Initial tests are routine haematobiochemistry, blood and sputum cultures and chest X-ray. Urine rapid testing for pneumococcal and legionella antigens may be useful in severe pneumonia but there is no robust evidence of improved outcome.

What would be your empirical first-line antibiotic for CAP?

Local guidelines vary and evolve quickly. Generally, amoxicillin remains the preferred choice for patients without severe pneumonia and without penicillin hypersensitivity. Hospitalised patients may receive seven days of oral amoxicillin together with a macrolide, doxycycline or a fluoroquinolone (enhanced pneumococcal activity may be provided by levofloxacin or moxifloxacin). A β-lactam antibiotic or non-first-generation cephalosporin, with a macrolide, are indicated in severe pneumonia, when therapy should be intravenous initially and for at least 10 days in total. Rifampicin may be added in legionella infection. The new 'Gram-positive' fluoroquinolones (levofloxacin, moxifloxacin) should not be used in the community or as first-line but may be useful in penicillin allergy or if there is local concern regarding *Clostridium difficile* diarrhoea with β-lactam use.

When should a patient be discharged from hospital following pneumonia?

When clinically stable, and without signs of clinical instability (Box 1.10). Radiographic resolution occurs in 50% at two weeks and 70% at six weeks and is slower in older people. All patients should be reviewed six weeks after discharge. Smokers, those over 50 or those with persistent symptoms should have a follow-up chest X-ray, with bronchoscopy considered for persisting changes.

Box 1.10 Signs of clinical instability in pneumonia

- Temperature > 37.8°C
- Heart rate > 100 beats/min
- Respiratory rate > 24 breaths/min
- Systolic blood pressure < 90 mmHg
- Oxygen saturation < 90%
- Abnormal mental state
- Inability to take oral medication

These features are all associated with a high readmission rate and mortality.

Which individuals should have the pneumococcal vaccine?

Current Department of Health recommendations include those over 65 years of age, asplenic patients or those with splenic dysfunction (e.g. coeliac disease), patients with chronic respiratory, heart, renal or liver conditions, immunosuppressed patients, those with cochlear implants and those with cerebrospinal fluid leaks.

Which individuals should receive the influenza vaccine?

Target groups based largely on increased susceptibility to infection include those in institutional care, those with chronic disease (e.g. heart disease, lung disease, cancer, immune deficiency, renal disease, diabetes, liver disease) and those aged over 65 years. In addition, vaccination of health-care workers and those caring for the elderly is recommended.

How does atypical pneumonia present?

The spectrum of disease ranges from asymptomatic infection to severe hypoxic respiratory failure requiring ventilatory support. Atypical pneumonia often affects young adults and there may be a travel history. It tends to produce insidious constitutional symptoms and a paucity of respiratory symptoms after a 10- to 20-day incubation period. Despite this, chest signs may be present and chest radiography may be impressive, often with bilateral infiltrates. Extrapulmonary features are common (Table 1.6).

List some differential diagnoses of unresolving pneumonia

- Bronchial carcinoma
- Empyema
- Lung abscess
- Pulmonary oedema
- Fibrotic lung disease
- Pulmonary emboli

What is a parapneumonic effusion and how does it differ from empyema?

These two entities are discussed in Case 1.21.

What cavitating lung conditions do you know?

A lung abscess causes cavitation with an air–fluid level. Common cavitating organisms include *Staphylococcus aureus*, *Klebsiella pneumoniae* and *Mycobacterium tuberculosis*. Other causes of cavitation include carcinoma, vasculitis and pulmonary infarction.

What is the differential diagnosis of a possible lung abscess on chest X-ray?

- Emphysema with consolidation ('tatty lungs')
- Bronchiectasis with air–fluid levels ('cystic bronchiectasis')
- Empyema
- Pulmonary infarction with secondary cavitation

Table 1.6 Features of atypical pneumonias

Extrapulmonary features shared by atypical pneumonias	Specific organism	Epidemiology	Clinical features
Arthralgias and myalgias Autoimmune haemolytic anaemia (usually mild) due to cold agglutinins, common in *Mycoplasma*	*Mycoplasma pneumoniae*	Younger adults Epidemics every few years	Non-productive cough (paroxysms common) invariable Paucity of signs compared to symptoms and chest X-ray appearances
Maculopapular rash, erythema multiforme, Stevens–Johnson syndrome, erythema nodosum	*Legionella pneumophila*	Gram-negative bacillus preferring stagnant water Legionnaire's disease more common with pre-existing lung disease	Pontiac fever – acute self-limiting febrile illness) Legionnaire's disease – diarrhoea, abdominal pain, abnormal liver function and headaches before respiratory symptoms Peripheral cytopenias Renal failure
Bullous myringitis (*Mycoplasma*) Sterile meningitis, meningoencephalitis, transverse myelitis, cranial neuropathies, peripheral mononeuropathies, Guillain–Barré syndrome	*Chlamydia pneumoniae*	Older adults	Extrapulmonary features less common
Myocarditis/pericarditis Hepatitis	*Chlamydia psittaci*	Classically transmitted from birds Human to human transmission possible	Often presents with severe headache
	Coxiella burnettii	Usually transmitted from farm animals (lambs and calves in spring)	Rare Q fever, ranging from asymptomatic infection to severe pneumonia

- Vasculitis
- Hiatus hernia
- Carcinoma
- An old tuberculosis cavity with an aspergilloma

How might a lung abscess be differentiated from carcinoma?

An abscess is thin-walled, with a marked fluid level, and is often central. A carcinoma is thick-walled, with an eccentric cavity.

Which organisms can cause a lung abscess?

These include *Staphylococcus*, *Streptococcus*, *Mycobacterium*, *Legionella*, Gram-negative bacteria (especially post-aspiration) and anaerobes (especially post-aspiration). 'Compost', with multiple types of bacteria, is common.

List some factors associated with the development of a lung abscess

- Increasing age
- Long duration of symptoms
- Influenza A epidemic (staphylococcal pneumonia)
- Source of metastatic infection (shunts, intravenous drug use)
- Aspiration (right lower lobe – always think aspiration in older people or inhaled foreign body in children – due to the more vertical orientation of the right main bronchus)

- Immune compromise
- Underlying lung disease

How is a lung abscess treated?

Drainage, aided by posture and physiotherapy, is important, but specialist care is needed because patients might have to lie in one position for hours and there is a danger of pus draining elsewhere. Antibiotics may include amoxicillin and flucloxacillin in an influenza epidemic, and metronidazole in patients with halitosis.

CASE 1.5

LUNG CANCER

Instruction

This 67-year-old gentleman has had a persistent cough. Please examine his respiratory system and discuss your findings.

Recognition

There may be one or a combination of clinical signs.

- *Cachexia* (Fig. 1.8)
- *Finger clubbing* (Fig. 1.12)
- *Chest signs* – consolidation, collapse or pleural effusion

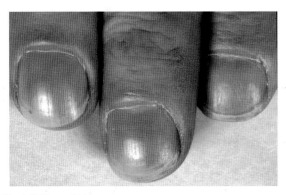

Fig. 1.12 Finger clubbing.

- Cervical or supraclavicular *lymphadenopathy*
- *Horner's syndrome* ± evidence of *brachial plexopathy* secondary to a Pancoast's tumour
- Signs of superior *vena cava obstruction*

Interpretation

Confirm the diagnosis

The differential diagnosis of lung cancer is wide:

- Slowly resolving pneumonia (consolidation)
- Lobar collapse by mucus plug
- Other causes of pleural effusion
- Benign tumour
- Metastases from alternative primary site
- Lymphoma
- Pulmonary embolism
- Tuberculosis (weight loss, haemoptysis)
- Vasculitis (haemoptysis)

Management is directed at excluding serious and immediately threatening diagnoses (malignancy, pulmonary embolism, vasculitis, tuberculosis).

What to do next – assess other systems

Tell the examiners that you would ask about:

- *Endobronchial symptoms* (cough, dyspnoea, haemoptysis), *systemic symptoms* (weight loss, anorexia) and *pain* (e.g. infiltration of brachial plexus; metastatic bone pain)
- *Hormonal/metabolic symptoms* suggesting a paraneoplastic syndrome (Box 1.11)

Hypertrophic pulmonary osteoarthropathy is a very rare, extreme form of clubbing associated with wrist and ankle swelling and characterised radiologically by subperiosteal new bone separating from the cortex; it is most commonly associated with squamous cell carcinoma. A hoarse voice may represent recurrent laryngeal nerve palsy, and although typically the result of lung cancer, other causes are sometimes the culprit, such as left atrial enlargement or an aortic arch aneurysm.

Box 1.11 Lung cancer paraneoplastic syndromes

- Parathyroid hormone-related peptide (PTHrp)-induced hypercalcaemia, often the result of squamous cell carcinoma; hypercalcaemia is, however, mostly a consequence of bone metastases
- Ectopic secretion of numerous hormones including adrenocorticotrophic hormone (ACTH) (Cushing's syndrome) and antidiuretic hormone (SIADH), commonly due to small-cell lung cancer, which is neuroendocrine derived
- Lambert–Eaton myasthenic syndrome (LEMS)

Table 1.7 WHO/Zubrod performance status scale in lung cancer

Stage	Features
0	Asymptomatic
1	Symptomatic but ambulatory
2	In bed < 50% of day (unable to work but living at home with assistance)
3	In bed > 50% of day (unable to care for self)
4	Bedridden

Consider severity/decompensation/complications

Tell the examiners that you would look for signs of distant metastases, e.g. brain, bone, liver or skin.

Tell the examiners that persistent haemoptysis, stridor or signs of superior vena cava obstruction would warrant immediate referral to a chest physician.

Consider function

Performance status in lung cancer may be assessed by numerous scales, e.g. WHO/Zubrod (Table 1.7), Karnofsky.

Discussion

Is lung cancer incidence increasing?

It is the most common malignancy in developed countries, the incidence increasing in developing countries because of smoking.

What are the causes of lung cancer?

Smoking is implicated in > 90% of cases. The risk is cumulative. Environmental/occupational exposure to asbestos, silicosis, arsenic, nickel, chromium, aromatic hydrocarbons and radon are rarer causes. The incidence is also increased in various medical disorders including idiopathic pulmonary fibrosis and dermatomyositis.

Which investigations would you consider when trying to establish a diagnosis of lung cancer?

An algorithm for lung cancer diagnosis is given in Fig. 1.13.

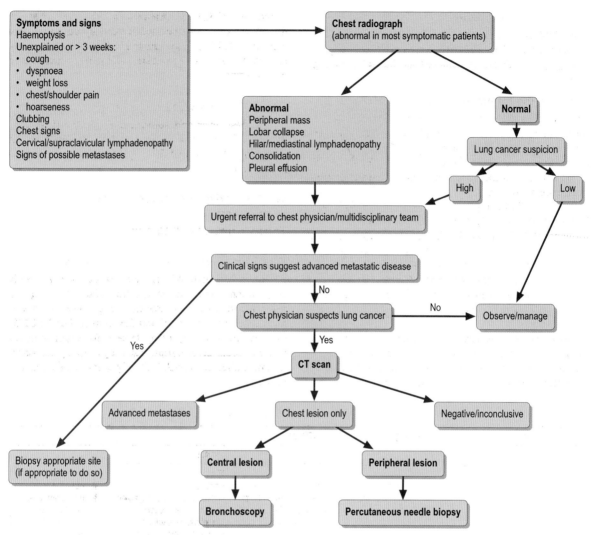

Fig. 1.13 Diagnosis of lung cancer.

What is the role of positron-emission tomography (PET) scanning in lung cancer?

Computed tomography (CT) scanning has limitations. Mediastinal and hilar nodes > 1 cm are assumed to be malignant, but some < 1 cm are malignant and some larger ones are benign. Some metastases are clinically silent and invisible on CT and so patients relapse after surgery. Some of these inaccuracies explain why five-year survival after surgery is only around 40%. PET is a radionuclide technique that exploits the fact that tumour cells take up glucose more avidly than other cells. ^{18}F-labelled fluoro-deoxyglucose (FDG) is an isotopically labelled glucose analogue containing positron (proton) emitting fluorine that is not cleared from tumour cells. FDG-PET is more sensitive and specific than CT in detecting metastases in nodes and distant organs and is very useful for assessing questionably large lymph nodes. PET combined with CT

(PET-CT) is now the definitive staging technique, especially to rule out metastases if radical treatment is planned, although even PET cannot resolve nodules < 1 cm in diameter nor detect cerebral metastases. Other indications for PET are:

- CT inconclusive or negative when lung cancer is still suspected
- Bronchoscopy or biopsy inconclusive
- The patient is not fit for bronchoscopy or biopsy and is CT inconclusive (where diagnosis would make a difference)

How is lung cancer classified?

About 20% is small-cell lung cancer (SCLC). About 80% is non-small-cell lung cancer (NSCLC) – squamous cell (primary disease often in main bronchus), adenocarcinoma (often peripheral) or large cell.

How is NSCLC classified?

The TNM staging classification is used for NSCLC to produce subsets that help direct treatment (Table 1.8).

Staging of NSCLC is achieved as illustrated in Fig. 1.14.

What are the treatment options for NSCLC?

Surgery offers the best chance of cure and is considered for fit patients with early disease (Table 1.8). It may comprise lobectomy or pneumonectomy. Recurrence rates after segmentectomy are higher. Generally, FEV_1 should be > 1 litre to consider lobectomy and > 1.5 litres to consider pneumonectomy.

Radical radiotherapy, potentially curative, is indicated in patients with stage I, II or III NSCLC with a good performance status (WHO 0, 1). Fractionation regimens such as continuous hyperfractionated accelerated radiotherapy (CHART) offer higher two-year survival and are offered to patients with stage I or II NSCLC who are medically inoperable but suitable for radical radiotherapy or patients with stage III NSCLC who cannot tolerate or who decline chemotherapy.

Chemotherapy is offered to patients with stage III or IV (distant metastases) NSCLC. Combinations of a platinum-based drug (carboplatin, cisplatin) with a third-generation drug (docetaxel, gemcitabine, paclitaxel, vinorelbine) control disease and improve survival and quality of life. Pemetrexed may be used for locally advanced and metastatic NSCLC. Biologics inhibiting epidermal receptor growth factor and vascular endothelial growth factor are emerging.

How is SCLC classified and treated?

CT of chest, liver and adrenals and additional selected imaging of symptomatic areas can determine if disease is limited or extensive, and this helps to determine treatment (Table 1.9).

What palliative options are available in lung cancer?

These are outlined in Table 1.10.

What do you know about lung cancer prognosis?

Prognosis for both NSCLC and SCLC is poor, with only around one-third being potentially localised at presentation. In a 1995 Scottish lung cancer audit the median survival for SCLC was 3.6 months. For NSCLC, five-year survival may be up to 60% for small tumours without nodal involvement, but drops rapidly for more extensive disease. Overall, 6–7% of patients are alive at five years.

Table 1.8 Staging classification of non-small-cell lung cancer (NSCLC)

		Tumour			
		T1 <3 cm Confined to lobar bronchus	**T2** >3 cm In main bronchus > 2 cm distal to carina invades viscera pleura	**T3** Any size Invades chest wall, diaphragm, mediastinal pleura or parietal pericardium In main bronchus < 2 cm distal to carina	**T4** Any size Invades other local structures, e.g. mediastinum, heart, oesophagus Malignant effusion
Nodes	**N0** No nodes	IA[a]	IB[a]	IIB[b]	IIIB[c]
	N1 Ipsilateral peribronchial, hilar or intrapulmonary nodes	IIA[a]	IIB[a]	IIIA[b]	IIIB[c]
	N2 Ipsilateral mediastinal or subcarinal nodes	IIIA[b]	IIIA[b]	IIIA[c]	IIIB[c]
	N3 Contralateral mediastinal or hilar nodes Any scalene or supraclavicular nodes	IIIB[c]	IIIB[c]	IIIB[c]	IIIB[c]

Key

a Offered surgery if fit.
b Surgery may be suitable.
c Surgery unsuitable.

Table 1.9 Staging and treatment of small-cell lung cancer (SCLC)

Stage (defined by possibility of encompassing all detectable tumour within a 'tolerable' radiotherapy field)	Limited Confined to one hemithorax Involves ipsilateral hilar nodes Involves ipsilateral and contralateral supraclavicular or mediastinal nodes With or without ipsilateral pleural effusion	Extensive Includes metastases in contralateral lung or distant metastases
Radiotherapy	Yes	No
Chemotherapy	Multi-drug platinum-based regimen offered to all patients, response excellent but short-lived	
Surgery	Surgery has almost no role, micrometastatic spread invariable at diagnosis	

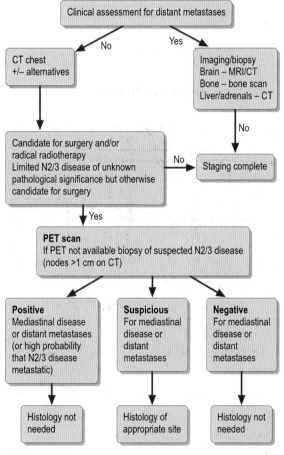

Fig. 1.14 How non-small-cell lung cancer (NSCLC) staging is achieved.

Table 1.10 Palliation of lung cancer symptoms

Symptom	Management
Breathlessness	Radiotherapy Debulking bronchoscopic procedures Endobronchial photodynamic therapy or brachytherapy Endobronchial stenting Pleural aspiration and pleurodesis
Cough/haemoptysis	Radiotherapy
Superior vena cava obstruction	Radiotherapy/chemotherapy Stenting
Brain metastases or spinal cord compression	Dexamethasone Radiotherapy
Bone metastases	Radiotherapy

Recognition

A tumour at the lung apex may invade locally to provoke Pancoast's syndrome (Fig. 1.15) with:

- Brachial plexus symptoms and signs, e.g. ipsilateral pain in the shoulder, upper anterior chest wall or between the scapulae, spreading to the arms and hands; unilateral *wasting of the intrinsic muscles of the hand*
- An ipsilateral *Horner's syndrome* (small pupil, ptosis, absence of sweating)

Interpretation

Confirm the diagnosis

Signs of apical consolidation and a chest X-ray confirm the apical tumour.

What to do next – assess other systems

See Case 1.5.

Consider severity/decompensation/complications

See Case 1.5.

Consider function

See Case 1.5.

CASE 1.6

PANCOAST'S SYNDROME

Instruction

This patient cannot abduct his shoulder. Please examine his respiratory system and discuss your findings.

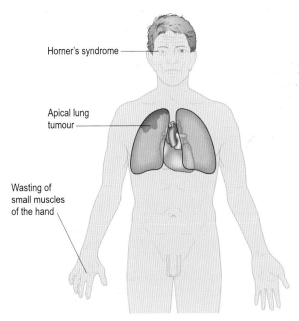

Horner's syndrome

Apical lung tumour

Wasting of small muscles of the hand

Fig. 1.15 Pancoast's syndrome.

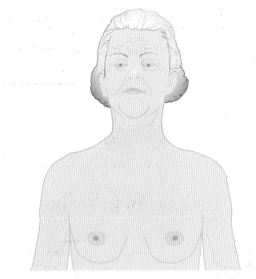

Fig. 1.16 Superior vena cava obstruction (SVCO).

Discussion

How are Pancoast's tumours treated?

The three considerations are radiotherapy, chemotherapy and palliation.

CASE 1.7

SUPERIOR VENA CAVA OBSTRUCTION

Instruction

This elderly lady has been progressively breathless over the last few weeks. Please examine her hands, mouth, neck and chest and report your findings.

Recognition

There is *marked venous distension in the neck* (Fig. 1.16) and the jugular venous pulse is *raised and fixed*. There is also *distension of veins* in the *hands*, on the underside of the *tongue* and on the *chest wall* (Fig. 1.17).

Interpretation

Confirm the diagnosis

A chest X-ray may confirm a bulky mediastinum.

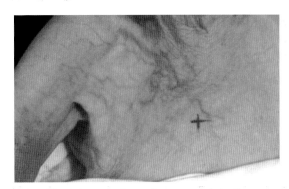

Fig. 1.17 Dilated chest veins in superior vena cava obstruction.

What to do next – assess other systems

See Case 1.5.

Consider severity/decompensation/complications

See Case 1.5.

Consider function

See Case 1.5.

Discussion

List some other causes of superior vena cava obstruction (SVCO)

- Lymphoma
- Aortic aneurysm
- Mediastinal mass
- Mediastinal fibrosis

How is SVCO managed?

Radiotherapy, chemotherapy or stenting are used.

What are the main causes of an anterior mediastinal mass?

- Thymoma
- Thyroid goitre
- Lymphoma
- Teratoma
- Lymph node spread from carcinoma

CASE 1.8

COLLAPSE/PNEUMONECTOMY/ LOBECTOMY

Instruction

This patient is breathless. Please examine his respiratory system and discuss your findings.

Recognition

There is *tracheal deviation* (to the affected side). *Decreased chest expansion, dullness to percussion* and *decreased breath sounds* occur *on the affected side* (Fig. 1.18). There may be a *thoracotomy scar* (Fig. 1.19) indicating previous lobectomy/pneumonectomy.

Interpretation

Confirm the diagnosis

Consolidation causes dullness to percussion, bronchial breath sounds and increased vocal resonance; it may coexist with collapse.

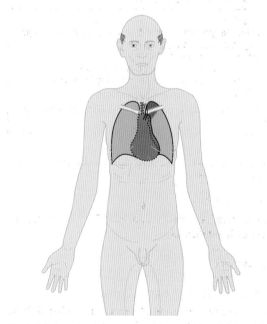

Fig. 1.18 Lobar collapse.

What to do next – consider causes

Collapse is commonly the result of pneumonia or lung cancer. Common reasons for previous lobectomy/pneumonectomy are lung cancer, tuberculosis, localised bronchiectasis or bullae.

Consider severity/decompensation/complications

This depends on the underlying cause e.g. pneumonia (CURB score), lung cancer (operability). Obstruction causing collapse may predispose to pneumonia or segmental bronchiectasis.

Consider function

Tell the examiners you would establish the limitations caused by breathlessness.

Discussion

List some causes of bronchial obstruction that can lead to collapse

- Carcinoma of bronchus
- Extrinsic compression, e.g. mediastinal lymph nodes
- Benign tumour
- Mucus plugs, e.g. asthma
- Foreign body
- Granulomata, e.g. tuberculosis, sarcoid

CASE 1.9

BRONCHIECTASIS

Instruction

This young man has been troubled by recurrent chest infections. Please examine his respiratory system and discuss possible causes.

Recognition

There is a *large volume* of *sputum* in the sputum pot beside the bed in this *underweight, dyspnoeic* and *cyanosed* patient with finger *clubbing*. Auscultation reveals *coarse, late inspiratory crackles* ± inspiratory clicks (audible with the unaided ear) and wheeze (mucus obstructing distal airways) (Fig. 1.20).

Interpretation

Confirm the diagnosis

The differential diagnosis of clubbing and crackles includes idiopathic pulmonary fibrosis. Tell the examiners that large sputum volumes suggest bronchiectasis.

What to do next – consider causes

Tell the examiners that you would consider the causes of bronchiectasis (Box 1.12).

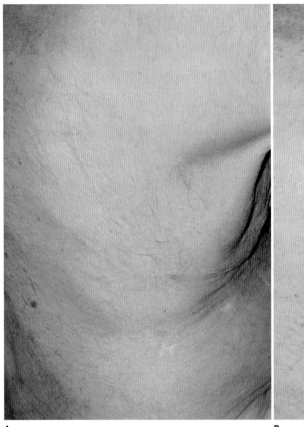
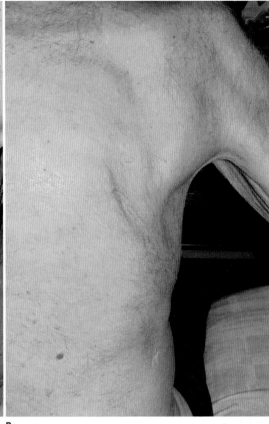

A   **B**

Fig. 1.19 (A,B) Thoracotomy scar.

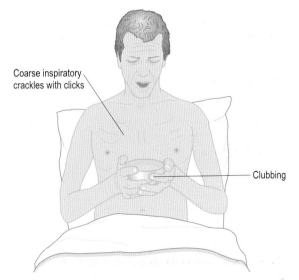

Coarse inspiratory
crackles with clicks

Clubbing

Fig. 1.20 Bronchiectasis.

> **Box 1.12 Causes of bronchiectasis**
>
> - Cystic fibrosis
> - Postinfective (pneumonia, tuberculosis, measles, whooping cough)
> - Allergic bronchopulmonary apergillosis (APBA)
> - Hypogammaglobulinaemia
> - Primary ciliary dyskinesia or Kartagener's syndrome
> - Localised/segmental bronchiectasis secondary to bronchial obstruction
>
> Many patients have no obvious cause but localised bronchiectasis is common in COPD.

Consider severity/decompensation/complications

Look for signs of cor pulmonale.

Consider function

Tell the examiners you would establish the limitations caused by breathlessness.

Discussion

What is meant by the term bronchiectasis?

This is a chronic infection of permanently dilated distal airways (often a self-perpetuating cycle).

List some potential complications

- Empyema/abscesses
- Cor pulmonale
- Secondary amyloidosis

Which investigations might be helpful in diagnosing bronchiectasis?

The chest X-ray may show tramline shadows indicating thickened bronchial walls; ring shadows and fluid levels may be present. A high-resolution CT scan is often helpful.

CASE 1.10

CYSTIC FIBROSIS

Instruction

This young man has recurrent chest infections. Please examine his respiratory system and discuss your findings.

Recognition

There is a *large volume* of *sputum* in the sputum pot beside the bed in this *underweight*, *dyspnoeic* and *cyanosed* patient with finger *clubbing*. Auscultation reveals *coarse*, *late inspiratory crackles* ± inspiratory clicks (audible with the unaided ear) and wheeze (mucus obstructing distal airways).

Interpretation

Confirm the diagnosis

Tell the examiners you wonder if cystic fibrosis transmembrane regulator (CFTR) gene testing has been performed.

What to do next – assess other systems

Tell the examiners you would ask about symptoms (Table 1.11).

Consider severity/decompensation/complications

Tell the examiners that:

Table 1.11 Cystic fibrosis symptoms

System	Problems	
Respiratory	Chronic sinusitis	
	Nasal polyps	
	Thick sputum, chronic cough, wheeze	
	Recurrent infection – pneumonia, bronchitis, chronic low grade infection with periodic relapses	
	Bronchiectasis	
	Pneumothoraces or severe haemoptysis	
Intestinal	Chronic liver disease	
	Biliary cirrhosis	
	Gallstones	
	Pancreatic failure with malabsorption	
	Intussusception and distal intestinal obstruction	
Infertility	Male infertility due to failure of development or obstruction of the vas deferens and seminiferous tubules	
	Female subfertility due to altered cervical mucus and menstrual irregularity	
Multiple joints	Arthropathy	

- Infection is inevitable – *Staphylococcus aureus* tends to affect infants, *Haemophilus influenzae* and *Klebsiella pneumoniae* appear through childhood, and *Pseudomonas aeruginosa* is ultimately almost inevitable. Chronic *S. aureus* and *P. aeruginosa* colonisation are almost impossible to eradicate. *Burkholderia* (*Pseudomonas*) *cepacia* infection can cause rapid decline; allergic bronchopulmonary aspergillosis (ABPA) and tuberculosis are also more common in cystic fibrosis (CF).
- Pneumothoraces, cor pulmonale and respiratory failure are common.
- Malabsorption leads to steatorrhoea and osteoporosis.
- A baby born with CF might now be expected to live past their fortieth birthday so diabetes, biliary cirrhosis and arthropathies are more likely.

Consider function

The psychological and social consequences of CF are often overlooked, but huge. Teenagers find that CF interferes with friendships and school, adults may find work challenging, and low self-esteem is common.

Discussion

Discuss the pathophysiology of CF

CF is autosomal recessive with a gene carriage rate of around 1 in 20 in whites and a disease incidence of around 1 in 2000. Most CF is the result of a mutation in chromosome 7 at position 508 where the codon for phenylalanine is deleted, although many mutations in the same gene have been described. The result is that the cystic fibrosis transmembrane regulator (CFTR) protein, a cAMP-regulated channel for chloride, is not produced in its normal form. CFTR normally permits chloride efflux from the luminal surface of airway epithelial cells; some sodium influx parallels this. In CF, chloride fails to escape but this is associated, strangely, with excess sodium influx. It is thought that this may seduce water from the lumen, resulting in viscous secretions, the water level at the surface being critical to mucus secretion. CF is pathophysiologically a complex disease because affected epithelial surfaces have different actions in their native state – airways and intestinal epithelial surfaces are volume absorbing, sweat ducts are salt absorbing and the pancreas is volume secreting – causing diverse clinical sequelae.

How is CF diagnosed?

It often starts with clinical suspicion in a child with unknown carrier parents. Chronic productive cough, poorly responsive 'asthma', chronic sinusitis, nasal polyps, chronic diarrhoea or failure to gain weight may raise suspicion. A sweat sodium concentration > 60 mmol/l is traditional, but modern techniques may allow detection of the voltage across airway cells produced by chloride and

sodium; this is normally – 20 mV, but in CF may be around 50 mV. Genetic testing is now also used.

What are the treatment options for CF?

These are outlined in Table 1.12.

Does gene therapy offer the potential for cure?

This has great potential in the next few years. CFTR nebulised alone into the airway is ineffective because it is unable to get into the epithelium. Thus, two options are viral or liposomal (fat globule) carriage of CFTR. Viral carriage has the advantage of 200–300 million years of evolution, and Sendai virus carriage has been shown to cure CF; unfortunately, this cure lasts for about a week because gene expression falls rapidly, and 'infection' cannot be repeated because the effect wanes rapidly as viral immunity develops. Thus, a non-viral approach seems mandatory. Importantly, CF carriers with 50% CFTR have no lung disease, and indeed patients with congenital absence of vas deferens who have very little CFTR do not have lung disease. Thus, a little CFTR, if capable of being delivered and retained, gives a lot, the likely requirement being 5% of CFTR mRNA in only 5% of cells to 'cure' CF. There are hundreds of potential gene transfer agents,

Table 1.12 Treatments for cystic fibrosis (CF)	
Treatment	**Comments**
Physiotherapy	Daily chest percussion and physiotherapy with postural drainage reduces respiratory exacerbations
Antibiotics	Early high-dose, broad-spectrum, long-duration (minimum 2–3 weeks) antibiotics minimise lung damage in infective exacerbations. Oral or intravenous fluoroquinolones (intravenous preferred for exacerbations in chronically infected patients), combined with nebulised antibiotic often the initial choice; resistance and chronic carriage needs intravenous combinations. CF nurses can administer therapy at home. Specialist antibiotics for less common organisms, mycobacterial infection, or APBA. Proplaylactic antibiotics increasingly used
Bronchodilators	Symptomatic relief
DNase-α mucolytics administered as an aerosol spray	Interferes with sputum neutrophil DNA, helping to liquefy sputum and encourage expectoration, reducing cough
Pancreatic enzyme replacement	Helps avoid malabsorption
Immunisation	Routine pneumococcal and influenza vaccination
Lung transplantation	Considered if pulmonary function < 30% with chronically infected, purulent bronchiectasis Side effects of immunosuppression significant ≥ 70% of patients survive > 1 year and 50% > 5 years
Palliative care	Advanced CF

but only a small number are non-toxic and give reproducible results and one liposome, lipid 67, has already worked in sheep. Results are inconsistent, but the stage is set for industry product development – current treatment would be prohibitively costly at a few million pounds per patient per year. The other limiting factor is the clinical trial; the cost of the sample size of a few hundred patients that would be needed to power it would be prohibitive, and the question arises as to what would be an appropriate outcome measure in such a trial.

CASE 1.11

KARTAGENER'S SYNDROME

Instruction

This patient has a frequent productive cough and breathlessness. Please examine his respiratory system and discuss your findings.

Recognition

There is a *large volume* of *sputum* in the sputum pot beside the bed in this *underweight, dyspnoeic* and *cyanosed* patient with finger *clubbing*. Auscultation reveals *coarse, late inspiratory crackles* ± inspiratory clicks (audible with the unaided ear). The *apex beat* is on the *right*.

Bronchiectsis + dextrocardia = Kartagener's syndrome (Box 1.13).

Interpretation

Confirm the diagnosis

The combination of bronchiectasis and dextrocardia suggests Kartagener's syndrome (Box 1.13).

What to do next – assess other systems

Tell the examiners that you would ask about sinus problems and fertility.

Consider severity/decompensation/complications

Look for signs of cor pulmonale.

Consider function

Tell the examiners you would establish the limitations caused by symptoms.

Box 1.13 Kartagener's syndrome

- Bronchiectasis (ciliary dysmotility)
- Dextrocardia
- Situs invertus
- Infertility
- Frontal sinus dysplasia
- Sinusitis
- Otitis media

Discussion

List some more common causes of bronchiectasis
- Cystic fibrosis
- Post-infective (pneumonia, tuberculosis, measles, whooping cough)
- Allergic bronchopulmonary aspergillosis
- Hypogammaglobulinaemia
- Localised bronchiectasis secondary to bronchial obstruction

CASE 1.12

TUBERCULOSIS

Instruction

Please examine this patient's chest and comment on your findings.

Recognition

Whilst the incidence of active tuberculosis (TB) is rising, you may still see the legacy of surgical treatments for TB. The broad aims were to render affected lung hypoxic (to kill the organism) and to close cavities. The results of these aims may include:

- *Thoracotomy scarring* posteriorly/previous rib resections. There is *chest deformity*. The *trachea deviates to the same side*, where there is *decreased expansion* and *breath sounds are reduced*.
- Scarring from iatrogenic pneumothoraces.
- *Supraclavicular fossae scarring* indicating previous phrenic nerve crush procedures. Again, there may be *diminished chest expansion*.

Interpretation

Confirm the diagnosis

Former TB may also be suggested by apical flattening and upper lobe crackles from fibrosis. Thoracoplasty was a common treatment for TB before the days of antimicrobial therapy. This may be associated with a 'white-out' of lung collapse on the chest radiograph. Pneumothoraces may leave calcified or thickened pleura radiologically. A raised hemidiaphragm may be seen radiologically in patients who underwent a phrenic nerve crush procedure.

What to do next – assess other systems

Tell the examiners that TB may be pulmonary or extrapulmonary. Extrapulmonary manifestations, in approximate order of frequency, are listed in Table 1.13.

Table 1.13 Extrapulmonary tuberculosis (TB)

Region		Clinical features	Usual mode of spread
Pleural		Effusion Empyema (rare)	Direct
Lymph-node (tuberculous lymphadenitis)		Painless lymphadenopathy (cervical or supraclavicular)	Direct
Pericardial		Pericarditis Pericardial effusion Tamponade	Direct
Genitourinary		Haematuria Dysuria Flank pain Pelvic pain Infertility	Haematogenous
Skeletal		Osteomyelitis Septic arthritis	Haematogenous
Gastrointestinal		Terminal ileum/caecum (abdominal pain, diarrhoea) Fever, weight loss, night sweats	Swallowing of sputum Haematogenous
Miliary (disseminated)	Acute ('classic') Pulmonary miliary (millet seed) pattern rather than infiltrate ± meningitis, lymphadenopathy, pleural disease Cryptic Extrapulmonary, e.g. hepatosplenomegaly, choroidal	Depend on region involved Fever, weight loss, night sweats Cryptic miliary TB often presents in older people with weight loss and a normal chest X-ray and can be rather covert	Haematogenous
Meningeal		Meningitis	Haematogenous
Less common	Eyes	Chorioretinitis Uveitis Painful hypersensitivity phlyctenular conjunctivitis (grey nodules near the limbus)	Haematogenous
	ENT	Simulation of Wegener's granulomatosis	Direct Haematogenous
	Skin	Erythema nodosum Erythema induratum Scrofularosum/abscesses Lupus vulgaris Chronic ulcers	Direct inoculation Haematogenous
	Adrenals	Hypoadrenalism	Haematogenous

Consider severity/decompensation/complications

List some complications to the examiners. Note that adult respiratory distress syndrome (ARDS) is a rare, acute, life-threatening complication of TB.

Consider function

Tell the examiners that the social situation is important from a public-health perspective.

Discussion

What is happening to the prevalence of TB?

Mycobacterium tuberculosis is increasing in prevalence worldwide, infecting previously healthy and immunosuppressed (HIV-infected relative risk 100) individuals with increasingly multidrug-resistant (MDR) strains. In the UK, 70% of TB affects ethnic minority groups and most TB in white people occurs in middle-aged to elderly patients.

What is primary TB?

The first infection with the tubercle bacillus is termed primary TB and this is usually respiratory TB. *Mycobacterium tuberculosis* can remain airborne for minutes to hours after people with pulmonary or laryngeal TB cough. The primary infection site is usually subpleural, but occasionally it is the tonsils or ileocaecum. Bacteria are taken up by alveolar macrophages, leading to a cascade of events resulting in:

- Containment, or
- Progression to active disease (primary progressive TB)

After macrophage ingestion, *M. tuberculosis* replicates slowly but continuously at the primary site and spreads via the lymphatics to regional, often hilar, lymph nodes. In most people, vigorous proinflammatory immunity develops within two to eight weeks. The primary infection site and regional lymph nodes are termed the primary complex, where macrophages and activated T lymphocytes form granulomata that aim to limit further replication and spread. The *M. tuberculosis* inhabits the centre of these characteristic necrotic (caseating or cheese-like) granulomata, and is usually not viable. Unless there is a defect in cell-mediated immunity, infection should remain contained and active disease may never occur. Thus, the primary complex may result in one or more of four potential outcomes (Table 1.14).

What is meant by tuberculin sensitivity?

After two to eight weeks, sensitisation to tuberculin protein develops due to the cell-mediated immune response. This gives rise to a positive tuberculin skin test (below). At the cellular level, infected macrophages release interleukins 12 and 18, which stimulate T helper lymphocyte release of interferon-γ, which in turn stimulates macrophage phagocytosis.

What is post-primary TB?

This is reactivation of TB, or re-infection. Like primary progressive TB, it is more common in children and immunocompromised patients, and in conditions of overcrowding. TB usually progresses within an unhealed lesion within the first 12 months, but reactivation of older lesions may occur at any time, usually decades later. There may be direct progression or haematogenous spread (Fig. 1.21), often with fever, anorexia, weight loss or night sweats.

Why does TB tend to affect the upper lobes?

These are the most highly oxygenated, sustaining the organism.

How is TB diagnosed?

Tuberculin skin tests inject purified protein into the volar aspect of the forearm. The Mantoux test is an intradermal injection of purified protein derivative (PPD), usually 100 units/ml. Induration diameter is measured at 72 hours and a diameter < 6 mm is negative and > 10 mm positive for past or present TB (> 15 mm if previous bacillus Calmette–Guérin or BCG vaccination). The Heaf test is the screening test, no longer in routine use. False-negative tuberculin tests occur in immunocompromised patients where the cell-mediated immunity is impaired (anergy).

Chest radiography may show patchy or nodular (usually bilateral upper lobe) opacification, calcification, volume loss or cavitation. Disease inactivity cannot be inferred from X-ray.

Microbiological isolation of the acid-fast bacillus confirms the diagnosis but in 50% of cases the bacterium is never isolated. Sputum is usually negative because bacilli in lesions tend not to communicate with bronchi. Morning gastric washings are sometimes helpful. Other options include pleural aspiration or biopsy, lymph node biopsy, bone marrow biopsy, bronchial lavage, early morning urine specimens or cerebrospinal fluid examination. Sputum, if necessary by lavage, is essential for diagnosing reactivated TB.

Is BCG immunisation useful?

BCG is given intradermally and protection is still considered useful but is under constant review. It is now only administered to those deemed at risk rather than through a national schools programme, e.g. occupational risk factors, infants in areas where incidence ≥ 40/100 000 or whose relatives were born in such an area, and previously unvaccinated immigrants from countries where prevalence is high. BCG is a live vaccine and should be avoided in immunosuppressed people. It can cause local abscess formation, regional lymphadenitis and keloid scarring.

Which drugs are used to treat TB?

For active TB a standard recommended regimen is isoniazid and rifampicin for six months with pyrizinamide and ethambutol during the first two months. For active meningeal TB

Table 1.14 Four potential outcomes of primary pulmonary tuberculosis (TB)	
Outcome	**What happens**
1. Asymptomatic infection	Discovered as incidental X-ray finding (90% of primary TB heals, with calcification, leaving its legacy, the Ghon focus, as spread is arrested)
2. Local symptoms	Persistent cough or compression of bronchus by primary complex
3. An overt cell-mediated immune response	Fever Erythema nodosum Phlyctenular conjunctivitis
4. Primary progressive TB Direct progression Haematogenous spread	Replication cannot be contained Common in children and the immunosuppressed Pulmonary or extrapulmonary features (Table 1.15)

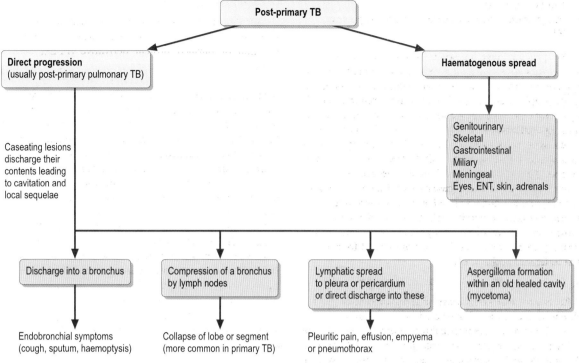

Fig. 1.21 Post-primary tuberculosis.

a 12-month regimen with glucocorticoid is used. Variations in the standard regimen, some including glucocorticoid, depend upon the site affected. The choice of regimen and monitoring should be provided by a chest physician.

IDIOPATHIC PULMONARY FIBROSIS AND DIFFUSE PARENCHYMAL LUNG DISEASE

Instruction

This 60-year-old man has been increasingly short of breath on exertion. Please examine his hands and chest and discuss your findings.

Recognition

There may be *finger clubbing* (25–50% of patients). There are *bilateral, fine, late inspiratory* ('*Velcro*') *crackles at the lung bases*, which do not clear with coughing.

Interpretation

Confirm the diagnosis

Bilateral, fine, basal, late inspiratory crackles characterise idiopathic pulmonary fibrosis (IPF), asbestosis and left ventricular failure. Bronchiectasis crackles are coarser, and earlier in inspiration.

What to do next – consider causes

There are many types of diffuse parenchymal lung disease (DPLD; see Table 1.15), and differential diagnoses of DPLD. Tell the examiners you would ask about symptoms (Box 1.14).

Note any signs of connective tissue disease in the face or hands, e.g. scleroderma, rheumatoid hands, malar rash, (Fig. 1.22).

Box 1.14 Symptoms suggesting a possible cause of diffuse parenchymal lung disease (DPLD) or its differential diagnoses

- Most DPLDs cause breathlessness
- Cough is common but diagnostically unhelpful
- Idiopathic pulmonary fibrosis invariably produces breathlessness, occasionally cough and seldom pleurisy
- Wheeze is not a feature except in pulmonary eosinophilia associated with asthma, and occasionally left ventricular failure
- Haemoptysis is common in pulmonary haemorrhage and vasculitis
- Large sputum volumes suggest bronchiectasis
- Chest pain is rare except in systemic lupus erythematosus
- Pneumothorax is common in rare cystic DPLDs
- Fever suggests infection, vasculitis or malignancy
- Weight loss suggests malignancy but can occur in any severe DPLD

Table 1.15 Classification of diffuse parenchymal lung disease (DPLD)

Classification of DPLD		Examples
Acute (< 3 weeks)		Infection Allergy Toxin Pulmonary haemorrhage or vasculitis, e.g. Wegener's granulomatosis, Goodpasture's syndrome, idiopathic pulmonary haemosiderosis
Episodic		Eosinophilic pneumonia Cryptogenic organising pneumonia Vasculitis, e.g. Churg–Strauss syndrome
Chronic, secondary to	**Occupation** (often termed pneumoconiosis if inorganic dust inhaled)	Asbestosis Silicosis Coal worker's pneumoconiosis
	Environmental agent (often termed extrinsic allergic alveolitis or hypersensitivity pneumonitis if occupational or recreational organic dust)	Farmer's lung Bird fancier's lung Radiotherapy
	Drug (drugs causative but also patients with pre-existing DPLD much more likely to develop severe disease)	Cytotoxics, e.g. methotrexate, cyclophosphamide Amiodarone Sulfasalazine, gold Antibiotics, e.g. sulphonamides, nitrofurantoin
Chronic, secondary to systemic disease		Sarcoidosis Systemic sclerosis Systemic lupus erythematosus Rheumatoid arthritis Ankylosing spondylitis Vasculitis Neurofibromatosis/tuberose sclerosis Ulcerative colitis (very rare)
Chronic – unknown cause		Refers to idiopathic pulmonary fibrosis

Tell the examiners you would take a detailed history of duration of symptoms, occupation and environmental risk factors (pneumoconiosis or extrinsic allergic alveolitis) and drugs.

Consider severity/decompensation/complications

Tell the examiners that:

- Crackles become more widespread and may extend into expiration as disease progresses.
- Pulmonary hypertension is particularly common with systemic sclerosis.
- In any advanced DPLD there may be central cyanosis and signs of cor pulmonale, again particularly common in systemic sclerosis.

Consider function

Tell the examiners you would establish the limitations caused by breathlessness.

Discussion

What is meant by the term diffuse parenchymal lung disease?

DPLD refers to a heterogeneous group of over 200 largely inflammatory diseases of the alveolar wall, often with alveolar transudates or exudates, characterised by breathlessness and interstitial shadows on chest X-ray.

How is DPLD classified?

DPLD has been classified by the British Thoracic Society into five groups (Table 1.15).

What is meant by the term interstitial pneumonia?

Pulmonary fibrosis is a clinical syndrome of bibasal late inspiratory crackles, bilateral interstitial shadows on chest X-ray and restrictive lung function. It may occur alone, known as idiopathic pulmonary fibrosis (IPF) – formerly cryptogenic fibrosing alveolitis – or with a systemic disorder. The syndrome was classified in 2003 by the British Thoracic Society into seven histological subtypes with differing appearances on high-resolution CT and different prognostic implications (Table 1.16). Usual interstitial pneumonia (UIP) is by far the commonest (6 to 14 per 100 000), followed by non-specific interstitial pneumonia (NSIP).

What causes IPF?

This is unknown. The modern hypothesis of IPF is that a repeated stimulus provokes sequential lung damage with aberrant wound healing and fibrosis. Imbalance between

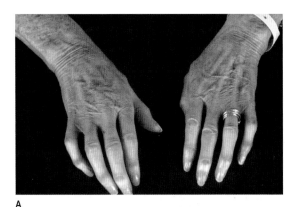

A

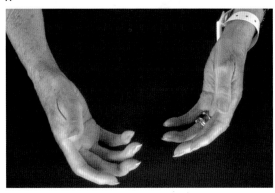

B

Fig. 1.22 (A,B) Scleroderma.

Box 1.15 Conditions with similar X-ray changes to diffuse parenchymal lung disease (DPLD)
• Pneumonia (bacterial, viral, fungal) • Miliary tuberculosis • Bronchiectasis • Left ventricular failure • Lymphangitis carcinomatosis • Broncheoalveolar cell carcinoma

T helper type 1 and type 2 responses, genetic factors and environmental agents augment or pacify this response. Exposure to wood and metal dusts may be a risk factor to those who are genetically predisposed and there is an association with an interleukin-1 receptor antagonist and a genetic variant of transforming growth factor-β. IPF is strongly associated with smoking.

What is adult respiratory distress syndrome (ARDS)?

This is acute alveolar wall inflammation with protein-rich oedema that is common in many insults including multi-organ failure. It causes acute respiratory failure that usually requires intensive-care management.

Which conditions produce similar chest X-ray changes to DPLD?

These are listed in Box 1.15.

Do clinical signs correlate with chest X-ray changes in IPF?

In IPF profuse crackles and a highly abnormal high-resolution CT may be associated with an almost normal chest X-ray, although the chest X-ray is invariably abnormal in at least subtle ways. Conversely, in sarcoidosis, also common, signs may be absent with widespread radiographic changes.

What do pulmonary function tests reveal in DPLDs?

A restrictive defect on spirometry with reduced vital capacity, total lung capacity (measured by body plethysmography) and transfer factor (may be raised in pulmonary haemorrhage) typify DPLD. Vital capacity (VC) and diffusing capacity of the lung for carbon monoxide (DL_{CO}) are best for monitoring progression.

How might blood tests further the diagnosis in DPLD?

Polycythaemia is rare despite hypoxia. A high titre for rheumatoid factor or antinuclear antibody (>1:160) suggests connective tissue disease but low titres are common in IPF. Positive serum precipitins suggest extrinsic allergic alveolitis (EAA). A positive antinuclear antibody suggests small vessel vasculitis. Serum angiotensin-converting enzyme (ACE) is raised in around 50% with sarcoidosis but has poor sensitivity and specificity. Eosinophilia occurs in pulmonary eosinophilia.

What is the role of lung biopsy in DPLD?

Biopsy is considered when the diagnosis remains unclear, with careful patient selection. Biopsy of honeycomb late disease only demonstrates fibrosis. Bronchoscopic transbronchial biopsy is useful when diagnosis can be made on small samples, e.g. sarcoidosis, malignancy, EAA. Video-assisted thoracoscopic surgery (VATS) or open-lung biopsy may be needed for most other DPLDs.

Is bronchoalveolar lavage helpful in DPLD?

This may be useful when infection is considered. Predominantly lymphocytic fluid suggests EAA or sarcoidosis. Asbestos bodies confirm asbestos exposure. Lipoproteinaceous material in alveolar proteinosis and intracellular bodies in Langerhans' histiocytosis on electron microscopy are diagnostic of these rare diseases. Haemosiderin-containing macrophages suggest pulmonary haemorrhage.

What treatments are there for IPF?

Corticosteroids improve symptoms in 50% and lung function in 25% and with azathioprine they improve survival. UIP has a poor prognosis but if NSIP is suspected responses to treatment are much more likely. The median survival in IPF is three years but older studies tended not to identify pure IPF.

40

Table 1.16 Interstitial pneumonias

Histological classification	Histology	High-resolution CT	Features	Treatment	Prognosis
Usual interstitial pneumonia (UIP)	Heterogeneous features within the same field – normal lung alternating with interstitial inflammation and fibrosis	Patchy Peripheral Lung bases Subpleural Reticular If severe, progresses to traction bronchiectasis and honeycombing Ground-glass opacification less common and correlates with active inflammation and cellularity (but fine intralobular fibrosis can give the same appearance)	UIP is the histological correlate of IPF, which has major and minor diagnostic criteria **Major criteria** 1. Exclusion of other causes 2. Typical pulmonary function 3. Typical HRCT 4. No alternative diagnosis on biopsy or bronchoalveolar lavage **Minor criteria** 1. > 50 years 2. Insidious 3. Present for > 3 weeks 4. Bibasal inspiratory crackles	No evidence for steroids but high-dose steroids often used for 2–4 months followed by objective response testing, e.g. exercise capacity, pulmonary function Azathioprine used but no benefit from other immunosuppression Immunomodulation may be a future strategy e.g. interferon-γ, pirfenidone	Relentlessly progressive without spontaneous remission Poor prognosis – mean survival 2–4 years (30–50% 5-year survival) Better prognosis if young, female, predominant ground-glass opacification on CT, improvement in first 6 months or smoker at diagnosis (not known why)
Non-specific interstitial pneumonitis (NSIP)	Uniform inflammation and fibrosis	Ground-glass opacification and consolidation, often linear Site depends on disease, e.g. sarcoidosis mid and upper zones	Middle age with slight female preponderance Usually associated with systemic disease, infection or drugs		Better prognosis than UIP (70% 5-year survival) but worse than RBAILD and DIP
Cryptogenic organising pneumonia (COP) Also called bronchiolitis obliterans organising pneumonia (BOOP)	Buds of granulation tissue and inflammation in alveoli	Non-segmental, often bilateral, sometimes flitting patchy consolidation	Fifth and sixth decade preponderance Subacute (75% present with symptoms for < 2 months) Breathlessness Cough Systemic, flu-like upset High ESR Restrictive defect	Rapid response to corticosteroids	May relapse
Acute interstitial pneumonia Also called Hamman–Rich syndrome	Histologically identical to ARDS	Ground-glass opacification and consolidation	Acute and rapidly progressive Usually previously healthy	Poor response to steroids and immunosuppression	High mortality
Respiratory bronchiolitis-associated interstitial lung disease (RBAILD)	Macrophage infiltration around bronchioles	Patchy ground-glass opacification	Smokers Extension of the inflammatory bronchiolitis that is a usual feature of COPD	Good response to smoking cessation Seldom need steroids	Good
Desquamative interstitial pneumonia (DIP)	Like RBAILD but alveoli affected	Patchy ground-glass opacification	Rare (< 3% this subtype) Younger smokers Male predominance Insidious Clubbing in 50%	Good response to smoking cessation Good response to steroids (70% 10-year survival)	Good
Lymphocytic interstitial pneumonia	Dense lymphoid infiltrate	Ground-glass opacification	Associated with autoimmune disease		

ARDS, adult respiratory distress syndrome; ESR, erythrocyte sedimentation rate; IPF, idiopathic pulmonary fibrosis.

Mention some rare causes of DPLD

Langerhans' cell histiocytosis and lymphangioleiomyo-matosis are nodular and cystic lung diseases. The former is more common in young male smokers, characterised by excessive Langerhans' cells, and may require corticosteroids. The latter is more common in young women, sometimes associated with tuberose sclerosis, characterised by smooth muscle cell proliferation and infiltration and causes irreversible damage without effective treatment. Alveolar proteinosis refers to the accumulation of protein-rich and lipid-rich material in alveoli and is sometimes associated with silica exposure or haematological disorders with immunodeficiency.

What eosinophilic lung diseases do you know of?

Eosinophils are predominantly tissue leucocytes, differentiating in bone marrow under the influence of interleukins 5 and 3 and granulocyte–macrophage colony-stimulating factor (GM-CSF) and seduced to tissues from blood by chemokines, including eotaxins. Eosinophilic disorders occur when excess eosinophils release toxic granular contents, prostaglandins and platelet-activating factor and stimulate mast cell degranulation leading to vascular permeability changes, mucus production and smooth muscle contraction. Eosinophilic lung diseases are outlined in Table 1.17.

Some other lung diseases are sometimes accompanied by eosinophilia e.g. sarcoidosis, fibrosing alveolitis, lung cancer, leukaemia, lymphoma.

Table 1.17 Eosinophilic lung diseases

Category	Diseases	Descriptions
Atopy	Asthma	Eosinophilia modest ($< 1.5 \times 10^9$/l)
	Allergic bronchopulmonary aspergillosis (ABPA)	Common Caused by a ubiquitous fungus (also causes aspergilloma in cavities and invasive aspergillosis in the immunocompromised) Inhaled spores cause eosinophilic bronchial and alveolar inflammation with breathlessness Chest X-ray infiltrates are dynamic (change over weeks) Positive skin test for *Aspergillus fumigatus*, immunoglobulin G antibody to *A. fumigatus* and high immunoglobulin E Treated with long-term or intermittent corticosteroids and sometimes systemic antifungals Tends to improve
Infection	Helminths and parasites	Eosinophilia usually modest
Drugs	e.g. nitrofurantoin, NSAIDs, antibiotics, sulfasalazine, methotrexate	
Idiopathic	Simple pulmonary eosinophilia (Loeffler syndrome)	Eosinophilia modest ($< 1.5 \times 10^9$/l) Transient bilateral infiltrates and few symptoms Resolves without treatment
	Chronic eosinophilic pneumonia	Insidious cough, breathlessness, fever, weight loss Respiratory failure possible More common in middle-aged females 50% have asthma 80% have peripheral blood eosinophilia Peripheral patchy consolidation in upper and mid zones on chest X-ray ± cavitation Treated with long-term corticosteroids
	Acute eosinophilic pneumonia	Rare Acute version of chronic eosinophilic pneumonia
	Idiopathic hypereosinophilic syndrome	Rare (may be due to a gene deletion activating tyrosine kinase) Eosinophilia $> 1.5 \times 10^9$/l and may be very high Lungs and heart affected e.g. heart failure
	Churg–Strauss syndrome	Established asthma Eosinophilia $> 1.5 \times 10^9$/l; may be very high Flitting or dynamic pulmonary infiltrates Multisystem, usually ANCA-associated, small vessel vasculitis, e.g. upper respiratory tract, skin, peripheral nerves, gastrointestinal, cardiovascular, renal PANCA-positive 50%

NSAIDs, non-steroidal anti-inflammatory drugs.

CASE 1.14

RHEUMATOID LUNG

Instruction

This patient is breathless. Please examine her respiratory system and discuss your findings.

Recognition

There are *fine crackles* in *both lungs* in this patient with *rheumatoid arthritis* and *rheumatoid nodules* (Fig. 1.23).

Interpretation

Confirm the diagnosis

Rheumatoid hands and nodules strongly suggest rheumatoid lung.

What to do next – assess other systems

Tell the examiners that rheumatoid nodules are associated with many other extra-articular manifestations of rheumatoid arthritis (Table 5.31, Case 5.16).

Consider severity/decompensation/complications

Rheumatoid lung fibrosis does not usually cause respiratory failure.

Consider function

Tell the examiners you would establish the limitations caused by breathlessness.

Discussion

List some lung manifestations of rheumatoid arthritis

- Pleuritic pain
- Pleural effusions
- Pulmonary fibrosis
- Pulmonary nodules

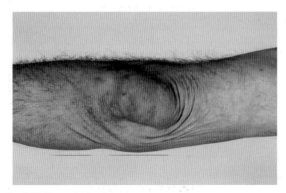

Fig. 1.23 Rheumatoid nodule.

- Methotrexate-induced fibrosis or nodules
- Caplan's syndrome

CASE 1.15

EXTRINSIC ALLERGIC ALVEOLITIS

Instruction

This patient is breathless. Please examine his respiratory system and discuss your findings.

Recognition

There may be *clubbing* (rare). There are *inspiratory crackles* and squeaks in the *mid-zones*.

Interpretation

Confirm the diagnosis

Tell the examiners you would ask about occupation and hobbies.

What to do next – consider causes

Extrinsic allergic alveolitis (EAA) refers to a group of diseases triggered by hypersensitivity to inhaled organic dusts and animal proteins. A vast array of types of EAA have been described (Fig. 1.24).

Consider severity/decompensation/complications

EAA can cause type 1 respiratory failure.

Consider function

Tell the examiners you would explore the impact of symptoms on work and of work on symptoms.

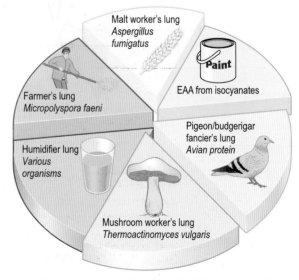

Fig. 1.24 Causes of extrinsic allergic alveolitis (EAA).

Discussion

What are the patterns of disease in EAA?

There are two clinical patterns (Table 1.18).

CASE 1.16

ASBESTOS-RELATED LUNG DISEASE AND PNEUMOCONIOSIS

Instruction

This man has an occupational cause of exertional breathlessness. Please examine his respiratory system and discuss your findings and possible causes.

Recognition

There are *fine inspiratory crackles* affecting both *lower zones*.

Interpretation

Confirm the diagnosis

Tell the examiners you would ask about asbestos exposure. Lower zone fibrosis on chest X-ray, often with benign pleural disease, is typical. Sputum analysis or bronchoalveolar lavage may reveal asbestos bodies (asbestos fibres are naturally occurring fibrous mineral silicates) but histological diagnosis is not necessary.

What to do next – consider causes

Asbestos causes most occupational dust diseases or pneumoconioses, but consider the other causes listed in Fig. 1.25.

Consider severity/decompensation/complications

Tell the examiners that:

- Finger clubbing is an adverse prognostic sign.
- Asbestosis increases the risk of lung cancer and mesothelioma.

Consider function

Tell the examiners you would establish the limitations caused by breathlessness.

Discussion

What are the effects of asbestos on the lung?

Patients with asbestos-related disease may have a history of work in shipbuilding, lagging, building, docks, or factories engaged in the manufacture of asbestos products. Effects are detailed in Table 1.19.

Table 1.18 Acute and chronic extrinsic allergic alveolitis		
	Acute	**Chronic**
Immune response	Early (within hours of high-concentration exposure) Immune complex (type III hypersensitivity) + T cell-mediated acute alveolitis	Prolonged exposure Delayed cell mediated chronic alveolitis (type IV hypersensitivity)
Pathology	Alveolar inflammation – early neutrophils and later lymphocytes on bronchoalveolar lavage Non-caseating granulomata	Chronic inflammation
Symptoms	Cough, breathlessness, fever, myalgia	Exertional breathlessness
Signs	Inspiratory crackles Hypoxia	Inspiratory crackles and squeaks Clubbing rarely
Blood tests	Neutrophilia May be immunoglobulin precipitins (present in some asymptomatic farmers and bird-keepers)	Appropriate precipitins in 90%
Chest X-ray	Small (1–3 mm) nodules lower zones or diffuse infiltrates	Upper and mid-zone fibrosis
Pulmonary function tests	Restrictive defect Reduced lung volumes Reduced gas transfer	Restrictive defect Reduced lung volumes Reduced gas transfer
High-resolution CT	Ill-defined nodules Patchy ground-glass shadows	Fibrosis Lower zones often predominant in contrast to chest X-ray
Progress	Settles within a few days May progress if antigen is not removed	Poorly reversible
Treatment	Not needed	One-month trial of prednisolone

Pneumoconioses							
Asbestos 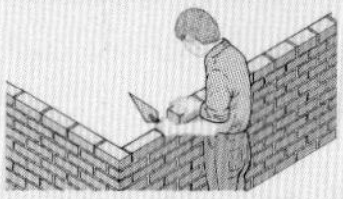			**Coal dust** 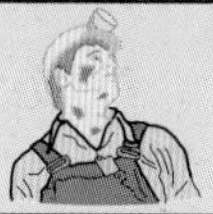		**Silicon dioxide** 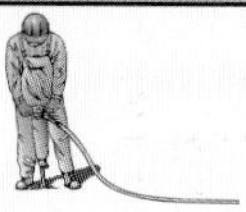		**Other**
Benign pleural disease	Asbestosis	Mesothelioma	Simple coal worker's pneumoconiosis	Complicated coal worker's pneumoconiosis	Simple silicosis	Accelerated silicosis	Acute silicosis	Siderosis (iron oxide) Stannosis (tin) Baritosis (barium) Berylliosis (beryllium)
See Table 1.19.					Similar to simple CWP	More rapid and diffuse than simple silicosis	Like pulmonary oedema Associated with massive exposure	

Fig. 1.25 Types of pneumoconiosis.

What do you know about coal worker's pneumoconiosis (CWP)?

This is related to total coal dust exposure. It is characterised by small or large rounded opacities on chest X-ray with or without focal emphysema, the latter more likely in smokers. There are two types of CWP. Simple CWP refers to asymptomatic small opacities, usually in the upper lobes. Complicated CWP usually occurs on a background of simple CWP and is associated with progressive, upper lobe mass formation (progressive massive fibrosis) causing cough, dyspnoea and sometimes progressive respiratory failure. Lesions may cavitate, mimicking tuberculosis or Wegener's granulomatosis. In Caplan's syndrome, multiple rounded pulmonary nodules develop in patients with rheumatoid arthritis and CWP. There is no effective treatment.

What do you know about silicosis?

This is caused by silicon dioxide, which is highly fibrogenic. High-risk occupations include foundry work, rock tunnelling, coal mining and refractory brick manufacturing. Silicosis is further discussed in Case 2.1.

CASE 1.17

PULMONARY SARCOIDOSIS

Instruction

This 62-year-old gentleman has been increasingly short of breath on exertion. Please examine his chest, neck and axillae and report your findings.

Recognition

There are *bilateral fine inspiratory* ('*Velcro*') *crackles throughout the lung fields* that do not clear with coughing, together with marked *lymphadenopathy*. There may also be obvious skin (*lupus pernio*; Fig. 1.26) or eye (*uveitis*) disease.

Interpretation

Confirm the diagnosis

The most common presentation in white patients is asymptomatic bilateral hilar lymphadenopathy (BHL) on routine chest X-ray or as part of Löfgren's triad (BHL + erythema nodosum + arthritis); fever is common. The second most common presentation is breathlessness or cough but signs may be minimal relative to the pulmonary infiltrates seen on chest X-ray.

What to do next – assess other systems

Check for hepatosplenomegaly and skin or eye lesions. Less common extrapulmonary features are listed in Table 1.20.

Consider severity/decompensation/complications

Situations mandating corticosteroid treatment include:

- Symptomatic pulmonary sarcoidosis
- Critical organ involvement
- Granulomatous vasculitis
- Systemic metabolic effects, e.g. hypercalcaemia, fever
- Local pressure effects

Consider function

Tell the examiners you would establish the limitations caused by breathlessness.

Discussion

What causes sarcoidosis?

Sarcoidosis is a multisystem granulomatous disease of unknown cause. It affects young adults and has a high

Table 1.19 Effects of asbestos on the lung

	Benign pleural disease			Asbestosis	Mesothelioma		
	Pleural plaques	Diffuse pleural thickening	Asbestos pleurisy ± effusion	Diffuse interstitial fibrosis	Pleural	Peritoneal (rare)	Pericardial or tunica vaginalis of testes (very rare)
Relationship with asbestos exposure	Usually > 20 years after low intensity exposure			Usually > 20 years after exposure; Severity linked to exposure intensity	Usually latent period > 30 years (incidence expected to rise over next two decades); May occur with minimal exposure but risk is dose-related; Almost always due to asbestos – crocidolite (blue) > amosite (brown) > chrysolite (white); Genetic susceptibility to fibre carcinogenesis		
Pathology	Fibrosis			Fibrosis – incomplete phagocytosis of fibres by macrophages with cytokine fibrogenesis	Malignancy; Asbestos bodies in lung but seldom pleura		
Clinical features	Pleural plaques asymptomatic; Diffuse pleural thickening may cause breathlessness; Asbestos pleurisy causes pleuritic pain and occasionally affects the pericardium			Exertional dyspnoea; Dry cough; Fine late inspiratory crackles in lower zones; Finger clubbing 40% (adverse prognostic sign)	Breathlessness and pleuritic pain, often with pleural effusion; Weight loss		
Chest X-ray	Pleural plaques discrete raised areas on parietal pleura (and sometimes pericardium and mediastinum) ± calcification; Diffuse pleural thickening of visceral pleura, usually starting at costophrenic angles (high-resolution CT may be needed to exclude other causes of a mass); Effusion			Scattered, irregular opacities in lower zones, mostly subpleural; Benign pleural disease common	Usually effusion; Diagnosis confirmed by high-resolution CT and pleural biopsy		
Pulmonary function tests	Normal with pleural plaques; Restrictive defect with diffuse pleural thickening			Restrictive defect with reduced transfer factor	Normal		
Treatment	Not needed			No effective treatment but corticosteroids and immunosuppression considered if rapidly progressive	No effective treatment; Radiotherapy, chemotherapy and biological therapies may modestly reduce tumour bulk		
Prognosis	Good; Pleural plaques not precursors to mesothelioma			Progressive; Lung cancer risk increased synergistically with smoking; 40% die of lung cancer, 10% of mesothelioma	Poor; Median survival 12–18 months		
Eligibility for industrial injury benefit	Usually ineligible			Eligible	Eligible		

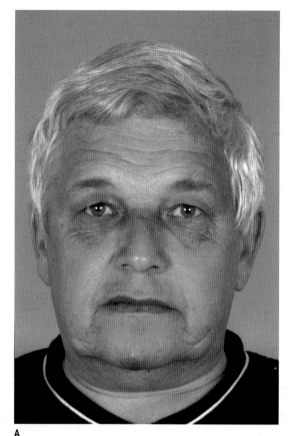

A

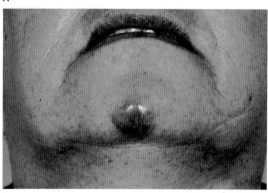

B

Fig. 1.26 (A,B) Lupus pernio.

Table 1.20 Extrapulmonary features of sarcoidosis	
System	Features
Skin	Erythema nodosum Lupus pernio Itch
Lymphoreticular	Lymphadenopathy (usually painless but can be bulky) Hepatosplenomegaly Deranged liver enzymes Portal hypertension
Eyes	Uveitis Retinitis/choroidal granulomata Sicca
Glands	Parotid, salivary or lacrimal involvement
Neurological	Facial nerve palsy (may be bilateral) Lymphocytic meningitis Seizures
Cardiac	Cardiomyopathy Heart block
Renal/metabolic	Interstitial nephritis Nephrolithiasis Hypercalcaemia Hypopituitarism Hypothyroidism Tumour necrosis factor-pyrexia
Musculoskeletal	Nasal septum perforation Myositis Polyarthritis Cystic dactylitis Bone sclerosis

prevalence in black Americans and West Indians. There is a seasonal spring peak in Europe with BHL and erythema nodosum. Postulated infectious causes include atypical mycobacteria and pneumonias, herpes virus 8 and *Propioibacterium acnes*, possibly interacting with polygenic disposition.

What is the pathogenesis of sarcoidosis?

The unknown antigen is presented by an antigen-presenting cell to activate T helper lymphocytes. This can lead to the release of interleukin-12 (IL-12) and thence interferon-γ (IFN-γ) and tumour necrosis factor-α (TNF-α) via the proinflammatory T helper type 1 (Th1) pathway. Chemokines that facilitate leucocyte attraction and adhesion in sarcoidosis include CCR2 and CCR5. Some patients have an exuberant inflammatory response that will progress unchecked to fibrosis, while in others it will switch off with spontaneous resolution, and this may relate to differences in levels of IL-8, IL-12, TNF-α, fibronectin and collagenase. Granulomata are the classic lesions, containing macrophages, lymphocytes, epithelioid cells and histiocytes, fused to form multinucleate giant cells.

How do the skin manifestations of sarcoidosis differ?

Acute sarcoidosis (granulomatous 'jelly') commonly presents with erythema nodosum as part of Löfgren's triad. This is benign, resolving over weeks, and tends to occur in white people. It involves an exuberant Th1 mediated proinflammatory response. Chronic sarcoidosis (granulomatous 'shoe leather') commonly presents as pulmonary fibrosis or lupus pernio, and is immunologically more 'anergic'.

What are the important differential diagnoses of sarcoidosis?

These are usually tuberculosis (TB), which can also cause erythema nodosum, or lymphoma. Treating sarcoid as TB is less dangerous than treating TB as sarcoid!

How would you manage sarcoidosis?

Investigations and treatments are listed in Table 1.21.

When would you treat sarcoidosis with corticosteroids or immunosuppression?

Treatment should be instituted for persistent symptoms, important complications or asymptomatic decline in lung function. Whilst there is a tendency to overtreat sarcoidosis (it generally resolves spontaneously) there is also a tendency to undertreat and either not monitor lung disease or assume that fibrosis is irreversible when it may in fact coexist with active alveolitis. Corticosteroids are very effective. Treatment is for at least two years if there is organ dysfunction, with regular pulmonary function tests, chest X-ray and serum angiotensin-converting enzyme (ACE) to monitor improvement and for signs of relapse. Many patients relapse up to many years later. Steroid-sparing agents include azathioprine, methotrexate and hydroxychloroquine. Cytokine modulation may evolve as a therapeutic strategy.

CASE 1.18

PULMONARY HYPERTENSION

Instruction

This young lady is breathless. Please examine her respiratory system and discuss your findings.

Recognition

There may be one or more of a sequence of signs (Fig. 1.27).

Interpretation

Confirm the diagnosis

This requires investigation, but a loud P2 is helpful.

What to do next – consider causes

Tell the examiners possible causes of pulmonary hypertension, classified, based on the World Health Organization classification, in Table 1.22.

Consider severity/decompensation/complications

Tell the examiners that severity may be determined by:

- Symptoms and adverse features, e.g. syncopal episodes, extremes of age, rapid progression
- Exercise capacity, e.g. the 'six-minute walk' test
- Haemodynamics – pulmonary artery oxygen saturation, cardiac index and right atrial pressure all provide objective haemodynamic information on severity, as does the lack of response to vasodilators at angiography

Cor pulmonale is right-sided heart failure secondary to pulmonary disease (the final common trigger being pulmonary hypertension).

Consider function

Tell the examiners you would establish exercise capacity.

Discussion

What is normal pulmonary artery pressure (PAP)?

Normal PAP is less than one-fifth of systemic arterial pressure and is defined as < 25 mmHg at rest and < 30 mmHg on exercise. Pulmonary hypertension is often progressive, and pressures generated by the right side of the heart may

Table 1.21 Management of sarcoidosis		
	BHL/Löfgren's triad	**Pulmonary infiltration**
Blood tests	Normal	Raised serum ACE reflecting granulomatous burden (50%) Hypercalcaemia (10%)
Chest X-ray	BHL	BHL BHL + inflitrates Infiltrates Fibrosis
CT scan	Mediastinal lymph nodes	Reticulonodular pattern with perilymphatic bronchovascular distribution
Pulmonary function tests	Normal or near normal	Restrictive defect
Biopsy	Only needed if lymphoma or TB suspected (absence of triad)	Transbronchial unless skin lesion or lymph node
Treatment	None NSAIDs for erythema nodosum Corticosteroid eye drops for uveitis Occasionally systemic corticosteroids	Corticosteroid trial
ACE, angiotensin-converting enzyme; BHL, bilateral hilar lymphadenopathy; NSAIDs, non-steroidal anti-inflammatory drugs.		

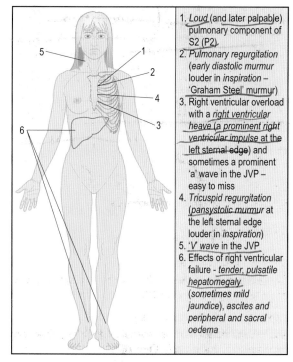

1. _Loud_ (and later palpable) pulmonary component of S2 (P2)
2. _Pulmonary regurgitation_ (early diastolic murmur louder in _inspiration_ – 'Graham Steel' murmur)
3. Right ventricular overload with a _right ventricular heave_ (a prominent right ventricular impulse at the left sternal edge) and sometimes a prominent 'a' wave in the JVP – easy to miss
4. _Tricuspid regurgitation_ (_pansystolic murmur_ at the left sternal edge louder in _inspiration_)
5. '_V_ wave in the JVP
6. Effects of right ventricular failure - _tender, pulsatile hepatomegaly_ (sometimes mild jaundice), ascites and peripheral and sacral oedema

Fig. 1.27 Signs of pulmonary hypertension. JVP, jugular venous pulse.

Table 1.22 Classification of pulmonary hypertension

Type	Subtypes
Pulmonary artery hypertension (PAH)	Idiopathic (IPAH) and a subgroup now known to be familial (both formerly known as primary pulmonary hypertension) Related to collagen vascular disease (notably scleroderma, where there is narrowing of small vessels in the lung peripheries), congenital heart disease, portal hypertension (mechanism uncertain), HIV infection or drugs/toxins (e.g. fenfluramine/dexfenfluramine). Pulmonary veno-occlusive disease
Left-sided heart disease	Left ventricular failure (leading to pulmonary venous congestion and pulmonary hypertension) – may cause pulmonary hypertension but it is seldom severe Mitral or aortic valve disease
Lung disease ± hypoxia	COPD – can lead to pulmonary hypertension (but seldom as severe as IPAH) and cor pulmonale
Chronic thromboembolic disease	Unresolved pulmonary embolism – persistent exertional dyspnoea despite anticoagulation following acute pulmonary embolism prompt concern; covert, recurrent small pulmonary emboli are probably under-recognised and may cause stepwise breathlessness
Miscellaneous	e.g. sarcoidosis, histiocytosis X, schistosomiasis

COPD, chronic obstructive pulmonary disease; HIV, human immunodeficiency virus.

even exceed systemic arterial pressure. The pressure over-loaded right ventricle initially hypertrophies, and eventually dilates and fails. PAP may paradoxically fall when a failing right ventricle becomes unable to elicit hitherto higher pressures.

What do you know about the pathophysiology of pulmonary artery hypertension (PAH)?

The causes share a similar pathophysiology but have widely different prognoses. Idiopathic PAH (IPAH) is most prevalent in young to middle-aged women, and the familial form is known to be due to a _BMPR2_ mutation leading to an abnormal transforming growth factor-β receptor. The pathophysiological process starts with environmental factors (e.g. hypoxia, inflammation, toxins, hormones, viruses, shear stresses) and genetic factors (e.g. _BMPR2_ mutation, endoglin, ALK-1) conspiring to trigger vascular injury. Vascular injury comprises:

- At the endothelial level, decreased nitric oxide (and other vasodilator molecules such as PG12) and increased endothelin-1 (and other vasoconstrictor molecules such as thomboxanes)
- Inflammation, with production of pro-inflammatory cytokines, e.g. IL-1, IL-6, RANTES
- Smooth muscle cell dysfunction, with smooth muscle cell proliferation, and an increase in many types of molecule, including elastase

What are the symptoms of pulmonary hypertension?

Exertional dyspnoea is often the only symptom. Other symptoms include lethargy, syncope and sometimes nausea.

Which investigations may help to confirm pulmonary hypertension?

Diagnosis or screening starts with a low index of suspicion. Early signs are easy to miss. The commonest misdiagnosis is asthma, and patients may be prescribed increasing doses of inhaled asthma therapy in the absence of spirometry suggesting lung disease. Eighty per cent of patients with IPAH have an abnormal ECG (right axis deviation, 'p pulmonale', dominant R in right precordial leads, RBBB) or chest X-ray (enlarged proximal pulmonary arteries, cardiomegaly), and if suspected, echocardiography is essential. Echocardiography may be normal in IPAH (and is operator dependent), but this is unusual. Nevertheless, angiography is a more accurate determinant of pulmonary artery pressure and continues to diagnose some patients with IPAH and normal echocardiograms. One approach is to use echocardiography and DCLO as a screening tool, PAP < 30 and DCLO > 50% implying low probability prompting tests for alternative diagnoses, PAP 30–40 implying intermediate probability prompting further investigation for PAH if DCLO is low, and PAP > 40 warranting further investigation for PAH.

How might you decide if a patient with normal left ventricular systolic function on echocardiography has diastolic dysfunction or an alternative diagnosis, such as IPAH?

Patients with diastolic dysfunction often have left atrial dilatation.

What treatments are there for pulmonary hypertension?

For left-sided heart causes and lung causes, treatment is directed at the underlying cause. Pulmonary thromboembolism is treated in the standard way with thrombendarterectomy contemplated if pulmonary hypertension remains refractory to warfarin. The best responders to specific drug treatments for pulmonary hypertension are those with IPAH. Patients with collagen vascular disease, congenital heart disease, portal hypertension, HIV or chronic thromboembolism may also respond. IPAH is generally diagnosed after angiography with assessment of response to vasodilators. Most patients without contraindications are anticoagulated. Around 20% respond to vasodilators, and calcium channel blockers are then appropriate therapy. For the 80% who do not respond to vasodilators or for those with an initial response who then fail on calcium channel blockers the following are options:

- prostacyclin analogues – continuous infusion of epoprostenol has been superseded by subcutaneous (treprostinil) or nebulised (iloprost) therapy; oral beraprost is disappointing; treatments may even provoke regression of vessel hypertrophy
- endothelin antagonists – bosentan, which acts on endothelin A and B receptors
- atrial septostomy or lung transplantation in refractory cases.

Newer potential treatments include antiproliferative therapies, phosphodiesterase inhibitors, newer endothelin antagonists and agents targeting intracellular signalling pathways at the endothelial level.

CASE 1.19

COR PULMONALE

Instruction

This gentleman is breathless. Please examine his respiratory system and discuss your findings.

Recognition

There is evidence of chronic obstructive pulmonary disease (COPD; see Case 1.1) and cor pulmonale secondary to pulmonary hypertension (see Case 1.18) (Fig. 1.28).

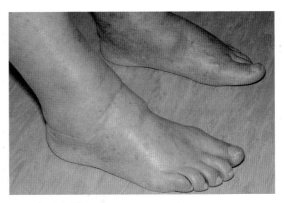

Fig. 1.28 Lower limb oedema in cor pulmonale.

Interpretation

Confirm the diagnosis

Cor pulmonale is invariably a clinical diagnosis, and exceedingly common in COPD.

What to do next – consider causes

Tell the examiners of other possible causes of pulmonary hypertension, described in Case 1.18.

Consider severity/decompensation/complications

Tell the examiners that central cyanosis and cor pulmonale imply decompensating lung disease.

Consider function

Tell the examiners you would establish exercise capacity.

Discussion

What is cor pulmonale?

This is right-sided heart failure secondary to pulmonary disease (the final common trigger being pulmonary hypertension).

How is it treated?

Oxygen and diuretics remain unsatisfactory in the treatment of what is an advanced condition.

CASE 1.20

PULMONARY EMBOLISM

Instruction

This 72-year-old lady reports pain on inspiration. Please examine her chest and report your findings.

Recognition

There is *tachypnoea* at rest with a respiratory rate of (state) and *tachycardia* with a *loud pulmonary component* to the *second heart sound* (P2). A *pleural rub* is audible at (state location). No other signs are present (Fig. 1.29).

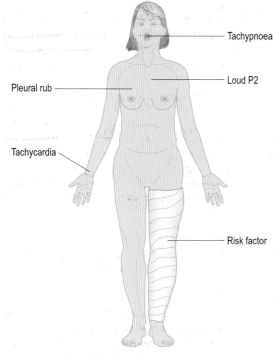

Tachypnoea

Loud P2

Pleural rub

Tachycardia

Risk factor

Fig. 1.29 Pulmonary embolism.

Table 1.23 Presentation of acute pulmonary embolism (PE)	
Presentation	**Features**
Pulmonary infarction syndrome (60%)	Typically pleuritic pain ± haemoptysis Pleural rub may be present
Isolated dyspnoea (25%)	Acute breathlessness without haemorrhage or circulatory collapse Typically sudden onset in presence of risk factors
Collapse, poor reserve (10%)	Usually older patients with limited cardiorespiratory reserve in whom a small PE can be catastrophic
Circulatory collapse (5%)	Hypotension ± syncope Usually due to massive PE with acute right-sided heart failure

Box 1.16 Risk factors for pulmonary embolism

Major (relative risk 5–20)
- Major and abdominal surgery
- Lower limb orthopaedic surgery
- Obstetric causes – late pregnancy, Caesarean section, pre-eclampsia
- Malignancy – pelvic, abdominal, metastatic
- Lower leg fracture or varicose veins
- Previous proven venous thromboembolism (VTE)

Minor (relative risk 2–4)
- Cardiovascular – heart failure, hypertension, congenital heart disease, central venous access
- Oestrogens – oral contraceptive pill, hormone replacement therapy
- Other – occult malignancy, chronic obstructive pulmonary disease, neurological disability, obesity, thrombotic and myeloproliferative disorders, nephrotic syndrome, inflammatory bowel disease

Recent studies show a risk of VTE in hospital inpatients with a wide variety of acute medical conditions comparable with that seen after major surgery – hence prophylactic LMWH in many older, bed-bound or sedentary in-patients.

Interpretation

Confirm the diagnosis

Tell the examiners that you would ask about symptoms. Dyspnoea and tachypnoea (respiratory rate > 20/minute) are the most common. The haemodynamic effects depend upon the area of the vascular tree involved and on the pre-existing cardiorespiratory state. Acute pulmonary embolism (PE) presents in one of four main ways (Table 1.23).

Chronic, covert thromboembolic disease typically presents with insidious breathlessness over weeks to months due to the increasing burden of recurrent small clots. It is under-recognised.

What to do next – consider causes

Risk factors for venous thromboembolism (VTE) are listed in Box 1.16.

Consider severity/decompensation/complications

Circulatory collapse indicates massive PE.

Consider function

Tell the examiners you would establish exercise capacity.

Discussion

Why is PE important?

The annual incidence is 60–70 per 100 000. Untreated mortality is about 30% and it is the commonest cause of death

after elective surgery and the commonest cause of maternal death in the UK.

What causes PE?

PE refers to obstruction of part of the vascular tree, usually because of a thrombus from a distant site, usually a deep vein thrombosis (DVT) in the leg and pelvis. Up to 50% of patients with a clinically obvious DVT have a high probability V/Q scan and around 70% of patients with proven PE have a proximal DVT. Rare causes include air, amniotic fluid and fat embolisms.

Does smoking increase the risk of VTE?

There is, surprisingly, little evidence for this.

What about 'economy class syndrome' as a risk factor?

Long-distance sedentary travel is a risk factor for VTE. A 2001 study of 135.29 million passengers showed an incidence of 4.8 cases per million for travel over 10 000 km, 1.5

per million for travel over 5000 km and up to 10 000 km and 0.01 per million under 5000 km. Air quality may have a bearing since watching television for an equivalent time period seems to carry less risk of PE (although a higher risk of obesity!).

What do you know about inherited thrombophilias?

These are discussed in Case 2.37; 25–30% of patients with PE have an identifiable inherited thrombophilia that must usually interact with an acquired risk factor to provoke VTE.

When might you consider thrombophilia testing?

The two main situations are listed in Box 1.17.

When are investigations for occult malignancy justified?

Occult cancer is present in 7–12% of patients with idiopathic VTE. Screening is currently recommended only when suspected clinically, or on chest X-ray or routine blood tests. These patients are more likely to have a poor prognosis because of regional or distant metastases. Earlier identification of malignancy is possible with screening but it is not known whether this impacts on survival.

Why does hypoxia occur in PE?

This is the result of reduced cardiac output, low mixed venous pO$_2$ and higher perfusion to the remaining alveoli, leading to mismatching of ventilation and perfusion (V/Q). Hypoxia is greater in those with a larger pre-morbid V/Q spread, e.g. pre-existing lung disease; a hitherto healthy person may thus not be hypoxic. Hypoxia is often disproportionate to the degree of lung affected, however, and this may be because of hitherto ill-understood inflammatory responses to PE, or sometimes due to showers of sub-radiographic emboli causing wider micro-damage. This said, if there is marked hypoxia with haemodynamic stability, the question must arise as to the possibility of a patent foramen ovale causing right to left shunting of blood.

How would you determine the clinical probability of PE?

The prevalence of PE in people in whom the diagnosis is suspected is only about 10%. PE cannot be safely diagnosed or excluded by history and examination; it is necessary to combine clinical (pre-test) probability with investigations. Criteria adapted from Wells (risk factors, consideration of alternative diagnosis, scoring of respiratory points and decision as to whether symptoms are atypical, typical or severe) are pooled into Table 1.24 and may

be used to determine clinical probability. In 1995, Wells *et al* developed a clinical prediction rule for likelihood of PE, revised in 1998 and further revised and simplified during a validation in 2000 (also in Table 1.24). Wells subsequently proposed two different scoring systems using three (2001) or two (2006) categories. Note that this differs from the Wells score used in diagnosing deep vein thrombosis.

This scheme is not easy to memorise! The 2003 British Thoracic Society guidelines offer a simplified model for determining clinical probability (Table 1.25), although the Wells score is commonly used in clinical practice.

The vast majority of patients with PE have at least one of dyspnoea, chest pain or hypoxia. Experienced clinicians and their instinct are as accurate as the pre-test clinical probability score.

How may suspected acute PE be confirmed?

The diagnosis of acute PE embraces the pre-test clinical probability score and several investigations.

D-dimer testing

D-dimers are released as a result of fibrinolysis and indicate intravascular thrombosis. D-dimer testing should not be used to screen for PE. A properly validated D-dimer test determines which tests are ordered and how they are interpreted. Validated D-dimer assays include the SimpliRED agglutination test (used when there is low clinical probability) and the Vidas ELISA test or MDA latex test (used when there is low or intermediate clinical probability). Interpretation of D-dimer testing is outlined in Box 1.18.

D-dimer testing becomes less useful with increasing duration of hospital stay (venepuncture and venous stasis from bed rest).

Computed tomography pulmonary angiography (CTPA)

CTPA (spiral CT) has emerged as the first-line imaging technique for non-massive PE. CTPA can diagnose PE, establish possible alternative diagnoses and exclude significant PE with similar accuracy to a normal V/Q scan or a negative pulmonary angiogram. The ability of CTPA to detect isolated subsegmental PE is improving. In patients with a high clinical probability but a negative CTPA it may be reasonable to conclude that PE has been excluded, consider further imaging such as leg ultrasound or invasive angiography, or seek specialist advice. However, many physicians would not be dissuaded by a negative CTPA (which may miss 5% of such PEs) with high clinical suspicion, and consider bilateral leg ultrasound or venography and anticoagulation. Leg ultrasound is an alternative to lung imaging in patients with clinical evidence of deep vein thrombosis (DVT) and suspected PE. Identification of DVT may be sufficient to confirm VTE, but compression ultrasound is of limited accuracy in detecting asymptomatic proximal DVT and should not be relied on for excluding subclinical DVT. Massive PE may be diagnosed by CTPA or echocardiography.

Box 1.17 When to test for thrombophilia

- Patients under 50 with recurrent idiopathic pulmonary embolism (50% have an identifiable thrombophilia)
- Patients with a strong family history (several family members in more than one generation) of proven pulmonary embolism

Table 1.24 Clinical probability of pulmonary embolism (PE)

Symptoms	Low probability	Intermediate probability	High probability
Score for the following respiratory points • Dyspnoea or worsening chronic dyspnoea • Pleuritic chest pain • Non-retrosternal and non-pleuritic chest pain • Arterial oxygen saturation < 92% in room air that corrects with 40% oxygen • Haemoptysis • Pleural rub			
Atypical symptoms Do not meet criteria for typical	Alternative diagnosis No risk factors*	No alternative diagnosis Risk factors*	
Typical symptoms Two or more respiratory points and any of heart rate > 90, leg symptoms, low-grade fever or chest X-ray compatible with PE	Alternative diagnosis No risk factors*	Any other combination	
Severe symptoms *Either* typical symptoms and all of syncope, systolic blood pressure (SBP) < 90 mmHg and heart rate > 100 and need for oxygen > 40% or assisted ventilation *or* typical symptoms and new right-sided heart failure *or* all of syncope, SBP < 90 mmHg and heart rate > 100, need for oxygen > 40% or assisted ventilation and new right-sided heart failure		Alternative diagnosis	No alternative diagnosis

*Risk factors are:
Previous venous thromboembolism
Recent immobilisation (leg paralysis; surgery or fracture in last 12 weeks; bedridden > 3 days in last 4 weeks)
Post-partum
Active cancer
Strong family history of venous thromboembolism (two or more family members; first-degree relative with hereditary thrombophilia)

The Wells score
Clinically suspected deep vein thrombosis (DVT)   3
Alternative diagnosis is less likely than PE   3
Tachycardia   1.5
Immobilization/surgery in previous 4 weeks   1.5
History of DVT or PE   1.5
Haemoptysis   1
Malignancy (treatment for within 6 months, palliative)   1
Interpretations of the Wells score   > 6 High probability
                                                         2–6 Moderate probability
                                                         < 2 Low probability
                                                         OR
                                                         > 4 PE likely
                                                         ≤ 4 PE unlikely

---

Table 1.25 Simplified model for determining clinical probability of pulmonary embolism (PE)

Symptoms or signs compatible with PE	Is another diagnosis unlikely?	
	No	**Yes**
Is there a major risk factor? No	Low risk	Intermediate risk
Yes	Intermediate risk	High risk

Box 1.18 Interpretation of D-dimer testing (post-test probability)

- A negative D-dimer combined with a low (intermediate with some assays) clinical probability is usually sufficient to exclude a PE (92% sensitivity for low and intermediate clinical probability).
- A raised D-dimer does not imply the presence of VTE because it may be raised in many clinical settings, that is only a negative result is of value (D-dimers have only negative predictive value).
- D-dimer testing should not be performed if clinical probability is high, when imaging should be the next step.

Isotope ventilation/perfusion (V/Q) scan

Isotope V/Q scanning may be considered as the initial imaging investigation if there is no significant concurrent cardiopulmonary disease and the chest X-ray is normal (or, more importantly, no history of lung disease), but this method has largely been superseded by CTPA. A low-probability scan combined with a low clinical probability excludes PE. A high-probability scan combined with a high clinical probability diagnoses PE (a significant minority of high-probability results are false-positives; therefore, a high-probability scan in the absence of high clinical probability warrants further investigation). All other combinations (i.e. non-diagnostic scan or discordant clinical and scan probability) require CTPA.

What might the ECG show in acute PE?

The ECG may show non-specific changes, sinus tachycardia most commonly, or atrial fibrillation, right axis deviation, right bundle branch block, anterior T-wave inversion (indicating right ventricular strain) or, uncommonly, the $S_1Q_3T_3$ pattern.

Is syncope a common presenting feature of PE?

Syncope used to be considered the presenting feature only in massive PE but is increasingly recognised as a possible presentation of smaller PEs. Possible mechanisms include interruption of right ventricular flow, induction of arrhythmias or induction of neurocardiogenic vagal tone, the latter often exacerbated by straining, explaining the reason for PE being a first consideration when people collapse 'in the toilet'. Dyspnoea is not invariable, and pleuritic pain is only present if the PE is peripheral, irritating the parietal pleura. Hypoxia is likely, and the ECG may show evidence of right heart strain. A CTPA is recommended in these circumstances.

What might the chest X-ray show in acute PE?

Non-specific changes are common, and small pleural effusions occur in about 40% of patients.

What might the arterial blood gases show in acute PE?

Hypoxia and hypocapnia are common.

When would you consider echocardiography?

This is diagnostic in massive PE, and is a useful bedside test.

When is low-molecular-weight heparin (LMWH) started in PE?

LMWH has revolutionised the early treatment of non-massive PE, and allows some patients to be discharged with daily outpatient investigation and treatment. Dosing and administration are simple, and monitoring is not required except in obesity, pregnancy and renal failure. LMWH should be instituted in patients with intermediate or high clinical probability before imaging. The efficacy and safety of LMWH in massive PE has not yet been established, and unfractionated heparin should be considered.

For how long should warfarin be administered following a diagnosis of PE?

Oral anticoagulation with a target International normalised ratio (INR) of 2.0–3.0 is administered for three to six months for a first idiopathic PE. Whilst duration of treatment is uncertain, emerging evidence suggests that six months provides no more benefit than three months, but increases the risk of serious bleeding. The prevention of recurrent VTE (PREVENT) and extended low-intensity anticoagulation for TE (ELITE) trials have shown that low-intensity warfarin significantly protects against recurrent VTE but there is no consensus as to which patients to treat. No guidelines exist for length of treatment for recurrent idiopathic PE but it depends upon individual risk of recurrence and risk of bleeding on warfarin. D-dimers may be useful in determining duration of therapy. Lifelong anticoagulation may be recommended for patients with persisting risk factors.

Should there be an overlap between warfarin introduction and heparin withdrawal?

Yes. Heparin should be continued for a few days after warfarin has been introduced (at least where anticoagulation is treating active clots as in VTE or mural thrombus, though not when warfarin is being started to prevent clots as in atrial fibrillation). Warfarin inhibits hepatic synthesis of prothrombotic factors II, VII, IX and X, but also inhibits the production of the natural anticoagulant promoter protein C and its cofactor protein S. The half-life of proteins C and S is short, and thus in the first few days of warfarin therapy a state of procoagulation may be induced, especially in patients with underlying protein C or S deficiency.

Is warfarin used in patients with cancer?

The CLOT study showed that LMWH was superior to warfarin over six months in preventing recurrent VTE in patients with acute PE in the setting of cancer.

What is recommended for prophylaxis of PE for long haul flights?

Mobility should be encouraged. Aspirin or LMWH is supported by limited evidence.

What is the role of direct thrombin inhibitors (DTIs)?

Ximelagatran has been withdrawn because of liver toxicity and the future of other DTIs, which had looked promising as alternatives to anticoagulation, now remains uncertain.

What is the place of inferior vena cava filters in PE?

This is limited to a very small number of cases of recurrent PE despite adequate anticoagulation. Clotting of the filter is common.

What is the place of thrombolytic therapy in PE?

Thrombolysis is the first-line treatment for massive PE (circulatory collapse). This makes intuitive sense, although evidence of survival benefit is minimal. A 50-mg bolus of alteplase may be instituted on clinical grounds if cardiac arrest seems imminent, and CTPA or bedside echocardiography is the urgent investigation of choice; a patient stable enough for a CTPA is often not clinically compromised enough to warrant consideration of thrombolysis. Since thrombolysis carries a fatal haemorrhage rate of around 2.1%, it should not be used in patients with non-massive PE. Invasive approaches such as thrombus fragmentation and inferior vena cava filter insertion may be considered.

How does management of suspected and confirmed PE differ in pregnancy?

Standard pre-test clinical probability should be determined in the same way, recognising that pregnancy is a major risk factor. D-dimer testing is of no value because it rises after about six weeks' gestation and is elevated until about three months post-partum. A chest X-ray is mandatory, and should not be delayed by concerns about fetal radiation. V/Q scanning and CTPA carry greater risks but the risk to mother and unborn child of delayed diagnosis is greater. A lone Q scan may be safest. Warfarin is contraindicated in pregnancy. LMWH is used from diagnosis until 6–12 weeks post-partum.

CASE 1.21

PLEURAL EFFUSION

Instruction

This 70-year-old lady is breathless. Please examine her chest and report your findings.

Recognition

The *trachea* is *deviated to the opposite side* (if large pleural effusion). There is *stony dullness* to percussion. *Breath sounds* and *vocal resonance* are *reduced* (Fig. 1.30).

Interpretation

Confirm the diagnosis

Consider the other causes of dullness at the lung base (Case 1.3).

What to do next – consider causes

Tell the examiners that it may be an exudate or transudate (Table 1.26).

Consider severity/decompensation/complications

This depends largely on the underlying cause.

Consider function

Tell the examiners you would establish exercise tolerance.

Discussion

Which drugs may cause a pleural effusion?

Many drugs have been reported as causal, and tend to cause exudates. Drugs for which over 100 cases of pleural

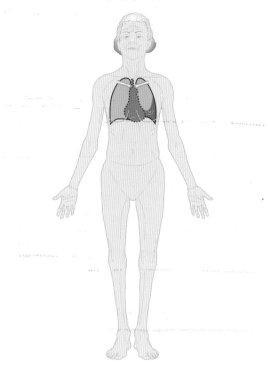

Fig. 1.30 Pleural effusion.

Table 1.26 Causes of transudates and exudates	
Transudates (< 30 g/l protein) **Tend to be bilateral**	**Exudates (> 30 g/l protein)** **Tend to be unilateral**
Left ventricular failure (*raised jugular venous pulse, pulmonary oedema, third heart sound*); chronic effusions may become exudates Nephrotic syndrome (*generalised/facial/periorbital oedema*) Hepatic failure (*signs of chronic liver disease*); in addition to hypoproteinaemia, right-sided diaphragmatic lymphatic channels may open secondary to ascites and contribute to the effusion Hypothyroidism (*myxoedematous*) Peritoneal dialysis Meigs' syndrome, with benign ovarian fibroma Constrictive pericarditis Superior vena cava obstruction	Bronchial carcinoma/mesothelioma (*cachexia, clubbing, tar staining*) Pneumonia (*consolidation*) Parapneumonic effusion and empyema Tuberculosis Pulmonary embolism (*pleural rub, deep vein thrombosis*) – 10–20% are transudates Connective tissue disease Subphrenic abscess Benign asbestos effusion Post-coronary artery bypass graft Pancreatitis Drug-induced Yellow nail syndrome (yellow nails and lymphatic hypoplasia) Fungal infection

effusion have been reported include amiodarone, nitrofurantoin, phenytoin and methotrexate.

How might pleural fluid analysis aid diagnosis of a unilateral pleural effusion?

Most unilateral pleural effusions are exudates. If a transudate is suspected pleural fluid analysis is generally only considered if the effusion does not resolve with treatment of the underlying cause. Table 1.27 displays common findings.

What are Light's criteria?

Protein concentration may be relied upon if pleural protein is < 25 g/l or > 35 g/l. For values between these, Light's criteria may be used (Box 1.19).

Which investigations may aid management of a unilateral pleural effusion?

Exudates or non-resolving pleural effusions require further investigation. Ultrasound can guide pleural aspiration if an effusion is small and can confirm any loculation. Contrast-enhanced CT scanning helps delineate the size and position of loculated effusions, identify associated lung pathology and differentiate between benign and malignant pleural thickening. Pleural biopsy may be helpful in suspected carcinoma, mesothelioma (with post-biopsy site irradiation) or tuberculosis (histopathological examination and culture). Thoracoscopy may be indicated if there is no diagnosis from less invasive tests. In an undiagnosed exudative effusion a thoracoscopic biopsy is the gold standard. Bronchoscopy is reserved for endobronchial symptoms. In immunocompromised patients the differential diagnosis is wide and more specialised investigations may be indicated.

In practice, how would you proceed when investigating a unilateral pleural effusion with suspected underlying malignancy?

Large unilateral pleural effusions are usually the result of malignancy – lung cancer, metastatic cancer or mesothelioma; diagnostic aspiration has only a 60% sensitivity for malignancy (blind pleural biopsy slightly increases diagnostic yield) and if cytology is negative then CT scanning should be performed before aspiration or drainage because it has a high sensitivity for malignancy. Pleural fluid should initially only be aspirated for symptom relief, leaving some fluid for safe image-guided biopsy or thoracoscopy, these tests having high diagnostic yields for malignant pleural disease. CT-guided biopsy should be used when pleural thickening is present, with only a small volume of pleural fluid; open thoracotomy and biopsy may be needed where CT-guided biopsy is inconclusive. Thoracoscopy (e.g. video-assisted thoracoscopy) should be used with more substantial fluid volumes, if no nodularity is revealed on CT, and where both diagnostic and therapeutic (talc pleurodesis) effects are needed. The decision about CT-guided biopsy versus thoracoscopy is often best made at a respiratory multidisciplinary meeting attended by a respiratory physician, cardiothoracic surgeon, radiologist and oncologist. Small catheters that may remain in situ (*Pleurex*) and be used for future drainage are now inserted routinely by cardiothoracic surgeons.

Should all pleural effusions associated with sepsis or a pneumonic illness be sampled?

Generally, yes. Ultrasound guidance is sensible to sample small effusions but if < 1 cm in thickness it may be reasonable to sample only if the effusion enlarges. Drainage is urgently required if an empyema is diagnosed.

Box 1.19 Light's criteria (≥ one of these favours an exudate)

- Pleural fluid protein: serum protein > 0.5
- Pleural fluid LDH: serum LDH > 0.6
- Pleural fluid LDH more than two-thirds the upper limit of normal serum LDH

Table 1.27 Pleural fluid analyses and diagnostic uses

Appearance	Odour	Biochemistry	Microbiology	Cytology
Serous	Putrid (anaerobic empyema)	Protein concentration (transudate or exudate)	Gram stain	Malignant cells may be identified in 60% of malignant pleural effusions
Blood tinged	Food particles (oesophageal rupture)	Amylase if acute pancreatitis or oesophageal rupture possible (may be raised in malignancy)	AAFB stain	Haematocrit may aid diagnosis of a haemothorax
Frankly bloody	Bile-stained (chylothorax)		Culture	
Purulent	Milky (chylo/pseudochylothorax)			Neutrophils may be raised in acute pleural inflammation with opacification on chest X-ray (parapneumonic effusions, pulmonary embolism) or with normal chest X-ray (pulmonary embolism, viral, acute tuberculosis, benign asbestos disease)
Turbid or milky (should be centrifuged; if supernatant is clear then cell debris and empyema are likely but if still turbid a high lipid concentration is likely)	'Anchovy sauce' (amoebic abscess rupture)	Lipid analysis if chylothorax suspected		
		LDH (Light's criteria)		
		pH and glucose (low because of bacterial or tumour metabolism in parapneumonic effusion, empyema, tuberculosis or malignancy)		Lymphocytes may be raised in malignancy and tuberculosis

What is a parapneumonic effusion and how does it differ from empyema?

The differences between these, and their diagnosis and treatment, are outlined in Table 1.28.

What are the common causes of empyema?

Empyema usually occurs with pneumonia, but surgery, trauma and extension of suppuration from elsewhere are possible causes. Sixty per cent of causative organisms are aerobic (e.g. streptococcus, staphylococcus, Gram-negatives) and *Pseudomonas* should be considered in hospitalised patients. Anaerobes and mixed growths are common.

What are the principles of managing a malignant pleural effusion?

Massive pleural effusions are most commonly the result of malignancy. Management may include simple observation if asymptomatic and with no recurrence after simple thoracocentesis, and recurrent aspiration and/or pleurodesis if recurrent. Generally no more than 1.5 litres should be aspirated on one occasion (risk of re-expansion pulmonary oedema).

But, as alluded to above, if malignancy is suspected a common error on admission is to drain to dryness; initial management should in fact aspirate only to relieve symptoms, leaving fluid present for diagnostic reasons, thoracoscopy and definitive insertion of a small indwelling (*Pleurex*) catheter organised through respiratory physicians.

How should a haemothorax be managed?

These may be secondary to trauma or disease, usually malignancy, and cardiothoracic surgeons should be consulted. Any significant haemothorax may require thoracoscopy (e.g. video-assisted thoracoscopic surgery) to ensure adequate evacuation and reduce the risk of subsequent empyema. Haemodynamic instability suggests ongoing bleeding.

CASE 1.22

PLEURAL RUB

Instruction

This 46-year-old lady reports pain on inspiration. Please examine her chest and report your findings.

Recognition

There is a superficial *scratching/grating/creaking sound on deep inspiration* (like the crackle of leaves underfoot on an autumn forest floor, or the crunching underfoot of freshly fallen snow). This is a pleural rub.

Table 1.28 Parapneumonic effusion and empyema				
Problem	**Parapneumonic effusion**	**First stage of empyema ('complicated parapneumonic effusion')**	**Macroscopically purulent empyema**	**More advanced**
Frequency	Up to 57% of people with pneumonia	Much less common Around 10% of parapneumonic effusions become infected with bacteria	Minority of patients with infected parapneumonic effusions progress to this	Small proportion of patients
What it is	Following dry pleuritis, pulmonary interstitial fluid crosses visceral pleura, accompanied by pro-inflammatory cytokine cascade	Infection of pleural space	Pus in pleural space	Thick pus, often with fibrin strands ± loculation After about 8 weeks pleura thickens and pleural 'cortex' ('peel' or 'rind'), an inelastic membrane adherent to lung, develops
Diagnosis (pleural fluid analysis)	pH normal Lactate dehydrogenase (LDH) normal Glucose normal	pH < 7.2 LDH > 1000 IU/l Glucose < 2.2 mmol/l (in practice unreliable) Neutrophils Culture	Pus Culture	CT scanning may help define
Treatment	Simple aspiration (need not be to dryness)	Aspiration to dryness with antibiotics (medical team) Historically large-bore (24–32 French) chest tube Small-bore (8–14 French) good if flushed 6-hourly with 30 ml saline	Possible 'medical' drainage Surgical input valued Place of surgery not well defined; common indication is failed medical management with persistent fever	Effective drainage of pleural space Usually surgical with video-assisted thoracoscopic surgery (VATS) Loculation requires thoracotomy The effectiveness of fibrinolytics in empyema is not compelling

Interpretation

Confirm the diagnosis

A pleural rub sounds 'close to the stethoscope' and does not change with coughing.

What to do next – consider causes

The two common causes are pulmonary embolism (tachypnoea, tachycardia, loud P2) and pneumonia (signs of consolidation).

Consider severity/decompensation/complications

Tell the examiners that you would urgently assess haemodynamic stability in suspected pulmonary embolism and the CURB score in suspected pneumonia.

Consider function

Tell the examiners you would establish exercise capacity.

Discussion

How might you distinguish a pleural friction rub from a pericardial friction rub?

The latter continues if the patient holds her breath.

CASE 1.23

PNEUMOTHORAX

Instruction

This young man was brought to hospital with sudden breathlessness. Please examine his chest and report your findings.

Recognition

There may be *reduced chest movement* on the affected side, associated with *tracheal deviation* to the affected side. On the affected side *breath sounds are reduced* and *vocal resonance is increased* (Fig. 1.31).

Interpretation

Confirm the diagnosis

With collapse of a lobe, vocal resonance is not increased. Remember that large bullae in chronic obstructive pulmonary disease (COPD) can resemble pneumothoraces radiographically.

What to do next – consider causes

Causes of pneumothorax are listed in Box 1.20.

Consider severity/decompensation/complications

Clinical assessment is unreliable at estimating pneumothorax size. Size is assessed radiologically (Box 1.21).

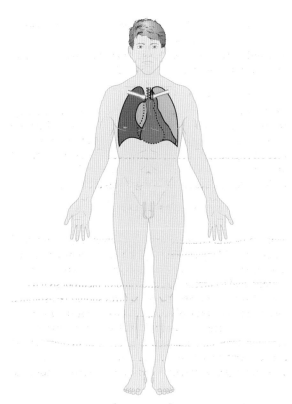

Fig. 1.31 Pneumothorax.

Box 1.20 Causes of pneumothorax

- Spontaneous (otherwise healthy young adults, often tall smokers)
- Marfan's syndrome
- Asthma/chronic obstructive pulmonary disease
- Pneumonia
- Cystic fibrosis
- HIV infection
- Iatrogenic (lines, mechanical ventilation)
- Trauma
- Catamenial (associated with menstruation)
- Rare cystic/nodular lung diseases
- Lung cancer
- Mechanical ventilation

Box 1.21 Pneumothorax size

Small

Visible rim < 2 cm between lung margin and chest wall

Large

Visible rim ≥ 2 cm between lung margin and chest wall (a 2-cm rim of air equates to 50% of the hemithorax)

Tell the examiners that you would be alert to the possibility of a tension pneumothorax (airflow through a 'one-way' valve into the pleural space causes rapid cardiorespiratory compromise demanding immediate drainage).

Consider function

Determine how limited the patient is by breathlessness.

Discussion

What probably predisposes to pneumothoraces in otherwise healthy young adults?

Subpleural blebs or bullae, which are more common in smokers.

Why might tall people be more at risk of a pneumothorax?

The gradient in pleural pressure increases from base to apex, and alveoli in tall people are subject to higher distending pressures and, theoretically, development of subpleural blebs.

Which investigations may aid diagnosis?

An inspiratory and lateral chest X-ray may be useful if clinical suspicion is not confirmed with a posterior–anterior (PA) film. CT scanning if necessary to differentiate a pneumothorax from complex bullous disease, when aberrant tube placement is suspected or when surgical emphysema obscures the lung-fields on chest X-ray.

What are the management principles for primary spontaneous pneumothoraces (PSP)?

Patients with a small (< 2 cm) closed pneumothorax without significant breathlessness may be observed. Patients who are breathless and/or have a large pneumothorax may be managed by simple aspiration and repeat chest X-ray and hospitalisation may be unnecessary. If unsuccessful, repeat aspiration may be considered if < 2.5 litres has been aspirated at the first attempt. If still unsuccessful, an intercostal drain is needed. If successful, the drain should be removed after 24 hours of full re-expansion/cessation of air leakage without clamping.

The British Thoracic Society (BTS) and American College of Chest Physicians (ACCP) both agree on the management of small asymptomatic PSP (observation and outpatient review) and clinically unstable PSP (intercostal drain insertion and admission), but differ on the management of symptomatic small PSP and clinically stable large PSP. The ACCP advise that simple aspiration is rarely appropriate, the BTS suggest simple aspiration with the management sequence above. A 2007 Cochrane report concluded that there was no difference in the immediate success rate, early failure rate or one-year success rate between the two guidelines but that aspiration resulted in a lower number of admissions and decreased

hospital stay. Current evidence supports the 2003 BTS guidelines.

What are the management principles for secondary pneumothoraces?

Persistent leaks are common with secondary pneumothoraces and the lung may be harder to expand and so guidelines suggest admission and aspiration of even small pneumothoraces. Simple aspiration may be considered in asymptomatic patients under 50 years of age who have a small (< 2 cm) pneumothorax. All others need intercostal drainage. Administration of oxygen can speed up spontaneous reabsorption of air.

Should an intercostal tube be clamped?

Only under specialist supervision. It should never be clamped if bubbling, and seldom even when not bubbling. A clamp should be removed immediately in a patient who becomes breathless or who develops surgical emphysema.

What size of intercostal drain would you use?

A small tube (10–14 F) should be adequate. Small-bore pleural catheters are as effective as larger bore intercostal drains in spontaneous pneumothorax but small-bore catheters may not be suitable in the presence of pleural fluid (where they could block) or a large or persistent air leak (owing to inadequate re-expansion). Suction should only be considered 48 hours after insertion, with specialist advice, to limit development of re-expansion pulmonary oedema. High-volume, low-pressure (-10 to -20 cmH$_2$O) suction systems are recommended.

Where should an intercostal drain be inserted?

The area of safety for intercostal drain insertion is between the third and fifth intercostal spaces in the mid-axillary line.

When would you consider referral to a respiratory specialist?

If, within 48 hours of unsuccessful intercostal drainage, there is persistence of symptoms, a persistent air leak or failure of the lung to re-expand. Suction may be considered but only under specialist observation, and referral to a cardiothoracic surgeon may be needed.

When might you consider surgery/pleurodesis?

This is for recurrent or bilateral pneumothoraces and for those with occupational risk; generally surgical treatment (open thoracotomy and pleurectomy, video-assisted thoracoscopic surgery, surgical talc pleurodesis) is preferable to medical pleurodesis.

Thoracic surgical opinion is indicated with a persistent air leak, or if the lung fails to re-expand after three to five days. Surgical options include video-assisted thoracoscopic surgery (VATS), pleural abrasion, surgical talc pleurode-sis, pleurectomy and open thoracostomy.

What discharge plans would you make for a patient after simple treatment of a pneumothorax?

A patient with a primary pneumothorax without need for intervention should have a repeat chest X-ray within two weeks. A patient with a primary pneumothorax treated with simple aspiration may be discharged after a period of observation with a follow-up plan. A patient with a secondary pneumothorax treated with simple aspiration should be admitted for 24 hours to ensure no recurrence.

What advice should be given about air travel and diving?

Air travel should not be permitted until at least six weeks after chest X-ray confirmation of resolution. A longer period may be needed for a secondary pneumothorax. Diving should be permanently avoided unless a patient has had bilateral surgical pleurectomy.

CASE 1.24

OBSTRUCTIVE SLEEP APNOEA–HYPOPNOEA SYNDROME

Instruction

This 34-year-old lady was recently involved in a road traffic accident. Please examine her and discuss your findings and management.

Recognition

There may be *plethora*. The patient is *overweight*. Consider underlying causes, e.g. obesity, acromegaly, Cushing's syndrome (Fig. 1.32). Tell the examiners that you would wish to know the body mass index.

Interpretation

Confirm the diagnosis

Obstructive sleep apnoea–hypopnoea syndrome (OSAHS) refers to recurrent episodes of complete or partial airway

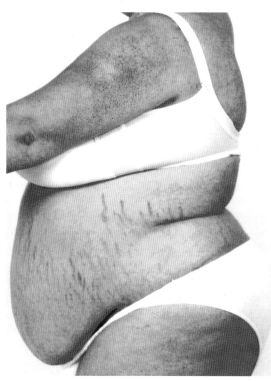

A

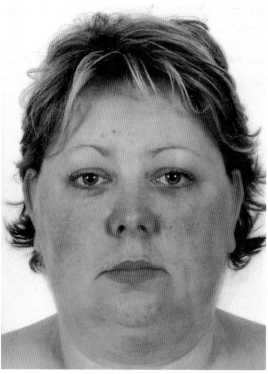

B

Fig. 1.32 (A,B) Cushing's disease.

obstruction during sleep. Apnoea is defined by cessation of airflow for > 10 seconds with continued respiratory effort; hypopnoea refers to reduction, rather than cessation, of airflow. Tell the examiners you would ask about symptoms suggesting OSAHS (Box 1.22) and ask if continuous positive airway pressure (CPAP) is used at night.

What to do next – consider causes

These include pharyngeal crowding, nasal obstruction and other craniofacial predisposing features; heavy snoring can lead to a reddened and oedematous uvula and soft palate.

Consider severity/decompensation/complications

Systemic hypertension with an increased risk of myocardial infarction and stroke is a feature of OSA; ask for the blood pressure.

Cor pulmonale is associated with OSAHS with chronic obstructive pulmonary disease (COPD); look for ankle swelling. Type 2 respiratory failure only occurs with very severe nocturnal hypoventilation.

The increased risk of road traffic accidents in OSAHS is significant.

Consider function

Tell the examiners you would ask about:

- Impaired cognition (OSAHS particularly affects sustained attention and vigilance, information-processing speed and visual and psychomotor performance or reaction times)
- Mood and irritability
- Sleeping in specific circumstances

Discussion

What is the place of a sleep study?

Full polysomnography, which includes detailed recordings of electroencephalography and electromyography, oxime-try, oronasal airflow, respiratory effort and snoring, has been the gold standard. In practice more limited nocturnal recording is sufficient for diagnosis. Oximetry alone is insufficient because of the high false-negative rate (in patients with partial obstruction but without hypoxia) and the high false-positive rate (in patients with coexisting lung disease such as COPD). Snoring per se is insufficient evidence for OSAHS and not an indication for a sleep study. An additional symptom, such as daytime somnolence, nocturnal choking or witnessed apnoeas, is an indication.

What management options are available for OSA?

General measures include weight reduction, smoking cessation and alcohol reduction. An ENT opinion may be sought if nasopharyngeal pathology is contributory. CPAP is the most effective therapy to date.

CASE 1.25

LUNG TRANSPLANT

Instruction

Please examine this lady's chest and report your findings.

Recognition

There is *evidence of major surgery for a presumed severe chronic lung condition*. There is *no breathlessness or tachypnoea*. There is a *mid-sternotomy scar*. Chest expansion is symmetrical and normal and percussion, breath sounds and vocal resonance are normal (Fig. 1.33).

Interpretation

Confirm the diagnosis

Tell the examiners you would ask the patient!

What to do next – consider causes

List some reasons to the examiners for lung transplantation (Box 1.23). Heart and lung transplantation is performed in some conditions.

Box 1.22 Symptoms suggesting obstructive sleep apnoea–hypopnoea syndrome (OSAHS)

- Heavy snoring
- Excessive daytime somnolence (measured by Epworth score), this correlating with the amount of sleep fragmentation rather than nocturnal hypoxia; this is because apnoeic episodes are associated with arousal (demonstrated by electroencephalography) and impede entry into deeper phases of refreshing sleep; partial collapse of the pharynx may also occur in the absence of apnoea, sufficient to disrupt sleep but not trigger hypoxia
- Witnessed apnoeas
- Nocturnal choking or reflux
- Restless sleep
- Nocturia
- Morning headaches
- Dry throat/mouth
- Unrefreshing sleep

Box 1.23 Indications for lung transplantation

- Cystic fibrosis and suppurative lung disease
- Obstructive lung disease, e.g. emphysema with or without α1-antitrypsin deficiency
- Restrictive lung disease, e.g. idiopathic pulmonary fibrosis, fibrosis secondary to connective tissue disease, chronic allergic alveolitis and sarcoidosis
- Pulmonary vascular disease, especially idiopathic pulmonary arterial hypertension and congenital heart disease
- Rare diseases, e.g. Langerhans' cell granulomatosis and lymphangioleiomyomatosis

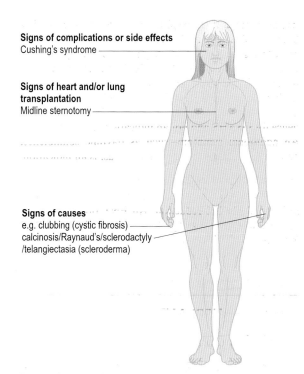

Signs of complications or side effects
Cushing's syndrome

Signs of heart and/or lung transplantation
Midline sternotomy

Signs of causes
e.g. clubbing (cystic fibrosis)
calcinosis/Raynaud's/sclerodactyly
/telangiectasia (scleroderma)

Fig. 1.33 Lung transplantation.

Consider severity/decompensation/complications

Mention some common complications, e.g. surgical graft problems, graft rejection, infection and side effects of immunosuppression.

Consider function

Tell the examiners you would explore pre- and post-transplantation quality of life.

Discussion

Is rejection common in lung transplantation?

Most patients have one or two episodes of acute rejection within the first few months.

What do you know about bronchiolitis obliterans syndrome?

This is a difficult complication of lung transplantation with rapidly progressive lung degeneration, irreversible airway obstruction and high mortality despite continuous oxygen therapy and enhanced immunosuppression. Symptoms include cough, dyspnoea and malaise. This is an entirely different entity to bronchiolitis obliterans organising pneumonia (BOOP; Case 1.13) a fibrotic lung condition with a good prognosis on corticosteroid treatment.

ABDOMINAL SYSTEM

Examination of the abdominal system

Inspection

General

- The patient should be lying comfortably supine, one pillow supporting the head, arms rested at the sides, exposed from xiphisternum to pubic symphysis.
- Introduce yourself, ensure that the patient is comfortable and then stand back.
- Note any cachexia.

Skin

- Look at the skin, especially for jaundice, pallor or pigmentation. Some skin signs of gastrointestinal disease are given in Table 1.29.

Face

- Look at the face, notably the sclera for jaundice, the eyelids for xanthelasmata (primary biliary cirrhosis) and the mouth for telangiectasia, pigmentation or signs of Crohn's disease.

Trunk

- Look for gynaecomastia and spider naevi.

Hands

- Look for other signs of chronic liver disease (Case 1.26) and feel for a flapping tremor (better felt than observed).

Abdomen

- Look for scars (Fig 1.34).
- Look for localised or generalised swellings.
- Look for abnormal pulsation (visible pulsation of the abdominal aorta is normal in thin people).
- Look for distended veins. Caput medusa refers to veins radiating from the umbilicus (Fig. 1.35) and suggests portal hypertension leading to portal to systemic flow via the umbilical veins. In inferior vena cava obstruction, collateral veins open up to channel blood to the heart (Fig. 1.35).

Palpation

Initial palpation

- Ask if there is any pain or tenderness.
- Palpate with your arm at the level of the patient's abdomen. With the palmar aspect of the fingers of your right hand (fingers flexed gently at the metacarpophalangeal joints, finger pads rather than

Table 1.29 Some skin signs of gastrointestinal pathology		
Sign	**Description**	**Disease**
Jaundice	Yellow sclera and skin	Liver disease
Anaemia	Pallor	Liver disease Gastrointestinal blood loss Malabsorption (iron, vitamin B12 or folate deficiency)
Pigmentation	Slate grey (haemosiderin stimulating melanin production by melanocytes)	Haemochromatosis
	Freckle-like macules around mouth and on buccal mucosa, fingers and toes	Peutz–Jeghers syndrome (associated with hamartomatous polyps, bleeding and, rarely, gastrointestinal adenocarcinoma)
	Addisonian-like pigmentation	Addison's disease Malabsorption
	Acanthosis nigricans (brown or black velvety papules due to confluent axillary papillomas)	Diabetes mellitus Rarely associated with gastrointestinal adenocarcinoma
Telangiectasia	Telangiectasia of lips and mouth	Hereditary haemorrhagic telangiectasia
	Telangiectasia and sclerodactyly	Systemic sclerosis
Other	Erythema nodosum	Inflammatory bowel disease
	Pyoderma gangrenosum	Inflammatory bowel disease
	Clubbing	Inflammatory bowel disease
	Mouth ulcers	Inflammatory bowel disease
	Fragile vesicles	Porphyria cutanea tarda (associated with liver disease)
	Flushing	Carcinoid syndrome
	Red, scaly lesions	Zinc deficiency (nutritional deficiencies cause various rashes)

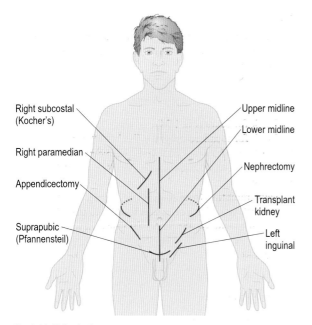

Right subcostal (Kocher's)
Upper midline
Lower midline
Right paramedian
Nephrectomy
Appendicectomy
Transplant kidney
Suprapubic (Pfannensteil)
Left inguinal

Fig. 1.34 Abdominal scars.

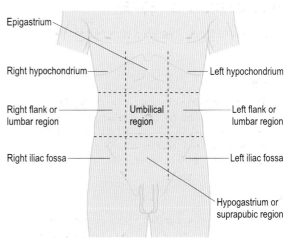

Epigastrium
Right hypochondrium
Left hypochondrium
Right flank or lumbar region
Umbilical region
Left flank or lumbar region
Right iliac fossa
Left iliac fossa
Hypogastrium or suprapubic region

Fig. 1.36 Regions of the abdomen.

tips making contact), palpate the four quadrants or nine regions of the abdomen (Fig. 1.36) for masses. Gentle, superficial palpation often yields more than deeper palpation. Palpate more deeply to detect deeper masses and define any masses. Guarding with rigidity and rebound tenderness is a sign of peritonitis and should not appear in PACES. Palpate specifically for liver, spleen or kidney enlargement (Fig. 1.37).

Liver

*   Start palpation at the right iliac fossa so as not to miss a massively enlarged liver. An enlarging liver enlarges downwards. Use the radial border of your index finger or finger pads. A normal liver may be palpable 2 cm below the costal margin. The liver displaces downwards on deep inspiration to meet your fingers. Keep your fingers stationary as the patient breathes in to feel the downward movement of the liver. If you feel the liver edge lower than expected, determine if it is displaced downwards (hyperinflated lungs) or enlarged, through percussion (below). Measure enlargement in centimetres from the costal margin. Remember that Reidel's lobe is a promontory of the right lobe's inferior aspect that very infrequently extends as far as the right iliac fossa.
*   If you detect a liver edge, note its surface and edge (smooth or irregular), whether or not it is tender and whether or not it is pulsatile.

Spleen

*   The spleen is not normally palpable and generally must be one and a half to twice normal size to be palpable. Start at the right iliac fossa as an enlarging spleen enlarges towards the right iliac fossa. Rolling the patient onto the right side may detect mild to moderate splenomegaly. Bimanual palpation of the spleen is preferred, although the purpose of the left

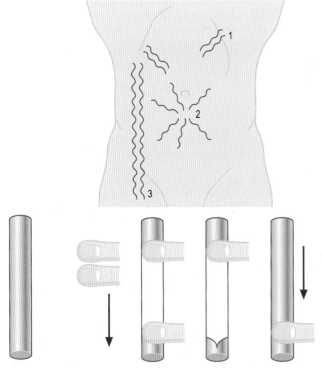

Fig. 1.35 Prominent abdominal wall veins. 1, thin veins at the costal margin (normal); 2, caput medusae (rare); 3, inferior vena caval obstruction. Detecting the direction of flow of a vein: (a) place two fingers firmly on the vein; (b) move the second finger to empty it and keep it occluded; (c) the second finger is removed but the vein does not refill; (d) at repeat testing and removing the first finger, filling occurs indicating the direction of flow. Below the umbilicus: in caput medusae, flow is towards the legs; in inferior vena cava obstruction, flow is towards the head.

63

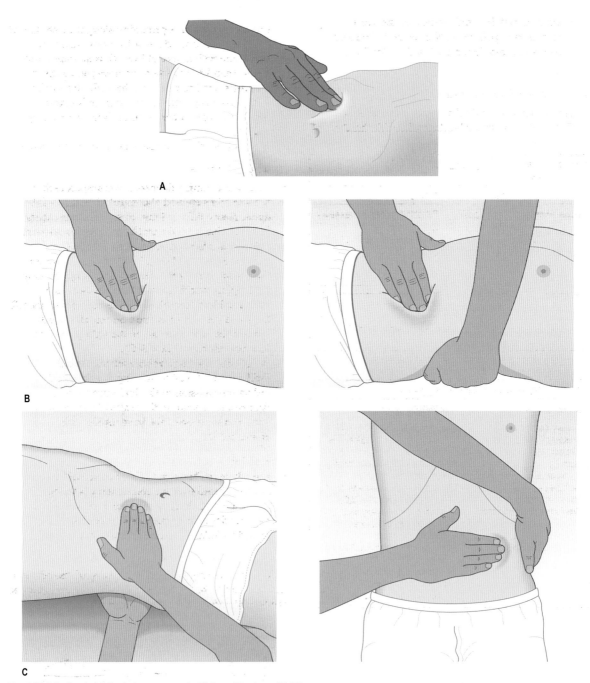

Fig. 1.37 Palpation for abdominal organomegaly: (A) liver, (B) spleen, (C) kidneys.

hand is more to steady the patient than to feel the spleen, which is protected largely by the ribs posterolaterally.

Kidneys

- Palpate for these bimanually and by ballottement. Ballottement refers to a 'flicking' movement in which the lower hand, in the renal angle, pushes the kidney towards the upper hand anteriorly. The kidneys are

normally only palpable in thin subjects. They move with respiration and may appear resonant because of overlying bowel. A common dilemma is in distinguishing a large left kidney from splenomegaly (Table 1.30).

Masses

- Attempt to describe any mass with respect to site, size, shape, surface, edge, consistency (hard or soft), fixation or mobility (with respect to the skin), tenderness and pulsatility. Normal and abnormal masses sometimes found are listed in Box 1.24.

Percussion

Percussion over liver and spleen

- Percuss from the right iliac fossa towards the liver. The level of the upper border varies with the phase of

Table 1.30 Distinguishing a large left kidney from a large spleen		
	Spleen	**Kidney**
Upper border	Not palpable	Palpable (you can 'get above it')
Medial notch	Yes	No
Movement with inspiration	Downwards and medially	Downwards only
Ballotable	No	Yes (because of retroperitoneal position)
Percussion	Dull over spleen	Often resonant over kidney

Box 1.24 Types of mass found on palpation	
Normal masses	**Abnormal masses**
Liver edge (including a large Reidel's lobe or left lobe) Kidneys Aorta Rectus abdominis Hard faeces Distended bladder Small inguinal lymph nodes	Carcinoma of sigmoid colon (left iliac lobe or the fossa)/caecum (right iliac fossa) Carcinoma of stomach or pancreas (epigastrium) Secondary lymphadenopathy or lymphoma (hard, often bulky masses arising at any site) Abscesses, e.g. appendiceal, diverticular, psoas Inflammatory masses, e.g. Crohn's disease Ovarian cysts or tumours Abdominal aortic aneurysm (pulsatile and, if leaking, may be expansile)

respiration but when percussing along the right lateral chest wall the lower three or four ribs are dull to percussion with a normal liver. Normal span should be less than 12.5 cm when percussing along the mid-clavicular line (from around the sixth rib superiorly to the lower edge inferiorly) but there is notorious observer error and measurement is not mandatory in PACES.

- Percuss from the right iliac fossa towards the spleen.

Examining for ascites

- Percuss for shifting dullness if you suspect ascites because of generalised abdominal distension – fat, flatus, faeces, fluid or fetus. Firstly, confirm ascites by percussing from the umbilicus, which is resonant unless ascites is massive and tense, to the flanks, which are stony dull (Fig. 1.38A,B). Secondly, ask the patient to roll onto their left side while marking (or keeping your finger over) the resonant–dull interface. Fluid from the right side further fills the left flank and the area of dullness on the left extends towards the umbilicus but on the right percussion becomes resonant (Fig. 1.38C).
- In patients with large volume ascites, a fluid thrill may be elicited by tapping one flank and feeling transmission of the fluid wave to the other. An assistant's hand on the centre of the abdomen limits transmission of the wave through the abdominal wall.

Auscultation

- Auscultate for bowel sounds, bruits (renal bruits are often heard over the epigastrium), a venous hum (rare, but almost pathognomonic of portal hypertension) and friction rubs (exceedingly rare, caused by inflamed peritoneal surfaces).

Completion of abdominal examination

Palpate for lymph nodes. Completion of examination includes, not to be performed in PACES, examination of the hernial orifices, genitalia and rectum.

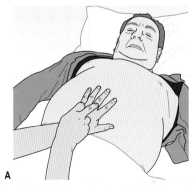 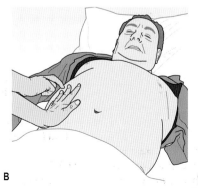 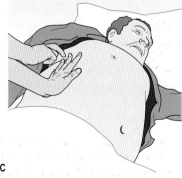

A   B   C

Fig. 1.38 (A–C) Percussing for shifting dullness.

Summary

A summary of the abdominal system examination sequence is in the Summary Box.

SUMMARY BOX – ABDOMINAL SYSTEM EXAMINATION SEQUENCE

- From a distance look for bedside clues.
- Look for cachexia.
- Look at the skin for jaundice, pallor or pigmentation.
- Look at the face for jaundice, xanthelasmata, telangiectasia, pigmentation or mouth ulcers.
- Look at the trunk for gynaecomastia and spider naevi.
- Look at the hands for signs of chronic liver disease.
- Look at the abdomen for scars, swellings, pulsation or distended veins.
- Gently palpate all regions of the abdomen.
- Feel for an enlarged liver, starting at the right iliac fossa and noting its downward displacement with inspiration; note its size and surface characteristics.
- Feel for an enlarged spleen, starting at the right iliac fossa.
- Bimanually palpate the kidneys.
- Feel for masses.
- Percuss over the liver and spleen.
- Examine for shifting dullness ± the fluid trill of ascites.
- Listen for bowel sounds and bruits.

Table 1.31 Childs–Pugh score

	1 point	2 points	3 points
Bilirubin (μmol/l)	< 34	34–51	> 51
Albumin (g/l)	> 35	28–35	< 28
Prothrombin time (seconds prolonged)	1–3	4–6	> 6
Ascites	None	Slight	Moderate
Encephalopathy grade	None	1–2	3–4

Box 1.25 Model of end-stage liver disease (MELD) score

MELD score is given by:
3.8 (ln serum bilirubin mg/dl) + 11.2 (ln INR) + 9.6 (ln serum creatinine mg/dl) + 6.4
where: ln is the natural logarithm; INR is International normalised ratio
Any score < 1.0 is set to 1.0
MELD scores between 6 and 40 are considered for transplant allocation in the USA.
With TIPSS the best outcomes may be with scores < 14, with poor outcomes > 24.

CASE 1.26

CHRONIC LIVER DISEASE

Instruction

Please examine this patient's abdominal system. Discuss your findings and comment on possible causes.

Recognition

There are many signs of chronic liver disease. It may be useful to group these into three categories (Fig. 1.39).

Palmer erythema and spider naevi are shown in Figs 1.40 and 1.41 respectively.

Interpretation

Confirm the diagnosis

Spider naevi offer the best initial confirmation of chronic liver disease (CLD).

What to do next – consider causes

These are listed in Fig. 1.39. Tell the examiners you would ask about:

- Alcohol intake
- Previous jaundice, transfusions or drug use (viral hepatitis)
- Medications, including complementary therapies
- Family history (genetic haemochromatosis, Wilson's disease, α1-antitrypsin deficiency)
- Occupational history
- Travel history
- Sexual history (viral hepatitis)

Consider severity/decompensation/complications

Severity as a determinant of prognosis

Prognosis correlates with the severity of hyperbilirubinaemia, encephalopathy, ascites, hypoalbuminaemia (g/l), prothrombin time prolongation, renal disease, shock or anaemia and comorbidity, notably sepsis. Tell the examiners that the Childs–Pugh score (Table 1.31) has been used to monitor disease progression and, though not so designed, to help determine referral to a transplant centre when the score approaches 10.

The model of end-stage liver disease (MELD) score (Box 1.25) is now often preferred to Childs–Pugh scoring in assessing the severity of liver disease. Advantages include a measure of renal function, and removal of subjective measurements for ascites and encephalopathy. It is used to prioritise transplant allocation in the USA.

Hepatic decompensation

Signs of hepatic decompensation are described in Table 1.32.

Consider function

Well-being relates both to severity of disease and the underlying cause.

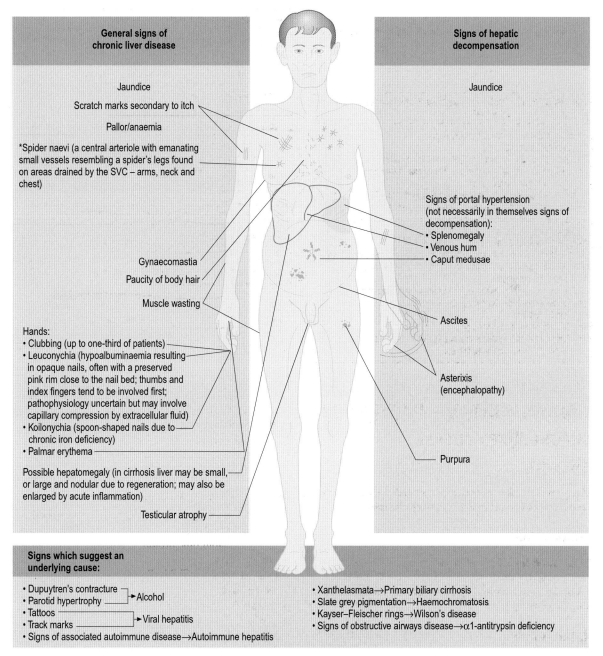

General signs of
chronic liver disease

Jaundice

Scratch marks secondary to itch

Pallor/anaemia

*Spider naevi (a central arteriole with emanating
small vessels resembling a spider's legs found
on areas drained by the SVC – arms, neck and
chest)

Gynaecomastia

Paucity of body hair

Muscle wasting

Hands:
• Clubbing (up to one-third of patients)
• Leuconychia (hypoalbuminaemia resulting
  in opaque nails, often with a preserved
  pink rim close to the nail bed; thumbs and
  index fingers tend to be involved first;
  pathophysiology uncertain but may involve
  capillary compression by extracellular fluid)
• Koilonychia (spoon-shaped nails due to
  chronic iron deficiency)
• Palmar erythema

Possible hepatomegaly (in cirrhosis liver may be small,
or large and nodular due to regeneration; may also be
enlarged by acute inflammation)

Testicular atrophy

Signs of hepatic
decompensation

Jaundice

Signs of portal hypertension
(not necessarily in themselves signs of
decompensation):
• Splenomegaly
• Venous hum
• Caput medusae

Ascites

Asterixis
(encephalopathy)

Purpura

Signs which suggest an
underlying cause:

• Dupuytren's contracture ┐
• Parotid hypertrophy ────┼─►Alcohol
• Tattoos ─────────────┐
• Track marks ─────────┴─►Viral hepatitis
• Signs of associated autoimmune disease→Autoimmune hepatitis

• Xanthelasmata→Primary biliary cirrhosis
• Slate grey pigmentation→Haemochromatosis
• Kayser–Fleischer rings→Wilson's disease
• Signs of obstructive airways disease→α1-antitrypsin deficiency

Fig. 1.39 Possible signs in chronic liver disease. *Differential diagnosis includes Campbell de Morgan spots (common, harmless flat or slightly elevated non-blanching red circular lesions on anterior chest and abdomen) and venous stars (2–3 cm lesions on lower chest and body caused by elevated venous pressure).

Discussion

What do you understand by the terms hepatic failure and hepatic decompensation?

Histologically, the liver is made up of lobules, each containing a central hepatic vein, a peripheral portal 'triad' comprising bile duct and branches of portal vein and hepatic artery, and hepatocytes between the two. Functionally, the liver comprises acini, centred the portal triad. The zone around the central vein sustains injury in venous congestion, as in right heart failure, while in hepatitis and cirrhosis damage starts at the portal triads.

The liver's job is to metabolise carbohydrate, fat and protein. While liver enzymes are useful in assessing causes of jaundice, serum bilirubin, albumin and prothrombin time better reflect synthetic liver function.

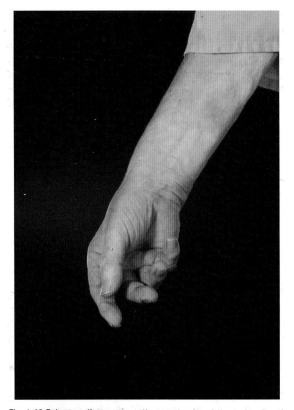

Fig. 1.40 Palmar erythema.

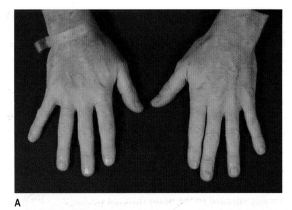

A

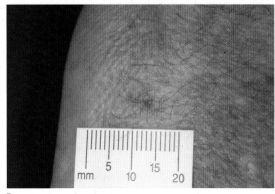

B

Fig. 1.41 (A,B) Spider naevi.

Table 1.32 Hepatic decompensation

Feature	Signs
Jaundice	Yellow sclera and skin
Hepatic encephalopathy	The clinical picture is complex and may be classified by the Wes Haven criteria into four grades: Grade 1: Subtle loss of awareness, reduced attention, impaired addition or subtraction Grade 2: Apathy, disorientation in time or place, behavioural change Grade 3: Somnolence but responsive to stimuli, confusion, gross disorientation Grade 4: Coma
Ascites	Shifting dullness Fluid thrill
Bleeding	Purpura Bleeding varices
Portal hypertension	Splenomegaly (but size correlates poorly with portal pressure) Secondary hypersplenism (can cause peripheral blood cytopenias) Caput medusa (distended veins radiating from the umbilicus) Venous hum

Most hepatic insults bring the threat of necrosis and failure of liver function or hepatocellular failure. The end result of a wide range of causes, from causes of fulminant and acute liver damage to causes of chronic liver disease, are similar – decompensation of liver function. Circulatory changes (hyperdynamic circulation, peripheral vasodilatation) and a propensity to sepsis also occur.

The extraordinary capacity for hepatic regeneration must be overcome if these changes are to occur. Jaundice is common in acute hepatitis because the speed of onset does not allow time for regeneration, but tends only to occur in chronic liver disease either when reserve is exhausted or when acute damage compromises the pre-existing limited reserve.

What do you understand by the term cirrhosis?

This is a diffuse process of fibrosis and regenerative nodule formation. It can be the end result of many insults to the liver; the response of the liver to such insults has been initially, and often recurrently, activation of an acute pro-inflammatory immune response, with chronic progression to fibrosis mediated by fibrogenic cytokines, and repair. The stages of cirrhosis (by no means always a sequence) are liver cell necrosis, inflammation, fibrosis and nodular regeneration. Cirrhosis starts at the portal triads, rippling outwards to form bridges of necrosis that progress to fibrosis and fibrous bands termed septae. In advanced disease there is more fibrosis than regenerated liver. Regenerating liver grows between septae, and the septa–regeneration junction is called the limiting plate. Tightly compacted septal bands with small islands of regeneration equate to micronodular cirrhosis; macronodular cirrhosis involves larger islands of regeneration.

How does hepatic encephalopathy arise?

The pathogenesis is multifactorial. Gut-derived substances inadequately cleared in hepatocellular failure may be directly shunted to the brain through portosystemic veins, which open up when portal vein pressure is high; impaired protein metabolism produces toxins to neurotransmission; ammonia probably affects the glutamate–glutamine cycle. That metabolic changes account for hepatic encephalopathy is supported by a tendency for reversibility.

List some reversible factors leading to acute decompensation of hepatic encephalopathy

- Gastrointestinal bleeding
- Drugs, e.g. sedatives
- Sepsis, e.g. spontaneous bacterial peritonitis
- Other catabolic states, e.g. surgery, trauma
- Transjugular intrahepatic portosystemic shunting
- Fluid and electrolyte disturbance, e.g. vomiting, diuretics, renal failure, large volume paracentesis
- Constipation
- High protein intake

What are the causes of bleeding in liver disease?

These are listed in Box 1.26.

How does portal hypertension arise?

The portal vein enters the liver at the porta hepatis and sends a branch to each lobe. It receives blood from all veins draining the abdominal part of the gastrointestinal tract and is formed from the union of the superior mesenteric vein and the splenic vein. Normal portal flow rate is about 1–1.5 l/min with a pressure of 5–10 mmHg. When portal flow is obstructed, either from within or outwith the liver, collateral circulation develops to carry blood into systemic veins (portosystemic shunting, although cyanosis occasionally occurs in liver disease as a result of pulmonary venous shunts). Two problems then arise – the liver's metabolic function is bypassed and increasing pressure in

collaterals (termed *varices*) causes bleeding. Varices are commonly oesophageal, derived from the left gastric vein; there are multiple layers of veins in the oesophagus and varices usually develop in the deep intrinsic layer. They occur at other sites including the stomach, colon and rectum. Hyperdynamic circulation accompanies portal hypertension and may in part develop to maintain portal flow as collaterals lower the pressure.

What are the causes of portal hypertension?

These may be:

- Prehepatic, e.g. portal vein thrombosis, extrinsic compression
- Hepatic, e.g. cirrhosis, acute hepatitis, congenital hepatic fibrosis
- Posthepatic, e.g. Budd–Chiari syndrome, constrictive pericarditis

What is Budd–Chiari syndrome?

This refers to hepatic vein thrombosis giving rise to ascites, hepatomegaly and pain. It may be acute and fulminant, or chronic. A thrombophilic disorder underlies most cases. Ascitic fluid has high protein content and a liver biopsy often shows centrilobar necrosis and sinusoidal congestion. Treatment is by shunting in a specialist centre (it can induce hepatic failure) and transplantation if that fails. Thrombolytic therapy is ineffective because the clot is not usually recent, but long-term anticoagulation is indicated.

What is the most important complication of portal hypertension?

Portal hypertension is a major complication of cirrhosis (not necessarily decompensated), and signs of portal hypertension such as caput medusa and splenomegaly are not in themselves signs of hepatic decompensation. Variceal bleeding is the most important complication of portal hypertension, usually presenting with haematemesis and diagnosed endoscopically. Decompensation with variceal bleeding may be the first sign of portal hypertension.

How are varices managed?

Management is outlined in Table 1.33. The risk of bleeding in cirrhosis from oesophageal varices that have not bled relates to the variceal size, red signs at endoscopy and the severity of liver dysfunction. Risk indicators for gastric varices are unknown. Varices bleed from the lower 5 cm of the oesophagus, because of high pressure, and so are explosive rather than erosive. The re-bleeding rate is 70% and only modestly correlates with severity of liver dysfunction.

How is hepatorenal syndrome (HRS) treated?

Renal failure in cirrhosis has a grave prognosis. Terlipressin plus intravenous albumin is established for type 1 HRS, and extacorporeal albumin dialysis has promise. Transjugular intrahepatic portosystemic shunt (TIPSS) and

---

Box 1.26 Causes of bleeding in liver disease

- Prolonged prothrombin time (PT) due to impaired synthesis of prothrombin and other coagulation factors (II, VII, IX, X)
- Thrombocytopenia due to splenomegaly and hypersplenism
- Portal venous bleeding in portal hypertension
- Gastritis and peptic ulceration associated with alcohol-induced liver disease

Table 1.33 Management of varices

Primary prevention of bleeding	Endoscopic variceal ligation (banding) reduces bleeding and mortality compared to propranol Protein pump inhibition is an important adjunct to reduce post-banding ulceration
	Non-selective beta blockers reduce variceal pressure by reducing cardiac output (blocking β_1) and allowing unopposed splanchnic vasoconstriction (blocking β_2); there is no additional benefit when combined with banding in primary prevention of bleeding but beta blockers may prevent recurrence of varices
	Beta blockers are still the first-line treatment for small varices because they may decrease progression to larger varices and hence reduce bleeding risk
	There is no evidence for pre-primary prophylaxis with beta blockers in cirrhosis without varices
Management of acutely bleeding varices	Resuscitation with blood and initial restoration of circulating volume with colloid and 5% dextrose are vital but overfilling exerts pressure on varices and may worsen bleeding; saline may aggravate ascites
	Vitamin K 10 mg i.v. should be given routinely; fresh frozen plasma may be indicated
	Terlipressin 2 mg i.v. 6-hourly (synthetic vasopressin) is the vasoactive drug of choice with a 34% mortality relative risk reduction (Cochrane meta-analysis); it is contraindicated in ischaemic heart disease
	Balloon tamponade can control bleeding in > 90% of patients and is indicated when ensanguination seems likely and transfusion cannot match blood loss; it cannot be applied for more than 12 hours because of mucosal ischaemia
	Endoscopic sclerotherapy – injection of sclerosant into a bleeding varix or overlying mucosa, the former obliterating the varix lumen by thrombosis, the latter inducing inflammation and fibrosis – controls bleeding in 70% after a first injection and 85% after a second Endoscopic band ligation is an alternative to sclerotherapy
	Antibiotics are administered routinely (quinolone or third-generation cephalosporin) as these reduce spontaneous bacterial peritonitis and mortality
	Alcohol withdrawal should be anticipated
	A transjugular intrahepatic portosystemic shunt (TIPSS) placed radiologically links the hepatic vein and intrahepatic portal vein and replaces emergency surgery when sclerotherapy fails
Secondary prevention	Early endoscopic variceal ligation (banding), with initial frequent endoscopic surveillance, is important
	Non-selective beta blockers are as effective as band ligation
	TIPSS is not a good long-term preventive strategy

transplantation are the only effective treatments. Prevention of renal failure in cirrhosis with spontaneous bacterial peritonitis is aided by prophylactic intravenous albumin.

Should intravenous albumin be used in liver disease?

Two clear indications are in spontaneous bacterial peritonitis to prevent renal failure and as volume replacement in high-volume paracentesis.

Which patients with liver disease may be suitable for liver transplantation?

Where the benefits of transplantation outweigh the risks of surgery and are likely to improve prognosis, indications for transplantation are listed in Box 1.27.

When is transplantation referral considered?

This is generally when disease reaches a certain severity in potential candidates and/or trigger events occur, e.g. diuretic-resistant ascites, spontaneous bacterial peritonitis, hepatorenal failure, hepatic encephalopathy or portal hypertensive bleeding.

Box 1.27 Possible indications for liver transplantation

- Acute liver failure (commonest cause worldwide is viral hepatitis but in UK is paracetamol)
- Alcoholic liver disease (if patient demonstrates ability to abstain)
- Hepatitis B or C virus-induced cirrhosis (but frequently recurs)
- Primary biliary cirrhosis
- Genetic haemochromatosis
- Wilson's disease
- Hepatocellular carcinoma
- Cholangiocarcinoma

How should hepatocellular carcinoma (HCC) be identified and treated?

The British Society of Gastroenterology recommends screening with six-monthly abdominal ultrasound and serum α-fetoprotein in high-risk individuals (cirrhosis due to hepatitis B or C, genetic haemochromatosis, alcoholic cirrhosis in patients likely to be concordant, cirrhosis from primary biliary cirrhosis). Transplantation is considered for single lesions under 5 cm and up to three lesions up to

3 cm without metastases. Other treatments include radio-frequency ablation, embolisation and chemotherapy.

JAUNDICE

Instruction

Please look at this patient's skin and examine his/her abdomen. Discuss your findings.

Recognition

Jaundice is present. (Jaundice is most apparent in fluid/tissues with high protein concentration such as cerebrospinal/ocular fluid and elastic tissue – skin, sclera (Fig. 1.42), blood vessel walls. Conjugated hyperbilirubinaemia tends to produce more intense jaundice because of its water solubility.)

Interpretation

Confirm the diagnosis

Jaundice may reflect acute liver disease or chronic liver disease (CLD). Look for signs of CLD.

What to do next – consider causes

Tell the examiners that the history might suggest a cause of CLD (Case 1.26) and that jaundice may be prehepatic, hepatic or cholestatic (Table 1.34).

Consider severity/decompensation/complications

Look for other signs of hepatic decompensation (Case 1.26) and tell the examiners you would aim to determine the severity of liver disease (Case 1.26).

Consider function

Well-being relates both to severity of disease and the underlying cause.

Discussion

How does bilirubin metabolism explain Gilbert's syndrome and other genetic causes of jaundice?

This is illustrated in Fig. 1.43. Bilirubin is the end product of haem metabolism, bound to haptoglobin in serum. Most

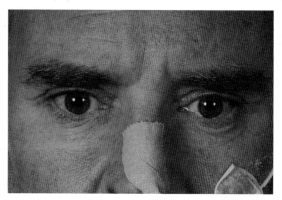

Fig. 1.42 Jaundiced sclera.

Table 1.34 Causes of jaundice				
	What to do	**What it is**	**Causes**	**Further assessment**
Prehepatic	Look for anaemia	Increased bilirubin load on hepatocytes	Usually haemolysis	Elevated reticulocyte count Unconjugated hyperbilirubinaemia Liver enzymes and synthetic liver function tests otherwise normal
Hepatic (hepatocellular)	Look for signs of chronic liver disease	Failure of liver cell to take up, metabolise or excrete bilirubin	Gilbert's syndrome or other enzymopathies Acute liver disease (viral, drugs, alcohol) CLD	Unconjugated and conjugated hyperbilirubinaemia Transaminase rise more pronounced than alkaline phosphatase rise; may be very high in acute hepatitis on a background of a normal liver, but low in cirrhosis where fewer hepatocytes remain to be destroyed Deranged synthetic liver function Liver 'screen' for causes of CLD
Posthepatic (cholestatic)	Look for cachexia Tell the examiners you would ask about symptoms with fatty meals	Obstruction to bilirubin excretion	Cholelithiasis Carcinoma of the pancreas or cholangiocarcinoma Lymphadenopathy Drugs	Conjugated hyperbilirubinaemia Alkaline phosphatase rise more pronounced than transaminase rise

Frequently, an insult causes a combination of hepatocellular failure and cholestasis (e.g. primary biliary cirrhosis) and the biochemical abnormalities in any of the above states may precede jaundice.
CLD, chronic liver disease.

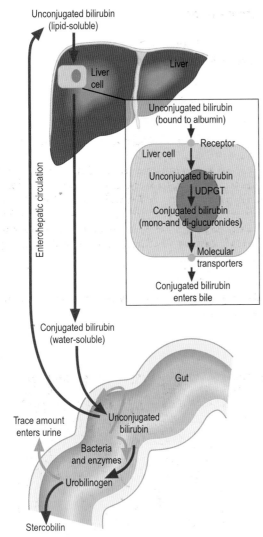

Fig. 1.43 Bilirubin metabolism (insert: conjugation process) and jaundice. UDPGT, uridine diphosphate glucuronosyl transferase.

of remanufactured unconjugated bilirubin and urobilinogen are reabsorbed through the enterohepatic circulation. A trace of reabsorbed urobilinogen ends up in the urine.

Gilbert's syndrome

Gilbert's syndrome is a common, harmless, autosomal dominant defect of the TATAA sequence leading to reduced levels of UDPGT. It results in mild, intermittent unconjugated hyperbilirubinaemia, occasionally with mild jaundice. Episodes may be precipitated by stress, fasting or intercurrent infection. It does not give rise to other abnormalities in liver function. Reassurance is all that is needed. Crigler–Najjar syndrome is a very rare and severe autosomal recessive defect in which UDPGT is absent.

Dubin–Johnson syndrome

Dubin–Johnson syndrome is a benign, autosomal recessive defect of molecular transporters responsible for transporting conjugated bilirubin out of liver cells. It gives rise to conjugated hyperbilirubinaemia and green-black liver pigmentation at autopsy.

Which types of bilirubin might be detected in the urine and under which circumstances?

Normally bilirubin is not present in urine except as traces of urobilinogen. In unconjugated hyperbilirubinaemia or prehepatic jaundice (overuse of normal pathways) it is detectable as increased urobilinogen. In conjugated hyperbilirubinaemia (outflow to gut obstructed) it enters urine in its conjugated water-soluble form producing dark urine; the stools are pale because urobilinogen, and hence stercobilin, is absent.

Which blood tests would you consider as part of a 'liver screen'?

These are listed in Box 1.28.

How would you investigate cholestatic jaundice?

This starts with ultrasound scanning to determine whether or not the bile ducts are dilated. Dilated ducts suggest extrahepatic cholestasis. Normal ducts suggest intrahepatic cholestasis. Extrahepatic causes include gallstones, tumours, strictures and parasites. Intrahepatic causes include primary biliary cirrhosis, sclerosing cholangitis, sepsis and drugs. Endoscopic retrograde cholangiopancreatography (ERCP) or magnetic resonance cholangio-

bilirubin comes from destroyed red cells. Unconjugated bilirubin is bound to albumin and lipid-soluble and transported to liver cell receptors before entering the liver cell. It is conjugated in the endoplasmic reticulum by uridine diphosphate glucuronosyl transferase (UDPGT). Different forms of UDPGT exist but UDPGT$_1$ is predominant. Expression of the *UDPGT* gene sequence is promoted by a 'transcription promoter region' in a nearby exon containing the nucleotide sequence TATAA. Conjugation converts unconjugated to conjugated bilirubin mono- and diglucuronides, transported out of the cell by molecular transporters. Conjugated bilirubin glucuronides are water-soluble and so poorly reabsorbed when they reach the intestine. Most are hydrolysed back to unconjugated bilirubin and reduced to urobilinogen by gut enzymes, and subsequently converted to stercobilin. Small amounts

pancreatography (MRCP) is an appropriate next step for extrahepatic disease, and for intrahepatic disease a liver biopsy is appropriate.

CASE 1.28

ASCITES

Instruction

Please examine this patient's abdomen and discuss your findings.

Recognition

There is *generalised swelling* (differential diagnosis fluid, fat, faeces, flatus, fetus) of the abdomen with *shifting dullness*. There may be a *fluid thrill* in tense ascites, and the umbilicus may be everted (Fig. 1.44). To palpate organs in the presence of ascites you must use a 'dipping' technique, pressing quickly, flexing at the wrist.

Interpretation

Confirm the diagnosis

Shifting dullness is pathognomonic.

What to do next – consider causes

These are listed in Table 1.35.

Consider severity/decompensation/complications

Look for other signs of hepatic decompensation (Case 1.26) and tell the examiners you would aim to determine the severity of liver disease (Case 1.26). Uncomplicated ascites that is not infected and not associated with hepatorenal syndrome may be classified as grade 1 (mild) only detectable by ultrasound, grade 2 (moderate) with moderate distension or grade 3 (large) with gross distension. Refractory ascites is that which cannot be shifted easily or which recurs rapidly.

Consider function

Well-being relates both to severity of disease and the underlying cause.

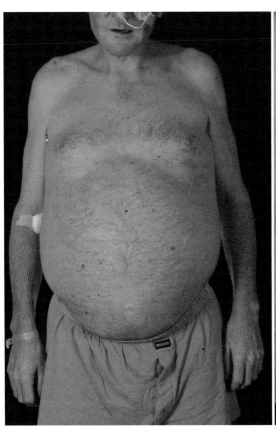
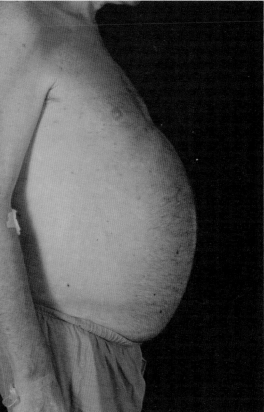

A   B

Fig. 1.44 (A,B) Ascites.

Table 1.35 Causes of ascites

Cause	What to do
Chronic liver disease (CLD)	Look for signs of CLD (Case 1.26) Tell the examiners that the history might suggest a cause of CLD
Malignancy (especially gastric, ovarian and liver metastases, and peritoneal mesothelioma or metastases)	Look for cachexia
Right/biventricular failure	Look for a raised jugular venous pulse and peripheral oedema
Nephrotic syndrome	Tell the examiners you would check a urinalysis
Rare causes, e.g. hypothyroidism, constrictive pericarditis, Meigs' syndrome, serositis in familial Mediterranean fever	Consider if other diagnoses are excluded

Discussion

What is the mechanism of ascites formation?

Over 75% of ascites is due to liver disease. The pathogenesis is uncertain but contributing factors include hypoalbuminaemia, portal hypertension and peripheral vasodilation promoting sodium and water retention by stimulating the renin–angiotensin–aldosterone system.

What laboratory analysis would you request on ascitic fluid?

This should include a cell count and differential protein, albumin and amylase concentration, cytology and Gram-stain and culture. The macroscopic appearance of ascitic fluid is also important – straw-coloured (most causes), turbid (pyogenic, tuberculosis), bloody (malignancy, tuberculosis), chylous (pancreatitis). In chronic liver disease spontaneous bacterial peritonitis should be considered, diagnosed by paracentesis, with microscopy and culture and excess neutrophils. Ascites may be minimal and detectable only by ultrasound.

What is the value of the serum:ascites albumin gradient?

Most causes of ascites are transudates (< 25 g/dl), malignancy and peritoneal tuberculosis being notable exceptions. Because diuresis affects the total ascitic protein concentration, the serum:ascites albumin gradient (SAG) is sometimes a preferred method of characterising ascites. The SAG correlates directly with portal pressure. Patients with normal portal pressures have a gradient < 1.1 g/dl. Conditions causing exudative ascites also tend to have a gradient < 1.1 g/dl, whereas ascites associated with heart failure, nephrotic syndrome or cirrhosis with portal hypertension usually has a gradient > 1.1 g/dl.

Is the chest X-ray ever abnormal as a consequence of ascites?

It may show a right pleural effusion because diaphragmatic channels open up and transmit fluid.

How would you manage ascites?

Any underlying remediable cause is identified and treated. Moderate ascites may be managed in the outpatient setting if without other complications of cirrhosis. Salt restriction and diuretics, especially the aldosterone antagonist spironolactone (50–200 mg daily), are important; the most common reason for diuretic 'failure' is inadequate salt restriction – < 40–60 mmol (1–1.5 g) of salt daily is ideal but unpalatable and difficult to achieve but < 80 mmol daily is practical. Weight loss of up to 500 g daily is desirable, up to 1 kg daily if there is peripheral oedema. Therapeutic paracentesis may be necessary for tense ascites, with concurrent administration of albumin; albumin prevents paracentesis-induced circulatory dysfunction (PICD) with risks of hypotension, recurrent ascites, hepatorenal syndrome and death, which are all more likely if more than 5 litres of fluid is removed.

CASE 1.29

ALCOHOLIC LIVER DISEASE

Instruction

Please examine this patient's abdominal system. You may briefly look for other signs you think may help determine an underlying cause. Discuss your findings and the likely cause.

Recognition

General *signs of chronic liver disease* may be present (Case 1.26) in this cachectic patient with signs of under-nutrition.

Interpretation

Confirm the diagnosis

Tell the examiners you would ask about alcohol intake. Remember that two or more causes of chronic liver disease may coexist.

What to do next – consider causes/assess other systems

Tell the examiners that you would ask about alcohol consumption, previous jaundice, previous transfusions, drug use, occupation, travel and sexual history.

Dupuytren's contractures (Fig. 1.45; not always due to alcohol!) and *parotid enlargement* may be present (parotid enlargement is also a feature of sarcoidosis, Sjögren's

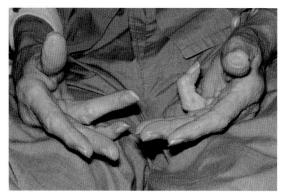
Fig. 1.45 Dupuytren's contractures.

syndrome and obstructed drainage). Other accompaniments to alcohol excess include cerebellar signs (*past pointing, broad-based gait*), Wernicke's encephalopathy (*ophthalmoplegia*) and evidence of dilated cardiomyopathy (*displaced apex ± signs of heart failure*).

Consider severity/decompensation/complications

Look for signs of hepatic decompensation (Case 1.26) and tell the examiners you would determine the severity of disease (Case 1.26).

Consider function

Well-being relates both to severity of disease and the underlying cause.

Discussion

How would you classify alcohol-induced liver damage?

Fatty change can be seen within days of ingestion on ultrasound. Alcohol-induced hepatitis ensues with continued exposure, the liver is swollen, smooth and tender, with ultimate progression to typically micronodular cirrhosis.

List some abnormal laboratory indices that may accompany alcohol misuse

- Raised γ-glutamyl transferase (GGT), due to enzyme induction
- Raised aspartate aminotransferase (AAT) and transaminases (and raised bilirubin, raised alkaline phosphatase and low albumin)
- Raised mean corpuscular volume (MCV), due to alteration in the red blood cell membrane lipid profile
- Thrombocytopenia (haematinic deficiency, hypersplenism, marrow toxicity)
- Low urea due to nutritional deficiency
- Raised white cell count

How would you treat alcoholic hepatitis?

Adequate enteral nutrition and corticosteroids are important in treating severe alcoholic hepatitis, although sus-

tained bilirubin levels after one week suggest non-response and poor outcome and the risk of corticosteroid side effects becomes unwarranted. Anti-tumour necrosis factor-α therapy (pentoxifylline) has shown survival in corticosteroid responsive patients through protection against hepatorenal syndrome but some tumour necrosis factor-α antibodies (infliximab) are in fact associated with higher mortality. Chlordiazepoxide or other benzodiazepines, thiamine and multivitamins are important in any patient presenting with alcohol withdrawal.

List some complications of alcohol misuse as well as chronic liver disease

- Dyspepsia, peptic ulcer disease
- Pancreatitis
- Hypertension, cardiomyopathy
- Withdrawal – delirium tremens, seizures
- Psychiatric disease
- Malignancy – increased risk of oral, pharyngeal, laryngeal, oesophageal, liver and breast cancer
- Social difficulties

What do you know about non-alcoholic fatty liver disease (NAFLD)?

This is now recognised as a massive problem. Of the adult population in the USA, 34% have a fatty liver and these patients have increased mortality with an overall increase in liver-related, as well as non-liver-related, death, a 5% occurrence of cirrhosis and an increased risk of hepatocellular carcinoma. Severity and progression correlate with body mass index (BMI).

Non-invasive imaging remains poor at determining disease extent but there is no clear guidance as to when to biopsy. Proponents of biopsy would argue that 10% of patients with abnormal liver function tests (LFTs) and a negative 'liver screen' who are assumed to have NAFLD have an alternative diagnosis, that LFTs do not predict fibrosis and cirrhosis and that diagnosing cirrhosis identifies the need for screening for complications such as hepatocellular carcinoma; opponents argue that there is significant error in biopsy specimens, it is not without risk and there are few data to support the idea that it changes outcome.

Treatment is with metformin and thioglitazones, usually as part of treatment for the metabolic syndrome.

CASE 1.30

VIRAL HEPATITIS

Instruction

This 45-year-old man has a history of intravenous drug misuse. Please examine his abdominal system and discuss your findings.

Recognition

General *signs of chronic liver disease* (CLD) may be present (Case 1.26).

Interpretation

Confirm the diagnosis

Tell the examiners you would explore risk factors for chronic viral hepatitis. Remember that two or more causes of CLD may coexist.

What to do next – consider causes

Tell the examiners that the history might also suggest other causes of CLD (Case 1.26).

Consider severity/decompensation/complications

Most viral hepatitis morbidity and mortality are the result of cirrhosis and hepatocellular carcinoma (HCC). Look for signs of hepatic decompensation (Case 1.26) and tell the examiners you would determine the severity of disease (Case 1.26).

Consider function

Well-being relates both to severity of disease and the underlying cause.

Discussion

What are the phases of hepatitis B virus (HBV) infection?

The virus

The virion comprises a surface envelope bearing the surface antigen (sAg) and a core containing the core antigen (cAg). A further antigen, eAg, arises from the same gene (C gene) as cAg. The C gene has two initiation codons, a precore and a core region. When translation is initiated at the precore region, the protein product is HBeAg, which has a signal peptide that facilitates its secretion into the serum. When translation is initiated at the core region, the protein product is HBcAg, which lacks a signal peptide, is not secreted and is not detectable in serum.

The natural history

An intact immune system is vital to HBV clearance; the more vigorous the response (and florid the clinical picture), the greater the chance of clearance. Most offspring of affected mothers progress to chronic carriage, whereas only a small minority of adults are chronic carriers. HBV infection has four phases (Table 1.36). Factors influencing the natural history through the four phases include host factors (age, immune status, concurrent infection with other virus and alcohol) and virus factors (HBV genotype and genome mutants).

What is meant by HBV chronic carriage and what are the markers of high and low infectivity in carriers?

Chronic carriers may still be in phase 2 disease pre-seroconversion and generally of higher infectivity, or in phase 3 disease post-seroconversion and generally of lower infectivity. HBV DNA detectability is the best test of ongoing infectivity. The markers are summarised in Table 1.36.

What are the markers of past HBV infection?

Anti-HBs must be positive before complete recovery from HBV infection and immunity can be inferred. Anti-HBe and Anti-HBc immunoglobulin G (IgG) positivity persists. All other markers are negative.

What is HBV pre-core mutant disease?

A variant C gene fails to produce HBeAg capable of secretion into the serum but otherwise causes typical viral replicating disease. The negative HBeAg test is a misleading false negative and HBV DNA is necessary to detect the presence of disease activity. Pre-core mutant strains may develop late in the disease process and lead to reactivation of disease – increasing viraemia and hepatitis even in stage 4 in the absence of HBe antigenaemia reflects the emergence of a pre-core mutant stain.

What do you know about treatment of acute HBV infection?

Most episodes of symptomatic HBV infection resolve without the need for treatment. However, acute HBV infection is associated with high serum HBV DNA, reflecting high viral replication and the potential for infection of non-infected cells and antiviral nucleoside or nucleotide analogues may have a role for early treatment of some patients – those with severe acute hepatitis with a prolonged INR (International normalised ratio), a protracted course with high transaminases or those at increased risk of chronicity, such as immunosuppressed patients.

Why is treatment of chronic HBV infection important?

Chronic HBV infection is probably under-recognised in the UK, and the prevalence is increasing, largely through migration. Most patients acquire infection in early life, often as newborns. It may be associated with serious extra-hepatic manifestations such as vasculitis or nephritis, but most morbidity and mortality is the result of progression to cirrhosis and HCC.

Which patients with chronic HBV infection should be treated?

Most patients with chronic HBV infection do not develop clinically significant liver disease, and have low levels of viral replication with HBeAg negativity and low levels of HBV DNA ($< 10^4$ IU/ml). These patients were formerly termed 'healthy carriers' but serum titres can subsequently

Table 1.36 Phases of hepatitis B virus (HBV) infection (in patients infected with HBe-positive virus)

	Phase 1 Incubation/active viral replication	Phase 2 Continued replication of virus and inflammatory response	Phase 3 Post-seroconversion	Phase 4 Clearance
Clinical features	Usually asymptomatic Lasts a few weeks	Widely varied time-course – from a few weeks to many years **Acute disease** Asymptomatic (70%) or symptomatic (30%) acute hepatitis illness; very rarely fulminant hepatitis **Chronic disease** Around 5–10% of adults progress to chronic carriage, which may persist for years (400 million chronic carriers worldwide!)	Begins once immune response eliminates or greatly diminishes infected cell load. Essentially infection is cleared but HBsAg remains positive because sAg gene has been inserted into host's genome	Resolved or cured
HBsAg	Positive	Positive	Positive	Negative (most eventually reach this stage)
Anti-HBs	Negative	Negative	Negative	Positive (also positive after HBV vaccination)
HBeAg	Positive	Positive Still secreted by infected liver cells	Negative	Negative
Anti-HBe	Negative	**Seroconversion** refers to loss of HBeAg, usually with the appearance of anti-HBe May be early after acute hepatitis In chronic HBV infection spontaneous seroconversion rate is only a small percentage per year	Positive	Positivity persists life-long (negative in HBV-vaccinated individuals who are only anti-HBs positive)
Anti-HBc	IgM positive IgG negative	IgM negative/low titre IgG high titre	IgM negative IgG moderate titre	IgM negative IgG positivity persists life-long (negative in HBV-vaccinated individuals who are only anti-HBs positive)
Serum HBV DNA	Positive (indicating active viral replication)	Positive but significant decline with seroconversion	May still be detectable in some by polymerase chain reaction (PCR)	Undetectable by PCR (implies reactivation or reinfection unlikely)
Transaminases	Normal	Raised	Normal	Normal
Histology	Chronic persistent hepatitis	Chronic active hepatitis Cirrhosis more likely if seroconversion is delayed	Inactive or minimal hepatitis or inactive cirrhosis	No significant disease, especially if seroconverted before cirrhosis Chronic active hepatitis if reactivation or emergence of HBV variant Hepatocellular carcinoma

rise causing inflammation and fibrosis, necessitating life-long surveillance.

Antiviral treatment can alter the natural history, as suppression of HBV replication delays or prevents fibrosis and cirrhosis, enables recovery from decompensation and reduces the risk of HCC.

There is a clear correlation between serum HBV titres and the risk of liver damage; low titres ($< 10^4$ IU/ml) are unlikely to be associated with progressive liver damage but high titres appear to be a prerequisite for liver damage (although a few young HBeAg-positive patients with high titres have little inflammation and are said to be in an immunotolerant phase). Thus, high serum HBV titres are an essential but insufficient indication for antiviral treatment, and likely candidates also have biochemical or histological evidence of inflammatory disease. Significant liver disease and need for transplantation are also more likely in males.

High serum HBV titres may be associated with HBeAg positivity or negativity and HBeAg-negative hepatitis is not uncommon, especially in older patients who may have advanced fibrosis or cirrhosis and who will inevitably have experienced a period of HBeAg-positive hepatitis in the past.

Which antiviral drugs are used?

Drugs include interferon-α (IFN-α), lamivudine (a nucleoside analogue) and adefovir dipivoxil (a nucleotide analogue); IFN-α has immunomodulatory and antiviral effects. Nucleos(t)ides inhibit HBV DNA transcription.

Is there a difference between treatment for HBeAg-positive and HBeAg-negative hepatitis?

This is described in Box 1.29.

What are the key methods of prevention of chronic HBV infection?

All of this highlights the importance of prevention through education, vaccination (which may ultimately become universal in the UK) and screening of newborn babies.

What do you know about the epidemiology of the hepatitis C virus (HCV)?

HCV infection is a major public-health concern, globally much more prevalent than human immunodeficiency virus (HIV) infection. The UK prevalence is unknown but estimated at around 0.5%. Infection is usually silent but is associated with a high chronic carrier state (80%), progression to cirrhosis in many chronic carriers and a 1–4% annual risk of HCC in those with cirrhosis. Acute HCV is usually asymptomatic (transaminases would be elevated) but sometimes occurs with jaundice.

How is HCV transmitted?

HCV is a single-stranded RNA virus of six genotypes (and many subtypes) with differences in pathogenicity, treatment response and prognosis. The two most important

---

Box 1.29 Treatment for chronic hepatitis B virus (HBV) infection

HBeAg-positive hepatitis

- Reflecting the importance of seroconversion on the natural history of chronic infection, this is an appropriate endpoint and has been used in most antiviral trials of HbeAg-positive hepatitis. Treatment increases seroconversion approximately by a factor of 2–3 over 6–12 months.
- With short-term antiviral treatment, IFN produces better seroconversion rates ($\times$ 3) than a nucleos(t)ide ($\times$ 2).
- For nucleos(t)ides, treatment should be sustained for at least six months after anti-HBe appears. Viral suppression, monitored by HBV DNA, without seroconversion, may still be beneficial, and prolonged nucleos(t)ide may be more feasible and better tolerated, and enhanced seroconversion does occur with prolonged treatment.
- There is no apparent benefit of combining IFN and a nucleos(t)ide.
- There is poor consensus as to whether to use IFN or a nucleos(t)ide, but a nucleos(t)ide is preferred in cirrhosis, HBV/HIV co-infection and immunosuppressed patients.
- Combination nucleos(t)ide treatments are under evaluation. Emergence of drug-resistant HBV species is well recognised with prolonged nucleos(t)ide treatment.

HBeAg-negative hepatitis

- Treatment aims to suppress HBV replication and is indicated for patients with serum HBV titres $> 10^4$ IU/ml with significant liver damage. HbsAg seroconversion is an appropriate, but rarely achieved, endpoint.
- Again, IFN may have a slight seroconversion advantage for short-term treatment, and a nucleos(t)ide for prolonged suppression of replication, and there is no value in combining the two treatments.

---

routes of transmission are sharing of needles or equipment by injecting drug users and transfusion of blood and blood products (now virtually eliminated in the UK since screening of donors in 1991). Potential routes include sharing of toothbrushes and razors, tattooing, body piercing, electrolysis and acupuncture. Sexual transmission and maternal vertical transmission rates appear to be low. Occupational risk in health-care workers is significant because HCV may be transmitted in many body fluids. The risk of transmission from an HCV needlestick injury is about 1 : 30.

How is HCV diagnosed?

The HCV antibody test is positive at six months after exposure but the RNA virus can be detected by polymerase chain reaction (PCR).

How is HCV disease severity assessed?

Liver biopsy is the only satisfactory way to assess severity, because serum transaminases may fluctuate disproportionately with activity.

Should acute HCV infection be treated?

Treatment may not be needed, and IFN has a higher incidence of side effects than for HBV infection. A substantial proportion of patients with symptomatic hepatitis clear the virus without treatment, and delaying treatment for three months seems not to compromise the very high rates of clearance produced at that stage with IFN-α with or without ribavirin. Pegylated rather than conventional IFN (PEG-IFN) for 24 weeks is probably as good as any treatment.

Which patients with chronic HCV infection should be treated?

Selection should consider:

- The predicted natural history of untreated infection, principal determinants of which are age when infected, duration of infection, gender and alcohol consumption. HCV is more aggressive in immunosuppressed patients. Liver biopsy may aid decisions.
- The predicted life expectancy if HCV were not present.
- Comorbidity that may compromise antiviral therapy.
- The predicted efficacy of antiviral therapy, patient concordance and HCV genotype being the main determinants, the latter also determining duration of treatment. Efficacy is greatest in type 2 (> 80% success) followed by type 3 (up to 80%) and type 1 (35–40%).

Some criteria for treatment are shown in Box 1.30.

What is the treatment for chronic HCV infection?

Combination treatment enhances efficacy and reduces resistance. Optimal treatment combines subcutaneous IFN-α (now once weekly if polyethylene glycol is added to the molecule as PEG-IFN) with oral ribavirin for 12 months in those with genotype 1 and for six months in patients with non-genotype 1. Rapid early viral response (EVR) rates are a marker of likelihood of successful eradication and patients should definitely complete treatment proto-cols. Sustained viral response (SVR), defined as PCR nega-tivity at six months, usually leads to continued clearance at 10 years.

List some causes of acute viral hepatitis

These include hepatitis A, hepatitis B and hepatitis C viruses, Epstein–Barr virus, parvovirus and atypical pneu-monia organisms.

Box 1.30 Criteria for treatment of chronic hepatitis C virus (HCV) infection

- Age > 18 years
- Persistently raised transaminases
- Compensated liver disease – biliribin normal, prothrombin time < 1.5, albumin normal, acceptable platelet count, no encephalopathy, no ascites, no bleeding, no varices
- Biopsy consistent with chronic hepatitis and at least portal fibrosis with moderate inflammation
- Absence of significant comorbidity, e.g. malignancy, chronic kidney disease

---

CASE 1.31

AUTOIMMUNE HEPATITIS

Instruction

Please examine this 45-year-old lady's abdominal system and comment on possible diagnoses.

Recognition

General *signs of chronic liver disease* (Case 1.26) may be present, e.g. spider naevi (Fig. 1.46).

Interpretation

Confirm the diagnosis

Criteria, proposed by the International Autoimmune Hepatitis Group, exist for diagnosing autoimmune hepatitis (AIH; Box 1.31) although you cannot determine this from clinical examination. Even where criteria are fulfilled, additional causes of chronic liver disease should be excluded as these alter management.

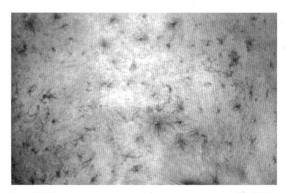

Fig. 1.46 Spider naevi, common in type 1 autoimmune hepatitis (AIH).

Box 1.31 Criteria for the diagnosis of autoimmune hepatitis (AIH)

Major

- Hypergammaglobulinaemia (preferentially IgG) on serum electrophoresis with immunoglobulin subtypes
- Autoantibodies (ANA – antinuclear antibody and antibodies to: SMA – smooth muscle antigen, SLA/LP – soluble liver antigen, LKM – liver–kidney–microsomal antigen)
- Absence of viral hepatitis
- Portal hepatitis (with lymphoplasmacellular infiltrates) on biopsy

Minor (give further support to diagnosis but not essential)

- Personal or family history of autoimmune disease
- Spontaneously fluctuating course
- Arthralgia
- Presence of HLA-DR3 or DR4

What to do next – consider causes/assess other systems

Causes

Consider the causes of chronic liver disease (Case 1.26). Tell the examiners that you would ask about alcohol consumption, previous jaundice, previous transfusions, drug use, occupation, travel and sexual history. Look for signs of other autoimmune diseases, especially thyroid disease (face) and rheumatoid arthritis and scleroderma (hands).

Symptoms

Tell the examiners that you would ask about symptoms. AIH is a relatively uncommon diagnosis that often affects young women. The usual presentation is non-specific, with fatigue, slight right upper quadrant pain, polymyalgia/arthralgia and abnormal liver function tests. The female:male ratio is 3:1. Other autoimmune conditions are present in up to 60% of patients – notably keratoconjunctivitis sicca, renal tubular acidosis, peripheral neuropathy, Hashimoto's thyroiditis, ulcerative colitis and rheumatoid arthritis. AIH can produce transient jaundice or may be detected serendipitously as an isolated transaminase rise. It may remain subclinical and undetected until cirrhosis provokes hepatic decompensation.

Consider severity/decompensation/complications

Look for signs of hepatic decompensation (Case 1.26) and tell the examiners you would determine the severity of disease (Case 1.26). AIH may progress rapidly to cirrhosis.

Consider function

Well-being relates both to severity of disease and side effects of treatment.

Discussion

What types of AIH do you know of?

AIH is a chronic inflammatory disease of the liver associated with hypergammaglobulinaemia and autoantibodies. Types of AIH are described in Table 1.37, but not all authors use this differentiation because some patients will be autoantibody negative at presentation and the autoimmune status tends not to affect management.

How would you investigate a patient with an isolated transaminase rise?

AIH illustrates the importance of investigating patients with 'incidental' raised transaminase levels in whom no clear diagnosis is apparent. Biochemical and serological tests ('liver screen') for causes of chronic liver disease are important, as is a liver ultrasound, but liver biopsy is often needed to secure the diagnosis.

How important is treatment for AIH?

Treatment of AIH switches a dismal prognosis to an excellent one with a normal life expectancy in the vast majority. The difficulty is that presentation is often delayed because of subclinical disease.

What is the treatment for AIH?

Immunosuppression with corticosteroids produces prompt induction of remission (1 mg/kg initially). Azathioprine is the drug of choice for maintenance of remission (50–100 mg daily). Regimens vary. Treatment is continued for at least three years but often life-long as relapse is common if treatment is stopped. Mycophenylate mofetil is the treatment of choice for patients who are intolerant of azathioprine (myelosuppression, hepatotoxicity, pancrea-

Table 1.37 Types of autoimmune hepatitis (AIH)			
	Type 1	Type 2	Type 3
Epidemiology	Classic type Around 80% of AIH	Around 10% of AIH, more prevalent in children	Small subgroup
Clinical features	Chronic or acute Palmar erythema and spider naevi common		Similar to type 1
Autoantibodies	Both ANA and SMA (directed at actin) antibodies present in 40–50% SLA/LP antibodies in 20% – in half of these the only demonstrable antibody (ANA/SMA/LKM antibodies may be found in other diseases; SLA/LP antibodies highly specific for AIH but missed on routine immunofluorescence)	LKM antibodies directed at cytochrome P450IID6	SLA antibodies directed at UGA-suppressor and tRNA-associated protein
Other tests	Polyclonal (especially IgG) hypergammaglobulinaemia	Type 2b associated with LKM antibodies and HCV infection	ANA/SMA/LKM antibodies not present No significant hypergammaglobulinaemia
Treatment	Corticosteroids	Corticosteroids (rapidly progressive without treatment)	Corticosteroids (rapidly progressive without treatment)

ANA, antinuclear antibody; HCV, hepatitis C virus; LKM, liver–kidney–microsomal antigen; SLA/LP, soluble liver antigen; SMA, smooth muscle antigen; UGA, uracil–guanine–adenine

titis). Late-diagnosed AIH is an indication for considering transplantation.

What is the AIH overlap syndrome?

Between 10% and 20% of patients have overlap with primary biliary cirrhosis or primary sclerosing cholangitis.

CASE 1.32

PRIMARY BILIARY CIRRHOSIS

Instruction

Please examine this lady's skin and abdomen. Discuss your findings.

Recognition

General *signs of chronic liver disease* (Case 1.26) may be present, e.g. xanthelasmata (Fig. 1.47).

Interpretation

Confirm the diagnosis

Consider the causes of chronic liver disease (Case 1.26). Tell the examiners that you would ask about alcohol consumption, previous jaundice, previous transfusions, drug use, occupation, travel and sexual history. In primary biliary cirrhosis (PBC) there may be prominent scratch marks (due to itch). Xanthelasmata affect 5–10% of patients.

What to do next – assess other systems

Tell the examiners that you would ask about symptoms:

- Fatigue and pruritis (20–70%) are the most common presenting symptoms, preceding jaundice by months to years.

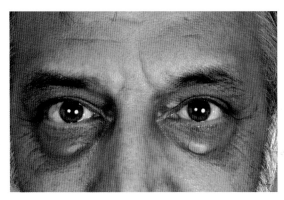

Fig. 1.47 Xanthelasmata.

- Right upper quadrant discomfort affects a small number of patients. PBC may first present as variceal bleeding, illustrating the importance of pre-emptive investigation of patients with isolated alkaline phosphatase elevation, but portal hypertension, variceal bleeding, ascites or hepatic encephalopathy are usually late features.

Other common findings in PBC are osteopenia, hyperlipidaemia and coexisting autoimmune diseases, notably hypothyroidism, Sjögren's syndrome, scleroderma, rheumatoid arthritis and thyroid disease. Less common are interstitial lung disease, coeliac disease, sarcoidosis, renal tubular acidosis and autoimmune blood disorders.

Consider severity/decompensation/complications

Look for signs of hepatic decompensation (Case 1.26) and tell the examiners you would determine the severity of disease (Case 1.26). In addition to hepatic decompensation, steatorrhoea and malabsorption may lead to osteomalacia with bone pain, but this tends to be late in the course of disease.

Consider function

Well-being relates both to severity of disease and side effects of treatment.

Discussion

What causes PBC?

PBC is a slowly progressive autoimmune disease of the liver primarily affecting women, with a peak incidence in the fifth decade. The cause is not known, but genetic or environmental factors likely trigger anti-mitochondrial antibodies (AMA) which target 2-oxo-acid dehydrogenase complexes that participate in oxidative phosphorylation, especially the pyruvate dehydrogenase E2 complex (PDC–E2). T lymphocytes infiltrating the liver are specific for PDC–E2 and intensely populate the portal tracts, with biliary epithelial destruction. The paradox in PBC is that mitochondrial proteins are present in all nucleated cells but disease is specific to the bile ducts, suggesting that PDC-E2 processing during apoptosis in bile duct cells may differ crucially from PDC-E2 processing elsewhere.

What diagnostic tests are there for PBC?

Diagnosis of PBC is outlined in Box 1.32.

What is the treatment for PBC?

Ursodeoxycholic acid may slow disease progression. It is more useful in early disease, delaying fibrosis and variceal evolution. Other drugs have been used, such as colchicine and methotrexate, but a drug panacea for all of the facets of PBC is elusive. PBC is one of the more common indications for liver transplantation.

What is primary sclerosing cholangitis (PSC)?

PSC is characterised by chronic fibrosis of intra- and extra-hepatic ducts and is associated with other autoimmune diseases. Seventy per cent of PSC occurs in the presence of ulcerative colitis. Secondary sclerosing cholangitis follows numerous insults including bacterial cholangitis and graft versus host disease.

Box 1.32 Diagnosis of primary biliary cirrhosis (PBC)

- Antimitochondrial antibody (AMA) – M₂ subtype – positivity (ANA often, but not invariably, positive)
- Elevated liver enzymes for more than six months
- Diagnostic histology – liver not affected uniformly but four general stages are portal triad inflammation, bile duct depletion, extending inflammation and cirrhosis.

  Diagnosis is probable with two of the three features, although AMA positivity to various PDC-E subtypes (notably PDC-E2) is highly specific and virtually diagnostic of PBC, as is an increasingly recognised ANA to a nuclear pore protein gp210 (although this only occurs in around 15% of patients); some authors suggest that all patients with PBC become AMA positive but others recognise AMA-negative PBC and call it autoimmune cholangitis.

CASE 1.33

GENETIC HAEMOCHROMATOSIS

Instruction

Please examine this 55-year-old man's skin and abdomen and proceed as you think appropriate.

Recognition

There may be *slate greyish pigmentation*. There is *firm, smooth hepatomegaly* ± splenomegaly. General *signs of chronic liver disease* may be present (Case 1.26).

Interpretation

Confirm the diagnosis

Consider the causes of chronic liver disease (Case 1.26). The dusky pigmentation in genetic haemochromatosis is characteristic and affects most patients, although some candidates fall into the trap of considering silvery amiodarone skin changes, which affect sun-exposed areas (Fig. 1.48). Generally, the disease presents in middle age, women

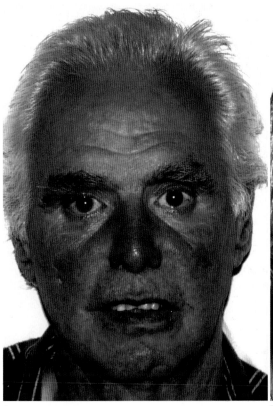
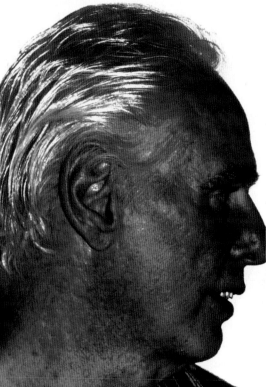

A   B

Fig. 1.48 (A,B) Amiodarone skin changes.

tending to be diagnosed later than men because of the protection afforded by menstruation. Tell the examiners that a liver biopsy is diagnostic. Secondary iron overload occurs in patients requiring repeated transfusion.

What to do next – assess other systems

The clinical manifestations of genetic haemochromatosis result from iron deposition in major organs, notably the skin, pancreas, heart, liver and anterior pituitary. Tell the examiners you would assess for these (Fig. 1.49).

Consider severity/decompensation/complications

Look for signs of hepatic decompensation (Case 1.26) and tell the examiners you would determine the severity of disease (Case 1.26). Hepatocellular carcinoma is the most

common cause of death, the relative risk being some 200-fold times that of the normal population. Tell the examiners that ultrasound screening is important.

Consider function

Well-being relates both to severity of disease and to organs involved.

Discussion

What do you know about the genetic basis of genetic haemochromatosis?

It is an autosomal recessive disorder of excessive absorption of dietary iron leading to deposition in several organs and organ failure. The genetic defect responsible for 90% of cases in the UK is homozygosity for a single base mutation (cytosine to tyrosine, C282Y) in the *HFE* gene, closely associated with *HLA A3* on the short arm of chromosome 6p. *HFE* encodes a class 1 human leucocyte antigen (HLA) protein which, when associated with β2-microglobulin, is transported to the cell surface where it binds with transferrin receptor-1. The C282Y mutation prevents HFE from associating with β2-microglobulin but how this leads to iron overload is uncertain. Less common mutations affect the transferrin receptor-2 gene and ferroportin gene. Variable penetrance of the common genotype suggests that other genes modify iron loading. A recently identified peptide, hepcidin, is thought to control iron absorption and macrophage iron release but hepcidin abnormalities probably contribute to only a very small proportion of haemochromatosis cases.

How is genetic haemochromatosis diagnosed?

Early symptoms are non-specific and may include fatigue, arthralgia, loss of libido, erectile dysfunction, amenorrhoea and increased skin pigmentation. Diabetes mellitus, cardiomyopathy, arrhythmias, cirrhosis and anterior pituitary failure ensue if the condition remains undetected. Clinical manifestations usually become overt by age 40–50. Diagnosis may be suggested by a high transferrin saturation (> 55% in > 90%), and confirmed by liver biopsy (excessive iron storage) or genetic testing. Transferrin saturation may be falsely positive in patients taking iron therapy. Serum ferritin may be falsely positive in inflammatory states.

What is the treatment for genetic haemochromatosis?

Regular venesection is needed, at least initially (e.g. 500 ml once or twice weekly until serum ferritin is in the normal range), and early treatment improves outcome, an argument in favour of screening.

What are the arguments for and against screening?

Patients do not usually develop symptoms until they are over 40 years of age, by which time iron deposition in

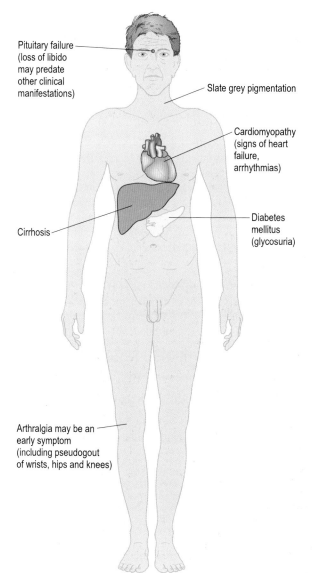

Pituitary failure (loss of libido may predate other clinical manifestations)

Slate grey pigmentation

Cardiomyopathy (signs of heart failure, arrhythmias)

Cirrhosis

Diabetes mellitus (glycosuria)

Arthralgia may be an early symptom (including pseudogout of wrists, hips and knees)

Fig. 1.49 Organ involvement in haemochromatosis.

affected organs may have caused irreversible tissue damage and incipient organ failure. Treatment in early disease can restore normal life expectancy. Although detectable at a presymptomatic stage, and treatable, genetic haemochromatosis does not fulfil all of the criteria for screening. It is relatively uncommon (although many would argue that its homozygous incidence of around 1:300 justifies screening), and the optimal test is contentious. Transferrin saturation only detects expressed disease. Further, the genetic test is not as useful as initially thought. C282Y is not the only mutation, and it is increasingly realised that many people are autosomal recessive for this gene yet are asymptomatic. Thus, the phenotype is not predicted by the genotype. To further complicate matters, asymptomatic autosomal recessive people do seem to be at increased risk if they carry an additional liver insult, notably carriage of the hepatitis C virus.

A suitable compromise is to screen anyone in whom symptoms or signs suggest possible disease, relatives of patients with disease and anyone with unexplained abnormal liver biochemistry (especially those with diabetes).

CASE 1.34

WILSON'S DISEASE

Instruction

Please examine this patient's abdominal system, then look briefly at his eyes before discussing your findings.

Recognition

General *signs of chronic liver disease* may be present (Case 1.26). Wilson's disease is very uncommon, but might appear in PACES. The clue from the instruction is to look for *Kayser–Fleischer rings* (Fig. 1.50).

Interpretation

Confirm the diagnosis

Kayser–Fleischer rings are rusty brown deposits of copper within Desçemet's membrane of the cornea and are pathognomonic of Wilson's disease. They start at 6 and 12 o'clock, are not always present, and sometimes only detectable with a slit-lamp.

What to do next – assess other systems

Extra-hepatic features of Wilson's disease are described in Box 1.33.

Consider severity/decompensation/complications

Look for signs of hepatic decompensation (Case 1.26) and tell the examiners you would determine the severity of disease (Case 1.26) and that it is important to recognise and treat before neuropsychiatric disease develops.

Consider function

Well-being relates both to severity of disease and side effects of treatment.

Discussion

What is the cause of Wilson's disease?

It is an inherited disorder caused by mutations in the gene *ATP7B* on chromosome 13. Different mutations run in different families. It is autosomal recessive with an average population prevalence of 30 per million and a carrier rate of 1:90. Copper cannot be incorporated into caeruloplasmin (the copper-carrying protein) within hepatocytes and hepatocytes are unable to excrete copper efficiently into bile because of the mutated copper-transporting ATPase.

When is Wilson's disease typically diagnosed?

Diagnosis is typically in children or young adults (5–45 years) but older presentations occur, and there is increasing evidence for under-recognition in older patients.

What hepatic manifestations occur in Wilson's disease?

These include asymptomatic hepatomegaly, hepatitis, chronic liver disease and, rarely, fulminant hepatic failure

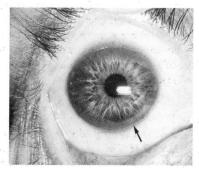

Fig. 1.50 Kayser–Fleischer ring.

> **Box 1.33 Extra-hepatic features of Wilson's disease**
>
> - Kayser–Fleischer rings (much less commonly sunflower cataracts)
> - Neurological features due to basal ganglia deposition – tremor, chorea, rigid dystonia, cramped handwriting, poor coordination
> - Psychiatric features – depression, neurosis, antisocial behaviour, emotional lability, poor memory, difficulty with abstract thinking
> - Fanconi's syndrome due to copper infiltration disrupting renal tubular exchange
> - Arthritis
> - Cardiac arrhythmias
> - Hypoparathyroidism

Box 1.34 Biochemical abnormalities in Wilson's disease

- Serum caeruloplasmin low
- Serum copper high, low or normal
- 24-hour basal urinary copper excretion high

liberating free copper into the bloodstream, whose toxicity destroys red cell membranes and damages renal tubules.

What biochemical abnormalities would you expect in Wilson's disease?

These are shown in Box 1.34.

What treatments are available for Wilson's disease?

Penicillamine may be effective. Treatment should be life-long because stopping treatment in stable patients often leads to rapid, irreversible deterioration. Other treatments include trientene, zinc and vitamin E. Liver transplantation is sometimes considered. Asymptomatic siblings should be screened.

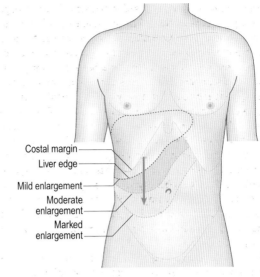

Fig. 1.51 Hepatomegaly.

CASE 1.35

HEPATOMEGALY

Instruction

Please examine this patient's abdomen and discuss your findings.

Recognition

There is *hepatomegaly* (Fig. 1.51), the liver enlarged to (state in cm) below the costal margin. The spleen is not enlarged.

Interpretation

Confirm the diagnosis

Hepatomegaly has numerous causes.

What to do next – consider causes

Look for the signs in Table 1.38.

Consider severity/decompensation/complications

Look for signs of hepatic decompensation (Case 1.26).

Consider function

This depends upon the cause.

Discussion

List some infective causes of hepatomegaly

- Pyogenic liver abscess
- Amoebic liver abscess
- Hydatid disease

Table 1.38 Signs of common causes of hepatomegaly

Causes (the three 'C's)	Signs
Cirrhosis	Signs of chronic liver disease (Case 1.26)
Cancer	Liver often hard, with nodular edge. Cachexia
Cardiac (right-sided heart failure)	Liver firm, with smooth, tender edge; may be pulsatile; liver tenderness suggests recent stretching of capsule due to heart failure or acute hepatitis. Raised jugular venous pulse. Peripheral oedema

From where might a pyogenic liver abscess arise?

Sources include a subphrenic abscess, biliary sepsis, diverticulitis, appendicitis, Crohn's disease and bacterial endocarditis.

What causes an amoebic abscess?

Entamoeba histolytica is transmitted by the faecal–oral route by ingestion of protozoal cysts. Ten per cent of the world's population is chronically infected. Cyst walls degrade in the small bowel to release trophozoites, which migrate to the large bowel and, assuming a pathogenic strain, cause colitis and invasive disease. Symptoms include right upper quadrant pain and fever.

What is hydatid disease?

This is caused by the dog tapeworm, *Echinococcus granulosus*. The life cycle involves ingestion by the dog of hydatid cysts from sheep liver. The dog, the definitive host, harbours the adult tapeworm in its small bowel, from which eggs are passed into its faeces and reingested by sheep.

Humans may be inadvertent intermediate hosts. Eggs hatch in the sheep's small bowel into larvae, which penetrate into the bloodstream, travel to the liver and form cysts.

CASE 1.36

SPLENOMEGALY

Instruction

Please examine this patient's abdomen and discuss your findings.

Recognition

There is *splenomegaly* (Fig. 1.52), the spleen enlarged to (state in cm) below the left costal margin towards the right iliac fossa. The liver is not enlarged.

Interpretation

Confirm the diagnosis

Splenomegaly has numerous causes.

What to do next – consider causes

These are similar to hepatosplenomegaly (Case 1.37), but an important additional cause is infective endocarditis (Case 3.11). Look for splinter haemorrhages, Osler's nodes or Janeway lesions.

Consider severity/decompensation/complications

Look for petechiae or purpura (hypersplenism).

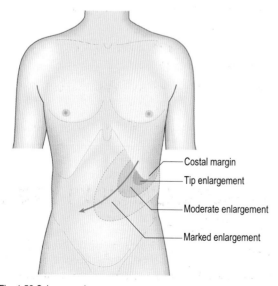

Fig. 1.52 Splenomegaly.

Labels: Costal margin / Tip enlargement / Moderate enlargement / Marked enlargement

Consider function

This depends upon the cause.

Discussion

What are the causes of a very large spleen?

These include chronic myeloid leukaemia, myelofibrosis and visceral leishmaniasis.

CASE 1.37

HEPATOSPLENOMEGALY

Instruction

Please examine this patient's abdomen and discuss your findings.

Recognition

There is *hepatomegaly*, the liver enlarged to (state in cm) below the right costal margin. There is *splenomegaly*, the spleen enlarged to (state in cm) below the left costal margin towards the right iliac fossa.

Interpretation

Confirm the diagnosis

Hepatosplenomegaly has numerous causes.

What to do next – consider causes

These include:

- Cirrhosis with portal hypertension (congestive splenomegaly)
- Lymphoproliferative disorders (Cases 1.46, 1.47)
- Myeloproliferative disorders (Case 1.45)
- Infection/infiltration

Consider severity/decompensation/complications

Look for signs of hepatic decompensation (Case 1.26) and for petechiae or purpura (hypersplenism).

Consider function

This depends upon the cause.

Discussion

List some infective and infiltrative disorders of the liver and spleen

- Glandular fever
- Brucellosis
- Leptospirosis
- Sarcoid
- Amyloidosis
- Glycogen storage disorders

CASE 1.38

FELTY'S SYNDROME

Instruction

Please examine this patient's abdomen and discuss your findings.

Recognition

There is *splenomegaly*, the spleen enlarged to (state in cm) below the left costal margin towards the right iliac fossa. The liver is not enlarged. The patient also has signs *of rheumatoid arthritis* in the hands (Fig. 1.53).

Interpretation

Confirm the diagnosis

Felty's syndrome is the triad of rheumatoid arthritis, splenomegaly and neutropenia.

What to do next – assess other systems

Tell the examiners that you would look for extra-articular signs of rheumatoid disease (Case 5.16). Lymphadeno-pathy may occur.

Consider severity/decompensation/complications

Tell the examiners that you would screen for neutropenia and sepsis.

Consider function

This depends upon the severity of the rheumatoid arthritis.

Discussion

Is rheumatoid factor positive or negative in Felty's syndrome?

Positive.

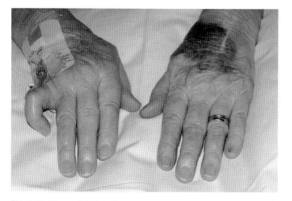

Fig. 1.53 Rheumatoid hands.

CASE 1.39

ABDOMINAL MASS

Instruction

Please examine this patient's abdomen and discuss your findings.

Recognition

There is an *abdominal mass* – describe it with respect to site, size, shape, surface, edge, consistency (hard or soft), fixation or mobility (with respect to the skin), tenderness and pulsatility.

Interpretation

Confirm the diagnosis

There are many causes. If there is not obvious organome-galy (liver, spleen, kidney), consider other causes.

What to do next – consider causes

Consider the causes in Fig. 1.54.

Consider severity/decompensation/complications

Tell the examiners that this relates to cause, e.g. a ruptured aortic aneurysm might become expansile (see Fig. 1.54) with abdominal pain and haemodynamic compromise.

Consider function

This depends on the cause.

Discussion

What are the causes of hepatomegaly?

These are discussed in Case 1.35.

What are the causes of splenomegaly?

These are discussed in Case 1.36.

What are the causes of hepatosplenomegaly?

These are discussed in Case 1.37.

List some other causes of an abdominal mass

These are illustrated in Box 1.24.

CASE 1.40

CROHN'S DISEASE

Instruction

Please examine this patient's abdominal system and discuss your findings.

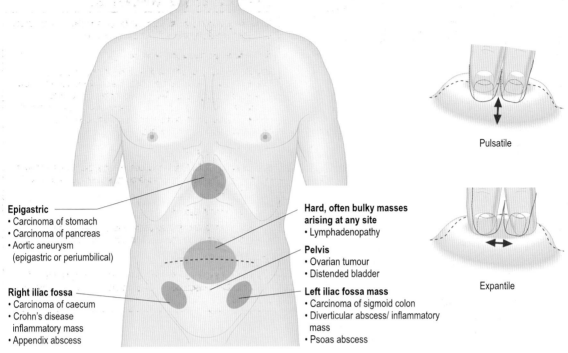

Epigastric
- Carcinoma of stomach
- Carcinoma of pancreas
- Aortic aneurysm
  (epigastric or periumbilical)

Right iliac fossa
- Carcinoma of caecum
- Crohn's disease
  inflammatory mass
- Appendix abscess

Hard, often bulky masses arising at any site
- Lymphadenopathy

Pelvis
- Ovarian tumour
- Distended bladder

Left iliac fossa mass
- Carcinoma of sigmoid colon
- Diverticular abscess/ inflammatory mass
- Psoas abscess

Pulsatile

Expantile

Fig. 1.54 Abnormal adbominal masses other than enlarged organs.

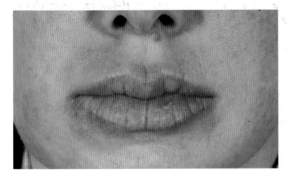

Fig. 1.55 Perioral Crohn's disease.

Recognition

There is *perioral aphthous ulceration* (Fig. 1.55). There is a *mass* in the right iliac fossa with evidence of previous surgery from a *midline laparotomy scar*. There may be *erythema nodosum* (Fig. 1.56).

Interpretation

Confirm the diagnosis

Tell the examiners there may be a history of diarrhoea, abdominal pain and bleeding and that diagnosis is histological.

What to do next – assess other systems

Extra-intestinal associations can arise in both Crohn's disease (CD) and ulcerative colitis (UC) and may be unrelated or related (most) to disease activity (Table 1.39).

Consider severity/decompensation/complications

Symptoms and complications of the subtypes of CD are outlined in Box 1.35.

Tell the examiners that colorectal cancer and toxic megacolon are two complications but that their incidence should be reduced with modern surveillance and treatment.

Consider function

Tell the examiners that inflammatory bowel disease (IBD) is a chronic, relapsing, often debilitating disease that can have profound psychological as well as physical effects.

Discussion

What do you know about the epidemiology of CD?

Both CD and UC are idiopathic chronic relapsing and remitting disorders. They are increasing in prevalence, more common in North America and Europe. CD usually presents at 20–60 years of age, and tends to be more common in women.

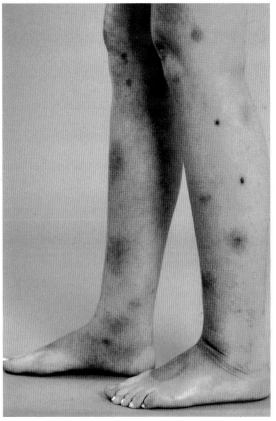

Fig. 1.56 Erythema nodosum.

Box 1.35 Clinical subtypes of Crohn's disease

Common symptoms are diarrhoea (70–90%), pain (50%), anal lesions (50–80%), rectal bleeding and systemic symptoms.

Active ileal and ileocaecal disease

Pain is a central feature of ileal and often ileocaecal disease, sometimes with a right iliac fossa inflammatory mass, with or without diarrhoea and weight loss. The pain is constant if caused by inflammation or abscess formation, and colicky with borborygmi and abdominal distension if the result of small bowel obstruction (strictures). Malabsorption may occur.

Active Crohn's colitis

Symptoms are similar to active ulcerative colitis, but frank bleeding is less common. Extra-intestinal manifestations are more common with colonic disease.

Perianal Crohn's disease

There may be fissuring, fistulae or abscesses, and perianal manifestations are more common with colonic disease.

Other

The rectum may be the only site of disease in elderly patients and very rarely Crohn's disease may be confined to the mouth, stomach or duodenum.

Table 1.39 Extra-intestinal associations of inflammatory bowel disease (IBD)

Unrelated to disease activity	Joints	Sacroiliitis (18% but usually asymptomatic) Ankylosing spondylitis (rare)
Related to disease activity	Perioral	Aphthous ulceration (20% with CD)
	Skin	Erythema nodosum (5–10%) Pyoderma gangrenosum (more common in UC)
	Joints	Acute arthritis
	Eyes	Uveitis (up to 10%) Episcleritis
	Liver and biliary tract	Gallstones (CD) Primary sclerosing cholangitis (UC) Cholangiocarcinoma Fatty change (CD) Amyloidosis (CD) Granulomata (CD)
	Kidneys	Ureteric calculi (oxalate in CD, urate in UC)

CD, Crohn's disease; UC, ulcerative colitis.

What causes IBD?

The cause is unknown. There is a 10-fold increased relative risk in first-degree relatives. Between 15% and 20% of patients with CD have a relative with CD or UC. Mutations in the *CARD15* (*NOD2*) gene on chromosome 16 have been found in around one-third of patients with CD, especially associated with ileal disease. Environmental associations include non-smoking (UC), smoking (CD), enteric infection (UC), other infections, drugs [including non-steroidal anti-inflammatories (NSAIDs), antibiotics and oral contraceptives], and high-refined-sugar/low-fibre diets (CD).

What is known about the immunological basis of CD?

Immunological responses (Case 2.46) that colonic bacterial antigens might normally stimulate, including B-lymphocyte-mediated antibody production and T-helper-lymphocyte-mediated production of pro-inflammatory cytokines [tumour necrosis factor-α (TNF-α) is increased in CD, together with nuclear factor-κB and mitogen-activated protein kinases], are normally balanced by down-regulatory cytokines, enhanced apoptosis in the lamina propria and absence of co-stimulatory second signals leading to tolerance. It may be that such tolerance mechanisms are deficient in CD.

What do you know about the pathology and distribution of CD?

CD is a chronic inflammatory disease with a T-helper-type 1-mediated proinflammatory response at its core. It may affect the entire gastrointestinal tract from mouth to anus, especially the terminal ileum (35%), ileocaecal region (40%) and anus. It is confined to the colon in 20%. The rectum is characteristically spared. There may be skip lesions, with normal mucosa between affected areas. Aphthous ulceration is common, but inflammation tends to be transmural (although predominantly submucosal), often with deep ulceration, fissuring and abscess formation. Histologically, glands are preserved, non-caseating granulomata may occur and the cellular infiltrate tends to comprise lymphocytes, plasma cells and macrophages.

What are the differential diagnoses of IBD?

If there is a clear history of inflammatory symptoms (blood, mucus, pus or slime) that are not of infective origin (history and stool culture), IBD is very likely. Sometimes, a non-specific diagnosis of 'colitis' will be made, but the underlying cause will probably be IBD. Other possibilities include ischaemic colitis, microscopic colitis (watery rather than bloody diarrhoea), radiation colitis, drug-induced colitis (usually due to NSAIDs, symptoms similar to UC but settling when withdrawn), rectal mucosal prolapse and colorectal cancer.

Should particular drugs be avoided in CD?

NSAIDs and antibiotics may provoke relapse.

Is there a role for dietary advice in managing CD?

Elemental diets (containing amino acids and glucose) and polymeric diets may be effective in treating active disease, but are unpalatable. Vitamin supplementation may be necessary in malabsorption.

Are there any non-drug strategies that aid maintenance of remission in CD?

Not smoking improves maintenance of remission.

How is active ileocaecal CD managed?

It usually responds to oral or, if severe, intravenous corticosteroid regimens similar to those used in UC. Controlled, ileal release budesonide at a daily dose of 9 mg is as effective as prednisolone, with fewer side effects. Metronidazole may be helpful in patients with sepsis or bacterial overgrowth.

Are salicylates as beneficial in CD as they are in UC?

Sulfasalazine, 1 g twice daily, may have a role in active colonic disease, but has no role in maintaining remission. Mesalazine may have a role in both active and relapsing CD. However, 5-aminosalicylic acid compounds are generally less beneficial for active CD than for active UC and evidence for maintaining remission is not good.

What is standard maintenance therapy in CD?

Patients with continually relapsing disease or those dependent on low-dose corticosteroids should be considered for azathioprine or 6-mercaptopurine or methotrexate. Benefit may not be apparent for some weeks.

Is immunotherapy beneficial in CD?

Two-thirds of patients with chronic active disease who are resistant to corticosteroids and immunosuppression respond to infliximab, an immunoglobulin G1 chimeric antibody to TNF-α. Relapses begin at two to three months but can be managed by further infusion. Concerns are of reactivation of latent tuberculosis, malignancy and a lupus-like syndrome. Other potential emerging 'biological' therapies include alternative anti-TNF antibodies and receptors, anti-interferon-γ antibodies, antibodies to interleukins 2, 6 and 12, anti-leucocyte trafficking using antibodies to chemokines such as integrin and intercellular adhesion molecule, and antibodies to CD3.

Are there any other options for perianal disease?

Tacrolimus is sometimes used.

What surgical procedures are common for CD?

Right hemicolectomy is the most common operation, but some patients need panproctocolectomy with a permanent ileostomy. Seton insertion for perianal fistulae involves a suture through the fistula track that is tied around the anus to keep the fistula open and prevent abscess formation. As well as entero-cutaneous fistulae, fistulae may be entero-enteral, entero-vesical or entero-vaginal. Improving medical therapy, earlier use of immunosuppressives and anti-TNF agents, and conservative surgical strategies, are reducing the need for radical surgical procedures and improving quality of life.

CASE 1.41

ULCERATIVE COLITIS

Instruction

Please examine this patient's abdomen and discuss your findings.

Recognition

There is an *ileostomy* in the *right iliac fossa* in this patient with signs of Cushing's syndrome. There may be *pyoderma gangrenosum* (Fig. 1.57).

Interpretation

Confirm the diagnosis

Tell the examiners there may be a history of diarrhoea, abdominal pain and bleeding and that diagnosis is histological.

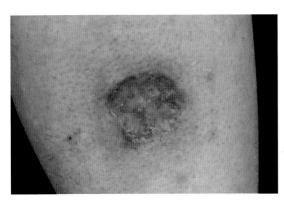

Fig. 1.57 Pyoderma gangrenosum.

What to do next – assess other systems

Extra-intestinal associations arise in either Crohn's disease (CD) or ulcerative colitis (UC) or both and may either be unrelated or related (most) to disease activity (see Table 1.39, Case 1.40).

Consider severity/decompensation/complications

Bloody diarrhoea is the central feature of UC, although proctitis may present with rectal bleeding and constipation. Truelove and Witt's objective criteria for stratifying UC severity are helpful in defining management (Box 1.36).

Consider function

Tell the examiners that inflammatory bowel disease (IBD) is a chronic, relapsing, often debilitating disease that can have profound psychological as well as physical effects.

Discussion

What do you know about the epidemiology of UC?

Unlike CD, UC shows a bimodal distribution with a major peak between 20 and 40 years and a lesser one between 60 and 80. It presents more commonly in winter.

What causes UC?

UC is 'idiopathic' but there is complex interplay between components of the innate immune system and environmental factors, notably microflora in the gut mucosa, which is dysregulated in UC.

What do you know about the pathology and distribution of UC?

UC is confined to the large bowel and always affects the rectum. A third of patients have pan-colitis, a third rectal (proctitis) or sigmoid disease only and a third colitis to the splenic flexure. Ulceration is usually superficial (mucosal). Granulomata are not a feature, and glands tend to be destroyed with crypt abscess formation, and the cellular infiltrate tends to comprise neutrophils, plasma cells and eosinophils.

How would you treat mild to moderate UC?

In active UC, prompt treatment can reduce the symptoms rapidly and reduce the risk of complications (Box 1.37).

What is standard maintenance therapy in UC?

This is described in Box 1.38.

How would you manage severe colitis in UC?

This is described in Box 1.39.

Box 1.38 Standard maintenance therapy in ulcerative colitis (UC)

- The relapse rate is reduced from 80% to 20% at one year with salicylates. 5-ASA inhibits pro-inflammatory eicosanoid release from colonic epithelial cells, but nephrotoxicity is a potential side effect when absorbed.
- Salicylate choice depends on efficacy, side effect profile, serum concentration of 5-ASA and cost. The original was sulfasalazine (e.g. 2 g daily), but side effects include headaches, nausea and occasionally agranulocytosis and Stevens–Johnson syndrome. Newer salicylates are better tolerated and not associated with male infertility. Mesalazine in a coated preparation such as Asacol (1.2 g daily) or Pentasa microspheres (1.5 g daily) is most commonly used, but with caution in renal disease. Olsalazine (1 g daily) may cause watery diarrhoea but is useful if there is proximal constipation with distal disease.
- Corticosteroids have no role in maintenance of remission.

Box 1.39 Management of severe colitis in ulcerative colitis (UC)

- Severe colitis (more than six stools daily with one other criterion) warrants admission for intravenous and rectal hydrocortisone, intravenous fluids, potassium monitoring and thromboembolic prophylaxis. Antibiotics are not beneficial.
- Other rescue treatments (which should be prescribed only by IBD specialists) include ciclosporin and infliximab.
- Antidiarrhoeal drugs (loperamide, opioids) and smooth muscle relaxants (buscopan) may provoke acute colonic dilatation and should be avoided. NSAIDs can worsen colonic inflammation.
- Toxic dilatation is treated medically for up to 24 hours but if no improvement occurs in stool frequency, colonic diameter and heart rate, urgent colectomy is indicated to avoid a 30% mortality rate associated with the risk of perforation.
- After five to seven days, approximately 40% will have a complete response, 30% an incomplete response treated thereafter as moderate colitis, and 30% may need colectomy (considered if more than eight stools daily or C-reactive protein > 45 mg/l after three days of intensive therapy).

What options are there for patients who have had an episode of severe colitis?

Patients who have had severe colitis should start azathioprine (2–2.5 mg/kg daily), e.g. for three to five years. Refractory severe colitis may be an indication for ciclosporin.

What options are there for patients with refractory UC?

Patients with moderate colitis who relapse with a dose of prednisolone reduced to under 15 mg or within six weeks of stopping prednisolone should start azathioprine as above. Thiopurine methyltransferase levels should be checked before starting azathioprine because in those with genetically low levels there is a much greater risk of profound myelosuppression. An alternative is 6-mercaptopurine. Metho-trexate is ineffective in UC, unlike CD. Refractory distal disease may respond to mesalazine sup-

positories (Pentasa 1 g at night) continued thrice weekly to maintain remission.

What are the indications for surgery in UC?

These include chronic symptoms (largest group), emergency surgery for severe disease and dysplasia or colorectal carcinoma. Surgical options include subtotal colectomy with a remnant rectal stump and ileostomy, colectomy with ileoanal pouch to avoid the need for ileostomy and panproctocolectomy with a permanent ileostomy.

When should colonoscopic surveillance be contemplated?

Colorectal cancer is more common with extensive and long-duration disease. The risk in patients with pancolitis is 5–10% at 15–25 years. Surveillance usually starts at 10 years. Long-term maintenance with aminosalicylates reduces the carcinoma risk.

Should any drugs be avoided in UC?

Antidiarrhoeal, antispasmodic and anticholinergic drugs may provoke colonic dilatation.

What is microscopic colitis?

This is defined as a triad of chronic watery diarrhoea with normal colonoscopy and characteristic microscopic inflammation of the lamina propria. It is more common in older people. The term embraces collagenous colitis and lymphocytic colitis, and there is overlap between the two. Microscopic colitis has a mean age of incidence of 55–68 years and is uncommon (each entity 1 to 5 per 100000/year) but is the final diagnosis in 10–15% of patients with chronic diarrhoea who present to specialist units. The cause is unclear, but luminal bacterial antigens may be important. Loperamide is useful for mild disease but budesonide and occasionally immunosuppression with azathioprine are needed for more severe disease.

CASE 1.42

ENTERIC AND URINARY STOMAS

Instruction

Please examine this patient's abdomen and discuss your findings.

Recognition

There is a *percutaneous endoscopic gastrostomy (PEG) tube* in situ in this patient with obvious hemiparesis and dsyphasia (Fig. 1.58).

Interpretation

Confirm the diagnosis

This depends on the type of stoma.

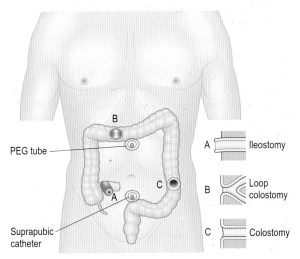

PEG tube

Suprapubic catheter

A — Ileostomy

B — Loop colostomy

C — Colostomy

Fig. 1.58 Percutaneous endoscopic gastrostomy (PEG) tube and other surgical stomas.

What to do next – consider causes

The underlying diagnoses are wide. Most PEG tubes are inserted in patients with chronic neurological disorders, notably stroke.

Consider severity/decompensation/complications

The risks and complications of PEG tubes are discussed in Case 4.32.

Consider function

Tell the examiners you would assess functional status following stroke rehabilitation.

Discussion

In which circumstances might a PEG tube be considered?

These are discussed in Case 4.32.

CASE 1.43

CARCINOID SYNDROME

Instruction

Please examine this patient's abdomen and briefly any other systems you think relevant before discussing your findings.

Recognition

There is *hepatomegaly* and *flushed skin*.

Interpretation

Confirm the diagnosis

Tell the examiners you would ask about flushing and diarrhoea.

What to do next – assess other systems

Listen to the heart for right-sided murmurs.

Consider severity/decompensation/complications

Tell the examiners that the peptides causing carcinoid syndrome may cause:

- Bronchoconstriction – wheeze
- Increased gut motility – diarrhoea
- Endocardial fibrosis (a direct toxic effect of serotonin), notably right-sided valvular lesions, e.g. pulmonary stenosis, tricuspid regurgitation

Carcinoid and other neuroendocrine tumours may also be part of multiple endocrine neoplasia (MEN) type 1.

Consider function

Carcinoid syndrome, unless specifically considered, can take considerable time to diagnose, promoting uncertainty and anguish.

Discussion

What are carcinoid tumours?

These are the most common neuroendocrine tumours of enterochromaffin-like cells, and may arise from the foregut (stomach, pancreas, bronchus), midgut (duodenum to transverse colon) or hindgut (remaining colon); most commonly they are appendiceal.

What is carcinoid syndrome?

Most carcinoid tumours are non-functioning and asymptomatic. They may be found incidentally, e.g. in appendicectomy specimens. Their products, if functional, are metabolised by the liver. Symptoms are produced by release of serotonin, tachykinins and other vasoactive peptides into the circulation, known as carcinoid syndrome.

Why are liver metastases invariably present in carcinoid syndrome?

Efficient metabolism of peptides from the portal circulation by the liver usually suppresses symptomatic carcinoid syndrome. Hepatic metastases or situations where peptides are released directly into the systemic circulation as in bronchial carcinoid lead to symptoms.

How is carcinoid syndrome diagnosed?

This is by collection of at least three 24-hour urine collections for detection of elevated 5-hydroxyindoleacetic acid (5-HIAA), a metabolite of serotonin. Other hormones may be elevated, e.g. vasoactive intestinal peptide.

What may cause false-positive results?

Certain foods (e.g. banana, avocado, pineapple, plum, walnut, vanilla, aubergine) and certain drugs (e.g. paracetamol, naproxen, caffeine).

What investigations are needed if carcinoid syndrome is confirmed?

Imaging (CT or MRI) is the next step. Bowel imaging may be needed. Somatostatin receptor scintigraphy is a highly sensitive and specific way of localising many neuroendocrine tumours.

How would you manage carcinoid syndrome?

Antihistamines and loperamide may give symptomatic relief. Niacin supplementation may assuage tryptophan deficiency from the excessive serotonin synthesis in carcinoid syndrome that might otherwise cause pellagra. The mainstay of treatment if the tumour expresses somatostatin receptors is a somatostatin analogue such as octreotide. Resection of a primary tumour or debulking of metastases may be considered. Debulking of tumour might also be achieved by transarterial embolisation, radiofrequency ablation or radiolabelled somatostatin analogues. Unhappily, the overall prognosis tends to be poor although the tumours are very slow growing.

What are multiple endocrine neoplasia (MEN) syndromes?

These are tumours involving two or more endocrine glands. Diagnosis and management of each tumour are similar to those in non-MEN patients. MEN syndromes are outlined in Table 1.40.

Who should be screened for MEN syndromes?

By measurement of calcium, parathyroid hormone and anterior pituitary hormones, people who should be screened for MEN1 are any patient with two or more MEN1-associated tumours, a young adult with a single MEN1 tumour or relatives of a patient with MEN1. People who should be screened for MEN2 are any patient with medullary thyroid carcinoma, any patient with two or more MEN2-associated tumours, a young adult with a single MEN2 tumour or relatives of a patient with MEN2.

Table 1.40 Multiple endocrine neoplasia (MEN) syndromes

MEN1 Chromosome 11q13 – probable tumour suppressor gene	MEN2 Chromosome 10cen – 10q11.2 containing c-ret proto-oncogene		
	MEN2a Most common MEN2	MEN2b	Medullary thyroid carcinoma only
Parathyroids (95%) – primary hyperparathyroidism	Medullary thyroid carcinoma – calcitonin	Medullary thyroid carcinoma – calcitonin	Medullary thyroid carcinoma – calcitonin
Pancreatic islets (40%) Gastrinoma – gastrin and gastric acid Insulinoma – insulin and hypoglycaemia Glucagonoma – glucogen and glucose intolerance VIPoma – VIP and watery diarrhoea with hypokalaemia			
Pituitary (30%) Prolactinoma – prolactin GH-secreting – growth hormone ACTH-secreting – cortisol	Phaeochromocytoma – catecholamines	Phaeochromocytoma – catecholamines	
Associated Carcinoid – 5-HIAA Adrenal corticol – cortisol Lipoma	Parathyroids – primary hyperparathyroidism	Associated Mucosal abnormalities Marfanoid habitus Medullated corneal nerve fibres Megacolon	

CHRONIC MYELOID LEUKAEMIA

Instruction

Please examine this patient's abdominal system and discuss your findings.

Recognition

The spleen *is markedly enlarged* (Fig. 1.59). *Lymphadenopathy* may be present. Signs of bone marrow failure (*anaemia, petechial rash, signs of sepsis*) may be present.

Interpretation

Confirm the diagnosis

Confirm splenomegaly. The spleen enlarges towards the right iliac fossa and has a medial notch and it is not possible to feel its upper border. Measure enlargement in centimetres from the costal margin. Look for a bone marrow aspiration/trephine dressing or bruising over the iliac crest.

What to do next – assess other systems

Tell the examiners that you would ask about weight loss, fever, night sweats or abdominal pain (splenomegaly or splenic infarction), and request a peripheral blood film.

Consider severity/decompensation/complications

Look for evidence of bone marrow failure (anaemia, fever, petechiae) (Fig. 1.60) or signs of immunosuppression from chemotherapy such as herpes zoster infection (Fig. 1.61).

Consider function

This very much depends on the stage of disease and its treatment, comorbidity and individual strategies for coping with it.

Discussion

What is the underlying genetic abnormality in chronic myeloid leukaemia (CML)?

In around 90% of patients there is a reciprocal translocation between chromosomes 9 and 22 to form a shortened chromosome 22 (Philadelphia chromosome), which contains the chimeric gene *BCR/ABL*. *ABL*, an oncogene encoding a tyrosine kinase, is translocated from chromosome 9 to a specific breakpoint cluster region *BCR* on chromosome 22. Chimeric *BCR/ABL* mRNA encodes a protein with aberrant tyrosine kinase activity, which accelerates growth and differentiation of the myeloid line. This cytogenetic defect arises as a somatic defect within a single pluripotent haemopoietic stem cell from which the clones of leukaemic cells are born. The defect usually arises spontaneously but radiation (e.g. radiotherapy) is a known risk.

What is the difference between a somatic and a germline mutation?

Somatic mutation refers to mutation of genetic material within a particular cell and its clonal offspring. Germline

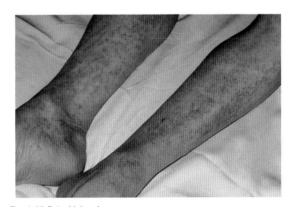

Fig. 1.60 Petechial rash.

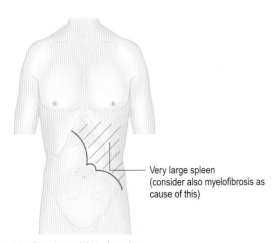

Very large spleen (consider also myelofibrosis as cause of this)

Fig. 1.59 Chronic myeloid leukaemia.

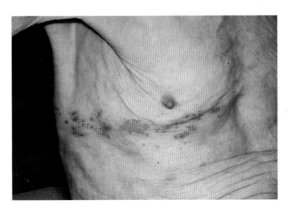

Fig. 1.61 Herpes zoster.

mutation implies that every cell in the body carries the mutation. Somatic mutations underlie leukaemias and many malignancies.

What is the natural history of CML?

An initial chronic phase of clonal myelopoiesis (> 5% blasts) progresses inevitably to an accelerated phase with new cytogenetic changes and ultimately a terminal blastic phase. The natural history is to evolve within three to five years from the chronic phase to the advanced stage (accelerated phase or blastic transformation), which is rapidly fatal – some 6–24 months for the accelerated phase and under six months for the blastic phase, and the accelerated phase is sometimes even bypassed.

How may CML be diagnosed?

CML is more common in middle-aged people. Around 50% of patients present when an abnormal blood film is detected as a chance finding, others often with non-specific symptoms. In the chronic phase a markedly raised white cell count (20×10^9 to $400 \times 10^9/l$) is typical. The peripheral blood film shows immature granulocytes with myelocytes and blasts. Basophils and platelets are often prominent. Vitamin B12 levels may be high. The bone marrow is hypercellular with loss of fat spaces. The *BCR/ABL* gene may be detected by fluorescence in situ hybridisation (FISH) with specific fluorescent probes or by reverse transcriptase polymerase chain reaction (RT-PCR). In the accelerated phase the white cell count increases, with anaemia, thrombocytosis or thrombocytopenia. In the blast phase, blasts or blasts and promyelocytes take over the bone marrow and spill liberally into the blood.

How is CML treated?

Treatments target the chronic phase, because normal stem cells are replaced by Philadelphia-positive stem cells as CML progresses, and are outlined in Box 1.40.

How are patients with CML monitored?

Patients responding to imatinib or in complete remission after stem cell transplantation are best monitored by measuring *BCR/ABL* transcripts using RT-PCR. This allows detection of minimal residual disease, early detection of relapse and assessment of cytogenetic responsiveness to treatment. Further, modern cytogenetic techniques can monitor cytogenetic changes heralding blast transformation.

What are haemopoietic stem cells (HSCs) and how do they become mature cells?

HSCs have the capacity for self-renewal and are pluripotent. They live in the bone marrow where they divide and differentiate into populations of progenitor cells committed to each of the main marrow cell lines.

Cell differentiation is directed by haemopoietic growth factors such as granulocyte colony-stimulating factor (G-

---

Box 1.40 Treatment of chronic myeloid leukaemia (CML)

- Imatinib is an oral inhibitor of BCR-ABL, acting through its ability to bind to the region of the ATP binding site of the BCR-ABL protein.
- Treatment options before imatinib were limited to long-term administration of interferon (IFN)-α or allogeneic (from an HLA-identical donor) stem cell transplantation (SCT).
- In 1999 imatinib was demonstrated to induce cytogenic and clinical remission in patients who failed to respond to IFN-α.
- Compared with allogeneic SCT, persistent leukaemia, as detected by PCR presence of BCR-ABL transcripts is evident in most patients treated with imatinib. This led to fears about the durabilty of cytogenetic and clinical responses, but time is showing durabiltiy in the great majority of patients in the chronic phase, although not the accelerated phase. Thus imatinib is standard treatment for most patients newly diagnosed with CML. Potential cure is possible with SCT, but it carries significant morbidity and mortality.
- Second-generation tyrosine-kinase inhibitors (e.g. dasatinib, nilotinib), with much greater ability to inhibit BCR-ABL, are now available.
- Alkylating agents may be used for CML resistant to imatinib and hydroxyurea, and combination chemotherapy, as for acute leukaemias, is appropriate for patients presenting in the accelerated phase, sometimes after imatinib.

CSF), thrombopoietin (TPO) and erythropoietin (EPO), all lineage specific.

Proerythroblasts are large with dark blue cytoplasm and primitive nuclear material or chromatin. As they differentiate they become smaller, with increasing amounts of haemoglobin and polychromatic cytoplasm as chromatin condenses. The nucleus is eventually extruded, giving rise to a reticulocyte. Reticulocytes still contain RNA and are capable of haemoglobin synthesis, but spend only a few days in the marrow before travelling to the spleen where they lose RNA and become fully-fledged erythrocytes.

Whilst the marrow is the primary site of granulocyte (neutrophil, eosinophil, basophil) and lymphocyte formation, most circulating mature lymphocytes are produced after migration to peripheral secondary lymphoid tissue (lymph nodes, spleen, thymus and gastrointestinal associated lymphoid tissue). Lymphocytes normally comprise < 10% of marrow cells. Plasma cells are typically basophilic cells with a blue tinge and eccentric nucleus. Large numbers of neutrophils are held in reserve in the marrow. Those that enter the circulation spend only hours within it before adhesion and migration into the tissues under the influence of chemokines. Of the circulating pool, about half are loosely adherent to the endothelium, a phenomenon called margination. Monocytes may survive for months or even years in tissues as macrophages or as antigen-presenting cells.

How may bone marrow examination aid diagnosis in haematological disease?

Bone marrow aspirates may be examined for morphology of cells and differential counts, the presence of abnormal cells such as leukaemic, metastatic or infective cells, and organisms and iron status. Bone marrow trephines provide cores of bone and marrow for histological assessment, useful for examining marrow architecture and cellularity and are the most reliable way of detecting marrow infiltrates.

List some causes of neutrophilia and neutropenia

Neutrophilia is common in bacterial infection and physiological stress (e.g. acute coronary syndrome); corticosteroids induce demargination – removal of marginated or adhered neutrophils on the endothelium, the latter a normal situation such that the normal laboratory range for neutrophils underestimates the real number. Neutropenia may be seen in overwhelming sepsis, chemotherapy, myelodysplasia and bone marrow infiltration from leukaemia, myeloma, lymphoma, myelofibrosis or secondary carcinoma. All cytopenias may be classified into either increased peripheral destruction/utilisation (there may be a compensatory bone marrow response as in sepsis, when the bone marrow response causes a left-shifted peripheral blood film) or deficient marrow production.

What is demargination?

This is the process in which neutrophils adherent to the endothelium slip off it, commonly induced by corticosteroid therapy to cause an approximate doubling in the laboratory neutrophil count.

What is leucoerythroblastic change?

This refers to the presence of nucleated red cells and white cell precursors in peripheral blood. It is seen in severe illness such as sepsis or trauma and in marrow infiltration.

How do acute leukaemias differ from chronic leukaemias?

Acute leukaemias are characterised by their rapid onset and their high proportion of undifferentiated blast cells compared with chronic leukaemias. Aberrant myeloid or lymphoid precursors arise in the bone marrow after somatic mutation of a single cell and spill into the blood. Blast cells on a peripheral blood film often provide initial evidence of suspected acute leukaemia. Clinical features of acute leukaemias result from the consequences of bone marrow failure (neutropenia, thrombocytopenia, anaemia) and organ infiltration [lymph nodes, spleen, liver, meninges, testes (especially acute lymphoblastic leukaemia), skin and gums (some acute myeloid leukaemias)]. Chronic lymphocytic leukaemia arises from mature lymphocyte precursors. CML is a stem cell disorder in which differentiation is possible. Acute myeloid leukaemia (AML) represents a more mature but arrested stage.

How is AML classified?

AML may be classified morphologically using the French American British (FAB) classification (Table 1.41) to distinguish subtypes based on cell appearance and cytochemistry staining, immunologically using monoclonal antibodies to cell surface markers, or cytogenetically. It is evident that the most important prognostic indicator is the specific mutation within a leukaemic clone and increasingly cytogenetic methods are used to define specific subtypes and guide treatment.

What are Auer rods?

Auer rods are aggregates of granules seen in M1, M2 and especially M3 stages of AML.

What is acute promyelocytic leukaemia (APML)?

APML is the result of the fusion of the *PML* gene on chromosome 15 with the *RARα* gene on chromosome 17 to form a chimeric fusion protein that interferes with factors essential for normal differentiation of myeloid precursors. APML cells contain procoagulant 'junk' material. Cell lysis can cause disseminated intravascular coagulation (DIC) but all-*trans* retinoic acid may be used to induce remission in the absence of chemotherapy without causing DIC. Postinduction chemotherapy is needed to maintain remission.

FAB classification	Subtype	Features
Table 1.41 FAB classification of acute myeloid leukaemia (AML)		
M0	Acute myeloblastic leukaemia with minimal differentiation	Least differentiated, with large, agranular myeloblasts
M1	Acute myeloblastic leukaemia without maturation	Blasts comprise ≥ 90% of nucleated (non-erythroid) cells
M2	Acute myeloblastic leukaemia with maturation	Blasts 30–89% but definite promyelocyte differentiation
M3	Acute promyelocytic leukaemia	Mostly abnormal promyelocytes, containing granules of procoagulant material
M4	Acute myelomonocytic leukaemia	An eosinophilic subtype is recognised
M5	Acute monocytic/monoblastic leukaemia	Monoblasts, promonocytes or monocytes comprise > 80% of nucleated cells
M6	Erythroleukaemia	Erythroid component of marrow comprises > 50% of cells
M7	Megakaryoblastic leukaemia	

FAB, French American British.

What are the treatment principles in AML?

Remission induction followed by consolidation therapy (better than low-dose maintenance), stem cell transplantation and supportive therapy (blood products, antimicrobials for febrile neutropenia, haemopoietic growth factors). In contrast to CML, the molecular complexity of AML means that targeting molecular therapies against tyrosine kinases and other pathways is more challenging, other than treatment for APML.

What are the principles of bone marrow or haemopoietic stem cell transplantation (HSCT)?

HSCT involves harvesting stem cells from donor marrow or more commonly peripheral blood (the stem cell content of blood being augmented by chemotherapy and G-CSF before harvest) and using these to repopulate and regenerate recipient marrow, thus rescuing the recipient from aplasia. HSCT relies on the fact that stem cells infused into the peripheral vein of a recipient 'home' to the marrow to re-establish haemopoiesis. Donors may be autologous (same patient) or allogeneic (HLA-matched relative or unrelated donor).

A specific concern with autologous transplantation is the potential for tumour cells to contaminate the graft, and numerous purging techniques have been used in attempts to reduce rates of disease relapse. HSCT, in conjunction with intensive supportive therapy until the infused stem cells are able to produce adequate numbers of red and white cells and platelets, allows the use of high-dose chemotherapy in recipients. Supportive therapy includes blood products, growth factors and antimicrobials.

In which conditions is HSCT considered?

HSCT can be used in AML, acute lymphoblastic leukaemia, CML, chronic lymphoblastic leukaemia, myelodysplasia, lymphoma, myeloma and non-malignant disorders including severe aplasia. HSCT for breast cancer has not proven beneficial and there is not yet evidence for benefit in other solid tumours.

What is graft versus host disease?

In allogeneic transplants donor and recipient are not immunologically identical and so activation of donor lymphocytes occurs against host antigens. This may cause immune damage to the skin, gut and liver of the recipient. However, a graft versus tumour effect may also occur, donor lymphocytes recognising and eliminating residual malignant cells in the recipient. This has led to interest in donor lymphocyte infusion for antimalignancy effects, notably in CML.

Do stem cells from other tissues have a role in medicine?

Of emerging interest is the use of stem cells from other tissues to repair diseased or degenerating tissue. Stem cells may have the ability to transdifferentiate ('plasticity'), and it may be possible to redirect stem cells from muscle, brain, skin, liver and other sites to differentiate into tissue different from that originally intended.

POLYCYTHAEMIA VERA, MYELOPROLIFERATIVE DISORDERS AND MYELODYSPLASIA

Instruction

This gentleman reports pruritus after a hot bath. Please examine his abdomen and report your findings.

Recognition

There is *moderate splenomegaly*. There may be facial plethora, suffusion of the conjunctivae and engorgement of retinal vessels.

Interpretation

Confirm the diagnosis

The median age of presentation is 55–60 years. Polycythaemia vera (PV) may present with the symptoms listed in Box 1.41. Tell the examiners that you would ask about these symptoms but in fact the classic presentation of splenomegaly and itch is uncommon.

What to do next – consider causes

Tell the examiners about differentiating the types of polycythaemia (erythrocytosis):

- Erythrocytosis is defined as a packed cell volume (PCV) > 0.51 in men and > 0.48 in women, and these, or haemoglobin concentrations respectively of > 17 and > 15 g/dl, warrant further evaluation.
- A red cell mass (RCM) study determines if erythrocytosis is absolute (increased RCM) or apparent (normal RCM, reduced plasma volume). Absolute may be assumed if PCV is > 0.60 in men or > 0.56 in women.
- If absolute, further tests are needed to differentiate between PV, secondary erythrocytosis and idiopathic erythrocytosis (Fig. 1.62). Exclusion of secondary causes may include oximetry, chest X-ray, serum ferritin (low levels more common in PV than secondary causes), renal and liver function tests, serum erythropoietin levels, abdominal imaging and sleep studies.

Box 1.41 Possible symptoms of polycythaemia vera
• Headaches   • Lethargy   • Dyspnoea   • Weight loss   • Night sweats   • Pruritus (exacerbated by a hot bath)   • Left upper quadrant pain (splenomegaly)

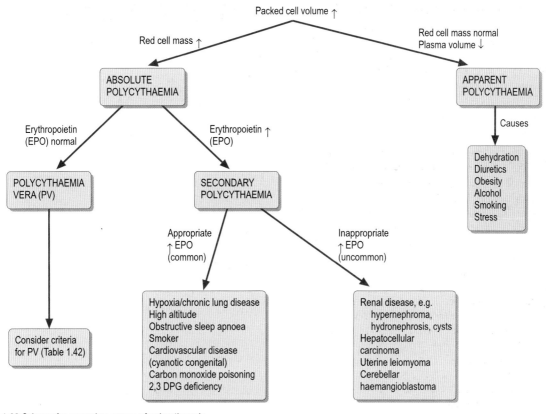

Fig. 1.62 Scheme for assessing causes of polycythaemia.

To confirm PV, the PV Study Group (in guidelines prepared by the British Committee of Standards in Haematology 2005) proposes the criteria listed in Table 1.42 and the World Health Organization (WHO) proposes similar criteria.

Diagnosis may now be furthered more precisely with bone marrow studies, cytogenetics and the finding of a specific *JAK2* mutation in PV.

Consider severity/decompensation/complications

Vascular thromboses, particularly arterial, and occasionally bleeding, are the major clinical events. Tell the examiners that you would ask about strokes and priapism. Other complications include erythromelalgia (red, burning feet and fingers), hepatosplenomegaly, peptic ulceration, gout and leukaemic transformation.

Classically there are two phases of PV, an initial proliferative polycythaemic phase and a spent or postpolycythaemic phase in which cytopenias are associated with ineffective haemopoiesis, marrow fibrosis, extramedullary haemopoiesis and splenomegaly.

Consider function

The symptoms and complications can be very disabling. Tell the examiners that it is imperative to

recognise and treat PV before thrombotic complications ensue.

Discussion

How is PV managed?

Thrombosis is the leading cause of death, with a median survival of 18 months in untreated patients extended to 8–15 years with treatment. Control of the elevated PCV is by venesection or cytoreductive therapy (especially if thrombocytosis) with hydroxyurea. The latter might increase the risk of leukaemia, but not as much as the previously used phosphorus and busulfan. Interferon-α and anagrelide are emerging new treatments, without leukaemogenic risk. The target PCV is 0.45 and platelets $400 \times 10^9/l$. Antiplatelet agents (aspirin) are beneficial if there are no contraindications such as bleeding or a very high platelet count ($> 1500 \times 10^9/l$), which can cause paradoxic bleeding.

What may PV transform to?

PV may transform to myelofibrosis (spent phase, occurring in 15–20% of patients at 10 years) characterised by progressive splenomegaly and pancytopenia and generally treated supportively, or AML (5% at 10 years), a terminal

Table 1.42 Criteria for polycythaemia vera (PV): PV diagnosed by A1 and A2, plus A3 or A4 or any two of B

Major criteria	Minor criteria
A1 RCM absolute increase or if RCM unavailable haematocrit ≥ 0.60 in males or ≥ 0.56 in females (WHO guidelines allow haemoglobin concentration)	B1 Thrombocytosis (50% of patients)
A2 No secondary cause	B2 Neutrophil leucocytosis (two-thirds of patients)
A3 Palpable spenomegaly (WHO guidelines do not stipulate palpable)	B3 Splenomegaly detected by scanning (WHO guidelines suggest marrow biopsy)
A4 Clonality marker (acquired abnormal marrow karyotype) other than Ph chromosome or *bcr/abl* fusion gene	B4 Characteristic growth of burst-forming units, erythroid, or reduced serum erythropoietin

Box 1.42 Myeloproliferative disorders

- Polycythaemia vera (PV)
- Essential thrombocythaemia (ET)
- Idiopathic myelofibrosis (IMF)
- Chronic myeloid leukaemia (CML)

feature of any myeloproliferative disorder and refractory to treatment.

What are myeloproliferative disorders (MPDs)?

These are clonal stem cell disorders characterised by proliferation of one or more of the erythroid, granulocytic or megakaryocytic cell lines with excess red cells, white cells or platelets in peripheral blood. There is often overlap of erythropoietic, granulopoietic and megakaryocytic expansion, lending support to the notion of a clonal stem cell defect. Cells are morphologically normal, although the World Health Organization classification now recognises overlap with myelodysplastic syndromes. The main MPDs are listed in Box 1.42.

Rare MPDs include chronic neutrophilic and eosinophilic leukaemia.

What do you know about essential thrombocythaemia (ET)?

ET causes clustering of megakaryocytes in marrow and persistent thrombocytosis ($> 600 \times 10^9/l$ is generally accepted for diagnosis). It results in thrombosis and bleeding and, longer term, myelofibrosis (10% at 10 years) or AML (1–2% at 10 years). Diagnosis is by exclusion of other MPDs and reactive thrombocytosis (iron deficiency anaemia, bleeding, inflammation, malignancy). The JAK-2 mutation is found in around 50% of patients. Most patients benefit from aspirin and hydroxyurea. Anagrelide is an emerging treatment.

What do you know about idiopathic myelofibrosis (IMF)?

IMF may arise de novo, or as a late phase of PV or ET. Fibrosis may occur because diseased megakaryocytes release mitogens such as growth factors directly stimulating fibroblast proliferation. Median presentation is at 50–60 years with symptoms relating to marrow failure or splenomegaly. Diagnosis is by splenomegaly, marrow histology (coarse parallel reticulin and later osteomyelofibrosis), a leucoerythroblastic blood film, often with tear drop cells, absence of other MPDs and exclusion of secondary myelofibrosis. Progression to AML occurs in 25% of patients.

What are myelodysplastic syndromes (MDSs)?

It has long been known that some leukaemias smoulder for a long time before becoming clinically apparent, and that some unusual anaemias transform to acute leukaemia. Myelodysplasia refers to a group of clonal disorders of haemopoietic stem cells, which retain the ability to differentiate into mature cells, but do so in a disordered and ineffective manner. This leads to hypercellular bone marrow and peripheral blood cytopenia.

How do MDSs arise?

They are caused by cumulative acquisition of cytogenetic errors, e.g. deletions of tumour suppressor genes on chromosomes 5 and 7 have been implicated. This causes the neoplastic clone to divide more rapidly, but the resultant haemopoiesis is ineffective with a high rate of apoptosis. As cytogenetic errors accumulate, the clone becomes less stable, myeloblasts accumulate and acute leukaemia ensues.

How are MDSs classified?

A new classification devised by the WHO (Table 1.43) differs from the FAB classification notably in that patients with > 20% blasts in marrow are now considered to have leukaemia.

How are MDSs diagnosed?

They are uncommon before 60 years of age. Patients are usually asymptomatic but may present with anaemia, bleeding, recurrent infections or mouth ulcers. Chronic myelomonocytic leukaemia may cause hepatosplenomegaly and when monocytes are too abundant and become tissue macrophages this can lead to gum hypertrophy, pleural or pericardial effusions, arthritis or skin lesions. Peripheral blood abnormalities in MDSs may include the presence of the following cells or phenomena: macrocytes,

Table 1.43 WHO classification of myelodysplastic syndromes

MDS	MDS/MPD
Refractory anaemia	Chronic myelomonocytic leukaemia
with ring sideroblasts	Atypical chronic myeloid leukaemia
without ring sideroblasts	Juvenile myelomonocytic leukaemia
Refractory cytopenia with	Unclassifiable
multi-lineage dysplasia	
Refractory anaemia with	
excess blasts	
type I (5–9% blasts)	
type II (10–19% blasts)	
5q-syndrome	
Unclassifiable	

MDS, myelodysplastic syndrome; MPD, myeloproliferative disorder.

Box 1.43 Treatments for myelodysplastic syndromes

- Supportive care (blood transfusion for symptomatic anaemia with iron chelation – without chelation 60 units usually leads to iron overload and 100 units leads to cardiac damage, platelet transfusions for bleeding and prompt treatment of febrile neutropenia)
- Erythropoietin 150–300 U/kg subcutaneously three to seven times weekly as an alternative ± G-CSF
- Allogeneic stem cell transplantation
- Chemotherapy
- Immunosuppression (some evidence for an immune process in pathogenesis)

aniso-poikilocytes, a dimorphic picture, polychromasia, basophilia, normoblasts, reticulocytopenia, hypogranular neutrophils, hypersegmented neutrophils, mono- or bilobed neutrophils, monocytosis, promonocytes, agranular platelets, giant platelets and megakaryocyte fragments. Marrow abnormalities may include erythroid hyperplasia, multinuclear red cell precursors, ring sideroblasts, hypogranularity of myeloid precursors, increased promonocytes, blasts and abnormal megakaryocytes. Cytogenetic chromosomal analysis is helpful. Serum B12 levels may be high. The differential diagnosis includes other causes of cytopenias, e.g. acute leukaemia, aplastic leukaemia, immune thrombocytopenia, marrow infiltration, acquired immunodeficiency syndrome.

What is the treatment for MDSs?

Treatments are listed in Box 1.43.

What is the prognosis in MDSs?

Several prognostic scoring systems have been devised, and > 5% blasts associated with shorter survival. Around a third of patients die from acute leukaemia, a third from cytopenia and a third from unrelated causes.

What do you understand by the term bone marrow failure?

Bone marrow failure refers to primary failure, at a haemopoietic stem cell level, to produce one or more cell lineages.

The term usually excludes pancytopenia associated with marrow infiltration as in leukaemias and cytopenias. Bone marrow failure may be acquired or congenital.

What causes acquired aplastic anaemia?

This is unknown except where a specific drug (there are many!), virus (e.g. parvovirus B19) or unusual association (e.g. paroxysmal nocturnal haemoglobinuria) can be implicated. An immune pathogenesis probably results in suppression of recovery of damaged cells; cytokines such as tumour necrosis factor-α and interferon-γ up-regulate the expression of stem cell receptors that trigger apoptosis.

How is aplastic anaemia investigated?

Anaemia, bleeding or infection can bring it to attention. It is classified as:

- Very severe (neutrophils $< 0.2 \times 10^9$/l, platelets $< 20 \times 10^9$/l, reticulocytes $< 20 \times 10^9$/l, transfusion dependent)
- Severe (neutrophils 0.2×10^9 to 0.5×10^9/l, otherwise as for very severe)
- Non-severe (neutrophils 0.5×10^9 to 1.5×10^9/l, platelets 20×10^9 to 100×10^9/l, reticulocytes 20×10^9 to 60×10^9/l)

Lymphocyte numbers may be preserved and neutrophils are heavily granulated. Bone marrow examination reveals hypocellularity and a 'lacy' appearance, but changes are patchy. Cytogenetic studies on marrow aspirates may show abnormal but stable clones, previously thought to indicate MDSs, although distinction between aplastic anaemia and hypoplastic MDSs can be difficult. Peripheral blood lymphocytes may be examined for chromosome breaks characteristic of Fanconi's anaemia.

How is aplastic anaemia managed?

Supportive measures may be followed by immunosuppression with antithymocyte globulin via a central vein together with ciclosporin. Allogeneic stem cell transplantation may be considered.

What other bone marrow failure syndromes are there?

These include pure red cell aplasia (often associated with viruses, drugs or autoimmune diseases), amegakaryocytic thrombocytopenia and cyclical neutropenia.

CASE 1.46

CHRONIC LYMPHOCYTIC LEUKAEMIA

Instruction

Please examine this 75-year-old gentleman's lymphoreticular system and discuss your findings.

Recognition

There is widespread *lymphadenopathy* and moderate *splenomegaly/hepatosplenomegaly* (Fig. 1.63). Lymph nodes are often markedly enlarged, painless and rubbery.

Interpretation

Confirm the diagnosis

Tell the examiners that you would request a peripheral blood film. This would demonstrate an excess of small, mature lymphocytes with smear/smudge cells (broken in vitro by slide preparation), pathognomonic of chronic lymphocytic leukaemia (CLL) and differentiating it from other lymphoproliferative disorders.

What to do next – assess other systems

Tell the examiners that you would ask about symptoms. B symptoms such as sweats and weight loss are uncommon.

Consider severity/decompensation/complications

The CLL clone invades the lymph nodes, liver, spleen and bone marrow (failure causing sepsis, bruising/bleeding and anaemia). Look for *petechial haemorrhages* and *pallor*. You could tell the examiners any of the following:

*   Cytopenias may also occur due to autoimmune phenomena.
*   Autoimmune haemolysis and thrombocytopenia are common.
*   The leukaemic B lymphocyte clone suppresses the normal B lymphocyte population, causing immune deficiency, but T-cell dysregulation also contributes.
*   Transformation of lymph node tissue to Richter's large cell lymphoma is a rare but serious complication.
*   Epstein–Barr virus-related transformation is more common now because of immunosuppression induced by purine analogue treatment, and herpes zoster virus reactivation remains very common (Fig. 1.64).

Staging

Clinical staging is important for prognosis, and assesses organ involvement and cytopenias. The Rai classification is shown in Box 1.44.

The alternative Binet classification considers three stages, A if between zero and two organs are involved, haemoglobin > 10 g/dl and platelets > 100×10^9/l, B if three

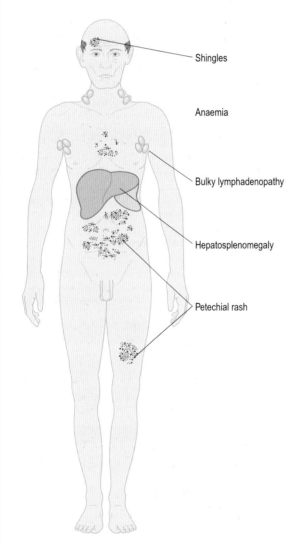

Fig. 1.63 Chronic lymphocytic leukaemia.

Labels on figure: Shingles, Anaemia, Bulky lymphadenopathy, Hepatosplenomegaly, Petechial rash

Box 1.44 Rai classification	
• 0	lymphocytosis
• I	lymphocytosis + lymphadenopathy
• II	lymphocytosis + splenomegaly and/or hepatomegaly
• III	lymphocytosis + anaemia (haemoglobin < 11 g/dl)
• IV	lymphocytosis + thrombocytopenia (platelets < 100×10^9/l)

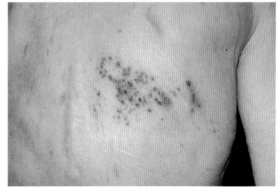

Fig. 1.64 Herpes zoster.

to five organs are involved with the same blood parameters and C if blood parameters are low.

Consider function

This very much depends on the stage of disease and its treatment and comorbidity (CLL tends to affect older people).

Discussion

What is the underlying defect in CLL?

CLL is the most common chronic leukaemia in the Western world, and tends to occur in older people, more so in men. A range of mutations is possible, arising in mature B lymphocyte precursors, with differing prognoses. The pathogenesis is uncertain. Trisomy 12 and chromosome 13 deletions are common but secondary to the primary event. In some young patients a deletion in chromosome 11 is associated with CLL and ataxia–telangiectasia. Around half of patients with CLL have somatic mutations in the immunoglobulin heavy-chain variable region genes and half do not, suggesting that CLL starts with disease in a germinal centre cell that has encountered an antigen in the former and in a naïve cell in the latter.

How is diagnosis confirmed?

Immunophenotyping for the cluster designation (CD) surface marker profile of blood or bone marrow clonal cells is diagnostic. CLL cells express CD23 and CD5. Routine investigations in the work-up of CLL and exclusion of differential diagnoses include haemobiochemistry, bone marrow examination, immunoglobulins, Coomb's test and abdominal CT scan.

When should CLL be treated?

Treatment is for symptomatic disease, aiming to decrease tumour cell load, because CLL is not curable. The long natural history means that many patients remain asymptomatic and die from an unrelated problem.

How is CLL treated?

Treatments are listed in Box 1.45.

Box 1.45 Treatment of chronic lymphoblastic leukaemia (CLL)

- First-line treatment is with alkylating agents (chlorambucil), fludarabine (a purine analogue) or combination chemotherapy. Fludarabine seems to have better response rates but this has not translated to improved survival. Prednisolone improves marrow reserve and is given if there is cytopenia.
- Campath-1H or rituximab may be used as second line.
- Splenectomy, splenic irradiation and leukapheresis may be used for bulky splenomegaly or cytopenias.
- Allogeneic stem cell transplant is considered in younger patients.
- Supportive treatments include antimicrobials, intravenous immunoglobulin, iron and folate supplements, allopurinol and haemopoietic growth factors.

CASE 1.47

LYMPHADENOPATHY AND LYMPHOMA

Instruction

Please examine this patient's abdomen and discuss your findings.

Recognition

There is *painless lymphadenopathy* (often widespread and not necessarily contiguous) and *hepatosplenomegaly*.

Other features may be present (Fig. 1.65).

Interpretation

Confirm the diagnosis

This is not possible clinically. Common abnormalities on blood tests are normochromic normocytic anaemia, neutropenia, thrombocytopenia, autoimmune cytopenia, and raised C-reactive protein (CRP) and erythrocyte sedimentation rate (ESR). Hypercalcaemia may be seen in adult T-cell lymphoma/leukaemia and any advanced non-Hodgkin's lymphoma (NHL). Circulating lymphoma cells (large cell, follicular and mantle cell lymphomas) are occasionally detected. Liver and renal dysfunction may reflect organ involvement. Serum or urine paraproteins are more common in indolent lymphomas. Normal immunoglobulins may be reduced.

Immunophenotyping on circulating lymphoma cells, fine-needle aspirates or fixed tissue sections from lymph nodes or other sites is essential for diagnosis and classification, aided by cytogenetic studies. Clonality may be demonstrated by Southern blot or polymerase chain reaction to detect immunoglobulin and T-cell receptor gene rearrangements. Specific translocations occur in certain subtypes, e.g. clonal integration of Epstein–Barr virus.

What to do next – assess other systems

Tell the examiners you would consider the differential diagnosis of lymphadenopathy (Box 1.46).

Consider severity/decompensation/complications

Tell the examiners that prognosis in NHL depends on the subtype. For example, there are two distinct prognostic

---

Box 1.46 Differential diagnosis of lymphadenopathy

- Infection, e.g. Epstein–Barr virus, cytomegalovirus, toxoplasmosis, tuberculosis, HIV, brucellosis
- Lymphoproliferative disease, e.g. non-Hodgkin's lymphoma, Hodgkin's lymphoma
- Carcinoma
- Sarcoidosis
- Autoimmune disease

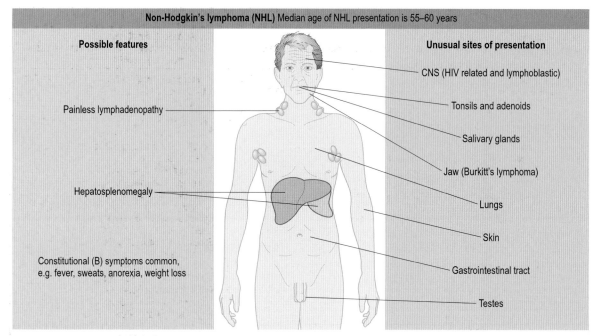

Non-Hodgkin's lymphoma (NHL) Median age of NHL presentation is 55–60 years

Possible features

Painless lymphadenopathy

Hepatosplenomegaly

Constitutional (B) symptoms common, e.g. fever, sweats, anorexia, weight loss

Unusual sites of presentation

CNS (HIV related and lymphoblastic)

Tonsils and adenoids

Salivary glands

Jaw (Burkitt's lymphoma)

Lungs

Skin

Gastrointestinal tract

Testes

Fig. 1.65 Non-Hodgkin's lymphoma (NHL).

groups in diffuse large B-cell NHL. The following are also associated with a poor prognosis:

- Stage III/IV
- Age > 60 years
- WHO classification performance status 2–4
- Raised lactic dehydrogenase (LDH)
- More than one extranodal site
- Raised β2-microglobulin
- Bulky disease (> 10 cm)
- Transformation from low-grade to high-grade NHL
- AIDS-related disease

Consider function

Tell the examiners that constitutional symptoms can be very debilitating, as can chemotherapy, and that there is a WHO classification for performance status.

Discussion

What is NHL?

NHL is a heterogeneous group of malignant diseases characterised by replacement of normal lymphoid structure with diffuse and nodular collections of abnormal lymphocytes.

What causes NHL?

The incidence increases with age, and has increased with human immunodeficiency virus (HIV). Some histological types have geographical associations reflecting environmental factors such as human T-cell lymphotropic virus 1

(HTLV-1) causing adult T-cell lymphoma/leukaemia (ATLL), Epstein–Barr virus and Burkitt's lymphoma, and *Helicobacter pylori* and mucosa-associated lymphoid tissue (MALT). Immunodeficiency, autoimmune disorders, poisons and some inherited disorders are associated with some lymphomas.

How is NHL classified?

The WHO classification of tumours of haemopoietic and lymphoid tissue in 2001 divided haematological malignancies according to cell lineage (myeloid, lymphoid or miscellaneous) and subcategories according to morphology, immunophenotype, genetics and clinical features (Table 1.44).

Some specific types of NHL have unique epidemiology, causation, presentation and management.

How is NHL staged?

Staging (Ann Arbor) is similar to that for Hodgkin's disease but less relevant because prognosis in NHL is based largely on histology. Investigations usually include chest X-ray and CT of chest, abdomen and pelvis and biopsy of an appropriate site, and may include bone marrow aspiration and trephine, gastrointestinal investigation, lumbar puncture in high-grade NHL and liver biopsy.

How is NHL managed?

Low-grade NHL is usually disseminated at diagnosis, with bone marrow involvement in 75%, and is often incurable, although single-site disease may be cured in 30–50% with

Table 1.44 WHO classification of lymphoid neoplasms with examples of immunophenotyping			
B-cell neoplasms Mature B-cell neoplasm > 85% of all NHL (large B cell and follicular B cell accounting for 50%)		**T- and NK-cell neoplasms** Relatively uncommon; more prevalent in Far East and developing countries	
Precursor (lymphoblastic) B lymphoblastic leukaemia/lymphoma	CD79a$^+$, CD19$^+$, CD10$^\pm$	**Precursor (lymphoblastic)** T lymphoblastic leukaemia/ lymphoma	CD2$^+$, CD3$^+$
Peripheral (mature) Chronic lymphocytic leukaemia B-cell prolymphocytic leukaemia Lymphoplasmocytic lymphoma/Waldenström's macroglobulinaemia Splenic marginal zone lymphoma Hairy cell leukaemia Plasma cell neoplasms – myeloma, plasmacytoma, heavy-chain disease Extranodal marginal zone B-cell lymphoma (MALT lymphoma) Nodal marginal zone B-cell lymphoma Follicular lymphoma (20% of NHL) Mantle cell lymphoma Diffuse large B-cell lymphoma (30% of NHL) Mediastinal (thymic) large B-cell lymphoma Intravascular large B-cell lymphoma Primary effusion lymphoma Burkitt's lymphoma/leukaemia Lymphomatoid granulomatosis	Ig$^+$, CD19$^+$, CD3$^-$	**Peripheral (mature)** T-cell prolymphocytic leukaemia T-cell large granular lymphocytic leukaemia Aggressive NK cell leukaemia Adult T-cell leukaemia/lymphoma Extranodal NK/T-cell lymphoma, nasal type Enteropathy-type T-cell lymphoma Hepatosplenic T-cell lymphoma Subcutaneous panniculitis-like T-cell lymphoma Blastic NK-cell lymphoma Mycosis fungoides/Sezary syndrome Primary cutaneous CD30$^+$ T-cell lymphoproliferative disease Angio-immunoblastic T-cell lymphoma Peripheral T-cell lymphoma unspecified Anaplastic large cell lymphoma	Ig$^-$, CD19$^-$, CD3$^+$, CD4$^+$ or CD8$^+$
Hodgkin's lymphoma (30% of lymphoma) Specific lymphoma Bimodal age distribution Typically peripheral (especially cervical) and mediastinal lymphadenopathy Reed–Sternberg cell pathognomonic Lymphocyte predominant, mixed cellularity, nodular sclerosing or lymphocyte deplete			
MALT, mucosa-associated lymphoid tissue; NK, natural killer.			

field radiotherapy. It has a long natural history, relapsing and remitting, with a median diagnosis of nine years. Indications for treatment are B symptoms, bone marrow failure, bulky disease or progression. Treatment is usually with a single alkylating agent (e.g. chlorambucil, cyclophosphamide) or fludaribine with a response rate of 80% for 18–24 months. Interferon-α prolongs remission but does not improve survival. Splenectomy may be curative in splenic lymphoma. Anti-CD20 monoclonal antibodies and high-dose therapy with autograft may have a place.

Diffuse large B-cell lymphoma in its early stage is treated with combination chemotherapy, sometimes with field radiotherapy. Mantle cell and peripheral T-cell lymphomas respond poorly to treatment.

Extranodal lymphomas may respond well to unique treatments, e.g. *H. pylori* eradication in MALT lymphoma, cutaneous therapies in cutaneous T-cell lymphoma.

Which patients should be considered for central nervous system prophylaxis?

Systemic or intrathecal methotrexate is considered in lymphoblastic, HIV-associated lymphoma, Burkitt's lymphoma or T-cell lymphoma.

Is haemopoietic stem cell transplantation (HSCT) of benefit in NHL?

High-dose chemotherapy and HSCT may benefit younger, high-risk patients with multiple poor prognostic factors. The advantages of allogeneic over autologous HSCT are uncontaminated stem cells and graft versus leukaemia effect.

Do molecular therapies have a place in treating NHL?

Monoclonal antibodies such as anti-CD20 (rituximab) are of emerging interest.

CASE 1.48

POLYCYSTIC KIDNEY DISEASE

Instruction

Please examine this patient's abdomen and discuss your findings.

Recognition

The *kidneys are palpable* (confirmed by bimanual palpation and ballottement, but often large enough to cause loin distension) (Fig. 1.66). The *liver may also be enlarged with an irregular surface*, also affected by polycystic disease. There may be a transplanted kidney in the right or left iliac fossa. Bulky polycystic kidneys are usually excised at transplantation.

Interpretation

Confirm the diagnosis

Bilateral flank masses make the diagnosis very likely. Ensure that you can 'get above' the masses. This may be challenging on the right if the liver is also polycystic.

What to do next – assess other systems

Tell the examiners that you would like to take the blood pressure, ask about a family history and ask about haematuria.

Consider severity/decompensation/complications

Renal manifestations

Polycystic kidney disease (PKD) may present with haematuria, hypertension, renal failure, large kidneys/loin pain or urinary sepsis. Approximately one-third of patients develop renal failure, one-third develop hypertension

without renal failure, and one-third remain asymptomatic through life. Look for evidence of current or previous renal failure (arteriovenous fistula in one or both forearms, scarring at internal jugular or subclavian haemodialysis catheter sites, renal transplantation).

Extra-renal manifestations

Tell the examiners that numerous extra-renal complications may occur (Box 1.47)

Consider function

The flank masses are sometimes uncomfortably bulky. The key is to prevent or delay progression of chronic kidney disease.

Discussion

What do you know about the genetics of PKD?

PKD is one of the more common genetic diseases. It may be autosomal dominant (ADPKD) or autosomal recessive (ARPKD, usually presenting in childhood). ADPKD can present at any age, but often in the fourth or fifth decades, and there may be a highly variable phenotype within families. In some families it may become more severe over successive generations (anticipation).

Most patients (85%) with ADPKD have mutations at chromosome 16p (*PKD-1*). *PKD-2* is the next most common genotype. These genes encode polycystin-1 and polycystin-2. *PKD-1* is associated with a more severe phenotype and a higher risk of end-stage renal disease at an earlier age, hypertension and urinary sepsis.

PKD-1 may also be associated with phenotypes of Marfan syndrome, tuberous sclerosis, familial intracranial aneurysm and polycystic liver disease.

The gene mutated in ARPKD encodes fibrocystin, a protein of unknown function.

List some other causes of renal cysts

* Simple cysts, which are extremely common and benign
* Medullary cystic disease, which causes chronic kidney disease
* Acquired cystic disease, which may be found in any scarred kidney
* Von Hippel–Lindau syndrome

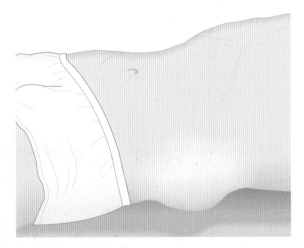

Fig. 1.66 Polycystic kidney disease.

Box 1.47 Extra-renal complications of polycystic kidney disease (PKD)
<ul><li>Hepatic, pancreatic or ovarian cysts. These are commonly asymptomatic</li><li>Loin pain or abdominal pain from bleeding into renal or extra-renal cysts/infected cysts</li><li>Mitral valve prolapse</li><li>Anaemia of chronic kidney disease</li><li>Polycythaemia (increased erythropoietin activity)</li><li>Cerebral aneurysms and subarachnoid haemorrhage</li></ul>

List some other renal diseases which have a genetic basis

A wide range of cystic, glomerular (e.g. Alport's syndrome) and tubular transport disorders are know known to correlate with pathogenic gene disturbances. In many of these, multiple different mutations may give rise to the same disease or the same spectrum of disease with slightly differing phenotypic expression. Tubular disorders include:

- Genetic renal glycosuria
- Aminoacidurias, e.g. Hartnup's disease, homocystinuria, cystinuria
- Cytinosis
- Bartter syndrome
- Gitelman syndrome
- Nephrogenic diabetes insipidus
- Proximal renal tubule acidosis
- Distal renal tubule acidosis
- Liddle's syndrome
- Glucocorticoid remediable excess
- Apparent mineralocorticoid excess
- Pseudohypoaldosteronism
- Hypophosphataemic rickets
- X-linked hypercalciuric nephrolithiasis (Dent's disease)

CASE 1.49

NEPHROTIC SYNDROME

Instruction

Please examine this patient's abdomen, nails and ankles and discuss your findings.

Recognition

There is *fluid overload* as evidenced by *sacral* and *peripheral oedema*. There may be *periorbital* or *facial oedema*. There may be *leuconychia*. Pulmonary oedema is less common.

Interpretation

Confirm the diagnosis

Tell the examiners that you would like to perform urinalysis to check for proteinuria. Nephrotic syndrome is outlined in Fig. 1.67.

What to do next – consider causes

The two common primary causes of nephrotic syndrome are minimal change disease and membranous nephropathy. Minimal change disease is usually primary but occasionally it is associated with Hodgkin's disease. Membranous nephropathy is usually primary but secondary causes include non-Hodgkin's lymphoma, carcinoma, melanoma, gold, penicillamine, diabetes, systemic lupus

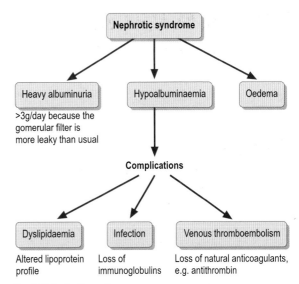

Fig. 1.67 Nephrotic syndrome.

> **Box 1.48 Principles of management of nephrotic syndrome**
>
> - Recognition of histopathological subtype (Case 2.27)
> - Identification and specific treatment of any secondary cause
> - Salt restriction and diuretics for oedema
> - Angiotensin-converting enzyme inhibitors for proteinuria
> - Statin therapy for hypercholesterolaemia
> - Antithrombotic therapy for prothrombotic tendency (controversial)
> - Early recognition and treatment of sepsis (often cellulitis)

erythematosus, amyloid, malaria, hepatitis B virus infection, syphilis and HIV infection. Tell the examiners that you would take a history and investigate for these.

Consider severity/decompensation/complications

Tell the examiners that you would ask about infection and venous thromboembolism.

Consider function

This depends on the underlying cause.

Discussion

What are the principles of management of nephrotic syndrome?

These are listed in Box 1.48.

CASE 1.50

RENAL TRANSPLANT

Instruction

Please examine this patient's abdomen and discuss your findings.

Recognition

There is a *palpable renal transplant in the right/left iliac fossa with an overlying scar*. There may be arteriovenous fistulae at the forearms and internal jugular/subclavian scarring from dialysis catheters or scarring from peritoneal dialysis catheters (Fig. 1.68).

Interpretation

Confirm the diagnosis
Refer to Fig. 1.68.

What to do next – consider causes/assess other systems
Refer to Fig. 1.68. Note that some patients with diabetes receive a kidney and pancreatic transplant.

Consider severity/decompensation/complications
Refer to Fig. 1.68 and Table 1.45.

Consider function
Renal transplantation carries the burden of long-term immunosuppressive treatment but allows the possibility of a relatively normal life, unlike long-term dialysis, a state of chronic ill-health.

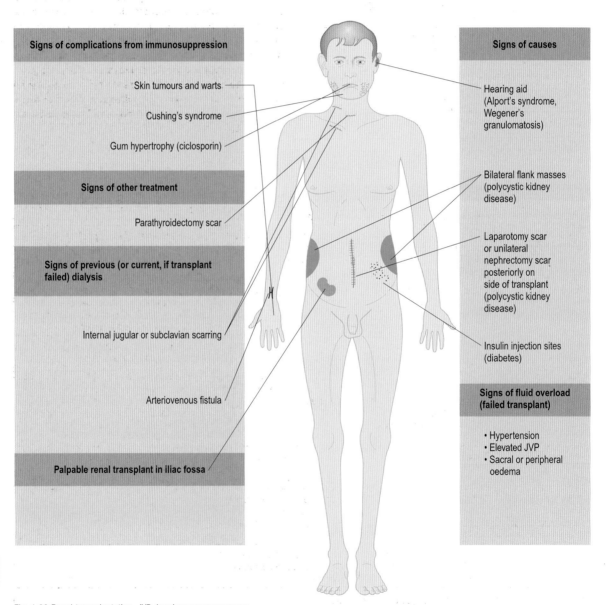

Fig. 1.68 Renal transplantation. JVP, jugular venous pressure.

Table 1.45 Complications of renal transplantation

Timing	Complications
Immediate	Hyperacute rejection – may occur within minutes or hours due to preformed antibodies; graft nephrectomy is necessary Acute tubular necrosis Surgical complications, e.g. renal artery stenosis, renal arterial or venous thrombosis, ureteric stenosis, ureteric leak, infection
Early	Acute rejection – occurs in the first few weeks or months due to host alloreactive T cells which enter the graft Infection, e.g. bacterial, cytomegalovirus – very common, *Pneumocystis carinii*, candidiasis (prophylaxis with ganciclovir if seronegative for cytomegalovirus, cotrimoxazole and antifungal therapy routine)
Late	Chronic rejection – caused partly by alloreactive T cells but immunosuppressive drugs probably contribute Accelerated vascular disease (reflecting underlying disease and drug therapy) Infection Malignancy – warts, skin cancers and lymphoproliferative disorders markedly increased

Discussion

What types of renal transplant are there?

Donor transplants may be cadaveric or live. Live transplants have a better outcome and are now used predominantly.

What therapeutic strategies are there to prevent rejection?

In both acute and chronic rejection, the initial reaction is between recipient T-cell receptors and donor human leucocyte antigen (HLA) molecules bearing foreign peptides. This leads to a cascade of intracellular and extracellular events, central to which is the production of interleukin-2 (Case 2.46). Recipient–donor matching to reduce rejection involves HLA typing, blood grouping and lymphocytotoxic cross-matching. Renal transplantation is highly immunogenic (unlike cornea, bone and artery grafts), so that immunosuppressive drugs are mandatory for graft survival. Prednisolone, azathioprine and ciclosporin-based triple therapy is a well-established regimen. Newer drugs and regimens aim to reduce rejection and limit side effects (Table 1.46).

Table 1.46 Drugs to prevent rejection

Treatment	How it works	Indication	Comment
Corticosteroids	Inhibits nuclear regulatory proteins – powerful anti-inflammatory actions	Maintenance treatment to prevent rejection Treatment of acute rejection	Doses tapered to 5–10 mg daily as maintenance and sometimes stopped altogether High doses to treat acute rejection
Azathioprine	Inhibits purine metabolism and lymphocyte DNA synthesis	Maintenance treatment to prevent rejection	Allopurinol contraindicated with azathioprine as combination may induce aplasia TPMT levels should be checked before starting and dose adjusted accordingly
Mycophenolate mofetil	Inhibits purine metabolism	Maintenance treatment to prevent rejection Post-rejection rescue	More potent than azathioprine Gastrointestinal side effects
Ciclosporin	Inhibits calcineurin – pivotal molecule in signalling cascade for IL-2 synthesis and hence T-lymphocyte activation and proliferation	Maintenance treatment to prevent rejection	Narrow therapeutic window Nephrotoxic Hypertension Hirsutism Gingival hyperplasia
Tacrolimus	Inhibits calcineurin	Maintenance treatment to prevent rejection Rejection rescue	More potent than ciclosporin May induce diabetes
Anti-T-cell antibodies (OKT3 – monoclonal, ATG – polyclonal)	T-cell inhibitor	Treatment of acute rejection not responding to steroids May be used at induction to prevent rejection	
IL-2 receptor antibodies	Inhibits IL-2, common mediator of Th1 pro-inflammatory pathway	Reduce episodes of acute rejection when added to a ciclosporin regimen	

IL-2, interleukin-2; Th1, T helper type 1; TPMT, thiopurine methyl transferase.

Which diseases recur in a transplanted kidney?

These are listed in Box 1.49.

Box 1.49 Some diseases which can recur in a transplanted kidney

- Focal and segmental glomerulosclerosis
- Diabetes (but reasonable prognosis for graft survival)
- Immunoglobulin A nephropathy
- Haemolytic uraemic syndrome/thrombotic thrombocytopenic purpura
- Anti-glomerular basement membrane disease rarely recurs but linear staining for immunoglobulin G is found in around 50% of biopsies
- Oxalosis

What do you know about post-transplantation lymphoproliferative disease (PTLD)?

PTLD is largely due to the Epstein–Barr virus (EBV), which infects and incorporates itself into the host genome of B lymphocytes. Cytotoxic lymphocytes normally suppress B-lymphocyte polyclonal proliferation but immunosuppressive regimens limit cytotoxic lymphocyte activity and allow B-lymphocyte proliferation. Further unharnessed genetic changes in B lymphocytes may lead to the escape of a malignant monoclonal line. PTLD is less common in patients previously exposed to EBV (immunoglobulin G positive) because some cytotoxicity will already be afforded.

References and further reading

Respiratory system

Chronic obstructive pulmonary disease
Heightman M, Bellingan G. Acute respiratory medicine. Clin Med 2007; 7:267–271

National Institute for Health and Clinical Excellence. Chronic obstructive pulmonary disease. Thorax 2004; 59(Suppl. 1):1–232

Pauwels RA, Buist AS, Calverley PM et al. GOLD Scientific Committee. Global strategy for the diagnosis, management and prevention of chronic obstructive pulmonary disease. NHLBI/WHO Global initiative for chronic Obstructive Lung Disease (GOLD). Workshop summary. Review. Am J Respir Crit Care Med 2001; 163:1256–1276. www.goldcopd.com

Vestbo J. Outpatient management of chronic obstructive pulmonary disease. Clin Med 2004; 4:220–224

Pneumonia
Lim WS. Community acquired pneumonia. Clin Med 2004; 4:224–228

Lung cancer
National Institute for Clinical Excellence. Lung cancer: the diagnosis and treatment of lung cancer. Clinical Guideline 24, 2005. Online. Available www.nice.org.uk

Tuberculosis
National Institute for Health and Clinical Excellence. Tuberculosis Clinical Guideline, 2006. Online. Available www.nice.org.uk

Asbestos-related lung disease and pneumoconiosis
Doll R, Peto J. Asbestos: effects on health of exposure to asbestos. London: HMSO; 1985

Pulmonary hypertension
Elliot C, Kierly DG. Pulmonary hypertension: diagnosis and treatment. Clin Med 2004; 4:211–215

Humbert M, Sirborn O, Simonneau G. Treatment of pulmonary arterial hypertension. N Engl J Med 2004; 351:1425–1436

Pulmonary embolism
British Thoracic Society. British Thoracic Society guidelines for the management of suspected acute pulmonary embolism. Thorax 2003; 58:470–483

Palareti G, Cosmi B, Legnani C et al; PROLONG Investigators. D-dimer testing to determine the duration of anticoagulation therapy. N Engl J Med 2006; 355:1780–1789

Robinson GV. Pulmonary embolism in hospital practice. BMJ 2006; 332:156–160

Roy PM, Colombet I, Durieux P et al. Systematic review and meta-analysis of strategies for the diagnosis of suspected pulmonary embolism. BMJ 2005; 331:259–263

Wells P, Anderson D, Rodger M et al. Derivation of a simple clinical model to categorize patients probability of pulmonary embolism: increasing the models utility with the SimpliRED D-dimer. Thromb Haemost 2000; 83:416–420

Wells PS, Anderson DR, Rodger M et al. Excluding pulmonary embolism at the bedside without diagnostic imaging: management of patients with suspected pulmonary embolism presenting to the emergency department by using a simple clinical model and D-dimer. Ann Intern Med 2001; 135:98–107

Pleural effusion
Chapman SJ, Davies RJO. Pleural effusions. Clin Med 2004; 4:207–210

Davies CWH, Gleeson FV, Davies RJO. BTS guidelines for the management of pleural infection. Thorax 2003; 58:ii18–28

Maskell NA, Butland RJA. BTS guidelines for the management of a unilateral pleural effusion in adults. Thorax 2003; 58:ii8–17

Rahman NM, Davies RJO, Gleeson FV. Investigating suspected malignant pleural effusion. BMJ 2007; 334:206–207

Pneumothorax
Henry M, Arnold T, Harvey J. BTS guidelines for the management of spontaneous pneumothorax. Thorax 2003; 58:ii39–52

Obstructive sleep apnoea
SIGN guideline/BTS. Management of obstructive sleep apnoea/hypopnoea syndrome in adults. Guideline no.73, Edinburgh: Scottish Intercollegiate Guidelines Network; 2003

Abdominal system

Chronic liver disease
Bernard B, Grange JD, Khac EN, Amiot X, Opolon P, Poynard T. Antibiotic prophylaxis for the prevention of bacterial infection in cirrhotic patients with gastrointestinal bleeding. A meta-analysis. Hepatology 1999; 29:1655–1661

Groszmann RG, Garcia-Tsao G, Makuch R, et al. Multicenter randomised placebo-controlled trial of non-selective beta-blockers in the prevention of the complications of portal hypertension: final results and identification of a predictive factor. Hepatology 2003; 38:(Suppl.1):206A

Jutabha R, Jensen DM, Martin P, Savides T, Han SH, Gornbein J. Randomized study comparing banding with propranolol to prevent initial variceal haemorrhage in cirrhotics with high-risk esophageal varices. Gastroenterology 2005; 128:870–881

Kamath PS, Wiesner RH, Malinchoc M, et al. A model to predict survival in patients with end-stage liver disease. Hepatology 2001; 33:464–470

Merkel C, Marin R, Angeli P, et al. A placebo controlled clinical trial of nadolol in the prophylaxis of growth of small esophageal varices in cirrhosis. Gastroenterology 2004; 127:476–484

Psilopoulos D, Galanis P, Goulas S, et al. Endoscopic variceal ligation vs propranolol for prevention of first variceal bleeding: a randomised controlled trial. Eur J Gastroenterol Hepatol 2005; 17:1111–1117

Saich R, Chapman R. What's new in . . . Liver disorders. Medicine 2006; 34:1–4

Shaheen NJ, Stuart E, Schmitz SM, et al. Pantoporazole reduces the size of postbanding ulcers after variceal band ligation: a randomised, controlled trial. Hepatology 2005; 41:588–594

Sharma BC, Tyagi P, Agarwal SR, Wadhawan M, Sarin SK. Endoscopic variceal ligation plus propranolol versus endoscopic variceal ligation alone in primary prophylaxis of variceal bleeding. Am J Gastroenterol 2005; 100:797–804

Sherlock S, Dooley J. Diseases of the liver and biliary system, 11th edn. Oxford: Blackwell Science; 2002

Alcoholic liver disease

Maturin P, Abdelnour M, Ramond M-J, et al. Early change in bilirubin levels is an important prognostic factor in severe alcoholic hepatitis treated with prednisolone. Hepatology 2003; 38:1363–1369

Saich R, Chapman R. What's new in . . . Liver disorders. Medicine 2006; 34:1–4

Viral hepatitis

Aggarwal R, Ranjan P. Preventing and treating hepatitis B infection. BMJ 2004; 329:1080–1086

Mutimer D. The role of antiviral agents in the management of viral hepatitis. Clin Med 2006; 6:29–34

Patel K, Muir AJ, McHutchinson JG. Diagnosis and treatment of chronic hepatitis C infection. BMJ 2006; 332:1013–1017

Autoimmune hepatitis

Krawitt E. Autoimmune hepatitis. N Engl J Med 2006; 354:54–66

Leuth S, Lahse AW. Autoimmune hepatitis. Clin Med 2006; 6:25–28

Primary biliary cirrhosis

Kaplan MM, Gershwin ME. Primary biliary cirrhosis. N Engl J Med 2005; 353:1261–1273

Crohn's disease

British Society of Gastroenterology. Guidelines for the management of inflammatory bowel disease in adults. Gut 2004; 53(Suppl. 5)

Jewell DP. Crohn's disease. Medicine. 2007; 35:283–289

Rampton D. A GP guide to inflammatory bowel disease. Practitioner 2001; 245:224–229

Rampton D. Management of Crohn's disease. BMJ 1999; 319:1480–1485

Ulcerative colitis

British Society of Gastroenterology. Guidelines for the management of inflammatory bowel disease in adults. Gut 2004; 53(Suppl. 5)

Gwo-Tzer H, Lees C, Satsangi J. Ulcerative colitis. Medicine 2007; 35:277–282

Hanauer S, Schwartz J, Robinson M, et al. Mesalazine capsules for treatment of active ulcerative colitis. Results of a controlled trial. Am J Gastroenterol 1993; 88:1188–1197

Rampton D. A GP guide to inflammatory bowel disease. Practitioner 2001; 245:224–229

Sutherland LR, Roth D, Beck P et al. Oral 5-aminosalicylic acid for maintenance of remission in ulcerative colitis (Cochrane review). Cochrane library, 1, 2002

Travis SPL. Therapy update: which 5-ASA? Gut 2002; 51:548–549

Travis S. Ulcerative colitis. Medicine 2003; 31:70–75

Chronic myeloid leukaemia

Craddock C. Molecular targeted therapies in myeloid leukaemias. Clin Med 2007; 7:635–635.

Druker BJ, Talpaz M, Resta DJ et al. Efficacy and safety of a specific inhibitor of the BCR-ABL tyrosine kinase in chronic myeloid leukaemia. N Engl J Med 2001; 344:1031–1037

Goldman JM, Melo JV. Chronic myeloid leukaemia. N Engl J Med 2003; 349:1449–1462

Hoffbrand AV, Pettit JE. Color atlas of clinical hematology. London: Mosby-Wolfe; 1994

Jandl JH. Blood. Textbook of hematology, 2nd edn. Boston: Little, Brown; 1996

Johnson PWM, Orchard K. Bone marrow transplants. BMJ 2002; 325:348–349

Polycythaemia vera

Hamblin TJ, Killick SB. Myelodysplastic syndromes. Medicine 2004; 32:61–64

Harrison C. Myeloproliferative disorders. Medicine 2004; 32:58–61

Kumar R, Prem S. Polycythaemia: diagnosis and management. J R Coll Physicians Edinb 2006; 36:49–54

Murray J. Myeloproliferative disorders. Clin Med 2005; 5:328–332

Chronic lymphocytic leukaemia

Binett JL, Auquier A, Dighiero G et al. A new prognostic classification of chronic lymphocytic leukaemia derived from a multivariate survival analysis. Cancer 1989; 48:198–206

Matutes E, Dearden C. Chronic lymphocytic leukaemia. Medicine 2004; 32:72–74

Rai KR, Sawtisky A, Cronkite E, et al. Clinical staging of chronic lymphocytic leukaemia. Blood 1975; 46:219–234

Lymphoma

Patten PEM, Devereux S. Lymphoma diagnosis: an update. Clin Med 2007; 7:620–624.

Polycystic kidney disease

Igarish P, Somlo S. Genetics and pathogenesis of polycystic kidney disease. J Am Soc Nephrol 2002; 13:2384–2398

Kalatzis V, Antignac C. Cystinosis: from gene to disease. Nephrol Dial Transplant 2002; 17:1883–1886

Morello JP, Bichet DG. Nephrogenic diabetes insipidus. Annu Rev Physiol 2001; 63:607–630

Scheinmann SJ, Guay-Woodford LM, Thakker RV et al. Genetic disorders of renal electrolyte transport. N Engl J Med 1999; 340:1177–1187

Renal transplant

Adu D, Cockwell P, Ives NJ, Shaw J, Wheatley K. Interleukin-2 receptor monoclonal antibodies in renal transplantation. Meta-analysis of randomised trials. BMJ 2003; 326:789

Margreiter R, European Tacrolimus vs Ciclosporin Microemulsion Renal Transplantation Study Group. Efficacy and safety of tacrolimus compared with ciclosporin microemulsion in renal transplantation: a randomised multicentre study. Lancet 2002; 359:741–746

Station 2
History-taking skills

INTRODUCTION TO HISTORY-TAKING SKILLS
Clinical reasoning 114
The traditional medical history model 114
Incorporating the patient's perspective – ideas,
    concerns and expectations 114
History-taking skills – the communication skills that
    make history taking effective 116
The traditional model and communication skills –
    putting these together 119
Cases
RESPIRATORY PROBLEMS
2.1   Breathlessness 121
2.2   Asthma 125
ABDOMINAL PROBLEMS
2.3   Dyspepsia 129
2.4   Dysphagia 133
2.5   Abdominal pain 136
2.6   Altered bowel habit 139
CARDIOVASCULAR PROBLEMS
2.7   Prevention of cardiovascular disease and
      weight gain 144
2.8   Chest pain and angina 151
2.9   Acute coronary syndrome 155
2.10 Heart failure 161
2.11 Palpitations 166
2.12 Atrial fibrillation 170
2.13 Dyslipidaemia 175
2.14 Hypertension 182
NEUROLOGICAL PROBLEMS
2.15 Headache 188
2.16 Transient ischaemic attack 192
2.17 Weakness and wasting 196
2.18 Multiple sclerosis 198
2.19 Tremor 202
LOCOMOTOR PROBLEMS
2.20 Back pain and osteoporosis 205
2.21 Joint pain 211

EYE PROBLEMS
2.22 Visual loss 213
ENDOCRINE PROBLEMS
2.23 Type 1 diabetes mellitus 215
2.24 Type 2 diabetes mellitus 220
RENAL AND METABOLIC PROBLEMS
2.25 Acute renal failure 228
2.26 Chronic kidney disease and renal replacement
      therapy 233
2.27 Glomerulonephritis 239
2.28 Systemic vasculitis 244
2.29 Hypercalcaemia 248
2.30 Hyponatraemia 252
2.31 Poisoning and metabolic disturbance 256
HAEMATOLOGICAL PROBLEMS
2.32 Anaemia 260
2.33 Sickle cell disease and thalassaemia 264
2.34 Purpura 267
2.35 Haemophilia 271
2.36 Deep vein thrombosis 273
2.37 Thrombophilic tendency 276
2.38 Myeloma 279
INFECTIOUS DISEASE PROBLEMS
2.39 Human immunodeficiency virus infection 284
**OTHER GENERAL MEDICAL AND ELDERLY CARE
      PROBLEMS**
2.40 Falls and rehabilitation 291
2.41 Syncope 295
2.42 Seizures 300
2.43 Acute confusion 304
2.44 Mild cognitive impairment and dementia 307
2.45 Incontinence 314
2.46 Raised inflammatory markers 317
2.47 Polymyalgia and giant cell arteritis 325
2.48 Pyrexia and sepsis 327
2.49 Weight loss 333
2.50 Tiredness 334

References and further reading 336

INTRODUCTION TO HISTORY-TAKING SKILLS

Clinical reasoning

What it is

Clinical or diagnostic reasoning is about:

- Identifying relevant clinical information
- Interpreting its meaning
- Establishing a working diagnosis

The traditional medical history model (see Box 2.1) aims, through many questions, to gradually converge towards a diagnosis. Alternative models tend to be based upon, or at least incorporate, communication skills.

Clinical reasoning strategies

Various strategies can be used to get to the diagnosis. Three main ones are hypothetico-deductive reasoning, scheme-inductive reasoning and pattern recognition. Imagine three

---

Box 2.1 The traditional medical history model
Presenting complaint or complaints
• Identification of the main symptoms – what is wrong and why the patient is in hospital
History of presenting complaint or complaints
• Eliciting symptoms (and consideration of possible causes for each symptom or possible risk factors and complications if a diagnosis is likely)
• Enquiring about investigations and treatments to date
Past medical history
• Eliciting a list of active and past problems
Drug and allergy history
• Drugs past and present
Family history
• Often neglected, but often relevant
Personal and social history
A personal and social history might explore such details as:
• Marital status and health of spouse or partner
• Other family members and relevant medical problems
• Involvement of family and external support services
• Description of accommodation, e.g. flat with lift, house with stairs
• Current and past occupation(s) and effects of work on symptoms and effects of symptoms on work
• Support from friends
• Interests and hobbies, including the effects of illness on the quality of life
• Alcohol intake, cigarette smoking and recreational drug use
• Quality of life
• Major effects of illness viewed by patient
• Activities of daily living, e.g. bathing, dressing, shopping, cooking and sleep
Systems review
• Excluding other symptoms through a systems review

---

diagnosticians presented with a four-legged animal. Diagnostician 1 thinks it is a zebra because it looks like one. Diagnostician 2 agrees it is a zebra because it has hooves and stripes and weighs around 300 kg. Diagnostician 3 is from the North Pole and has only ever seen Arctic animals before. He agrees it might be a zebra but also thinks it might be a giraffe because of its hooves or a tiger because of its stripes.

Hypothetico-deductive reasoning

Diagnostician 3 will take some time reaching the diagnosis. He has little knowledge, and would approach the problem by identifying all relevant information, interpreting it, generating hypotheses and testing these. It is the traditional history-taking–examination–investigation approach, converging to the diagnosis. It emphasises depth of data collection at the expense of more focused enquiry.

Scheme-inductive reasoning

Diagnostician 2 arrived at the diagnosis through logic. He has some relevant knowledge and used a scheme or structure that reflected it. It is often an algorithmic approach.

Pattern recognition

Diagnostician 1 arrived at the diagnosis quickly, through experience. She has relevant knowledge. The 'problem' led to the diagnosis; turning upside down the pyramid that is hypothetico-deductive reasoning. With experience, data are gathered more selectively from the unstructured mass of information. However, the evidence is that it takes around 10 years in any field to move from novice to expert, and that experts use pattern recognition successfully most of the time, but when it does not work they must default to a framework.

In PACES, you probably lie somewhere between novice and expert, but closer to expert. What is not in doubt is that you should be thinking about the data you are gathering during history taking, and relating it to the patient's problem.

The traditional medical history model

The traditional model

The traditional model is an essential checklist of the content to be covered in a medical history (Box 2.1).

Limitations of the traditional model

The traditional model does not ensure that history taking is effective. Effective history taking is more than asking a checklist of questions, noting responses and formulating a diagnosis at the end.

Incorporating the patient's perspective – ideas, concerns and expectations

Understanding what patients are thinking

In PACES you have 15 minutes to take a history, witnessed by examiners examining your *history-taking skills*

– the *communication skills that make history taking effective*.

Fifteen minutes may seem a short time in which to take a medical history, although general practitioners regularly have less than 10 minutes, relying on focused questions incorporating the patient's perspective. In PACES, as in practice, feeling pressured because you are short of time and trying to extract the 'facts' at all costs from the patient is ultimately less effective than demonstrating these skills. Patients often report things in what seems a chaotic order, dodging from one area of the history to another; candidates might prefer patients to quickly and simply answer questions rather than volunteer extra information. Yet this extra information often contains vital elements of the real problem.

History taking is a way of guiding what patients say. The best way to understand how history-taking skills can guide patients is to understand what patients are thinking.

Scenario

A PACES scenario is shown in Box 2.2.

The patient's perspective – ideas, concerns and expectations (ICE)

Having taken such a history, you should of course consider the possibility of deep venous thrombosis (DVT). DVT is the most serious of the differential diagnoses, although intuitively you may have some doubts; the duration of symptoms is long and the flight two months ago is probably irrelevant. Hypothesis testing (pursuing possibilities in turn until they are either excluded or warrant further testing) may also bring a popliteal cyst and muscle strain into the differential diagnosis. You may also wonder whether as a nurse she might be particularly worried about a DVT. She will have seen DVTs on the surgical wards and know them to be dangerous. She might also be aware of the risks of air travel, but unaware that two months is a long time to 'harbour' a thrombosis. She is probably apprehensive. Being a patient in hospital or clinic – as a health-care professional to a greater or lesser extent – is being in an alien environment amidst other unwell and sometimes dying people. Many patients have strong preconceptions about doctors and hospitals learned from relatives, friends or the media; doctors seem not to tell patients much, and what they do tell can be difficult to understand; they make mistakes, sometimes with fatal outcomes. This patient might have already decided that she has a blood clot in her leg until proven otherwise. She may know that blood clots can travel to the lung and prove fatal. Much convincing evidence to the contrary may be needed if, for example, her grandmother died from a blood clot (albeit after a fractured hip). She might have seen patients on warfarin, a dangerous drug sometimes taken for life. She may be scared that she has a serious condition requiring dangerous treatment.

These types of thoughts going through her mind may be summarised as her ideas (beliefs), concerns and expectations about what her symptoms may represent. She might:

- *believe* she has a blood clot
- be *concerned* about why it has happened and what needs to be done about it
- and *expect* the worst if nothing is done.

A 30-year-old athlete with similar symptoms might believe them to represent a strained muscle, have very few concerns and expect them to go away.

But don't just assume!

Patients do not present just with symptoms, but with thoughts about their symptoms. Some patients volunteer their thoughts. When patients do not volunteer their thoughts, asking is much better than assuming:

> *What have you been told before/so far about this?*
> *What thoughts have gone through your mind about this?*
> *Are you worried about anything in particular?*

Without asking such a question, you will not discover (as the candidate here failed to discover) that the patient was worried she might have multiple sclerosis. Her sister in Australia had presented two years earlier with a painful left leg, later diagnosed as multiple sclerosis. She in fact:

- *believed* that she had multiple sclerosis and that it had happened because it ran in her family
- was *concerned* about needing a lumbar puncture
- and *expected* to become wheelchair-bound as her sister had.

Failing to establish a patient's thoughts can mean that doctor and patient are looking at the same problem from different angles, or even at two different problems. Discovering a patient's thoughts and any hidden agenda is important. For all sorts of reasons patients do not always report their concerns, and a simple question can confirm:

> *Your asthma has obviously been troubling you a lot recently. How do you feel we could best help you? By trying to improve the sleepless nights, or something else?*

Box 2.2 PACES scenario

You have taken a history from a 52-year-old woman with a painful left calf and mild swelling in the region of the popliteal fossa. You discover that she has had worsening pain for three weeks, exacerbated when going up and down stairs, and that sometimes it is so painful it reduces her to tears. She has had to stop work. You discover that she is a nurse on a surgical ward, married, with two children. She has no significant past medical history but two months ago was on a long-haul flight, returning from a visit to her sister in Australia. You are told that examination confirms mild swelling in the popliteal fossa and calf tenderness but is otherwise unremarkable.

ICE in practice

Overt doctor centredness (pure information gathering) and overt patient centredness (purely addressing the patient's perspective) are extremes of a spectrum. History taking naturally undulates within the spectrum, generally starting with patient-centred open questions:

> *Your GP says you have had a painful leg. Would you be able to tell me more about that?*
>
> *Well, yes, I noticed it a week or two ago, but didn't do anything about it.*
>
> *Why not?*
>
> *I hoped it would go away. I hoped it wasn't anything serious.*
>
> *And what has happened since then?*

Patient-centred history taking aims to identify a patient's ideas, concerns and expectations. The following questions are examples of this patient-centred approach:

> *I expect you've been thinking about this for a while. Are you worried about anything in particular?*
>
> *I was wondering what thoughts you'd had yourself about this?*
>
> *What were your own thoughts about this problem?*
>
> *Have you had any thoughts yourself about what may be causing this?*
>
> *What did you think might be causing it?*
>
> *Were you worried it might be due to something in particular?*
>
> *Some people might have thought it might be due to blood pressure. Did that worry you at all?*
>
> *When you hear the word . . . , what does that mean to you?*
>
> *Tell me what you have heard about . . .*
>
> *What types of . . . have you heard of?*
>
> *You mentioned a family history of stroke. Is that what really worries you at the moment?*
>
> *Which part of this bothers you most – is it what the surgeon said or what your wife might think or something else?*
>
> *What exactly is it about the operation that worries you most of all?*

Patient centredness taken too far can render history taking just as ineffective as pure doctor centredness. History taking should certainly involve guiding a patient back on track if the account starts to wander into areas you feel will not yield useful information; it is perfectly acceptable to say something like:

> *That is obviously important to you and perhaps we could return to it later, but didn't you say that the main problem you were having was . . .*

How it all affects the patient

Exploring the patient's perspective fully should explore not just ideas, concerns and expectations, but how the illness or problem(s) affects that patient. This overlaps significantly with the social history. The principle is that it is as important to understand the person who has the disease, as it is to understand the disease itself, and it can be helpful to encourage the patient to express their feelings. Opening questions could be:

> *How is this affecting you at work?*
>
> *How are you coping at home with this?*

History-taking skills – the communication skills that make history taking effective

Communication skills training is now a core component of medical education, and there is good evidence that these skills can be acquired. Important communication skills include:

- listening skills
- use of appropriate questions
- 'eliciting' or facilitating skills
- recognising and responding to cues
- use of appropriate language
- summarising.

Listening skills

As with examining patients and starting with inspection, good history-taking candidates are alert to how patients look, talk and behave. The patient may be relaxed or anxious, waiting for questions, may have already started talking or may pre-empt your opening question:

> *I don't know where to start.*
>
> *I don't like hospitals.*
>
> *I don't know what I'm going to do about my breathing.*

The important thing is not to rush in with questions, suppressing information that may provide a valuable insight into what the patient is thinking. Useful opening questions might be:

> *What seems to be the problem?*
>
> *Your GP says you have had a painful leg. Could you tell me about that?*
>
> *Could you tell me why you have come into hospital?*

The response might be:

> *It's my heart, doctor.*
>
> *I just don't seem to have any energy any more.*

Again, it is very important to continue listening. Many candidates respond immediately with questions, for example by asking about cardiac symptoms or by assuming the problem to be tiredness and asking about thyroid symptoms. Remember that asking *a direct question usually only gives you the answer to that question!* Careful listening for a minute or two, encouraging the patient to elaborate, will help you form a much more accurate assessment of what the problem is likely to be about:

I just don't seem to have any energy any more . . . It all started last October when I began to get short of breath . . . I'd never been in hospital in my life before that . . . now I seem to be here every few weeks. I first noticed it when I was out walking my dog. He's always full of energy but I was beginning to find that I couldn't keep up with him any more. I went to see my own doctor because you hear about people suddenly dropping down with heart attacks at my age, don't you? I'd had a few pains in my chest as well. He said that the heart tracing was okay but thought I should have an X-ray – that was when he sent me into hospital.

Your thoughts may now be quite different. Heart failure? Angina? Pulmonary emboli? Chronic obstructive pulmonary disease? Pulmonary fibrosis? The point is that listening, giving a little time for the patient to tell you what has been happening in their words, will give you a clearer idea of the direction you need to take.

Active listening

Active rather than passive listening is showing that you are interested in what the patient is saying. Active listening skills include:

- An attentive manner (it helps to sit forward – not slouching! – and make eye contact)
- Not interrupting (at least, not immediately)
- Encouraging noises, posture and gestures, or the skilful use of silence
- Reflecting back answers to create follow-up questions – *What do you mean by dizzy?*

Use of appropriate questions

Open questions

These are particularly important if you are to avoid jumping to conclusions. They are essential early in the medical interview:

Can you describe the pain in more detail?
Can you tell me a little more about that incident?
And what has been happening since then?
So you're worried about what this pain says about your health?
Have you noticed if the pain is brought on by anything in particular?
May I ask some general questions about your health?
What has been the result of all of this?

Closed questions

These help to clarify what a patient has said or to obtain factual information that has not been volunteered:

Have you coughed up any blood?

In general, save closed questions until the patient has had the chance to tell their story. A relevant systems enquiry is, of course, an appropriate series of closed questions.

Eliciting or facilitating skills

Disclosure of relevant medical information and information important to a patient needs to be facilitated. Some patients need little encouragement to talk, and their account should be guided towards what you see as clinically relevant. Some patients are reserved, and need encouragement. Probably the two most important eliciting skills are active listening and the use of appropriate questions. As well as asking open and closed questions, remember that some questions may seem irrelevant to patients and it is important to explain why you are asking them. This may be especially important for sensitive issues:

Some of my patients with emphysema get quite depressed. I often ask patients with emphysema if they have been feeling depressed.

Encouragement

There are many ways of encouraging a patient to continue their account. The simplest, yet very effective, methods are silence with encouraging facial gestures (smiling and showing concern), nodding, saying *Mmn* or *Yes* and *echoing* what is said:

I have this headache sometimes.
Headache?
Not all the time, but I get it a lot.
Which part of your head gets sore?
This bit. It comes and goes. I wondered if it was serious.
What do you mean by serious?
Well you hear about headaches.
What have you heard?

Interpretation

Reframing or recounting information for patients can help encapsulate information into meaningful 'packages' and show that you understand:

I don't know how best to say it. I'm not depressed exactly.
No, I understand. But I would think you are lonely since your wife died.

Clarification

Sometimes it is necessary to clarify statements that are unclear or need amplification:

Could you explain what you mean by . . .

'Questions in disguise'

Questions that are not actually questions can be very useful for eliciting information.

A statement may be used as question:

It sounds as though that incident alarmed you.

Conjecture may be used as a question:

I was wondering whether . . .
Sometimes people with headaches worry that it might be something serious . . .
Sometimes when women have pain like this they worry they might be pregnant . . .

Sharing an experience or examples can be used as a question:

I had a patient recently who went through a similar . . .

Legitimising

Legitimising feelings can help a patient to talk openly:

This is clearly worrying you a great deal.
You have a lot to cope with; I think most people would feel the same way.

Recognising and responding to cues

A cue is hard to define, and more easily recognisable. It could be defined as a signpost to an area in the history you might otherwise ignore but which may be very important to the patient. Cues are very common. They are often not consciously presented by patients, but offer an insight into undeclared concerns.

Verbal cues

Examples of verbal cues are:

I hoped it wasn't anything serious.
I don't get paid when I don't work.
It's my chest again.
I just seem to be losing it.
Of course it could just be stress.
Of course it could be my heart.
I'm not worried . . . after all a lot of those TV programmes just show the worst cases.
It doesn't help that my sisters aren't here.
I hope this won't mean lots of tests. I've got a lot on my plate at the moment.

There may also be cues in the pace, pitch, volume, rhythm or modulation of speech and there may be cues in censored speech – *in what is not said*. Patients frequently hesitate or appear to omit information you intuitively feel should be included:

It's no better (what's no better?)
Something will have to be done (what will have to be done?)
I'm worried (about what?)
I feel worse (worse than what or when?)
I'm suffering (from what?)
I feel a failure (why?)

Sometimes, patients use generalisations to express their concerns:

I don't like hospitals.
No one understands.
I always get headaches.
It never seems to get any better.

Non-verbal cues

Cues may be non-verbal, expressed through body language, facial expression or affect. A patient may look sad or anxious and it might be appropriate to respond:

You look worried about that.

Furthermore, not all cues need an immediate response. Sometimes storing a piece of information and returning to it later is effective:

You mentioned earlier that you hadn't wanted to come into hospital. Was there anything worrying you in particular about hospital?

You will not detect all cues and you do not need to act on all cues that you detect. But examiners will notice if you ignore what seems to be an important cue.

Use of appropriate language

Most importantly, use clear and concise language that you think the patient will understand, and avoid technical terms or jargon that might not be understood, or at least explain any necessary jargon. It can sometimes help to 'match' a patient's verbal and non-verbal behaviour. Patients often speak in visual or auditory terms or in concepts and might say:

I don't see a way out.
It sounds like bad news to me.
It's all a bit much.

Sometimes harnessing the patient's language in this way can enhance rapport and you may find yourself doing it naturally:

I see what you mean but while it may look that way . . .
It sounds bad and not what you wanted to hear but . . .
I can imagine what you must be going through.

Sometimes, in subtle ways, it is possible to match body language as well as speech. Matching is a two-way process. Speaking loudly and clearly will often encourage a patient to do the same.

Summarising

Summarising periodically

Summarising periodically, as well as at the end of the interview, can be useful in verifying your understanding and in inviting the patient to correct any misinterpretation or add information.

Summarising at the end

Always give your patient a chance to add information or ask questions before concluding. You might ask:

> *Is there anything you would like to ask?*
> *Is there anything else you feel I should know?*
> *Is there anything that is important to you that you feel I have left out?*

It is good practice to confirm shared understanding:

> *May I take a moment to summarise what you've told me so I can check that I've understood everything that is important to you.*

Finish by thanking the patient.

The traditional model and communication skills – putting these together

Content versus process

The traditional history model describes the *content* of the interview – what to cover. Communication models describe the *process* of the interview – how to do it. Doctors often revert to closed questions and a tightly structured history directed towards gathering medical information. This is understandable because most doctors learned this model, and doctors are seldom observed taking histories but are often observed presenting their findings, engendering the erroneous belief that the format for presenting information is the same as that for gathering information. Furthermore, doctors document their findings using the traditional model, augmenting this belief. Communication skills have previously been taught on courses that are separate to the content skills taught at the bedside so the belief that 'real' doctors take 'histories' and that communication skills disregard the clinical history is all too

```
┌─────────────────────────────────────────────┐
│ Box 2.3 Common faults in history taking      │
├─────────────────────────────────────────────┤
│ • Poor introduction                          │
│ • Inappropriate questions                    │
│ • Avoiding personal issues                   │
│ • Lack of warmth or empathy                  │
│ • Repetition                                 │
│ • Poor clarification                         │
│ • Poor control                               │
│ • Poor facilitation of patient disclosure    │
│ • Premature or restricted focus              │
└─────────────────────────────────────────────┘
```

common. Yet the traditional model fails to elicit much of the information needed to understand and manage a patient's problems. Indeed, studies of patient satisfaction, concordance, recall and physiological outcomes validate the need to combine the traditional model with communication skills models. Many communication models exist, such as the Calgary–Cambridge guides. Communication models provide alternative frameworks and lists of skills that are the means by which doctors get through the medical interview, develop rapport, gather information and then discuss their findings and management options with patients.

Content plus process

Because content and process are different frameworks it is easy to see them as alternatives and use only one. Indeed, if not learned and practised together, the tendency is to allow one (usually the traditional model) to inhibit the other. This can lead to many of the common faults in history taking (Box 2.3).

Comprehensive clinical methods that explicitly integrate the traditional model with effective communication skills have been proposed. Table 2.1 is a summary of content working with process.

Table 2.1 Putting it together – the traditional history model (content) and communication skills (process)

Content		Process (tasks and communication skills)	
GATHERING INFORMATION	**STRUCTURING THE INTERVIEW**	**INTRODUCTION**	**CREATING GOOD DOCTOR–PATIENT RELATIONSHIP**
Problem(s)	Following a logical sequence and keeping on track (doctor's agenda)	Establishing initial rapport by greeting patient, introducing yourself, and showing respect and interest	Demonstrating appropriate non-verbal behaviour, e.g. sitting at same level as patient, making good eye contact
Exploration of problem(s)		Identifying the problem(s), best through open questions and listening	
Medical perspective (disease) *Patient perspective (illness)*		**GATHERING INFORMATION**	Not letting note-keeping disturb flow
Sequence of events ICE		Encouraging the patient's narrative	Developing rapport by an empathetic and supportive attitude, and legitimising
Symptom analysis Effects on life	Summarising periodically	Listening	
		Appropriate use of questions	
Background information (context)		Eliciting or facilitative skills	Continuing to respond to cues
Past medical history		Recognising and responding to cues	
Drug and allergy history		Appropriate use of language	Demonstrating confidence
Family history		Summarising periodically	Involving the patient, e.g. sharing thoughts, explaining why you are asking a question
Personal and social history	Timekeeping	Exploring ICE and effects on patient	
Review of systems			
CLINICAL EXAMINATION		**CLINICAL EXAMINATION**	
Not possible at this Station in PACES		Not possible at this Station in PACES	
SUMMARY – ASSESSMENT AND PLAN		**EXPLANATION AND PLANNING**	
A precise plan may not be possible without examination findings, but it may be possible to say:		(This is assessed in more detail in Station 4; summarising and agreeing a plan of action is enough for Station 2)	
From what we have discussed, it is possible that your symptoms could be due to (problem or differential diagnoses). I think we should consider the following test(s) to help confirm this/treatments		Providing right amount and type of information –	
		– Assessing prior knowledge and extent of patient's wish for information	
		– Giving information in manageable chunks	
		– Using patient's responses to guide how to proceed	
		Promoting accurate understanding –	
		– Using appropriate language	
		– Organising information (e.g. discrete sections, logical sequence, explicit categorisation: *There are three important points I think we should discuss*)	
		– Repetition and summarising to reinforce information	
		– Visual aids (e.g. drawings)	
		– Checking understanding and clarifying as necessary	
		Achieving shared understanding and incorporating patient's perspective –	
		– Relating explanations to previously elicited ICE and encouraging patient contribution and questions	
		Planning by shared decision making –	
		– Sharing your thought processes and dilemmas and encouraging patient to contribute ideas	
		Inviting questions	
		CLOSURE	
		Forward planning, agreeing with patient next steps and casting a safety net for unexpected outcomes (what to do if plan not working and how and when to seek help)	
		Summarising session and plan briefly and finally checking patient agrees and is comfortable	

ICE, ideas, concerns and expectations.

RESPIRATORY PROBLEMS

CASE 2.1

BREATHLESSNESS

Candidate information

Role

You are a doctor in the medical outpatient clinic. Please read the following letter from the patient's general practitioner. You may make notes on the paper provided. When the bell sounds, enter the examination room to begin the consultation.

Scenario

> Dear Doctor
>
> Re: Mr John Thorn, aged 56
>
> Thank you for seeing this man who has become progressively breathless over six months. Three months ago he developed a lower respiratory tract infection that responded to amoxycillin and clarithromycin but he continues to be breathless, particularly on exertion. He smokes and I wonder if he is developing chronic obstructive pulmonary disease (COPD). His peak flow is slightly lower than predicted at 420 l/min, although salbutamol and ipratropium inhalers appear to have made little difference. A course of prednisolone did not improve his breathing. Your assessment is appreciated.
>
> Yours sincerely

Please take a history from the patient (you may continue to make notes if you wish on the paper provided). Your examiners will warn you when 12 minutes have elapsed. You have 14 minutes to take a history from the patient followed by 1 minute of reflection. There will then follow 5 minutes of discussion with the examiners. Be prepared to discuss solutions to the problems posed by the case and how you might reply to the GP's letter. You are not required to examine the patient.

Patient information

Mr John Thorn is a 56-year-old man who has been troubled by progressive breathlessness on exertion for the past six months, with a dry cough. He saw his GP three months ago when he developed purulent sputum and although this settled over about two weeks with two different courses of antibiotics, his breathlessness and dry cough persisted. He is not breathless at rest, or lying down. He thinks he may have lost a little weight, but has no other notable symptoms. He has smoked 20 cigarettes a day since he was a young man and attributes his symptoms to this. He has no other past medical history of note. He has worked for 30 years as a road-builder. He has never worked in shipyards or building construction and to his knowledge has not been exposed to asbestos. He is not prone to allergies. He has owned the same parrot for the last eight years and has no other pets. Inhalers have not helped his breathlessness. A course of steroids helped his breathing only marginally. He is worried that if his breathing deteriorates he will no longer be able to visit his brother, who lives in California.

How to approach the case

Data gathering in the interview and interpretation and use of information gathered

Presenting problem(s) and symptom exploration

■ **Elicit details of breathlessness** Find out:

- If it is chronic, and if so, if it is progressive
- If it came on suddenly or insidiously
- If it is continuous, discrete or with stepwise episodes of worsening (pulmonary emboli; infective exacerbations of COPD)
- If it is present only on exertion, or also at rest, and if there is orthopnoea (left ventricular failure)

■ **Ask about trigger factors** Ask about exercise, cold, smoking and allergens.

■ **Explore associated symptoms** Ask about:

- Cough, with sputum (characteristics and volumes – large volumes suggest bronchiectasis) or dry (interstitial lung disease)
- Haemoptysis (lung cancer, pneumonia, pulmonary tuberculosis, bronchiectasis, pulmonary embolus, vasculitis, pulmonary haemorrhage)
- Wheeze (asthma, COPD)
- Symptoms suggesting a cardiac cause (exertional chest pain, orthopnoea, paroxysmal nocturnal dyspnoea, ankle swelling – which may also be due to cor pulmonale)
- Alarm symptoms for malignancy such as weight loss, anorexia, haemoptysis or hoarseness

Patient perspective

Explore his concerns about the limitations caused by breathlessness, and reassure him that you will do all you can to improve his breathing to enable him to fly.

Past medical history

Ask breathless patients about previous respiratory diseases, such as tuberculosis or asthma, cardiovascular disease or risk factors, and atopy (personal or family history of asthma, eczema or allergic rhinitis).

Drug and allergy history

Many drugs may contribute to dyspnoea, cough or wheeze; specifically ask about non-steroidal anti-inflammatory drugs (NSAIDs) and angiotensin-converting enzyme (ACE) inhibitors.

Family history

Ask about atopy or respiratory disease.

Social history

Ask about:

- Smoking (including passive smoking and pipe smoking – when started/stopped, quantity and pack years)
- Occupations past and present (specifically about the shipyard and building industries for asbestos exposure and road-building for silicosis)
- Travel (atypical pneumonia)
- Pets (cats and dogs commonly trigger asthma, and birds can trigger atypical pneumonia and extrinsic allergic alveolitis)

Consider the effects of symptoms on daily activities and the effects of daily activities on symptoms.

SUMMARY – ASSESSMENT AND PLAN

- COPD seems likely in a smoker, but pulmonary fibrosis should always be suspected in a patient with progressive exertional dyspnoea and early on it may be the only feature of disease, with examination and chest X-ray unremarkable; the occupation is important here. Pneumonia that fails to resolve in a smoker should always prompt investigation for possible lung cancer. Exertional dyspnoea also has cardiac causes including ischaemic and valvular heart disease.
- Chest X-ray and spirometry are mandatory initial investigations in suspected COPD or fibrosis.
- Spirometry would confirm obstructive or restrictive lung disease (Table 2.2).
- Exertional breathlessness can be the result of cardiac rather than respiratory disease; coronary disease may present as exertional dyspnoea rather than chest pain and if no persuasive respiratory cause is found then exercise tolerance testing is advised.

Discussion

What is silicosis?

Silicosis is a pneumoconiosis caused by inhalation of crystalline silicon dioxide (quartz), which is highly fibrogenic. Many occupations (e.g. stonemasons, road-builders) still involve exposure to quartz dust, which is concentrated in rocks such as granite and sandstone. Particles are engulfed by macrophages and swept to the hilar nodes where inflammation, fibrosis and blockage to lymphatic drainage occur. A similar process can occur in the lungs, provoking small fibrotic nodules. Silicosis does not usually occur with brief exposure; most patients have been exposed for years or decades. With high exposure, small lung nodules can coalesce into large, destructive masses with surrounding bullae. Nodules continue to grow and merge, even after exposure has ceased, causing dyspnoea. Very high expo-

sure occasionally causes an acute inflammatory destructive process with respiratory failure in the absence of nodules. The chest X-ray usually shows 'eggshell' hilar calcification and small (< 5 mm) diffuse nodules. The history, chest X-ray and workplace inspection by an occupational physician usually suffice for diagnosis. Biopsy is seldom necessary, but reveals quartz particles.

What is meant by the terms total lung capacity (TLC), vital capacity (VC) and residual volume (RV)? (Fig. 2.1)

- TLC is the total volume of air in the lungs at full inspiration. TLC is limited by the elasticity of the thoracic cage and the fibrous and elastic tissues of the lungs, and by inspiratory muscle strength. TLC varies little with age in healthy people.
- VC is the volume of air expired from full inspiration to full expiration. VC varies widely between healthy people depending upon height, gender and race (3–6 litres) and tends to decrease with age.
- RV is the volume always left in the lung after breathing out the vital capacity. RV is reached when the ribs cannot move closer together. It tends to increase with age and in obstructive lung disease when airways close early in expiration.

Which dynamic volumes are helpful in pulmonary function testing?

The above are static volumes. What we measure mostly in practice are dynamic volumes (volumes which change) because patients are breathing!

- *Forced vital capacity* (FVC) is the forced maximal volume of air expired from full inspiration (TLC) to full expiration (RV), the patient breathing out as hard and long as they can.
- *Forced expiratory volume over one second (FEV$_1$)* is the amount of air expired over the first second of FVC. FEV$_1$ is normally > 75–80% of normal VC. FEV$_1$ depends on effort, lung elastic recoil and the positive pressure applied by expiratory muscles. It is a useful indicator of the severity of obstructive lung

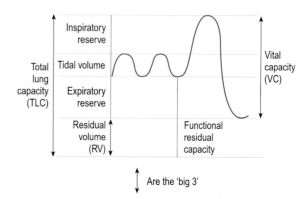

Fig. 2.1 Useful lung volumes.

disease and a screening test for cardiorespiratory health as it correlates with maximal exercise capacity.

The normal FEV_1/FVC ratio is around 70–80%, > 70% for males and > 75% for females. It is highest in young non-smokers. Spirometry measures this and differentiates two major groups of lung disease, obstructive or restrictive (Table 2.2).

What happens to flow rates and flow rate curves in obstructive and restrictive lung diseases?

As well as plotting expiratory flow rate on a volume/time curve, it is possible to plot flow rate (e.g. expiratory flow rate during a FVC manoeuvre) against lung volume (which changes as a person breathes out) as shown in Fig. 2.2.

It may seem from Fig. 2.2 that the expiratory flow rate in restrictive lung diseases is decreased but if we correct this for the decreased lung volume in restrictive lung diseases, then it is normal or even increased. This is because a fibrotic lung provides more traction than usual on airways, holding them open. Nevertheless, lungs are shrunken and airways are narrowed, increasing their resistance and hence the work of breathing and sensation of inspiratory effort or breathlessness.

In obstructive lung disease, expiratory flow rates are decreased. Although the lungs are hyperinflated, inflammation, oedema and mucus in the smaller airways cause these to close earlier than usual despite normal traction from the lung parenchyma attempting to keep them open.

Note from Fig. 2.2 that expiratory flow rates in normal and diseased lungs vary according to lung volume. For example, in normal lungs the maximum flow rate, about 6 litres per second, occurs when about 4 litres of air are left in the lungs. This *peak expiratory flow rate* (PEFR) is normally 300–700 litres/min, varying between people as for vital capacity, but reproducible to within 5% for an individual. PEFR reflects airway calibre and respiratory effort, and is most useful for monitoring asthma.

Sometimes, rather than plotting flow rate against volume, flow rate is plotted against percentage vital capacity. This is essentially the same thing, simply plotting flow rate through the various stages of exhaling the vital capacity. For example, when 75% of the vital capacity has been exhaled, the flow rate is called V_{max75}, or forced expiratory flow $(FEF)_{75}$.

Note from Fig. 2.3 that in healthy individuals the maximal expiratory flow rate (MEFR) decreases steadily throughout forced expiration – as the lungs empty, the airways decrease in size. Note also that the flow rate is low in obstructive lung disease at all stages of exhaling the vital

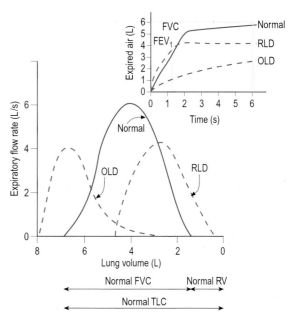

Fig. 2.2 Expiratory flow rate plotted against lung volume-normal. FEV, forced expiratory volume over 1 second; FVC, forced vital capacity; OLD, obstructive lung disease; RLD, restrictive lung disease; RV, residual volume.

Table 2.2 Obstructive lung disease (OLD) and restrictive lung disease (RLD)		
	OLD	**RLD**
Diseases	COPD Asthma	Interstitial lung disease Lung or lobe resection Thoracic deformity or inspiratory muscle weakness
Static volumes	There is air trapping or hyperinflation TLC preserved or ↑ RV ↑ (early small airway closure and VC ↓) Tidal volume can vary widely	The lungs are small and fibrotic TLC ↓ RV ↓ (alveoli obliterated) Tidal volume often ↓
Dynamic volumes	FEV₁ markedly ↓ (< 80% of predicted in COPD) FVC normal or ↓ (because small airways close early in expiration) FEV₁/FVC ↓ (< 70% diagnostic)	FEV₁ ↓ FVC ↓ FEV₁/FVC normal or high (> 80–85%)
Expiratory flow rates	↓	Normal
Transfer factor	↓ in COPD, normal in asthma	Normal or ↓

COPD, chronic obstructive pulmonary disease; FEV, forced expiratory volume over 1 second; FVC, forced vital capacity; TLC, total lung capacity; RV, residual volume.

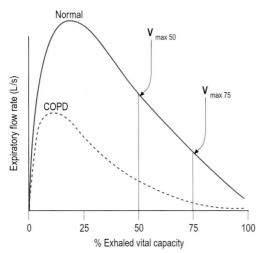

Fig. 2.3 Flow rate variation in normal lung and in chronic obstructive pulmonary disease (COPD).

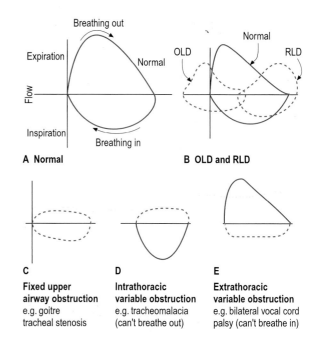

Fig. 2.4 Flow–volume loops (maximal flow). (A) Normal. Normally, maximal expiratory flow rate (MEFR) decreases during expiration (above), but inspiration is more rapid. Maximal flow rates are much greater than those of tidal breathing (not shown). (B) Obstructive lung disease (OLD) and restrictive lung disease (RLD). In OLD, MEFR decreases during the middle of forced expiration (above) because the small airways collapse just after the onset of forced expiration. For this reason, forced expiration may be less effective than quiet breathing. (C) Fixed upper airway obstruction (e.g. goitre, tracheal stenosis, glottis problems, laryngeal problems). Here, MEFR and maximal inspiratory flow rate (MIFR) are reduced and essentially equal. (D) Intrathoracic variable obstruction (e.g. tracheobronchial collapse as a consequence of emphysema, tracheomalacia, rare bronchial cartilage disorders). Here, the main problem is with 'breathing out', MEFR being reduced from the start of expiration (MEFR may be constant for the first few hundred millilitres of expiration, after which it behaves like fixed upper airway obstruction). (E) Extrathoracic variable obstruction (e.g. bilateral vocal cord palsy). Here, the main problem is with 'breathing in', MIFR being reduced from the start of inspiration.

capacity, in other words at all lung volumes. Also note that in obstructive lung disease the curve is scooped out. This dip in MEFR during the middle of forced expiration is one of the earliest signs of small airway damage and is seen in young smokers before clinical features of disease, often with a normal FVC and FEV_1.

What do you understand by compliance and elastic recoil?

Compliance is essentially a measure of the 'give' of the lung when expanding, and elastic recoil is a measure of its ability to shrink to its original size again, like a deflating balloon. Obstructive lung disease lungs are very compliant, but have too little elastic recoil because there is too much airspace and not enough parenchyma. In emphysema elastic recoil is particularly reduced, and FEV_1 is reduced even when the airways are patent. Restrictive lung disease lungs are not very compliant (they are too stiff), having too much recoil, if anything.

What are flow volume loops?

Complex mathematics has been applied to produce the shapes of the expiratory flow curves for normal and diseased lungs. Fortunately, physicians do not need to understand the maths but need merely to recognise the shapes of certain curves and what they imply. Curves have been created not just for expiration, but also for inspiration. Therefore, as well as flow–volume curves, flow–volume loops (Fig. 2.4) tracking the full inspiration–expiration cycle can be plotted, and these too have characteristic shapes.

What do you understand by the term transfer factor and which diseases affect it?

The transfer factor (TLCO) measures total transfer of carbon monoxide across the lung during 10 seconds of breath holding after full inspiration. It is a measure of alveolar–capillary exchange (surface area and thickness) or effective ventilation/perfusion (V/Q) matching. TLCO is also known as diffusing capacity (DLCO). The KCO, or transfer coefficient, corrects TLCO for lung volume. For example, a TLCO that is half that predicted may occur after a pneumonectomy but the KCO will be normal.

A decreased TLCO (and KCO) occurs in COPD, interstitial lung disease, pulmonary vascular disease (pulmonary emboli, pulmonary hypertension, pulmonary oedema), right to left shunts and anaemia. In emphysema, TLCO is misleadingly elevated because CO lingers in the bullae, when in fact the obliterated alveoli cause markedly diminished gas exchange.

CO has a high affinity for blood cells, and so transfer is apparently increased in pulmonary haemorrhage, e.g. in the setting of pulmonary vasculitis. TLCO and KCO are also increased in polycythaemia, left to right shunts and exercise.

A decreased TLCO and normal KCO is the result of extrapulmonary restriction or 'functional' volume loss, e.g. neuromuscular disease, or volume loss post-pneumonectomy.

What is respiratory failure?

Arterial pCO_2 (p_aCO_2) is normally about 5 kPa (40 mmHg) and is regulated by chemoreceptors. Arterial pO_2 (p_aO_2) is more variable, between 10 and 16 kPa (80–120 mmHg). In type 1 respiratory failure, p_aO_2 is < 8 kPa (60 mmHg) and p_aCO_2 is normal or decreased. Causes include interstitial lung disease, pulmonary vascular disease, asthma and COPD. In type 2 (hypoventilatory) respiratory failure, p_aCO_2 is increased to > 6 kPa (50 mmHg). Causes include COPD, asthma in a tiring patient, and neuromuscular disease.

CASE 2.2

ASTHMA

Candidate information

Role

You are a doctor in the respiratory clinic. Please read the following letter from the patient's general practitioner. You may make notes on the paper provided. When the bell sounds, enter the examination room to begin the consultation.

Scenario

Dear Doctor

Re: Mrs Claire Pickles, aged 30

Thank you for seeing this lady with episodes of cough, breathlessness, wheeze and chest 'tightness' for the last few months. Although her symptoms seem to be responding to salbutamol and steroid inhalers I am always a little apprehensive about making a new diagnosis of asthma in adults. I am grateful for your advice as to the likelihood of the diagnosis.

Yours sincerely

Please take a history from the patient (you may continue to make notes if you wish on the paper provided). Your examiners will warn you when 12 minutes have elapsed. You have 14 minutes to take a history from the patient followed by 1 minute of reflection. There will then follow 5 minutes of discussion with the examiners. Be prepared to discuss solutions to the problems posed by the case and

how you might reply to the GP's letter. You are not required to examine the patient.

Patient information

Mrs Claire Pickles is a 30-year-old lady who has had episodes of cough, breathlessness, wheeze and chest 'tightness' for the last four months, partially responsive to a blue 'treatment' and a brown 'prevention' inhaler. She had eczema as a child but no history of apparent asthma until now and has no other significant past medical history. She moved into a country cottage six months ago with her husband and two sons. The cottage is extremely dusty and they are in the process of renovating and rebuilding some of it. Local cats tend to wander in. During house moving she injured her knee and has taken regular ibuprofen for a few months. She cannot understand why she has asthma, as she does not smoke.

How to approach the case

Data gathering in the interview and interpretation and use of information gathered

Presenting problem(s) and symptom exploration

The history should cover similar points to Case 2.1. The differential diagnosis of asthma includes pulmonary emboli, primary pulmonary hypertension, COPD, interstitial lung disease, cardiac disease, tumours (laryngeal/tracheal/lung), vocal cord dysfunction, foreign body aspiration, bronchiectasis and hyperventilation. However, asthma not uncommonly starts in adults, and not always with identifiable triggers, and here symptoms are characteristic. She should be asked about diurnal variation of cough (often worse at night), wheeze and shortness of breath.

▧ **Explore precipitating factors** These include pollens, dust (house dust mite), animals (cats!), exercise, viral infection, chemicals (fumes, sprays and perfumes) and irritants (including cigarettes!). Has she, for example, from recently moving house, come into increased contact with more house dust mites? Has she bought a new pet? Has she taken up a new form of exercise? Has she come into contact with any new materials at work? Has she moved in with a smoker?

▧ **Seek red flags** Specialist opinion is often sought in the following situations:

- Diagnosis unclear
- Symptoms persistent rather than episodic
- Wheeze unilateral or fixed, or stridor
- Other atypical symptoms, such as chest pain or weight loss
- Clinical findings suggest an alternative cause (e.g. clubbing, crackles, cyanosis)

- Spirometry does not suggest asthma
- Occupational asthma is possible

Patient perspective

Explore her ideas about asthma precipitants.

Past medical history

Ask about previous hospital admissions and particularly whether or not assisted ventilation has ever been needed.

Drug and allergy history

Sometimes symptoms appear or worsen with aspirin/NSAIDs or beta blockers. Ask specifically about cumulative oral steroid use with consideration of the need for osteoporosis prophylaxis.

Family history

Ask about a personal or family history of asthma or atopy (eczema, allergic rhinitis).

Social history

In addition to a full home and work history, The Royal College of Physicians document *Measuring Outcomes in Asthma* suggests the following three questions be specifically asked about the last week/month:

1. *Have you had difficulty sleeping because of your asthma symptoms (including cough)?*
2. *Have you had your usual asthma symptoms during the day (cough, wheeze, chest tightness or breathlessness)?*
3. *Has your asthma interfered with your usual activities (e.g. housework, work, school)?*

SUMMARY – ASSESSMENT AND PLAN

- She almost certainly has adult onset asthma.
- She should be asked to monitor her morning and evening peak flow (demonstrated to her later) in a peak flow diary. A single normal peak flow measurement does not exclude asthma!
- She should be managed according to British Thoracic Society guidelines. She should have a self-management plan, with long-term follow up by her GP/asthma nurse. An attempt to wean/withdraw her steroid should be made when identifiable triggers are removed.

Discussion

What is asthma?

Asthma is characterised by airway inflammation (often failing to settle between attacks and now appreciated as a core problem in asthma) giving rise to reversible airway narrowing, and airway hyperreactivity giving rise to cough, wheeze and dyspnoea.

What do you know about the pathophysiology of asthma?

Asthma and allergic diseases are increasing in prevalence in the Western world. Atopy refers to the predisposition to generate allergic antibodies (i.e. immunoglobulin E; IgE) in response to environmental triggers. The immune system responds to foreign antigens by their being presented to naïve T helper (Th) lymphocytes which differentiate either to a Th1 response driving intense inflammation or a Th2 response driving B lymphocytes to switch to IgE production. The optimal scenario is a well-balanced ability to produce Th1 and Th2 responses. Allergy is associated with a Th2-weighted imbalance.

Atopic predisposition may start in early life, with impaired interferon-γ (IFN-γ) production leading to impaired suppression of Th2 activity involved in IgE-mediated allergy. Healthy neonates have a weak Th2-based immune response that is subsequently suppressed in early life. Exposure to bacteria in early life may increase IFN-γ levels, lending weight to the 'hygiene' hypothesis, which suggests that reduced exposure to bacteria together with antibiotics and modern infant diets result in the persistence of a dominant Th2 pathway. Mycobacterial species are known to stimulate powerful IFN-γ production and research has considered bacterial vaccines to promote switching from Th2 to Th1 pathways.

How is asthma diagnosed?

Asthma is most commonly diagnosed by the peak expiratory flow rate (PEFR) exhibiting $> 20\%$ diurnal variation on ≥ 3 days in a week for two weeks. An increase in forced expiratory volume over one second (FEV_1) $\geq 15\%$ (and 200 ml) after a short-acting β-agonist (e.g. salbutamol 400 μg by MDI + spacer or 2.5 mg by nebuliser) or steroids (prednisolone 30 mg/day for 14 days) is also diagnostic. No significant reversibility suggests COPD. A decrease in $FEV_1 \geq 15\%$ after six minutes of exercise (running) or a histamine or metacholine challenge may help in difficult cases.

What do you know about the British guidelines for the management of chronic asthma in adults?

Pharmacological aims are to control symptoms (including nocturnal and exercise-induced symptoms), prevent exacerbations, achieve best possible pulmonary function and minimise side effects. Treatment is stepwise (Table 2.3), starting at the most appropriate step to achieve early control, stepping up as necessary and down when control is good. Patients should be maintained at the lowest possible doses of inhaled steroid, but reductions should be slow, by around 25–50% at three-monthly intervals.

Rescue courses of steroid may be used at any time.

Table 2.3 Stepwise approach to asthma in adults

Step 1: Mild intermittent asthma	Inhaled short-acting β_2-agonist as required
Step 2: Regular prevention therapy	Add inhaled steroid 200–800 µg/day (beclometasone or equivalent)
Step 3: Add-on therapy	Add inhaled long-acting β_2-agonist (LABA): if good response continue, if benefit but incomplete control increase inhaled steroid dose to 800 µg and if no response stop and increase inhaled steroid to 800 µg; if control remains inadequate consider other therapies such as a leukotriene receptor antagonist or SR theophylline.
Step 4: Persistent poor control	Consider trials of increasing inhaled steroid to 2000 µg daily or addition of a fourth drug such as a leukotriene receptor antagonist, SR theophylline or a β_2-agonist tablet
Step 5: Continuous or frequent use of oral steroids	Daily steroid tablets in lowest dose possible

Table 2.4 Features of asthma of varying severity

Moderate exacerbation of asthma	Increasing symptoms PEF 50–75% of best or predicted No features of ASA
Acute severe asthma	Any one of: PEF 33–50% of best or predicted Respiratory rate $\geq$ 25/min Heart rate $\geq$ 110/min Inability to complete sentences in one breath
Life-threatening asthma	PEF < 33% of best or predicted SpO_2 < 92% Respiratory failure on arterial blood gases (rising p_aCO_2 a sign of near-fatal asthma) Silent chest Cyanosis Feeble respiratory effort Bradycardia, dysrhythmia, hypotension Exhaustion, confusion, coma

Box 2.4 Indications for referral to ITU in acute asthma

This is indicated if ventilatory support is needed or if ASA or life-threatening asthma is failing to respond, as evidenced by any of the following:

- Deteriorating PEF
- Persistent or worsening hypoxia
- Hypercapnia, acidosis
- Exhaustion
- Feeble respiration
- Drowsiness
- Confusion
- Coma
- Respiratory arrest

How would you explain to a patient how to use a metered dose inhaler (MDI)?

Instructions are as follows:

- *Shake the inhaler and remove the dust cap.*
- *Breathe out gently and fully.*
- *Place the mouthpiece between your teeth and seal your lips around it.*
- *Breathe in steadily, and at the moment you start breathing in . . .*
- *Press the inhaler to release the dose immediately after beginning to breathe in and keep breathing in to full inspiration (until your lungs are full).*
- *Remove the inhaler from your mouth and hold your breath for 10 seconds or as long as is comfortable.*
- *If a second dose is needed, wait for 30–60 seconds.*

How would you recognise acute severe asthma (ASA) and life-threatening asthma?

Features of moderate exacerbations, ASA and life-threatening asthma are listed in Table 2.4.

How would you manage acute asthma?

High-flow oxygen and β_2-agonist bronchodilators by nebuliser are administered to all patients. Nebulised ipratropium bromide (0.5 mg four- to six-hourly) may be added to the β_2-agonist for ASA or life-threatening asthma or when initial response to β_2-agonists is poor. Systemic steroid (e.g. prednisolone 40–50 mg daily) is administered to all patients. A single dose of intravenous magnesium sulphate (1.2–2 g by 20 minute infusion) is considered in ASA without a good initial response or in life-threatening asthma. Referral to the intensive therapy unit (ITU) should be made in those circumstances outlined in Box 2.4.

Does asthma management differ in pregnancy?

The β_2-agonists, steroids and theophyllines are each used as normal, but leukotriene receptor antagonists have not been adequately researched. Poorly controlled asthma is worse for the baby than any risk from oral steroids. ASA management is unchanged.

When would you consider it safe to discharge a patient from hospital after ASA?

Discharge is appropriate under those criteria listed in Box 2.5.

Box 2.5 Criteria for safe discharge following acute severe asthma

- Identification and modification of trigger factors achieved where possible
- Patient on discharge medication for at least 24 hours
- PEF > 75% of predicted or best and preferably PEF diurnal variability < 25%
- Patient on steroids in addition to bronchodilators
- Patient has individualised management plan, and, where possible, is able to self-monitor their PEF
- GP and specialist follow-up arranged with good communication between all parties

List some factors you might consider when a patient has chronic asthma that is difficult to control

- Persistence of trigger factors
- Poor concordance with treatment
- Poor technique/patient education
- Alternative diagnosis, e.g. heart failure, Churg–Strauss syndrome (severity may be masked by steroids)

ABDOMINAL PROBLEMS

CASE 2.3

DYSPEPSIA

Candidate information

Role

You are a doctor in the medical outpatient clinic. Please read the following letter from the patient's general practitioner. You may make notes on the paper provided. When the bell sounds, enter the examination room to begin the consultation.

Scenario

> Dear Doctor
>
> Re: Mrs Elizabeth Richards, aged 67 years
>
> Thank you for seeing this lady who is anaemic with a haemoglobin of 10 g/dl. She has lost 7 kg in weight over a few months. Four years ago she had grade 3 oesophagitis diagnosed on biopsy and has been on omeprazole 40 mg daily since. Her routine biochemistry is normal. Her ferritin is 30 µg/l. I would value your assessment and advice on further investigation.
>
> Yours sincerely

Please take a history from the patient (you may continue to make notes if you wish on the paper provided). Your examiners will warn you when 12 minutes have elapsed. You have 14 minutes to take a history from the patient followed by 1 minute of reflection. There will then follow 5 minutes of discussion with the examiners. Be prepared to discuss solutions to the problems posed by the case and how you might reply to the GP's letter. You are not required to examine the patient.

Patient information

Mrs Elizabeth Richards is a 67-year-old lady who is anaemic. She has lost around one stone in weight over the last few months and feels that her abdomen is getting 'fuller'. She has a little discomfort in her chest after eating but no vomiting or alteration in bowel habit. She has type 2 diabetes, which is controlled by diet. Four years ago she had heartburn and endoscopy revealed moderately severe oesophagitis and she has taken omeprazole since. She takes no other medications, and in particular has not taken non-steroidal anti-inflammatory drugs (NSAIDs). She does not drink alcohol nor smoke. She has a family history of breast cancer, her mother and sister both being affected. She feels well, apart from the above, and wonders why she cannot simply take iron tablets to correct the anaemia. She will ask the doctor why further tests are necessary and has not considered malignancy as a possibility needing exclusion.

How to approach the case

Data gathering in the interview and interpretation and use of information gathered

Presenting problem(s) and symptom exploration

- **Consider the causes of dyspepsia**   Dyspepsia refers to a group of symptoms arising from the upper gastrointestinal tract including epigastric or upper abdominal discomfort, heartburn, nausea and bloating. The symptoms may indicate one of four possibilities (Box 2.6).
- **Consider the differential diagnoses of dyspepsia**   A cardiac history is essential because cardiac pain and dyspepsia can be difficult to distinguish. Other causes of upper abdominal pain include aerophagy, biliary disease, abdominal wall pain, chronic pancreatitis, mesenteric ischaemia, diabetes and hypercalcaemia.

Patient perspective

Explore her ideas and expectations about simply treating anaemia with iron and explain the reasons for wanting to investigate further.

Past medical history

The history of oesophagitis is important, even though she has taken a proton pump inhibitor, because it can transform to oesophageal malignancy.

Box 2.6 The causes of dyspepsia

Gastro-oesophageal reflux disease (GORD) with or without oesophagitis

Heartburn is the primary symptom of GORD; some gastroenterologists restrict the term dyspepsia to epigastric discomfort, which excludes heartburn. Symptoms are typically after meals, on bending or lying flat. Other symptoms include nausea and vomiting, dental enamel erosion, dysphonia and hoarseness (posterior pharyngitis, contact ulceration or subglottic stenosis), globus hystericus, odonyphagia (painful swallowing), recurrent aspiration, nocturnal and postprandial cough, and chest pain mimicking angina.

Peptic ulcer disease

Symptoms include epigastric pain and a history of haematemesis or melaena. The common causes are *Helicobacter pylori* and NSAIDs.

Upper gastrointestinal malignancy

Ask about alarm features

- **A**   anaemia
- **L**   loss of weight (a worry, prompting check of inflammatory markers) or anorexia
- **A**   abdominal mass
- **R**   recent onset of progressive symptoms
- **M**   melaena or haematemesis
- **D**   dysphagia or vomiting

'Functional' dyspepsia

At least two-thirds of patients have no structural explanation for their symptoms. The cause is often unclear, and although around half may test positive for *H. pylori* this approximates the prevalence in asymptomatic individuals.

Drug and allergy history

Ask specifically about NSAIDS or corticosteroids (often for chronic inflammatory conditions such as asthma, inflammatory bowel disease and connective tissue disease).

Family history

The family history of breast cancer may be relevant because it may link with ovarian cancer. The latter must be in the differential diagnosis as a cause of weight loss, abdominal fullness and unexplained anaemia that may not be iron deficient.

Social history

Ask about alcohol and smoking, both risk factors for peptic ulceration.

SUMMARY – ASSESSMENT AND PLAN

- Recurrence of oesophagitis or oesophageal malignancy must be excluded. Other possibilities include malignancy elsewhere including colorectal cancer and ovarian cancer.
- A full examination including a rectal examination would be mandatory.
- Initial blood tests should include a full blood count, haematinics, inflammatory markers, renal and liver function, calcium and thyroid function.
- An urgent oesophagogastroduodenoscopy (OGD) and ultrasound scan of abdomen and pelvis would seem sensible initial investigations.

Discussion

What do you know about GORD and oesophagitis?

Gastro-oesophageal reflux disease (GORD) refers to symptomatic or asymptomatic mucosal damage (oesophagitis) resulting from exposure of the lower oesophagus to refluxed gastric contents. It is potentially (although rarely) serious. It is associated with transient lower oesophageal sphincter (LOS) relaxation unrelated to swallowing or to failed swallows – those not followed by normal peristalsis. The LOS comprises oesophageal smooth muscle and diaphragmatic striated muscle, the latter being incompetent in a hiatus hernia. GORD can lead to the complications listed in Box 2.7.

A clear history of heartburn (a rising feeling from the stomach to the neck) is unlikely to be caused by anything else and quality of life is affected in proportion to the frequency and severity of this, irrespective of the presence or severity of oesophagitis. Traditionally, oesophagitis was seen as a continuous spectrum of disease, with endoscopy-negative symptoms labelled as mild and Barrett's oesophagus labelled as very severe. However, progression from normal to erosive oesophagitis to Barrett's oesophagus is seldom seen and symptoms are tending to replace mucosal findings in determining severity.

Box 2.7 Complications of GORD

- Oesophagitis (various grades)
- Barrett's oesophagus (upward propagation of columnar epithelium, replacing squamous epithelium)
- Benign strictures
- Oesophageal carcinoma (the majority are squamous, but adenocarcinoma is a complication of Barrett's oesophagus)

What is the relationship between a hiatus hernia and GORD?

A hiatus hernia does not diagnose GORD. The majority of hiatus hernias are asymptomatic (rarely, a hiatus hernia may undergo torsion to cause acute pain and vomiting) although 90% of patients with severe oesophagitis will have a hiatus hernia.

Why is Barrett's oesophagus important and how is it managed?

It can be a precursor to adenocarcinoma of the oesophagus (relative risk around 80-fold). Cancer is heralded by high-grade dysplasia and is more likely with a long segment (> 7 cm) of Barrett's oesophagus. Endoscopic surveillance is appropriate every one to two years if there is no significant dysplasia. There is no evidence that proton pump inhibitors or antireflux surgery lead to regression of Barrett's oesophagus.

Is there a role for endoscopy in patients with GORD?

Many gastroenterologists believe it to have a limited diagnostic role because most patients do not have endoscopically visible lesions. There is no consensus as to which patients merit endoscopy. Indications include alarm symptoms, exclusion of other causes (especially if symptoms are refractory to treatment) or assessment for GORD complications (Barrett's oesophagus, stricture, very rarely ulcer). Barrett's oesophagus confers an increased risk of oesophageal adenocarcinoma, but optimal practice for endoscopic detection and surveillance remains unclear. Free reflux on barium swallow is specific but poorly sensitive for GORD. The most accurate test is ambulatory oesophageal pH monitoring.

What proportion of patients with GORD have a normal endoscopy?

Around 50% have a normal endoscopy, 40% erosive oesophagitis and 10% a metaplastic (columnar lined) oesophagus.

What treatments might you recommend for a patient with GORD?

These are outlined in Box 2.8.

Other than GORD, what other causes of oesophageal pain are there?

GORD is the most common cause, but motility disturbances, increased or decreased – as in achalasia – can occur, as can hypersensitivity and often an overlap of these problems. Oesophageal spasm, relieved with nitrates, is very rare.

What do you know about *Helicobacter pylori*?

Helicobacter pylori is a Gram-negative bacillus that colonises only the mucus layer of the human stomach. Most infected people (> 70%) are asymptomatic. However, there is strong evidence that *H. pylori* has an important causative role in > 90% of duodenal ulcers and a role in benign gastric ulcers that are not attributable to NSAIDs. There is evidence of a causative role in gastric cancer and gastric lymphoma. It may have a role in functional (non-ulcer) dyspepsia (NUD). Although *H. pylori* initially causes an inflammatory gastritis the immunological response is not sufficient to clear it and it becomes chronic. Polyclonal strains are common. It is, however, decreasing in prevalence.

What do you know about the pathophysiology of peptic ulceration and gastric cancer, and their links with *H. pylori*?

Normal gastric secretion

The stomach comprises a proximal fundus, a body and a distal antrum. Parietal (oxyntic) cells in the body and fundus produce hydrochloric acid and intrinsic factor. Chief (peptic) cells secrete pepsinogen, a pepsin precursor. Stimulation of these and other gastric secretions has neuronal (vagal), hormonal (gastrin) and histamine (stimulated by gastrin) inputs. Inhibition of secretion is mediated by sympathetic nerve activity, low pH and negative feedback from small bowel enzymes. Gastrin is produced from G cells in the antrum. Its secretion is stimulated by food, distension, vagal input and high pH. Gastrin promotes acid, intrinsic factor and pepsin secretion (the H_2 receptor being the final common pathway), gastric emptying, pancreatic bicarbonate release and secretin release. Somatostatin in the antrum inhibits gastrin release. The pieces of information important here to the development of peptic ulceration and gastric cancer are that:

- acid is produced from the body and fundus of the stomach;

- gastrin, which stimulates acid, is produced in the antrum; and
- somatostatin, which inhibits gastrin, is also produced in the antrum.

How peptic ulceration develops

Patients with duodenal ulcers have excessive numbers of parietal cells with acid hypersecretion. That acid hypersecretion is virtually always due to *H. pylori* is evidenced by the fact that secretion returns to normal when *H. pylori* is eradicated. A predominantly antral gastritis due to *H. pylori* occurs in *H. pylori*-provoked duodenal ulcers (the vast majority are *H. pylori* provoked). This tends to cause suppression of somatostatin cells and a consequent increase in gastrin release from G cells leading to acid hypersecretion. Further, areas of gastric metaplasia in the duodenum can be colonised by *H. pylori*, causing duodenitis; gastric metaplasia increases with the amount of acid entering the duodenum and tends to be lowest in pernicious anaemia (in which acid-producing areas are destroyed) and highest in patients with gastrin-secreting tumours (Zollinger–Ellison syndrome). Unlike patients with duodenal ulcers, patients with gastric ulcers and functional dyspepsia have normal numbers of parietal cells and acid secretion, and the link with *H. pylori* is variable.

How gastric cancer develops

H. pylori also predisposes to gastric cancer, but patients have acid hyposecretion. This was once thought to be due to gastric body gastritis leading to atrophy and loss of acid-producing parietal cells. However, acid hyposecretion can in part be reversed by *H. pylori* eradication, suggesting that *H. pylori* causes gastric body gastritis/inflammation rather than permanent cell loss. Acid hyposecretion may be self-perpetuating because it supports the presence of *H. pylori* in the gastric body and so worsening gastric body gastritis, maintaining suppression of acid secretion. Acid hyposecretion predisposes to cancer by several mechanisms including impaired vitamin C absorption and overgrowth of bacteria in the stomach.

Is the location of *H. pylori* therefore important in determining clinical outcome?

Given the above, the location of *H. pylori* (together with environmental, bacterial and host factors) thus determines whether a person with *H. pylori* infection tends towards a state of acid hypersecretion (predominantly antral gastritis) or acid hyposecretion (predominantly gastric body gastritis) and therefore the clinical outcome – asymptomatic infection, duodenal ulceration, gastric ulceration or gastric cancer.

Are there any implications from the presence of *H. pylori* for the use of proton pump inhibitors?

Acid normally protects the gastric body from *H. pylori* colonisation. A proton pump inhibitor (PPI), by reducing acid production in the gastric body, can allow *H. pylori* to shift from the antrum to the gastric body, causing gastric body gastritis. PPIs thus have the potential to improve symptoms by reducing 'acid' symptoms but promote an increased risk of gastric cancer. Eradicating *H. pylori* should therefore be considered concurrently, although in practice this theoretical risk has not appeared to translate to substantial concern, and the widespread empiric use of PPIs appears to be relatively safe provided guidelines for when to test for *H. pylori* and when to contemplate endoscopy are followed.

List some causes of duodenal and gastric ulceration

These are listed in Table 2.5.

What is Zollinger–Ellison syndrome?

This is peptic ulcer disease resulting from a gastrin-secreting adenoma, usually of pancreatic origin. It may be part of multiple endocrine neoplasia type 1 (MEN1) syndrome.

How is *H. pylori* diagnosed?

Endoscopically, histology is very useful, culture is unreliable and urease tests (CLO test) indicate only the presence or absence of infection. Serology is non-invasive – *H. pylori* elicits a local and systemic antibody response and circulating immunoglobulin G (IgG) antibodies can be detected but individuals vary in antibody responses and titres fall slowly after eradication so serology cannot distinguish eradication from re-infection (there are no reliable IgM tests). The urea breath test has a sensitivity and specificity > 90% – urea is hydrolysed by *H. pylori* urease to carbon dioxide and ammonia and following ingestion of carbon radio-labelled urea, radio-labelled carbon dioxide is detected in the breath of patients harbouring *H. pylori*. The faecal antigen test has a similar sensitivity and specificity to the urease breath test.

When is *H. pylori* eradication indicated?

Triple therapy eradication is indicated for duodenal ulcers, gastric ulcers that are not the result of NSAIDs and mucosa-associated lymphoid tissue (MALT) lymphoma. It is not indicated in peptic ulcers caused by NSAIDs. The

situation with GORD, functional dyspepsia and gastric cancer remains unclear.

What do you know about *H. pylori* eradication and anti-secretory treatment for GORD?

The interaction between *H. pylori*, antisecretory treatment and GORD is complex and contentious. *H. pylori* may be no more prevalent in GORD than in the general population, and indeed may be less prevalent, suggesting a protective role of *H. pylori*, perhaps by producing gastric body gastritis and decreasing acid output. Furthermore, acid suppression with PPIs promotes *H. pylori* spread from the antrum to the gastric body and fundus causing a chronic active pangastritis that may progress to atrophic gastritis and, over time, gastric adenocarcinoma.

When is endoscopy indicated in patients with dyspepsia?

The *British Society of Gastroenterology* guidelines suggest, for first presentation of dyspepsia, that patients < 55 years without alarm symptoms should have *H. pylori* serology checked (or breath tested). Patients who test positive should receive a triple therapy eradication regimen, and patients with symptoms that persist after eradication therapy or patients who test negative whose symptoms persist after anti-secretory treatment should proceed to endoscopy. No action is required for patients rendered asymptomatic. For patients with persistent or recurrent symptoms who tested positive for *H. pylori* and received eradication therapy, the optimum first step to confirm successful eradication is breath testing. Patients aged 55 years or over or patients with alarm symptoms should proceed to endoscopy.

How would you manage persistent symptoms after endoscopically proven peptic ulcer disease treated with eradication triple therapy?

Urea breath testing for *H. pylori* more than four weeks after triple therapy is appropriate for an uncomplicated duodenal ulcer. If positive, an alternative eradication regimen could be used. If negative, alternative causes should be considered. Eradication of *H. pylori* should always be confirmed in cases where a duodenal ulcer has

Table 2.5 Causes of duodenal and gastric ulceration	
Duodenal ulceration	**Gastric ulceration**
H. pylori infection (> 90%) NSAIDs Zollinger–Ellison syndrome Hypercalcaemia Granulomatous disease (Crohn's disease, sarcoidosis, Wegener's granulomatosis) Neoplasia (carcinoma, lymphoma, leiomyoma, leiomyosarcoma) Infection (tuberculosis, syphilis, herpes simplex, cytomegalovirus, candida) Ectopic pancreatic tissue	*H. pylori* infection (non-atrophic gastritis, although the latter is usually autoimmune) NSAIDs Neoplasia (carcinoma, lymphoma, leiomyosarcoma) Granulomatous disease (Crohn's disease, sarcoidosis, Wegener's granulomatosis) Infection (tuberculosis, syphilis, herpes simplex, cytomegalovirus, candida) Radiotherapy
NSAID, non-steroidal anti-inflammatory drugs.	

bled to ensure complete epithelialisation of the crater. The main difference is the need to exclude malignancy in a gastric ulcer. Endoscopy is mandatory, with targeted biopsies of the rim and base, and a repeat endoscopy should be performed eight weeks later to confirm healing and obtain biopsies from the original ulcer site.

List some causes of upper gastrointestinal bleeding

Causes and frequencies are shown in Table 2.6. Small bowel (e.g. angiodysplasia, investigated by wireless capsule endoscopy or CT angiography) and right-sided colonic disease may present with melaena.

How should peptic ulcer bleeding be managed?

PPIs appear not to significantly reduce re-bleeding or need for surgery. Several endoscopic modalities are available to achieve haemostasis for bleeding ulcers. Combination therapy of adrenaline injection with mechanical methods of haemostasis reduce rebleeding compared with a single treatment. A minority of patients with refractory bleeding need surgical oversewing of an artery or partial gastrectomy.

How might you assess risk in a patient who presents with upper gastrointestinal bleeding?

Haematemesis (bright red, dark clots or coffee-ground) or melaena indicate an upper gastrointestinal bleed. The Rockall score is a clinical and endoscopic predictor of risk of re-bleeding and death (Table 2.7). Blatchford proposed an alternative risk score that does not rely on endoscopy (Table 2.7); its place is more to predict the need for intervention than to predict mortality, and so has greater emphasis in less severe bleeding.

Can bradycardia be a sign of acute haemorrhage?

A normal or low heart rate and hypotension may occur in acute haemorrhage, often after gastrointestinal surgery. The first response to maintain arterial pressure despite a falling cardiac output involves tachycardia and baroreceptor reflex vasoconstriction. A second phase, however, occurs when about a third of circulating volume has been lost, in which sympathetically mediated vasoconstriction and cardiac drive fall abruptly and cardiac vagal drive increases.

Table 2.6 Causes of upper gastrointestinal bleeding

Cause	Frequency (%)
Peptic ulceration	35–50
Oesophagitis	20–30
Erosive disease (duodenitis, gastritis, erosions)	10–20
Varices	5–10
Mallory Weiss tear	2–5
Neoplasm	2–5
Vascular malformations	2–3%
Aorto-gastrointestinal fistula	< 1%

CASE 2.4

DYSPHAGIA

Candidate information

Role

You are a doctor in the gastroenterology clinic. Please read the following letter from the patient's general practitioner. You may make notes on the paper provided. When the bell sounds, enter the examination room to begin the consultation.

Scenario

Dear Doctor

Re: Mr James Morton, aged 62 years

Thank you for seeing this gentleman who reports difficult swallowing over the last three months. He is now frequently vomiting and his routine blood tests show he has a sodium of 130 mmol/l and potassium of 2.9 mmol/l. His renal function tests are normal and he is not anaemic. A routine chest X-ray is reported as showing a hugely dilated oesophagus. Please see and advise on urgent management.

Yours sincerely

Please take a history from the patient (you may continue to make notes if you wish on the paper provided). Your examiners will warn you when 12 minutes have elapsed. You have 14 minutes to take a history from the patient followed by 1 minute of reflection. There will then follow 5 minutes of discussion with the examiners. Be prepared to discuss solutions to the problems posed by the case and how you might reply to the GP's letter. You are not required to examine the patient.

Patient information

Mr James Morton is a 62-year-old retired, rather stoical farmer with a history of reflux symptoms treated by his GP with omeprazole for the last 12 months (although he has taken it sparingly). He takes no other medications. For the last three months he has had difficulty swallowing and some vomiting to the extent that he can become dehydrated. He has lost around 10 kg in weight, but attributes this to not being able to eat. He is otherwise previously well. He wishes to avoid further investigation or treatment if possible because he believes 'treatment does more harm than good and these things are best left to nature to heal'.

Table 2.7 The Rockall and Blatchford scores

The Rockall score

	0	1	2	3		Score
Age	< 60	61–79	≥ 80	–	Pre-endo-scopy score (maximum 7)	0–2 low risk (endoscopy routine)
Shock	SBP ≥ 100 HR ≤ 100	SBP ≥ 100 HR ≥ 100	SBP ≤ 100 HR ≥ 100	–		3–5 moderate risk (endoscopy within 24 hours)
Co-morbidity	Nil	Nil	e.g. ischaemic heart disease	e.g. liver or renal disease, malignancy		6–7 high risk (endoscopy with 8 hours)
Diagnosis	Nil or Mallory Weiss tear	All other diagnoses	Malignancy		A post-endoscopy score can now be derived (maximum 11, 2 predicting 0.1% mortality and 8 predicting 41% mortality)	
Major endoscopic stigmata of recent haemorrhage	Clean base or dark spots	–	Ooze, adherent clot, non-visible bleeding vessels, active spurting	–		

The Blatchford score*

Variable	Score
Urea (mmol/l)	
> 6.5, < 8	2
≥ 8, < 10	3
≥ 10, < 25	4
≥ 25	6
Haemoglobin (g/dl)	
Men Women	
≥ 12, < 13 ≥ 10, < 12	1
≥ 10, < 12	3
< 10 < 10	6
SBP	
100–109	1
90–99	2
< 90	3
Pulse > 100	
Melaena	1
Syncope	2
Liver disease	2
Cardiac failure	2

*A score of 5 or more predicts need for intervention. HR, heart rate; SBP, systolic blood pressure.

How to approach the case

Data gathering in the interview and interpretation and use of information gathered

Presenting problem(s) and symptom exploration

Dysphagia refers to delay in the passage of solids or liquids from mouth to stomach. It should be distinguished from odonyphagia, which is discomfort or pain on swallowing hot or cold liquids. The history should take a similar approach to that of dyspepsia, in particular asking about alarm features:

- **A**naemia
- **L**oss of weight (a worry, prompting check of inflammatory markers) or anorexia
- **A**bdominal mass
- **R**ecent onset of progressive symptoms
- **M**elaena or haematemesis
- **D**ysphagia

Although attempted localisation can be misleading clinically, it is useful to separate those causes that predominantly affect the pharynx and proximal oesophagus (high dysphagia) from those that affect the oesophageal body and oesophago-gastric junction (Table 2.8).

Table 2.8 Causes of dysphagia

Type of dysphagia	Causes	Pointers in history to possible causes
Low (oesophageal)	Oesophageal or oesophago-gastric junction malignancy GORD with or without stricture Oesophagitis secondary to *Candida*, cytomegalovirus or herpes simplex virus (consider AIDS) Oesophageal motility disorders, e.g. achalasia, diffuse oesophageal spasm	Malignancy suggested by alarm symptoms and short history with dysphagia for solids more than liquids Otherwise, achalasia more likely, patients often describing chest pain and minor dysphagia Reflux-induced strictures common, often without a history of GORD Barrett's oesophagus often characterised by diminished oesophageal sensitivity and lack of pain
High (pharyngeal)	Stroke Parkinson's disease Bulbar palsy, e.g. motor neurone disease, myasthenia gravis Oropharyngeal malignancy Crico-oesophageal spasm Pharyngeal pouch	Known neurological disease, e.g. multiple sclerosis, motor neurone disease Tendency for spillage into trachea on eating, causing coughing or choking

GORD, gastro-oesophageal reflux disease.

■ **Swallowing assessment**   Ask about the following factors that can influence swallowing:

- Medications
- Nutritional intake
- Teeth
- Posture
- Neck problems, e.g. cervical spondylosis
- Neck or limb weakness
- Respiratory problems

Patient perspective

Explore his reasons for preferring to avoid treatment and explain the possible causes, and risks if left untreated.

Past medical history

The history of oesophagitis is important, even though he has taken a proton pump inhibitor, because it can transform to oesophageal malignancy.

Drug and allergy history

Ask specifically about non-steroidal anti-inflammatories (NSAIDs) or corticosteroids.

Family history

Relevance here is unlikely.

SUMMARY – ASSESSMENT AND PLAN

- Malignancy must be excluded. Achalasia, however, is very likely given the distended oesophagus on chest X-ray.
- A full examination is important; ear, nose and throat (ENT) specialist opinion is often indicated.
- Initial tests for dysphagia should always include a full blood count, haematinics, inflammatory markers, renal and liver function, calcium and thyroid function and a chest X-ray.
- Assessment by a speech and language therapist should be requested.
- An oesophagogastroduodenoscopy (OGD) should be arranged urgently.

Social history

Ask about alcohol and smoking, both risk factors for peptic ulceration.

Discussion

What are the phases of swallowing?

Swallowing has cortical input and is mediated in the brainstem, which receives sensory information from the tongue, fauces and pharynx. Following pre-oral anticipation of food there are three phases of swallowing:

Oral phase

This involves propulsion of the bolus backwards along the tongue past the fauces and into the pharynx, triggering the swallow reflex and initiation of the pharyngeal phase. The tongue tip and blade press the bolus against the hard palate, the sides of the tongue rising in smooth progression from front to back to force the bolus along a central groove, and swallowing is triggered when the bolus reaches the tongue base, the soft palate rising to occlude the nasopharynx and avoid nasal regurgitation. In the oral phase the airway is open and the cricopharyngeal sphincter is closed. The timing from the start of lingual peristalsis to trigger of swallow is normally less than one second. Once swallow is triggered, voluntary control is surpassed.

Pharyngeal phase

This is rapid, also less than one second. It involves movement of the bolus through the pharynx by pharyngeal muscle contraction, with elevation of the larynx to fit under the tongue base, the vocal cords coming together and the epiglottis covering the laryngeal opening. All of this is seen externally as the Adam's apple rising to protect the airway. The bolus may sit transiently in the valleculae then pharyngeal peristalsis squeezes it downwards as the cricopharyngeal sphincter relaxes to admit the bolus into the oesophagus. The soft palate and larynx are then lowered and breathing recommences.

Oesophageal phase

This is reflexic, not under voluntary control, and no longer a speech and language therapist's territory.

Outline your approach to managing dysphagia

This is outlined in Box 2.9.

What is the role of speech and language therapists in a swallow assessment?

Bedside screening (e.g. water swallow test) to identify patients at risk of aspiration can be carried out by any doctor. It can miss silent aspiration and pharyngeal function can only be inferred. Referral to a speech and language therapist is appropriate in patients who are alert, able to sit upright for at least 15 minutes, have a stable chest status and in whom there is evidence of oral or facial weakness or sensory disturbance, a wet/gurgly voice or drooling.

Speech and language therapists more fully assess swallow stages and safety and may recommend videofluoroscopy (the gold standard for identifying aspiration and features of dysphagia).

A full history takes account of the normal level of independence with feeding to avoid overly optimistic expectations. Problems with cooperation and cognition (e.g.

awareness of spoons, cups and straws in patients with dyspraxia or dementia or volition to eat or swallow in dementia), communication (dysphasia, dysarthria, dysphonia), vision, hearing, dentition and gross motor function of head and neck and upper limbs are all relevant. Fatiguability is important to elicit. Respiratory function and clearance of secretions are important in assessing risk of aspiration (e.g. immediate or delayed reflexive cough, audible pharyngeal crackles, wet/gurgly vocal quality, respiratory difficulty), as is oral hygiene.

Manual assessment of the pharyngeal phase can be performed observing initiation of tongue movement and feeling the rise, forward motion and fall of the larynx.

If considered safe to proceed, oral handling of fluid and diet is assessed. Some patients who aspirate thin fluids may not with thickened fluids.

In Parkinson's disease, for example, there is a prolonged oral phase with considerable rocking and rolling of the bolus in the mouth. Multiple swallows may be needed to clear each mouthful with retention of bolus in the mouth. Pharyngeal motility, cricopharyngeal opening and oesophageal motility may all be reduced.

Overall, a decision is made as to whether swallow is safe or poses a risk of aspiration.

Therapeutic measures include advice on food type, texture, consistency, size and preferences and positions for feeding. Nasogastric or gastrostomy feeding may be necessary.

Box 2.9 Management of dysphagia

Low (oesophageal) dysphagia

- Endoscopy is the investigation of choice. Where endoscopy is normal, ambulatory pH studies and oesophageal manometry and occasionally oesophageal provocation tests are indicated.
- A benign stricture is confirmed histologically and managed by dilation if possible and maintenance treatment with a proton pump inhibitor. Oesophagitis caused by infection warrants specific treatment.
- An oesophageal or gastric tumour is managed operatively by resection in fit patients where there is no evidence of metastases, stenting or laser treatment, or pure palliation.
- Achalasia may be detected as a widened oesophagus on chest X-ray and is characterised by absent distal oesophageal peristalsis and abnormal relaxation of the lower oesophageal sphincter; it may be managed by pneumatic balloon dilatation, often repeatedly, or, failing this, Heller's myotomy of the lower oesophageal sphincter.
- Diffuse oesophageal spasm is rare and is characterised by simultaneous contractions seen on barium swallow as a 'corkscrew' oesophagus.

High (pharyngeal) dysphagia

- Radiology is generally more rewarding than endoscopy. Most problems are the result of failure of pharyngeal contraction or cricopharyngeal relaxation or both and cineradiography with barium (liquid or bread soaked in) can give functional as well as anatomical information.
- A pouch or pharyngeal bar can be managed by surgical myotomy of the overactive cricopharyngeus, sometimes with pouch excision.
- Neuromuscular problems (e.g. post-stroke) may require consideration of percutaneous endoscopic gastrostomy feeding.

CASE 2.5

ABDOMINAL PAIN

Candidate information

Role

You are a doctor in the emergency medical admissions unit. Please read the following letter from the patient's general practitioner. You may make notes on the paper provided. When the bell sounds, enter the examination room to begin the consultation.

Scenario

Dear Doctor

Re: Mr Edward Bertram, aged 80 years

Mr Bertram has developed subacute abdominal pain over the past few days. I phoned the surgical team, but because he has a complex history, they would prefer you to take the patient and advise on his medical management. They are happy to be consulted about his pain if you suspect a surgical cause.

Yours sincerely

Please take a history from the patient (you may continue to make notes if you wish on the paper provided). Your examiners will warn you when 12 minutes have elapsed. You have 14 minutes to take a history from the patient followed by 1 minute of reflection. There will then follow 5 minutes of discussion with the examiners. Be prepared to discuss solutions to the problems posed by the case and how you might reply to the GP's letter. You are not required to examine the patient.

Patient information

Mr Edward Bertram is an 80-year-old gentleman who has just been admitted to hospital because of worsening episodes of abdominal pain over the past few days. Over the past few months he has noticed dull pain after meals centred on the umbilicus. Sometimes this is associated with blood-tinged diarrhoea. The pain tends to occur mostly with bigger meals, and not with snacks, although he has not noticed any association with particular types of food. He has a past medical history of ischaemic heart disease, atrial fibrillation and type 2 diabetes. He gets angina about twice weekly. He also has Crohn's disease, having had a terminal ileal resection eight years ago, but the disease has not been symptomatically active for two years. He takes aspirin 75 mg daily, bisoprolol 5 mg daily, simvastatin 40 mg daily, perindopril 4 mg daily and mesalazine. He is an ex-heavy smoker. He lives with his wife, who has advanced dementia, and he is her only carer. He is very worried about who will look after her because no other family members are nearby and he was rushed into hospital by ambulance before care could be arranged. He has good neighbours, and needs to contact them.

How to approach the case

Data gathering in the interview and interpretation and use of information gathered

Presenting problem(s) and symptom exploration

▪ **Determine the type of abdominal pain**   There are two types of acute abdominal pain (Table 2.9).

▪ **Determine the site of abdominal pain**   These two types of pain may occur at one of three main sites in the abdomen because the brain receives visceral pain impulses from each of the three embryological components of the gut (Table 2.10).

▪ **Integrate the above two pieces of information to form likely diagnoses**   This knowledge of types and sites of pain can direct you towards common causes. *Colicky epigastric pain* is frequently the result of biliary colic. *Continuous epigastric pain* is more likely to be the result of peptic ulcer disease or pancreatitis. *Colicky periumbilical pain* in an elderly patient with weight loss and anaemia is right-sided colonic cancer unless proven otherwise. In a young patient with episodic diarrhoea, constipation and bloating, without alarm symptoms, it may well be irritable bowel syndrome. *Continuous periumbilical* pain may be caused by peritonitis resulting from a perforated viscus, mesenteric ischaemia or visceral peritoneal irritation in appendicitis. *Colicky suprapubic pain* with alteration in bowel habit may be the result of colorectal cancer, inflammatory bowel disease or irritable bowel syndrome. *Continuous pelvic pain* in a young woman may be caused by pelvic inflammatory disease, an ovarian cyst or ovarian torsion. *Visceral pain* is often a vague, colicky midline pain, because it arises from visceral peritoneum in communication with a viscus. Continuous pain may be of visceral or parietal origin or both. *Parietal pain* tends to be more localised because the parietal peritoneum is innervated by spinal nerve roots that have specific sensory cortical representation. Hence, appendicitis, biliary colic and diverticulitis may all start as midline visceral pain but further localise to the right iliac fossa, right hypochondrium and left iliac fossa, respectively, if the parietal peritoneum becomes inflamed. The kidneys and ureters (retroperitoneal structures) have parietal or spinal innervation from T8 to L1; hence ureteric colic may be perceived as progressing from the loin (T8 dermatome) to the groin (L1 dermatome). Pain may also arise from structures outside the abdominal cavity such as the abdominal wall or in a nerve root as in shingles.

Table 2.10 Sites of abdominal pain	
Derivation	**Site of pain**
Foregut (stomach, proximal duodenum, gallbladder, biliary tree and pancreas)	Epigastric
Midgut (distal duodenum to two-thirds across the transverse colon)	Periumbilical
Hindgut (last third of transverse colon to rectum, and gynaecological areas of the pelvis, derived from the cloacal sac)	Suprapubic/pelvic

Table 2.9 Two types of acute abdominal pain	
Type of pain	**Cause**
Colicky (gripping, often severe and comes in waves)	Abnormally strong peristalsis of a hollow viscus triggered either by obstruction (e.g. stone, tumour, hernia) or irritation (e.g. gastroenteritis)
Continuous (present lying still and exacerbated by movement)	Inflammation, triggered by infection, ulceration, peritonitis or ischaemia

Table 2.11 Common causes of abdominal pain and their symptoms

Biliary colic	Intense, right upper quadrant pain With fever and tenderness indicates acute cholecystitis
Pancreatitis	Epigastric/central abdominal pain radiating to the back Such pain could also represent ruptured abdominal aortic aneurysm
Bowel obstruction, e.g. volvulus	Constipation Colicky abdominal pain Distension Vomiting
Perforated viscus	Progressive pain exacerbated by minimal movement Rebound tenderness
Mesenteric ischaemia/infarction	Pain with or without rectal bleeding Usually vascular risk factors
Diverticulitis	Left iliac fossa discomfort ± fever History of constipation
Ureteric colic	Intense, intermittent pain from loin to groin Often haematuria
Abdominal aortic aneurysm rupture	Leaks may be either acute, with an expansile pulsatile mass, or slow

■ **Be alert to typical patterns of common conditions**   These are outlined in Table 2.11.

Patient perspective

Explore any ideas, concerns and expectations.

Past medical history

Take a full history about the Crohn's disease and its treatments.

Drug and allergy history

He is taking aspirin rather than warfarin for atrial fibrillation. Determine if there are reasons for this.

Family history

The family history of familial Mediterranean fever is probably irrelevant.

Social history

The level of care required by his wife should be explored, and, crucially, whether care needs to be put in place immediately for her own safety.

SUMMARY – ASSESSMENT AND PLAN

- The symptoms and risk factors are in keeping with mesenteric ischaemia. A flare-up of Crohn's disease is possible.
- He should have a full examination and a full set of haematobiochemistry tests, including glucose and inflammatory markers. A raised serum lactate may suggest infarcted tissue, but may be normal in ischaemia. Chest and abdominal radiographs are important, as is an ECG to determine the rhythm.
- A surgical opinion should be sought unless it is very clear that he has a flare-up of Crohn's disease.

Discussion

What are the major arteries supplying the small intestine and colon?

The superior mesenteric artery (SMA) supplies the small intestine and ascending and transverse colon via the ileo-colic, jejunal, ileal, right colic and middle colic arteries. The inferior mesenteric artery (IMA) supplies the left colic artery, marginal artery and sigmoid arteries.

What is meant by the term acute mesenteric ischaemia?

Acute mesenteric ischaemia or infarction implies impaired blood flow in the mesenteric arterial or venous systems and is most often caused by thrombotic or embolic disease (Table 2.12).

How does acute mesenteric ischaemia present?

It often presents non-specifically, with abdominal pain. Classically, the abdominal pain is disproportionately exaggerated relative to signs and persists and may evolve into an acute abdomen with distension, guarding (rigidity), tenderness, fever and signs of circulatory compromise. Blood loss per rectum occurs in a minority of patients.

How does chronic mesenteric ischaemia present?

Chronic mesenteric ischaemia ('intestinal angina') is often characterised by postprandial pain, sitophobia (fear of eating) and weight loss. Pain may be minimal at the outset but progress over weeks. Obstruction of at least two or three major splanchnic arteries usually occurs before symptoms are evident. When thrombosis affects the portal or splenic veins, the initial presentation may be variceal bleeding, ascites or splenomegaly.

Table 2.12 Causes of acute mesenteric ischaemia

Arterial occlusion (50%)	Superior mesenteric artery embolus (mural thrombus, atrial fibrillation, valve lesion, cholesterol embolus)
	Thrombotic (atherosclerosis, acute obstruction on background of chronic mesenteric ischaemia)
	Dissecting aortic aneurysm
	Vasculitis
	Fibromuscular dysplasia
	Trauma
	Endotoxic shock
Non-occlusive (20–30%)	Cardiac failure
	Septic shock
Venous occlusion (5–15%) (usually small intestine)	Prothrombotic disorder
	Inflammation
	Neoplasm
	Drugs
Extravascular causes	Incarcerated hernia
	Volvulus
	Adhesions

What do you know about ischaemic colitis?

Ischaemic colitis results from hypoperfusion or thrombotic or embolic occlusion (although the cause is often not identified) and is the most common ischaemic injury to the gastrointestinal tract. In younger patients, vasculitis, sickle cell disease, prothrombotic disorders and drugs including cocaine may all be causes. Blood supply to the colon arises from branches of the SMA and IMA, and the rectum also receives a supply from the haemorrhoidal arteries, branches of the internal iliac.

Which investigations may aid diagnosis of intestinal ischaemic disorders?

Metabolic (lactic) acidosis may be a clue to severe ischaemia. Plain X-rays are usually non-specific but can help exclude perforation or obstruction; the classic thumbprinting of submucosal haemorrhage or oedema resulting in focal mural thickening is a late sign. Intramural pneumatosis may be seen in advanced infarction. Ultrasound may detect mesenteric stenosis. Computed tomography and magnetic resonance angiography are non-invasive ways to diagnose mesenteric ischaemia.

What treatments are available?

Surgical revascularisation remains the treatment of choice for mesenteric ischaemia, but thrombolytic therapy and vascular interventional radiography have a growing role. Indications for surgical management of ischaemic colitis include peritoneal signs, massive haemorrhage, sepsis, stricture formation and persistent symptoms.

How should biliary sepsis be managed?

Appropriate antibiotics for suspected biliary sepsis include ciprofloxacin or tazocin. It should be suspected with pain in the right upper quadrant, fever and deranged liver enzymes but may be covert. An ultrasound scan is important, and an ERCP may be considered if any underlying obstructive lesion is suspected.

CASE 2.6

ALTERED BOWEL HABIT

Candidate information

Role

You are a doctor in the medical outpatient clinic. Please read the following letter from the patient's general practitioner. You may make notes on the paper provided. When the bell sounds, enter the examination room to begin the consultation.

Scenario

> Dear Doctor
>
> Re: Ms Louise Musgrove, aged 30 years
>
> This lady has a four-month history of watery diarrhoea. There is associated mucus. She was previously well. I would be grateful for your further assessment and append her laboratory results.
>
> Yours sincerely
>
> Full blood count (FBC) normal except for mild hypochromic microcytic anaemia, liver function tests (LFTs) including albumin normal, erythrocyte sedimentation rate (ESR) 45, stool microscopy and culture negative for bacteria, ova, cysts and parasites.

Please take a history from the patient (you may continue to make notes if you wish on the paper provided). Your examiners will warn you when 12 minutes have elapsed. You have 14 minutes to take a history from the patient followed by 1 minute of reflection. There will then follow 5 minutes of discussion with the examiners. Be prepared to discuss solutions to the problems posed by the case and how you might reply to the GP's letter. You are not required to examine the patient.

Patient information

Ms Louise Musgrove is a 30-year-old lady who has had watery diarrhoea, passing at least six stools per day, sometimes with mucus, for four months. She is usually well. Ten months ago she travelled through Australia and the Far East with friends, but her trip was punctuated by a three-week episode of gastroenteritis for which she took a self-administered course of doxycycline. Symptoms seemed to settle, recurring transiently a month or two later, but then she was well for a few months before symptoms re-curred with more severity than previously. Her GP has checked stool cultures (negative) and tried a further course of doxycycline but this time without effect. She has lost around 8 kg in weight since before travelling. Before travelling she was very well. She works as a solicitor. She does not smoke. Her sister has type 1 diabetes, an aunt has coeliac disease and a cousin undergoes regular surveillance after treatment for colon cancer diagnosed at an early age.

How to approach the case

Data gathering in the interview and interpretation and use of information gathered

Presenting problem(s) and symptom exploration

▪ **Determine the type of diarrhoea**   Diarrhoea is difficult to define. Definitions sometimes refer to > 200 ml of stool per day or to increased stool frequency and decreased consistency. It may be acute (less than two weeks in duration), subacute (two to four weeks) or chronic (more than four weeks), and is predominantly a result of small bowel disease (often large volume, pale, with steatorrhoea) or large bowel disease (often smaller volume with blood or mucus). Small bowel causes of diarrhoea may be classified as secretory (e.g. infectious, malabsorptive), osmotic (e.g. osmotic laxatives) or the result of altered motility (e.g. hyperthyroidism, autonomic neuropathy). Secretory symptoms tend to persist with fasting.

▪ **If symptoms suggest a small bowel cause**   Consider the common causes of malabsorption in the UK (Box 2.10).

▪ **If symptoms suggest a large bowel cause**   Consider inflammatory bowel disease (ask about blood, mucus, pus, slime) and colorectal cancer, and ask about alarm symptoms. Remember that irritable bowel syndrome is characterised by episodes of constipation and diarrhoea with abdominal bloating in a younger adult without alarm symptoms. In older patients, diverticular disease and mesenteric ischaemia are common. Candida can cause diarrhoea on a prolonged antibiotic course in hospital.

Patient perspective

Ascertain her ideas, concerns and expectations.

Past medical history

Ask about thyroid disease, coeliac disease, diabetes and previous surgery.

Drug and allergy history

Ask about recent antibiotics.

Family history

Note the family history of colorectal cancer at an early age.

> **Box 2.10 Malabsorption**
>
> **Symptoms**
>
> Malabsorption typically causes steatorrhoea, weight loss and fatigue, together with symptoms resulting from deficiency of essential nutrients and vitamins such as iron, folate and calcium.
>
> **Causes**
>
> Common causes in the UK include:
>
> - Coeliac disease (a range of other presentations are common)
> - Cystic fibrosis (diagnosed in childhood)
> - Post-enteritis enteropathy
> - Giardiasis
> - Chronic pancreatitis, e.g. alcohol; autoimmune form increasingly recognised
>
>   Broadly, malabsorption may be the result of a lack of pancreatic enzymes (cystic fibrosis, chronic pancreatitis), lack of solubilising bile salts causing failure of micelle formation (obstructive liver disease, small bowel bacterial overgrowth), decreased transit time (post-gastrectomy, 'short gut syndrome', thyrotoxicosis), small bowel mucosal pathology impeding absorption (coeliac disease, post-infectious enteropathy, Whipple's disease, Crohn's disease, intestinal lymphangiectasia, lymphoma) or intestinal infestation (giardiasis). Small bowel bacterial overgrowth may be secondary to diverticulae, blind loops, obstruction (Crohn's disease), infiltration (systemic sclerosis), poor motility (pseudo-obstruction, diabetes) or immunodeficiency (IgA deficiency).

Social history

Ask about alcohol intake (chronic pancreatitis, often presenting as relapsing steatorrhoea and back pain). Ask about foreign travel or unwell contacts (infectious causes).

> **SUMMARY – ASSESSMENT AND PLAN**
>
> - Post-enteritis enteropathy is a leading contender given that she was previously well and that her symptoms started with gastroenteritis overseas; persistent infection due to, for example, *Giardia*, should be excluded with multiple stool cultures.
> - Coeliac disease should be considered given the strong family history of autoimmune disease.
> - Haematobiochemistry should include thyroid function and markers of malabsorption.
> - Colonoscopy should be considered relatively urgently to exclude inflammatory bowel disease and, given the family history, colorectal cancer.

Discussion

List some investigations for diarrhoea with a suspected small bowel cause

These are listed in Box 2.11.

What are the infectious causes of acute watery diarrhoea?

This is usually the result of small bowel disease, often viral, such as norovirus with an incubation period of 24–48

- Full blood count for anaemia, with iron, folate and vitamin B12 levels
- Inflammatory markers, e.g. erythrocyte sedimentation rate (ESR), C-reactive protein (CRP)
- Urea, electrolytes, liver function tests (especially albumin) and calcium (hypocalcaemia and concurrent hypomagnesaemia is a very important cause–effect vicious cycle of diarrhoea)
- Stool microscopy and culture for bacteria, ova, cysts and parasites
- Tests for bacterial overgrowth (sometimes jejunal aspirates for bacterial quantification)
- Endoscopy and jejunal biopsy; wireless capsule endoscopy is now possible for small bowel visualisation

hours, or the result of *Escherichia coli*. Enterotoxigenic *E. coli* is a common cause of 'traveller's diarrhoea'. Cholera is a very important cause worldwide. Preformed toxins in food also cause acute watery diarrhoea, such as toxins from *Staphylococcus aureus* or *Bacillus cereus* provoking symptoms within six hours (tending to provoke vomiting more than diarrhoea) or toxins from *Clostridium perfringens* within 8–12 hours.

What are the infectious causes of acute bloody diarrhoea?

This implies invasive disease, usually colitis. The broad term for this presentation is 'dysentery'. The most common causes in the UK are non-typhoidal *Salmonella* spp., *Campylobacter jejuni* and *Shigella*, with incubation periods of one to five days. The enteric fevers *Salmonella typhi* and *Salmonella paratyphi* should be considered following travel to an area of risk. *Vibrio parahaemolyticus* should be considered with a history of shellfish ingestion.

What are the infectious causes of chronic watery diarrhoea?

This is most commonly caused by *Giardia lamblia* (giardiasis). Cryptosporidiosis, microsporidiosis and isosporiasis should be considered in immunosuppressed patients. Non-infectious causes, especially coeliac disease, must be considered.

What are the infectious causes of chronic bloody diarrhoea?

This may be caused by amoebic dysentery. The commonest non-infectious cause is inflammatory bowel disease.

Are there any advances in antimicrobial treatment of diarrhoea?

Diagnosis still falls heavily on stool microscopy and culture, but faecal antigen- and DNA-based tests are advancing. Whilst rehydration remains the most important treatment step, quinolones may be used in traveller's diarrhoea, the non-absorbable antibiotic rifaximim is very effective in traveller's diarrhoea and the broad-spectrum antimicrobial nitazoxanide useful in cryptosporidiosis,

and sometimes in giardiasis, amoebiasis and *Clostridium difficile* infection. There is increasing evidence for probiotics and prebiotics in treating and preventing a range of intestinal infections.

Why is Shiga-toxin-producing *E. coli* (STEC) important?

Although infrequent, STEC carries the potentially serious complication of haemolytic uraemic syndrome (HUS).

Why is norovirus important?

Norovirus is the most common cause of institutional, particularly health-care-associated, outbreaks of gastroenteritis and is difficult to contain.

What is *Clostridium difficile*?

Clostridium difficile is a Gram-positive, spore-bearing anaerobe that is widely distributed in the environment. It dies rapidly in the air but its spores can survive indefinitely (for a thousand years or more). It has two toxins, toxin A an enterotoxin, and toxin B a cytotoxin, the latter causing inflammation.

Why is *C. difficile* important?

C. difficile is increasing in incidence, with increasingly virulent strains. It is carried asymptomatically by 2% of healthy adults and up to 10–20% of older hospitalised patients. The clinical spectrum is diverse. It is frequently ingested from soil, beaches or rivers, dies rapidly in gastric acid, but may asymptomatically colonise the gut or cause diarrhoea, colitis or pseudomembranous colitis. Protective factors include carriage on admission to hospital, high serum antibody titres to toxin A, and good health.

When is *C. difficile* likely to become more pathogenic?

It is more likely to become pathogenic with mucosal damage, often induced by antibiotics or foods containing antibiotics.

Which haematobiochemical disturbances are common with *C. difficile*-associated diarrhoea (CDAD) and how is it diagnosed?

It tends to cause a very high white cell count ($> 15 \times 10^9$/l common and $> 30 \times 10^9$/l in 25% of patients), decreased serum albumin and altered electrolytes. Diagnosis is by detection of toxin, most commonly by immunoassay, which has an 85–95% sensitivity for toxins A or B. Two negative results should cast doubt on the diagnosis. Culture of *C. difficile* is not specific for disease because of asymptomatic carriage and non-toxicogenic strains. Typing, if needed, may be confirmed by polymerase chain reaction, 001 the most common.

How is *C. difficile*-associated diarrhoea treated?

Precipitating antibiotics should be stopped where possible. Anti-motility agents should be avoided. Fluid and electrolyte balance correction is often needed. Surgery is occasionally needed, if toxic megacolon occurs. The first-line antibiotic is oral metronidazole (400 mg t.d.s.), with a response rate of 75–98% and recurrence rate of 5–50%. Resistance is low. The second-line antibiotic is oral vancomycin 125 mg t.d.s., larger doses not superior, with a response rate of 80–97% and recurrence rate of 10–40%. Other options include rifampicin, fusidic acid, teicoplanin and nitazoxanide. Recurrence is not usually because of resistance, and so the same treatment may be used as for the original episode. Many measures have observational but not rigorously evidence-based value; these include adjunctive probiotics, intravenous immunoglobulin and faecal donation per rectum or via a long jejunal line. Stool toxin positivity persists for weeks to months after treatment.

How is *C. difficile* controlled?

Hygiene, isolation of symptomatic patients and antibiotic control are important. Alcohol hand-rub does not kill spores, and so hand washing with soap and water after removal of apron and gloves is very important.

Where are the major nutrients absorbed, including iron, vitamin B12 and folate?

The small bowel is the main site of absorption of nutrients, notably carbohydrates, fats (triglycerides split into fatty acids and glycerol by pancreatic lipase and fatty acids are solubilised by bile salts from the liver to form water-soluble micelles) and proteins, which enter the circulation via the portal vein. Iron is absorbed in the upper small bowel, folate in the duodenum and jejunum and vitamin B12, bound to intrinsic factor, mainly in the terminal ileum.

What do you know about coeliac disease?

Coeliac disease is discussed in Box 2.12.

How is constipation managed?

After consideration and assessment for underlying causes, options include stimulants such as senna, softeners such as lactulose, and sodium docusate or Movicol. Fybogel is a bulking agent.

What do you know about the molecular basis and genetics of colorectal cancer (CRC) risk?

More than 70% of CRCs develop from sporadic adenomatous polyps. The most common well-defined hereditary syndromes are the familial adenomatous polyposis (FAP) and hereditary non-polyposis colon cancer (HNPCC)/Lynch syndromes. Peutz–Jehgers syndrome is rare.

FAP is an autosomal dominant disorder in which there is a germline mutation in the tumour suppressor gene for adenomatous polyposis coli (*APC*) on chromosome 5. It accounts for < 1% of all CRC. Patients often have hundreds of pedunculated colonic polyps. Extracolonic manifestations may occur (previously referred to as Gardner and Turcot syndromes), including duodenal adenomas and cerebral and thyroid tumours. In HNPCC there are germline mutations in DNA mismatch repair

---

Box 2.12 Coeliac disease

Cause

Coeliac disease is the result of sensitivity to the gliadin component of gluten causing villous atrophy in genetically susceptible individuals. Tissue transglutaminase (TTG) may modify gliadin and act as an autoantigen. Coeliac disease has a wide range of presentations, is more common than previously recognised and confers an increased risk of malignancy, especially small bowel lymphoma.

Symptoms

Coeliac disease may cause diarrhoea, malabsorption with steatorrhoea, weight loss and growth retardation. A wide spectrum of disease activity has been recognised. Covert symptoms include malaise and recurrent aphthous ulceration. It may cause hyposplenism. It may also present as unexplained folate or iron deficiency anaemia (now the commonest presentation). It is important to ask about itchy rashes (dermatitis herpetiformis is rare, however) and bone pain (osteomalacia).

Diagnosis

The gold standard test is jejunal biopsy for villous atrophy. Patients should undergo re-endoscopy after a period of gluten exclusion to confirm villous regeneration. Other causes of villous atrophy include Whipple's disease and small bowel lymphoma. Antiendomysial and anti-TTG antibodies are highly specific and nearly always positive. Antigliadin and antireticulin antibodies may be positive.

Treatment

A strict diet with complete exclusion of gluten-containing flour from wheat, rye, oats and barley is essential. Folate, iron and calcium supplements may be needed. Lifelong annual review should include assessment of symptoms, body mass index, haemoglobin, ferritin, folate, albumin, autoantibodies and osteoporosis risk (with bone densitometry for postmenopausal females and males aged over 55 years).

---

genes giving rise to pedunculated and flat polyps, predominantly in the proximal colon.

The proportion of CRC attributable to HNPCC is unclear, but HNPCC probably accounts for a significantly higher proportion than FAP. Associations include endometrial, ovarian, gastric and other cancers.

Clusters of CRC also occur in some families without a recognisable syndrome, suggesting a genetic origin. The immediate family members of a patient with CRC have a two- to three-fold relative risk of developing the disease.

Ulcerative colitis is unequivocally associated with increased CRC risk, high-risk factors including disease > 10 years, extensive disease and the presence of primary sclerosing cholangitis.

Factors which may promote the adenoma to CRC sequence include *APC* gene mutations, k-*ras* mutations, deleted in colon cancer (*DCC*) mutations and *p53* gene mutations.

Which factors determine a higher risk of malignant transformation within a polyp?

These include large size, a sessile or flattened appearance, severe dysplasia or squamous metaplasia, villous rather than tubular architecture and multiplicity (e.g. FAP).

What do you know about CRC screening?

CRC is a major public health challenge. Outcome is directly related to histological staging and patients with Dukes' A lesions have a five-year survival of up to 90%. Early detection is imperative, and this includes prompt investigation of patients with symptoms, selective screening of high-risk patients and population screening.

Patients at increased risk of CRC should be considered for surveillance. This group includes patients with a positive family history and patients with longstanding inflammatory bowel disease. The lifetime risk of CRC is 1:50, rising to 1:17 if one first-degree relative is affected and >1:10 if two or more first-degree relatives are affected. Patients with a family history of CRC should be offered screening if one first-degree relative is affected under 45 years of age or if two first-degree relatives have been affected at any age. Screening should be by colonoscopy at presentation or at age 35–40 years, whichever is later. If negative, further colonoscopy is advised at 55 years. For people with more than two affected first-degree relatives a clinical geneticist should be consulted because of the possibility of FAP or HNPCC, and those with a known family history of such a genetic syndrome HNPCC should be screened.

The arguments for a national screening programme are that CRC is common, with a known premalignant lesion (adenoma). As it takes a long time (years) for adenomas to undergo malignant change, intervention is likely to significantly reduce the morbidity and mortality burden of CRC.

The two problems faced by population screening are which patients to target and by which method. Faecal occult blood testing is non-invasive, cheap and simple. It is relatively insensitive and non-specific, but has the potential to save many lives at an acceptable cost, reducing CRC mortality by 15–33%; it is proposed to screen people between the ages of 60 and 69 years biannually in the UK. Flexible sigmoidoscopy detects up to 80% of CRC as it examines the entire left colon and rectum, although even when combined with faecal occult blood testing this combined strategy misses 24% of CRC. Colonsocopy is the gold standard diagnostic test, but three times more costly than faecal occult blood testing and twice that of flexible sigmoidoscopy, and inconvenient. Virtual colonoscopy using spiral CT or MRI scanning are non-invasive alternatives, and may be superior for large polyps. Stool DNA analysis may have a role.

How is CRC managed?

CRC is a curable disease with over 90% of patients alive at five years after surgical removal of a Dukes' A lesion. Despite this, it remains the second most common cause of cancer death in the UK.

Important associations of CRC with diet, obesity and exercise suggest prevention is often possible, and screening is considered for those with HNPCC, FAP and others at high risk.

The two-week wait system under the 2000 NHS Plan is important for those with symptoms. A total of 35 000 people develop CRC each year in the UK, most sporadic. The majority affect the rectum or rectosigmoid and may present with rectal bleeding or an increase in stool frequency; right-sided cancers are more likely to be detected through anaemia. Colonscopy is the standard investigation. If CRC is confirmed, staging involves CT imaging of chest, abdomen and pelvis, but for rectal cancers MR imaging gives better information about local pelvic disease burden and nodal status and helps inform decisions about pre-operative chemotherapy. All CRCs should be discussed at multidisciplinary meetings to decide the optimum treatment strategy. As well as traditional surgical approaches, rectal cancer has seen a variety of new surgical approaches, minimally invasive procedures are on the increase, and multimodal treatments include neoadjuvant therapy; 5-fluorouracil is often used in combination with other chemotherapeutic agents.

CARDIOVASCULAR PROBLEMS

CASE 2.7

PREVENTION OF CARDIOVASCULAR DISEASE AND WEIGHT GAIN

Candidate information

Role

You are a doctor in the medical outpatient clinic. Please read the following letter from the patient's general practitioner. You may make notes on the paper provided. When the bell sounds, enter the examination room to begin the consultation.

Scenario

Dear Doctor

Re: Mrs Anna Shirley, aged 38 years

Thank you for seeing this lady, who is seeking a specialist opinion about her weight. She has a body mass index (BMI) of 32 kg/m² and a strong family history of obesity and type 2 diabetes. She has a random blood glucose of 10.9 mmol/l and a blood pressure of 160/90. Her total cholesterol is 5.6 mmol/l. Her thyroid function is normal. I recently commenced ramipril and have asked the practice nurse to review her diet.

Yours sincerely

Please take a history from the patient (you may continue to make notes if you wish on the paper provided). Your examiners will warn you when 12 minutes have elapsed. You have 14 minutes to take a history from the patient followed by 1 minute of reflection. There will then follow 5 minutes of discussion with the examiners. Be prepared to discuss solutions to the problems posed by the case and how you might reply to the GP's letter. You are not required to examine the patient.

Patient information

Mrs Anna Shirley is a 38-year-old nurse who has problems with her weight. She has always tended to be overweight but despite dietary advice has put on approximately 5 kg over the past year. Her current BMI is 32 kg/m². She is increasingly shy about undressing and no longer goes swimming or to the gym. Her occupation is stressful but does not lend itself to fitness. She suffers from chronic back pain, and has had other complications probably related to her weight, including gallstones and a deep vein thrombosis in pregnancy. She has impaired fasting glucose. She has a strong family history of type 2 diabetes and her mother died at the age of 56 from a myocardial infarction. She is a non-smoker. She has slightly erratic menstrual periods but is otherwise well. She has resigned herself to not ever being 'thin' but is desperately keen to ensure that no secondary cause is being missed, to lose some weight, and to optimise primary prevention of cardiovascular disease (CVD) as she wants to 'see her two children grow up'.

How to approach the case

Data gathering in the interview and interpretation and use of information gathered

Presenting problem(s) and symptom exploration

■ **Consider causes**   Secondary causes of obesity should always be considered but are much less common. Secondary causes are listed in Box 2.13.

Weight gain and obesity are largely a result of eating too much and not taking enough exercise. Despite a drive to reduce calorie intake, physical exercise by people in the Western world has diminished, the nefarious edge of a double-edged sword that brings safer, easier lives. Around 90% of Western people are predisposed to developing the 'abdominal' phenotype. We put on 0.9 grams every day from around ages 25 to 55! This contrasts with 'wild-type' humans, who no longer exist, but whose weight would plateau in adulthood. We are, on average, 15 kg heavier than 100 years ago (although a little taller, by approximately 1 cm/decade). Between 13% and 14% of the UK population is obese, and over 20% of the US population have incipient 'diabesity'. In the 1970s a survey showed that American women would rather be married to a convicted rapist than an obese man! Ironically, 50% of American women are now married to the latter (and an alarming number to the former). Social class is a factor. Television makes us obese, and people in social class 5 watch the most. 'Cocacolarisation' is very evident in communities recently exposed to Western lifestyles, exemplified by Aboriginals where the 'thrifty gene' hypothesis has been postulated – that our ancestors were predisposed to diabetes because those predisposing mechanisms allowed survival during famine. But perhaps in reality, all people have this 'thrifty' potential.

Box 2.13 Secondary causes of obesity

- Hypothyroidism
- Cushing's syndrome
- Polycystic ovarian syndrome
- Insulinoma
- Hypothalamic or pituitary disease
- Drugs
- Genetic syndromes, e.g. Laurence–Moon–Biedl syndrome
- Leptin deficiency or leptin receptor defects

Box 2.14 Risks of obesity

- Low self-esteem and depression
- Discrimination
- Type 2 diabetes
- Cardiovascular disease
- Worsening of chronic obstructive pulmonary disease and asthma
- Obstructive sleep apnoea
- Venous thromboembolism
- Biliary disease
- Intertrigo
- Soft tissue infection
- Varicose veins
- Back pain
- Osteoarthritis
- Hepatic steatosis (fatty liver)
- Increased risk of falls
- Stress incontinence
- Oligomenorrhoea and infertility
- Risks from the contraceptive pill
- Pregnancy complications
- Anaesthetic risks
- Increased risk of some cancers (now strong evidence for strong association)

■ **Consider risks** Risks from weight gain and obesity are outlined in Box 2.14.

Patient perspective

The effects on self-esteem should not be underestimated. Expectations should not be destroyed. Rather than focusing on past 'failure' to lose weight, focus on what can be done:

- A short list of tests to exclude secondary causes and build in reassurance
- Referral to a dietitian
- Gradual but sustained weight loss through adjustments in diet and exercise routines (see Summary box)
- Reassurance that such measures can halt the development of diabetes
- Consideration of anti-obesity drugs if necessary
- Exploration of possible depression and consideration of treatment

Past medical history

All of her past medical problems could be explained by obesity.

Drug and allergy history

Drugs commonly provoking weight gain include corticosteroids, antithyroid drugs, sulphonylureas and antipsychotics.

Family history

A family history of obesity is often present.

Social history

Explore fully what she eats, and physical exercise undertaken.

SUMMARY – ASSESSMENT AND PLAN

The following are important to establish – weight and height to derive the body mass index, waist circumference, blood pressure, urinalysis for glycosuria, thyroid function, lipid profile, fasting plasma glucose.

Body Mass Index (BMI) (kg/m^2)

< 18.5 = underweight
18.5–24.9 = normal range
25–29.9 = overweight/pre-obese
≥ 30 = obese

- Other hormonal tests (e.g. for polycystic ovarian syndrome) are usually directed by the history, but only a very small proportion of people have a secondary cause
- A dietitian should be consulted
- Weight loss of 0.5–1 kg/week is an ideal, but frequently not attainable, goal
- She should be advised to avoid food with more than 2–3 g fat/100 g.
- Exercise such as brisk walking, swimming or cycling is recommended for 30–40 minutes a day on at least five days of the week
- Drug therapy is considered only as an adjunct for patients with a BMI over 30 when other measures have failed.
- Surgery, for example gastric stapling, may be considered for patients with very high BMIs.

Discussion

What are the objectives of the Joint British Societies' guidelines (JBS 2) on prevention of CVD in clinical practice?

The JBS 2, developed by the British Cardiac Society, British Hypertension Society, Diabetes UK, HEART UK, Primary Care Cardiovascular Society and the Stroke Association, promote a consistent multidisciplinary approach to managing established atherosclerotic CVD and those at high risk of developing symptomatic atherosclerotic disease. The objectives are to reduce the risk of a non-fatal or fatal atherosclerotic cardiovascular event, including the need for a percutaneous or surgical revascularisation procedure in any artery territory, and to improve quality and length of life.

Which groups of people should be prioritised for CVD prevention?

JBS 2 recommends that CVD prevention should focus equally on those groups listed in Box 2.15.

Who should have a CVD risk assessment?

All adults aged 40–80 years without a history of CVD or diabetes or not already on treatment for blood pressure or lipids or not in the lower list in Box 2.15 (all of whom should receive professional intervention to achieve JBS 2 targets) should be considered for an opportunistic comprehensive risk assessment in primary care. Younger adults with a family history of premature CVD should also be assessed, arbitrarily defined in relation to coronary heart disease (CHD) as a male first-degree relative < 55 years or

---

Box 2.15 People at high cardiovascular disease (CVD) risk (thresholds for treatment)

1. People with established atherosclerotic CVD
2. Asymptomatic, apparently healthy individuals without established CVD who have a combination of risk factors which puts them at high total risk (estimated multifactorial CVD risk ≥ 20% over 10 years) of developing symptomatic atherosclerotic CVD
3. People with diabetes mellitus (type 1 or 2)

These three groups require professional lifestyle and multifactorial risk factor management to define lifestyle and risk factor targets. In addition, other people with particularly elevated single risk factors also need CVD prevention because they are at high CVD risk regardless of other risk factors:

- Elevated blood pressure ≥ 160 mmHg systolic or ≥ 100 mmHg diastolic, or lesser degrees with target organ damage – retinopathy, micro/macroalbuminuria, raised creatinine, left ventricular hypertrophy
- Elevated total cholesterol (TC) to high-density lipoprotein (HDL) cholesterol ratio ≥ 6.0
- Renal disease
- Familial dyslipidaemia, such as familial hypercholesterolaemia (FH) or familial combined hyperlipidaemia (FCH)

Box 2.16 Five risk factors and total risk prediction

1. Age (< 50, 50–59, ≥ 60 years)
2. Sex
3. Smoking habit history
4. Systolic blood pressure
5. TC : HDL-C ratio (HDL-C assumed to be 1.0 if unavailable)

The estimated probability (percentage chance) of developing CVD over 10 years is referred to as total CVD risk, synonymous with the epidemiological term absolute risk; a total CVD risk ≥ 20% over 10 years is defined as high risk, implying that at least 20 in 100 people with the same risk factors would be expected to develop CVD over the next 10 years.

Box 2.17 Risk factors not included in cardiovascular disease (CVD) risk prediction charts

- Younger adults with a family history of premature CVD (men < 55 years, women < 65 years)
- Obesity (BMI ≥ 30 kg/m²) and especially central/abdominal obesity (waist circumference in whites ≥ 102 cm in men and ≥ 88 cm in women and in Asians ≥ 90 cm in men and ≥ 80 cm in women); this increases the risk of diabetes and CVD
- Low HDL-C (< 1.0 mmol/l in men and < 1.2 mmol/l in women)
- Raised fasting triglycerides (≥ 1.7 mmol/l)
- Impaired glucose regulation (below)
- Premature menopause

In some ethnic groups the charts can under-estimate, or even over-estimate, risk; in people from the Indian subcontinent it is reasonable to assume risk 1.4 times higher than predicted.

---

a female first-degree relative < 65 years. Assessment should be repeated within five years for those found not to be at high risk. Women are at equal risk of CVD as men; it simply tends to present later.

How is risk estimated for people already on treatment for blood pressure or lipids?

Estimating risk is more complicated and on-treatment values tend to underestimate risk. Attempts to do so should be based on pretreatment values or, if unavailable, these should be assumed to have been at least 160 mmHg systolic or at least 6.0 for the total cholesterol (TC) : high-density lipoprotein cholesterol (HDL-C) ratio, rendering risk estimation unnecessary because such individuals qualify as high risk.

Why is total CVD risk preferable to considering single risk factors?

The concept of medical intervention based on estimated total CVD risk in asymptomatic people is now widely accepted in the UK and internationally because CVD is multifactorial, risk factors tend to cluster and co-existent risk factors tend to have a multiplicative effect on CVD risk. Single risk factors in isolation are an inadequate guide to overall CVD risk and the potential benefit from lifestyle and therapeutic interventions. There are exceptions, e.g. when blood pressure is particularly high treatment is required regardless of total CVD risk.

How is CVD risk estimated?

JBS 1 in 1998 used the concept of total CHD risk. JBS 2 replaced CHD with CVD risk – a combined endpoint of CHD (fatal and non-fatal myocardial infarction and new angina) plus stroke (fatal and non-fatal stroke and cerebral haemorrhage) and transient cerebral ischaemia.

Some primary cardiovascular events such as aortic aneurysm and lower limb ischaemia are not included but are a small proportion of all CVD events. The stroke endpoint is based on occlusive cerebral infarction (related to blood pressure and lipids) and intracerebral haemorrhage (related to blood pressure). The JBS 2 prediction chart estimates the total risk in an asymptomatic individual of developing CVD based on five risk factors (Box 2.16).

In the charts, CVD risks of ≥ 10%, ≥ 20% and ≥ 30% are highlighted, equivalent to CHD risks of about ≥ 8%, ≥ 15% and ≥ 23% respectively. Those at highest risk are thus identified and management of blood pressure and lipids is addressed in this overall context such that, for example, the same TC value might qualify for treatment in one individual but not another. Risk factors not included in the CVD risk prediction charts should be considered in assessing and managing a person's overall CVD risk (Box 2.17).

Risk assessment should be repeated within five years in people not found to be at high risk.

What are the advantages of estimating total CVD risk over isolated risk factors?

These are as follows:

- The physician asks 'What is this person's CVD risk?' rather than 'does this person have hypertension or hypercholesterolaemia warranting treatment?'

- The threshold of total CVD risk is based on an integral of scientific evidence
- The absolute benefits of treatments will always be greatest
- Inappropriate treatment of single risk factors in those at low total CVD risk is avoided
- It is consonant with clinical practice, treating the whole person

Are there any potential disadvantages of estimating total risk?

Treatments will tend to focus on older people, especially those aged over 70 years in whom CVD risk is usually $\geq 20\%$, especially for men. Younger people will always be at low total CVD risk over the short term, although may be at relatively high risk relative to peers of the same age. Considering only short-term CVD risk for younger people ignores potential life-years to be gained by treating someone earlier when they are on track to become high risk later in life. Younger people with adverse risk profiles will have a higher CVD risk than predicted when they reach 49 years of age because blood pressure, TC and glucose all rise, and HDL-C falls, with age.

The charts are for three age ranges: < 50, 50–59, ≥ 60 years; however, risks for these are based on ages 49, 59 and 69 respectively. Thus, in the lower two bands, except for those aged 49 and 59, risk will be overestimated, and in the upper band risk will be overestimated for those aged under 69 and underestimated for those aged 70 or over. So projecting CVD risk to 49 years in younger people projects intervention to those at higher risk in this younger age group, while a decision to intervene in older persons requires individual judgement.

Why are JBS 2 guidelines based on Framingham (US) rather than European data?

It might seem logical to base UK guidelines on European rather than US data. But the HEARTSCORE CVD risk estimation based on the SCORE project and on which the Joint European Societies' guidelines are based only predicts fatal CVD, which underestimates the true burden of total CVD based on non-fatal and fatal CVD events.

What are the lifestyle interventions and targets in people with high CVD risk?

Lifestyle targets for all people (not just high CVD risk) are outlined in Box 2.18.

Saturated fat is positively associated with CVD. Polyunsaturated fatty acids of n-6 and n-3 classes are inversely proportional to risk. Linoleic acid is the main n-6, found mainly in vegetable oils. Alpha-linoleic acid is a precursor of the n-3 group, its main source certain vegetable oils – soybean, safflower, linseed oils. Plant stenols or sterols are beneficial. People who regularly eat fish have a lower risk of fatal CHD, including sudden death. A Mediterranean diet is recommended, inclusive of oily fish, but there is no

---

Box 2.18 Lifestyle targets in all people (not just high CVD risk)

- Do not smoke
- Maintain ideal body weight (BMI approximately 20–25 kg/m²) and avoid central obesity
- Keep dietary intake of fat to ≤ 30% of total energy intake
- Keep saturated fats to a minimum (≤ 10% of total fat intake)
- Keep intake of dietary cholesterol to < 300 mg/day
- Replace saturated fats with monounsaturated fats
- Increase fruit and vegetable intake to at least five portions per day
- Aim for a regular intake of fish and other sources of omega 3 fatty acids (at least two servings of fish per week or 70 g; tablets may be considered in those not achieving this following myocardial infarction)
- Limit alcohol to < 21 units/week for men and < 14 units per week for women
- Limit salt intake to < 100 mmol/l per day (< 6 g sodium chloride or < 2.4 g sodium per day)
- Aim for regular aerobic physical activity of at least 30 minutes per day, most days of the week, e.g. fast walking, swimming

---

evidence for supplementation of beta-carotene, antioxidants, vitamins C or E or folic acid.

Energy intake and expenditure balance must be adjusted to achieve a normal BMI. In clinical practice, however, realistic and individual targets should be set for weight loss. With an exercise programme, weight loss of 1–2 kg/month can be achieved by reducing the caloric intake by less than 500 kcal/day below that required for weight maintenance.

Caloric intake is most efficiently reduced by reducing the consumption of high-energy dense foods, especially saturated fats, refined carbohydrates and some alcoholic drinks, and for obese people it is necessary to restrict calories as well. Fat intake should be less than 30% total intake. Foods with high fat content should be replaced with vegetables, fruit and cereal products.

Increasing physical activity can make an important contribution to weight loss, in preserving a stable weight and in preventing weight gain. Most people begin to gain weight again a few months afterwards, and motivation is needed! Although a study confirmed that 30 minutes of moderate-intensity exercise on most days was associated with a reduction in blood pressure and TC and triglyceride levels, 60–75 minutes was required to reduce weight, waist circumference, fasting glucose and low-density lipoprotein cholesterol (LDL-C), increase HDL-C and reduce overall CVD risk.

Anti-obesity drugs include pancreatic lipase inhibitors reducing intestinal fat absorption and those acting in the central nervous system to suppress appetite, reduce food intake, increase satiety or increase thermogenesis. Clinical trials of these medicines are short term and long-term meta-analysis of CVD risk is not known. Research into novel therapeutic targets has produced good news for rats but it may be another 15–20 years before humans benefit.

Obesity guidelines currently recommend that drug therapy be considered in obese people (BMI ≥ 30 kg/m²) or a BMI 27–30 kg/m² with one or more obesity-related disorders.

In short, we need to 'move a little more and eat a little less'.

Is unaccustomed exercise risky?

Platelet activation during unaccustomed exercise causes a 50-fold increase in the risk of sudden death and a 100-fold increase in the risk of acute myocardial infarction.

What are the blood pressure targets in people with high CVD risk?

Targets for blood pressure are shown in Box 2.19.

Lowering systolic or diastolic blood pressure by 10 mmHg or 5 mmHg respectively reduces the risk of CHD by about 25% at age 65.

What are the lipid targets in people with high CVD risk?

Targets for lipids are shown in Box 2.20.

Some statins achieve larger reductions in cholesterol, but that does not mean they are preferred. Simvastatin 40 mg and atorvastatin 40 mg are safe and well tolerated

---

Box 2.19 Targets for blood pressure in people at high risk

- < 140 mmHg systolic *and* < 85 mmHg diastolic
- < 130 mmHg systolic *and* < 80 mmHg diastolic in selected high-risk people (established atherosclerotic disease, diabetes and chronic kidney disease)

Box 2.20 Targets for lipids in people at high risk

- Total cholesterol (TC) < 4.0 mmol/l *and* low-density lipoprotein cholesterol (LDL-C) < 2.0 mmol/l, or a 25% reduction in TC *and* a 30% reduction in LDL-C, whichever achieves the lowest value

  As TC, LDL-C and high-density lipoprotein cholesterol (HDL-C) may fall after an acute CVD event, and triglycerides rise, a random TC is all that is warranted immediately; a full fasting lipoprotein profile should then be obtained after eight weeks.

---

and equivalent in efficacy. Atorvastatin 80 mg and rosuvastatin 40 mg reduce LDL-cholesterol by up to 2.6 mmol/l, but the risk of side effects is greater (e.g. as well as muscle and liver effects, there is concern with high-dose atorrastatin promoting cerebral haemorrhage).

What are the definitions of diabetes mellitus, impaired fasting glucose and impaired glucose tolerance?

Glycaemia is continuously related to the risk of developing CVD. Diagnostic definitions of diabetes mellitus, impaired fasting glucose (IFG) and impaired glucose tolerance (IGT), endorsed by the World Health Organisation (2000), are given in Table 2.13.

Currently, there are no CVD risk assessment models that incorporate glycaemia with other CVD risk factors. A pragmatic strategy is to measure random glucose as part of initial CVD risk assessment. If ≤ 6.0 mmol/l, lifestyle advice is appropriate. If ≥ 6.1 mmol/l, a fasting plasma glucose (FPG) should be checked:

- If FPG is ≤ 6.0 mmol/l, lifestyle advice is appropriate.
- If FPG is ≥ 6.1 mmol/l and ≤ 7.0 mmol/l, it should be repeated or an OGTT performed to confirm IFG or IGT respectively as per the definitions in Table 2.13. Appropriate therapeutic management of blood pressure, lipids and glucose and a repeat CVD assessment in one year are the next steps.
- If FPG is ≥ 7.0 mmol/l, it should be repeated or an OGTT performed to confirm diabetes as per the definitions in Table 2.13. Appropriate therapeutic management of blood pressure, lipids and glucose are the next steps.

What are the blood glucose targets in people with high CVD risk?

Targets for plasma glucose are shown in Box 2.21.

Which drugs reduce CVD risk?

These are outlined in Table 2.14.

Table 2.13 Diagnosis of diabetes mellitus, impaired fasting glucose (IFG) and impaired glucose tolerance (IGT)

	Fasting plasma glucose (FPG)	Random plasma glucose	Oral glucose tolerance test (OGTT)
	The preferred test of the three. Fasting = no calories for at least 8 hours; water is allowed	Plasma glucose at any time	75 mg anhydrous glucose load dissolved in water with plasma glucose two hours later
Diabetes	≥ 7.0 mmol/l plus symptoms (polyuria, polydipsia, weight loss)	≥ 11.1 mmol/l plus symptoms	≥ 11.1 mmol/l
Impaired glucose regulation ('pre-diabetes' or dysglycaemia)	IFG ≥ 6.1 and < 7.0 mmol/l (American Diabetes Association recommends ≥ 5.6 mmol/l)	(if ≥ 6.1 mmol/l check FPG)	IGT ≥ 7.8 and < 11.1 mmol/l
Normal	≤ 6.0 mmol/l		< 7.8 mmol/l

In the absence of unequivocal hyperglycaemia with acute metabolic decompensation or symptoms, one of the three tests should be repeated on a different day to confirm diagnosis.

Why might older patients be at increased risk of CVD?

As well as the higher prevalence of atherosclerosis, ageing is associated with proinflammatory (increase in inflammatory markers, e.g. C-reactive protein, interleukin-6) and prothrombotic (increase in fibrinogen, clotting factors and D-dimer) tendencies.

Should statins be available over the counter?

People at high CVD risk are a medical responsibility, and all drugs, including statins, should be prescribed and monitored by physicians. There is clinical evidence for benefit from statins in people at moderate (10–20%) CVD risk and clinical evidence for as low as 8% CVD risk. So there is benefit in taking an over-the-counter statin for moderate risk, although absolute benefits will be small, but for low

---

Box 2.21 Targets for plasma glucose in people at high risk

- In all high-risk people the optimal fasting plasma glucose is ≤ 6.0 mmol/l and HbA$_{1c}$ is ≤ 6.1%
- In diabetes the optimal targets are 4.0–6.0 mmol/l for fasting or pre-prandial glucose and HbA$_{1c}$ < 6.5%

Table 2.14 Drugs to reduce CVD risk

Strategy	Indication		Therapy
Antithrombotic therapy	Coronary and peripheral atherosclerotic disease		Aspirin 75 mg daily Clopidogrel 75 mg daily if aspirin is contraindicated or side effects Anticoagulation in selected people at high risk, e.g. at risk of systemic embolisation from large myocardial infarction, heart failure, left ventricular aneurysm or paroxysmal tachyarrhythmias
	Cerebral atherosclerotic disease (non-haemorrhagic) – cerebral infarction or transient ischaemic attack	Sinus rhythm	Aspirin 75–150 mg once daily plus dipyridamole M/R 200 mg twice daily, the latter for two years following initial event
		Atrial fibrillation	Anticoagulation if moderate risk (60–75 years without additional risk factor) or high risk (> 75 years, or > 60 years with other risk factors such as hypertension, diabetes or left ventricular dysfunction)
	High risk without established CVD	Total risk ≥ 20% over 10 years	Aspirin 75 mg daily ≥ 50 years (if blood pressure < 150 mmHg systolic and < 90 mmHg diastolic)
		Diabetes (≥ 50 years or disease > 10 years or on blood pressure treatment)	Aspirin 75 mg daily (if blood pressure < 150 mmHg systolic and < 90 mmHg diastolic)
Blood pressure-lowering therapy	Heart failure Left ventricular systolic dysfunction (ejection fraction < 40%) Coronary artery disease if blood pressure not below target of < 130 mmHg systolic and < 80 mmHg diastolic		ACE inhibitor Angiotensin receptor blocker (ARB) possible alternative if side effects with ACE inhibitor
	Stroke Angina or post myocardial infarction unless contraindications, especially if complicated by heart failure or ventricular arrhythmias		ACE inhibitor/thiazide combination (stroke) Beta blocker
	If blood pressure not below target		Calcium channel blocker Diuretic
Lipid-lowering therapy	Established atherosclerotic disease		Statin to achieve targets
	Diabetes	Type 1, or 2 ≥ 40 years	
		Type 1, or 2 18–39 years with at least one of retinopathy, nephropathy, poor glycaemic control (HbA$_{1c}$ > 9%), elevated blood pressure on therapy, TC ≥ 6.0 mmol/l, features of metabolic syndrome or family history of premature CVD	
	Asymptomatic people at high total risk of CVD		
	If targets not achieved		Other lipid-lowering agents considered

risk (< 10%) benefit is not established and must not detract from the importance of a healthy lifestyle. Furthermore, the dose of statin required to significantly impact on CVD risk reduction is simvastatin 40 mg or equivalent, much higher than over-the-counter doses.

What are the indications for angiotensin-converting enzyme inhibitors in CVD?

The role of angiotensin-converting enzyme (ACE) inhibitors in CVD is discussed in Box 2.22.

Can these benefits of ACE inhibitors in CVD be extrapolated to angiotensin receptor blockers?

The place of angiotensin receptor blockers (ARBs) in heart failure and hypertension is discussed in Cases 2.10 and 2.14, respectively. The valsartan antihypertensive long-term use evaluation (VALUE) trial looked at reducing blood pressure in patients at high risk. Valsartan produced a statistically significant (19%) increase in fatal and non-

---

Box 2.22 The role of ACE inhibitors in cardiovascular disease

Angiotensin-converting enzyme (ACE) inhibitors have had proven benefit in chronic heart failure for many years, and also left ventricular dysfunction following myocardial infarction. The vasodilatory and haemodynamic effects (which help prevent remodelling following myocardial infarction, for example) may not be the only benefits. ACE inhibitors may also improve endothelial structure and function with beneficial effects on cytokine profiles, inflammation and oxidative stress, with reduced proliferation of vascular smooth muscle cells, lower risk of plaque rupture and enhanced fibrinolysis.

Heart failure

ACE inhibitors in heart failure are discussed in Case 2.10.

High risk of cardiovascular events

In view of beneficial results in a range of high-risk patients (including those with heart failure, myocardial infarction, hypertension, diabetes, peripheral vascular disease, stroke), the EUROPA trial examined people with stable coronary artery disease (positive exercise tolerance test, angiographic evidence, previous myocardial infarction, coronary revascularisation) otherwise considered to be at low risk and without heart failure. It showed gradual onset and progressive benefit of ACE inhibitors (reduction in cardiovascular death, myocardial infarction or cardiac arrest by 20%), consistent with the ramipril HOPE study, establishing antiatherosclerotic as well as antihypertensive properties of perindopril.

Hypertension

ACE inhibitors in hypertension are discussed in Case 2.14. They may be especially beneficial in younger patients whose hypertension tends to have a high renin–angiotensin–aldosterone drive.

Diabetes

There were 3577 patients with diabetes in the HOPE study and the improvements in microvascular outcomes in HOPE are consistent with other evidence that ACE inhibitors reduce diabetic nephropathy in type 1 and type 2 diabetes and retinopathy in type 1 diabetes (Cases 2.23 and 2.24, respectively). EUROPA showed similar benefits in patients with diabetes.

Stroke

The benefits of ACE inhibitors in secondary stroke prevention were shown in the PROGRESS study (Case 3.27).

---

fatal myocardial infarction and a 13% increase in stroke compared with amlodipine and raised concerns that ARBs might be neutral or even harmful on myocardial infarction rates despite a reduction in blood pressure. Furthermore, the CHARM-alternative heart failure trial showed a significant 36% increase in myocardial infarction with candesartan, the study on cognition and prognosis in the elderly (SCOPE) a non-significant increase and the LIFE study no protection against myocardial infarction despite blood pressure benefits. However, to infer that these drugs may be harmful may be incorrect. In the absence of a placebo in VALUE, it was not possible to say if amlodipine was better or valsartan worse; both drugs could be protective. Other large trials such as OPTIMAAL and VALIANT in patients post myocardial infarction or with heart failure did not show excessive cardiovascular events and a systematic review did not show statistically increased risk with ARBs. However, results from one drug should never be extrapolated to another without caution. However, in ONTARGET (25,620 patients), telmisartan, a modern ARB, was as protective as ramipril (HOPE study) in reducing cardiovascular death, myocardial infarction, stroke, and hospitalisation for heart failure in a broad range of high-risk patients and with better tolerability; patients were already receiving standard care e.g. antiplatelet therapy, statins, antihypertensives.

Can type 2 diabetes be prevented?

Impaired glucose regulation is associated with increased risk of developing diabetes and death from atherosclerotic CVD and all causes. Progression to diabetes can be prevented or postponed by lifestyle intervention, and intensive lifestyle intervention has been shown to be superior to metformin alone. Other measures that thwart progression include acarbose in impaired glucose tolerance and orlistat in obese people with normal or impaired glucose tolerance.

Why do we not all become obese?

The reasons why some people become obese and others do not are complex, but genetics plays a role. Adipose tissue produces the satiety hormone leptin, which stimulates the hypothalamus to produce anorexogenic hormones that in turn decrease appetite and fat mass and interact with various other systems, including the sympathetic nervous system, the thyroid and the gonadal axis. Gene defects such as the OB4 defect impair leptin synthesis and promote obesity but intriguingly therapeutic leptin failed as an elixir for weight loss. Other peptides including ghrelin, adiponectin and resistin have hitherto unknown complex roles in weight homeostasis.

Have you heard of the Polypill?

This combination of three low-dose antihypertensives, a statin, aspirin and folic acid, advocated for all (without contraindications) over the age of 55, all with diabetes over the age of 35 and all with known CVD, could reduce the

---

Box 2.23 Clinical diagnosis of metabolic syndrome

National Cholesterol Education Program (NCEP) guidelines

- Central obesity: waist circumference > 88 cm (women) and > 102 cm (men)
- Blood pressure ≥ 130 mmHg / ≥ 85 mmHg
- Fasting glucose ≥ 6.1 mmol/l
- Serum triglycerides ≥ 1.7 mmol/l
- High-density lipoprotein cholesterol < 1.3 mmol/l (women) and < 1.0 mmol/l (men)

---

risk of CVD events by over 80%. It is not a substitute for lifestyle measures.

What do you know about abdominal obesity and the hypertriglyceridaemic phenotype?

Abdominal obesity, which is closely associated with intra-abdominal or visceral fat (which can be distinguished from subcutaneous fat by imaging) and measured by waist circumference (male > 102 cm, female > 88 cm) or waist:hip ratio, predicts coronary artery disease better than the BMI. Furthermore, abdominal obesity is associated with insulin resistance and predicts the development of type 2 diabetes. High waist and fasting triglyceride measurements – the hypertriglyceridaemic waist – are markers for the metabolic syndrome (Box 2.23).

Homeostasis refers to constancy of the internal environment (negative feedback). Allostasis refers to adaptation of the internal environment to changing conditions (positive feedback). This is the problem with obesity. It engenders the nasty cascade of insulin resistance, hyperinsulinaemia, hypertension, hyperglycaemia, dyslipidaemia and vascular disease and the trouble is that it is too late to treat the end stage, which is when we see it in outpatient clinics and hospitals.

Type 1 diabetes, characterised by loss of beta cell function and endogenous insulin production, carries a two- to three-fold increase in risk of developing CHD and stroke in later life, notably increased if there is diabetic nephropathy. Type 2 diabetes, characterised by insulin resistance and eventual beta cell failure, often occurs in the context of the metabolic syndrome and all patients are at increased risk of CVD, even in the absence of nephropathy.

CASE 2.8

CHEST PAIN AND ANGINA

Candidate instructions

Role

You are a doctor in a rapid access chest pain clinic. Please read the following letter from the patient's general practitioner. You may make notes on the paper provided. When the bell sounds, enter the examination room to begin the consultation.

Scenario

Dear Doctor

Re: Mr John Aubrey, aged 49 years

Thank you for seeing Mr Aubrey, who has type 2 diabetes, used to smoke and has a family history of ischaemic heart disease. His blood pressure is 160/94. His TC:HDL ratio is > 6 mmol/l. He reports recent worsening episodes of chest pain that I suspect are angina and I would appreciate your urgent investigation.

Yours sincerely

Please take a history from the patient (you may continue to make notes if you wish on the paper provided). Your examiners will warn you when 12 minutes have elapsed. You have 14 minutes to take a history from the patient followed by 1 minute of reflection. There will then follow 5 minutes of discussion with the examiners. Be prepared to discuss solutions to the problems posed by the case and how you might reply to the GP's letter. You are not required to examine the patient.

Patient information

Mr John Aubrey is a 49-year-old gentleman who has had chest pains of increasing frequency and severity over the last month. Pains are central and crushing in nature, and have increased in frequency from once or twice a week to almost every day. They always occur on exertion but recently have been provoked by minimal activity such as walking up a few stairs at home. He has a history of diet-controlled diabetes, high cholesterol and high blood pressure, and currently takes aspirin 75 mg, simvastatin 40 mg, perindopril 4 mg and atenolol 50 mg, all daily. He has a sedentary occupation as a cinema projectionist. He lives with his wife and two children, and has not smoked for 20 years. His mother died of a heart attack aged 62 and his father from a stroke aged 78. He is not very concerned about these pains, believing them to be indigestion, as they often seem to come on when he gets up and walks around after a heavy meal.

How to approach the case

Data gathering in the interview and interpretation and use of data gathered

Presenting problem(s) and symptom exploration

▪ **Elicit details of chest pain** Elicit the details listed in Table 2.15.

Ask about rest pain and nocturnal pain.

▪ **Ask about associated symptoms** Ask about dyspnoea, orthopnoea, paroxysmal nocturnal dyspnoea and ankle swelling. Syncope or presyncopal symptoms are unusual

Table 2.15 Details of chest pain

	Suggest ischaemia
Site	Poorly localised retrosternal discomfort
Character	Often described as heavy, pressing, dull, tight or band-like Often patients deny pain and refer to it as 'just a discomfort'
Radiation	May radiate to arms, neck, jaw, gums or abdomen (sometimes these may be the only sites)
Onset	Builds up over minutes
Duration	Episodic rather than constant
Precipitating factors	Exertion Walking uphill Cold air Meals
Relieving factors	Rest Nitrate spray Not relieved by posture or movement

Box 2.24 Canadian Cardiovascular Society classification of angina

1. Angina only on strenuous, rapid or prolonged exercise
2. Slight limitation of ordinary activity (e.g. angina on rapidly climbing stairs or walking uphill)
3. Marked limitation of ordinary activity
4. Inability to carry out physical activity without discomfort (includes unstable angina)

but could represent aortic stenosis or non-sustained arrhythmias or conduction block.

■ **Explore risk factors** These include family history (especially at an early age), smoking, hypertension, dyslipidaemia, diabetes, obesity and a sedentary lifestyle. Emerging risk factors include psychosocial, plasma homocysteine concentration and infection (but no evidence for antibiotic prophylaxis) and inflammation with concomitant fibrinogen production.

■ **Consider the severity of angina** If angina seems likely, consider its severity (Box 2.24).

■ **Consider the differential diagnosis of chest pain** This includes dissecting aortic aneurysm (classically radiating to the back), pulmonary embolus, pericarditis, pneumonia, dyspepsia, cholecystitis, shingles and musculoskeletal pain (including viral disease and costochondritis).

Patient perspective

New angina is often perceived by patients to be 'indigestion', especially if induced by meals.

Past medical history

He has the typical constellation of risk factors for ischaemic cardiac pain.

Drug and allergy history

He is taking appropriate drug therapy to modify cardiovascular disease (CVD) risk but this could be enhanced if unstable angina seems likely, and urgent assessment may well include coronary angiography.

Family history

Family history is very relevant in CVD.

Social history

The sedentary lifestyle is a risk factor.

SUMMARY – ASSESSMENT AND PLAN

- He probably has ischaemic cardiac pain, and the rapid evolution and minimal provocation suggest unstable coronary anatomy.
- If unstable angina is suspected, he should be admitted to hospital.
- An urgent ECG is mandatory, but even if normal, coronary angiography to visualise coronary anatomy with consideration of revascularisation may be preferable to investigations such as exercise tolerance testing.
- He should take a combination of aspirin and clopidogrel, initially 300 mg and then 75 mg daily. Low-molecular-weight heparin is also indicated where clopidogrel is indicated, i.e. for unstable angina or a suspected non-ST elevation myocardial infarction.

Discussion

What is atherosclerosis?

Atherosclerotic lesions or atheromata are asymmetric focal thickenings on the arterial intima comprising cells (blood-borne inflammatory and immune cells, endothelial cells and smooth muscle cells), connective tissue, lipids and debris.

Is atherosclerosis an inflammatory disease?

Inflammation plays a key role in coronary artery disease. Immune cells dominate early atherosclerotic lesions, their effector molecules accelerate progression of these lesions and activation of inflammation can elicit acute coronary syndromes. The inflammatory process may lead to elevated blood levels of inflammatory cytokines and acute-phase reactants including C-reactive protein and interleukin-6 (IL-6).

How do atherosclerotic lesions evolve?

Endothelial activation

Chronic minimal injury to the endothelium is physiological. It occurs at bends and bifurcations of vessels and results from turbulent blood flow. It is enhanced by hypertension and induced by hypercholesterolaemia, tobacco toxins, advanced glycation end products in diabetes and possibly infection. But this minimal injury, sometimes referred to as endothelial dysfunction, encourages low-density lipoprotein (LDL), laden with cholesterol, to enter the subendothelial space and bind to subendothelial extracellular matrix. Here, LDL becomes trapped and subject to oxidation or enzyme attack by resident cells, including endothelial and smooth muscle cells and macrophages.

Chemokines and adhesion molecules

Modified LDL particles stimulate monocyte chemotactic protein 1 (MCP-1) synthesis and release from resident cells. MCP-1 is a chemokine that attracts circulating monocytes; these adhere to the endothelial wall facilitated by adhesion molecules such as vascular-cell adhesion molecule 1 (VCAM-1) before entering the subendothelial space.

Macrophages in the developing plaque

Modified LDL also stimulates macrophage colony stimulating factor (M-CSF) production by resident cells, enabling monocytes to differentiate into macrophages. Macrophages take up the modified LDL, apolipoprotein B100 on LDL being recognised by macrophage scavenger receptors, and become foam cells; these are so named because they have a foamy appearance when laden with fat. This process is critical for development of atherosclerosis. Toll-like receptors also bind with pathogen-like material but, in contrast to scavenger receptors, they can initiate cell activation and may be important in plaque inflammation.

T-cell activation and vascular inflammation

Antigens presented by macrophages and antigen-presenting cells trigger the activation of antigen-specific T lymphocytes in the artery, most of which produce T helper type 1 (Th1) cytokines (e.g. interferon-γ), which activate macrophages and vascular cells, leading to inflammation. Some counter-regulatory Th2 and anti-inflammatory cytokines are also activated (e.g. IL-10, transforming growth factor-β), but atherosclerosis is dominated by a Th1-mediated proinflammatory response. The proinflammatory versus anti-inflammatory balance dictates progression of atherosclerosis.

Types of atherosclerotic lesion

Early lesions, containing foam cells, are common from the first decade. Foam cells eventually undergo necrosis and discharge their fat, together with necrotic debris, into the extracellular space. The earliest atherosclerotic lesion, the fatty streak, has the beginnings of an extracellular connective tissue matrix streaming through extracellular fat, and represents a dynamic balance between entry and exit of lipoprotein, and between development and breakdown of matrix. Essentially, if more lipoprotein exits the fatty streak than enters (e.g. by risk modification), scarring with minimal risk results; if more lipoprotein enters than exits, vulnerable lesions form. These occur as early as the third decade. Vulnerable atheromatous lesions are soft with a core of foam cells and extracellular lipid and a thin fibrous cap. Macrophages and T cells are abundant, particularly in the 'shoulder region' (between evolving plaque and vessel wall), where atheroma grows. More mature lesions contain increasing amounts of connective tissue, derived from proliferating smooth muscle cells migrating from the media to the intima, forming a firmer fibrous cap.

Does infection contribute to atherosclerosis?

Numerous studies have linked infections to coronary artery disease (e.g. *Chlamydia pneumoniae*). It is likely that these are not causative but that the total burden of infection at various sites from various organisms may influence progression of atherosclerosis.

How do atherosclerotic plaques rupture?

Angiographically, small plaques are often the most vulnerable to disruption, provoking thrombus formation with stenosis or total vessel occlusion. Plaque disruption may be passive, in which the thin fibrous cap mechanically erodes, fissures or ruptures, frequently at the plaque's shoulder, or active, in which several cells, including macrophages and T cells, destabilise lesions by producing proteolytic enzymes such as matrix metalloproteinases (MMPs) and cysteine proteases, inflammatory cytokines, coagulation factors, radicals and vasoactive molecules.

How do acute coronary syndromes arise?

Tissue factor (TF) is exposed after plaque rupture and initiates the extrinsic coagulation pathway, and thrombus forms on the disrupted plaque to occlude the vessel. Platelet-induced vasoconstriction can exacerbate vessel occlusion. Angina results when myocardial oxygen demand outweighs the supply that stenosed vessels can provide. Angina may occur when a plaque produces a > 50% diameter stenosis (or > 75% reduction in cross-sectional area). In acute coronary syndromes there is invariably some degree of plaque disruption with superimposed thrombosis and vasoconstriction. The type of acute coronary syndrome depends upon the lesion, the degree of natural reversibility from spontaneous thrombolysis and the degree of safety netting from collateral vessels. Myocardial infarction in patients with no antecedent ischaemia is often more catastrophic.

What mechanisms normally protect against myocardial ischaemia?

Arteriole dilatation (in response to increased energy consumption, mediated by metabolic signals from the myocardium and amplified by nitric oxide), collateral blood vessel formation stimulated by angiogenic signals from the myocardium, arterial pressure (increasing in diastole when most subendocardial coronary perfusion occurs) and possibly preconditioning are all protective mechanisms. This preconditioning refers to the protective effect of brief (minutes) periods of ischaemia in limiting the adverse effects of subsequent ischaemia.

What do you understand by the terms stunning and hibernation?

Contractile recovery from brief ischaemia is usually rapid. Stunning refers to delayed contractile recovery, and represents the combined insults of ischaemia and reperfusion, which itself releases damaging bursts of oxygen free radicals. Patients are at risk of ventricular arrhythmias and heart failure. Hibernation refers to a reduction in contractile performance due to postulated downregulation of myocardial metabolism. In contrast to stunning, it may be protective, limiting the heart's metabolic needs in response to ischaemia. Hibernating myocardium is viable and its contractility can improve following coronary revascularisation.

What do you understand by the terms stable and unstable angina?

Stable angina is characterised by a pattern of symptoms occurring predictably on exertion.

Unstable angina refers to symptoms of recent onset, symptoms increasing in frequency, severity or duration, or symptoms occurring at rest. It suggests plaque instability, and is a medical emergency. All patients with newly diagnosed cardiac pain should presumptively be considered to have unstable disease and be referred for objective assessment of myocardial ischaemia.

Which investigations can identify myocardial ischaemia?

These are listed in Table 2.16.

What are the indications for an exercise tolerance test (ETT)?

These are listed in Box 2.25.

Which features on an ETT indicate a positive test?

An ETT is interpreted in terms of achieved workload, symptoms and ECG response. A 1-mm depression in the horizontal ST segment is the usual cut-off point for significant ischaemia. Poor exercise capacity, an abnormal blood pressure response and overt ischaemic changes are associated with a poor prognosis. Features indicative of a strongly positive test are listed in Box 2.26.

When might a myocardial perfusion scan be indicated?

It may be an initial diagnostic tool for suspected coronary disease in patients for whom an ETT may be less sensitive (e.g. females) or difficult to interpret (e.g. left bundle branch block; LBBB) and for patients unable to exercise. It may also be part of the investigation strategy in patients who remain symptomatic following myocardial infarction or reperfusion intervention.

What are the indications for coronary angiography?

These are listed in Box 2.27.

Which angiographic lesions tend to pose a higher risk?

Certain features suggest higher risk. These include diffuse rather than discrete lesions, eccentric rather than concentric lesions, proximal tortuosity rather than a readily accessible lesion, moderate or heavy calcification and involvement of major side branches.

Box 2.25 Indications for an exercise tolerance test

- Confirmation of suspected angina
- Evaluation of extent of myocardial ischaemia
- Risk stratification after myocardial infarction (but increasingly patients 'go straight to angiography')
- Detection of exercise-induced arrhythmias
- Evaluation of outcome of intervention

Box 2.26 Features of a positive exercise tolerance test

- Exercise limited by angina to < 6 minutes of Bruce protocol
- Failure of systolic blood pressure to increase > 10 mmHg, or a fall with evidence of ischaemia
- Widespread marked ST depression > 2 mm (down-sloping or planar more predictive than up-sloping)
- Prolonged recovery of ST changes (> 6 minutes)
- Ventricular tachycardia

Box 2.27 Indications for coronary angiography

- Coronary artery disease cannot be excluded by non-invasive tests
- Positive exercise tolerance test
- Angina despite maximal therapy
- Prolonged angina with ECG changes
- Post non-ST elevation myocardial infarction
- ST elevation myocardial infarction

Table 2.16 Investigations for myocardial ischaemia	
Exercise tolerance testing	Standardised treadmill
Myocardial perfusion imaging	With radioisotope such as thallium; area of reduced perfusion at stress that normalises with rest indicates ischaemia, while fixed perfusion defect indicates permanent damage
Stress echocardiography	May show wall motion abnormalities under dobutamine stress
Coronary angiography	Gold standard for demonstrating coronary anatomy
Emerging methods	Cardiac magnetic resonance imaging to assess function, mass and volume, and detect infarction and fibrosis Computed tomography to score coronary calcium Myocardial perfusion scintigraphy single photon emission computed tomography (SPECT)

What are the arguments for medical treatment, coronary artery bypass grafting (CABG) and percutaneous coronary intervention (PCI) in chronic stable angina?

Treatment of stable angina aims to limit chest pain and prevent cardiovascular events. Treatment principles are given in Box 2.28.

Do you know of any new drugs in the treatment of chronic stable angina?

I$_f$ inhibitors (ivabridine) block the sinus node directly via an inward depolarising current to produce pure reduction in heart rate. There are no beta-blocking side effects but visual disturbance may occur because I$_f$ receptors are present in the retina.

Fatty acid oxidation inhibitors are still experimental, the rationale being that during ischaemia the heart switches from glucose-based metabolism to energy derived from free fatty acids, which is far less efficient.

Do NSAIDS and COX-2 inhibitors pose a risk in ischaemic heart disease?

Within the lumen, platelet cyclooxygenase 1 (COX-1)-dependent prothrombotic thromboxane-A2 and endothelial COX-2-dependent antithrombotic prostacyclin are balanced and so prevent coagulation. This balance may be disturbed by non-steroidal anti-inflammatory drugs or COX-2 inhibitors and these drugs may be associated with an increased risk of adverse cardiovascular events.

Do you know of any non-pharmacological, non-direct coronary intervention approaches to managing refractory angina?

'Self-management' strategies include cognitive–behavioural therapy, which may induce more favourable cardiovascular physiology, and neuromodulation techniques such as transcutaneous electrical nerve stimulation and spinal cord stimulation. These are, however, expensive and available only in some specialist centres. One technique – enhanced external counterpulsation – applies a series of pneumatic cuffs that sequentially compress the calves and thighs and appears to reduce exercise-induced ischaemic symptoms, but requires up to 30 treatments over a few weeks.

Box 2.28 Treatments for chronic stable angina

- Antiplatelet therapy, beta blockers and statins reduce cardiac events, but only beta blockers also have antianginal effects.
- ACE inhibitors benefit patients at high CVD risk.
- Beta blockers, calcium channel blockers and nitrates provide symptomatic benefit. Verapamil and diltiazem are the first-choice calcium channel blockers in patients in whom beta-blockade is not possible because they are rate limiting, but diltiazem should be used with caution in heart failure, and under cardiologist supervision with beta blockers (verapamil avoided here) because the combination may impair left ventricular function and cardiac conduction. Amlodipine and nifedipine do not limit heart rate and may precipitate reflex tachycardia and angina (especially during exercise) but may be used safely in combination with a beta blocker. Tolerance is a major limitation to the use of nitrates. Nicorandil has nitrate-like properties and activates potassium channels, thereby acting as a balanced coronary and peripheral vasodilator, and reduces both cardiac preload and afterload. It may also reduce coronary events.
- Statins have endothelial stabilising as well as lipid-lowering benefits and should be considered for all patients. They may also promote very moderate regression of atheromatous lesions.

Coronary artery bypass grafting (CABG)

- Trials in the 1970s showed CABG to be more effective in symptom relief than medical therapy. CABG provides a better prognosis in high-risk patients with left main stem or triple-vessel disease or two-vessel disease involving the proximal left anterior descending artery.

Percutaneous coronary intervention (PCI)

- PCI, which includes percutaneous transluminal coronary angioplasty (PTCA) and stenting, is less invasive than CABG but confers a higher rate of angina recurrence (although advances in PCI are continuously improving outcomes and vastly reducing indications for CABG). The re-stenosis rate is lower with stents (10–20%), than with PTCA.
- Adjunctive glycoprotein IIb/IIIa inhibitors have reduced the risk of acute vessel occlusion and the need for rescue CABG. Clopidogrel has been widely used following PCI, with the combined use of aspirin and clopidogrel (in the short term at least) reducing thrombotic complications after stenting.
- Patients with chest pain post stent insertion should be readmitted for ECG and troponin analysis and possible angiography.
- PTCA provides better antianginal effects than medical therapy, but neither PTCA nor medical therapy has a clear advantage over the other in terms of outcome. Future meta-analyses will need to take account of more widespread use in recent years of both statins and stents.

CASE 2.9

ACUTE CORONARY SYNDROME

Candidate instructions

Role

You are a doctor in the emergency medical admissions unit. Please read the following letter from the patient's general practitioner. You may make notes on the paper provided. When the bell sounds, enter the examination room to begin the consultation.

Scenario

Dear Doctor

Re: Mr William Harwood, aged 62 years

Thank you for admitting Mr Harwood, who has had two hours of chest pain this morning. This came on while gardening and did not settle with his usual glyceryl trinitrate (GTN) spray but has now settled with morphine 5 mg at the surgery. He had a coronary stent inserted in his right coronary artery six weeks ago and I am clearly concerned about unstable coronary disease. I have given him aspirin 300 mg. I have taken an ECG which shows T-wave inversion in the inferior leads but I think this may be old.

Yours sincerely

Please take a history from the patient (you may continue to make notes if you wish on the paper provided). Your examiners will warn you when 12 minutes have elapsed. You have 14 minutes to take a history from the patient followed by 1 minute of reflection. There will then follow 5 minutes of discussion with the examiners. Be prepared to discuss solutions to the problems posed by the case and how you might reply to the GP's letter. You are not required to examine the patient.

Patient instructions

Mr William Harwood is a 62-year-old gentleman who has just arrived at the hospital after experiencing angina-like chest pain for two hours this morning. This came on while gardening and did not settle with three sprays of GTN but it eventually settled with morphine at the GP's surgery, to where he managed to drive. He did not want to call an ambulance because he did not want to come to hospital. His wife has severe osteoporosis and has been troubled recently with severe back pain because of a vertebral compression fracture rendering her immobile; she is awaiting a review by the orthopaedic specialist. Mr Harwood is her main carer. He has had a previous heart attack and had a coronary stent inserted in his right coronary artery six weeks ago and knows in himself that there is very likely a problem with the stent because if anything his angina has been worse since it was inserted. He has tried to ignore it, hoping that his medications will work. He was told by the hospital doctor last time that the medications he takes should 'protect the heart' and he had hoped that this would be the case even if he were experiencing pain. He does not smoke. His medications are aspirin 75 mg, clopidogrel 75 mg, simvastatin 40 mg, atenolol 50 mg, ramipril 10 mg, all daily, and GTN.

How to approach the case

Data gathering in the interview and interpretation and use of data gathered

Presenting problem(s) and symptom exploration

The definition of an acute coronary syndrome is given in Box 2.29.

▪ **Ask about the chest pain**   Ask about:

- The site, character (like his usual angina?) and radiation of chest pain
- Its evolution and the duration of symptoms (acute unrelenting pain or intermittent progression?)
- Any precipitating activity
- How it settled (did the GTN have any impact, or was it only the morphine, and has it now settled completely?)
- Its intensity (was this as bad as his original heart attack?)

> **Box 2.29 Acute coronary syndrome – definition**
>
> The term acute coronary syndrome (ACS) refers to a spectrum of presentations caused by myocardial ischaemia that includes unstable angina, non-ST elevation myocardial infarction (NSTEMI) and ST elevation myocardial infarction (STEMI). The embracing term reflects the common pathophysiology of plaque disruption, intravascular thrombosis and impaired myocardial blood supply. However, STEMI is the result of complete epicardial occlusion following plaque disruption and leads to propagation of thrombus and epicardial vasoconstriction but NSTEMI is incomplete and transient epicardial occlusion with platelet-rich thrombus and phasic distal embolisation occurs. Troponin assays have confirmed that many patients with what might have formerly been attributed to unstable angina do in fact sustain myocardial damage and have had a NSTEMI.

▪ **Ask about associated symptoms**   Ask about:

- Dyspnoea, orthopnoea, paroxysmal nocturnal dyspnoea and ankle swelling
- Syncope or presyncopal symptoms (aortic stenosis)

▪ **Ask about progress**   Ask about details of any action/treatment en route to hospital by the ambulance crew and ask what he has been told so far about what is suspected to be wrong.

▪ **Consider the differential diagnosis of acute chest pain**   The differential diagnosis includes all causes of chest pain (Case 2.8), not least dyspepsia from aspirin and clopidogrel. If aortic dissection is considered in the differential diagnosis, immediate imaging with computed tomography/magnetic resonance imaging is needed, a chest radiograph being unhelpful in this context.

Patient perspective

Reassure him that he did the right thing in agreeing to come to hospital, and that while the medications are somewhat protective, if he is having pain it may well mean that there is a problem with one of the arteries that needs urgent attention.

Past medical history

His CVD risk factors will need to be reviewed to ensure optimal medical therapy is on board but immediately he needs exclusion of and presumptive treatment for an acute coronary syndrome.

Drug and allergy history

His medications are all very reasonable.

Family history

There may or may not be a family history of coronary disease, but the relevance of that is historical; he has coronary disease and is by definition at high risk.

Social history

Explore who might be in a position to care for his wife if he is in hospital for a few days.

SUMMARY – ASSESSMENT AND PLAN

- He has had an acute coronary syndrome until proven otherwise.
- He should have routine blood tests, serial ECGs and a troponin level taken at least 12 hours after the time of maximal pain.
- He should be commenced on low-molecular-weight heparin.
- Early liaison with his cardiologist is needed for consideration of repeat coronary angiography.

Discussion

What are the management principles in ACS without persistent ST elevation (non-ST elevation myocardial infarction – NSTEMI)?

Risk stratification and management are outlined in Fig. 2.5.

'Conservative' management involves intensive medical treatment followed by non-invasive risk stratification

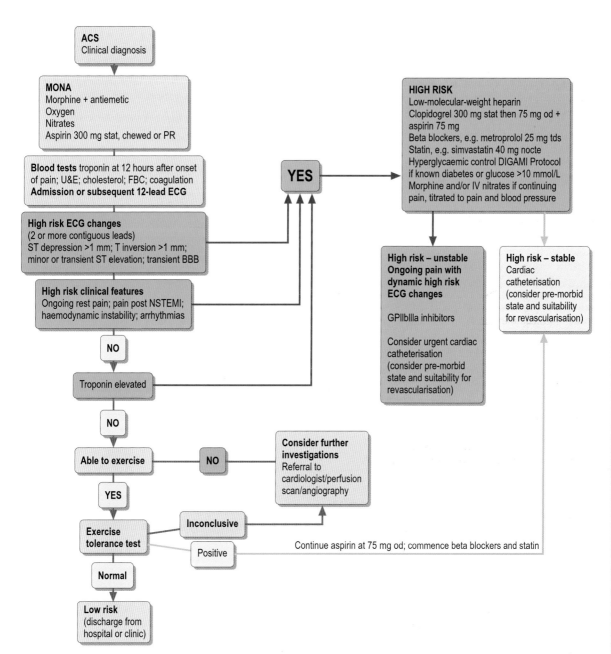

Fig. 2.5 Management of an acute coronary syndrome (ACS) without persistent ST elevation. DIGAMI, diabetes mellitus, insulin glucose infusion in acute myocardial infarction; ECG, electrocardiogram; GPIIb, glycoprotein IIb; FBC, full blood count; NSTEMI, non-ST elevation myocardial infarction; U&E, urea and electrolytes.

investigation (stress testing) to identify patients who may need coronary angiography. Based on TIMI IIIB and VANQWISH data, there was no outcome benefit when an early invasive strategy was used routinely, compared to a selective approach. However, later evidence from trials such as FRISC 2 (Fragmin and fast Revascularisation during Instability in Coronary artery disease 2), TACTICS-TIMI 18 (Treat Angina with Aggrastat and Determine Cost of Therapy with an Invasive or Conservative Strategy – Thrombolysis In Myocardial Infarction 18) and RITA 3 have demonstrated the advantages of an invasive strategy in high-risk patients and no advantage of such a strategy for low-risk patients. It is still not fully clear which patients should proceed to coronary angiography (all or those at high risk) or when coronary angiography should be undertaken (immediately or after a period of 'cooling down' conservative treatment).

What is the Thrombolysis In Myocardial Infarction (TIMI) score (or do you know of any other systems for stratifying ACS risk)?

This is an objective means of risk stratification intended for acute 'through the door' decision-making based on seven variables (Box 2.30). Other scoring systems include the Global Registry of Acute Coronary Syndromes (GRACE) system. Predictors of death in the GRACE system are age, Killip class (heart failure), heart rate, blood pressure, ST deviation, cardiac arrest, raised creatinine or raised cardiac enzymes.

What are the indications for clopidogrel in acute coronary syndromes?

This is indicated with aspirin in high-risk unstable angina or NSTEMI, based on data from the CURE study. The CHARISMA study did not reproduce these results, but was flawed by the inclusion of patients following an acute coronary syndrome (who did benefit from clopidogrel) and those at high risk taking clopidogrel for primary prophylaxis (who did not benefit). Clopidogrel should be continued for 9–12 months at 75 mg daily (as well as aspirin

75 mg daily indefinitely) after the most recent acute coronary syndrome, although the exact timing is unclear. Clopidogrel in addition to aspirin is also recommended in patients as an adjunct to percutaneous coronary intervention (PCI) with stenting, administration of clopidogrel continuing until new endothelium has stabilised the stent (the optimum duration is not clear but 12 months is currently standard).

There is increasing evidence (CLARITY, COMMIT) for the benefit of clopidogrel following ST elevation myocardial infarction.

What are the indications for low-molecular-weight heparin (LMWH) in a NSTEMI?

LMWH is indicated in all NSTEMIs until symptoms have stabilised.

How do antiplatelet agents work?

Aspirin inhibits platelet isoenzyme cyclo-oxygenase 1 (COX-1) leading to suppression of thromboxane production, a potent platelet activator. This action is irreversible but platelet lifespan is approximately 10 days and new recruits continuously exit their bone marrow barracks, hence the need for daily dosing. Thienopyridines like clopidogrel induce irreversible changes in platelet receptor $P2Y_{12}$, a receptor for adenine nucleotides; this mediates inhibition of adenylcyclase activity by adenosine diphosphate, which inhibits platelet aggregation. Since clopidogel and aspirin act on different platelet receptors, dual use may be expected to have additive effects.

Why is LMWH better than unfractionated heparin?

LMWH is as effective, more practical, does not require monitoring and the side effects, such as heparin-induced thrombocytopenia (HIT), are fewer. A mild self-limiting form of HIT is common and a more dangerous immune-mediated form occurs infrequently in patients exposed to treatment for longer than five days.

What are the indications for GPIIbIIIa inhibitors?

GPIIbIIIa inhibitors inhibit the platelet receptor for fibrinogen and hence prevent sandwiching of fibrinogen between platelets and the final common pathway of aggregation. Oral GPIIbIIIa inhibitors have not been shown to be very effective. The drugs in current use are abciximab, eptifibatide and tirofiban. Indications are adjunctively to elective PCI in chronic stable angina, and in high-risk patients with NSTEMI scheduled for PCI. The place of GPIIbIIIa inhibitors in all patients with NSTEMI or unstable angina remains debatable.

What do you understand by the term drug-eluting stent?

PCI drug-eluting stents (DES) reduce the rate of in-stent stenosis and the overall need for further revasularisation. However, they do this at the price of an increased risk of

---

Box 2.30 TIMI Score

1. Age ≥ 65
2. Three or more risk factors for coronary disease
3. More than 50% coronary stenosis on angiography
4. ST segment change > 0.5 mm
5. Two or more anginal episodes in 24 hours before presentation
6. Elevated serum cardiac markers
7. Use of aspirin in seven days before presentation

One point is scored for each variable. The score is interpreted as:

- 0–2: low risk
- 3–4: intermediate risk
- 5–7: high risk

The situation can clearly change in subsequent days; furthermore, some think that troponin concentrations should qualify for more than one point.

stent thrombosis, not seen in bare metal stents. The risk of DES thrombosis is much increased by the premature cessation of dual antiplatelet therapy (DAPT); DAPT is currently recommended for 12 months after DES implantation, and does not seem associated with excessive bleeding, although thrombotic risk appears to continue after 12 months. Stent technology is ever changing.

What issues might be relevant in older patients being considered for PCI?

This is a more heterogeneous population in terms of disease, comorbidity and functional status. Technical issues include the fact that diffuse, multi-vessel disease of calcified, tortuous arteries is more likely. As with many diseases in older people there may be more to gain but more risk.

Why are patients with diabetes at higher risk of an acute coronary syndrome?

Diabetes is associated with risk factors for accelerated CVD and risk of acute coronary syndrome. These include a prothrombotic state mediated by increased plasminogen activator inhibitor 1 and increased GpIIbIIIa receptors, and increased endothelial dysfunction mediated by hyperglycaemia and dyslipidaemia.

What are the causes of a raised cardiac troponin level?

Cardiac causes include myocardial infarction, arrhythmias, coronary vasospasm, cardiomyopathy, myocarditis, amyloidosis, contusion, PCI, surgery and cardioversion/implantable cardioverter defibrillator shocks. Non-cardiac causes include critical illness, chemotherapy, primary pulmonary hypertension, pulmonary embolism, renal failure, subarachnoid haemorrhage, sepsis, stroke and ultra-endurance exercise.

Are other markers of myocardial damage on the horizon?

Troponin testing has improved identification of high-risk patients but there is room for refinement of markers. The vascular inflammation that occurs at the time of an acute coronary syndrome may yield new markers and the CD40 ligand is a marker of future events in acute coronary syndromes. In the MIRACL (Myocardial Ischaemia Reduction with Aggressive Cholesterol Lowering) study patients with a high CD40 ligand level had an event rate similar to those with a low level if they received high-dose atorvastatin.

Which ECG leads are affected in each type of myocardial infarction?

II, III, aVF (inferior leads) indicate right coronary artery (RCA) territory disease. I, aVF, V5, V6 (lateral leads) indicate left circumflex artery (LCA) territory disease. V1–V5 (anterior leads) indicate left anterior descending (LAD) territory disease. Posterior STEMIs can produce reciprocal ST depression in V1–V4 with prominent R waves and/or ST elevation in leads V7–V9 placed horizontally under the left scapula at the level of V4–V6.

What are the immediate management principles in a STEMI?

Immediate management is outlined in Fig. 2.6.

Non-enteric aspirin 300 mg should be given immediately to all patients and continued indefinitely except in those with aspirin allergy who should receive 300–600 mg clopidogrel immediately. Intravenous beta-blockade does not seem beneficial in the revascularisation stage. In the absence of contraindications, reperfusion therapy should be instituted without delay if there is ST elevation, new left bundle branch block or evidence of posterior infarction. Either thrombolysis or primary percutaneous coronary intervention (PPCI) are acceptable. For thrombolysis, a door to needle time of under 30 minutes and for PCI a door to balloon time of under 90 minutes are the aims.

All trials comparing thrombolysis to primary angioplasty (primary PCI), even those involving the transfer of patients to a tertiary treatment centre, have shown superior results with PCI. The benefits may not be so great when compared to pre-hospital thrombolysis. Advantages of PCI include a higher patency rate of the artery, reduced short- and long-term mortality, re-infarction and stroke rates, shorter hospital stay and likely cost-effectiveness.

The REACT (Rescue Angioplasty versus Conservative Treatment or Repeat Thrombolysis) trial has shown that patients do worse with repeat thrombolysis compared with an invasive approach.

Early PCI in cardiogenic shock is also beneficial.

Clopidogrel 300–600 mg initially followed by 75 mg once daily is essential prior to PPCI and is also likely to improve prognosis with thrombolysis therapy.

Are there other causes of ST elevation?

Causes of ST elevation are listed in Box 2.31.

What do you know about right ventricular infarction (RVI)?

The V4R lead and other chest leads placed on the right side of the chest symmetrical to where they are usually placed may help diagnose RVI. V4R should be performed in the setting of an acute inferior territory infarct when it may

---

Box 2.31 Causes of ST elevation

- Normal in 90% of healthy young males – concave elevation 1 – 3 mm in V2 especially or early repolarisation marked in V4 with notching of the J point and tall upright Ts (± reciprocal ST depression aVR); some of these changes are sometimes referred to as high take-off
- Normal variant
- Left ventricular hypertrophy
- Left bundle branch block
- Pericarditis (diffuse)
- Hyperkalaemia
- Brugada syndrome
- Pulmonary embolism
- Cardioversion (transient)

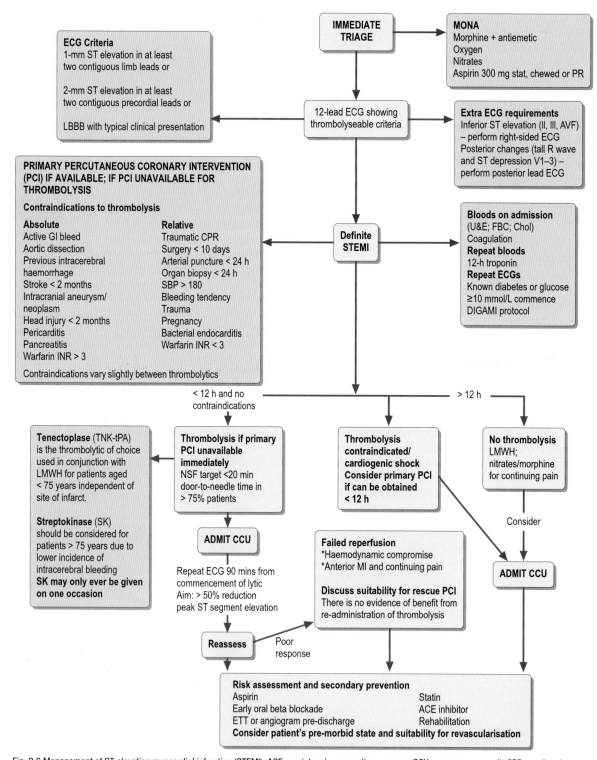

IMMEDIATE TRIAGE

MONA
Morphine + antiemetic
Oxygen
Nitrates
Aspirin 300 mg stat, chewed or PR

ECG Criteria
1-mm ST elevation in at least
two contiguous limb leads or

2-mm ST elevation in at least
two contiguous precordial leads or

LBBB with typical clinical presentation

12-lead ECG showing
thrombolyseable criteria

Extra ECG requirements
Inferior ST elevation (II, III, AVF)
– perform right-sided ECG
Posterior changes (tall R wave
and ST depression V1–3) –
perform posterior lead ECG

PRIMARY PERCUTANEOUS CORONARY INTERVENTION (PCI) IF AVAILABLE; IF PCI UNAVAILABLE FOR THROMBOLYSIS

Contraindications to thrombolysis

Absolute	Relative
Active GI bleed	Traumatic CPR
Aortic dissection	Surgery < 10 days
Previous intracerebral	Arterial puncture < 24 h
haemorrhage	Organ biopsy < 24 h
Stroke < 2 months	SBP > 180
Intracranial aneurysm/	Bleeding tendency
neoplasm	Trauma
Head injury < 2 months	Pregnancy
Pericarditis	Bacterial endocarditis
Pancreatitis	Warfarin INR < 3
Warfarin INR > 3	

Contraindications vary slightly between thrombolytics

Definite STEMI

Bloods on admission
(U&E; FBC; Chol)
Coagulation
Repeat bloods
12-h troponin
Repeat ECGs
Known diabetes or glucose
≥10 mmol/L commence
DIGAMI protocol

< 12 h and no contraindications

> 12 h

Tenectoplase (TNK-tPA)
is the thrombolytic of choice
used in conjunction with
LMWH for patients aged
< 75 years independent of
site of infarct.

Streptokinase (SK)
should be considered for
patients > 75 years due to
lower incidence of
intracerebral bleeding
**SK may only ever be given
on one occasion**

**Thrombolysis if primary
PCI unavailable
immediately**
NSF target <20 min
door-to-needle time in
> 75% patients

**Thrombolysis
contraindicated/
cardiogenic shock
Consider primary PCI
if can be obtained
< 12 h**

No thrombolysis
LMWH;
nitrates/morphine
for continuing pain

ADMIT CCU

Repeat ECG 90 mins from
commencement of lytic
Aim: > 50% reduction
peak ST segment elevation

Failed reperfusion
*Haemodynamic compromise
*Anterior MI and continuing pain

Discuss suitability for rescue PCI
There is no evidence of benefit from
re-administration of thrombolysis

Consider

ADMIT CCU

Reassess   Poor
response

Risk assessment and secondary prevention

Aspirin	Statin
Early oral beta blockade	ACE inhibitor
ETT or angiogram pre-discharge	Rehabilitation

Consider patient's pre-morbid state and suitability for revascularisation

Fig. 2.6 Management of ST elevation myocardial infarction (STEMI). ACE, angiotensin-converting enzyme; CCU, coronary care unit; CPR, cardiopulmonary rescuscitation; DIGAMI, diabetes mellitus, insulin glucose infusion in acute myocardial infarction; ECG, electrocardiogram; FBC, full blood count; GPIIb, glycoprotein IIb; LMWH, low-molecular-weight heparin; NSTEMI, non-ST elevation myocardial infarction; U&E, urea and electrolytes.

Table 2.17 Secondary preventive measures following an acute coronary syndrome

Treatment	Comment
Antiplatelet therapy (aspirin 75–150 mg daily)	Continued indefinitely unless contraindications (plus clopidogrel for 9–12 months after moderate- to high-risk NSTEMI and at least 4 weeks if started after a STEMI)
Beta blocker	Continued indefinitely unless contraindications
Statin	Continued indefinitely unless contraindications Intensive lipid-lowering more beneficial than moderate
ACE inhibitor	All patients indefinitely unless contraindications (angiotensin receptor blockers not used routinely) All should have echocardiogram to assess left ventricular function and exclude mural thrombus
Blood pressure, lipid and glycaemic targets	As for all patients at high CVD risk (Case 2.7)
Mobilisation	Days 2–3, with risk factor modification, lifestyle assessment and introduction to cardiac rehabilitation
Aldosterone antagonists	All patients with LVSD post MI, preferably after institution of ACE inhibitor, from day 3 to 14 indefinitely (spironolactone greatest evidence in heart failure and inexpensive, epleronone some evidence post-MI)
Anticoagulation	Considered for patients with AF, large anterior wall myocardial infarction, severe left ventricular dysfunction or echocardiographic evidence of mural thrombus or left ventricular aneurysm
Implantable cardiac defibrillator (ICD)	Considered for patients at risk of sudden cardiac death (specific indications listed in Case 3.10) Antiarrhythmic drugs other than beta blockers exhibit harm or no benefit.

reveal ST segment elevation that is absent in its usual V4 placement. RCA occlusion usually threatens the inferior wall of the heart. Unlike LAD territory, which supplies much of the anterior wall (scarring of which impairs left ventricular function), RCA territory supplies the AV node in 80% of cases (the circumflex artery supplying it in the remaining 20%) and RCA infarcts tend to cause brady-arrhythmias. Temporary pacing is often life saving but because these arrhythmias often represent reversibly isch-aemic penumbrae, long-term pacing is not inevitable. ST elevation in right-sided leads implies involvement of the right ventricular branch (RVB) of the RCA. This occurs if the RCA occlusion is proximal to its RVB offshoot. An infarcted right ventricle will impair left heart filling and cause hypotension. Bradyarrhythmias will also cause hypo-tension, as will a more extensive infarct with left ventricular involvement, as will hypotensive drugs such as beta block-ers. Unlike most causes of hypotension in the setting of acute myocardial infarction, RVI demands high filling pressures. Fluids, rather than diuretics, are needed to main-tain right ventricular output and left ventricular filling.

Which complications may follow myocardial infarction?

These are listed in Box 2.32.

What are the important secondary preventive measures after an acute coronary syndrome?

Secondary preventive measures are described in Table 2.17.

'Uncomplicated' patients may be discharged from hos-pital at day 5. Patients should mobilise at home for the following week, and gradually increase their exercise there-

Box 2.32 Complications of myocardial infarction

- Arrhythmias (heart block especially in inferior infarction)
- Heart failure/acute pulmonary oedema (especially in anterior infarction)
- Papillary valve rupture and mitral regurgitation
- Septal rupture
- Thromboembolism (AF or mural thrombus)
- Pericarditis/Dressler syndrome (pericarditis, pleurisy and pyrexia)

after. Cardiac rehabilitation programmes are now well developed. An outpatient visit at four to six weeks with consideration of an exercise tolerance test (ETT) is increas-ingly giving way to early coronary angiography before discharge from hospital. Those with ongoing symptoms definitely proceed to angiography.

CASE 2.10

HEART FAILURE

Candidate information

Role

You are a doctor in the medical outpatient clinic. Please read the following letter from the patient's general practi-tioner. You may make notes on the paper provided. When the bell sounds, enter the examination room to begin the consultation.

Scenario

> Dear Doctor
>
> Re: Mrs Julie Havelock, aged 78 years
>
> This lady has become increasingly dyspnoeic over the last six months. She has no cough. She has been sleeping with extra pillows for two months and her exertional tolerance has worsened. She gets occasional angina, relieved with a GTN spray. Her full blood picture, urea and electrolytes, glucose and liver and thyroid function tests are normal. Creatinine is slightly elevated at 128 µmol/l and total cholesterol is 5.3 mmol/l. She takes aspirin, frusemide 40 mg daily and ramipril 5 mg daily. I would appreciate your further assessment.
>
> Yours sincerely

Please take a history from the patient (you may continue to make notes if you wish on the paper provided). Your examiners will warn you when 12 minutes have elapsed. You have 14 minutes to take a history from the patient followed by 1 minute of reflection. There will then follow 5 minutes of discussion with the examiners. Be prepared to discuss solutions to the problems posed by the case and how you might reply to the GP's letter. You are not required to examine the patient.

Patient information

Mrs Julie Havelock is a 78-year-old lady whose main symptomatic problem is shortness of breath. This has been progressive over the past six months, initially just on exertion but now she feels breathless lying in bed without three pillows. She has found it increasingly difficult to walk to the shops over the past six months. She gets very occasional angina on exertion that is rapidly relieved with a spray. This is a problem for her because she does not drive on account of visual impairment from age-related macular degeneration and her husband, who is 10 years older than she, suffers from dementia. She is his main carer. They live in a house with stairs, which she still manages to climb. She has never smoked, but has a family history of 'heart trouble'. There is a parrot at home, which they have had for four years. She is otherwise well but takes a substantial amount of ibuprofen for longstanding back pain.

How to approach the case

Data gathering in the interview and interpretation and use of data gathered

Presenting problem(s) and symptom exploration

▪ **Elicit details of symptoms**   Try to confirm that symptoms are consistent with heart failure rather than other common causes of dyspnoea such as chronic obstructive

pulmonary disease (COPD), recurrent pulmonary emboli, lower respiratory tract infection and pleural effusion/malignancy. Left ventricular systolic dysfunction (LVSD) on an echocardiogram does not exclude alternative causes or the possibility of multiple causes of breathlessness. Hypoalbuminaemia due to liver disease (impaired synthesis) or renal disease (e.g. nephrotic syndrome), lower limb venous insufficiency and drug-induced fluid retention [e.g. non-steroidal anti-inflammatory drugs (NSAIDS), dihydropyridine calcium channel blockers causing ankle swelling] may also masquerade as heart failure. Renal artery stenosis may cause 'flash floods' of pulmonary oedema.

Left ventricular failure (LVF) may result in dyspnoea, orthopnoea, paroxysmal nocturnal dyspnoea, nocturnal cough or fatigue (signs include a third heart sound, tachycardia, hypotension, bibasal crackles). Remember that symptoms that are worse when lying flat do not necessarily imply LVF. Symptoms from gastro-oesophageal reflux disease, postnasal drip and bronchial secretions can also be worse supine.

Right ventricular failure may result in ankle swelling (signs include raised jugular venous pulse, pulsatile tender hepatomegaly, sacral and peripheral oedema).

Biventricular failure leads to both sets of symptoms.

▪ **Establish symptom severity**   The New York Heart Association (NYHA) classification is summarised in Box 2.33.

▪ **Consider causes**   There are many causes of heart failure, although the usual is ischaemic heart disease (Table 2.18).

Patient perspective

Explore her thoughts about the cause of symptoms and her expectations of treatment. What can she no longer do that she would like to do? The impact on the care for her husband is paramount.

Past medical history

This usually unveils some cardiovascular risk factors.

Drug and allergy history

Ask about NSAIDS.

Family history

It is unlikely that this is relevant in this case.

Social history

Exploring support from family, and any need for and her willingness to accept adjunctive support from social

---

Box 2.33 NYHA classification of heart failure symptoms

- I – no limitations
- II – slight limitation of physical activity
- III – marked limitation of physical activity
- IV – symptoms at rest

Table 2.18 Causes of heart failure

Causes		What to ask about
Ischaemic heart disease		Symptoms of angina Risk factors
Pressure overload, especially due to hypertension or aortic stenosis		High blood pressure Valve disease
Volume overload, especially due to aortic or mitral regurgitation		Valve disease
Arrhythmias, especially AF		Palpitations
Cor pulmonale (right heart failure secondary to lung disease)	COPD Parenchymal lung disease Pulmonary emboli	Recurrent multiple pulmonary emboli tend to be underdiagnosed – ask about stepwise deterioration/breathlessness
Cardiomyopathy	Hypertrophic cardiomyopathy Dilated cardiomyopathy, e.g. alcohol, haemochromatosis, diabetes Restrictive cardiomyopathy, e.g. sarcoid, amyloid	Ask if history suggests a possibility, e.g. alcohol
Myocarditis		Ask if history suggests a possibility, e.g. viral illness before symptoms, chemotherapy drugs
Pericardial disease		Ask if history suggests a possibility, e.g. viral illness, tuberculous, connective tissue disease, malignancy
High output failure		Ask if history suggests a possibility, e.g. thyrotoxicosis, anaemia, Paget's disease, left to right cardiac shunts

AF, atrial fibrillation; COPD, chronic obstructive pulmonary disease.

services, occupational therapy (e.g. stairlifts) and of course her GP is pivotal, as is a predictive approach to future care pathways for her husband, with the support of her GP, and possibly community psychiatric services.

SUMMARY – ASSESSMENT AND PLAN

- The blood tests her GP has obtained should be routine. Renal function and albumin should always be part of the assessment of patients with 'heart failure', because fluid overload leading to pulmonary oedema can be the result of renal failure or bilateral renal artery stenosis or, less commonly, hypoalbuminaemia. Urinalysis should also be performed, together with peak flow measurement or spirometry to exclude pulmonary causes.
- The NICE and European Society of Cardiology algorithms for heart failure diagnosis recommend ECG, chest X-ray and natriuretic peptide testing (BNP or N-terminal pro-BNP, where available) if heart failure is suspected on the basis of symptoms or signs.
- If these tests are normal, heart failure is unlikely. If ECG or natriuretic peptide is abnormal, transthoracic Doppler two-dimensional echocardiography should be performed. This is a pivotal test, not just in confirming LVSD and determining the left ventricular ejection fraction (LVEF), but also in detecting/excluding valve disease, assessing cardiac dimensions and excluding intracardiac shunts. The LVEF is determined from the LV end diastolic and LV end systolic dimensions. Normally, it is around 65% or greater. In NYHA class IV disease it is generally < 35%. Frequently, echocardiography excludes heart failure, prompting a search for alternative causes of breathlessness and allowing cardiac drugs to be ceased.

Discussion

What is heart failure?

Heart failure is a complex syndrome resulting from any structural or functional cardiac disorder that impairs the ability of the heart to act as a pump to support physiological circulation, and is characterised by symptoms such as breathlessness and fatigue and signs such as fluid retention. It affects 1–2% of the population (10–20% of the very elderly) and has a poor prognosis with mortality up to 30% in the first three months and 10% per year thereafter. Treatment has the potential to double life expectancy.

What is the pathophysiology of heart failure?

The shape of the normal left ventricle is designed for maximal efficiency of ejection. Remodelling from scarring, hypertrophy (pressure overload) and dilatation (volume overload) compromises this ideal shape, and ushers in a vicious cycle of decreased cardiac output and compensatory neurohumoral stimulation (sympathetic nervous system and the renin–angiotensin–aldosterone system; RAAS) with positive ionotropy, salt and water retention and vasoconstriction. This leads to increased myocardial work, relative hypoxia, cell death and further left ventricular dysfunction. Arrhythmias are more likely. The role of natriuretic peptides (notably B natriuretic peptide – or N-terminal pro-B-type natriuretic peptide) in heart failure and their use as diagnostic markers are of ongoing interest.

Which pharmacological treatments improve the prognosis in LVSD?

Optimal treatments (Box 2.34) serve to modulate the RAAS and up-regulate or re-sensitise beta receptors.

How do angiotensin-converting enzyme inhibitors work?

Angiotensin-converting enzyme (ACE) inhibitors inhibit angiotensin-converting enzyme, which converts angiotensin I to angiotensin II (AII). AII has numerous actions including systemic vasoconstriction and stimulation of aldosterone. ACE inhibitors promote systemic vasodilation, which reduces afterload and preload. This reduces intracardiac pressures and unfavourable ventricular remodelling. Formerly, the combination of nitrates and hydralazine was used to respectively reduce preload and afterload.

Why are ACE inhibitors relatively contraindicated in aortic stenosis?

Reducing afterload increases the pressure drop or gradient across the aortic valve. Reducing preload limits the heart's capacity to compensate by increased cardiac output. Nitrates are thus also contraindicated in aortic stenosis, and antihypertensives other than ACE inhibitors/angiotensin receptor blockers (ARBs) such as calcium channel blockers need to be used with caution.

Box 2.34 Pharmacological treatments in left ventricular systolic dysfunction (LVSD)

Angiotensin-converting enzyme (ACE) inhibitors and angiotensin II receptor blockers (ARBs)

ACE inhibitors improve outcome and should be used in all patients unless there are contraindications (e.g. significant renal impairment or renal artery stenosis). ARBs may be alternatives for patients intolerant of ACE inhibitors. The combination of nitrates and hydralazine remains an alternative for the few patients intolerant of both. ACE inhibitors should be started at low dose and titrated upwards (e.g. at two-weekly intervals) to the target dose provided blood pressure and chemistry allow. Asymptomatic hypotension is usually acceptable if systolic blood pressure is above, say 90–100 mmHg, and symptomatic hypotension may be limited by limiting the use of other vasodilating antihypertensives. Cough occurs in about one-third of patients. A rise in urea, creatinine and potassium is to be expected. A rise in creatinine to 50% above baseline or to 200 μmol/l, whichever is smaller, is acceptable. A rise in potassium to ≤ 5.9 mmol/l is acceptable. Other potentially nephrotoxic drugs should be limited. If greater rises in creatinine or potassium occur the dose of the ACE inhibitor should be halved and stopped if subsequent chemistry shows an unsatisfactory response, and the ACE inhibitor should be stopped without further ado if creatinine rises by > 100% or to 350 μmol/l or potassium to 6.0 mmol/l and chemistry should be monitored until stable.

Loop diuretics

Everyday experience shows that these improve symptoms but there is no evidence for prognostic improvement. They are used for patients with signs of salt/water retention at any stage in the concomitant therapeutic ladder and as first-line in patients with acute pulmonary oedema. Bumetanide 1 mg is approximately equivalent to frusemide 40 mg, and may be metabolically 'cleaner' with a lower risk of gout and glucose disturbance. A thiazide such as metolazone for short-term use (days) may aid large volume fluid loss as adjunctive treatment but often with significant metabolic derangement.

Aldosterone antagonists

Low-dose spironolactone (25 mg, titrated to 50 mg) should be considered for patients who remain moderately to severely symptomatic in NYHA III–IV despite optimal therapy, with careful monitoring of blood chemistry because the combination with ACE inhibitors or ARBs can lead to dangerous hyperkalaemia. If potassium rises to ≥ 6.0 mmol/l or creatinine to > 200 μmol/l spironolactone should be stopped. Breast discomfort or gynaecomastia are potential complications. Eplerenone is beneficial in stable patients with an LVEF ≤ 40% and clinical evidence of heart failure after recent myocardial infarction.

Beta blockers

These improve outcome in patients who have already been treated with an ACE inhibitor but negative ionotropism has the potential for harm and treatment should only be considered in chronic, stable heart failure without clinical or radiological signs of decompensation. The rule is to 'start low and go slow'. Beta blockers may not improve symptoms despite improving prognosis, a fact that should be shared with patients. Bisoprolol starting at 1.25 mg titrating to a target of 10 mg once daily and carvedilol 3.125 mg twice daily titrated to 25 mg (50 mg if mild to moderate heart failure and > 85 kg) twice daily are licensed for treatment and metoprolol succinate also has an evidence base in heart failure. Doses should be doubled at not less than two-weekly intervals, carefully monitoring heart rate, blood pressure and fluid status. If heart rate is < 50 beats per minute the dose should be halved and if more severe deterioration it should be stopped. Drugs that compound bradycardia, such as digoxin or amiodarone, should be used with caution and rate-limiting calcium channel blockers are virtually contraindicated. Rebound worsening of ischaemia or arrhythmias may occur with beta blocker withdrawal.

Digoxin

This should be considered in all patients with heart failure and AF and in patients in sinus rhythm who are symptomatic despite optimal therapy. There is no significant evidence of a survival benefit, but it may reduce hospital admissions.

Aspirin and statin therapy

These are indicated if there is concomitant atherosclerotic arterial disease. There is no evidence for aspirin otherwise in heart failure, and the WATCH study examined aspirin, clopidogrel and warfarin in such patients and failed to find significant differences in endpoints other than a trend favouring warfarin in non-fatal stroke. Heart failure patients were excluded from many statin trials, and there is no evidence for statin use in heart failure, and indeed some data even suggests that cholesterol may be beneficial, perhaps by mopping up endotoxin. This illustrates the dangers of extrapolating results from trials to different populations. The CORONA trial will address statin use in heart failure.

Anticoagulation

This is indicated in AF and in sinus rhythm with a history of thromboembolism, left ventricular aneurysm or intracardiac thrombus.

Why are ACE inhibitors relatively contraindicated in renal artery stenosis?

Numerous molecules act on the afferent and efferent arterioles in the kidney to maintain glomerular filtration rate. Angiotensin II (AII) is activated by reduction in renal artery perfusion pressure, via the RAAS. AII promotes renal vasoconstriction (of the afferent and efferent arterioles, the efferent arteriole being especially important because it constricts to maintain intraglomerular pressure). ACE inhibitors (and ARBs) promote afferent and efferent arteriole vasodilation. In renal artery stenosis, the efferent arteriole dilates increasing 'run-off' in the setting of a reduced afferent supply. Blood effectively bypasses the glomerulus. This concept is explained more fully in Case 2.26.

When might you suspect renal artery stenosis clinically?

The presence of a renal bruit (epigastric or loin) is helpful. Peripheral vascular disease may be surrogate evidence.

How do ARBs work?

ACE inhibitors effectively act as a 'dam' to the production of AII, which gives rise to two potential problems:

- Accumulation of substrates such as bradykinin, which promote cough, potential angioedema and other side effects (it is unclear whether all substrates which build up are potentially harmful or whether indeed some may confer benefit).
- Alternative ways 'around the dam' to promote AII.

ARBs provide a molecular spanner limiting the effects of AII. However, numerous AII receptor sites have been identified in humans, including AT_1 and AT_2. Blocking AT_1 appears to be important in treating heart failure, whereas AT_2 may have important endothelial roles whose blockade may be best avoided. Selective ARBs may be developed in future. ACE inhibitors and ARBs may be used in combination, but with beta blockers the triple combination is potentially dangerous.

Should ACE inhibitors and ARBs be used in combination?

The CHARM study programme of 7601 patients using candesartan compared with placebo in a broad range of patients with heart failure irrespective of systolic function or background therapy, had three facets.

- In CHARM Alternative (LVEF ≥ 40%, patients intolerant of ACE inhibitors) there was unequivocal (23%) risk reduction in cardiovascular death or hospitalisation from heart failure.
- In CHARM Added (LVEF ≥ 40%, patients on ACE inhibitors for at least 30 days) there was a small but significant (15%) risk reduction in cardiovascular death or hospitalisation from heart failure, but no

effect on all-cause mortality. Benefit was also seen in patients taking a beta blocker, contrasting with previous data suggesting that the triple combination of ACE inhibitor, ARB and beta blocker was associated with adverse outcomes.

- In CHARM Preserved (LVEF > 40%, history of hospitalisation for a cardiac reason with or without current use of ACE inhibitor) there was a trend towards reduction in cardiovascular death or hospitalisation from heart failure.

There is general consensus that ARBs should be used in heart failure in patients intolerant of ACE inhibitors but combination therapy is more contentious.

How do beta blockers work in heart failure?

Beta blockers reduce sympathetic drive on the heart. In chronic heart failure, cardiac β-receptors are down-regulated, but $β_2$-receptors to a lesser extent than $β_1$. It might, therefore, be that $β_2$-receptors are relatively more active in heart failure than in the normal heart, and that non-selective beta blockers are preferable to $β_1$-selective drugs. The Carvedilol Or Metoprolol European Trial (COMET) compared metoprolol (a $β_1$-selective blocker) with carvedilol (a non-specific beta blocker that blocks both $β_1$ and $β_2$ and that has α-blocking effects). Carvedilol produced a striking reduction in all-cause mortality, favouring non-selective blockade, but there has been concern that the dose and formulation of metoprolol used in COMET was different to that in the MERIT-HF study, which showed the benefit of metoprolol. Bisoprolol is a selective $β_1$ blocker.

How does spironolactone work in heart failure?

Spironolactone inhibits aldosterone but also seems to reduce cardiac filling pressures and stiffness and enhance compliance. The RALES trial demonstrated the benefit of spironolactone in heart failure and EPHESUS showed that the aldosterone antagonist eplerenone improved outcome in LVSD following myocardial infarction.

List some non-pharmacological interventions you might consider for a patient with LVSD

- Management of other modifiable risk factors (smoking cessation, hypertension, diabetes)
- Stopping drugs which precipitate fluid retention (e.g. NSAIDs, corticosteroids, calcium channel blockers) or depress myocardial function
- Salt restriction (ready-to-cook meals and convenience foods have a high salt content)
- Fluid intake restriction to 1.5–2 litres daily in advanced heart failure
- Exercise
- Weight reduction (unless cardiac cachexia)
- Vaccination (influenza annually; pneumonococcal once only)

Table 2.19 Comparison of systolic and diastolic heart failure

	Systolic heart failure	Diastolic heart failure
Demographics	More often male, typically elderly	Frequently female, usually elderly
LV ejection fraction	Reduced	Normal, $\geq 40\%$
LV cavity size	Usually dilated	Usually normal
LV hypertrophy	Sometimes hypertrophy	Usually concentric hypertrophy
Gallop rhythm	S3	S4
Causes/ associations	Typically due to ischaemic heart disease with associated risk factors	As for systolic heart failure, but associated especially with LV hypertrophy (hypertension; aortic stenosis), hypertrophic cardiomyopathy, restrictive cardiomyopathy, obesity, chronic lung disease, sleep apnoea and long-term dialysis
LV, left ventricular.		

The role of CABG revascularisation in patients with heart failure from coronary disease is uncertain, and the HEART-UK study aims to further inform in the setting of angina and heart failure. Underlying precipitants such as anaemia may need to be corrected. Heart failure is frequently associated with anaemia of chronic disease.

What is the role of biventricular pacing in heart failure?

In many failing hearts, parts of the left ventricle contract after aortic valve closure, increasing oxygen demand without doing useful work. Pacing both ventricles can resynchronise contraction, an approach that may reduce mortality, as suggested in the COMPANION study. Further, it appears that pacing solely the right ventricular apex may be deleterious in patients with heart failure. Implantable cardioverter defibrillators (ICDs) can reduce mortality in survivors of cardiac arrest due to ventricular tachycardia or ventricular failure and in patients with arrhythmogenic poor left ventricular function (LVEF < 35%) and may be combined with atrio-biventricular pacing. However, such an approach is costly (and accessing the left ventricle is much more tricky than the right) and attempts to stratify those at higher risk are being made (e.g. those with T wave alterans may be at higher risk). NICE guidelines recommend cardiac resynchronisation therapy (CRT, see also Case 3.10) for patients with moderate to severe heart failure with LBBB and LVEF < 35% who are taking optimal drug therapy, sometimes in conjunction with an implantable cardiac defibrillator.

How might you differentiate between heart failure and cor pulmonale in a patient with significant peripheral oedema?

A history of COPD, a bounding pulse and warm peripheries favours the latter; heart failure is often associated with cool peripheries.

What is diastolic dysfunction or diastolic heart failure?

Heart failure usually involves left ventricular contractile or systolic dysfunction (LVSD). Diastolic dysfunction occurs when the ventricle resists filling. A stiff ventricle causes compensatory atrial hypertrophy with a fourth heart sound (S4). Causes of diastolic dysfunction include severe left ventricle hypertrophy (hypertension in the elderly the most common cause; aortic stenosis), hypertrophic cardiomyopathy and restrictive cardiomyopathy. A comparison of systolic and diastolic heart failure is given in Table 2.19.

Most patients, however, with a clinical diagnosis of heart failure but preserved LVSD will have an alternative explanation for their symptoms such as obesity, lung disease or myocardial ischaemia. Treatments suitable for LVSD cannot be extrapolated to diastolic heart failure.

CASE 2.11

PALPITATIONS

Candidate information

Role

You are a doctor in the medical outpatient clinic. Please read the following letter from the patient's general practitioner. You may make notes on the paper provided. When the bell sounds, enter the examination room to begin the consultation.

Scenario

Dear Doctor
Re: Mr Walter Cartwright, aged 74 years
Thank you for seeing this gentleman with a two-month history of intermittent, fast palpitations.

Episodes occur without warning, and during these he feels dizzy but has never lost consciousness. He has a history of ischaemic heart disease and I wonder if he is now describing paroxysmal atrial fibrillation. Past medical history comprises asbestosis with a mild restrictive picture (under annual review at the respiratory clinic) and giant cell arteritis diagnosed a year ago, under control on prednisolone 5 mg daily. He also takes aspirin, atenolol 50 mg daily (for infrequent angina), simvastatin 40 mg daily, alendronate and calcium/vitamin D. He lives with his wife and is an ex-smoker. On examination his heart rate is 44 beats per minute (his ECG shows sinus rhythm), blood pressure is satisfactory at 146/84, heart sounds are present with no murmurs and he has scattered chest crackles consistent with asbestosis. I would value your advice as to a need for a further investigation of his palpitations.

Yours sincerely

Please take a history from the patient (you may continue to make notes if you wish on the paper provided). Your examiners will warn you when 12 minutes have elapsed. You have 14 minutes to take a history from the patient followed by 1 minute of reflection. There will then follow 5 minutes of discussion with the examiners. Be prepared to discuss solutions to the problems posed by the case and how you might reply to the GP's letter. You are not required to examine the patient.

Patient information

Mr Walter Cartwright is a 74-year-old gentleman who for the last two months has experienced episodes of fast, regular palpitations. He also experiences light-headedness, but has never lost consciousness. These differing episodes do not always occur together, and can occur at any time of day, at rest or during exercise. He has even been aware of symptoms in bed. He has a past medical history of chronic stable angina and asbestos-related lung disease with minor reduction in lung capacity. An ex-smoker of 40 cigarettes per day, he seldom drinks alcohol, takes moderate caffeine and is fully independent, living with his wife in their two-bedroom house. He has no real concerns and will be happy to be 'dismissed' without further tests.

How to approach the case

Data gathering in the interview and interpretation and use of information gathered

Presenting problem(s) and symptom exploration

■ **Consider possible causes** Palpitations are common, and many patients do not have a proven cardiac arrhythmia.

Older patients are more likely to have structural heart disease provoking atrial fibrillation (AF) or (non-sustained) ventricular tachycardia (VT). An older man with ischaemic heart disease and left ventricular dysfunction with intermittent fast, regular palpitations is more likely to have VT. Irregular palpitations may indicate AF. A 40-year-old woman with irregular, fast palpitations at rest and on exertion, who also feels sweaty, should be checked for thyrotoxicosis.

Younger patients are more likely to be describing sinus tachycardia or supraventricular tachycardia (SVT). Symptomatic ventricular ectopic beats (VEBs) are extremely common. Sinus tachycardia may be the result of anxiety, thyrotoxicosis, phaeocromocytoma or sympathomimetic drugs. A 30-year-old woman with fast, regular palpitations lasting several minutes to several hours is most likely describing SVT, and the baseline ECG may show evidence of Wolff–Parkinson–White syndrome but will more likely be normal. Ambulatory ECG monitoring is indicated unless there is a clear precipitant such as caffeine or alcohol. A 25-year-old man with a history of feeling that his heart 'misses a beat', and whose episodes last a few seconds, often before falling asleep, is probably describing occasional ventricular or supraventricular ectopic beats, and can be reassured if there are no clinical signs of structural heart disease.

■ **Elicit details of the palpitations** Ask:

- If these are regular (sinus tachycardia, SVT, VT) or irregular (AF, VEBs); patients can sometimes tap out the beat
- If these are fast (sinus tachycardia, AF, atrial flutter, SVT, VT) or slow
- If these are intermittent or persistent; if intermittent, ask about the frequency of attacks, abruptness of onset of each attack and duration of each attack
- For how long attacks have been recurring (since childhood suggests SVT)
- If there are any trigger or relieving factors such as exercise, caffeine, alcohol or drugs

■ **Ask about associated symptoms** Ask about chest pain, dyspnoea and syncope.

■ **Ask about risk factors for AF** These include coronary heart disease, hypertension, valvular heart disease (history of rheumatic fever), alcohol intake and thyrotoxicosis.

Patient perspective

He may have no particular concerns but that should not dissuade you from recognising that he could be describing tachyarrhythmias with or without significant sinus pauses warranting an implantable cardiac defibrillator or pacemaker.

Past medical history

The history of ischaemic heart disease should alert you to episodes of AF or VT or a tachy–brady syndrome.

Drug and allergy history

Antihypertensive drugs, notably calcium channel blockers, may precipitate reflex tachycardia. Ask if any drug treatments have been tried for the palpitations.

Family history

This can be very relevant in younger patients with inherited structural heart disease (e.g. hypertrophic cardiomyopathy) or an inherited conduction disturbance.

Social history

Explore the impact of his symptoms on his daily routine, notably driving.

SUMMARY – ASSESSMENT AND PLAN

- When palpitations are the primary symptoms, the most useful tests are a 12-lead ECG and ECG monitoring (exercise ECG testing if symptoms are produced on exercise). Echocardiography is unlikely to add information if clinical examination and the ECG are normal.
- This patient should have routine blood chemistry including potassium, magnesium and calcium levels, a 12-lead ECG and an ambulatory ECG recording (a patient-activated event recorder if episodes are sufficiently infrequent that 24–48-hour measurement is unlikely to capture any disturbance).
- He is likely to have sick sinus or 'tachy–brady' syndrome, ischaemic disturbance of the sinus node and its pathways. Presyncopal episodes are more likely to be the result of bradyarrhythmias than AF, although non-sustained VT is a possibility. Sinus pauses of three or more seconds warrant a permanent pacemaker, as may shorter pauses that are symptomatic. Atenolol should be stopped but if there is combined tachy–brady disturbance beta blockers may be a necessary adjunct to a pacemaker.

Discussion

List some types of tachyarrhythmia

- Atrial fibrillation
- Atrial flutter
- Atrial ectopy (focal/multifocal)
- Atrioventricular re-entry tachycardia (overt accessory pathway as in Wolff–Parkinson–White syndrome/concealed accessory pathway)
- Atrioventricular nodal (junctional) re-entry tachycardia
- Ventricular tachycardia

How may SVT arise in Wolff–Parkinson–White (WPW) syndrome?

WPW syndrome is caused by an accessory conduction pathway that bypasses the atrioventricular node (AVN).

The accessory pathway may not always conduct and so the ECG may be intermittently normal. When it does conduct, impulses reach the ventricle from both the accessory pathway and the AVN. Impulses via the accessory pathway are faster than those through the AVN, giving rise to the delta wave on the ECG (pre-excitation). This does not usually provoke tachycardia.

There may, however, be retrograde conduction through the accessory pathway. This can arise during the transient window of opportunity when the accessory pathway is refractory (having delivered its impulses to the ventricle), and the slower AVN pathway is still conducting (an extrasystole is a common precursor, because it delays AVN conduction). At this time, AVN impulses may loop back up into the accessory pathway, setting up a loop of continuous conduction, which results in a re-entry SVT.

This antegrade conduction through the AV node and retrograde conduction through the accessory pathway is termed orthodromic conduction and produces a narrow complex tachycardia. Less commonly, conduction is down the accessory pathway, termed antedromic conduction, producing a broad complex tachycardia. These types of SVT are referred to as atrioventricular re-entrant tachycardias (AVRTs).

How may SVT be treated?

Vagal manoeuvres (carotid sinus massage, Valsalva manoeuvre) or adenosine (3 mg then 6 mg then 12 mg) may terminate SVT by transiently blocking the AV node. Adenosine should be used with caution in COPD and is contraindicated in asthma. Verapamil 5 mg intravenously over 1 minute, repeated once if necessary, is an alternative regimen. Beta blockers may be used.

Why is digoxin contraindicated in WPW syndrome?

AF occurs in up to 15% of patients with WPW. Digoxin must never be used because it decreases the refractory period of the accessory pathway and allows rapid antegrade conduction from atrium to ventricle. The very fast ventricular rate may degenerate to ventricular fibrillation.

What other types of SVT are there?

The AVN itself may contain both a slow and fast pathway and other SVTs may arise through the ability of the AVN to conduct in an antegrade direction down one of these and a retrograde along the other, giving rise to atrioventricular nodal re-entry tachycardias (AVNRTs).

SVT is common in patients without structural aberrations in whom there may be numerous triggers such as caffeine or alcohol.

Which clinical or ECG features can help to determine whether a broad complex tachycardia is the result of VT or SVT with aberrant conduction?

VT is suggested by:

- History of ischaemic heart disease (the strongest predictive factor)
- QRS > 140 milliseconds

- Capture or fusion beats (intermittent sinoatrial beats, or sinoatrial beats fused with ventricular beats)
- Concordance in precordial leads (all of the V lead complexes point in the same direction)
- Absence of bundle branch block on a previous ECG in sinus rhythm

How might you manage VT?

If well tolerated, amiodarone or lignocaine may terminate it. Urgent DC cardioversion is required in cardiogenic shock. Torsades de pointes VT should be distinguished from polymorphic VT with a normal QT interval, the latter treated as standard VT but QT prolonging anti-arrhythmics (class 1A, 1C and 3) contraindicated in torsades; intravenous magnesium, overdrive ventricular pacing and beta-blockade may be required. If VT continues, intra-aortic balloon counterpulsation/angiography/VT ablation may be necessary.

What may cause bradycardia?

Causes include acute ischaemia or chronic degeneration of conducting pathways, metabolic disturbances, hypothermia, hypothyroidism, beta blockers, digoxin, verapamil, diltiazem and Lyme disease.

What is meant by the term sudden cardiac death (SCD)?

SCD refers to death from a cardiac cause within one hour of symptoms without a known prior condition. Sixty per cent of all cardiac death is SCD, with a male to female ratio of 4:1. Causes include:

- Coronary heart disease (80%)
- Myocarditis
- Cardiomyopathies, e.g. hypertrophic cardiomyopathy
- Ventricular dysplasia, e.g. arrhythmogenic right ventricular cardiomyopathy (ARVC)
- Mitral valve prolapse
- Congenital heart disease
- Primary arrhythmias (below)
- 'Non-cardiac' causes (e.g. subarachnoid haemorrhage, aortic rupture, iatrogenic, drug overdose)

Athletes may develop left ventricular hypertrophy or dilatation that can be difficult to distinguish from a minor degree of hypertrophic cardiomyopathy.

What are the causes of SCD in young people?

The majority of these deaths are still the result of coronary heart disease. In some cases there is no evidence of a structural cardiac abnormality and the cause of death is unascertainable at autopsy. The term sudden arrhythmic death syndrome (SADS) is sometimes used, and the underlying causes of sudden death in individuals with morphologically normal hearts include WPW syndrome and the ion channelopathies:

- Long QT syndrome (LQTS), an inherited repolarisation disorder causing QT prolongation (QTc > 440 ms) and risk of ventricular arrhythmias (torsade de pointes 'twisting of points'). Torsade de pointes may also be caused by metabolic disturbances and drugs.
- Brugada syndrome, a disorder of abnormal potassium/sodium channelling within the sarcolemma causing right bundle branch block and ST elevation in V1–3 with a risk of polymorphic VT. Three types of Brugada syndrome may occur, and the ECG abnormality may only be evident with exercise.
- Progressive cardiac conduction disease, a disorder causing variable degrees of heart block.
- Catecholaminergic polymorphic ventricular tachycardia, a disorder of cellular calcium handling causing exertional ventricular arrhythmias.

These are potentially inherited disorders and relatives of affected family members may be at risk.

How might family members of victims of SCD be evaluated?

Investigations are largely to exclude coronary heart disease (CHD) and may include identification of risk factors (hypertension, dyslipidaemia, smoking, diabetes, early family history), exercise tolerance testing – the best predictors of CHD being chest pain, poor exercise duration (< 5 minutes) and typical ECG changes, echocardiography, nuclear cardiography, coronary angiography, electrophysiological studies, high-speed computed tomography scanning/magnetic resonance angiography/positron emission tomography scanning and coronary calcium scoring. Genotyping of families with LQTS, Brugada syndrome and hypertrophic obstructive cardiomyopathy may allow confirmation of diagnosis and clarification of carrier status, and may sometimes guide therapy – for example beta blockers and/or implantable cardiac defibrillators in LQTS. Limited knowledge of the full genetics of these disorders, however, renders negative results unhelpful.

Can coronary heart disease occur with angiographically normal coronary arteries?

Microvascular coronary artery disease may cause angina, and a syndrome, more common in females, giving rise to a functional change with small coronary arteries, is recognised. Coronary artery spasm (Prinzmetal's angina) is very rare.

What are the indications for an electrophysiological study?

Persistent palpitations, recurrent syncope or presyncope with impaired left ventricular function are symptoms suitable for investigation. Radiofrequency ablation – accessory pathways, junctional tachycardias, atrial flutter, atrial fibrillation, and investigation of narrow or broad complex arrhythmias, with or without radiofrequency ablation, are other indications.

Which treatments may be considered for patients at risk of SCD?

Treatments for coronary heart disease are by far the biggest intervention overall. Indications for implantable cardioverter defibrillators (ICDs) are outlined in Box 3.15, Case 3.10.

For patients with VT for whom ICD insertion is not contemplated, antiarrhythmic therapy (amiodarone or beta blocker) is a second choice. Prophylactic use of an ICD in high-risk patients (LVEF $\leq 35\%$ and impaired cardiac autonomic function manifested as depressed heart rate variability or an elevated average heart rate) who have recently had a myocardial infarction does not reduce overall mortality – reduction in arrhythmic death is offset by increased non-arrhythmic death.

Percutaneous interventional electrophysiology is an expanding cardiac subspecialty.

Cardiac surgery may be indicated, notably coronary artery bypass grafting (CABG) for coronary disease and valve replacement for valvular heart disease. Cardiac surgery carries a higher risk if there is left ventricular dysfunction, hypertension, renal failure or carotid disease. Patients aged over 80 years have a significant immediate risk of death from cardiac surgery (up to 10%), but, for example, a history of blackouts attributable to aortic stenosis may confer an 80% risk of death within the next year and patients with symptomatic valve disease and no significant co-morbidity should be referred for consideration of surgery. CABG benefit is harder to prove, except for left main stem disease, three-vessel disease and proximal left anterior descending artery disease (less evidence).

CASE 2.12

ATRIAL FIBRILLATION

Candidate information

Role

You are a doctor in the emergency medical admissions unit. Please read the following letter from the patient's general practitioner. You may make notes on the paper provided. When the bell sounds, enter the examination room to begin the consultation.

Scenario

Dear Doctor

Re: Mrs Dorothy Brooks, aged 78 years

This 78-year-old lady presents with fast palpitations and an irregular pulse. Her current ECG shows atrial fibrillation (AF) but she was in sinus rhythm last year when admitted with chest pain under your team's care. Her current medications are aspirin, atenolol 25 mg, simvastatin 20 mg and ramipril 5 mg, all daily. She experiences intermittent palpitations but is otherwise well. I wonder if she has paroxysmal AF and whether or not she should be considered for anticoagulation.

Yours sincerely

Please take a history from the patient (you may continue to make notes if you wish on the paper provided). Your examiners will warn you when 12 minutes have elapsed. You have 14 minutes to take a history from the patient followed by 1 minute of reflection. There will then follow 5 minutes of discussion with the examiners. Be prepared to discuss solutions to the problems posed by the case and how you might reply to the GP's letter. You are not required to examine the patient.

Patient information

Mrs Dorothy Brooks is a 78-year-old lady who has just been admitted to hospital with fast palpitations. She has had numerous episodes of irregular, fast palpitations over the last year since being admitted to hospital a year ago with a non-ST elevation myocardial infarction. She experiences no ongoing chest pains but does feel moderately breathless if the episodes last for more than an hour or so. Episodes have no diurnal pattern or obvious precipitant. She is usually well although sometimes has hot flushes during which she feels hot and sweaty. She takes aspirin 75 mg, atenolol 25 mg, simvastatin 20 mg and ramipril 5 mg, daily. Otherwise, she has no significant past medical history of note. She is widowed and lives with her cat. She smoked many years ago and does not drink. She has no particular concerns.

How to approach the case

Data gathering in the interview and interpretation and use of information gathered

Presenting problem(s) and exploration of symptoms

The history should follow similar lines to that in Case 2.11. In addition, explore the reasons AF matters to patients and physicians, namely its causes, symptoms and complications.

■ **Explore symptoms** Atrial fibrillation may result in any of the symptoms listed in Box 2.35.

These symptoms occur due to loss of atrial systole/atrioventricular asynchrony (which reduces left ventricular filling and so cardiac output by up to 50%), variable stroke volume (a slow rate allows a longer filling time and thus

Box 2.35 Symptoms of atrial fibrillation

- No/minimal symptoms
- Palpitations
- Dyspnoea (exertional or other)
- Fatigue/reduced exercise capacity
- Presyncope/syncope
- Complications

Box 2.36 Complications of atrial fibrillation

- Thromboembolism
- Impaired left ventricular systolic function (heart failure)

Box 2.37 Leading causes of atrial fibrillation

- Coronary heart disease
- Valvular heart disease
- Hypertensive heart disease
- Alcohol
- Thyrotoxicosis (but also any dysthyroid state)

    Other important causes are infection, chronic respiratory disease, pulmonary embolus, high caffeine supplements, sinus node disease due to fibrosis, Wolff–Parkinson–White syndrome, cardiomyopathy, myocarditis and really any structural heart defect. Where absolutely no cause can be identified, the condition is termed 'lone AF' (a term usually reserved for patients < 60 years of age).

Drug and allergy history

She is taking a range of secondary prophylaxis, but at suboptimal doses.

Family history

Relevance here is unlikely.

Social history

There are no obvious worries, but she lives alone and should be asked if things are all well at home.

SUMMARY – ASSESSMENT AND PLAN

- If AF is confirmed, an initial decision to rate control is probably best as it cannot be unequivocally established that this episode came on within the last 48 hours; further, she has likely had numerous previous episodes and asymptomatic paroxysmal AF is common. Digoxin loading at 500 µg followed by 500 µg six hours later and then 125 µg daily is appropriate, as would be increasing the dosage of beta blockade (safer to use a short-acting agent such as metoprolol in acute settings).
- A troponin assay as well as routine haematobiochemistry including potassium, magnesium and calcium levels, and thyroid function tests should be obtained, although troponin levels are sometimes elevated by atrial fibrillation alone.
- Low-molecular-weight heparin at a therapeutic dose for thromboembolic prophylaxis should be commenced, and warfarin subsequently considered.
- She should have an echocardiogram in the near future.
- Her simvastatin should be increased to 40 mg and her ramipril to 10 mg if there are no contraindications.

improved stroke volume, hence the importance of rate control in AF), the irregular ventricular rate (which patients can be aware of), dyschronotropy (usually fast, and related to activity), mitral regurgitation (ventricular systole may begin when the mitral valve is still open) or the underlying cause.

Consider potential complications Atrial fibrillation means atrial 'quivering' or disordered contraction and this predisposes to two important complications (Box 2.36).

Total mortality is doubled, largely due to stroke, which is increased six-fold, and up to 18-fold for those with rheumatic heart disease. Stasis leads to thrombus formation, especially in the left atrial appendage, and thrombi are often large such that strokes attributable to AF are often devastating. Morbidity relates to age and underlying cause, and based on Framingham data the annual stroke risk is 1.5% for patients aged 50–59 rising to 23.5% in patients aged 80–89.

Patient perspective

She has no particular concerns.

Past medical history

Atrial fibrillation alerts physicians to underlying disease. The leading causes are listed in Box 2.37.

Discussion

How common is AF?

The incidence is around 0.4–0.7% in those aged 50 rising to 1–2% in those aged 80 years.

How would you differentiate clinically between ventricular ectopic beats and AF?

Exercise decreases the frequency of 'benign' ventricular ectopic beats (VEBs) but has no effect on AF. Multiple or frequent VEBs on an ECG, which represent an 'irritable myocardium' with underlying ischaemia, may worsen with exercise or progress to ventricular tachycardia.

How is AF classified?

This classification is shown in Table 2.20.

A first episode of AF is not paroxysmal, which by definition is recurrent.

What is the mechanism of AF?

Several theories may be combined into two groups, a single focus hypothesis and a multiple focus hypothesis.

Single focus hypothesis

This asserts that AF is due to a single rapid macrore-entry circuit, with wavefronts emanating from a primary driver

Table 2.20 Classification of atrial fibrillation	
Paroxysmal	Duration < 7 days Terminates spontaneously
Persistent	Duration > 7 days Would be indefinite without cardioversion
Permanent	Duration > 7 days Sinus rhythm not possible

circuit (rotor, which may be fixed or moving) and breaking against regions of varying refractoriness; this gives rise to the irregular global activity that characterises the arrhythmia. It is a bit like a large mother wave breaking against rocks of all different shapes and sizes, producing all sorts of smaller, diversely directed waves. The single focus also fires at an automatic, regular but very rapid rate that cannot be followed by the rest of the atrial tissue in a 1:1 fashion, so producing fibrillatory conduction.

Multiple sources hypothesis

This asserts that multiple re-entrant circuits produce wavelets that are separated by lines of functional conduction block, generating irregular re-entrant activity occuring in a dyssynchronous fashion in various atrial regions.

A combination of single and multiple foci may be at play.

Wavelets usually arise in the myocardial sleeves extending from the left atrium to the proximal 5–6 cm of the pulmonary veins. Arrhythmogenic foci in the pulmonary veins may be amenable to ablation but access is difficult and through puncture of the atrial septum.

How AF is sustained

The electrical properties of the atria are altered by sustained AF, making the atria more susceptible to initiation and maintenance of AF. Sustained AF then induces further electrophysiological and structural alterations known as atrial remodelling:

- Tachycardia causes calcium overload in atrial myocytes; this alters gene expression leading to downregulation of one type of calcium current, a shortening of the refractory period and a decrease in wavelength, promoting multiple wave re-entry (electrical remodelling).
- Increased cell volume, sarcomere misalignment, proteolysis, loss of contractile elements and accumulation of glycogen lead to atrial myopathy (structural remodelling).

These factors explain why AF may recur early after electrical cardioversion, why paroxysmalAF may progress to chronic AF and why chronic AF is harder to treat.

Sequalae

All of these factors lead to an increasing tendency for irregular, often fast atrial activity, and thromboembolic risk due to stasis of blood flow and endothelial dysfunction. Around one in six ischaemic strokes are due to AF, most cardiogenic embolism from left atrial appendage thrombus.

List some predictors of recurrence of AF following cardioversion

- Duration more than three months
- Heart failure/structural heart disease
- Hypertension
- Age
- Left atrial diameter > 6.5 cm

When might you consider cardioversion in AF and which treatments can achieve it?

For stable patients, in whom AF onset is uncertain or of over 48 hours, anticoagulation for at least three weeks is needed before cardioversion to allow resolution of potential thrombi; because mechanical activity may not resume concurrently with electrical activity, anticoagulation should be continued for at least a further four weeks after cardioversion, and indefinitely if there is a high risk of recurrence. Transoesophageal echocardiography may exclude thrombus and facilitate earlier cardioversion but anticoagulation is still needed afterwards in the standard way. Prolonged anticoagulation is not needed for AF of duration < 48 hours.

Synchronised external DC cardioversion under sedation or anaesthesia, starting at 200 J but up to 360 J, has a success rate of 70–90%.

Class I or class III antiarrhythmics are commonly used for cardioversion and maintenance of sinus rhythm. Flecainide, propafenone and amiodarone may be effective in descending order, but class Ic drugs (flecainide and propafenone) should be avoided in ischaemic heart disease and impaired left ventricular function. Class Ic antiarrhythmics are also dangerous in atrial flutter. Flutter has an average atrial rate of 300 and with 2:1 block an average ventricular rate of 150. Class Ic antiarrhythmics may slow the atrial rate to, for example, 200, which can then be conducted via an intact atrioventricular node to produce a similar ventricular rate. Amiodarone can be used in such patients, although time to cardioversion may range from days to weeks. Dofetilide and ibutilide, newer pure class III drugs, are not currently licensed in the UK.

How might maintenance of sinus rhythm be achieved after cardioversion?

A high relapse rate after cardioversion (up to 50% at one year especially if there is comorbidity) often necessitates long-term rhythm control.

First-line treatment

Standard beta blockers are now frequently recommended as first-line treatment in all patients (structural or non-structural heart disease) without contraindications, to maintain sinus rhythm.

Second-line treatment

Sotalol is not effective for cardioversion but has some efficacy in maintaining sinus rhythm in patients with structural heart disease, including ischaemic heart disease and left ventricular dysfunction. Class Ic drugs (flecainide or propafenone) are better tolerated and more effective than class Ia drugs (quinidine and disopyramide) but are contraindicated in structural heart disease including ischaemic heart disease and left ventricular dysfunction.

Third-line treatment

Amiodarone may be more effective than sotalol and class I drugs but is limited in the long term by side effects (skin rash, thyroid function disturbance, pulmonary fibrosis, corneal deposits). Dronedarone, a new amiodarone derivative, may be a future alternative.

Fourth-line treatment

Acceptance of a rate control strategy may be the next step.

The above four steps are advocated in NICE guidelines, although in ACA/AHA/ESC guidelines more detail is given to antiarrhythmic selection based on the absence or presence of structural heart disease – flecainide or propafenone or sotalol for lone AF or AF associated with hypertension without significant left ventricular hypertrophy, sotalol in coronary artery disease and amiodarone in left ventricular dysfunction or heart failure or if other agents are ineffective. When single-drug therapy is ineffective, combinations (e.g. beta blocker, sotalol or amiodarone with class Ic agent) may be tried.

An alternative strategy in paroxysmal AF

An alternative to long-term antiarrhythmic therapy in paroxysmal AF, particularly if infrequent and of low thromboembolic risk but symptomatic, is a single oral dose of a drug at the start of palpitations. Flecainide or propafenone are suitable in patients without significant heart disease.

Future directions

There is increasing interest in novel antiarrhythmics acting on ion channels involved in atrial repolarisation (atrial repolarisation delaying agents or ARDAs) and in non-traditional antiarrhythmics which may have antiarrhythmic properties such as angiotensin blocking agents and statins.

When might you consider rate control in AF and what might you use?

Rate control is the only approach for permanent AF but has gained popularity for persistent AF. Numerous ran-

Table 2.21 Rhythm or rate control first	
Try rhythm control first	**Try rate control first**
Symptomatic	Age over 65 years
Younger	Coronary artery disease
First presentation of lone AF	Contraindications to antiarrhythmic
Secondary to a treated or	drugs
corrected precipitant	Unsuitable for cardioversion
Heart failure	

domised controlled trials, including the AFFIRM study, have demonstrated no difference in the endpoints of mortality or disabling stroke between rate versus rhythm control, with more side effects from drug treatment in the rhythm control groups. Furthermore, sinus rhythm is often not maintained and rhythm control does not lower the need for antithrombotic therapy. Rate control may now be considered for patients aged > 65 years; Table 2.21 lists factors that can aid decision-making about rhythm versus rate control. It is important to understand, however, that younger patients, especially, those with symptoms or heart failure, benefit more from rhythm control.

Infrequent, well-tolerated paroxysmal AF may require no treatment. Beta blockers and digoxin are otherwise first-line choices. Digoxin is ineffective in paroxysmal AF, exercise and states with a high sympathetic drive such as thyrotoxicosis and critical illness, and is potentially dangerous if there is underlying Wolff–Parkinson–White syndrome. In patients with good left ventricular function, beta blockers or non-dihydropyridine calcium channel blockers (verapamil and diltiazam) are the drugs of choice if there are no contraindications. Beta blockers with digoxin have the potential in elderly people to augment long sinus pauses, and beta blockers with rate-limiting calcium channel blockers are highly dangerous because of the risks of heart block and/or suppression of contractility and should not be prescribed. Adenosine agonists for rate control are being researched. In heart failure digoxin or amiodarone should be used. Target rates vary with age but are generally 60–90 at rest and 90–115 during exercise.

What might you be concerned about if the ventricular rate is very fast?

If the ventricular rate is very fast (200–300 bpm) or delta waves are seen, a rapidly conducting accessory pathway is likely and intravenous flecainide and/or DC cardioversion is recommended. AV node blockers (e.g. adenosine, digoxin, verapamil, diltiazem) are contraindicated as they potentially further accelerate the ventricular response.

What do you know about antithrombotic therapy for stroke prevention in AF?

The risk of stroke in non-valvular AF is around 5% per year, but varies according to specific risk factors. The risk in patients with rheumatic heart disease is much higher.

Pooled data from trials comparing antithrombotic therapy with placebo have shown that warfarin reduces stroke risk by 62% and aspirin by 22%. However, these data are based on trials comparing each treatment with placebo. In a systematic review of head-to-head comparison between aspirin and warfarin for non-rheumatic AF, the benefit of warfarin appeared to be less significant. Most physicians would advise warfarin where AF is present with one or more additional risk factors (and age is a strong risk factor) unless the balance of perceived risk is greater (dementia, recurrent injurious falls, high bleeding risk, very advanced age). An algorithm for antithrombotic therapy in AF is shown in Fig. 2.7, based on a wide body of evidence and supported by the NICE guideline.

The American College of Cardiology/American Heart Association/European Society of Cardiology (ACC/AHA/ESC) guidelines use different criteria for high, moderate and low risk:

- High-risk factors: previous stroke, TIA or systemic embolism, mitral stenosis, prosthetic valve
- Moderate-risk factors: age ≥ 75 years, hypertension, heart failure, left ventricular ejection fraction $\leq 35\%$, diabetes
- Less validated or weaker risk factors: female gender, age 65–74 years, coronary artery disease, thyrotoxicosis

The ACC/AHA/ESC guidelines recommend warfarin for any one high risk factor or more than one moderate risk factor and aspirin otherwise.

The CHADS$_2$ scoring system is another means of expressing stroke risk, each of congestive heart failure, hypertension, age ≥ 75 years, diabetes, stroke or TIA scoring 1 point; expressed as percentage risk per 100 patient years, a score of 0–1 gives a 1.9–2.8% risk, 2–4 a 4.0–5.95% risk and 5–6 a 12.5–18.2% risk.

Thyrotoxicosis is highly thrombogenic and patients should be given anticoagulants at any age until euthyroid and cardiac function is unimpaired. Many physicians regard those at moderate risk as candidates for warfarin on the basis that an additional risk factor is usually present 'if you look hard enough'.

The limitations of warfarin have prompted the development of new anticoagulants with predictable pharmacokinetics and without the need for monitoring. Ximelagatran, an oral direct thrombin inhibitor, was shown in the SPORTIF III and SPORTIF V trials to be as effective as warfarin, although around 6% of patients developed liver function abnormalities and it has subsequently been withdrawn. Idraparinux, a factor Xa inhibitor administered by once weekly subcutaneous injection was evaluated in AF in the AMADEUS trial, stopped early because of bleeding issues. The ACTIVE (Atrial fibrillation Clopidogrel Trial with Irbesartan for prevention of Vascular Events) failed to show equivalence of benefit of combined antiplatelet therapy with aspirin and clopidogrel over warfarin in 6706 high-risk AF patients. In patients with coronary disease requiring warfarin for AF, evidence does not support additional aspirin.

How much less protective is a subtherapeutic INR?

An INR of 1.5–1.9 in high-risk patients probably reduces the preventive efficacy of warfarin by a factor of 3.6 in

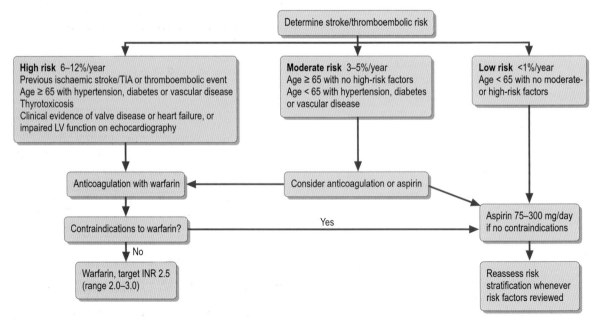

Fig. 2.7 Antithrombotic therapy in atrial fibrillation.

patients under 75 years and 2 in patients over 75 years compared with a therapeutic INR.

How much more risky is an above-therapeutic INR?

The overall risk of intracranial haemorrhage is around 0.3–0.5% per 100 patient-years but rises exponentially to 2.7% at INR values of 4.0–4.5 and 9.4% at INR values over 4.5.

Should patients with paroxysmal AF (PAF) be anticoagulated?

Decisions should be based on appropriate risk stratification (see Fig. 2.7) and not on the duration or symptoms of paroxysms. There is good evidence that anticoagulation should be considered for patients with PAF, even if rhythm control agents are used, the latter reducing episodes and symptoms but not obliterating risk. However, shorts bursts of AF (e.g. 6–10 beats) are common on ambulatory ECG recordings and evidence for cardioembolic risk with these is lacking and they are invariably asymptomatic; it may be preferable to ignore these or, if frequently occurring, to try to limit them with an agent such as a beta blocker, perhaps repeating the ambulatory ECG to see if they have been suppressed.

Should patients with acute onset AF (< 48 hours) be anticoagulated or immediately cardioverted?

They should generally be anticoagulated with heparin followed by warfarin, if there is any doubt about time of onset or if paroxysmal episodes are possible, which covers most cases. A history of intracerebral haemorrhage is a contraindication to anticoagulation (low-dose antiplatelet therapy is sometimes considered long after the episode, and antithrombotic therapy is more compelling where haemorrhage has been secondary to infarct). While cardioversion can be contemplated pharmacologically (e.g. flecainide 150–300 mg if no ischaemic or structural heart disease) if it is certain that an isolated episode started within the last 48 hours, electrical cardioversion is now seldom advised without transoesophageal echocardiography to exclude a left atrial appendage thrombus. Patients with a fast ventricular response and angina, heart failure, hypotension (systolic blood pressure < 90 mmHg) or impaired level of consciousness should undergo urgent synchronised DC cardioversion.

What non-pharmacological therapies are you aware of for AF?

These include radiofrequency catheter ablation of the AN node and permanent pacing ('ablate and pace', best reserved as a last resort), obliteration of the left atrial appendage and implantable atrial defibrillators. Pulmonary vein isolation to prevent induction of AF (by rapid repetitive pulmonary vein ectopic activity emanating from 'sleeves' of the atrial myocardium inside the pulmonary veins) has a success rate of over 75% and its impact and wider use remain to be seen.

How might you manage atrial flutter?

Recommendations for atrial flutter are similar to atrial fibrillation. Carotid sinus massage or adenosine may transiently slow atrioventricular conduction, making the flutter waves more obvious. Atrial flutter ablation, a definitive cure, should be considered at an early stage for recurrent atrial flutter.

CASE 2.13

DYSLIPIDAEMIA

Candidate information

Role

You are a doctor in the medical outpatient clinic. Please read the following letter from the patient's general practitioner. You may make notes on the paper provided. When the bell sounds, enter the examination room to begin the consultation.

Scenario

> Dear Doctor
> Re: Mrs Jean Buchanan, aged 64 years
> Thank you for advising on the treatment of this lady's lipid profile. She has type 2 diabetes and her total cholesterol six months ago was 7.5 mmol/l. She is now on the maximum dose of atorvastatin, and her cholesterol has fallen to 6.0 mmol/l with a high-density lipoprotein of 0.9 mmol/l and raised triglycerides. She is overweight. She also takes metformin, insulatard, perindopril, bendroflumethiazide and aspirin. She has a slightly raised thyroid-stimulating hormone (TSH) but a normal thyroxine (T4), which I am monitoring.
> Yours sincerely

Please take a history from the patient (you may continue to make notes if you wish on the paper provided). Your examiners will warn you when 12 minutes have elapsed. You have 14 minutes to take a history from the patient followed by 1 minute of reflection. There will then follow 5 minutes of discussion with the examiners. Be prepared to discuss solutions to the problems posed by the case and how you might reply to the GP's letter. You are not required to examine the patient.

Patient information

Mrs Jean Buchanan is a 64-year-old lady with raised cholesterol, 7.5 mmol/l, discovered at her diabetes check at the surgery six months ago. Her atorvastatin was increased to a higher dose of 80 mg and when rechecked recently her cholesterol was 6.0 mmol/l. She feels well in herself and is fully independent. She was diagnosed with diabetes 10 years ago and since then has developed numerous complications – she has had laser therapy for diabetic retinopathy and had to give up work as a secretary due to eye disease. She has proteinuria, recently discovered. She has numbness of both feet and a small diabetic foot ulcer. She has hypertension, treated with perindopril 4 mg once a day and bendroflumethiazide 2.5 mg once a day. She also takes aspirin 75 mg once a day, metformin 1 g t.d.s. and insulatard 20 units at night. She is overweight, despite advice from the practice on diet and exercise and eats three meals a day: breakfast of cereal and buttered toast, lunch of soup with bread and butter and dinner of meat, potatoes and vegetables. She snacks between meals, especially if she increases her insulin dose. Home blood glucose monitoring reveals levels of 9–14. Her HbA$_{1c}$ is 10 mmol/l. She does not smoke or drink alcohol. She is very concerned about reducing her cholesterol level, as she been told it is a risk factor for ischaemic heart disease and both her parents died of heart attacks.

How to approach the case

Data gathering in the interview and interpretation and use of information gathered

Presenting problem(s) and symptom exploration

Take a full history of her:

- Dyslipidaemia (many patients know their exact levels)
- Diabetes, including complications (retinopathy, nephropathy, neuropathy)
- Cardiovascular disease (CVD) risk (age and sex, level of diabetes control, hypertension, smoking status, family history, excess weight, alcohol intake, lack of exercise)

She very probably has dyslipidaemia secondary to diabetes but it is important to be aware of the types of dyslipidaemia (Table 2.22) and consider other potential contributors. The WHO numerical classification is largely superseded in practice by a descriptive one.

Patient perspective

Acknowledge and explore her concerns about ischaemic heart disease.

Past medical history

Explore all the usual CVD suspects, including her diabetes complications.

Drug and allergy history

Review her lipid-lowering, blood pressure and diabetes drugs.

Family history

Ask about the ages of family members when they suffered CVD events.

Social history

Explore her reasons for giving up work and the impact of this.

SUMMARY – ASSESSMENT AND PLAN

- Unfortunately, she is already taking a good range of evidence-based primary prophylaxis.
- Her diet should be reviewed, and although atorvastatin 80 mg is considered the highest dose, there may be an indication for considering a second lipid-lowering agent.
- Her overall CVD risk management is more important than focusing only on her cholesterol level.
- Tighter control of her diabetes is imperative in reducing her overall CVD risk, including its benefits on her lipid profile; she might be considered for a long-acting insulin analogue such as glargine and short-acting analogues.

Discussion

What are lipoproteins?

Lipoproteins are complexes of lipid and protein that carry hydrophobic plasma lipids, notably cholesterol and triglycerides. Abundance of larger, triglyceride-containing lipoproteins can turn plasma milky. Cholesterol and triglycerides form the core of lipoproteins and phospholipids and apolipoproteins form the surface; the latter are synthesised largely in the liver and are pivotal in lipid transport and metabolism. Lipoproteins are classified, through escalating density, as chylomicrons, very-low-density lipoprotein (VLDL), intermediate-density lipoprotein (IDL), low-density lipoprotein (LDL) and high-density lipoprotein (HDL).

What types of apolipoprotein are there?

Apo B100 is the major apolipoprotein of VLDL and LDL. It is the ligand for the removal of LDL by the LDL receptor, a cell surface molecule that binds and internalises lipoproteins containing apo B100 or apo E. Apo B48 is the major apolipoprotein of chylomicrons. Apo Cs are present in all plasma lipoproteins (traces in LDL) and tend to inhibit the removal of plasma chylomicrons and VLDL remnants by the liver. Apo CII activates lipoprotein lipase (LPL). LPL hydrolyses triglycerides in chylomicrons and VLDL. Deficiency causes severe hypertriglyceridaemia. Apo CIII inhibits LPL activity. Apo E is found in chylomicrons, VLDL and HDL and is a ligand for their uptake both by the LDL receptor and LDL-receptor-related protein (LRP). There are three major alleles, E2, 3 and 4; E2 binds most easily to the LDL receptor. Apolipoproteins AI, AII and AIV are found mostly on HDL. Apo AI is integral to HDL and its deficiency causes HDL deficiency. It also activates lecithin : cholesterol acetyltransferase (LCAT).

Table 2.22 Classification of dyslipidaemia

	Prevalence	Cause/ pathophysiology	Biochemical features	Clinical features
Familial hypercholesterolaemia (FH)	1 in 500 Much rarer homozygotes (around 1 in 10^6) develop childhood CVD	Autosomal dominant Mutation in LDL receptor prevents binding or internalising of LDL Very rarely abnormal apo B100	Definite diagnostic criteria TC > 7.5 mmol/l in adults over 16 years or LDL > 4.9 mmol/l *plus* Either tendon xanthomata in person or first- or second-degree relative and/or DNA evidence of LDL receptor mutation or defective apo B-100 Possible diagnostic criteria TC > 7.5 mmol/l in adults over 16 years or LDL > 4.9 mmol/l *plus one of* Family history of myocardial infarction < 50 years in second-degree relative or < 60 in first-degree relative Family history of raised TC > 7.5 mmol/l in first- or second-degree relative	Tendon xanthomata almost pathognomonic, commonly over Achilles, knuckles, tibial tuberosity at patellar insertion, elbows; overlying skin normal colour CVD events typically in men 30–50 years and women 50–70 years, with mortality at least 10 times expected
(Familial) combined hyperlipidaemia (FHC)	More common than FH	Many abnormalities, e.g. variations in LPL or its activators/ inhibitors apo CII/CIII or CETP	Raised TC, triglycerides (2–10 mmol/l), LDL, VLDL Low HDL, partly because of impaired LPL activity – LPL, in catabolising triglycerides from lipoproteins, generates HDL	High CVD risk
Polygenic hypercholesterolaemia	The common hypercholesterolaemia, representing the right side of the normal distribution curve and affecting 20–80% of the population, depending upon cut-off point	High saturated fat intake	Excess VLDL, converted quickly to LDL so that VLDL and triglyceride levels normal but LDL raised	CVD risk
Small dense LDL and hyperapobetalipoproteinaemia		Patients with hypertriglyceridaemia also susceptible to raised small, dense LDL	Standard laboratory LDL levels are normal Small, dense LDL particles (could be detected by the presence of apoB)	Even more susceptible than LDL to oxidisation and highly atherogenic High CVD risk
Type III hyperlipoproteinaemia (dysbetalipoproteinaemia or chylomicron – remnant – hyperlipidaemia)	Rare		Mixed TC (7–12 mmol/l) and triglyceride (5–20 mmol/l) lipidaemia	Striate palmar and tuberoeruptive xanthomata High CVD risk
Moderate and severe hypertriglyceridaemia	Many formerly considered to have isolated hypertriglyceridaemia now classified as combined as acceptable cholesterol thresholds have lowered Prevalence of severe probably around 1 in 1000	Familial LPL deficiency or heterozygous LPL mutation Sometimes associated secondary factor, e.g. obesity, diabetes, alcohol	Fasting triglycerides > 10 mmol/l Raised chylomicrons and VLDL (both compete for the same clearance mechanism, LPL) Chylomicronaemia can produce spectacularly raised triglycerides, e.g. > 100 mmol/l TC can be markedly elevated with normal LDL because chylomicrons and VLDL contain it	Eruptive xanthomata – yellow nodules extensor surfaces (elbows, knees, buttocks, back) in hypertriglyceridaemia Hepatosplenomegaly rarely Acute pancreatitis with triglyceride > 20–30 mmol/l Pseudohyponatraemia
Secondary hyperlipidaemia	Common	Diabetes Hypothyroidism Cholestasis Nephrotic syndrome	High triglycerides and low HDL in diabetes	High CVD risk

apo, apolipoprotein; CVD, cardiovascular disease; HDL, high-density lipoprotein cholesterol; LDL, low-density lipoprotein cholesterol; LPL, lipoprotein lipase; TC, total cholesterol; VLDL, very-low-density lipoprotein cholesterol.

What happens to dietary (exogenous) lipids?
(Fig. 2.8A)

Dietary triglycerides and cholesterol are incorporated into chylomicrons in gut mucosa. Chylomicrons are fat droplets with a very high triglyceride concentration. They enter the circulation via the thoracic duct, where HDL donates apo

CII molecules, activating hydrolysis of triglycerides by LPL to free fatty acids (FFAs) and glycerol on capillary endothelial cells in fat and muscle. FFAs are used for energy in adjacent tissue or stored as fat. Insulin helps stimulate LPL and so diabetes impairs triglyceride clearance, as can LPL deficiency. Most circulating LPL is asso-

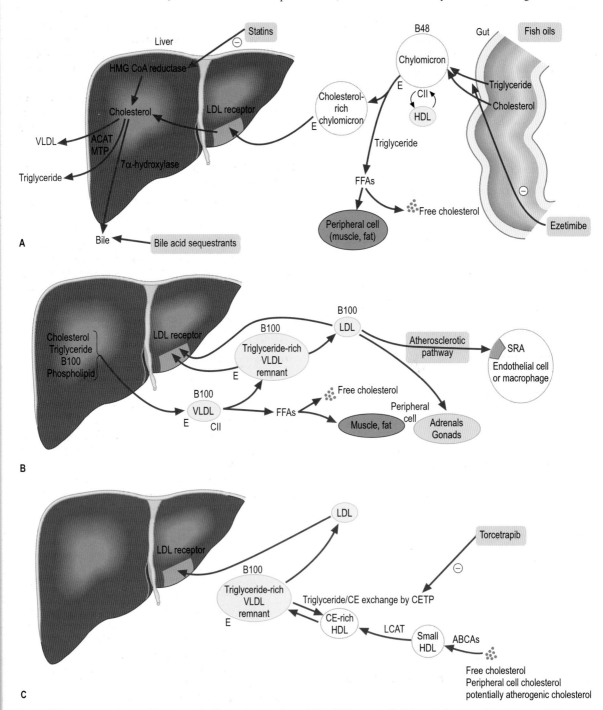

Fig. 2.8 Lipid transport and sites of drug action: (A) What happens to dietary lipids? (B) Transport of lipid from the liver to peripheral tissues. (C) Transport of lipid from peripheral tissues to the liver.

ciated with LDL. Apo E allows chylomicron remnants (after the triglyceride core has been hydrolysed and apo CII has recirculated back to HDL) to bind to hepatic LDL receptors (or LRP). The overall results are utilisation or storage of triglycerides and uptake of cholesterol by the liver. Cholesterol can also be synthesised de novo in the liver by the action of HMG CoA reductase. Liver cholesterol can be used for bile acid formation through the action of 7α-hydroxylase, excreted as cholesterol in bile, incorporated into membranes or resecreted into the circulation either directly as VLDL or by conversion to triglyceride by the action of acyl-coA : cholesterol acyltransferase (ACAT) and microsomal triglyceride transfer protein (MTP).

What is endogenous lipid transport and metabolism?

This refers to the transfer of lipids from the liver to the peripheral tissues and back.

How is lipid transported from the liver to peripheral tissues? (Fig. 2.8B)

This is via the apo B100 system, and concerns VLDL, IDL and LDL. In the liver, cholesterol is taken up from chylomicron remnants or synthesised de novo and triglycerides are made from FFAs taken up from plasma or synthesised de novo. These core lipids are packaged with apo B100 and phospholipid into VLDL and secreted into plasma where apolipoproteins C and E are added. VLDL is triglyceride-rich, even more so in states of triglyceride excess such as overeating, diabetes and alcohol consumption. In the plasma, LPL hydrolyses VLDL triglycerides to create smaller, denser VLDL remnants (also known as IDL). These can re-enter the liver via apo E binding to the LDL receptor or become LDL, apo B100 the only remaining surface protein on LDL. Most LDL is taken up by the liver via the LDL receptor. Some is delivered to tissues such as adrenals and gonads and used for steroid hormone synthesis.

What influences LDL levels as well as diet?

LDL levels are influenced by LDL receptor availability or activity; they are down-regulated when liver cholesterol is replete.

Why are increased LDL levels dangerous?

Increased LDL and apo B100 are risk factors for CVD, because excess LDL undergoes lipid peroxidation and becomes a ligand for alternative, scavenger receptor pathways (e.g. SRA, see Fig. 2.8B) present on endothelial cells and macrophages. Oxidised lipoproteins (often the cholesterol esters in LDL or chylomicron remnants) within macrophages transform these into foam cells, the first phase of the atherosclerosis mechanism (Case 2.8).

How is lipid transported from peripheral tissues to the liver? (Fig. 2.8C)

This is through the apo A1 system, and concerns HDL. It is known as the reverse cholesterol pathway. HDL particles are formed in the plasma from the coalescence of phospholipid–apolipoprotein complexes. Free plasma cholesterol is transferred by ATP binding cassette transporter A1 (ABCA1) to these small, cholesterol-poor HDL particles and esterified by LCAT, which is bound to HDL, to cholesterol ester (CE). This enables HDL to accept more cholesterol and larger HDL particles develop which can be metabolised in one of two ways. The entire HDL particle can be removed from plasma, or its CEs can be exchanged with triglyceride in VLDL, mediated by cholesterol ester transfer protein. The CEs are returned to the liver via VLDL conversion to LDL and LDL liver reception. The triglyceride transferred to HDL is a substrate for LPL and HDL particles are condensed down again to their smaller form. When apo B100 is removed by the liver, reverse cholesterol transfer is complete.

What is the association between CVD and cholesterol?

As total cholesterol (TC) (and LDL) increases so does CVD risk, the relative risks being similar for those with and without CVD. CVD risk is principally determined by the concentrations of LDL and HDL and to a lesser extent by triglycerides. Lowering cholesterol by diet, drugs or other means decreases CVD risk. A 1 mmol/l decrease in LDL reduces coronary death by 11% in the first year, 24% in the second, 33% in the third to fifth and 36% in the sixth and subsequent years. Of course, lipoproteins are only one part of overall CVD risk (Case 2.7).

How strong is the evidence for lipid-lowering therapy in reducing CVD risk?

The compelling evidence is with statins, with non-fatal and fatal endpoints. The early major statin trials in people with established CVD using simvastatin and pravastatin (4S, CARE, LIPID) and in asymptomatic people at risk of developing CVD (WOSCOPS, AFCAPS/TEXCAPS) showed significant reductions in coronary events, coronary mortality and often all-cause mortality. A meta-analysis of these five trials showed significant reductions of major coronary events by 31%, coronary mortality by 29% and all-cause mortality by 21%. There was no difference in non-CVD mortality.

Later statin trials with atorvastatin (GREASE, ASCOT, CARDS, PROVE-IT, TNT, IDEAL, 4D), fluvastatin (LIPS, ALERT), pravastatin (ALLHAT, PROSPER, PROVE-IT) and simvastatin (HPS, A to Z, IDEAL) extended the evidence base to many populations including women, older people, people with acute coronary disease, people with diabetes, renal transplantation, but not haemodialysis, and in populations hitherto thought to have low TC and LDL-C concentrations. The HPS randomised people with TC > 3.5 mmol/l.

The Cholesterol Trialists' Collaboration, in a meta-analysis of statin trials, showed safe reduction in the five-year incidence of major coronary events, coronary revascularisation and stroke by about one-fifth per mmol reduction in LDL-C.

Is the benefit of statin therapy as clear for stroke as for coronary heart disease (CHD)?

The relation between cholesterol and stroke (analysed in the HPS, MIRACL, PROSPER, ASCOT-LLA, ALERT and LIPS studies) is less clear than for CHD. The Cholesterol Trialists' Collaboration reported a 17% reduction in the incidence of first stroke and evidence for statin therapy in the primary prevention of stroke is strong, and this applies to people with CHD, hypertension, diabetes and others at high total CVD risk. In the secondary prevention of stroke evidence for statin therapy is less clear.

Might statins work in ways other than lipid lowering?

Accelerated atherosclerosis in chronic inflammatory conditions such as rheumatoid arthritis is not explained by traditional risk factors. Such patients may have increased levels of a CD4 subset of T cells that lack CD28 expression called CD4 null cells, which can also be activated by infection and are more abundant in older people. These cells express interferon-γ and may cause a number of effects including endothelial cell death via engagement of their Toll-like receptor TLR2. TLR2 may be regulated by statins and there is evidence for endothelial stabilisation and regression of atherosclerosis with statin therapy, the anti-inflammatory effects of which are being examined in a range of non-CVD conditions including rheumatoid arthritis.

Should muscle and liver enzymes be checked in people on statin therapy?

Baseline creatine phosphokinase (CK) and transaminases are often checked when starting therapy. Routine monitoring is not necessary in the absence of symptoms. Transaminases may be allowed to rise to three times and CK to five or even 10 times the upper limit of normal. Acute myositis is rare, and non-fatal or fatal rhabdomyolysis very rare.

What other lipid-lowering therapies are there?

A meta-analysis of fibrate trials showed a 25% reduction in major coronary events, although the largest trial, FIELD, showed no statistically significant reduction. A meta-analysis of nicotinic acid trials showed a 27% reduction in major coronary events. Lipid-lowering therapies are summarised in Table 2.23.

Should triglycerides and non-LDL cholesterol be considered to be as threatening as LDL?

Mixed dyslipidaemia with elevated triglycerides and low HDL is common. The main strategy is still a statin to treat LDL to target. Mixed dyslipidaemia represents the accumulation of atherogenic remnant lipoproteins, small, dense, LDL particles converted from triglyceride-rich VLDL remnants that are less rapidly cleared and more readily taken up by macrophages. As triglycerides rise, especially when HDL is low, so does CVD risk, especially above 1.7 mmol/l. Unfortunately statins have little effect on triglycerides and HDL; trials are ongoing with other agents that may improve non-LDL lipid profiles including the Heart Protection Study-2 (THRIVE).

How should we react to HDL levels on current evidence?

Low HDL (< 1.0 mmol/l in men, < 1.2 mmol/l in women) remains a strong independent risk factor for CVD. Levels may be improved by exercise and stopping smoking. High levels of HDL are often associated with elevated LDL. While the ratio of the two is often regarded as a useful index of CVD risk, a normal ratio in the setting of raised HDL and LDL has been shown to increase risk, and the efficacy of statins in the Heart Protection Study was independent of HDL levels. The combination effect of statins and torcetrapib may have additive effects on lowering LDL and raising HDL.

Do any drugs raise HDL?

Torcetrapib (an emerging drug) raises HDL by inhibiting cholesteryl ester transfer protein (CETP). Statins increase HDL by about 3–10%. Fibrates increase HDL moderately. Nicotinic acid may raise HDL. Fish oils (n-3 fatty acids; DHA/EPA) may raise HDL and reduce triglycerides.

Is HDL cholesterol always good?

HDL-mediated reverse cholesterol transport is thought to be the major mechanism by which HDL protects against atherosclerosis, and plasma levels of HDL and Apo AI are inversely proportional to CVD risk. Almost 40% of HDL variation between individuals is genetically determined, one-quarter of which is attributable to polymorphisms of the *CETP* gene. Lower CETP levels mean higher HDL levels (or at least higher levels of large, cholesterol-rich HDL). Evidence as to whether these mutations are protective is conflicting. Some studies have shown increased CVD risk. Adverse effects of CETP deficiency may be attributable to impairment of reverse cholesterol transport and loss of the antiatherogenic properties of HDL resulting from its increased cholesterol content and larger size. A few studies have even shown CVD reduction with increased HDL particle size.

Are there other ways of assessing dyslipidaemia as well as serum lipid profiles?

Computed tomography scan calcification scoring is one way of further assessing risk in asymptomatic people.

Is hypolipidaemia a problem?

It may be secondary to malabsorption. Primary hypoalphalipoproteinaemia (low HDL) is a common correlate of hypertriglyceridaemia (prevalence 10–25%). Isolated low

Table 2.23 Lipid-lowering therapies

Class of drug	How they work	What they do	Compelling indications	Possible indications	Caution	Compelling contraindications
Statins, e.g. simvastatin, atorvastatin	HMG-CoA reductase inhibition	Lower TC and LDL (40 mg simvastatin lowers LDL by 25% – therefore atorvastatin if TC very high)	Atherosclerotic CVD Total CVD risk ≥ 20% Diabetes	Total CVD risk 10–20% TC:HDL > 6 LDL > 5 mmol/l	Non-alcoholic steatohepatitis Untreated hypothyroidism Significant kidney disease Excessive grapefruit juice (metabolised through P450)	Gemfibrozil (gemfibrozil interferes with statin metabolism)
Fibrates, e.g. gemfibrozil	Modulation of nuclear receptors in various tissues (liver, muscle, fat)	Raise HDL Lower triglycerides	Type III hyperlipoproteinaemia Severe hypertriglyceridaemia (> 10 mmol/l) with risk of pancreatitis	Type 2 diabetes (specialist) Moderate to severe hypertriglyceridaemia with controlled LDL and very high CVD risk (specialist)	Kidney disease Statin	Statin (gemfibrozil interferes with statin metabolism)
Bile acid sequestrants/anion exchange resins, e.g. cholestyramine, cholestipol	Bind bile acids in intestine	Increase LDL receptor activity in liver Increase LDL clearance from plasma	None (poorly tolerated)	Inadequate LDL on statin and ezetimibe (e.g. familial hypercholesterolaemia) Cholestasis with itching	Gastrointestinal disease Exacerbation of hypertriglyceridaemia	None
Nicotinic acids		Reduce triglycerides and cholesterol	Severe hypertriglyceridaemia with prior acute pancreatitis Severe hypertriglyceridaemia not responsive to fibrates	With other lipid-lowering drugs, most often in mixed hyperlipidaemia	Other lipid-lowering drugs Kidney disease Liver disease Diabetes Gout Peptic ulcer Flushing	Glucose intolerance
Cholesterol absorption inhibitors, e.g. ezetimibe	Block cholesterol absorption in the gut	Lower LDL by 15–20% when added to diet or by 20–25% when added to diet with statin Long-term trial data awaited	Familial sitosterolaemia	With statin where LDL not at target despite maximum statin or tolerated statin dose Monotherapy in statin intolerance	Liver disease Fibrates	None Well tolerated
Fish oils Omega-3 (n-3) fatty acids/ acid ethyl esters: Eicosapentaenoic (EPA), docosahexaenoic (DHA) and alpha-tocopherol as Omacor 2–4 g/day Omega-3-marine triglycerides as Maxepa 5–10 g/day			Severe hypertriglyceridaemia (Maxepa) CHD prevention (Omacor)	Hypertriglyceridaemia	Anticoagulants Haemorrhagic disorders Aspirin-sensitive asthma Diabetes	None

CHD, coronary heart disease; CVD, cardiovascular disease; HDL, high-density lipoprotein cholesterol; LDL, low-density lipoprotein cholesterol; TC, total cholesterol.

HDL due to, for example, *ABCA1* mutations, is very rare. Hypobetalipiproteinaemias are rare, but the very rare abetalipoproteinaemia with severe hypocholesterolaemia is associated with retinitis pigmentosa, fatty liver, acanthocytes and a Friedrich's ataxia-like syndrome. There is an uncertain but observational relationship between low cholesterol levels and cancer.

Who should receive lipid-lowering therapy, what are the targets and when should it be started?

People at high CVD risk should receive lipid-lowering therapy and targets for this are described in Case 2.7. The traditional approach was dietary advice first, but early initiation of therapy has been shown to be beneficial (MIRACL, A to Z, PROVE-IT). It should start early in acute atherosclerotic CVD (coronary, cerebral, peripheral) events because of evidence of benefit and because most patients will have levels above targets and acute blood tests tend to underestimate levels.

CASE 2.14

HYPERTENSION

Candidate information

Role

You are a doctor in the medical outpatient clinic. Please read the following letter from the patient's general practitioner. You may make notes on the paper provided. When the bell sounds, enter the examination room to begin the consultation.

Scenario

> Dear Doctor
>
> Re: Mr Thomas Roberts, aged 45 years
>
> Thank you for seeing Mr Roberts, who was diagnosed with hypertension two months ago at an insurance medical, urgently. Blood pressure then was 190/114 and baseline investigations revealed normal urinalysis, normal electrolytes and creatinine and a normal ECG. He did admit to occasional palpitations. His fasting blood glucose was normal and his cholesterol was 5.4 mmol/l. He was started on atenolol 50 mg and reviewed one month later at which time blood pressure was 180/110 and amlodipine was added. He has noticed intermittent headaches and sweats since then, and blood pressure today is 200/120. I am concerned that there may be a secondary cause for his hypertension and that the headaches may represent worsening incipient complications.
>
> Yours sincerely

Please take a history from the patient (you may continue to make notes if you wish on the paper provided). Your examiners will warn you when 12 minutes have elapsed. You have 14 minutes to take a history from the patient followed by 1 minute of reflection. There will then follow 5 minutes of discussion with the examiners. Be prepared to discuss solutions to the problems posed by the case and how you might reply to the GP's letter. You are not required to examine the patient.

Patient information

Mr Thomas Roberts is a 45-year-old solicitor recently diagnosed with hypertension at an insurance medical for a second mortgage as he and his wife were buying a new house for their expanding family of three children and two dogs. He has no past medical history of note but has seen his GP regularly over the last two months for first-line investigations (blood tests and ECG, which he has been advised are normal) and started treatment, initially atenolol, and now additional amlodipine. He has noticed occasional episodes of his heart racing over the last few months, which he has attributed to stress, and occasional sweats, which he has put down to being 'less fit than he used to be'. He has developed headaches since starting the amlodipine, and a small amount of ankle swelling. He is concerned about being on medication potentially lifelong and also being declined life assurance.

How to approach the case

Data gathering in the interview and interpretation and use of information gathered

Presenting problem(s) and symptom exploration

The objectives when evaluating hypertension are: assessment for possible causes, assessment for target organ damage and planning of appropriate investigation and treatment. Referral to secondary care is indicated in the following circumstances:

- A need for urgent treatment, as in accelerated or malignant hypertension (blood pressure > 180/110 with papilloedema or retinal haemorrhage)
- Suspected phaeocromocytoma (labile or postural hypotension, headache, palpitations, pallor or diaphoresis)
- Other symptoms suggesting a secondary cause
- Young age (< 20 years or needing treatment < 30 years)
- Sudden onset or worsening hypertension
- Resistance to a multidrug regimen (three or more drugs) or problems with intolerance or multiple contraindications

- Special situations such as unusual blood pressure variability, possible white-coat hypertension or pregnancy

■ **Consider causes**   Most hypertension is 'idiopathic', a conspiracy of nefarious and poorly understood genetics and a rogue environment. Secondary causes are listed in Table 2.24.

Patient perspective

Explore his concerns about hypertension and its effects on life assurance for a mortgage.

Past medical history

■ **Consider target organs**   Possible target organ damage in hypertension is listed in Box 2.38.
■ **Consider risk factors for cardiovascular disease**   The usual suspects include age and sex, smoking, diabetes, cholesterol and family history. Contributory factors include excess weight, excess alcohol (> 3 units/day for men, > 2 units/day for women), excess salt, lack of exercise and environmental stress.

Drug and allergy history

Ask about drugs exacerbating hypertension. These include non-steroidal anti-inflammatory drugs (NSAIDs), steroids and ciclosporin. Ask about possible side effects of antihypertensives (calcium channel blockers can cause headaches, flushing and ankle swelling).

Family history

Ask about renal disease (e.g. adult polycystic kidney disease).

Social history

Explore his concerns about hypertension and its effects on life assurance for a mortgage.

Box 2.38 Possible target organ damage in hypertension

- Cerebrovascular disease (history of transient ischaemic attacks or stroke)
- Coronary heart disease (history of angina or previous acute coronary syndrome, percutaneous coronary intervention or bypass grafting)
- Left ventricular hypertrophy or strain (ECG)
- Heart failure
- Renovascular disease (proteinuria or raised creatinine)
- Peripheral vascular disease (claudication)
- Aortic aneurysm in older patients
- Hypertensive retinopathy

SUMMARY – ASSESSMENT AND PLAN

- All hypertensive patients should have a thorough history and examination, urinalysis, serum creatinine and electrolytes, fasting blood glucose, lipid profile with a TC:HDL ratio (ideally fasted for evaluation of triglycerides) and an ECG.
- Further investigations in this case should include measurement of urinary catecholamines on three separate occasions to exclude phaeochromocytoma, screening for Conn's syndrome, measurement of thyroid function and possibly a renal ultrasound and echocardiogram. While a renal cause is less likely with a normal urinalysis, renal artery stenosis is possible and definitive exclusion might require magnetic resonance angiography.
- This patient's headaches may be the result of amlodipine.
- Assure him that investigations will determine the optimum treatment and that while hypertension needs to be declared in his application, it should not deny him life assurance.

Table 2.24 Secondary causes of hypertension

Secondary causes		Clinical clues
Renal		Haematuria Known history or family history of renal disease
Endocrine	Phaeochromocytoma	Sweats and palpitations Paroxysmal symptoms 90% have at least one of three symptoms – sweats, palpitations or anxiety Headaches The 10% 'rule' of these catecholamine-secreting tumours is that 10% are bilateral, 10% extra-adrenal, 10% malignant and 10% familial
	Conn's syndrome	Consider in this patient's age group Symptoms rare, but may include tetany, muscle weakness and polyuria Sodium retention increases the extracellular fluid volume but water retention is usually insufficient for development of oedema
	Cushing's syndrome	Unusual without other symptoms or signs
Aortic coarctation		Blood pressure discrepancy between right and left
Genetic		Defined genetic causes should be considered in young patients (e.g. aged 20) and include those in Box 2.39
Drugs		

Discussion

How would you screen for Conn's syndrome?

Hypertension in Conn's syndrome is associated with hypo-kalaemic alkalosis (usual in Conn's). While normal serum potassium does not exclude Conn's syndrome, many experts are satisfied with three normal results. Screening investigations reveal high aldosterone levels, usually markedly suppressed renin levels in response to aldosterone-mediated volume increase, and a low ambulant or erect renin–aldosterone ratio. These tests should be reserved for selected patients. Aldosterone may fail to suppress with salt loading, e.g. saline, salt tablets or fludrocortisone 0.2 mg daily for five days. Imaging is limited by the high incidence of adrenal 'incidentalomas' but adrenal vein sampling may detect hypersecretion from the adenoma. Calcium channel blockers are suitable antihypertensives pre-investigation as they do not interfere with the renin–angiotensin–aldosterone axis (RAAS); patients on other antihypertensives may need to have these stopped then be admitted for fludrocortisone suppression testing.

How may the RAAS contribute to the pathophysiology of hypertension?

Hypertension can result from raised peripheral resistance, excessive activation of the RAAS, excessive sympathetic nervous system activity or alteration in the balance of endothelial-derived vasoactive molecules. A range of genetic factors contributes.

Renin is released from the juxtaglomerular apparatus (JGA) of the kidney in response to low sodium or reduced renal perfusion. Renin converts angiotensinogen to angiotensin I (AI). AI is converted in the lung to angiotensin II (AII) by the action of angiotensin-converting enzyme (ACE). AII restores circulating volume via release from the adrenal cortex of aldosterone, which promotes sodium and water retention at the distal renal tubule in exchange for potassium and hydrogen, vasoconstriction and thirst. Aldosterone secretion is controlled almost exclusively by the RAAS and not by adrenocorticotrophic hormone. Numerous abnormalities of the RAAS can lead to hyperaldosteronism (Box 2.39).

How is phaeochromocytoma managed?

Clonidine suppression testing may be used for suspected phaeocromocytoma where urinalysis gives equivocal results. Where confirmed, phaeocromocytoma requires specialist management, including a search for the tumour with structural or functional imaging. Treatment with beta blockers is contraindicated without α-blockade (e.g. phenoxybenzamine) because unopposed α-blockade can cause severe vasoconstriction and pulmonary oedema; this is especially important perioperatively.

> **Box 2.39 Abnormalities in the renin–angiotensin–aldosterone system (RAAS)**
>
> **Primary hyperaldosteronism**
>
> This is usually caused by an aldosterone-secreting adenoma (Conn's syndrome). Rarely it can result from bilateral hyperplasia or carcinoma. Renin production is suppressed.
>
> **Secondary hyperaldosteronism**
>
> This is hyper-reninaemic, usually in response to low sodium or reduced renal perfusion. The kidney perceives low circulating volume, which may be apparent as in renal artery stensois or true as in dehydration.
>
> **Pseudohyperaldosteronism (Liddle's syndrome)**
>
> This occurs when the sodium channel (ENac) in the tubule normally stimulated by aldosterone is switched permanently 'on' in the absence of aldosterone by an autosomal dominant mutation in its gene. Renin is suppressed. Hypertension may respond to amiloride. Liddle's syndrome is one of a number of genetically determined causes of low renin hypertension. Two others are glucocorticoid remediable hypertension and apparent mineralocorticoid excess.
>
> **Glucocorticoid-remediable aldosteronism (GRA)**
>
> Two closely related enzymes, 11β-hydroxylase and aldosterone synthase, normally coordinate synthesis of glucocorticoid and mineralocorticoid in the adrenal gland. In GRA a chimeric gene (autosomal dominant), comprising the aldosterone synthase gene with an upstream ACTH-dependent promoter, results in expression of aldosterone synthase under ACTH regulation. Hypertension may respond to dexamethasone, which suppresses ACTH.
>
> **Apparent mineralocorticoid excess (AME)**
>
> Normally an enzyme called 11β-hydroxysteroid dehydrogenase (11β-OHSD) within the renal tubules converts cortisol, which has a high affinity for the minerocorticoid receptor, to cortisone, which does not. In AME the 11β-OHSD gene is mutated (autosomal recessive), leading to low enzyme activity and high cellular levels of cortisol which can then act as a potent mineralocorticoid. Liquorice inhibits 11β-OHSD, exposing the mineralocorticoid and hypertensive potential. Hypertension may be treated with amiloride, spironolactone or dexamethasone suppression of cortisol synthesis, as dexamethasone is a less potent mineralocorticoid than cortisol.
>
> **Primary hypoaldosteronism**
>
> This is due either to Addison's disease or to other conditions that damage the adrenal gland. Renin is elevated.
>
> **Pseudohypoaldosteronism**
>
> This occurs when ENac does not work and is a cause of type 4 renal tubular acidosis.

How does the British Hypertension Society (BHS) define hypertension?

The definitions in Table 2.25 equate with the European Society and World Health Organisation–International Society of Hypertension. Values are clinic, not ambulatory, for which 24-hour values are > 125/80 (and 135/85 for self/home monitoring). If systolic and diastolic blood pressures fall into different categories, the higher value should be taken for classification.

List some possible indications for ambulatory blood pressure monitoring

- Unusual blood pressure variability
- Possible 'white-coat' hypertension
- Informing equivocal treatment decisions
- Evaluating nocturnal hypertension
- Determining efficacy of drug treatment over 24 hours
- Pregnancy
- Evaluating symptomatic hypotension

What are the BHS thresholds for intervention with drug treatment?

These are given in Table 2.26.

Which lifestyle measures may limit hypertension?

The following are important:

- Maintaining a normal weight (BMI 20–25 kg/m^2)
- Reducing salt intake to < 100 mmol/day (< 6 g NaCl or < 2.4 g Na/day)
- Reducing alcohol intake to three or fewer units/day for men and two or fewer units/day for women
- Regular aerobic physical exercise (brisk walking rather than weightlifting) for ≥ 30 minutes/day, ideally on most days but at least three days/week
- Taking five or more portions/day of fresh fruit/vegetables
- Reducing intake of total and saturated fat

What are the BHS treatment targets?

Definitive evidence on optimal targets is lacking. The Hypertension Optimal Treatment (HOT) trial was under-powered but provides the best evidence to date, with an optimal blood pressure of 139/83 mmHg. However, below this value caused no harm, and patients with blood pressures between 139/83 and 150/90 were not disadvantaged. Thus, an audit standard of < 150/90 has been chosen by the BHS, although evidence from intervention trials in hypertensive people with diabetes, at high risk of cardiovascular disease (CVD) or after stroke supports a 'lower the better' policy. Benefit probably extends down to 115/75 after which there are no data. BHS optimal targets are:

- ≤ 140/85 for most patients; and
- ≤ 130/80 for patients with diabetes, chronic kidney disease or established CVD.

When ambulatory measurements are used, mean daytime pressures are preferred and the value would be expected to be approximately 10/5 mmHg lower than the clinic equivalent.

Which factors determine choice of antihypertensive therapy?

Benefits beyond blood-pressure lowering

There is overwhelming evidence that lowering blood pressure reduces cardiovascular risk, in particular stroke and myocardial infarction. There is much debate about the concept of 'beyond blood pressure' whereby different drug classes are believed to be advantageous over and above their blood-pressure-lowering effects. This is certainly true for targeted patients (e.g. ACE inhibitors if there is diabetic nephropathy) but until recently the evidence suggested that the major benefit on outcome was dependent on successful blood pressure lowering alone.

The Blood Pressure Lowering Treatment Trialist's Collaboration 2003 meta-analysis assessed data from 29 trials involving 162 341 patients and concluded that there was no significant difference in cardiovascular events or mortality between ACE inhibitors, beta blockers, calcium channel blockers or diuretics. A caveat was that ACE inhibitors might have more benefits than other agents in stroke. An

Table 2.25 BHS blood pressure definitions

	Systolic	Diastolic
Optimal	< 120	< 80
Normal	< 130	< 85
High normal	130–139	85–89
Grade 1 hypertension (mild)	140–159	90–99
Grade 2 hypertension (moderate)	160–179	100–109
Grade 3 hypertension (severe)	≥ 180	≥ 110
Grade 1 isolated systolic hypertension	140–159	< 90
Grade 2 isolated systolic hypertension	≥ 160	< 90

Table 2.26 Thresholds for intervention

≥ 180/110 (grade 3 hypertension)	Treat, but unless malignant phase of hypertensive emergency confirm over 1–2 weeks before treatment
160–179/100–109 (grade 2 hypertension)	If target organ damage, CVD complications or diabetes, confirm over 3–4 weeks then treat; if absent remeasure weekly and treat if blood pressure persists at these levels over 4–12 weeks
140–159/90–99 (grade 1 hypertension)	If target organ damage, CVD complications or diabetes, confirm over 12 weeks then treat; if absent remeasure monthly, treat if blood pressure persists at these levels and if estimated 10-year CVD risk is ≥ 20%, but reassess CVD risk yearly if < 20% and institute lifestyle measures
130–139/85–89 (high normal)	Reassess yearly
< 130/85 (normal)	Reassess in 5 years

independent National Institute for Health and Clinical Excellence (NICE) meta-analysis drew the same conclusions.

However, the ASCOT blood pressure trial was stopped early because of a reduction in all-cause mortality and additional cardiovascular and stroke benefits in favour of amlodipine and perindopril over atenolol and a thiazide. Amlodipine and perindopril did result in an overall slightly greater blood pressure reduction (2.9/1.8) suggesting again that blood-pressure lowering is key but compared with standard treatment reduction in stroke, coronary events, cardiovascular death and development of new diabetes were 25%, 15%, 25% and 30% respectively. ASCOT impacted significantly on the 2004 BHS guidelines, which had recommended an AB/CD rule giving beta blockers equal weight with other agents.

Prescribing sequence if no compelling indications or contraindications

Most people need more than one drug to control blood pressure. However, NICE guidance in 2006 concluded that beta blockers were usually less effective than a comparator drug at reducing cardiovascular events, particularly stroke, and less effective than an ACE inhibitor or calcium channel blocker at reducing the risk of diabetes. The guidance relegated the use of beta blockers and promoted the prescribing sequence outlined in Table 2.27.

Beta blockers, while no longer preferred as initial routine therapy, are not ineffective but may merely be less effective than other agents. There may still be compelling indications for their use as first-line treatment (see Table 2.28),

Table 2.27 Choosing drugs for patients newly diagnosed with hypertension

	Younger than 55 years	55 years or older or black patient of any age
Step 1	A	C or D
Step 2	A + C or A + D	
Step 3	A + C + D	
Step 4	Add further diuretic therapy or beta blocker or alpha blocker	

A, angiotensin-converting enzyme inhibitor or angiotensin receptor blocker; B, beta blocker; C, calcium channel blocker; D, diuretic (thiazide or thiazide-like).

Table 2.28 Choosing antihypertensive agents

	Compelling indications	Possible indications	Caution	Compelling contraindications
Alpha blocker	Benign prostatic hypertrophy		Postural hypotension Heart failure as monotherapy	Urinary incontinence
Angiotensin-converting enzyme (ACE) inhibitor	Heart failure Post-myocardial infarction CVD Type 1 diabetes Secondary stroke prevention	CKD Type 2 diabetic nephropathy Proteinuric renal disease	Renal impairment Peripheral vascular disease	Pregnancy Renovascular disease
Angiotensin II receptor blocker (ARB)	ACE inhibitor intolerance Type 2 diabetes Hypertension with LVH Heart failure in ACE inhibitor intolerant patients Post-myocardial infarction	LV dysfunction post myocardial infarction Intolerance of other antihypertensive drugs Proteinuric renal disease Chronic kidney disease	Renal impairment Peripheral vascular disease	Pregnancy Renovascular disease
Beta blocker	Angina, myocardial infarction	Heart failure	Heart failure (but increasingly used to treat heart failure under specialist supervision) Peripheral vascular disease Diabetes (except with CVD)	Asthma/COPD Heart block
Calcium channel blocker (dihydropyridine, e.g. amlodipine)	Elderly, isolated systolic hypertension	Angina		
Calcium channel blocker (rate limiting, e.g. diltiazem, verapamil)	Angina	Elderly patient	Combination with beta blocker	Heart block Heart failure
Thiazide	Elderly Isolated systolic hypertension Heart failure Secondary stroke prevention			Gout (but thiazide occasionally necessary, with allopurinol)

COPD, chronic obstructive pulmonary disease; CKD, chronic kidney disease; CVD, cardiovascular disease; LV, left ventricular; LVH, left ventricular hypertrophy.

and they may be preferable in younger patients, for women of childbearing age, patients with increased sympathetic overdrive and patients intolerant of ACE inhibitors or angiotensin receptor blockers. The combination of a beta blocker and diuretic may increase the risk of developing diabetes. Refractory hypertension not responsive to modern prescribing occasionally may be tackled with centrally acting sympatholytics such as moxonidine or methyldopa, or vasodilators such as hydralazine. The results of a new class of drug that inhibits renin directly (inhibition of the RAAS is desirable in hypertension and yet ACE inhibitors and ARBs may cause plasma renin levels to increase) remain to be seen.

Compelling and potential indications and contraindications

In many, particularly older, patients there are compelling reasons to choose or not to choose a drug that deviates from the prescribing sequence. These are shown in Table 2.28.

What is the place of aspirin and statin therapy in hypertensive patients?

All hypertensive patients could have their CVD risk reduced by 30% (and stroke by 25%) by the addition of statin therapy (ASCOT-LLA). The targets are total cholesterol ≤ 4.0 mmol/l and LDL cholesterol ≤ 2.0 mmol/l. Low HDL cholesterol or raised triglycerides (diabetes, glucose intolerance, obesity) may respond to exercise, weight loss, fibrates, nicotinic acid or Omacor as additional therapy. The BHS guidelines suggest:

- For secondary prevention (including patients with type 2 diabetes) aspirin should be used unless contraindicated plus a statin in sufficient doses to reach targets if aged up to at least 80 years with a total cholesterol ≥ 3.5 mmol/l.
- For primary prevention, aspirin 75 mg daily is indicated if aged ≥ 50 years with blood pressure controlled to < 150/90 and target organ damage, diabetes or a 10-year risk of CVD ≥ 20%, plus a statin in sufficient dose to reach targets if aged up to at least 80 years with a 10-year risk of CVD ≥ 20% and a total cholesterol ≥ 3.5 mmol/l.
- For primary and secondary prevention, targets are to lower total cholesterol by 25% or LDL by 30% or to reach ≤ 4.0 mmol/l or ≤ 2.0 mmol/l, respectively.

NEUROLOGICAL PROBLEMS

CASE 2.15

HEADACHE

Candidate information

Role

You are a doctor in the emergency medical admissions unit. Please read the following letter from the patient's general practitioner. You may make notes on the paper provided. When the bell sounds, enter the examination room to begin the consultation.

Scenario

Dear Doctor

Re: Ms Deborah Good, aged 23 years

Please see this young lady, who developed a severe headache over the weekend. I am concerned that it has not improved after two days and would appreciate your excluding serious causes before treating it as migraine. She is normally well and works at your hospital as a dietitian.

Yours sincerely

Please take a history from the patient (you may continue to make notes if you wish on the paper provided). Your examiners will warn you when 12 minutes have elapsed. You have 14 minutes to take a history from the patient followed by 1 minute of reflection. There will then follow 5 minutes of discussion with the examiners. Be prepared to discuss solutions to the problems posed by the case and how you might reply to the GP's letter. You are not required to examine the patient.

Patient information

Ms Deborah Good is a 23-year-old dietitian who developed a sudden headache two days ago which has not improved and now she has been admitted to hospital. The headache came on suddenly during a night out drinking with friends and felt like something 'popping' at the back of her head. She has a history of migraine headaches for which she takes occasional sumatriptan or over-the-counter tablets. Her migraines usually evolve over a few hours, tend to be unilateral, usually left-sided but occasionally right, and associated with photophobia and nausea, but this headache was more sudden and did not respond to medication. Her migraine headaches have worsened recently because of work stresses and she has had almost daily headaches for the last two months. Her daily headaches are band-like across both temples and tend to be worse in the afternoon. She has taken more over-the-counter paracetamol, ibuprofen and codeine because of these. She does not sleep well and finds work tiring. She does not smoke and has never taken illicit drugs. She seldom drinks alcohol but last weekend was an exception when she was 'drowning her sorrows' with friends. She is very afraid both of being admitted to the hospital where she works and of needles.

How to approach the case

Data gathering in the interview and interpretation and use of information gathered

Presenting problem(s) and symptom exploration

▪ **Elicit details of the headaches** She likely has two or three different types of headache and it is important to elicit the following details for each:

- How *recently* headaches began (days, weeks, months or years ago) and if they have *changed* over time
- *Frequency* of headaches – episodic (e.g. daily, weekly, monthly, cyclical) or unremitting. A headache diary is useful
- *Details about each headache* – presence or absence of aura, time of day, associated sleep disturbance, after intercourse or exertion
- *Duration* of each headache, with and without treatment
- *Character (quality and intensity)* of the headache (e.g. dull ache, lancing pain) and associated symptoms such as nausea, vomiting or photophobia, or focal neurological symptoms
- *Site and spread* of headache and whether unilateral or bilateral
- *Predisposing* or *trigger* or *aggravating factors* such as foods, work, sneezing, coughing or bending
- *Relieving factors* such as a darkened room
- What the patient *does during the attack* and what activities are limited by it
- State of health between attacks
- Interventions to date

▪ **Consider causes** A knowledge of causes of headache (Box 2.40), exclusion of serious causes (Box 2.41) and appreciation that multiple types of headache often overlap is essential. One approach to making the diagnosis is to consider three questions:

- Is there a recognisable syndrome, such as migraine?
- Could it be a serious headache, such as a subarachnoid haemorrhage (SAH), meningitis or the result of raised intracranial pressure?
- Could there be an alternative diagnosis?

Patterns of headache are important. Acute single headaches could be the result of a first migraine, SAH or meningitis. Recurrent headaches could be migraine, tension-type headache or cluster headache. Dull headache increasing in

Box 2.40 Causes of headache

The International Headache Society updated its headache classification in 2004 and it remains largely based on clinical features.

Primary headaches

1. Migraine, without or with aura
2. Tension-type headache (TTH), episodic or chronic
3. Cluster headache and other trigeminal autonomic cephalgias (TAC)
4. Other primary headaches, including stabbing, cough, exertional, sexual, hypnic and primary thunderclap headache, hemicrania continua and new daily persistent headache. Exertional and sexual headaches are repeated attacks of short-lived pain associated with activity; diagnosis cannot be made after one attack. Hypnic headaches are generalised headaches that wake from sleep, are brief (5–180 minutes) and may occur 2–3 times per night; they present exclusively in older people and are benign. Primary thunderclap headache has features of subarachnoid haemorrhage but with negative investigations.

Transformation from episodic migraine or TTH to chronic headache may be attributed to analgesics, hormones or depression. The most recent classification attempts to classify patients with chronic headache who improve after aggravating factors have been removed, e.g. probable medication overuse headache (MOH) – confirmation of this diagnosis is only if chronicity ceases during a two-month period without regular analgesics. Persistent headache, defined as pain > 15 days a month for > 3 months, is then considered chronic. Most patients with chronic headache, now termed 'new daily persistent headache', arise from episodic migraine or TTH, and as headache becomes more chronic there are fewer features that unequivocally distinguish migraine from TTH.

Secondary headaches

5. Headache associated with head and/or neck trauma including chronic post-traumatic headache
6. Headache attributed to cranial or cervical vascular disorders, including ischaemia, intracerebral haemorrhage, subarachnoid haemorrhage (SAH), giant cell arteritis, carotid or vertebral artery dissection and cerebral venous sinus thrombosis
7. Headache attributed to non-vascular intracranial disorders, including idiopathic intracranial hypertension and increased intracranial pressure from neoplasm and hydrocephalus
8. Headache attributed to a substance or its withdrawal, including acute alcohol-induced headache, food-related headaches and MOH; MOH is now known to be an important cause of headaches, daily TTH provoked by most analgesics and migraine by triptans
9. Headache attributed to infection
10. Headache attributed to a disorder of homeostasis including hypoxia or hypercapnia, metabolic disturbance, fasting, arterial hypertension (including phaeochromocytoma) and hypertensive encephalopathy
11. Headache or facial pain attributed to disorder of cranium, neck, eyes, ears, nose, sinuses, teeth, mouth or other facial or cranial structures, including headache of cervical spine origin, acute sinus headache, acute glaucoma and optic neuritis with visual loss
12. Headache attributed to psychiatric disorder
13. Cranial neuralgias and central causes of facial pain, including trigeminal neuralgia and occipital neuralgia

Box 2.41 Symptoms of some serious headaches

Sub-arachnoid haemorrhage (SAH)

- Sudden onset
- 'Worst headache ever' (explosive)
- Headache alone in 20%
- Vomiting
- Warning or sentinel bleeds possibly a myth
- The crucial step in the history is to establish how quickly the headache reached maximal intensity – a headache still increasing in severity after 15 minutes is unlikely to be an SAH (although it could still have a serious pathology, e.g. meningitis). For exactly how many minutes a headache may still crescendo and still be SAH is unknown, as is for how long an SAH headache may last, although most physicians would think SAH unlikely if it does not reach maximum intensity within a minute of onset and fully resolves within an hour or two.

Meningitis

- Onset over hours to days
- Fever
- Neck pain and stiffness
- Drowsiness

Raised intracranial pressure due to structural lesions

- Morning headaches
- Exacerbation by coughing or bending forward
- Seizures
- Personality change

severity is usually benign, but may be caused by medication overuse, the oral contraceptive pill, idiopathic intracranial hypertension, neck disease, giant cell arteritis or tumour. A dull, unchanging headache may be a chronic tension-type headache or as a result of depression.

Patient perspective

Explore any concerns she may have about the cause of the headache and appreciate her fear of being admitted to her workplace and of needles.

Past medical history

Explore her migraine symptoms. Patients with migraine without aura report recurrent headaches lasting 4–72 hours (untreated or unsuccessfully treated) with:

- A normal physical examination
- No other reversible cause
- At least two of unilateral location, pulsating or throbbing quality, moderate or severe intensity or aggravation by routine activity (as such, there may be marked restriction of usual activities)
- At least one of nausea or vomiting, or photophobia or phonophobia

Patients tend to prefer a quiet, dark room. Recently recognised features of migraine include cutaneous allodynia (tender skin/face/scalp) and autonomic symptoms such as nasal stuffiness. Patients with migraine with aura (10–20%) report, in addition, reversible focal neurological disturbances such as hemianopia, speech disturbance or unilateral paraesthesia of face, arm or hand. Many have ill-defined blurring of vision and/or photophobia. Occasionally there are more characteristic disturbances, including bright zigzags migrating across the visual field from the centre to the periphery over about 30 minutes with or without transient loss of vision. Some patients develop an aura without headaches. Migraine frequency varies widely – three to four attacks per week to but a few in a lifetime.

Tension-type headache has at least two of the following characteristics – bilateral band-like location, pressure/tightening (non-pulsating) quality, mild or moderate intensity and not aggravated by routine physical activity. It is rarely significantly disabling. Nausea or vomiting is not a feature but photophobia may occur. It may spread to or from the neck, and may be associated with stress or cervical or cranial musculoskeletal abnormalities. It seldom lasts more than a few hours and may be infrequent or frequent and episodic or chronic, the latter occurring on most days. Most never seek medical advice but many take analgesics daily and the headache often settles when these are withdrawn.

Depression and anxiety symptoms should be explored.

Drug and allergy history

Medication overuse headache is caused by a wide range of analgesics, which paradoxically exacerbate symptoms when used regularly.

Family history

A family history of migraine is common. Any family history of sudden unexplained death or confirmed aneurysmal leaks is important to elicit.

Social history

Ask about stresses at work and at home. Migraine can disrupt social life and employment to a great extent.

SUMMARY – ASSESSMENT AND PLAN

- Explain that she probably has a combination of tension-type headache and alcohol withdrawal headache on a background of migraine and stress. Explain that these are non-threatening and will get better.
- Explain that a small subarachnoid haemorrhage cannot be excluded but it is essential to exclude it by computed tomography (CT) brain scan and possible lumbar puncture, being sensitive to her fear of needles.

Discussion

How are migraine attacks treated?

Acute treatments include aspirin, non-steroidal anti-inflammatory drugs (NSAIDs) or triptans, orally then parenterally.

What different triptans are there?

The benefits of ergotamine are thought to be mediated by agonist activity at the serotonin $5\text{-}HT_{1B}$ and $5\text{-}HT_{1D}$ receptors and triptans are pure agonists of these without the side effects of ergotamine, which acts at other receptors such as $5\text{-}HT_2$. The pharmacological and clinical differences between sumatriptan, zolmitriptan, rizatriptan and probably eletriptan seem small, but naratriptan, almotripan and perhaps frovatriptan have longer duration of action and sometimes delayed onset of action and a lower incidence of short-term side effects and a lower recurrence rate. Triptans are contra-indicated in ischaemic heart disease. Side effects include paraesthesia and myalgia. Sumatriptan and zolmitriptan are available as nasal sprays and are suitable where vomiting is a major migraine feature.

How is migraine prevented?

Triggers should be avoided, e.g. cheese, chocolate, citrus, caffeine, many types of alcoholic drink. Be aware that the oral contraceptive pill or hormone replacement therapy can be triggers. Beta blockers (propranolol or atenolol) are the prophylactic treatment of choice in patients without asthma. Topiramate is a newer, well-tolerated, effective strategy for migraine prophylaxis at 100 mg daily and is a useful second-line treatment. Amitriptyline and sodium valproate have some prophylactic evidence. Gabapentin may be tried third line. Methysergide and pizotifen are now used much less frequently. It is recognised that a subtle persistently patent foramen ovale can cause migraine and this can be closed.

What are cluster headaches and other trigeminal autonomic cephalgias (TACs)?

Cluster headaches are more common in males and may occur from every other day to multiple times per day. They are characterised by severe and disabling unilateral orbital, supraorbital and/or temporal pain lasting 15–180 minutes associated with ipsilateral autonomic features such as conjunctival injection and lacrimation, nasal congestion and/or rhinorrhoea, eyelid oedema, facial sweating, miosis or ptosis.

Analgesia is difficult, but treatments include oxygen, subcutaneous sumatriptan or nasal sumatriptan or zolmitriptan, verapamil (current treatment of choice), lithium, gabapentin and corticosteroids.

Related disorders include paroxysmal hemicrania, shortlasting neuralgiform headache with conjunctival injection and tearing ('SUNCT') and TACs.

How is an SAH diagnosed?

Non-contrast CT detects > 90% of SAH if performed in the first 12 hours after onset of symptoms, but sensitivity decreases thereafter or if a small bleed is suspected. Lumbar puncture is mandatory if CT is negative and the history is typical, although many patients will have normal cerebrospinal fluid (thunderclap headache). Lumbar puncture should be performed after 12 hours from the onset of symptoms and the use of spectrophotometry should be used to detect xanthochromia.

What is xanthochromia?

Net bilirubin absorption (NBA) is calculated from spectrophotometric scanning. Xanthochromia is caused by the presence of bilirubin in the sample from the breakdown of red blood cells. Phagocytosis of the red cells releases oxyhaemoglobin (oxyHb), which is converted to bilirubin in vivo in a time-dependent manner. False-positives may be the result of increased cerebrospinal fluid (CSF) protein or jaundice and results may be interpreted as follows:

- No significant NBA and no oxyHb – no evidence of SAH
- No significant NBA but oxyHb present – SAH very unlikely and bloody tap possible (the absence of bilirubin in the presence of oxyHb suggests that red cells are fresh and have not yet broken down, which is not the case in SAH provided that a lumbar puncture has been performed after 12 hours); discuss with neurosurgeons if there are clinical concerns
- NBA present and no oxyHb – may be the result of jaundice (if serum bilirubin normal and CSF protein low then SAH is likely, usually in those presenting a week after symptom onset; if serum bilirubin is high then SAH is likely if the adjusted NBA is high and jaundice is probable if it is low and oxyHb is absent)
- NBA and oxyHb present – SAH very likely

List some causes of headache and fever

- Meningitis (bacterial or viral)
- Encephalitis
- Cerebral abscess
- Otitis media
- Mastoiditis
- Non-specific symptom of infection elsewhere, e.g. pneumonia, sinusitis, tonsillitis
- Non-infectious causes, e.g. SAH, cerebral venous sinus thrombosis, giant cell arteritis, pontine haemorrhage

List some warning signs in meningococcal disease

Warning signs of impending shock, respiratory failure or raised intracranial pressure in meningococcal disease are

---

Box 2.42 Warning signs in meningococcal disease

- Rapidly progressive rash
- Respiratory rate < 8 or > 30 breaths per minute
- Poor peripheral perfusion, capillary refill time > 4 seconds, oliguria or systolic blood pressure < 90 mmHg (hypotension often a late sign)
- Heart rate < 40 or ≥ 140 beats per minute
- Acidosis (pH < 7.3 or base excess > − 5)
- White cell count $< 4 \times 10^9$/l
- Markedly depressed [Glasgow Coma Score (GCS) < 12 or fluctuating (decrease in GCS > 2)] level of consciousness
- Focal neurology
- Persistent seizures
- Papilloedema

---

listed in Box 2.42. Most of these would be contraindications to lumbar puncture.

What are the findings of a normal CSF examination?

Fluid is clear with a normal pressure of 8–16 cmH$_2$O, fewer than five lymphocytes, a protein concentration of 0.1–0.45 g/l and a glucose concentration more than 50% that of blood glucose.

Should patients with suspected bacterial meningitis be scanned before lumbar puncture?

There is no evidence for this, and CT scanning is not reliable in excluding raised intracranial pressure. Generally, patients with suspected meningitis do not need neuroimaging prior to lumbar puncture, but indications to do so include diagnostic doubt (e.g. sudden headache and suspected intracranial haemorrhage), signs of raised pressure (e.g. severe vomiting, papilloedema), focal neurology, impaired consciousness or seizures.

What is the treatment of choice for bacterial meningitis?

The most common causes of community-acquired bacterial meningitis are *Neisseria meningitides* and *Streptococcus pneumoniae*. Cefotaxime 2 g six-hourly or ceftriaxone 2 g 12-hourly with vancomycin and/or rifampicin for suspected penicillin-resistant meningococci are recommended in the UK where third-generation cephalosporin resistance to *S. pneumoniae* is less prevalent. Adults over 55 years of age and anyone at risk (e.g. soft cheese consumers) should also receive amoxicillin 2 g four-hourly as *Listeria monocytogenes* is possible. Brain imaging is not necessary in most cases initially. Dexamethasone is now given with antibiotics unless there are contraindications.

When might you scan a patient with a headache?

Indications for a scan are given in Box 2.43.

What is idiopathic intracranial hypertension?

This causes a progressive headache more common in obese young women. It is associated with intracranial hypertension, the latter often characterised by any of papilloedema, an enlarged blind spot, a visual field defect or a sixth nerve palsy, together with increased CSF pressure (> 200 mmH$_2$O in non-obese, > 250 mmH$_2$O in obese). CSF chemistry is normal. Other disorders must be excluded, including venous sinus thrombosis, and the cause is uncertain although microthrombi (i.e. part of the venous sinus

---

Box 2.43 When to scan a patient with a headache

- First or worst headache, particularly of sudden onset
- Headaches of increasing severity or frequency
- Increasing frequency of vomiting or headache on waking
- Headache triggered by coughing or straining or change in posture (although many headaches are worse with these, including sinusitis)
- Persistent symptoms or signs after attacks
- Meningism, confusion, impairment of consciousness or seizures

thrombosis spectrum) have been postulated. Headache relates closely to intracranial pressure and improves after withdrawal of CSF to 120–170 mmH$_2$O.

What do you know about cerebral venous sinus thrombosis (CVST)?

Although uncommon, CVST is an important cause of headache. Predisposing factors include pregnancy, prothrombotic states, dehydration and sepsis, especially intracranial. Headache is usually generalised and acute or subacute. There may be signs of raised intracranial pressure, meningism, altered consciousness, seizures (often focal) and focal neurological deficit due to stroke (venous infarct). A non-contrast CT in the acute phase may show an 'empty delta' sign and hyperintensity in the sagittal, straight and transverse sinuses. CT or MR venography is useful. Initial treatment is with heparin followed by warfarin, duration dependent on persistence of the underlying cause. Secondary intracranial venous haemorrhage is common and does not necessarily contraindicate anticoagulation.

CASE 2.16

TRANSIENT ISCHAEMIC ATTACK

Candidate information

Role

You are a doctor in a rapid access transient ischaemic attack (TIA)/stroke clinic. Please read the following letter from the patient's general practitioner. You may make notes on the paper provided. When the bell sounds, enter the examination room to begin the consultation.

Scenario

> Dear Doctor
> Re: Mr Jack Middleton, aged 72 years
> Thank you for seeing Mr Middleton, who last week experienced an episode of expressive dysphasia. It lasted around five minutes. His vision, hearing and limb movements were unaffected. He is in sinus rhythm and blood pressure is currently around 160/90 mmHg. He takes amlodipine for hypertension. I would appreciate assessment in your rapid access stroke clinic.
> Yours sincerely

Please take a history from the patient (you may continue to make notes if you wish on the paper provided). Your examiners will warn you when 12 minutes have elapsed. You have 14 minutes to take a history from the patient followed by 1 minute of reflection. There will then follow 5 minutes of discussion with the examiners. Be prepared

to discuss solutions to the problems posed by the case and how you might reply to the GP's letter. You are not required to examine the patient.

Patient information

Mr Jack Middleton is a 72-year-old gentleman who last week had an episode of being unable to talk. He could hear what others were saying and knew how he wished to reply, but could not speak words which expressed his thoughts, or, if he began to, could not complete his sentences and found himself substituting incorrect words. It lasted around five minutes. He is usually well apart from high blood pressure, for which he takes amlodipine. He has also had two episodes in which his right hand became 'clumsy', during which he was unable to do up his shoelaces or grip objects properly. He is very concerned about the speech loss and weakness because he is a composer who not only plays piano but lectures on music.

How to approach the case

Data gathering in the interview and interpretation and use of information gathered

Presenting problem(s) and symptom exploration

■ **Elicit details of symptoms**   Establish handedness. The dominant hemisphere is usually the left, in right-handed individuals. Around 50% of left-handed individuals have a dominant right hemisphere. Then elicit details of symptoms (Box 2.44).

> **Box 2.44 Symptoms of transient ischaemic attacks (TIAs)**
>
> Symptoms attributable to a TIA relate to a specific area of the brain. Loss of consciousness, syncope and confusion do not have a focal origin and are *not* suggestive of a TIA. Diagnosing a TIA remains largely clinical and the following features are characteristic:
>
> • Symptoms are almost invariably of *sudden onset*.
> • The deficit tends to be *maximal at the onset* with progressive resolution over minutes or hours.
> • Attacks are *self-limiting*.
> • Symptoms are characteristically '*negative*' e.g. loss of movement, rather than unwanted movement.
> • Symptoms are *attributable to focal areas of brain* such as motor cortex or language areas. *Anterior circulation TIAs* may produce weakness or sensory symptoms in the contralateral upper limb, lower limb or face, dysphasia (especially dominant hemisphere, usually left) or amaurosis fugax. *Posterior circulation TIAs* may produce diplopia, ataxia, dysphagia, unilateral or bilateral weakness or sensory symptoms but usually more than one symptom.
> • Most patients do not experience significant headache but mild headache can occur. Severe headache during the attack should prompt an alternative diagnosis.
> • Loss of consciousness is highly unusual (perhaps 1:1000 to 1:10 000 patients), and almost always the result of a small proportion of basilar TIAs that disturb consciousness centres. It is surprising how frequently loss of consciousness or confusion remain cited as 'probable TIA' or 'probable stroke' in hospital admissions. It appears to be a myth that is hard to dispel.

■ **Consider other conditions that can produce focal neurological symptoms**

- Migraine (particularly acephalgic)
- Focal seizure or focal weakness (Todd's paresis) following a seizure
- Intracranial space-occupying lesion (haemorrhage, tumour)
- Disorders causing vertigo
- Metabolic disturbances (usually global)
- Demyelination

Patient perspective

Assure him that your purpose is to prevent further attacks. Tell him that his GP was very correct to arrange urgent referral because TIAs or 'mini-strokes' are possible warning signs of a more significant stroke, but that the risk can be markedly reduced with prompt investigation and appropriate treatment. Explain that a TIA or 'mini-stroke' is usually the result of a small blood clot or a piece of fatty material that has broken off into the circulation.

Past medical history

TIAs are usually caused by atherosclerosis or emboli. Patients frequently have a history of cardiovascular disease, hypertension (the single biggest risk factor for stroke) or atrial fibrillation.

Drug and allergy history

Ask about previous treatment for hypertension and any intolerance of drugs.

Family history

A family history is seldom relevant.

Social history

This is very important, particularly with respect to smoking, although in a rapid access stroke clinic it often gives way to the pressing arrangement of urgent investigations.

SUMMARY – ASSESSMENT AND PLAN

- The diagnosis is left anterior circulation TIAs.
- Brain imaging is not usually necessary with brief episodes, unless there are features of concern such as headache or a history of malignancy or if TIAs have recurred in a short time-frame.
- Carotid Dopplers are indicated urgently.
- A 24-hour ECG recording is desirable to look for paroxysmal atrial fibrillation (PAF).
- An echocardiogram may be indicated if there are murmurs or if a mural thrombus is possible (e.g. recent myocardial infarction).
- Aspirin 300 mg daily for two weeks (then 75 mg daily) and dipyridamole MR 200 mg b.d. are indicated, substituted by warfarin if an embolic source is discovered (usually PAF, less commonly mural thrombus).
- Statin therapy (simvastatin 40 mg) is almost invariably indicated.
- Blood pressure should be vigorously controlled (after a stroke treatment is usually not manipulated for 14 days but it should be controlled quickly after a TIA).

Discussion

Which investigations would you recommend for a patient following a suspected TIA?

Investigations are best undertaken via a rapid access TIA/stroke clinic but high-risk patients who may warrant immediate admission to hospital include those with crescendo TIAs. Investigations are directed at establishing a predisposing cause (Table 2.29).

What additional investigations might be indicated in selected patients?

These are outlined in Table 2.30.

How does carotid stenosis cause TIAs?

While dislodged fatty atheromatous material, particularly prevalent in smokers, was traditionally thought to be the major mechanism, evidence now suggests that the mechanism from such atheromatous plaques is the same as that in coronary syndromes; a plaque may rupture, fissure or erode, triggering platelet aggregation and formation of thrombus which leads to local occlusion or distal embolisation. Cap thickness in ruptured carotid plaques is generally thicker than ruptured coronary plaques, but rupture is still associated with relatively thin caps with dense macrophage infiltration.

Why do recurrent TIAs often give rise to identical symptoms?

Recurrent TIAs often have similar characteristics, implying that the same area of brain is rendered ischaemic. The cause is usually recurrent atherosclerotic embolism and emboli must therefore tend to lodge in the same small artery recurrently. As the point of origin of an embolus is far from its final lodging place, and with a potentially large number of other small arteries to choose from, the question of how so many emboli reach the same artery is at first intriguing. The probable explanation is the 'Poohsticks phenomenon', that currents and eddies in blood vessels are similar at different times, such that many emboli released from the internal carotid artery might be expected to reach the same destination, just as many 'Poohsticks' thrown into a stream from the same point on a bridge follow a similar course.

Why does dissection cause TIAs and strokes?

This is either by occlusion from the dissecting vessel or, more commonly, by thrombus forming within the dissected wall throwing off emboli.

Why might a patent foramen ovale lead to stroke?

While stroke is more likely in people with active venous thromboembolism, small clots may form in the circulation in healthy people that would otherwise be filtered and broken down in the pulmonary circulation.

Table 2.29 Routine investigations following a TIA

Investigation	Indications	Reason
Blood tests – full blood picture, urea and electrolytes, glucose, lipid profile, coagulation profile	All patients	Exclude diabetes Assess lipid profile
ECG	All patients	Exclude atrial fibrillation or recent myocardial infarction
Carotid Dopplers	All patients with anterior circulation symptoms, including amaurosis fugax, who would be considered fit for endarterectomy	Exclude carotid stenosis of at least 70% on appropriate side
24-hour ECG	Many patients (especially if history of palpitations)	Exclude paroxysmal atrial fibrillation
Echocardiography	Multi-territory symptoms Recent myocardial infarction Atrial fibrillation (if cardioversion might be contemplated) Murmurs	Assess left atrial size and assess for thrombus Exclude mural thrombus Exclude endocarditis (transoesophageal echocardiography if cardiac origin strongly suspected but not confirmed by transthoracic echocardiography)
	Heart failure Young patients (especially if history of or suspected venous thromboembolism)	Exclude significant hypokinesis Exclude patent foramen ovale
Brain imaging	Prolonged TIAs Features of concern, e.g. headache, history of malignancy	Exclude bleed Exclude tumour Exclude arteriovenous malformation

Table 2.30 Selected investigations following a transient ischaemic attack (TIA)

Investigation	Indications	Purpose
Erythrocyte sedimentation rate C-reactive protein Temporal artery biopsy	Headache Older patients	Exclude giant cell arteritis
Autoimmune screen Vasculitis screen	Other symptoms or signs suggesting autoimmune disease Raised inflammatory markers	Exclude systemic lupus erythematosus Exclude primary systemic vasculitis (seldom causes TIAs)
Thrombophilia screen	Young patient Recurrent	Exclude antiphospholipid syndrome (Protein C deficiency, protein S deficiency, activated protein C resistance and antithrombin III deficiency usually associated with venous and not with arterial thrombosis)
MR or CT angiography	History or trauma Progressive or 'crescendo' symptoms	Exclude carotid or vertebral dissection
CT angiography of aortic arch	Recurrent TIAs in same hemi-territory with normal carotid Dopplers	Exclude significant aortic arch atheroma
CT angiography of thorax	Sensory symptoms in arm with arm raised above head Cervical rib on chest X-ray	Exclude thoracic outlet syndrome
Echocardiogram (with 'bubbles')	History of venous thromboembolism	Exclude patent foramen ovale or other right to left shunt

Patent foramina ovales are not uncommon, perhaps as common as 10–20% in the adult population, and usually asymptomatic.

What are crescendo TIAs?

These are TIAs that rapidly increase in frequency or severity. They warrant urgent admission to hospital. They are not very common, and are usually the result of carotid stenosis or a stroke 'mimic' such as a tumour. Urgent brain imaging is needed.

What secondary prevention measures would you recommend for a patient after a suspected TIA?

The risk of stroke after a TIA is highest in the first year and patients remain at increased risk without secondary prevention. Measures are listed in Table 2.31.

Table 2.31 Secondary prevention after a suspected TIA

Management strategy	Indication
Carotid endarterectomy	Symptomatic carotid stenosis ≥ 70%
Aspirin and dipyridamole	Ischaemic stroke (ESPRIT study)
Clopidogrel	Considered alone instead of dual antiplatelet therapy with aspirin and dipyridamole if aspirin intolerance (aspirin plus clopidogrel benefits negated by bleeding risks in MATCH trial); however, if dipyridamole intolerance then aspirin preferred to clopidogrel
Anticoagulation	Embolic source (atrial fibrillation, mural thrombus)
Antihypertensive therapy	To achieve JBS-2 targets (Case 2.7)
Statin therapy	To achieve JBS-2 targets (Case 2.7)
Modification of other CVD risk factors (smoking cessation, increase exercise, meticulous glycaemic control)	All patients

Would you consider statin therapy in an 89-year-old following a TIA?

This is treatment 'outside the evidence-based box'. Although caution should be observed in extrapolating data from clinical trials to different patient groups, older people are under-represented in clinical trials and absence of evidence does not equate to absence of benefit and a treatment with evidence so compelling as statin therapy should be considered in an independent, free-living person 'outside the box'.

Would you consider referral for consideration of endarterectomy in a patient with asymptomatic carotid stenosis?

This is contentious, with emerging evidence of benefit balanced against a 1–2% of risk of a severe stroke due to the procedure itself as atheromatous material is dislodged and endothelium disturbed.

Would you consider referral for consideration of endarterectomy in a patient with less than 70% carotid stenosis and symptomatic territory?

Although the evidence for endarterectomy is for stenosis of at least 70%, compelling symptoms and severe stenosis that does not reach 70% may still warrant referral to vascular surgeons for consideration. Crescendo TIAs thought to be the result of carotid stenosis may also warrant consideration.

Do carotid stenoses merit treatment with warfarin, and when should endarterectomy be considered?

Dual antiplatelet therapy is the antithrombotic treatment of choice, rather than warfarin, together with modification of other risk factors and urgent consideration of endarterectomy if there is carotid stenosis of at least 70% on the relevant side.

How urgently should endarterectomy be performed in symptomatic carotid stenosis of at least 70%?

It should be performed as soon as possible; the risk of major stroke is up to 30% in the first month, falling rapidly with time, as does the benefit of endarterectomy – the number needed to treat to prevent one major event is five in the first two weeks but 125 after 12 weeks. The benefit may be particularly great after a small stroke compared with a TIA.

Would you anticoagulate a patient with recurrent TIAs despite antiplatelet therapy?

This is contentious. Recurrent TIAs should generally still be treated with dual antiplatelet therapy except where an embolic source has been identified, in which case warfarin is appropriate. In an acute situation, where TIAs are 'hotly' recurring, intravenous heparin may be considered, and is very important in atrial fibrillation or with clinically relevant carotid stenosis, following brain imaging that excludes alternative pathology, and with a plan for urgent or early consideration of carotid endarterectomy in the latter.

A patient with a non-STEMI and a recent stent has a small cerebral infarct. He is not in atrial fibrillation. His echocardiogram shows moderate hypokinesis but no mural thrombus. He must take aspirin and clopidogrel for cardiac reasons. Would you add warfarin at day 14?

Aspirin and clopidogrel are indicated for cardiac reasons (CURE study and stent survival), although the combination has been shown to be associated with a risk of haemorrhage that approximately negates any benefit in stroke (MATCH study). Aspirin and dipyridamole are safer and effective (ESPRIT). Additional anticoagulation is not without risk, and might be mandated were a mural thrombus demonstrated or were there an akinetic segment, for at least a few months. With moderate hypokinesis, it may be best to avoid warfarin. This is an example of a hole in the evidence, widened by conflicting evidence for two different conditions.

What if the same patient were found to be in atrial fibrillation?

In this situation warfarin at day 14 would ordinarily be important (see also Case 3.27). However, the cardiologists would doubtless recommend he stay on antiplatelet therapy, not least clopidogrel, much favoured to anticoagulation for prevention of stent stenosis. Evidence would not answer this question unequivocally. One option would be to continue aspirin and clopidogrel for the stent for 9–12 months, switching to aspirin and warfarin, or warfarin alone, thereafter. An alternative option would be early anticoagulation, perhaps retaining the clopidogrel alongside it but relinquishing the aspirin since three antithrombotic agents might prove to be a somewhat extravagant temper of fate; this might be a more com-pelling option were he to have severe hypokinesis with a mural thrombus.

How is carotid dissection managed?

It is usually managed with antithrombotic therapy, either anticoagulation or dual antiplatelet therapy. There is not a strong evidence base to guide.

Which patients with a TIA are at highest risk of subsequent stroke?

Two prognostic scores, the ABCD score to predict risk of stroke at 7 days and the California score to predict risk of stroke at 90 days, have been validated by a study by Johnston et al for predicting stroke risk after a TIA. The study also showed that a new unified score, ABCD based on five clinical factors, had greater predictive value. The validity of ABCD is also supported by studies identifying age, limb weakness, and diabetes as risk factors for stroke after a TIA. Aspects of ABCD (e.g. unilateral weakness, speech disturbance, prolonged TIA duration) may have prognostic value because they improve the diagnosis of TIA. Features that are important vascular risk factors (increasing age, high blood pressure, and diabetes) are likely to be relevant to the cause of future stroke.

The unified $ABCD^2$ score (range 0–7) is a summation of five independent risk predictors: age (≥ 60 years = 1), blood pressure (systolic > 140 mmHg or diastolic ≥ 90 mmHg = 1), clinical features (focal weakness = 2, speech impairment without focal weakness = 1), duration of symptoms (≥ 60 min = 2, 10–59 min = 1) and diabetes = 1. The prevalence of stroke is shown in Table 2.32.

Patients classified at higher risk (e.g. $ABCD^2 \geq 3$) should be managed within 24 hours (occasionally admitted) with neuroimaging (increasingly DW MRI, see also Case 3.27), carotid duplex/Doppler ultrasound, antiplatelet therapy and secondary prophylaxis. Referral for carotid endarterectomy in patients with a TIA or non-disabling stroke and consistent carotid stenosis of 70–99% (EST criteria) or 50–99% (NASCET criteria) should ideally be within 7 days. Patients at low risk should be managed similarly but first assessed within 7 days. Additional risk factors might augment the predictive accuracy of $ABCD^2$ (e.g. frequent TIAs, symptomatic large artery disease, new ischaemic lesions on imaging).

CASE 2.17

WEAKNESS AND WASTING

Candidate information

Role

You are a doctor in the emergency medical admissions unit. Please read the following letter from the patient's general practitioner. You may make notes on the paper provided. When the bell sounds, enter the examination room to begin the consultation.

Scenario

Dear Doctor

Re: Mr John Willoughby, aged 68 years

Thank you for admitting this man, who has been losing a dramatic amount of weight over the last three months (around 12 kg). He was seen recently in the outpatient clinic where it was noted that he had ataxia and postural hypotension. Normal blood tests included urea and electrolytes and renal function, liver function tests, calcium, C-reactive protein (CRP), full blood count, thyroid function and prostate-specific antigen (PSA). An urgent computed tomography (CT) brain scan was normal, as was a synacthen test, and he was started on fludrocortisone without effect. He has subsequently developed what appears to be a right radial nerve palsy, and possibly ulnar wasting of the hand together with fasciculation. He is due for clinic review soon but his ataxia has worsened considerably and I feel he needs urgent inpatient assessment.

Yours sincerely

Please take a history from the patient (you may continue to make notes if you wish on the paper provided). Your examiners will warn you when 12 minutes have elapsed. You have 14 minutes to take a history from the patient followed by 1 minute of reflection. There will then follow 5 minutes of discussion with the examiners. Be prepared to discuss solutions to the problems posed by the case and how you might reply to the GP's letter. You are not required to examine the patient.

Patient information

Mr John Willoughby is a 68-year-old gentleman who has just been admitted to hospital for investigation of weight loss, unsteadiness and light-headedness. His weight loss

Table 2.32 Prevalence of stroke (%) at 2, 7 and 90 days after a TIA using the unified $ABCD^2$ risk score

Risk group (score)	2-day stroke	7-day stroke	90-day stroke
Low (0–3)	1.0	1.2	3.1
Moderate (4–5)	4.1	5.9	9.8
High (6–7)	8.1	12	18

has been rapid, over two to three months. He has no significant past medical history other than rheumatic fever as a child. He takes no medications. He is an ex-builder, and has a past history of alcohol excess (up to 10 units per day but absolutely no alcohol in the past 12 months) and heavy smoking. There is no family history of balance problems. His balance is very unsteady, like being on a ship in rough seas, and he has a tremor of both arms that is worse with movement. He has recently developed weakness of his right hand, and noticed that his muscles are wasting quickly. He lives alone, and is not looking after himself very well, but is a little passive about this.

How to approach the case

Data gathering in the interview and interpretation and use of information gathered

Presenting problem(s) and symptom exploration

The differential diagnosis of subacute weakness and weight loss is wide (Table 2.33).

Patient perspective

Although he is not looking after himself and not eating well, his weight loss should not be attributed to this. Whether or not he is perturbed by his situation, he should be offered full social services, occupational therapy and physiotherapy assessments.

Past medical history

Infective endocarditis in the context of rheumatic heart disease must be considered, but the normal CRP would be very unusual.

Drug and allergy history

He appears not to be on any anorexogenic drugs.

Family history

A neurodegenerative disorder should always be considered such as a familial spinocerebellar disorder. Motor neuron disease is rarely hereditary.

Social history

Alcohol-induced cerebellar degeneration could account for ataxia, but the profound wasting, focal neurological signs and weight loss should not be attributed to alcohol alone. The heavy smoking history makes a search for cancer paramount.

SUMMARY – ASSESSMENT AND PLAN

- He should have an urgent chest X-ray, and will almost certainly need a CT of thorax, abdomen and pelvis and magnetic resonance imaging of his brain and brainstem.
- Electrophysiological tests should be performed for any evidence of anterior horn cell disease.
- In addition to a full screen of blood tests, paraneoplastic antibodies – Hu, Yo, ganglioside – are probably warranted.

Discussion

How might malignancy affect the nervous system?

Possible mechanisms are outlined in Box 2.45.

Table 2.33 Causes of subacute weakness and weight loss	
Cause	**Likelihood**
Malignancy, especially paraneoplastic syndromes	High given weight loss, ataxia and smoking history Subacute onset and speed of progression unusual for most conditions, even for motor neurone disease, but typical of a paraneoplastic syndrome
Primary neurodegenerative disease, e.g. motor neurone disease, multiple sclerosis	Possible given wasting and weakness, ataxia and postural hypotension (Creutzfeldt–Jakob disease remains rare but must be considered with rapid weight loss and ataxia)
Spinal cord pathology	Low Does not explain lower motor neuron signs unless spinoradicular disease, e.g. T1 given hand findings Does not explain ataxia unless part of spinocerebellar ataxia
Guillain–Barré syndrome/Miller–Fischer syndrome	Not typical
Myasthenia gravis	Not typical
Myositis	Low Does not explain ataxia or fasciculation
Autoimmune disease including vasculitis	Unusual with normal C-reactive protein (CRP)
Infection, e.g. tuberculosis, subacute bacterial endocarditis	Unusual with normal CRP and neurological signs
Alcohol	Possible given alcohol history and ataxia (vitamin B12 deficiency must also be considered)
Toxicity, e.g. lead poisoning, botulism	Should always be considered, but unlikely

Table 2.34 Paraneoplastic antibodies

Paraneoplastic antibody	Effects	Cause
Anti-Hu (ANNA-1)	Encephalomyelitis Cerebellar neuropathy Sensory neuropathy due to dorsal root ganglion disease Autonomic neuropathy	Small cell lung cancer
Anti-Yo (PLA-1)	Cerebellar neuropathy (severe gait ataxia, nystagmus, dysarthria, limb ataxia)	Breast cancer Ovarian cancer
Anti-Ma	Cerebellar involvement Brainstem encephalitis (vertigo, ataxia, abnormal eye movements, long tract signs, cranial nerve signs, life threatening)	Breast, lung or colorectal cancer
Anti-Ma2 (Ta)	Limbic encephalitis (amnesia, confusion, seizures) Brainstem encephalitis	Testicular cancer
Anti-Ri (ANNA-2)	Opsoclonus–myoclonus Brainstem encephalitis	Breast cancer Small cell lung cancer
Anti-recoverin	Retinopathy	Small cell lung cancer
Anti-voltage-gated calcium channel	Lambert–Eaton myasthenic syndrome	Small cell lung cancer
Anti-CV2 (CRMP-5)	Encephalomyelitis, chorea, uveitis, optic neuropathy	Small cell lung cancer Thymoma
Anti-amphiphysin	Encephalomyelitis Stiff person syndrome (axial muscle stiffness)	Small cell lung cancer Breast cancer

Box 2.45 Malignancy and the nervous system

- Direct invasion
- Spinal metastases
- Opportunistic infection
- Neoplastic meningitis (e.g. cortical signs, headache, cranial neuropathies)
- Radiotherapy – white matter necrosis, Lhermitte's phenomenon (transient), transverse myelitis (spastic paraparesis), localised cord necrosis with oedema
- Metabolic – ectopic hormone production
- Paraneoplastic neurological disorders (PND)

What are the characteristic features of paraneoplastic syndromes?

These are rapidly progressive, often fatal within a few months. Standard investigations are normal, although high protein and oligoclonal bands in cerebrospinal fluid suggest an immune rather than degenerative cause.

What types of paraneoplastic syndrome do you know of?

These are outlined in Table 2.34.

CASE 2.18

MULTIPLE SCLEROSIS

Candidate information

Role

You are a doctor in the emergency medical admissions unit. Please read the following letter from the patient's general practitioner. You may make notes on the paper provided. When the bell sounds, enter the examination room to begin the consultation.

Scenario

> Dear Doctor
>
> Re: Mr Keith Bertram, aged 40 years
>
> Mr Bertram has become very unsteady on his feet in the last few days and now has a markedly ataxic gait. Last year he had an episode of optic neuritis and the ophthalmologist suggested to him, when asked, that multiple sclerosis could be a possibility. I am obviously concerned that this is a second episode of demyelination and appreciate your urgent assessment.
>
> Yours sincerely

Please take a history from the patient (you may continue to make notes if you wish on the paper provided). Your examiners will warn you when 12 minutes have elapsed. You have 14 minutes to take a history from the patient followed by 1 minute of reflection. There will then follow 5 minutes of discussion with the examiners. Be prepared to discuss solutions to the problems posed by the case and how you might reply to the GP's letter. You are not required to examine the patient.

Patient information

Mr Keith Bertram is a 40-year-old gentleman who has become very unsteady on his feet in the last few days and now has a markedly lurching gait, rather like being on ship. Last year he had an episode of visual blurring with pain in the right eye and the ophthalmologist suggested to him, when asked, that multiple sclerosis could be a possibility. He took this rather well, and tends to be someone who lives from day to day, taking whatever life brings. He would not describe himself as an alcoholic, but does 'like a drink' and recently has drunk a little more than usual (a bottle of whisky a week) to celebrate passing an Open University degree in Aboriginal culture. He is Australian by birth, and his sister (his only surviving relative) lives in Melbourne. He is hoping to go back to live in Australia soon, and work as a tour guide. He did not ever know his father. A second sister committed suicide 10 years ago. His mother died at the age of 60 from an unexplained neurodegenerative illness. Apart from the visual symptoms last year and the current symptoms, he has had a number of episodes of tingling in the right arm. He has normal bladder, bowel and erectile function.

How to approach the case

Data gathering in the interview and interpretation and use of information gathered

Presenting problem(s) and symptom exploration

▪ **Elicit the range of symptoms** Symptoms in multiple sclerosis (MS) tend to emerge over days, plateau and then resolve slowly. Symptoms characteristically may reappear transiently or worsen with increased body temperature (Uhtoff phenomenon). Symptoms arise from plaques in white matter tracts and so symptoms of cortical dysfunction such as dysphasia, hemiparesis or hemianopia are uncommon. Common symptoms in MS are limb weakness (initial presentation in 40%), optic neuritis (initial presentation in 22%), sensory disturbance (initial presentation in 21%), spasticity, ataxia, diplopia (initial presentation in 12%), fatigue, neuropathic pain, mood disturbance, erectile dysfunction and bladder and bowel dysfunction. Symptoms are more easily recalled by considering the sites of demyelination in Table 2.35.

▪ **Consider the types of MS** About 85% of patients present with a relapsing–remitting form of MS and after many years most enter a secondary progressive phase; 15% of these have a mild course with minimal disability at 15 years. About 15% present with a slowly progressive pattern called primary progressive MS.

▪ **Consider differential diagnoses** The diagnosis is in doubt if the features in Box 2.46 are true. Possible differential diagnoses are listed in Box 2.47.

Patient perspective

His rather passive approach to his symptoms should not detract you from engaging and involving him in your thoughts and recommendations.

Past medical history

He is previously well.

Table 2.35 Sites of demyelination and possible clinical features	
Site of demyelination	**Possible clinical features**
Spinal cord	Limb weakness, e.g. spastic paraparesis Sensory symptoms, e.g. numbness, 'cold water' trickling feeling along a limb Lhermitte's phenomenon (neck flexion induces an 'electric shock' sensation running down the back because of a cervical plaque) Erectile dysfunction Urinary frequency or retention Constipation Spasticity of limbs, with flexor spasms, cramps or spontaneous clonus Pseudoathetosis (loss of sensory feedback from arm due to a cervical plaque causing involuntary writhing movements of fingers and wrist when eyes closed)
Brainstem	Ataxia Vertigo Diplopia (including internuclear ophthalmoplegia) Dysarthria Facial weakness or numbness Dysphagia
Cerebellum	Gait ataxia Limb ataxia Dysarthria
Optic nerve	Optic neuritis (pain, especially on movement, and dimming of vision in one eye, often described as looking through a murky window)
Cerebrum	Mood or memory disturbance

Drug and allergy history

Ask about prescription and non-prescription drugs.

Family history

His family history of suicide should alert you to possible depression. The relative risk of suicide in MS is also increased.

Social history

His social history should focus on his alcohol consumption, home circumstances, support network and travel plans.

Discussion

What is MS?

MS is an inflammatory demyelinating disease of the central nervous system (brain and spinal cord) that is dissemi-nated in time and space. Therefore, either a relapsing–remitting syndrome in one site or a monophasic syndrome in several areas cannot be diagnosed as MS, although a recent consensus statement allows MS to be diagnosed (McDonald criteria) if there is MRI evidence of new disease activity three months or more after one clinical episode. If the presenting MRI is abnormal, the likelihood of a second clinical attack in the next 14 years increases from 15% to 90%.

What do you know about the epidemiology of MS?

The UK prevalence is 100–150/100 000. It is twice as common in women. It is more prevalent at greater distances from the equator.

What is the pathogenesis of MS?

It used to be thought MS was an intermittent disease with inflammatory breakdown of myelin, but it is now evident that it is more continuous, with diffuse white and grey matter changes, breakdown of myelin and axonal damage. An acute MS plaque results from primed lymphocytes crossing the blood–brain barrier and activating macrophages. The resultant inflammation strips myelin from nerve axons, impairing conduction, but direct axonal damage occurs from inflammatory mediators such as nitric oxide. Acute attacks of inflammation cause irreversible damage although rapid resolution of symptoms can occur when the inflammation subsides. Secondary atrophic axonal damage from demyelination probably accounts for the secondary progressive phase of MS.

MS is thus a disease of two phases – an initially inflammatory, relapsing–remitting phase when anti-inflammatory drugs might be effective, and a neurodegenerative progressive phase. Remyelination and rearrangement of ion channels on persistently demyelinated axons contribute to recovery.

Weak associations with human leucocyte antigen (HLA) DR15 and DQ6 suggest a possible autoimmune basis to MS but an antigen is not known. There is a higher prevalence in identical twins, and in 20% of patients another family member is affected but a more extensive pedigree raises the possibility of another diagnosis, e.g. hereditary ataxia. Infective agents are also postulated.

Do you know of any diagnostic criteria for MS?

The Poser diagnostic criteria since the early 1980s relied on evidence of at least two relapses typical of MS and evidence of involvement of white matter in more than one site in the central nervous system, the concept of 'lesions scattered in time and space'. The more recent McDonald criteria allow earlier diagnosis of MS (Table 2.36) after one clinical attack if MRI criteria are also present, although recently it has been questioned as to whether MRI inaccuracy may lead to over-diagnosis.

Table 2.36 McDonald criteria for multiple sclerosis (MS) diagnosis

Clinical presentation	Additional data needed
Two or more attacks (relapses) Two or more objective clinical lesions	None
Two or more attacks One objective clinical lesion	Dissemination in space, demonstrated by: MRI or positive CSF and two or more MRI lesions consistent with MS or further clinical lesion at different site
One attack Two or more objective clinical lesions	Dissemination in time, demonstrated by: MRI or second attack
One attack One objective clinical lesion (monosymptomatic presentation)	Dissemination in space, demonstrated by: MRI or positive CSF and two or more MRI lesions consistent with MS and Dissemination in time, demonstrated by: MRI or second attack
Insidious neurological progression suggestive of primary progressive MS	Positive CSF and Dissemination in space, demonstrated by: MRI evidence of nine or more T2 brain lesions or two or more spinal cord lesions or four to eight brain and one spinal cord lesion or positive VEP with four to eight MRI lesions or positive VEP with less than four brain lesions plus one spinal cord lesion and Dissemination in time, demonstrated by: MRI or continued progression for one year

CSF, cerebrospinal fluid, MRI, magnetic resonance imaging; VEP, visual evoked potential.

How would you investigate a patient with possible MS?

The importance of MRI is demonstrated in Table 2.36. For every clinical relapse about 10 MRI lesions are seen. Serial MRI therefore demonstrates progression more rapidly than waiting for clinical relapses. In young patients, MRI appearances are characteristic but in older patients white matter high-signal changes are less specific and can be seen in healthy people or associated with cerebral ischaemia.

Unilateral delay in visual-evoked potentials (in which scalp electrodes record potentials generated in the cortex by a pattern reversing image) is the most sensitive indicator of previous subclinical optic neuritis.

Oligoclonal bands in cerebrospinal fluid but not serum indicate inflammation confined to the central nervous system and are seen in 95% of clinically definite MS, their absence raising diagnostic doubt, although they are present in other central nervous system inflammatory conditions such as vasculitis and paraneoplastic syndromes.

What symptomatic treatments are used in MS?

These are outlined in Box 2.48.

Box 2.48 Symptomatic treatments in multiple sclerosis

The most amenable symptoms to treatment are spasticity and urinary dysfunction.

- Spasticity often affects the legs. Baclofen, titrated slowly, is the most widely used treatment, acting on γ-aminobutyric acid receptors to suppress reflex arcs that have been released from higher inhibitory control. Side effects are sedation and weakness. Tizanidine acts via cord α_2-receptors to modulate pre-synaptic release of excitatory amino acids. Dantrolene and gabapentin have been used.
- Bladder problems are generally one or both of storage failure leading to frequency or emptying failure leading to hesitancy and retention. In the former, anticholinergic drugs such as oxybutinin may help and in the latter, confirmed by a post-micturition bladder volume of > 100 ml, intermittent self-catheterisation may be indicated.
- Erectile dysfunction is common in MS, and treated with phosphodiesterase inhibitors.
- Tremor, usually rubral, is difficult to treat.
- Fatigue is difficult to treat.
- Depression is common and should be proactively considered.

How are acute relapses treated?

Methylprednisolone 500 mg to 1 g p.o. or i.v. for three to five days is advocated by NICE guidelines.

What disease-modifying treatments are used in MS?

Interferon-β (IFN-β), a cytokine with widespread activity within the immune system, is available in three preparations – Betaferon (IFN-β1b), Avonex and Rebif (IFN-β1a) – and glatirimir acetate, which is chemically different but also used. There are no stringent comparative trials of these different preparations that differ in composition, dose and administration (s.c. or i.m.) and are generally given once to thrice weekly.

Relapsing–remitting disease

Early treatment has been shown to have better outcomes. All four drugs reduce relapse frequency by about one-third; in the average patient this means a reduction from three to two relapses over three years. They can also reduce the severity of attacks, the number of new lesions on MRI and progression. The Association of British Neurologists suggests treatment in ambulant patients with at least two relapses in the past two years. Treatment may be accompanied by a slowing of the accumulation of disability. Novel potential treatments in patients who continue to relapse include monoclonal antibodies such as rituximab, and natalizumab is an inhibitor of an integrin adhesion molecule that attenuates access of immune cells across the blood–brain barrier. Treatment late in disease when no relapses are occurring is of doubtful benefit.

Primary and secondary progressive disease

Evidence does not support benefit from IFN-β in primary progressive disease, and limited evidence of benefit in secondary progressive disease is rather outweighed by other trials failing to show benefit. Most neurologists do not advocate IFN-β in progressive disease because it is increasingly thought that neurodegeneration rather than inflammation is responsible.

What do you know about the course and prognosis of MS?

Initially, most patients experience relapses that resolve completely or partially, usually with one or two relapses per year. At 10 years 50% of patients have entered the secondary progressive phase (90% after 25 years) with continuous accrual of deficit with or without relapses. Primary progressive disease affects about 10% of patients, more commonly men.

Disabling paraparesis eventually affects one-third of patients, 25% are incontinent or catheterised and 15% are confined to a wheelchair. Fifty per cent of patients are unable to work at five years and after 15 years 50% need at least a stick to walk 100 yards. Ten per cent of patients remain minimally disabled at 10 years ('benign MS').

CASE 2.19

TREMOR

Candidate information

Role

You are a doctor in a care of the elderly clinic. Please read the following letter from the patient's general practitioner. You may make notes on the paper provided. When the bell sounds, enter the examination room to begin the consultation.

Scenario

> Dear Doctor
>
> Re: Mr Robert Matthews, aged 68 years
>
> Thank you for seeing Mr Matthews, who has a tremor affecting his right arm. He is new to our practice and tells me he has had the tremor for some years but that it is worsening. He has no bradykinesia or rigidity but I am wondering if he might have Parkinson's disease. I would appreciate your advice.
>
> Yours sincerely

Please take a history from the patient (you may continue to make notes if you wish on the paper provided). Your examiners will warn you when 12 minutes have elapsed. You have 14 minutes to take a history from the patient followed by 1 minute of reflection. There will then follow 5 minutes of discussion with the examiners. Be prepared to discuss solutions to the problems posed by the case and how you might reply to the GP's letter. You are not required to examine the patient.

Patient information

Mr Robert Matthews is a 68-year-old gentleman who has had a tremor affecting his arm for around five years. It can affect either arm and is worse on activity but especially so when he is aware of people watching. There has been some difficulty in the past on the part of physicians deciding whether he has essential tremor or Parkinson's disease. He once tried propranolol at a high dose but it made him feel 'washed out'. He takes atenolol 50 mg for mild hypertension (recent blood pressure 140/80 mmHg). He has recently changed his GP, having moved to a new area. He now has a prominent head tremor and sought a further referral because he would now like to receive some treatment. He does not have any slowness or rigidity, has a very steady gait and has no reduction in facial expression or blink frequency (he has acquaintances with Parkinson's disease who do). He has noticed an extremely good therapeutic response to quite small doses of alcohol but understandably avoids it as a therapeutic measure except in very special circumstances. He lives with his wife, is retired but chair of the 'Age Concern' organisation locally and has no other medical history of note. As a further problem, he has noticed a 'creepy crawly' sensation in his legs for the past two years that appears to be a separate problem entirely to his other symptoms.

How to approach the case

Data gathering in the interview and interpretation and use of information gathered

Presenting problem(s) and symptom exploration

Types of tremor are listed in Table 2.37.

Patient perspective

Establish his ideas and concerns about the tremor. Reassure him that you agree it does not look like Parkinson's disease.

Explore his reactions to propranolol, and his willingness or otherwise to reconsider this drug, assuring him of a more cautious introduction to it. If he is unhappy to reconsider it despite explanation, explain that other strategies are possible. Find out what he hopes to expect from treatment.

Past medical history

Ask about blood pressure readings.

Drug and alcohol history

Ask if he knows what dose of propranolol he was started on.

Family history

There is not infrequently a family history of essential tremor.

Social history

Clearly very important, as essential tremor can have significant social repercussions. The improvement with alcohol is significant.

Table 2.37 Types of tremor			
Type of tremor	**Causes**	**Features**	**Management**
Parkinsonian tremor	Parkinson's disease Other extrapyramidal disorders	Rest-predominant tremor, 5 Hz Pill-rolling Asymmetrical Other features of Parkinson's disease	Levodopa Dopamine agonists Enzyme inhibitors
Cerebellar tremor	Cerebellar disease	Action-predominant tremor, 3 Hz	Treat underlying cause
Essential tremor	Family history in 50% Autosomal dominant Identified genes *ETM1* (chromosome 3q13) and *ETM2* (chromosome 2q22–25)	Much more common than in Parkinson's disease Postural or action tremor Symmetrical Associated head tremor in 50% Tongue, lips and voice may be affected Anxiety accentuates Alcohol attenuates No other neurological features usual, although cerebellar and cognitive disturbances increasingly seen Slowly progressive but seldom severe	Beta blockers Primidone
Task-specific/ performance tremor	e.g. primary writing tremor	Appearance of localised essential tremor but with task specificity of the dystonia	Beta blockers Anticholinergics
Orthostatic tremor	Unknown	Affects legs and trunk Only when standing still	Clonazepam
Rubral tremor	Usually seen in multiple sclerosis (lesion in red nucleus, ipsilateral cerebellar dentate nucleus or superior peduncle of midbrain)	Severe tremor Marked worsening with movement	No effective treatment except treatment of underlying disease
Drug-induced tremor	e.g. Lithium	Various	Stop drug
Psychogenic	Anxiety	Various	Anxiety management
Physiological	Normal	Small oscillations	None

SUMMARY – ASSESSMENT AND PLAN

- A head tremor is never associated with Parkinson's disease; a jaw tremor is the most one might observe.
- Moreover, he has no other features of Parkinson's disease with a lively facial expression and lots of spontaneous movement and blink frequency.
- He has essential tremor, beyond doubt.
- Only two agents help a significant proportion with essential tremor – propranolol and primidone: all other agents have either not been exhibited to a formal controlled trial or have generally not seen success. The best strategy is to try to get the best out of these agents unless they have unequivocally not been tolerated before.
- Atenolol should be substituted with propranolol. Propranolol is started at 10 mg once daily and if tolerated in one week incremented to 10 mg b.d., then 20 mg b.d. a week later and finally 40 mg b.d. Other beta blockers are less effective; propranolol is lipid soluble and crosses the blood–brain barrier. However, some people just feel washed out and less well on propranolol and so it is worth incrementing very slowly to try to improve tolerability.
- If propranolol is not tolerated or ineffective, then primidone may be tried. It is seldom tolerated as a whole tablet and should be started as a quarter tablet (i.e. 62.5 mg) once daily for around two weeks then half a tablet for two weeks, three-quarters of a tablet and so on.
- For a 'no–no' tremor, botulinum toxin is sometimes effective.
- He may have restless leg syndrome as an additional diagnosis.

Discussion

Are there any tests that can help distinguish the tremor in essential tremor from that in Parkinson's disease?

A DaT scan (also known as single photon emission tomography) can help, and its uses are discussed in Case 3.32.

What is restless legs syndrome (RLS)?

This is common, affecting 5–15% of the population. There are no involuntary movements but a discomfort due to abnormal sensation (many varieties, e.g. a 'creepy-crawly' feeling) or pain that is relieved by movement. There is a family history in around 90%, with autosomal dominant inheritance. RLS is more common in females. Four essential criteria must be present for the clinical diagnosis – akathasia, wakeful motor restlessness, rest symptoms relieved by movement, and preponderance towards the end of the day. Secondary causes include pregnancy, iron deficiency, chronic kidney disease, B12 or folate deficiency, hypothyroidism, diabetes, drugs such as steroids and anti-depressants, and caffeine, chocolate or alcohol. Investigations should thus include renal function, ferritin, B12 and folate levels, and thyroid function. Iron concentrations may be decreased in the substantia nigra in a significant proportion of patients, the degree of depletion relating to severity, and mirrored by ferritin levels (< 50 usually associated with severe symptoms). There may be post-synaptic dopaminergic dysfunction with abnormal D2 receptor dopamine agonism, this receptor also the iron binder. Treatments include reassurance, avoidance of prolonged sitting, avoidance of precipitants, iron replacement and dopaminergic stimulation. Levodopa tends to cause morning rebound (simply delays onset of symptoms) or evening augmentation of symptoms. Dopamine agonists appear currently most favourable, once in the evening or thrice daily if symptom shifting occurs, but carry the risks of excessive daytime somnolence, obsessive behaviour and gambling. RLS occurs in Parkinson's disease but is not otherwise especially linked to it.

LOCOMOTOR PROBLEMS

CASE 2.20

BACK PAIN AND OSTEOPOROSIS

Candidate information

Role

You are a doctor in the medical outpatient clinic. Please read the following letter from the patient's general practitioner. You may make notes on the paper provided. When the bell sounds, enter the examination room to begin the consultation.

Scenario

> Dear Doctor
>
> Re: Mrs Catherine Bingley, aged 62 years
>
> Thank you for seeing this lady who has had back pain for two months. There is no history of injury and she is otherwise well. She had a relatively early menopause and I wonder if she might have osteoporosis and might merit a bone densitometry scan.
>
> Yours sincerely

Please take a history from the patient (you may continue to make notes if you wish on the paper provided). Your examiners will warn you when 12 minutes have elapsed. You have 14 minutes to take a history from the patient followed by 1 minute of reflection. There will then follow 5 minutes of discussion with the examiners. Be prepared to discuss solutions to the problems posed by the case and how you might reply to the GP's letter. You are not required to examine the patient.

Patient information

Mrs Catherine Bingley is a 62-year-old lady with a two-month history of backache. The pain is localised to the mid-thoracic region and is dull, but exacerbated by and sharper on coughing. It sometimes interferes with her sleep. It is not getting worse, but equally is not improving. There is no clear history of trauma or a fall although she did lift heavy garden rubbish about three days before the onset of symptoms. She has no joint or muscle symptoms. She has not lost weight and is systemically well. She has been postmenopausal for 20 years and there is a strong family history of early menopause and osteoporosis. There is no other significant family history and in particular no family history of breast cancer. She did not take hormone replacement therapy (HRT) because she had a deep vein thrombosis following childbirth 35 years ago and had been aware that HRT increased the risk of deep vein thrombo-

sis. She has been otherwise previously well. She is divorced and works as a solicitor's secretary. She used to smoke. She is concerned she may have osteoporosis, but has also read in a magazine of a woman with cancer whose initial symptom was back pain.

How to approach the case

Data gathering in the interview and interpretation and use of information gathered

Presenting problem(s) and symptom exploration

■ **Determine more about the back pain**   Back pain can be the result of a problem in the back or may be referred from elsewhere such as the genitourinary system. Whereas simple mechanical back pain is very common in young to middle-aged patients with lumbosacral, buttock or thigh symptoms, the 'red flags' in Box 2.49 should be considered.

■ **Consider osteoporosis symptoms**   Osteoporosis is silent until a fracture is sustained. The main clinical presentations are listed in Box 2.50.

Fractures of the wrist or spine occur in younger post-menopausal women, and the hip in older people. A Colles' fracture is often the first sign in women aged 45–65 years. Vertebral fractures may present with severe thoracic back pain, in up to two-thirds without recollection of trauma, but are often asymptomatic. The relative risk of a new vertebral fracture is more than doubled by a previous vertebral fracture and more than quadrupled by a previous vertebral fracture with low bone mineral density (BMD). New fractures tend to occur rapidly after the first – a one in five chance within 12 months. Hip fractures are often the presenting feature of osteoporosis in older people,

---

> **Box 2.49 Red flags to back pain**
>
> - Age > 55 years
> - 'Non-mechanical' back pain with no clear aggravation by movement or change with posture
> - Thoracic pain
> - Systemic symptoms such as weight loss or loss of appetite
> - Past history of carcinoma (especially colorectal, breast, renal, thyroid)
> - Patient with human immunodeficiency virus infection
> - Drug history, especially repeat prescriptions for corticosteroids
> - Neurological symptoms and signs; any history of bladder or bowel symptoms should also be elicited in determining whether or not back pain is a neurosurgical emergency

---

> **Box 2.50 Main clinical presentations of osteoporosis**
>
> - Overt fracture (wrist, spine, hip), often with low trauma, e.g. fall from standing height or less
> - Pain
> - Height loss
> - Incidental osteopenia noted on X-ray

most well over 70 years, and most are associated with osteoporosis. These may be intertrochanteric, femoral neck or subcapital. Mortality is 20%, 50% have long-term incapacity and 20% enter long-term care.

■ **Consider falls risk** Both prevention of falls and prevention of osteoporosis are crucial to prevention of osteoporotic fractures.

Patient perspective

Acknowledge her concerns about osteoporosis and explore her concerns about cancer. While malignancy can present with back pain, she has no alarm symptoms for malignancy but does have risk factors – family history, early menopause and smoking – for osteoporosis and may have sustained a compression fracture during heavy lifting.

Past medical history

■ **Explore osteoporosis risk factors** Risk factors for osteoporosis are listed in Box 2.51.

Drug and allergy history

Ask about drug treatments, in particular repeated courses of corticosteroids for conditions like asthma, chronic obstructive pulmonary disease or inflammatory bowel disease.

Family history

Elicit any family history of osteoporosis.

Box 2.51 Clinical indications for bone densitometry (presence of strong risk factors)

- Radiological evidence of osteopenia or vertebral deformity/collapse
- Previous fragility fracture of wrist, spine or hip
- Oral glucocorticoid therapy
- Oestrogen deficiency (premature menopause < 45 years, oophorectomy, prolonged secondary amenorrhoea, primary hypogonadism)
- Height loss/kyphosis
- Prolonged immobilisation
- Family history of osteoporosis, especially maternal hip fracture
- Low body mass index (≤ 19 kg/m²)
- Anorexia nervosa
- Malabsorption
- Hyperthyroidism
- Primary hyperparathyroidism
- Cushing's disease
- Transplantation
- Chronic kidney disease

  These risk factors are listed in the Royal College of Physicians guidelines for bone densitometry. Other risk factors include smoking, excess alcohol, low dietary calcium, vitamin D deficiency, physical inactivity, hypogonadism, high caffeine intake, heparin, malignancy (especially myeloma and lymphoma), osteogenesis imperfecta, Marfan syndrome, Ehlers–Danlos syndrome, rheumatoid arthritis, chronic liver disease and drugs (aromatase inhibitors, androgen deprivation therapy).

  The three most important factors independent of bone mineral density are age > 65, the presence or history of a fragility fracture and a strong family history of fracture.

Social history

Ask about smoking or heavy alcohol ingestion. Ask how she is coping at home.

SUMMARY – ASSESSMENT AND PLAN

- She has strong osteoporosis risk factors and may have sustained a thoracic compression fracture.
- There is nothing other than back pain, which is a very common symptom, to suggest malignancy.
- A full screen of blood tests including inflammatory markers should be requested, together with a thoracic spine X-ray.
- She merits a bone densitometry scan but treatment for osteoporosis should be considered empirically.

Discussion

What is the scale of the osteoporosis problem?

One in three women and one in five men over 80 years will suffer a hip fracture. By age 50, the lifetime risk of an osteoporotic fracture in white women is nearly 40% and in men is 13%. The incidence increases markedly with age. In women this increase is after 45 years and mainly in forearm fractures up to 65 years, hip fractures then rising exponentially. In men, fragility fractures increase after 75 years. There are marked geographic variations, osteoporosis most common in white and Asian populations.

What do you understand by bone remodelling?

Bone comprises collagen (mostly type 1), other proteins and minerals, mostly calcium and phosphate within hydroxyapatite crystals. There are two types – cortical bone (80%) is dense, envelops the marrow cavity and forms Haversian systems or concentric lamellae around a central canal of blood vessels; trabecular bone (20%) is 'spongy', less dense and forms the centre of long bones, flat bones and vertebrae as a meshwork of trabeculae and marrow-filled spaces and is more metabolically active. Bone provides structural support, is a reservoir for mineral exchange and is dynamic, about 10% being remodelled at any time.

Bone resorption

Remodelling begins with bone resorption. Osteoclast precursors in blood are attracted to skeletal micro-damage, where they differentiate into mature osteoclasts by activation of their RANK (receptor activator of nuclear factor-κB) receptors by RANK ligands (RANKL) expressed on osteoblasts and other bone cells. The interaction is inhibited by osteoprotegerin (OPG), a 'decoy' molecule that is analogous to RANK and also binds RANKL. RANK and OPG are members of the tumour necrosis factor (TNF) receptor family, and RANKL is part of the TNF family. Other important molecules include PU.1 (differentiation of stem cells in myeloid lineage), c-fos (differentiation of myeloid precursors to osteoclasts), macrophage-colony stimulating factor (differentiation of macrophages and osteoclasts) and TRAF6 (transduces differentiation signals from RANK to nucleus). Osteoclasts contain membrane pumps that release acid, which dissolves hydroxyapatite and allows proteolytic enzymes to degrade bone matrix. When resorption is complete, osteoclasts undergo apoptosis, heralding bone formation.

Bone formation

This begins with attraction of osteoblast precursors derived from marrow stroma to the resorption site. Osteoblasts mature in response to transcription factor Cbfa1, which binds to the promoter of osteoblast-specific genes such as osteocalcin, type-1 collagen and alkaline phosphatase. 'Bone morphogenic proteins' (BMPs) are thought to contribute to the formation and differentiation of osteoblast precursors and a protein seems to inhibit formation by inhibiting BMPs. Mature osteoblasts lay down uncalcified matrix (osteoid) on the bone surface, and this calcifies in about 10 days to form mature mineralised bone. Alkaline phosphatase, produced by osteoblasts, promotes mineralisation by degrading pyrophosphate, an inhibitor of mineralisation. During formation, some osteoblasts become trapped in bone matrix and differentiate into osteocytes, the most abundant cells in bone. Osteocytes produce signalling molecules in response to mechanical loading and have a role in sensing mechanical strain.

What regulates bone remodelling?

It is regulated by circulating hormones and local cytokines. Mechanical loading increases formation whereas pro-inflammatory cytokines such as interleukin-1 (IL-1) and TNF increase remodelling. Calciotropic hormones such as parathyroid hormone (PTH) and 1,25 hydroxy vitamin D increase remodelling to maintain plasma calcium homeostasis. Remodelling is increased by thyroid hormone and growth hormone and suppressed by oestrogen, androgens and calcitonin. Many hormones act by modulating the expression of local cytokines, e.g. sex hormone deficiency enhances the expression of IL-1 and IL-6. Ultimately, the final common pathway of regulation by hormones

and cytokines appears to be the RANKL-RANK-OPG system.

How do problems with bone remodelling lead to disease?

Most bone diseases result from abnormal remodelling (Table 2.38) that compromise its structure and strength and lead to pain, deformity, fractures and abnormal mineral homeostasis.

What is the pathophysiology of osteoporosis?

Bone mineral density (BMD)

Low BMD is one of the key predisposing factors for osteoporotic fractures. Adult BMD is determined both by *acquisition of peak bone mass* during adolescence and the *degree of subsequent bone loss*. These processes are regulated by genetic and environmental factors at the level of bone remodelling units (BMUs). Each remodelling cycle is balanced – resorption equalling formation – and lasts 90–130 days. Remodelling cycles can become imbalanced, invariably due to excess resorption, often because of changes in hormones, dietary intake or mechanical loading.

Acquisition of peak bone mass

Acquisition of BMD is most rapid at 12–15 years and peak BMD is attained by 20–30 years. Genetic factors, sex hormone status and dietary calcium are the main regulators of peak BMD. Impaired acquisition of peak BMD is responsible for 60–70% of the variance in BMD at any age.

Bone loss

Hormonal and environmental factors are the strongest determinants of bone loss after the fourth decade in men and women. During the menopause, oestrogen deprivation enhances bone loss, causing around 1% loss per year, but in a small proportion of women a loss of spine BMD up to 5% per year may occur. It is not possible to prospectively identify this group. Although formation accelerates in an attempt to match resorption around the menopause, it does not catch up. Young amenorrhoeic athletes are at

Table 2.38 Abnormal bone remodelling and disease	
Disease	**Bone remodelling problem**
Osteoporosis	Excessive resorption, usually associated with post-menopausal sex hormone deficiency, coupled with determinants of peak bone mass attained in earlier life
Paget's disease	Focal areas of excessive bone turnover
Bone metastases	Focal increases in osteoclast resorption stimulated by osteoclast-activating factors released by tumour cells, e.g. interleukin-1, tumour necrosis factor, parathyroid hormone-related protein
Osteopetrosis	Greatly increased bone maturation due to failure of osteoclasts to secrete acid, causing nerve compression and marrow failure
Inflammatory disease, e.g. rheumatoid arthritis	Proinflammatory cytokine excess enhances bone loss

greater risk of osteoporosis because of impaired acquisition of peak BMD and accelerated bone loss. In the elderly, there is chronic uncoupling or imbalance of resorption and formation – resorption normal or slightly increased and formation suppressed, normal or only slightly increased – together with oestrogen or androgen deprivation and often calcium and vitamin D deficiency (dietary, and reduced activation of vitamin D) and secondary hyperparathyroidism accounting for bone resorption at least equivalent to menopausal levels.

Fractures

An osteoporotic fracture occurs due to major or minor trauma to a bone of reduced quantity and quality. Fractures in virtually all sites in postmenopausal women can be considered osteoporotic excepting facial and compound road traffic accident trauma. Although there is a strong inverse relationship between BMD and fracture risk, other mechanical factors contribute to bone strength and absolute fracture risk and include the rate of turnover, cortical and trabecular thickness and bone shape; trabecular perforation occurs with increased turnover and leads to disproportionate loss of strength for the amount of bone lost. The lower the BMD, the less force needed to fracture.

How is osteoporosis defined?

The definition is based on the standard deviation of BMD, called a T score, in relation to the young adult normal mean BMD (Table 2.39).

Table 2.39 T score

T score	Bone disease	Fracture risk
> −1.0	None	Low
− 1 to −2.5	Osteopenia	Average
< −2.5	Osteoporosis	High
< −2.5 and fracture	Severe osteoporosis	Very high

How would you measure BMD?

Dual energy X-ray absorption (DEXA) employs two energy peaks of X-rays that are absorbed to different extents by bone and soft tissue, and BMD is calculated in g/cm^2 using simultaneous equations. The result is compared with two reference ranges – young adults and age-matched adults. Those at risk of osteoporosis (see Box 2.51) are targeted for DEXA scanning, and, if osteoporosis is confirmed, then they proceed to treatment. Some physicians start treatment before confirmation. Although osteophytes and aortic calcification may affect reliability, DEXA scanning is the most reliable test available for BMD. Calcaneal ultrasound is used in research.

Are there any other investigations you might consider in osteoporosis?

Over 90% of patients have no secondary cause. Investigations in selected patients in whom a secondary cause is suspected are listed in Table 2.40.

Do biochemical markers of bone turnover have a place?

They are not used in clinical practice. Markers of resorption include pyridinium cross-links of collagen, cross-linking telopeptides of type 1 collagen, serum tartrate-resistant acid phosphatase and urinary hydro-xyproline. Markers of formation include bone alkaline phosphatase, serum osteocalcin and serum type-1 procollagen peptides.

How is osteoporosis treated?

Antiresorptive agents

These include bisphosphonates (Box 2.52), raloxifene and HRT and mostly prevent menopausal and age-related loss. An initial increase in BMD caused by catch-up formation is followed by a plateau or, in the case of more potent antiresorptive agents such as alendronate, sustained by smaller increases in BMD caused by secondary mineralisation.

Raloxifene is a selective oestrogen receptor modulator (SERM); it is tissue specific, having both oestrogenic and

Table 2.40 Secondary investigations in osteoporosis

Investigation	Reason
Follicle-stimulating hormone (FSH)	Detects menopause in hysterectomised women with conserved ovaries – osteoporosis risk is higher despite ovarian presence
Erythrocyte sedimentation rate and immunoglobulin electrophoresis	Myeloma
Renal and liver function	Chronic kidney disease/liver disease
Calcium, phosphate, alkaline phosphatase	'Bone profile'
Thyroid function tests	Hyperthyroidism
Testosterone	Male hypogonadism
Full blood picture	Malabsorption
Parathyroid hormone	If hypercalcaemia

Box 2.52 Bisphosphonates

Bisphosphonates are used to prevent and treat osteoporosis in postmenopausal females, corticosteroid-induced osteoporosis (CIO) in males and females and (although without evidence) osteoporosis in males. They unequivocally reduce overall fracture rates. Alendronate and risedronate are more potent than etidronate.

In the vertebral arm of the Fracture Intervention (FIT) trial of approximately 2000 women with existing vertebral fracture, daily alendronate for three years halved the risk of a new vertebral fracture and reduced the risk of two or more fractures by 90%. The risk of hip and wrist fractures was reduced by around 50%. This was associated with a rise in bone mineral density (BMD) of 3.2% in the hip and 8% in lumbar spine. Alendronate in established osteoporosis produces rapid, significant reduction in spine and non-vertebral fractures. Women who benefit most are those at high risk, such as those over 65 years with previous fractures and very low BMD.

Two large multicentre trials of risedronate of more than 3600 postmenopausal women with at least one vertebral fracture demonstrated, after three years, almost 45% reduction in new vertebral fractures and significant reduction in non-vertebral fractures. No reduction in new hip fractures was shown but there was an increase in spine BMD of 5% and hip BMD of 3%. Anti-fracture efficacy was evident after a year. Reduction in hip fractures was demonstrated in another study of 5445 women aged 70–79 years with osteoporosis of the hip and at least one fall risk factor. Hip fracture incidence was 2.8% compared with 3.9% in the control group.

Bisphosphonates are generally poorly absorbed and need to be taken on an empty stomach with a full glass of water, the patient remaining upright and abstaining from food for 30 minutes. Alendronate and risedronate may both cause erosive oesophagitis and patients are advised to take these drugs with water and not to lie down afterwards. Bisphosphonates very occasionally cause jaw necrosis, but this side effect is almost exclusive to patients receiving intravenous bisphosphonate therapy in the setting of malignancy, often combined with corticosteroids. Alendronate and risedronate are available once weekly, a newer agent ibandronate can be taken monthly orally and three-monthly by intravenous bolus, and annual treatments such as intravenous zolendronate are now available.

---

antioestrogenic effects. It may confer BMD benefit without breast and uterine risk. It increases BMD at the spine and hip in postmenopausal women and reduces the risk of vertebral fractures, but there is no evidence for hip-fracture prevention.

HRT is effective for osteoporosis prevention and treatment but is reserved only for menopausal symptoms because it increases the risk of breast cancer, venous thromboembolism and cardiovascular disease.

Calcitonin, normally produced by the thyroid, increases calcium excretion by the kidney and inhibits bone resorption by acting at osteoclast receptors. Therapeutic preparations have side effects but are used in acute vertebral fractures for analgesia. Calcitriol may be useful in corticosteroid-induced osteoporosis. Testosterone is used in men with hypogonadism.

Stimulation of bone formation – teriparatide (recombinant human PTH peptide 1–34)

Continuous exposure to exogenous PTH causes bone resorption. Paradoxically, PTH stimulates bone formation when administered intermittently, increasing BMD, strength and connectivity. This anabolic effect is achieved both by de novo formation on resting bone surfaces and by a positive remodelling balance at the BMU. In a randomised controlled trial of 1637 women with osteoporosis, teriparatide 20 or 40 µg daily by subcutaneous injection over a mean treatment period of 18 months resulted in significant increases in BMD in the spine and proximal femur and significant reductions of 65–70% in vertebral fractures and 53–54% in non-vertebral fractures, but without evidence for reduction in hip fractures. The risk of two or more new vertebral fractures was reduced by 77% in the 20-µg group and 86% in the 40-µg group. PTH is very much reserved for cases where treatment with other agents has failed. Teriparatide is administered as a daily subcutaneous injection, 20 µg, and the full 1–84 peptide at a dose of 100 µg.

Dual action treatment – strontium ranelate

Results of two large Phase III studies, Spinal Osteoporosis Therapeutic Intervention (SOTI) and Treatment of Peripheral Osteoporosis (TROPOS), support a role for strontium. In SOTI 1649 postmenopausal women with osteoporosis were treated for three years leading to a 41% relative risk reduction for vertebral fractures with benefits seen after one year. In TROPOS treatment of 5091 postmenopausal women with osteoporosis led to a significant 16% reduction in all non-vertebral fractures after three years; for women at high risk of hip fracture there was a 36% risk reduction. Strontium is second-line treatment for patients intolerant of bisphosphonates (PTH, very costly, the only evidenced treatment for fractures on bisphosphonates) and carries a small but appreciable risk of venous thromboembolism. It is administered orally, 2 g once daily as a sachet dissolved in water.

Other measures for osteoporosis prevention and treatment

Smoking and excessive alcohol should be discouraged. Weight-bearing exercise such as walking is beneficial and non-weight-bearing exercise may also reduce fracture risk by improving strength and coordination and reducing the risk of falls. Loss of the effect of gravity on the skeleton (e.g. immobilisation) produces dramatic loss of BMD because of uncoupling – resorption increasing dramatically and formation is markedly suppressed – the evidence being greatest in younger people. Physiotherapy can help at-risk patients in reducing falls and help with pain management. Patients with osteopenia and a previous fracture may also be considered for these treatment options. Hip protectors may be used in institutionalised people but otherwise there is limited evidence of benefit, possibly because of poor compliance. Analgesia and vertebroplasty, the injection of 'cement', decrease pain and height loss but vertebroplasty may increase the risk of fracture above and below the treated site.

What is the place for calcium and vitamin D3 supplementation?

These should always be used with bisphosphonate therapy, at doses of around 1200 mg calcium and 800 IU vitamin D3/calcitriol daily, e.g. calcichew D3 forte, one tablet twice daily, in those at risk such as older patients.

How might you in practice approach the use of DEXA scanning and primary and secondary prevention of osteoporosis in post-menopausal women?

Despite RCP guidelines for DEXA scanning indications, NICE guidelines are more restrictive and suggest the following:

Primary prevention

Alendronate is recommended for post-menopausal women with DEXA confirmed osteoporosis older than 70 years with at least one of the following risk factors – family history, severe rheumatoid arthritis or at least 4 units of alcohol consumption per day; other risk factors listed that may be considered are a BMI < 22, ankylosing spondylitis, Crohn's disease, immobility, premature menopause, previous fracture and corticosteroid use. For women under 70 years a DEXA scan is recommended for severe rheumatoid arthritis, ankylosing spondylitis, Crohn's disease or immobility together with at least one other risk factor. For women over 75 years a DEXA scan is not necessary if there are at least two risk factors.

Secondary prevention

Alendronate is recommended in women under 75 years with a fragility fracture and a BMD of < −2.5. For women over 75 years a DEXA scan may not be required to confirm osteoporosis, treatment empirical. NICE guidelines now accept the need for second-line treatment, often as an alternative biphosphonate, parenteral biphosphonate therapy

for those with swallowing problems, or strontium. There is a paucity of data for drug therapy in men, but most physicians would treat as for women.

When does glucocorticoid-induced osteoporosis begin?

Glucocorticoids simultaneously suppress bone formation and increase resorption, and do so rapidly, within the first few months. Even small doses (< 7.5 mg prednisolone) cause some bone loss. Risk increases rapidly in the first three to six months and so bone protection with a bisphosphonate and calcium/vitamin D preparation should start as soon as long-term corticosteroids are started.

Is testosterone deficiency a wide problem?

It is an under-appreciated cause of osteoporosis and may be treated by patches, implants or intramuscular sustained-release preparations. The problem may not be simply decreased androgens but testicular or pituitary failure. Testicular ischaemia/infarction is not well understood but is very likely in patients with renal artery stenosis or aortic disease because the testicular arteries have a very long course. Hormone treatments for prostate cancer are another common cause of testosterone deficiency.

Does osteomalacia commonly compound osteoporosis?

Osteomalacia refers to defective bone mineralisation, and is mostly caused by vitamin D deficiency (Table 2.41). Although bone pain and raised alkaline phosphates are the traditional 'textbook' features of vitamin D deficiency, it has been appreciated in recent years that primary vitamin D deficiency is not uncommon, especially in older people, and serum biochemistry is frequently normal.

It has also been appreciated in recent years that vitamin D has a role not just in bone mineralisation but also in muscle stability, and that deficiency increases instability and the risk of falls.

Table 2.41 Causes of osteomalacia	
Primary (nutritional) vitamin D deficiency	Older people Housebound and institutionalised
Secondary vitamin D deficiency	Partial gastrectomy Small bowel malabsorption Liver disease (liver converts vitamin D3 or cholecalciferol CC to 25OHCC) Chronic kidney disease (kidney converts 25OHCC to 1,25 diOHCC)
Drugs and toxins	Anti-epileptic drugs Bisphosphonates Fluoride Phosphate-binding acids
Biochemical disturbances	Hypophosphataemia Calcium depletion Magnesium depletion Primary hyperparathyroidism
Hereditary	Hypophosphataemia (X-linked and autosomal recessive) Viitamin D-dependent rickets Renal tubular disorders

CASE 2.21

JOINT PAIN

Candidate information

Role

You are a doctor in the medical outpatient clinic. Please read the following letter from the patient's general practitioner. You may make notes on the paper provided. When the bell sounds, enter the examination room to begin the consultation.

Scenario

> Dear Doctor
>
> Re: Mrs Elaine Tilney, aged 52 years
>
> Mrs Tilney has been complaining of worsening polyarthralgia in her hands and wrists for six months. Her blood results are as follows: full blood count normal except for a borderline normochromic normocytic anaemia; creatinine of 135 mmol/l, otherwise urea, electrolytes and liver function tests are normal; rheumatoid factor is positive. I would be grateful for your further assessment.
>
> Yours sincerely

Please take a history from the patient (you may continue to make notes if you wish on the paper provided). Your examiners will warn you when 12 minutes have elapsed. You have 14 minutes to take a history from the patient followed by 1 minute of reflection. There will then follow 5 minutes of discussion with the examiners. Be prepared to discuss solutions to the problems posed by the case and how you might reply to the GP's letter. You are not required to examine the patient.

Patient information

Mrs Elaine Tilney is a 52-year-old lady who has had increasing pain in the joints of her hands for six months. The joints, especially the metacarpals (knuckles), also tend to become spongy and to swell. Pain, and in particular stiffness, is worse in the mornings and starts to subside after an hour or so. Before this started she had an episode of swelling in her right knee which lasted around three days. She has been increasingly fatigued over the last six months, and has taken many days off work. She works as a part-time secretary at the hospital. She lives with her husband and two 'grown-up' children in a small house, which she had been trying to improve before putting on the market for sale. However, she has increasingly had to stop work on the house, decorating and so forth, because her hands are too painful to use. Her husband works full time as a nurse on night shifts, and there are tensions at home. She feels he is seldom around, and is always too

tired because of his 'full-time job' to decorate or do the housework. Mrs Tilney feels she is trying to cope with her part-time job, home improvement, demanding children who should be out at work and a husband who is seldom there, against a backdrop of increasing pain and fatigue, and financial worries. If she does not work they will have to sell the house sooner rather than later.

How to approach the case

Data gathering in the interview and interpretation and use of information gathered

Presenting problem(s) and symptom exploration

■ **Determine if symptoms are localised to joints and the pattern and features of joint involvement**

- Ask if pain is localised to joints, and not diffuse. The latter could imply a chronic pain syndrome such as fibromylagia. Myalgic symptoms can occur in rheumatoid arthritis.
- Determine as precisely as you can which joints are affected.
- Determine if there is joint stiffness as well as pain. Morning stiffness, improving with exercise, characterises an inflammatory arthropathy. Mechanical pain is usually relieved by rest.
- It is essential to know if there is joint swelling (polyarthritis) as well as pain (polyarthralgia) and stiffness. Any soft tissue swelling is highly suggestive of inflammatory joint disease.

■ **Consider the differential diagnoses** The next step is to test each differential diagnosis in turn by asking about symptoms from the diagnostic criteria. In this lady you should consider rheumatoid arthritis (rheumatoid factor is positive) and systemic lupus erythematosus (SLE; given the raised creatinine) first. The presence of normochromic normocytic anaemia supports an inflammatory condition but does not help diagnostically. For rheumatoid arthritis, ask about morning stiffness for longer than one hour, hand joint involvement, symmetrical involvement and nodules. For SLE, ask about rashes, sunlight sensitivity, mouth ulcers and Raynaud's phenomenon.

Patient perspective

Clearly very relevant here is her fatigue, contributed to largely by active inflammatory disease but compounded by her stress and lifestyle. To her, what is going on at home and the impact her symptoms have had on her work are probably more significant than the symptoms themselves. Explore the huge impact her symptoms have had, and try to reassure her that you will try to confirm the diagnosis quickly and get her condition under good control with treatment, reducing symptoms and thereby hopefully improving everything else.

Past medical history

She is previously well.

Drug and allergy history

Ask about prescription and non-prescription medications.

Family history

Seek a family history of any autoimmune disease.

Social history

Explore her duties at home with her family and her work in detail.

SUMMARY – ASSESSMENT AND PLAN

- This is very likely to be rheumatoid arthritis.
- She should be considered for early disease-modifying antirheumatic drug treatment and referred to a rheumatologist.

Discussion

Patients, especially older patients, often present with non-specific aches and decreased mobility. Do you have an approach to the differential diagnosis?

An approach to the differential diagnosis of an older person with decreased mobility and painful joints or muscles is given in Fig. 2.9.

What do you know about septic arthritis?

Septic arthritis is extremely serious. It is often caused by entry of staphyloccocus from a breach in the skin, or sometimes from another source such as discitis, or sometimes from urine. Organisms tend to seed to damaged joints, as in rheumatoid arthritis, just as they may seed to damaged heart valves causing endocarditis. Multiple joints may be affected, and methicillin-resistant *S. aureus* (MRSA) septic arthritis has a very high mortality.

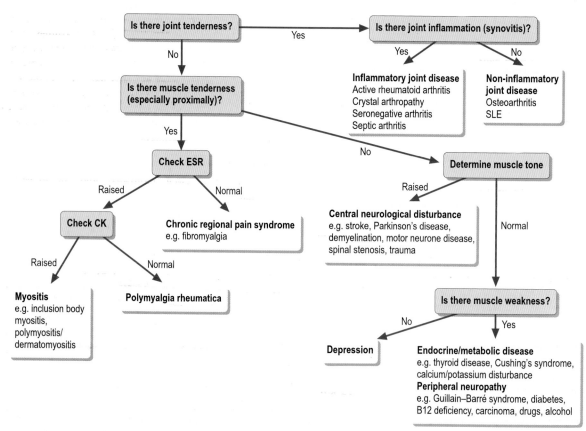

Fig. 2.9 Approach to the differential diagnosis of an older person with decreased mobility and painful joints or muscles. CK, creative kinase; ESR, erythrocyte sedimentation rate; SLE, systemic lupus erythematosus.

EYE PROBLEMS

CASE 2.22

VISUAL LOSS

Candidate information

Role

You are a doctor in the diabetes clinic. Please read the following letter from the patient's general practitioner. You may make notes on the paper provided. When the bell sounds, enter the examination room to begin the consultation.

Scenario

> Dear Doctor
>
> Re: Mr John Knight, aged 80 years
>
> Thank you for seeing this gentleman urgently. He has had several episodes of zig-zag vision over the last few months. He has type 2 diabetes for which he takes metformin, aspirin, simvastatin, perindopril and bendroflumethiazide. He had a stroke three years ago from which he made a full recovery. I wonder if he could have worsening diabetic retinopathy or if these are transient ischaemic attacks.
>
> Yours sincerely

Please take a history from the patient (you may continue to make notes if you wish on the paper provided). Your examiners will warn you when 12 minutes have elapsed. You have 14 minutes to take a history from the patient followed by 1 minute of reflection. There will then follow 5 minutes of discussion with the examiners. Be prepared to discuss solutions to the problems posed by the case and how you might reply to the GP's letter. You are not required to examine the patient.

Patient information

Mr John Knight is an 80-year-old widowed gentleman with type 2 diabetes mellitus who has experienced several episodes of disturbed vision over the past three months – sometimes blurred vision, sometimes glare while driving and sometimes indistinct letters when reading. Both eyes appear to be affected. Episodes resolve spontaneously and last for up to an hour. There is no associated limb weakness or speech difficulty or altered sensation. He feels his vision has generally become less distinct over the past year. He is still driving. He has a past medical history of type 2 diabetes but since a stroke with right arm weakness three years ago he has been very strict about keeping himself healthy. He made a full recovery from his stroke. He takes metformin 850 mg twice daily, aspirin 75 mg daily, simvastatin 40 mg daily, perindopril 4 mg daily and bendroflumethiazide 2.5 mg daily. He monitors his blood glucose and knows that his HbA_{1c} is 7.5%. He monitors his blood pressure and average readings are around 140/70 mmHg. His total cholesterol is 4.8 mmol/l. He has background diabetic retinopathy and at retinal screening six months ago the ophthalmology team were happy.

How to approach the case

Data gathering in the interview and interpretation and use of information gathered

Presenting problem(s) and symptom exploration

- **Explore visual loss**   Visual loss may be acute or gradual, and may affect one or both eyes. It is commonly the result of the causes listed in Table 2.42.
- **Ask about colours or shapes**   Patients frequently complain of *spots* in their vision. It is important to differentiate between *flashing lights* (a sign of incipient retinal detachment) and *floaters* (opacities in the vitreous). Haloes (a waterlogged cornea breaks up white light as does the sky after a rainstorm, and because of the shape of the cornea the 'rainbow' is round) may be a sign of incipient acute glaucoma. Wavy lines on a grid may be due to wet age-related macular degeneration.

Patient perspective

He is extremely well motivated and an excellent historian.

Table 2.42 Causes of visual loss

Type of visual loss	Causes
Gradual loss of central vision in one or both eyes	Cataract Age-related macular degeneration (ARMD)
Gradual loss of peripheral vision in one or both eyes	Primary open-angle glaucoma Retinal detachment Retinitis pigmentosa
Acute loss of central vision in one eye	Optic neuritis
Acute loss of vision (total or variable distribution) in one eye	Central/branch retinal vein occlusion Central retinal artery occlusion Retinal detachment Retinal haemorrhage Amaurosis fugax
Acute homonymous visual field loss	Stroke

Past medical history

His past medical history of stroke and diabetes immediately alert you to diabetic retinopathy or transient ischaemic attacks (TIAs) but the bilateral symptoms suggest alternative diagnoses.

Drug and allergy history

He is concordant with a good range of secondary vascular prophylaxis.

Family history

Relevance here is unlikely.

Social history

He should not drive until TIAs have absolutely been excluded and until his vision has been fully assessed.

SUMMARY – ASSESSMENT AND PLAN

- Likely diagnoses are cataracts (related or unrelated to his diabetes) or age-related macular degeneration or a combination of both. Glaucoma is possible. He should certainly be referred to an ophthalmologist.
- TIAs seem less likely, but if there is concern about focal neurological symptoms/amaurosis fugax then a carotid Doppler study should be undertaken promptly.
- Hypoglycaemic episodes are possible.

Discussion

What is glaucoma?

This is described in Case 5.38.

What are the visual requirements for driving?

These are described in Case 4.49.

ENDOCRINE PROBLEMS

CASE 2.23

TYPE 1 DIABETES MELLITUS

Candidate information

Role

You are a doctor in the emergency medical assessment unit. Please read the following letter from the patient's general practitioner. You may make notes on the paper provided. When the bell sounds, enter the examination room to begin the consultation.

Scenario

Dear Doctor

Re: Ms Jill Masters, aged 19 years

Thank you for admitting Ms Masters, who has been complaining of increasing thirst and polyuria over the last few weeks. Her blood glucose monitor reading is 28 and her urine is positive for ketones, although she is relatively well in herself. I have told her that I suspect she has diabetes and am grateful for your ongoing management.

Yours sincerely

Please take a history from the patient (you may continue to make notes if you wish on the paper provided). Your examiners will warn you when 12 minutes have elapsed. You have 14 minutes to take a history from the patient followed by 1 minute of reflection. There will then follow 5 minutes of discussion with the examiners. Be prepared to discuss solutions to the problems posed by the case and how you might reply to the GP's letter. You are not required to examine the patient.

Patient information

Ms Jill Masters is a 19-year-old medical student in her first year at medical school. She has been increasingly thirsty over the last four weeks, and passing larger volumes of urine, and her GP has just admitted her with a new diagnosis of diabetes. She has no past medical history of note and does not take any medications. She is usually very active, leading the university swimming team. Her mother has hypothyroidism but otherwise there is no clear family history of autoimmune disease.

How to approach the case

Data gathering in the interview and interpretation and use of information gathered

Presenting problem(s) and symptom exploration

■ **Initial priorities in assessing a patient with newly diagnosed diabetes** A decision as to whether immediate rehydration and insulin are needed should be made, determined by the presence of dehydration, vomiting or ketonuria. Thirst, polyuria and initial glucose levels correlate less well with the need for immediate insulin.

■ **Presentation of type 1 diabetes** Presentation varies according to the rate and degree of insulitis and beta cell failure. The classic presentation is outlined in Box 2.53.

Adult-onset type 1 diabetes is increasingly recognised, with a more indolent presentation, a lower incidence of osmotic symptoms and ketoacidosis and a lower prevalence of autoantibodies and genetic susceptibility. Latent autoimmune diabetes of adulthood (LADA) is a term for patients aged 25 years or more with type 1 diabetes often masquerading as type 2 diabetes with initial control obtained by diet or oral hypoglycaemic drugs; patients have lower levels of C-peptide (the cleavage product remaining after insulin has split from its precursor, proinsulin, with no biological activity) and are often positive for GAD antibodies. Elderly people can present with type 1 diabetes, often with weight loss and diarrhoea.

■ **Consider if admission to hospital is warranted** Admission can be a very negative first experience of newly diagnosed diabetes. Patients invariably proceed to insulin but this can be instituted in a diabetes clinic if there are no features to suggest that insulin is urgently needed and patients are not acutely unwell. Indications for admission are listed in Box 2.54.

Box 2.53 Classic presentation of type 1 diabetes

- Onset childhood/adolescence (peak incidence age 10–14 years)
- Lean
- Acute onset of osmotic symptoms (polyuria when renal threshold of plasma glucose 10 mmol/l reached, polydipsia, weight loss)
- Ketosis-prone
- High levels of islet autoantibodies
- High prevalence of susceptibility genotypes (HLA DR3, DR4, DQ2, DQ8)

Box 2.54 Indications for admission in newly diagnosed type 1 diabetes

- Acutely unwell
- Blood glucose > 30 mmol/l
- Ketones in blood
- Moderate to large ketones in urine
- Dehydration
- Vomiting

Patient perspective

She may initially be very afraid of a diagnosis that has important implications for lifestyle adjustment and carries long-term complications. Some of the skills for breaking bad news (Station 4) may be important, and it is important to emphasise the advances in monitoring and treatment that are less intrusive on lifestyle.

Past medical history

A new diagnosis in this age group is usually type 1 diabetes but rarer causes are listed in Table 2.43.

Drug and allergy history

Although certain drugs such as corticosteroids exacerbate hyperglycaemia, drug causes of diabetes are very rare.

Family history

A family history of autoimmune disease is common.

Social history

As well as asking about smoking (future cardiovascular disease risk) and alcohol (which can affect glycaemic control), enquire about university social life and sports activities.

SUMMARY – ASSESSMENT AND PLAN

The case may lead to an initial discussion with the examiners about management of diabetic ketoacidosis (DKA).

Referral to critical care while resuscitating

This may be appropriate if there is dehydration > 10%, coma, a pH < 7.1 or a plasma sodium < 120 mmol/l or > 160 mmol/l. Dehydration may be assessed as < 3% (no signs), 5% (dry mucous membranes and reduced skin turgor), 10% (sunken eyes, poor capillary return), > 10% (hypotensive, tachycardic).

Fluid resuscitation

Isotonic saline at a rate exceeding losses (e.g. 1 litre first hour, 1 litre next two hours, 1 litre next four hours, 1 litre six-hourly) is switched to 5% dextrose when plasma glucose is < 15 mmol/l. It is possible, but not proven, that faster rates than 1 litre in the first hour are associated with an increased risk of cerebral oedema and slower rates of correction of bicarbonate.

Insulin

Use 50 Units short-acting insulin in 50 ml saline delivered via syringe pump on a sliding scale:

Blood glucose (mmol/l)	Insulin (Units/hour)
< 4.0	0
4.1–6.0	1
6.1–12.0	3
12.1–17.0	5
> 17.1	8

Consider stopping sliding scale when no ketonuria, not acidotic, not dehydrated and eating and drinking. It is possible, but not proven, that rates of fall in plasma glucose > 5 mmol/hour may increase the risk of cerebral oedema.

Potassium

A suitable replacement is 40 mmol KCl/l if < 3.5 mmol/l, 20 mmol KCl/l if 3.5–5.5 mmol/l.

Table 2.43 Types of diabetes

Type 1	Pancreatic cell destruction, usually autoimmune	Various types as well as classic presentation in teens/ young adults such as latent autoimmune diabetes of adulthood (LADA) often diagnosed as type 2 diabetes but presenting with weight loss
Type 2	Complex metabolic disorder with beta cell dysfunction and insulin resistance; the latter also associated with hypertension, obesity and polycystic ovarian syndrome, often occurring in type 2 diabetes Genetic basis not fully understood	
Other/type 3	Genetic defects in beta cell function	MODY (maturity onset diabetes of youth) Mitochondrial DNA disorders
	Genetic defects in insulin action Exocrine pancreatic disorders	Pancreatitis Pancreatic carcinoma Haemochromatosis
	Endocrinopathies	Cushing's syndrome Acromegaly Glucagonoma Phaeochromocytoma Aldosteronoma Hyperthyroidism Somatostatinoma
	Drug- or chemical-induced Infection	
Gestational diabetes		

Discussion

How is diabetes defined?

Diabetes is not a single disorder but a range of metabolic conditions associated with hyperglycaemia caused by defects in insulin secretion or action that cause premature atherosclerosis with microvascular (retina, kidney, peripheral nerves) and macrovascular (coronary, cerebrovascular, peripheral vascular) complications. Diagnostic definitions of diabetes are given in Table 2.13, Case 2.7.

How is diabetes classified?

There are two main forms, type 1 and type 2, together with a range of rarer disorders (Table 2.43).

How does type 1 diabetes arise?

Type 1 diabetes involves autoimmune destruction of pancreatic beta cells resulting in insulin deficiency. A complex interaction occurs between genetic susceptibility and environmental factors. It is possible that susceptible human leucocyte antigen (HLA) molecules fail to react with pancreatic self-peptides; this leads to failed deletion of autoreactive T cells, amplified by environmental factors and beta cell antigens, which, coupled with immune dysregulation, allows autoimmune beta cell failure to proceed. A further hypothesis, the accelerator hypothesis, is that autoimmune reactivity occurs against up-regulated beta cells attempting to respond to insulin resistance.

Which autoantibodies may be detectable in type 1 diabetes?

Islet cell antibodies (ICA) are the most sensitive markers of future risk of type 1 diabetes. Autoantibodies to glutamic acid decarboxylase (GAD), IA-2 and IA-2β (phogrin) constitute a major part of ICA immunofluorescence. GAD is the best characterised beta cell autoantigen and is found in the pancreas and cerebellum. Insulin autoantibodies (IAAs) become less prevalent with age, as do IA-2, so that GAD is a better marker of late-onset type 1 diabetes. Most people with type 1 diabetes have multiple antibodies, and testing for a range of antibodies gives better sensitivity and specificity. A few patients do not have identifiable autoantibodies. Relatives often have autoantibodies, and three or more predicts a 70–100% chance of developing diabetes within 5–8 years. Autoimmunity heralding diabetes occurs in the first few years of life.

What is diabetic ketoacidosis?

Diabetic ketoacidosis (DKA) is defined as metabolic acidosis with plasma bicarbonate less than 15 mmol/l and a total ketone body concentration more than 5 mmol/l, but in practice it is identified by dehydration, hyperglycaemia, acidosis and ketonuria. It is caused by insulin deficiency and usually occurs in type 1 diabetes but can occur in type 2 diabetes. There may be precipitating causes such as infection or myocardial infarction, which all have a common denominator – an increase in catecholamines, glucagon, cortisol and growth hormone (all catabolic hormones) – which together with insulin (anabolic hormone) deficiency promote the problems listed in Table 2.44.

What do you know about glycaemic monitoring in diabetes?

Haemoglobin A_{1c} (HbA$_{1c}$), and even short half-life analytes like glycated albumin, can determine long-term glycaemic control. HbA$_{1c}$ should be measured from two- to six-monthly, but finger-prick glucose measurement remains the standard day-to-day monitoring tool, and should take account of mealtimes rather than specified clock times. A useful frequency is four times daily, before meals and at bedtime, and patients should ideally keep a diary.

What are the glycaemic targets in diabetes?

The Joint British Societies guidelines for prevention of cardiovascular disease recommend that optimal targets are 4.0–6.0 mmol/l for fasting or pre-prandial glucose and HbA$_{1c}$ < 6.5%. There are no clear evidence-based targets, but good control might reasonably be represented by four

Table 2.44 Diabetic ketoacidosis			
Hormone problem	**Resulting pathophysiology**	**Biochemical problem**	**Symptoms**
Insulin deficiency	Hepatic glucose mobilisation Decreased peripheral glucose storage	Hyperglycaemia	Polyuria Polydipsia Dehydration Confusion Drowsiness Coma
Catabolic hormone excess (often the result of precipitating cause)	Triglyceride breakdown delivering fatty acids to liver and ketogenesis – generation of ketone bodies 3-hydroxybutyrate and acetoacetate (these alternative energy pathways are also a consequence of insulin deficiency causing failure of incorporation of glucose into vital organs	Ketoacidosis	Vomiting Ketonuria Abdominal pain Kussmaul breathing 'Pear drop' or 'nail varnish' breath due to ketone body metabolism in lungs

out of five preprandial glucose readings in the range 4–10 mmol/l (it is not really possible to expect completely normal levels), poor control by one or no readings in the range and suboptimal control somewhere in between. Treatment aims to avoid symptomatic hyper- or hypoglycaemia, although exaggerated fear of hypoglycaemia makes unnecessary hyperglycaemia common. Plasma glucose can double after a meal and if insulin is withheld from a patient because their blood glucose level is normal it will not stay normal for long!

What different types of insulin regimen do you know of?

Insulin regimens are described in Box 2.55.

Box 2.55 Insulin regimens in type 1 diabetes

Insulin has a natural background basal release with prandial surges. Thus, glucose is normally tightly controlled. In the 1970s through to the 1990s human insulins and recombinant human insulins (*Escherichia coli* purified insulin without C-peptide) began to replace animal insulins and were available as short-, intermediate- or long-acting preparations.

Twice daily premixed (biphasic) regimens

- Pre-mixed combinations of short- and intermediate-acting insulin twice daily such as human *Mixtard 30/70* or *Humulin M3* (soluble *Actrapid* 30% and isophane 70% – ratios may be altered) are easy to administer and adequate for many patients with type 2 diabetes and for some with type 1 diabetes. However, they allow for a less flexible lifestyle, do not provide tight control and hypoglycaemia may occur late morning and overnight. They are being superseded by ultra-long-acting insulins that aim to tighten basal control (below). Weight gain can be minimised by combining with oral hypoglycaemic agents in type 2 diabetes.
- The ideal aim is a plasma glucose 5.1–7.0 (seldom achievable with any regimen). When starting insulin, a short-acting insulin sliding scale can determine the number of units needed over 24 hours, around two-thirds of the requirement administered in the morning and one-third at night.
- Blood glucose measurements always reflect previous insulin. For example, a measurement of 5.1 at 17.30 h means it is safe to give the teatime dose provided the patient will eat at 18.00 h. If there is concern about nocturnal hypoglycaemia, an 03.00 h measurement may be useful; if, for example, it is 3.5, teatime insulin should be reduced. As a general rule, insulin doses should generally be altered by at least 20% of total daily dose at a time.

Basal bolus regimens

- Short-acting insulin (e.g. *Actrapid*, *Humulin S*) before meals with a once daily longer, intermediate-acting insulin (isophane as *Insulatard* or *Humulin I*) should provide tighter glycaemic control than a twice-daily regimen and allow more flexible mealtimes and lifestyle.
- Doses may be estimated by dividing the number of units of short-acting insulin delivered by a sliding scale over 24 hours into four split doses – breakfast, lunch, teatime (short-acting insulin) and before bed (longer-acting insulin). Without a 24-hour guide, an empirical dose of around 6–8 units four times daily is sometimes used.
- Traditional short-acting insulins like *Actrapid* have an onset of action of around 30 minutes, a peak at around two hours (i.e. they do not act rapidly and mealtimes must be predicted) and last for around eight hours (i.e. missing a predicted meal can result in prolonged hypoglycaemia). Traditional intermediate- and long-acting insulins seldom provide 24 hours of continuous basal insulin. Isophane, for example, wanes at 12–16 hours. For these reasons, insulins like *Actrapid* and *Mixtard* are becoming more historical.

Insulin analogues

- In the late 1990s modified versions of insulin called insulin analogues started to appear.
- Short-acting analogues (SAAs) such as *Novorapid* (aspart) and *Humalog* (lispro) are rapidly absorbed subcutaneously and very rapid acting, with an onset of action between 1 and 2 minutes. They can

be administered at meal times (even during meals) to mimic endogenous prandial insulin release. They are metabolised from the system within 1–2 hours, reducing the risk of subsequent hypoglycaemia.

- Long-acting analogues (LAAs) such as *Lantus* (glargine) or *Levemir* (detemir) are more predictably absorbed long-acting insulins with prolonged activity profiles and no pronounced peaks in activity. They mimic endogenous, fasting, 24-hour basal insulin.
- Tight control can now be achieved with a combination of a once-daily LAA and SAAs at mealtimes, limiting blood glucose rises between meals and reducing the risk of hypoglycaemia between meals and overnight.
- Isophane is still more widely used than an LAA in basal bolus regimens containing SAAs but may need to be given twice daily with SAAs (i.e. five daily injections). LAAs are not used routinely in type 2 diabetes unless the patient's lifestyle is significantly restricted by hypoglycaemia. Indications for an LAA include a variable effect from isophane (variable absorption or poor mixing – glargine is premixed), basal waning by evening in a basal-bolus regimen or 03.00 h hypoglycaemic episodes. LAAs may also be useful in patients on isophane with morning hyperglycaemia where dose increases can produce nocturnal hypoglycaemia. The same number of units of glargine is used as once daily isophane but 20% less glargine if twice-daily isophane.
- Initial requirements can be estimated by calculating the total number of units of short-acting insulin given over 24 hours (e.g. 50 units); this number of units is then divided into fifths; two-fifths (20 units) is given as glargine and one-fifth (10 units) as *Novorapid* at each of breakfast, lunch and tea. A pre-breakfast blood glucose monitor reading can be monitored weekly and if > 7.0, glargine is increased (it is important to get the LAA step right first of all) and then the SAA can be adjusted by 2–4 units with each meal if the BM remains > 7.0.

Insulin pumps

Increasingly, tiny insulin pumps are used to deliver short-acting insulin; they have implantable glucose sensors.

Inhaled insulin

This was available between 2006 and 2008 but did not gain popularity; its re-emergence is uncertain.

Other regimens

- Premixed (biphasic) insulins containing SAAs (e.g. *Novomix 30*, *Humalog Mix 25* or *50*) combine SAAs with intermediate-acting insulins. They are convenient, without a need for a 30-minute gap before meals and may produce better post-prandial glucose control with less risk of hypoglycaemia. However, biphasic insulins are rather inflexible.
- Twice-daily isophane alone is sometimes used initially in type 1 diabetes before breakfast and evening meal, although a short-acting insulin is usually needed before long. It may be considered in very elderly people where avoidance of hypoglycaemia is more critical than tight glycaemia.
- Regimens in type 2 diabetes, in older people and combined with oral hypoglycaemic agents are discussed in Case 2.24.

What are the principles of nutrition in diabetes?

The old fashioned approach was a diet low in carbohydrate and high in fat. The modern trend is lower fat and higher carbohydrate, with the concept of knowing the carbohydrate content of foods and responding to carbohydrate units and adjusting insulin accordingly rather than limiting eating.

Does glycaemic control in type 1 diabetes reduce vascular complications?

The Diabetes Control and Complications Trial (DCCT) showed significant relative risk reductions with intensive treatment (HbA$_{1c}$ 7%) of 76% for the onset of retinopathy, 54% for retinopathy progression, 39% for nephropathy and significant reduction in neuropathy. Continuous benefit was suggested at lower levels but at the cost of a higher risk of hypoglycaemia. Evidence for microvascular benefit appeared greater than for macrovascular benefit, although because there were few macrovascular events in short-term follow-up, the study was underpowered in that respect. However, more recent follow-up has shown reduced macrovascular events.

Why does glycaemic control in diabetes tend to destabilise in hospital?

Stress causes a surge of counter-regulatory hormones including adrenaline, glucagon, cortisol and growth hormone. These cause the effects listed in Table 2.45.

Do you know of any potential future therapies in diabetes?

These include pancreatic islet cell transplantation, xeno-transplantation and inhaled, oral and nasal insulins.

Why is hypoglycaemia dangerous?

The brain depends on a constant supply of glucose to function, neuronal activity declining at levels < 3.5 mmol/l and cognitive function at < 3 mmol/l. Alternative fuels such as lactate and ketones cannot be mobilised in time during acute insulin-induced hypoglycaemia.

How is hypoglycaemia normally detected?

The hypothalamus and other areas of the brain normally sense hypoglycaemia, initiating a generalised autonomic (sympathetic) response.

What is the normal response to hypoglycaemia?

The autonomic response is protective both by producing counter-regulatory hormone release (glucagon and the catecholamine adrenaline, which stimulate hepatic glucose release and reduce glucose uptake by fat and muscle) and generating symptoms that alert the individual (Table 2.45). Growth hormone and cortisol, also produced during hypoglycaemia, play a relatively minor role during insulin-induced hypoglycaemia.

How problematic is hypoglycaemia in diabetes?

Hypoglycaemia is a potential problem when aiming for tight glycaemic control. Major hypoglycaemia was experienced by 27% of intensively treated patients in the DCCT and only 2% of patients in the UKPDS (Case 2.24) despite broadly similar levels of glycaemic control. In the UKPDS over the first 10 years, major hypoglycaemia rates varied depending upon treatment modality, but were highest at 2.3% for patients on insulin. Hypoglycaemia remains very common in older people in residential care, who may eat little and still take their tablets. Long-acting analogues reduce the risk of hypoglycaemia but cause sustained hypoglycaemia when it does occur and effects may occur days after the last dose.

What are hypoglycaemia-associated autonomic failure (HAAF) and hypoglycaemic unawareness?

Difficulty recognising hypoglycaemia affects about 25% of patients with type 1 diabetes and almost 50% who have had the disease for over 20 years. In insulin-deficient diabetes, exogenous insulin levels do not fall as glucose levels fall and the integrity of counter-regulatory hormones assumes greater significance. The glucagon response begins to fail within the first year or two of type 1 diabetes and is generally absent after five years, the adrenaline response becoming the crucial line of defence. The adrenaline response itself, however, is progressively blunted by antecedent hypoglycaemia (usually later in disease than glucagon failure), as is hypoglycaemic awareness because of loss of sympathetic symptoms. This combination of glucagon and adrenaline failure and unawareness because of antecedent hypoglycaemia is known as HAAF. By shifting glucose

Table 2.45 Normal responses to hypoglycaemia	
Approximate blood glucose (mmol/l) at which response starts	**Response**
3.7	Adrenaline release
3.5	Start of neuronal dysfunction Sweating, tremor, palpitations, hunger (autonomic symptoms)
3.0	Start of cognitive dysfunction
2.5	Confusion, loss of concentration, speech difficulty, odd behaviour, incoordination, occasionally focal neurological deficits (neuroglycopenic symptoms)
1.0	Coma or seizure
Sustained hypoglycaemia	Permanent brain damage

thresholds downwards for the symptomatic and sympatho-adrenal responses (to a level of around 2.5 mmol/l), antecedent hypoglycaemia creates a self-perpetuating cycle of recurrent hypoglycaemia without warning symptoms and further blunting of counter-regulation. The cycle can be broken by scrupulous avoidance of hypoglycaemia, which restores adrenaline (but not glucagon activity) and demonstrates that hypoglycaemic unawareness is not caused by autonomic neuropathy but rather HAAF.

How is hypoglycaemia treated?

A conscious patient should be given 10 g of quick-acting glucose (two teaspoons of sugar, three dextrose tablets, 50 ml original Lucozade, jam or honey) followed by long-acting carbohydrate such as bread, biscuits or milk. An unconscious patient should receive 50 ml of 50% dextrose intravenously or 1 mg of intramuscular glucagon.

Can hypoglycaemia be predicted and prevented?

Predictors include previous severe hypoglycaemia, recurrent asymptomatic hypoglycaemia (often nocturnal), diabetes of long duration and intensified insulin therapy. Education is vital. Hypoglycaemic awareness is more likely when patients have autonomic symptoms (sweats, shakes, palpitations) but less likely for patients relying on neuroglycopenic symptoms (confusion, dysarthria, unsteadiness). For those with impaired awareness, more physiological insulin and relaxation of glycaemic targets (e.g. pre-meal 4 mmol/l and pre-bed 7 mmol/l) may help, and scrupulous avoidance of hypoglycaemia may break the HAAF cycle.

How would you tackle nocturnal hypoglycaemia?

Nocturnal hypoglycaemia affects over 50% of people taking insulin, and more physiological replacement with insulin analogues and matching replacement to carbohydrate intake may lessen the problem, as may a bedtime snack. Snacking between meals may also help patients with non-physiological insulin profiles. Overnight insulin should be reduced after an overactive day. Alcohol should be avoided to excess, and overnight insulin should sometimes be reduced.

What is hyperosmolar non-ketotic coma (HONC)?

This is an insidious rise in glucose to often very high levels, that predisposes to thrombotic complications; it is more common in older people with unrecognised type 2 diabetes and may present with polydipsia, polyuria or confusion.

Ketones are absent or minimally present as insulin is not completely deficient, present in sufficient amount to incorporate some glucose into organs and thus prevent switching to alternative ketotic pathway sources of energy. However, glucose levels build up slowly in the bloodstream to impressive levels with a high osmolarity. Treatment is rehydration, insulin and anticoagulation.

Can type 1 diabetes be prevented?

Major trials of agents in antibody-positive relatives of people with type 1 diabetes failed to prevent development of type 1 diabetes.

CASE 2.24

TYPE 2 DIABETES MELLITUS

Candidate information

Role

You are a doctor in the diabetes clinic. Please read the following letter from the patient's general practitioner. You may make notes on the paper provided. When the bell sounds, enter the examination room to begin the consultation.

Scenario

> Dear Doctor
> Re: Mrs Lorna Fairlee, aged 60 years
> Thank you for seeing this lady urgently in clinic. She was diagnosed with type 2 diabetes 10 years ago and has a small ulcer on her right big toe that has now turned gangrenous. She has a history of sensory neuropathy. Her total cholesterol is 5.9 mmol/l despite statin therapy. Her current medications are metformin 1 g b.d., isophane insulin 20 units before bed, simvastatin 40 mg, aspirin 75 mg and atenolol 50 mg, all daily.
> Yours sincerely

Please take a history from the patient (you may continue to make notes if you wish on the paper provided). Your examiners will warn you when 12 minutes have elapsed. You have 14 minutes to take a history from the patient followed by 1 minute of reflection. There will then follow 5 minutes of discussion with the examiners. Be prepared to discuss solutions to the problems posed by the case and how you might reply to the GP's letter. You are not required to examine the patient.

Patient information

Mrs Lorna Fairlee is a 60-year-old retired pharmaceutical representative who was diagnosed with type 2 diabetes 10 years ago and has been on insulin at night for two years together with metformin. She now has a small ulcer on her right big toe, which has turned black and painful. She has a history of sensory neuropathy with numbness, and poor peripheral circulation, and is an ex-smoker of 20 cigarettes a day. She has high cholesterol despite simvastatin. Her previous history comprises angina on exertion and problems with obesity. She had laser eye surgery last year but has no visual impairment. She feels her diet is reasonable but admits that exercise is difficult on account of her neuropathy and that she spent much of her working life in the car. She is now horrified by the black toe. Her husband is unwell with back problems, and needs help with washing and dressing.

How to approach the case

Data gathering in the interview and interpretation and use of information gathered

Presenting problem(s) and symptom exploration

▪ **Elicit the range of symptoms and complications** Presentation of type 2 diabetes is usually with symptoms of hyperglycaemia or cardiovascular disease (CVD) complications after many years of silent development. The classic presentation and features are outlined in Box 2.56.

Type 2 diabetes is characterised by complications. Take a full history of events surrounding the foot ulcer, and for:

- Glycaemic control – home monitoring and knowledge of HbA_{1c}
- Blood pressure
- Lipid levels
- Previous CVD complications – myocardial infarction, stroke, peripheral vascular disease
- Retinopathy
- Nephropathy
- Peripheral neuropathy

Patient perspective

The Diabetes Education Self Management Ongoing Newly Diagnosed (DESMOND) Collaborative Project has set out an evidence-based structured education and self-management programme for type 2 diabetes that aims to develop understanding of diabetes, and promote the specific diabetes (e.g. monitoring) and general self-management (e.g. goal setting) skills needed for effective

---

Box 2.56 Classic presentation and features of type 2 diabetes

- Usually occurs in over 30s
- Gradual onset
- Diagnosis often missed; first presentation may be:
  - microvascular complication – retinopathy, nephropathy or neuropathy (25–30% have retinopathy at presentation, correlating with 7 years of antecedent hyperglycaemia)
  - macrovascular event – acute coronary syndrome, stroke or peripheral vascular disease
- Overweight or obese (> 80%)
- Not associated with ketoacidosis (usually)
- Family history often positive
- Autoimmune markers tend to be negative
- Diet and physical activity can often control disease

---

self-management. Areas included (that may prompt questions in the history) include: housekeeping; the patient's story; what diabetes is; main means of managing diabetes; consequences and personal risk; monitoring and taking action (including hypoglycaemic awareness); food choices; physical activity; stress and emotion; and screening and complication surveillance.

Past medical history

Explore the history of angina, investigations performed and treatment.

Drug and allergy history

Beta blockers and diuretics are associated with a significantly increased incidence of diabetes, and the former exacerbate peripheral vascular disease.

Family history

A family history of type 2 diabetes is common.

Social history

Enquire about the needs of her husband were she to be admitted to hospital.

SUMMARY – ASSESSMENT AND PLAN

- Explain that vascular studies will be needed to determine arterial flow, with care jointly by the diabetologists and vascular surgeons.
- Possible outcomes include discharge and medical management, admission for further investigations, toe amputation or, possibly electively, revascularisation surgery.
- An ABC approach for managing type 2 diabetes is summarised in Table 2.46.

Discussion

What is the scale of the problem of type 2 diabetes?

Type 2 diabetes accounts for about 90% of all diabetes. It is a worldwide epidemic, tripling in prevalence over the last 30 years and affecting 6–8% of middle-aged to older adults in the UK and USA. In the last 10 years there has been a shift towards incidence in younger adults and even children. It is strongly associated with obesity, physical inactivity and other risk factors for CVD, and may be part of the metabolic syndrome (Case 2.7, Box 2.24).

What causes type 2 diabetes?

There is a strong, albeit poorly understood, genetic susceptibility, and environmental factors crucial to development include excessive food intake, obesity and physical inactivity. Type 2 diabetes is a chronic, progressive metabolic disorder characterised by insulin resistance and impaired secretion.

Table 2.46 An ABC approach to managing type 2 diabetes

ABC ...	Strategies and targets
Advice	Education
	Support groups include 'Diabetes UK', and education and management may be coordinated by a specialist diabetic service with which patients are registered on a regional diabetic register; the level of integration of care between primary and secondary care varies from region to region.
	Self management
	Diet
	Carbohydrate > 50% of calorie intake, especially from complex carbohydrate foods rich in natural fibre such as fruit and vegetables (sucrose and other sugars < 10%)
	Fat < 35% of calorie intake (saturated fat to a minimum)
	Protein < 10% of intake or < 1 g/kg body weight
	Physical activity
	Weight reduction
	Optimum BMI 20–25 kg/m²
	Driving
	Patients on oral hypoglycaemic treatment or insulin have a responsibility to inform the DVLA
Blood pressure	< 130/80 mmHg
Cholesterol	TC < 4.0 mmol/l and LDL-C < 2.0 mmol/l or
	25% reduction in TC and 30% reduction in LDL-C
Diabetes control	$HbA_{1c} \leq 6.5\%$
Eye care	Yearly digital photography
Foot care	Yearly examination
'Guardian' drugs	Aspirin 75 mg daily if established CVD, ≥ 50 years or diabetes > 10 years or on treatment for hypertension
	Statin in most to achieve TC and LDL-C targets
	ACE inhibitor/ARB in microalbuminuria or proteinuria or diabetic nephropathy

ACE, angiotensin-converting enzyme; ARB, angiotensin receptor blocker; BMI, body mass index; CVD, cardiovascular disease; DVLA, Driver and Vehicle Licensing Agency; LDL-C, low-density lipoprotein cholesterol; TC, total cholesterol.

Insulin resistance

Insulin acts on cells in muscle, fat and liver by binding to membrane receptors and triggering a series of intracellular phosphorylation steps leading to glucose uptake, and effects on fatty acid and protein metabolism. In type 2 diabetes, basal hepatic glucose output is increased, suppression of hepatic glucose output after meals is impaired and insulin-induced glucose uptake in muscle and fat is reduced. Increased triglycerides and low-density lipoprotein cholesterol (LDL-C) and decreased high-density lipoprotein cholesterol (HDL-C), together with uric acidaemia and increased plasminogen activator inhibitor 1, are also effects of insulin resistance and increase CVD risk. Both the insulin molecule and cell receptors are normal, but intracellular pathways are aberrant after insulin binding. Insulin resistance leads to elevated insulin concentrations in contrast to type 1 and other forms of diabetes in which endogenous insulin is low or absent.

Beta cell failure

Despite hyperinsulinaemia, the beta cell response to hyperglycaemia is inadequate and insulin secretion is always abnormal once type 2 diabetes is fully established. Insulin secretory responses to meals are severely blunted, with post-prandial hyperglycaemia early in disease leading to fasting hyperglycaemia as disease progresses and insulin concentrations cannot overcome hepatic insulin resistance. Ultimately, hyperinsulinaemia gives way to beta cell failure and hypoinsulinaemia.

What is maturity onset diabetes of the young (MODY)?

MODY refers to a group of disorders with autosomal dominant inheritance usually presenting before 25 years of age and with primary defects in insulin secretion: MODY 1 [HNF-4α (hepatocyte nuclear factor 4α)], MODY 2 (glucokinase), MODY 3 (HNF-1α), MODY 4 [IPF-1 (insulin promoter factor 1)], MODY 5 (HNF-1β), MODY 6 (neuroD1 or BETA 2). Patients are not typically obese.

How is type 2 diabetes diagnosed?

Diagnostic definitions are given in Table 2.13, Case 2.7.

Does glycaemic control in type 2 diabetes reduce vascular complications?

Acute glycaemic management

Short-term glycaemic control in hospitalised patients might be expected to improve well-being, reduce infection rates, aid wound healing, prevent severe hyperglycaemia and reduce vascular complications. The Dextrose Insulin and Glucose in Acute Myocardial Infarction (DIGAMI) study showed that tight control at the time of infarction

Table 2.47 Effects of a 1% reduction in HbA$_{1c}$ on complications in type 2 diabetes

Complication	Risk reduction
Albuminuria at 12 years	33%
Retinopathy at 12 years	21%
Microvascular disease	25%
Myocardial infarction	16%
Any diabetes-related complication	12%

and for three months reduced three-year mortality by 11%. Some studies in critically ill patients without diabetes have also shown reductions in serious outcomes such as sepsis, others have been conflicting, and in DIGAMI 2 the benefits of DIGAMI were not replicated.

The UK Prospective Diabetes Study (UKPDS) and long-term control

The UKPDS was a 20-year study of over 5000 patients with type 2 diabetes. It showed that the intensive glycaemic control (average HbA$_{1c}$ 7.0%) produces considerably fewer microvascular complications (Table 2.47) than conventional control (average HbA$_{1c}$ 7.9%). Good glycaemic control also reduces the risk of stroke with a favourable trend towards lower myocardial infarction. There were no differences in glucose control or microvascular endpoints between patients treated with chlorpropamide, glibenclamide or insulin. Metformin, used as primary therapy for overweight patients, reduced microvascular and macrovascular endpoints at similar levels of glucose control to other therapies, and was the only therapy not associated with weight gain. Improving glycaemic control with insulin or a sulphonylurea had only marginal macrovascular benefit but an explanation for this may be similar to that of the Diabetes Control and Complications Trial (DCCT; Case 2.23) in type 1 diabetes. However, UKPDS did show that controlling hypertension had an important impact on macrovascular events. UKPDS also showed that HbA$_{1c}$ tended to rise every five years by around 1% even in tightly controlled patients, perhaps reducing the temptation to 'blame' patients or doctors for disease progression.

What do you know about the pathogenesis of diabetes complications?

Advanced glycation endproducts are of pathogenic importance. Glucose binds with protein to produce glycated proteins such as glycosylated haemoglobin HbA$_{1c}$. The property of these proteins is altered by, for example, crosslinks, and this is very important for molecules that are not readily renewed such as collagen, which become advanced glycation endproducts.

Can type 2 diabetes be prevented?

This is discussed in Case 2.7.

Which groups of oral hypoglycaemic agent are used in type 2 diabetes?

Diet control and weight loss are much more effective than oral hypoglycaemic agents, which are summarised in Table 2.48.

What other anti-hyperglycaemic agents are in development?

Glucagon-like peptide (GLP)-1 is a gut hormone that stimulates insulin secretion. Together with the related hormone, glucose-dependent insulinotropic polypeptide (GIP), it is responsible for the incretin effect, the augmentation of insulin secretion after oral administration of glucose. Patients with type 2 diabetes typically have little or no incretin-mediated augmentation of insulin due to decreased secretion of GLP-1 and loss of the insulinotropic effects of GIP. GLP-1 is rapidly degraded by the enzyme dipeptidyl peptidase 4 (DPP4); GLP-1 analogues and DPP4 inhibitors are emerging – exenatide, a GLP-1 analogue for type 2 diabetes inadequately controlled on metformin and sulphonylurea, and DPP4 tablets. Other agents studied are combined peroxisome proliferator-activated receptor γ- and α-agonists (the latter having fibrate effects) and endocannabinoid receptor blockers (thought to be overactive in obesity and smokers).

When is insulin indicated in type 2 diabetes?

Box 2.57 describes the indications for insulin and regimens used in type 2 diabetes.

Mrs Fairlee, two years after you have seen her, takes 32 units of a human *Mixtard* 30/70 before breakfast and 28 units before tea. She is admitted with gastroenteritis. Her vomiting settles, but she has not yet mobilised. Her total insulin dose over 24 hours has been 48 units. What would you do now about her insulin?

If she is normally well controlled she is likely to go back on her usual insulin at the day of discharge. However, as she may not have fully recovered, a short-acting insulin or short-acting analogue (SAA) before breakfast, lunch and dinner and a long-acting insulin before bed is appropriate. Splitting her usual insulin into four doses and rounding up to even numbers of units, 14 units at each of these time-points seems appropriate; 12 units seems too little even though it equates to the previous 24 hours whilst 14 units is closer to her usual dose. It is not possible to predict accurately her future requirements, so her blood glucose should be monitored four times daily and her insulin should be adjusted upwards or downwards as necessary. If she responds well, she could be discharged the following day, continuing the four times daily regimen to lunchtime and then resume her usual insulin at teatime, monitoring carefully and with diabetes specialist nurse support if needed. The management of insulin in hospital patients is outlined in Box 2.58.

Table 2.48 Oral hypoglycaemic agents (OHAs)

Drugs	Action	Indications	Dose	Advantages	Side effects
Metformin	Reduces hepatic gluconeogenesis Enhances peripheral utilisation of glucose Only effective in presence of endogenous insulin (some residual beta cell function)	First line in overweight or obese Suitable monotherapy	500 mg b.d. to optimum 850 mg t.d.s. if tolerated Available in modified-release formulation	No weight gain Seldom hypoglycaemia May be cardioprotective (UKPDS)	Gastrointestinal (20%) – diarrhoea, nausea – may arise after years of treatment Lactic acidosis (contraindicated if acutely ill, renal failure – creatinine > 150 µmol/l, decompensated liver disease, severe heart failure) Vitamin B12 deficiency
Sulphonylureas, e.g. gliclazide	Insulin secretagogues (potentiate insulin release) by binding receptors on beta cells and closing potassium channels Long or short acting	Normal/underweight (metformin may be considered) Suitable monotherapy		No lactic acidosis	Weight gain Hypoglycaemia (low incidence but dangerous and sometimes prolonged warranting hospital admission for 48 hours)
Prandial glucose regulators, e.g. repaglinide, netaglinide	Induce rapid post-prandial insulin release (target early phase insulin release) Ultra-short acting Taken with meals; may be useful if unpredictable lifestyle	Suitable monotherapy, or add on to metformin or insulin	Repaglinide 0.5 mg pre-meals to maximum 16 mg/day Netaglinide 60 mg t.d.s to maximum 180 mg t.d.s.	Early phase insulin release is one of the earliest malfunctions in type 2 diabetes Well tolerated Reduce HbA$_{1c}$	Hypoglycaemia
Thiazolidinediones 'Glitazones', e.g. rosiglitazone, pioglitazone	Activate nuclear peroxisome proliferator activated receptor γ (PPARγ) in liver, muscle and fat; this controls expression of genes regulating metabolism Improves insulin sensitivity, especially in skeletal muscle Slow onset of action	Place in treatment controversial but mechanism of action suggests may be appropriate in patients intolerant of metformin Not used with insulin	Pioglitazone 15–45 mg o.d. Rosiglitazone 4–8 mg o.d. or b.d.	Improve HbA$_{1c}$ by up to 1.5% Pioglitazone especially lowers triglycerides and raises HDL-C	Fluid retention (contraindicated in heart failure; caution in renal or liver disease)
α-glucosidase inhibitors, e.g. acarbose	Attenuate carbohydrate absorption by inhibiting mucosal enzymes that hydrolyse complex to simple sugars	Monotherapy or combined with metformin or sulphonylurea	25–100 mg t.d.s.	No metabolic side effects	Excessive abdominal bloating, flatulence and pain Less impact on HbA$_{1c}$ (UKPDS)

Box 2.57 Insulin in type 2 diabetes, older people and combined with oral hypoglycaemic agents (OHAs)

It is increasingly common to use OHAs and insulin in type 2 diabetes. Typically a patient may be on maximal OHA therapy (e.g. metformin 2 g with a sulphonylurea or thiazolinedione) and insulin is substituted for the sulphonylurea or thiazolinedione, the latter being contraindicated with insulin. Most patients with type 2 diabetes would probably ultimately benefit from insulin were they to live long enough. Insulin is probably underused, with the false perception that many patients would find it too difficult. Indications in type 2 diabetes include:

- Poor glycaemic control associated with marked symptoms and weight loss (suggests beta cell failure) – patients often respond very well and feel much better
- Poor glycaemic control (despite concordance with lifestyle change and combination therapy) without symptoms ($HbA_{1c} > 9.0\%$)
- Suboptimal glycaemic control with high risk of complications (young age or established vascular complications; insulin should only be used in the right context – a 10-year risk reduction may not be the aim in a 90-year-old with comorbidities, and there are practical considerations with administration)
- Intolerance of OHAs

Insulin may also be used temporarily in acute coronary syndromes, acute illness, surgery and short-term corticosteroid use.

Twice-daily pre-mixed regimens

Traditional regimens use biphasic preparations combining short- and intermediate- or long-acting insulin usually in a twice-daily regimen (e.g. *Mixtard 30/70*, *Humulin M3*, *Novomix*). A reasonable starting dose is 10 units twice daily.

Once-daily isophane or long-acting insulin with daytime OHAs

Once-daily intermediate-acting isophane, best given at bedtime, with daytime OHAs is another way of introducing insulin, aiming for a dose that produces a fasting glucose of around 6.0. Potential problems are a tendency to hyperglycaemia later in the day and nocturnal hypoglycaemia, especially with higher doses (> 30 units). An LAA, giving a very respectable level after about 2 hours and remaining so for 24 hours with predictable absorption, may be preferable to isophane if there is variable effect from isophane (variable absorption or poor mixing – glargine is premixed), basal waning by evening or 03.00 h hypoglycaemic episodes. Many diabetologists now regard metformin and an LAA as the regimen of choice. The same number of units of glargine is used as once-daily isophane but 20% less glargine as from a twice-daily isophane regimen; in general 10–12 units of LAA is a reasonable starting dose.

Twice daily isophane used as basal insulin

This may be tried if once-daily isophane fails to contain hyperglycaemia, instead of switching to an LAA.

Basal bolus regimens

Basal bolus regimens are usually reserved for type 1 diabetes but may be used in active, younger patients with type 2 diabetes, or in unwell patients with type 2 diabetes. Short-acting insulins or SAAs are useful with meals with isophane such as *Insulatard* at night (or with a LAA because SAAs are metabolised rapidly). A common starting regimen for an unwell patient in hospital not normally on insulin is 10 units of *Actrapid* with meals and 10 units of *Insulatard* before bed.

Box 2.58 Insulin – hospital patients

There are three levels of insulin intensity for hospitalised patients:

1. An intravenous insulin/glucose regimen for acutely ill patients who are not eating. Unless there is a need to limit fluid volume, patients usually receive isotonic dextrose with added potassium for the insulin to 'work against', which dampens swings in plasma glucose. Insulin is infused through a syringe driver and adjusted in rate to hourly near patient glucose measurements.
2. A four-times-daily basal bolus regimen for patients who are unstable but well enough to eat.
3. A maintenance regimen or a patient's usual insulin for all other patients. This is more commonly a twice-daily regimen of pre-mixed short- and intermediate-acting insulin in type 2 diabetes (some patients take a single basal dose combined with metformin) and a basal bolus regimen for motivated (usually type 1) patients.

Insulin can be thought of as anticipating or following the level of glycaemic control. A patient tailoring short-acting insulin doses before meals to the amount they expect to eat is anticipating the effect of food on plasma glucose. At the other extreme, infused insulin is chasing the tail of glucose excursions. Sliding-scale insulin would thus be inappropriate in unstable patients who are well enough to eat because it would chase its tail after meals. Here, an anticipating regimen is needed and the basal bolus regimen anticipates rises after meals but can also follow. Insulin doses may be varied on the experience of previous doses/meals both to anticipate insulin need and to correct hyper- or hypoglycaemia. In other words, it combines the anticipating and following principles, and is the logical choice for a patient coming off sliding-scale insulin. The first bolus is given 30 minutes after stopping the infusion. There is no evidence that sulphonylureas are unsafe in acutely ill patients but insulin is preferable because of its short half-life and responsiveness in rapidly changing situations. Metformin should not be used because of the risk of lactic acidosis.

What is the evidence for blood pressure lowering in type 2 diabetes?

Elevated blood pressure (> 140/90 mmHg) is twice as common in diabetes and greatly increases an already increased CVD risk. The combination of hypertension and diabetes doubles the risk of developing microvascular and macrovascular complications, and doubles mortality compared with non-diabetic people with hypertension. Evidence for blood pressure reduction is largely from trials that included people with diabetes, shown to reduce or prevent major cardiovascular events including heart failure, cardiovascular death and total mortality. There is also evidence of reduced progression to retinopathy and nephropathy in people with diabetes but without CVD. The UKPDS randomised people with diabetes and hypertension in a sub-study to intensive or less intensive antihypertensive therapy, intensive therapy significantly reduced stroke by 44% and myocardial infarction by 21%, the latter not reaching statistical significance (probably because the study was underpowered). Atenolol and captopril were equally effective.

What are the targets for blood pressure in diabetes and how might these be achieved?

The blood pressure targets are < 130/80 mmHg, possibly lower in diabetic nephropathy, the greater the reduction the greater the benefit and there appears to be no threshold below which risk no longer declines. Strict blood pressure control is the most important factor preventing diabetic nephropathy and stage 5 kidney disease. Almost all patients need a combination of drugs and the evidence for nephro-protection is greatest with renin–angiotensin system blockade.

What is the evidence for lipid-lowering in diabetes?

Diabetic dyslipidaemia is characterised by high LDL-C and triglycerides and low HDL-C. Covert hypothyroidism may coexist with diabetes and produce similar dyslipidae-mia. Evidence for lipid-lowering in diabetes reducing CVD is largely from sub-group analyses including people with diabetes. More recent trials exclusively in diabetes have shown significant reductions in coronary and cardiovascu-lar events in people with diabetes comparable with those without diabetes. The Heart Protection Study included more people with type 1 and type 2 diabetes than previous studies combined and showed that patients with type 2 diabetes, one other risk factor for CHD and a total cho-lesterol > 3.5 mmol/l had 33% fewer CVD events (coronary or stroke) with 40 mg simvastatin. ASCOT-LLA similarly had a large diabetes cohort and the 19% non-significant reduction in fatal coronary heart disease and myocardial infarction probably reflected reduced statistical power because it was stopped early. CARDS evaluated statin therapy exclusively in diabetic patients and compared atorvastatin 10 mg with placebo and was terminated early because the 37% reduction in CVD events (taken sepa-rately significant reductions in acute CHD events by 37% and stroke by 48%) was larger than that observed in the Heart Protection Study. All patients with diabetes should therefore be considered for statin therapy, with a minimum dose of simvastatin 40 mg or equivalent.

What are the targets for lipid-lowering in diabetes and how are these achieved?

Targets for people at high risk are outlined in Case 2.7; these people include those with type 1 or 2 diabetes ≥ 40 years of age and those with type 1 or 2 diabetes 18–39 years of age with at least one of retinopathy, nephropathy, poor glycae-mic control (HbA$_{1c}$ > 9%), elevated blood pressure on therapy, total cholesterol ≥ 6.0 mmol/l, features of meta-bolic syndrome or family history of premature CVD.

What is the definition of diabetic nephropathy?

By convention, this is an albumin excretion rate (AER) > 300 mg/24 hours in a person with diabetes of more than five years and concomitant retinopathy, in the absence of urinary tract infection, other renal disease or heart failure. Urinary AER in a timed collection should only be determined if urinary albumin concentra-tion or albumin : creatinine ratio exceed the normal range (Table 2.49), and then confirmed on two subsequent samples. All patients should be screened annually.

What types of diabetic nephropathy are there?

Diabetic nephropathy in type 1 diabetes is usually of classic type, rare in the first 10 years, peaking at 3% per year at 15 years and declining slowly thereafter such that after 40 years' duration it is only 1% per year. Those without it then are at low risk. In type 2 diabetes, the classic form with retinopathy and progression from microalbu-minuria to proteinuria is common, but an atypical form without retinopathy and with minimal or no proteinuria occurs.

Why is diabetic nephropathy important?

Increased glomerular filtration, renal blood flow and hypertrophy precede diabetic nephropathy and are revers-ible with good glycaemic control. Significant structural damage accompanies microalbuminuria, often with hyper-tension, and although the glomerular filtration rate (GFR) may not be affected until the high microalbuminuria range is reached, microalbuminuria is strongly predictive of death from CVD, especially in older patients with type 2 diabetes. In those with type 1 diabetes developing protein-uria after a very long duration, it more likely reflects CVD than diabetic nephropathy. Persistent albuminuria or overt diabetic nephropathy is usually accompanied by athero-sclerosis and, untreated, a relentless decline in GFR with death after an average 7–10 years. It is recognised that anaemia may occur earlier in diabetic nephropathy than other kidney diseases.

How is diabetic nephropathy treated?

Good glycaemic control can prevent diabetic nephropathy but there is less evidence that it prevents progression once established. Strict blood pressure control is the mainstay of treatment, with blockade of the renin–angiotensin system. In type 1 diabetes, angiotensin-converting enzyme

Table 2.49 Proteinuria quantification			
	Normal	Microalbuminuria	Persistent albuminuria
Urinary albumin concentration (mg/l)	< 20	20–200	> 200
Albumin : creatinine ratio (ACR) (mg/mmol)			≥ 30 mg/mmol (TPCR ≥ 50 mg/mmol)
Urinary albumin excretion rate (AER) (mg/24 hours)	< 30	30–300	> 300 (TPER > 500)

(ACE) inhibitors reduce progression from microalbumin-uria to overt nephropathy and from overt nephropathy to end-stage kidney disease. In type 2 diabetes, ACE inhibi-tors reduce mortality in those with microalbuminuria, and angiotensin receptor blockers (ARBs) reduce progression

Box 2.59 Diabetic neuropathies

- Chronic symmetrical (distal sensory causing chronic pain, sensorimotor with mild motor weakness, autonomic)
- Acute/reversible (acute painful neuropathy, diabetic amyotrophy, acute focal neuropathy)
- Compression
- Autonomic neuropathy

from microalbuminuria to overt nephropathy and progres-sion thereof. There is no evidence that ARBs reduce mor-tality, however, and so ACE inhibitors remain the first-line treatment for all forms of diabetic nephropathy in types 1 and 2 diabetes, although some favour ARBs in type 2 diabetes. The combination of an ACE inhibitor and ARB may be beneficial in thwarting nephropathy, but large studies are lacking.

What do you know about diabetic neuropathy?

Diabetic neuropathies are summarised in Box 2.59.

Complications of diabetic neuropathy in the foot include ulceration, callus formation, Charcot's joints and wasting.

RENAL AND METABOLIC PROBLEMS

CASE 2.25

ACUTE RENAL FAILURE

Candidate information

Role

You are a doctor in the emergency medical admissions unit. Please read the following letter from the patient's general practitioner. You may make notes on the paper provided. When the bell sounds, enter the examination room to begin the consultation.

Scenario

Dear Doctor

Re: Mr Philip Martin, aged 72 years

Thank you for admitting this gentleman who appears to be oligoanuric. He seems to be developing oedema in his ankles and his blood pressure, usually well controlled, is 190/110 mmHg. His blood tests show a creatinine of 750 µmol/l and a potassium of 6.7 mmol/l. Urinalysis shows a trace of protein but no blood. His creatinine was 130 µmol/l a year ago, at which time he also had a normal renal ultrasound. He has a past medical history of hypertension for which he takes ramipril and bendroflumethiazide, and benign prostatic hypertrophy under surveillance.

Yours sincerely

Please take a history from the patient (you may continue to make notes if you wish on the paper provided). Your examiners will warn you when 12 minutes have elapsed. You have 14 minutes to take a history from the patient followed by 1 minute of reflection. There will then follow 5 minutes of discussion with the examiners. Be prepared to discuss solutions to the problems posed by the case and how you might reply to the GP's letter. You are not required to examine the patient.

Patient information

Mr Philip Martin is a 72-year-old gentleman who for the last two weeks has noticed difficulty passing urine and gradual swelling of his ankles. He now feels uncomfortable suprapubically and has been admitted to hospital. He has a history of hypertension for which he takes ramipril 10 mg and bendroflumethiazide 2.5 mg, both daily. Last year he was investigated for possible prostate cancer, which turned out to be benign. He normally has a little trouble with urinary flow but nothing as problematic as this week. He feels generally weak and lethargic. He put off seeing his doctor because his wife has moderately severe Alzheimer's dementia and there is no one to look after her. He is a very active man who finally decided he must see his doctor because his symptoms had become so severe.

How to approach the case

Data gathering in the interview and interpretation and use of information gathered

Presenting problem(s) and symptom exploration

Most acute renal failure (ARF) is managed by general physicians; it is essential to be able to assess and treat ARF in the first few hours of admission and know when to seek nephrology input. The RIFLE (risk, injury, failure, loss and end-stage) classification of ARF proposed by the Acute Dialysis Quality Initiative (ADQI) Group classifies risk, injury and failure according to serum creatinine ($> 1.5 \times$, $> 2 \times$, $> 3 \times$ baseline respectively) or urine output (<0.5 ml/kg/hour for 6 hours, <0.5 ml/kg/hour for 12 hours, <0.3 ml/kg/hour for 24 hours or oliguria respectively). The principles of assessing and treating a patient in ARF are as follows.

▪ **Ensure safety**   Before full assessment, immediate management of hyperkalaemia (below), hypoxia (usually due to pulmonary oedema) or restoration of circulating volume may be needed.

▪ **Consider the effects of renal failure**   The next step is to consider the effects of renal failure. Three areas should be considered:

* Uraemic symptoms
* Fluid status
* Metabolic status

Uraemic symptoms Patients are usually asymptomatic until advanced stages. The syndrome of uraemia is complex and results from retention of multiple substances, many not yet established. The role of urea in uraemic syndrome is uncertain. Uraemic symptoms should be explored and are listed in Box 2.60.

Fluid status The history is a good guide to fluid status. A history of vomiting and diarrhoea suggests dehydration while shortness of breath or ankle swelling suggests fluid overload. The presence of any oedema suggests that a patient is at least a few litres overloaded. Assessment of fluid status is outlined in Box 2.61. Early chronic kidney disease (CKD) may cause nocturia (attempts to remove

Box 2.60 Uraemic symptoms
• Anorexia, nausea and vomiting
• Cramps and restless legs
• Peripheral neuropathy symptoms
• Cognitive disturbance and drowsiness
• Hiccups
• Itch
• Pericarditis symptoms
• Myoclonus

toxins), tubular dysfunction and sometimes polyuria. Oligoanuria is a late sign in CKD but usual in ARF.

Metabolic status Important renal blood tests (Box 2.62) establish haematobiochemical complications that can be life-threatening or clues to the severity of renal failure and its duration. Renal failure also causes platelet dysfunction, which may respond to synthetic antidiuretic hormone (DDAVP/desmopressin).

■ **Consider if acute or chronic, or acute on chronic and if stable or progressive**   The duration of renal disease, and whether stable or progressive, determines how quickly to investigate. The rate of change of serum creatinine is the best guide. Oliguria usually implies ARF but not all patients with ARF are oliguric. Anaemia suggests chronicity but can have other causes. Small smooth kidneys on ultrasound suggest chronicity.

■ **Consider the causes of renal failure**   Early consideration of causes is essential to identify those that may be reversible. Causes are listed in Box 2.63.

Patient perspective

Explore his concerns about his wife and establish her needs, assuring him that you can make all necessary

arrangements to secure her safety, for example by contacting relatives, the GP or social services.

Past medical history

The history of hypertension probably explains his CKD and obstruction from prostatic enlargement the acute presentation.

Drug and allergy history

The angiotensin-converting enzyme (ACE) inhibitor and bendroflumethiazide are now contributing to the mischief and must be stopped.

Family history

It is always important to ask about hereditary kidney disease, notably polycystic kidney disease, although it is unlikely here.

Social history

Establish more details about the care his wife needs and, if necessary, invoke the help of a social worker.

Discussion

What investigations are important in newly detected renal failure?

Tests aim to determine cause, whether acute or chronic, assess severity and monitor progress and may include:

- Urine sediment analysis (blood and protein = 'active', prompting microscopy for casts)
- Urine protein or protein : creatinine quantification (Table 2.49, Case 2.24)
- 'Renal blood tests' (Box 2.62)
- Autoimmune screen [antinuclear antibodies (ANAs), double stranded DNA, antineutrophil cytoplasmic antibodies (ANCAs), complement components, anti-glomerular basement membrane (GBM) antibodies]
- Paraprotein screen (immunoglobulin levels, serum electrophoresis, urine for light chains/Bence Jones proteins) with low threshold of suspicion
- Uric acid concentration
- Creatine kinase if tissue damage possible (rhabdomyolysis)
- Blood film for microangiopathic haemolytic anaemia
- Hepatitis B virus/hepatitis C virus/human immunodeficiency virus status if renal replacement therapy likely

Box 2.63 Causes of renal failure

Combinations of causes are common. Causes are pre-renal, renal and post-renal.

Pre-renal causes of renal failure

Pre-renal acute renal failure is an appropriate physiological response to:

- Hypovolaemia, e.g. haemorrhage, diarrhoea, vomiting
- Hypotension – cardiogenic shock or distributive shock, e.g. sepsis/the systemic inflammatory response syndrome, anaphylaxis
- Renal hypoperfusion, e.g. non-steroidal anti-inflammatory drugs (NSAIDs), angiotensin-converting enzyme (ACE) inhibitors, angiotensin receptor blockers, renal artery stenosis
- Oedematous states, e.g. cardiac failure, cirrhosis, nephrotic syndrome

The kidneys preserve sodium and water at the expense of reducing the glomerular filtration rate (GFR). Urea clearance is reduced more than creatinine clearance, largely due to the action of antidiuretic hormone (ADH). Pre-renal acute renal failure (ARF) may compound chronic kidney disease (CKD), as in heart failure and renovascular disease, where GFR may fall sharply due to worsening cardiac output or nephrotoxic drugs. Pre-renal ARF is reversible if the cause can be swiftly corrected.

Intrinsic causes of renal failure

The kidney comprises glomeruli, tubules and interstitium, and blood vessels. Disease in any of these can cause renal failure.

Glomerular disease

This may be inflammatory or non-inflammatory:

- Glomerulonephritis (GN) is discussed in Case 2.27. Most causes lead to CKD, but rapidly progressive GN because of vasculitis, systemic lupus erythematosus or Goodpasture's disease may cause ARF.
- Non-inflammatory glomerular disease includes disseminated intravascular coagulation and thrombotic thrombocytopenic purpura.

Tubular injury and interstitial nephritis

These may cause ARF or acute on chronic renal failure. Causes of tubular injury include:

- Ischaemia from prolonged hypoperfusion – acute tubular necrosis (ATN)
- Toxins, e.g. aminoglycosides, herbal remedies, radiological contrast
- Metabolic, e.g. hypercalcaemia, immunoglobulin light chains
- Crystals, e.g. urate, oxalate
- Rhabdomyolysis (crush injury, status epilepticus, drug overdose)

Causes of interstitial nephritis include:

- Drugs, e.g. NSAIDs, antibiotics
- Infiltrative – lymphoma
- Granulomatous – sarcoidois, tuberculosis
- Infection-related – post infective, pyelonephritis

Renovascular disease

This is a leading cause of CKD. Diabetes mellitus and hypertension are the two most common causes of CKD and renovascular disease is very common in people with macrovascular disease at other sites, such as coronary, peripheral and cerebrovascular disease.

- *Macrovascular renal artery disease* (renal artery stenosis) is usually atherosclerotic, and because the juxtaglomerular apparatus perceives low volume it stimulates hyper-reninaemic hyperaldosteronism. Fibromuscular dysplasia is a rare cause of distal, 'sausage string' renal artery stenosis, seen especially in younger females. Some patients experience 'flash floods' of pulmonary oedema. Clinical assessment may detect a renal artery bruit (commonly at the epigastrium) and investigations include MR angiography. Where hyperaldosteronism is refractory to medical therapy, angioplasty, stents, artery bypass or nephrectomy may be necessary.
- *Microvascular renovascular disease* may be atherosclerotic or embolic. The cause of chronic renal dysfunction in atherosclerotic renovascular disease (ARVD) is usually long-standing intra-renal vascular disease and parenchymal injury rather than reversible ischaemia, reflected in the variability in renal function outcome after revascularisation for renal artery stenosis. Thrombolysis, anticoagulants or invasive procedures shearing endothelial plaques occasionally trigger embolic showers which scatter through the renovascular system. Episodes of cholesterol emboli may be associated with eosinophilia. Occasionally a large renal embolism may result from infective endocarditis or cardiac thrombus.
- *Renal infarction* may be asymptomatic or induce loin pain with or without haematuria. A high serum lactate is a strong clue.
- The kidney may be involved in *systemic vasculitides*.
- *Renal artery dissection* can cause back pain.
- *Renal vein thrombosis* may occasionally complicate malignancy or nephrotic syndrome.

Whilst renal failure promotes hypertension, chronic inadequately controlled hypertension causes *nephrosclerosis*, which may prompt or accelerate CKD.

Post-renal causes of renal failure

Obstructive (urological) causes include:

- Prostatic hypertrophy
- Stones
- Transitional cell carcinoma of the bladder obstructing the ureters
- Ovarian and other pelvic masses obstructing the ureters
- Urethral strictures
- Retroperitoneal and radiation fibrosis

- Chest X-ray
- ECG
- Renal ultrasound

What do you understand by the term acute tubular necrosis or injury (ATN or ATI)?

ATN (injury rather than necrosis reflects potential reversibility) refers to ischaemic tubular damage that is a consequence of pre-renal ARF. Various mechanisms play a role, including intense renal vasoconstriction, formation of tubular casts and reperfusion injury.

How may pre-renal ARF be distinguished from established ATN or oliguric ARF?

In pre-renal ARF, the tubules can reabsorb and thus concentrate urine. In ATN, the tubules are damaged and 'everything leaks out' (Table 2.50). However, pre-renal ARF often leads to ATN and results become indeterminate. Diuretics also mislead by increasing urinary sodium excretion. Fractional excretion of urea, which is given by [(urine urea/plasma urea) / (urine creatinine/plasma creatinine) × 100%] is less affected by diuretics; values < 35% suggest pre-renal ARF.

Table 2.50 Features that distinguish pre-renal acute renal failure (ARF) from acute tubular necrosis (ATN)

	Pre-renal ARF	ATN
Urine osmolality	Increased (> 500 mosm/kg)	Decreased (< 350 mosm/kg)
Urine sodium	Low (< 20 mmol/l)	Normal/high (> 40 mmol/l)
Urine concentration	Normal	Dilute

Box 2.64 Management of the acute uraemic emergency

The facts of greatest importance are the urine output and serum creatinine (which has an approximate inverse relationship to urine output in the steady state).

1. Treat the effects

Both rate of deterioration and severity are proportional to the urgency of this response. Urgent attention may be needed for:

- Serum potassium
- Fluid status
- Encephalopathy
- Anaemia

Hyperkalaemia is discussed below. Volume status must be optimised urgently. Dopamine is of no value. A central venous line is seldom needed. A patient with hypotension, postural hypotension, decreased skin turgor and dry mucous membranes will be dry. A dry patient may develop acute tubular necrosis and need dialysis. The most important principle is to put fluid in and 'fill up the bath', and if too much is put in it can be removed and the 'plug pulled' with frusemide. Frusemide should otherwise be avoided. A patient with a raised jugular venous pulse and oedema will be overloaded.

2. Establish the cause

This depends on the setting, which may be expected as in septic shock or heart failure, or unexpected. Urinalysis for an active sediment with blood is an essential first step in considering vasculitis. An urgent renal ultrasound helps to distinguish between three possibilities:

- Obstruction, in which hydronephrosis is invariably present, with a normal ultrasound in < 2% of cases. Urological and sometimes oncological referral is needed.
- CKD with small smooth kidneys.
- Normal kidney appearances, indicating acute intrinsic renal failure. This is a situation where a normal result indicates an emergency, and immediate nephrology referral for consideration of a biopsy, especially if there is an active urinary sediment. Large kidneys occasionally result from infiltrative causes or renal vein thrombosis.

3. Establish reversibility

If this is not clear, a nephrologist should be consulted. Errors in managing an acute uraemic emergency include failure to identify the cause, delayed referral if renal function is deteriorating and fiddling with irrelevant issues such as watching urine output without acting.

What are the management principles in an acute uraemic emergency?

These are outlined in Box 2.64.

Obstruction is a common cause of ARF, typically in older men with prostatic disease. A bladder is often palpable but chronic retention is usually painless and patients still pass urine – obstruction may be unilateral or there may be a battle between antegrade and retrograde flow before the battle is lost. Chronic obstruction exerts abnormal pressure on tubules and impairs tubular function and this can lead to increased urine output as sodium and water reabsorption is impaired. Significant diuresis may follow relief of obstruction, requiring large volume fluid replacement.

How would you manage a patient with renal and heart failure who has pulmonary oedema but is hypotensive?

Cardiorenal failure is extremely common, with hypotension from left ventricular failure with or without pulmonary oedema, and renal failure from low cardiac output and often renovascular disease. Such patients are fluid overloaded, but the notion of being 'wet but intravascularly dry' is frequently mooted. Treatment of the situation depends upon the goal. To improve breathing, the patient will need to be dry, aided by loop diuretics, and if creatinine rises from, say, 150 to 210, then that is of course perfectly acceptable. But without respiratory symptoms of overload, adequate fluid replacement to maintain acceptable renal function is preferred. What is absolutely illogical and should not be instituted in combination is fluid replacement and diuretics. Occasionally, pure cor pulmonale without left ventricular failure is the cause. There is no evidence in this situation for augmenting treatment with ACE inhibitors when the position has stabilised.

What are the indications for urgent haemodialysis?

The indications for urgent haemodialysis via a temporary central venous catheter are given in Box 2.65.

When should an urgent renal biopsy be considered?

It should be considered in patients with normal-sized, unobstructed kidneys where ATN causing ARF does not seem likely, and without delay in patients in whom rapidly progressive glomerulonephritis due to vasculitis seems likely.

What do you understand by the term glomerular filtration rate (GFR)?

The glomerulus is a filter producing a cell-free and protein-free ultrafiltrate of plasma which enters the tubule. GFR is determined by the driving force of hydrostatic pressure from the heart and counteractive forces including Bowman's space hydrostatic pressure, oncotic pressures, filter permeability and surface area. GFR is greatly reduced in

Box 2.65 Indications for acute haemodialysis

- Pulmonary oedema in an anuric patient
- Life-threatening hyperkalaemia
- Symptomatic uraemia, e.g. nausea, drowsiness
- Serositis (now rare), e.g. pericarditis, pericardial rub, pleuritis
- Severe acidosis (e.g. bicarbonate < 12 mmol/l) if unwell or an additional indication is present

inflammatory glomerular disease. Normal GFR is around 125 ml/min (around 150–180 l of ultrafiltrate daily), most of which is reabsorbed by the tubules. GFR is tightly autoregulated by constriction or dilatation of the afferent or efferent arterioles in response to changes in renal artery perfusion. Measuring GFR is unhelpful in ARF because of rapidly changing function.

What do the renal tubules do?

Glomerular filtration and tubular transport (Case 2.31) are the two sequential mechanisms underlying renal function. Renal clearance of a substance refers to its net handling and is the sum of urine concentration × urine flow rate/plasma concentration (ml/min). Most reabsorptive processes occur in the proximal tubule and loop of Henle; the distal tubule and collecting duct are important in determining final urinary excretion of water and solutes. Most tubular transport processes are directly or indirectly coupled to reabsorption of sodium ions. Na^+ ions leave the lumen and passively cross the apical surface of the tubular cell down a concentration or electrochemical gradient via Na^+ channels or transporters and exit across the basolateral membrane via a Na^+/K^+-ATPase pump (ultimately required for most reabsorptive and secretory processes).

How is serum potassium concentration regulated and what are the causes of hypokalaemia and hyperkalaemia? (Table 2.51)

Acute changes in potassium concentration are usually the result of redistribution between the extracellular fluid (ECF) and intracellular fluid (ICF). Alkalosis, catecholamines (potassium is often slightly low in patients due to the stress response, which increases sympathetic drive and releases glucocorticoids and mineralocorticoids, e.g. after an acute coronary syndrome) and insulin and β_2-agonists tend to redistribute potassium ions into cells. The hypokalaemic and hyperkalaemic periodic paralyses are the result of redistribution abnormalities. Rapid cell growth (e.g. in the treatment of megaloblastic anaemia) may also cause shift of potassium ions into cells. Chronic regulation of

Table 2.51 Causes of hypokalaemia and hyperkalaemia					
Hypokalaemia			**Hyperkalaemia**		
Redistribution	Alkalosis Catecholamines Insulin β_2-agonists Periodic paralyses Rapid cell growth		**Redistribution or spurious**	Haemolysed sample Sample stored on ice Fist clenching Hyperventilation Inorganic acids Diabetic ketoacidosis Lactic acidosis Hyperkalaemic periodic paralysis Cell lysis, e.g. rhabdomyolysis, haemolysis, tumour lysis, chemotherapy	
Total body potassium depletion	Decreased intake, e.g. anorexia		**Total body potassium excess**	Increased intake, e.g. bananas, oranges	
	Increased loss	Gastrointestinal: urine K^+ < 20 mmol/day; Renal: urine K^+ > 20 mmol/day		Retention in renal failure	
Aldosterone role	Hyperaldosteronism with hypertension, fluid overload and urine K^+ > 20 mmol/day.	Primary, e.g. Conn's syndrome, Cushing's syndrome Secondary, e.g. renal artery stenosis, genetic syndrome of tubular dysfunction – pseudohyperaldosteronism (Liddle), glucocorticoid remediable hyperaldosteronism, apparent mineralocorticoid excess (Case 2.14)	**Aldosterone role**	Aldosterone deficiency e.g. Addison's disease (hyper-reninaemic hypoaldosteronism)	
	Aldosterone not primarily involved, with normotension and urine K^+ < 20 mmol/day	Acidosis (plasma bicarbonate low) e.g. types 1 or 2 renal tubular acidosis Alkalosis (plasma bicarbonate high) e.g. diuretics, Bartter's syndrome, Gitelman's syndrome, hypomagnesaemia		Aldosterone resistance: congenital, e.g. pseudohypoaldosteronsism; acquired, e.g. ACE inhibitors, potassium sparing diuretics (spironolactone, amiloride), renal tubular acidosis (SLE, amyloid, diabetes mellitus, obstructive uropathy)	

potassium concentration is undertaken by the kidney, in the distal tubule. Potassium disorders may be evaluated with three questions:

- Is redistribution likely?
- Is the kidney involved in the pathogenesis (by measurement of urinary potassium)?
- If the kidney is involved, what is the role of aldosterone?

How would you treat hypokalaemia?

Treatment depends upon duration. Chronic hypokalaemia may be associated with a total body potassium deficit > 100 mmol, which should be replaced orally. Intravenous potassium should not exceed 20 mmol/hour. If there is concurrent metabolic acidosis, then hypokalaemia should be treated first.

What level of serum potassium is life threatening?

There is no absolute level. Rate of change is more important, and chronic rises are better tolerated such that extreme levels up to 8 or 9 mmol/l are sometimes seen (although these should still be treated urgently). Fasting lowers insulin levels and may exacerbate hyperkalaemia in chronic kidney disease. Cardiac arrest is rare under 7 mmol/l but 6.5 mmol/l is dangerous and a level > 6 mmol/l warrants close consideration of treatment.

How would you treat hyperkalaemia?

- Calcium (calcium gluconate) is administered intravenously if there are ECG changes. This promotes intracellular shift of potassium and is cardioprotective. Tented T waves are usually not life threatening but may progress to immediately life-threatening broadening of QRS complexes and T-wave disappearance and a bizarre ECG. Calcium should be administered immediately with an immediate venous blood gas to urgently estimate serum potassium.
- Dextrose and insulin (50 mmol 50% dextrose with 10 units of actrapid intravenously over 15–30 minutes) shifts potassium intravenously and should also be given with or without ECG changes.
- Salbutamol 10–20 mg by nebuliser acts similarly but causes tachycardia and agitation and may not be necessary if intravenous treatment can be established quickly.
- Bicarbonate may help and is popular in some renal units, but evidence is weak.
- These measures are temporary, causing potassium shift but have no effect on total body potassium and levels can swing upwards again within a few hours. Definitive lowering of potassium requires a diuresis (fluid resuscitation if dehydrated, frusemide if fluid overload) but if oligoanuria persists then haemodialysis may be needed.

- Calcium resonium 1 g t.d.s. orally may sustain safe levels but evidence is weak. This is more likely where there is tissue damage (e.g. rhabdomyolysis) sustaining the problem.
- Stopping exacerbating drugs (e.g. ACE inhibitors, sprionolactone, angiotensin receptor blockers) and a low potassium diet are essential.

CASE 2.26

CHRONIC KIDNEY DISEASE AND RENAL REPLACEMENT THERAPY

Candidate information

Role

You are a doctor in the medical outpatient clinic. Please read the following letter from the patient's general practitioner. You may make notes on the paper provided. When the bell sounds, enter the examination room to begin the consultation.

Scenario

> Dear Doctor
>
> Re: Mrs May Russell, aged 68 years
>
> Thank you for seeing this lady whose creatinine is 175 µmol/l, haemoglobin 9.9 g/dl, albumin 32 and estimated glomerular filtration rate 24. She is otherwise well but her creatinine was 125 µmol/l 12 months ago and I wonder if she now merits a renal opinion. Her blood pressure is 160/92 mmHg and her total cholesterol is 5 mmol/l. Her myeloma screen is negative. She has proteinuria ++ but no blood, glucose or nitrites on urinalysis.
>
> Yours sincerely

Please take a history from the patient (you may continue to make notes if you wish on the paper provided). Your examiners will warn you when 12 minutes have elapsed. You have 14 minutes to take a history from the patient followed by 1 minute of reflection. There will then follow 5 minutes of discussion with the examiners. Be prepared to discuss solutions to the problems posed by the case and how you might reply to the GP's letter. You are not required to examine the patient.

Patient information

Mrs May Russell is a 68-year-old lady with chronic kidney disease (CKD). She feels well but has been referred to the hospital for an opinion as to whether further investigations are needed because her kidney function has deteriorated moderately since a year ago. Her past medical history comprises hypertension, angina and a possible transient ischaemic attack; she recently had an episode of transient loss of vision in one eye but did not mention this to her GP. She does not have diabetes. Her medications are aspirin 75 mg, simvastatin 20 mg, perindopril 4 mg and atenolol 50 mg, all daily. She also takes non-prescription ibuprofen for back pain, a problem she has had for 30 years since a road-traffic accident. She smokes 10 cigarettes per day. She is very afraid of ending up on 'dialysis' since her husband died of advanced kidney failure due to prostate disease.

How to approach the case

Data gathering in the interview and interpretation and use of information gathered

Presenting problem(s) and symptom exploration

A similar approach to considering causes to Case 2.25 should be taken.

Patient perspective

Harness her strong desire to avoid dialysis by emphasising the significant benefits of stopping smoking and explain that there are things you can do to modify her risk, including optimising her blood pressure and serum cholesterol.

Past medical history

The history of hypertension and cardiovascular disease imply likely renovascular disease.

Drug and allergy history

The angiotensin-converting enzyme (ACE) inhibitor can continue but an alternative to non-steroidal anti-inflammatory drugs (NSAIDs) should be sought.

Family history

Relevance here is unlikely.

Social history

She should stop smoking because this contributes to her coronary disease, likely renovascular disease and possible carotid atheroma.

SUMMARY – ASSESSMENT AND PLAN

- The cause of her CKD is likely to be vascular, particularly with isolated proteinuria, but the situation warrants a screen of blood tests and renal tract ultrasound.
- The drugs, including the ACE inhibitor, should continue, the simvastatin should be increased to its optimal dose of 40 mg and her hypertension control should be optimised with the addition of, for example, a calcium channel blocker.
- Further investigation for possible amaurosis fugax includes a carotid Doppler study and possibly ambulatory ECG monitoring.

Discussion

How is chronic kidney disease (CKD) classified and how does the classification aid management?

CKD (term replaces chronic renal failure) is classified by the US National Kidney Foundation (NKF), now adopted across the UK and Europe, as shown in Table 2.52. It is stratified by glomerular filtration rate (GFR), and the importance of albumin as a marker of kidney damage is emphasised, the latter being easily detected and quantified by the albumin : creatinine ratio in a spot urine specimen, or a total protein (mg/l) : creatinine (mmol/l) ratio (TPCR) in mg/mmol in more substantial proteinuria, these tests more accurate than 24-hour collections for protein (Table 2.49, Case 2.24). Stratifying CKD helps to identify patients in whom metabolic complications are likely to arise (stage 3) and so guides preparation of dialysis and transplantation. Patients should not be allowed to 'crash land' to haemodialysis; late referral is associated with a poorer outcome (central-line complications, sepsis, etc.) and higher cost.

Why is early detection of CKD important?

Renal disease is often progressive once GFR falls below 25% of normal. The haemodynamic changes (including angiotensin II activity), which sustain renal function initially in surviving nephrons, are ultimately detrimental. People at high risk should be evaluated for markers of CKD (albuminuria, abnormal urine sediment, elevated serum creatinine, decreased GFR) because of the potential to modify disease progression and because of the accelerated cardiovascular disease (CVD) associated with CKD.

What are the commonest causes of CKD?

These are diabetes (50% in the USA) and hypertension (27% in the USA). Glomerulonephritis is a relatively small group (13%).

How is GFR derived?

Isotope measurement of GFR is the gold standard measurement of renal function. Since measuring it is cumbersome, GFR is estimated by creatinine clearance, a correlate of GFR determined by either the Modification of Diet in Renal Disease (MDRD) or the Cockroft–Gault formula.

$$\text{Cr clearance} = [186 \times \text{creatinine (ml/min/1.73 m}^2)] / [88.4 - (1.154 \times \text{age})] \text{ (for male)}$$

$$\text{Cr clearance} = [186 \times \text{creatinine (ml/min/1.73 m}^2)] / [88.4 - (0.742 \times \text{age})] \text{ (for female)}$$

Estimated GFR (eGFR) is now calculated on all samples sent for creatinine measurement; information can also be obtained at www.renal.org.

Why is GFR a better marker of renal function than serum creatinine?

The kidneys have enormous reserve. Mildly elevated creatinine may imply that three-quarters of functioning renal

Table 2.52 Classification and management of chronic kidney disease (CKD)

Stage	GFR ml/min/1.73 m²	Description	Monitoring	Referral to nephrologist	Management
	As a general rule, estimated GFR (eGFR) is a measure of percentage of overall kidney function				
1	≥ 90	Kidney damage with normal or ↑ GFR	12-monthly	Generally managed in primary care Referral if: Proteinuria Microscopic/macroscopic haematuria (urologist if older, nephrologists if younger) Multisystem disease suspected, e.g. systemic lupus erythematosus Family history, e.g. polycystic kidney disease Uncontrolled hypertension GFR declining rapidly	Diagnosis Renoprotection (usually modification of CVD risk factors) Identification of comorbidity Monitoring for progression
2	60–89	Kidney damage with mild ↓ GFR	12-monthly	As for stage 1	As for stage 1
3 (approximately 4% of the population)	30–59	Moderate ↓ GFR	6-monthly	Referral if: Any of the conditions for Stage 1 or 2 above are met eGFR falls by at least 10% per year Anaemia Metabolic disturbance (calcium, phosphate, potassium)	Evaluation and treatment of CKD complications Anaemia correction Calcium and phosphate disturbance correction
4	15–29	Severe ↓ GFR	3-monthly	Urgent referral, especially if any of the conditions for Stage 3 are met, diabetes present, eGFR is falling rapidly or there are metabolic disturbances inclusive of a low bicarbonate or a raised parathyroid hormone (PTH) level	Preparation for renal replacement therapy (RRT) – likely to be needed in 6–8 months Diet assessment Immunisation – influenza, pneumococcus, hepatitis Correction of acidosis with bicarbonate (contentious) Stop metformin if on it
5	< 15 or dialysis	Established renal failure	3-monthly	Immediate	Renal replacement therapy
Notes		Established renal failure replaces the term end-stage renal disease	Also monitor people at high risk of CKD: Obstructive kidney disease Diabetes Hypertension Cardiovascular disease Heart failure Nephrotoxic drugs, e.g. NSAIDs, ACE inhibitors, ARBs, diuretics Multisystem disease	Refer with normal GFR if: Malignant hypertension Hyperkalaemia Proteinuria with oedema/hypoalbuminaemia Abnormal urine sediment, e.g. microscopic haematuria without a urological cause	

235

tissue is lost. Because of the reciprocal relationship between GFR and creatinine concentration, a small GFR change close to the normal range will have much less effect on creatinine than a small change when the GFR is markedly reduced. Further, changes in creatinine lag behind changes in GFR. Serum creatinine alone is a poor indicator of the degree of renal failure because it is influenced by muscle mass, age, sex, weight, diet and drugs. An elderly patient with a small body mass index and creatinine of 300 might have uraemic symptoms while a young muscular patient with a creatinine of 1000 might not. Creatinine may also exhibit a modest decrease because of haemodilution in rapid fluid resuscitation and increase with trimethoprim.

How may acute renal failure (ARF) be distinguished from CKD?

History and knowledge of previous blood test results are most valuable. Hypocalcaemia suggests renal osteodystrophy (CKD) and anaemia may be the result of erythropoietin deficiency. On ultrasonography, small kidneys, thinning of cortices and increased echogenicity favour a diagnosis of CKD.

What strategies can slow the rate of progression of CKD?

Factors causing progressive decline in renal function and strategies to slow progression are outlined in Table 2.53.

How should hypertension be managed in CKD?

The British Hypertension Society Guidelines are very much applicable (Case 2.14), but with a tendency towards angiotensin blockade treatment strategies. In CKD stages 3 and 4 there is good evidence for slowing the rate of progression of renal disease and reducing cardiovascular morbidity and mortality, and evidence suggests reducing blood pressure to less than 130/80. In CKD stage 5, evidence of benefit is more controversial, and the aim is usually to reduce cardiovascular morbidity and mortality, several studies showing worse outcomes in patients with low blood pressure. In renal transplant recipients additional factors need to be considered such as corticosteroid and calcineurin sparing to reduce hypertension, and blood pressure lowering as in CKD stages 3–4 reduces cardiovascular morbidity and mortality and prolongs graft survival.

What is the rationale for using ACE inhibitors or angiotensin II receptor blockers (ARBs) in diabetic nephropathy?

The strong rationale is discussed in Case 2.23.

What is the rationale for using ACE inhibitors or ARBs in non-diabetic nephropathy?

ACE inhibitors slow the progression of non-diabetic nephropathy. In the Ramipril Efficacy in Nephropathy (REIN) studies, ramipril was so effective in slowing the rate of GFR decline in patients with nephrotic-range proteinuria that the trial was stopped early; in patients with

Table 2.53 Strategies to slow progression of CKD	
Factors causing progressive decline in renal function	**Strategies to slow progression**
Persistent activity of underlying cause	Treat cause
Hypertension	Meticulous blood pressure control – the most important intervention to slow progression < 130/80 mmHg (< 125/75 mmHg if proteinuria or diabetes) ACE inhibitor or angiotensin receptor blocker (in diabetes use even if normotensive) (Aspirin also advocated in CKD if 10-year risk of CVD ≥ 10%)
Persistent proteinuria, the best predictor of decline (unusual without hypertension, and the threshold for defining hypertension may be different in proteinuria)	ACE inhibitor or angiotensin receptor blocker
Poor glycaemic control	Meticulous glycaemic control
Dyslipidaemia	Lipid lowering (TC < 4.0 mmol/l, LDL < 2.0 mmol/l)
Smoking	Smoking cessation
High phosphate or protein diet	But maintain good nutrition and avoid low-protein diet because malnourishment leads to a poorer outcome with dialysis
Hyperphosphataemia	Phosphate binders
Anaemia (may cause high cardiac output and left ventricular hypertrophy)	Erythropoietin
ACE, angiotensin-converting enzyme; LDL, low-density lipoprotein; TC, total cholesterol.	

1–3 g/day of proteinuria the median time to established renal failure almost doubled, benefit seen across a wide range of initial GFRs. A meta-analysis by Jafar et al. confirmed the benefit and the COOPERATE trial showed that combination of ACE inhibitors and ARBs safely slows the progression of non-diabetic nephropathy.

How do ACE inhibitors and ARBs delay progression of CKD?

In CKD perfusion of the glomerulus is often maintained by angiotensin II (AII)-mediated efferent arteriole vasoconstriction. Whilst this is immediately beneficial, it is ultimately destructive as it raises pressure in the glomerulus and predisposes to glomerular sclerosis. Decreasing AII-mediated vasoconstriction with ACE inhibitors or ARBs lowers glomerular pressure and is ultimately beneficial but does cause a reversible rise in serum creatinine or fall in GFR.

Why might ACE inhibitors or ARBs be dangerous in renal artery stenosis (RAS)? (Fig. 2.10)

Numerous molecules act on the afferent and efferent arterioles in the kidney to maintain GFR. Angiotensin II is activated by reduction in renal artery perfusion pressure. This occurs in situations that would cause pre-renal renal failure (hypovolaemia, left ventricular failure, sepsis), which lead to a fall in glomerular hydrostatic pressure, a fall in GFR and in renin release from the juxtaglomerular apparatus. Angiotensin II promotes aldosterone action and promotes systemic vasoconstriction and renal vasoconstriction (the efferent arteriole is particularly affected and constricts to maintain intraglomerular pressure).

ACE inhibitors and ARBs cause afferent and efferent arteriole vasodilatation. In renal artery stenosis, the affer-

ent arteriole cannot effectively dilate but the efferent arteriole can. Blood then effectively bypasses the glomerulus.

However, decreased GFR or elevated creatinine do not necessarily occur, even with bilateral renal artery stenosis, and decreased GFR or elevated creatinine often occur with ACE inhibitors in people without RAS. In any low blood pressure state, GFR becomes angiotensin-II-dependent and thus ACE-inhibitor-sensitive (RAS a perceived low volume state where blood pressure is usually high), ACE inhibitors removing the partially protective effect of angiotensin-II-mediated efferent arteriolar vasoconstriction.

Furthermore, in CKD of any cause there is an overall drop in GFR because of nephron loss triggering angiotensin-mediated compensatory increased GFR in surviving nephrons; this increase in GFR seldom exceeds 30%.

Should ACE inhibitors or ARBs be stopped if serum creatinine rises?

Given the above, in CKD creatinine may rise by up to 30% on these treatments but if it subsequently plateaus and serum potassium is within safe limits then ACE inhibitors and ARBs should be continued with close monitoring.

What are the problems with anaemia in CKD?

It causes angina, decreased exercise tolerance or fatigue and cognitive disturbance. High cardiac output and left ventricular hypertrophy are potential complications and anaemia may be independently associated with increased CVD in CKD.

How is anaemia in CKD managed?

Folate or vitamin B12 abnormalities should be excluded. If the degree of anaemia is proportional to the degree of CKD and is not microcytic, ferritin levels are normal and there are no features of blood loss, seeking a gastrointestinal source of bleeding is unlikely to be necessary. Treatments for anaemia in CKD include iron, recombinant human erythropoietin (EPO) and erythropoietin-stimulating agents. Intravenous iron (Venofer) 200 mg twice or thrice weekly may be considered if ferritin is < 150 g/dl and haemoglobin (Hb) < 12 g/dl. If iron is replete, EPO is considered. The threshold varies, the aim being to maintain Hb at a level at which patients are unimpeded in their daily activities but below that which may result in excessive thrombotic risk. The NKF recommends evaluation of anaemia if Hb is < 11 g/dl and consideration of EPO to maintain Hb > 11 g/dl; some renal physicians use a threshold of 10 g/dl. Red cell aplasia is a recognised side effect of EPO caused by anti-EPO antibodies. Treatment can be administered as Neorecorom 20 iu/kg thrice weekly via a prefilled syringe, Eprex or Aranesp (darbepoetin-α) once weekly. Doses may be titrated monthly. Hypertension is a side effect of EPO. Resistance to EPO-stimulating agents may occur in hyperparathyroidism, haematinic deficiency, infection, malignancy or with ACE inhibitors.

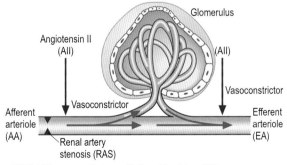

- ACE inhibitors normally cause dilation of the AA and EA
- In RAS, the AA cannot (functionally*) dilate but the EA can; blood preferentially bypasses the glomerulus
- * the obstruction is really in the trunk artery but the effect is the same – the ratio of supply to EA run off is reduced and the glomeruli are deprived of blood

Fig. 2.10 Why angiotensin-converting enzyme (ACE) inhibitors are contraindicated in renal artery stenosis (RAS).

What do you understand by renal osteodystrophy?

CKD is associated with various types of bone disease, collectively known as renal osteodystrophy.

Secondary hyperparathyoidism

In early CKD a slightly raised phosphate (retention) is associated with mild hypocalcaemia. Decreased 1,25-dihydroxycholecalciferol (calcitriol) production by the kidney leads to reduced gut calcium and phosphate absorption and secondary hyperparathyroidism, which normalises serum calcium but increases phosphate. Alkaline phosphatase may be raised. Osteitis fibrosa cystica refers to the effect of secondary hyperparathyroidism on trabecular bone, with accelerated turnover and fibrosis of marrow; excessive osteoblast and osteoclast activity is driven by parathyroid hormone (PTH) and cytokines, in severe cases the latter causing bone cysts. Radiological correlates of hyperparathyroidism are osteopenia and areas of sclerosis ('rugger jersey spine', 'pepper-pot skull') and subperiosteal erosions (starting in the phalanges).

Tertiary hyperparathyoidism

As CKD progresses, insensitivity of the parathyroids to calcium and skeletal resistance to PTH worsen the situation, ultimately with parathyroid hyperplasia and autonomous PTH secretion – tertiary hyperparathyroidism – provoking hypercalcaemia.

Osteomalacia

Osteomalacia (reduced bone mineralisation) is more readily induced by hypophosphataemia, hypocalcaemia, chronic acidosis and aluminium toxicity.

Mixed renal osteodystrophy

This refers to the combination of increased osteoid (due to hyperparathyroidism) and reduced mineralisation (due to osteomalacia).

Adynamic bone disease

This is characterised by reduced trabecular bone formation and resorption, with thinned trabeculae.

Other skeletal problems in kidney disease include osteoporosis (especially post-transplantation), dialysis associated amyloid and metastatic calcification.

When does renal osteodystrophy occur?

Renal osteodystrophy can start early in CKD (stage 2), and is common in stage 3.

How are mineral disturbances corrected?

Hyperphosphataemia is generally corrected first of all, and agents include aluminium hydroxide, calcium carbonate, calcium acetate and lanthanum carbonate. Aluminium toxicity is generally of lesser concern in older people but calcium-based phosphate binders are traditionally first choice, e.g. calcium carbonate or calcium acetate two tablets thrice daily. Concerns about increasing the calcium phosphate product (below), however, have led to the increasing use of lanthanum carbonate and sevelamer.

Vitamin D levels are seldom measured, and vitamin D replacement in the form of alfacalcidol tends to be given after phosphate correction if PTH levels, measured six-monthly, are raised. If vitamin D does not correct PTH levels then parathyroidectomy may need to be considered.

These measures are generally instituted in stages 3 or 4 CKD.

Why is CKD associated with accelerated CVD?

CVD is the main cause of death in CKD. Traditional risk factors are common but do not explain an independent very substantial increased risk. Possible mechanisms for increased vascular calcification and CVD risk include hyperphosphataemia and increased calcium-phosphate product (Ca-PP) with a high calcium intake. Hyperphosphataemia is associated with increased death rates in dialysis patients. Vascular smooth muscle cells exposed to high phosphate enhance osteoblast gene expression. Arteriosclerosis and calcification increase pulse wave velocity and left ventricular hypertrophy with reduced coronary flow in diastole. Concerns about hyperphosphataemia and a high calcium intake leading to cardiovascular calcification have prompted a shift from traditional management of secondary hyperparathyroidism in CKD and a move away from calcium-based phosphate binders. Calcitriol (dihydroxycholecalciferol) can elevate the serum Ca-PP by increasing gut calcium and phosphate absorption; calcimimetic agents that are vitamin D analogues that reduce PTH release by direct action on calcium-sensing receptors in the parathyroid glands may provide future, less calcaemic and less phosphataemic alternatives to calcitriol. Calcium citrate augments aluminium absorption and is contraindicated.

Is lipid-lowering therapy beneficial in CKD?

Renal functional decline was significantly higher in patients with dyslipidaemia in the Physician's Health Study. In those with normal renal function in the Helsinki Heart study, lowering elevated cholesterol slowed progression. The ALERT study showed a reduction in proteinuria and progression with lipid-lowering therapy, predominantly statin therapy, in renal transplant recipients. Currently lipids are treated as per JBS targets but further evidence for lipid-lowering therapy with statins and ezetimibe in CKD will emerge from the Study of Heart and Renal Protection (SHARP) trial.

Why is dialysis use increasing?

There is large variation in dialysis prevalence between countries, even across Europe. Dialysis is increasing as a mode of treatment because of an ageing population (now being considered for people in their 80s and 90s) and a result of strategies designed to slow progression of CKD also tending to treat CVD, leading to improved survival from CVD. The context to this is also an increase in diseases that cause CKD, notably diabetes.

What forms of dialysis are there?

There are haemodialysis and peritoneal dialysis.

What are the forms of vascular access?

A temporary double-lumen catheter may be inserted into the internal jugular or subclavian vein (the femoral vein is acceptable in an emergency but is suboptimal). Permanent haemodialysis requires an arteriovenous fistula (AVF) or gortex graft. An AVF is an anastomosis created surgically between an artery and vein, commonly at the forearm, which dilates over a number of weeks to become suitable for twin-needled dialysis access. By convention, the 'out' line is termed the 'A' line and the 'in' line the 'V' line. The needles point in opposite directions to minimise mixing of outgoing and incoming blood and hence the dialysing of freshly dialysed incoming blood.

Discuss the principles of haemodialysis (Fig. 2.11)

From the point of vascular access, blood leaves the body and runs to a pump and thence to the dialyser ('artificial kidney'). The pump is designed not to crush blood cells. In the dialyser, blood enters thousands of semi-permeable microtubules, not dissimilar in diameter to a capillary. Between these microtubules and running in the opposite direction is *dialysis fluid*, against which the blood is dia-lysed. Dialysis fluid contains concentrations of substances such that an osmotic or ionic gradient is set up from blood to dialysis fluid. Since most patients with CKD are acidotic, dialysis fluid is alkaline and contains bicarbonate, thus allowing correction of acidosis in the blood. However, it is desirable to avoid large ionic shifts. Equally, dialysis fluid contains a low concentration of potassium (1–2 mmol/l) to draw potassium from the blood and usually a low concentration of calcium. Sodium and glucose concentrations are usually normal. Dialysed blood returns to the body via a separate lumen. The *dialysate* is discarded. The transmembrane pressure gradient from blood to dialysis fluid is proportional to the rate and force of the pump. Adjusting the pump settings determines the amount of fluid removed at dialysis. The net amount of fluid removed is called the *ultrafiltrate*. Sometimes, patients are fluid overloaded but metabolically stable. In such cases, pure ultrafiltration, rather than dialysis, is indicated. Adjunctive treatments for dialysis patients are as for any patient with CKD.

What complications of haemodialysis may occur?

These include access problems, sepsis, haemodynamic instability and β_2-microglobulin accumulation. β_2-microglobulin is a non-dialysed molecule which, over many years, forms amyloid deposits in musculoskeletal tissues.

When should dialysis be started?

Improved modification of progression of CKD has made predicting the time for dialysis more challenging. Clinical pointers such as appetite, nutrition and cognition are often more helpful than numerical parameters.

When might dialysis be considered inappropriate?

The main reason is when patients are dying with, rather than because of, renal failure. Evidence suggests that over the age of 75 years with comorbidity, dialysis is of more questionable mortality benefit. Dialysis is not a true form of renal replacement; typically it might improve GFR from 5% to 12%, and thus maintains a state of chronic ill health.

CASE 2.27

GLOMERULONEPHRITIS

Candidate information

Role

You are a doctor in the medical outpatient clinic. Please read the following letter from the patient's general practitioner. You may make notes on the paper provided. When the bell sounds, enter the examination room to begin the consultation.

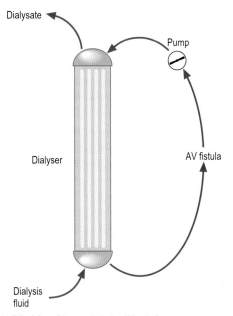

Fig. 2.11 Principles of haemodialysis. AV, arteriovenous.

Scenario

Dear Doctor

Re: Mr Sam Spider, aged 48 years

Thank you for seeing Mr Spider who has had three episodes of painless macroscopic haematuria recently. His creatinine is mildly elevated at 135 μmol/l and urinalysis continues to show a trace of blood and protein. Otherwise he is a well gentleman. I would value your advice on further investigation.

Yours sincerely

Please take a history from the patient (you may continue to make notes if you wish on the paper provided). Your examiners will warn you when 12 minutes have elapsed. You have 14 minutes to take a history from the patient followed by 1 minute of reflection. There will then follow 5 minutes of discussion with the examiners. Be prepared to discuss solutions to the problems posed by the case and how you might reply to the GP's letter. You are not required to examine the patient.

Patient information

Mr Sam Spider is a 48-year-old long-haul airline pilot. In the last three months he has had three episodes of macroscopic haematuria. On the first occasion he had a mild, concurrent sore throat. All episodes have been without loin or abdominal pain. His GP told him that his blood pressure was very slightly high and that his kidney blood test was slightly raised. He has no other past medical history. He is divorced, does not smoke, drinks occasional alcohol and enjoys keeping active. He is concerned about the possibility of cancer.

How to approach the case

Data gathering in the interview and interpretation and use of information gathered

Presenting problem(s) and symptom exploration

▪ **Establish the range of symptoms** Establishing these often leads to consideration of differential diagnoses of each symptom then looking for a diagnosis common to each. Here the combination of symptoms points immediately to the unifying diagnosis of a glomerulonephritis (GN), possibly immunoglobulin A (IgA) nephropathy. It is nevertheless imperative to keep an open mind, consider all possibilities and obtain a reasonably thorough but succinct systematic enquiry.

▪ **Consider possible causes of haematuria** These include nephritic syndrome, renal cell carcinoma and ureteric calculi. Occasionally foods and chemicals can produce red urine mimicking haematuria.

Patient perspective

Tell him that you think a form of kidney inflammation, perhaps provoked by the initial sore throat illness, to be much more likely than cancer but that your tests will look at all possibilities.

Past medical history

He is previously well, typically the case in many types of GN.

Drug and allergy history

He appears not to be taking any medications but a history taken from anyone with renal disease should ask specifically about non-steroidal anti-inflammatory drugs (NSAIDS) and non-prescription drugs.

Family history

A family history of renal disease should be sought, especially polycystic kidney disease.

Social history

His occupation is important, and he should be advised to consult with his occupational medical team, who will be familiar with Civil Aviation Authority regulations, to establish his fitness for flying.

SUMMARY – ASSESSMENT AND PLAN

- The combination of blood and protein on urinalysis, hypertension and mildly impaired renal function suggests nephritic syndrome, and the syn-pharyngitic (sore throat concomitant with renal effects) history and episodes of macroscopic haematuria strongly suggest IgA nephropathy.
- The next steps are to arrange examination of urine for casts and dysmorphic red cells, up-to-date renal function and a renal tract ultrasound.
- The ultrasound occasionally suggests an alternative diagnosis such as renal cell carcinoma; if symptoms suggest ureteric calculi (pain) then an intravenous pyelogram and referral to a urologist might also be indicated.
- If microscopy reveals casts or dysmorphic red cells or the renal ultrasound and history do not suggest an alternative cause then he should be referred to a nephrologist for early consideration of a renal biopsy to confirm the type of GN.

Discussion

How may GN be classified?

GN is confusing because nomenclature attempts to encapsulate aetiology, pathology and clinical presentation. Aetiology descriptions refer to primary causes (unknown but thought to be autoimmune) or secondary causes (associated with autoimmunity, infection, malignancy or metabolic disturbance). Pathological descriptions address glomerular involvement, cell involvement and changes in non-cellular components. Although each clinical presentation can be the result of several types of GN as defined by aetiology or pathology, clinical classification best directs management (Table 2.54).

Table 2.54 Classification of glomerulonephritis (GN) by clinical presentation and management principles

Clinical presentation of GN	Management principles
Asymptomatic urinary abnormalities Subnephrotic-range proteinuria and/or microscopic haematuria without renal impairment, oedema or hypertension.	Referral to nephrologist if > 1 g protein/24 hours or glomerular haematuria or abnormal creatinine. Non-urgent renal biopsy in some cases or close observation in others. Referral to urologist if non-glomerular haematuria for ultrasound, X-ray of kidneys/ureters/bladder, intravenous pyelogram, flexible cystoscopy
Chronic GN Persistent proteinuria ± haematuria with slowly progressive renal impairment.	Non-urgent biopsy and treatment to slow progression of chronic kidney disease
Nephritic syndrome – *the glomerular filter is damaged but inflammation renders it less leaky than normal* Recent onset of haematuria and proteinuria, renal impairment (often oliguric acute renal failure) and salt and water retention causing hypertension.	Usually urgent biopsy to guide management and prognosis
Nephrotic syndrome – *the glomerular filter is damaged and more leaky than usual. This leads to hypoalbuminuria and oedema* Nephrotic-range proteinuria (> 3.5 g in 24 h), hypoalbuminaemia, oedema and hyperlipidaemia, sometimes with predisposition to venous thrombosis and bacterial infection. The selective nature of the proteinuria tends to alter lipoprotein profiles causing loss of natural anticoagulant proteins and immunoglobulin subtypes.	Usually urgent biopsy to guide management and prognosis
Rapidly progressive GN Progression to renal failure over days to weeks, usually within a nephritic presentation.	Emergency demanding urgent tissue diagnosis (typically extensive crescenteric GN) and treatment

How is glomerular haematuria detected?

Glomerular haematuria arises from diseased glomeruli and red cells are typically dysmorphic and form red cell casts in the tubule. Non-glomerular haematuria arises distal to the glomerulus and red cells are normal in appearance.

What are casts?

Casts are cylinders of material extruded from the renal tubule. Hyaline casts are formed from Tamm Horsfall protein and physiologically secreted in fever and exercise and do not imply disease. Granular casts indicate renal disease but are non-specific and common in acute tubular necrosis. White cell casts are found in pyogenic conditions.

What types of proteinuria are there?

Persistent proteinuria usually implies renal disease. Glomerular proteinuria is usually > 500 mg/24 h and comprises mostly albumin. True orthostatic proteinuria (no proteinuria early morning, proteinuria with ambulation) and tubulointerstitial disease are usually associated with minor proteinuria.

How prevalent is GN?

The overall incidence and prevalence of GN is unknown because it often causes mild, asymptomatic, unrecognised illness. Population studies have shown that evidence of kidney damage – proteinuria, haematuria, low GFR or combinations of these – affects around 16% of adults in Australia and the USA. Diabetic and hypertensive nephropathy are two major causes, but GN is likely the cause in a substantial proportion.

What are the common types of GN?

IgA nephropathy is the most common GN, followed by focal and segmental glomerulosclerosis and vasculitis. Defined populations are at increased risk of types of GN. Australian Aboriginals are at increased risk of infection-associated GN after streptococcal throat or skin infections, now rare in developed countries. Chronic infections, notably hepatitis B or C viruses or human immunodeficiency virus increase the risk of several types of immune-mediated GN.

Which types of GN tend to progress to stage 5 chronic kidney disease?

Most patients incur chronic kidney disease (CKD) with risks of accelerated cardiovascular disease. GN is the commonest cause of stage 5 (end-stage) CKD in Australia, and the third most common, after diabetes and hypertension, in the USA. Types that can progress to stage 5 include IgA nephropathy, FSGS, rapidly progressive GN with crescents (vasculitis and anti-glomerular basement membrane disease), membranous nephropathy and lupus nephritis. Male sex, hypertension, heavy proteinuria and reduced GFR tend to carry a worse prognosis for most types of GN.

What treatments are there for GN?

Recent understanding of the types of pathology, locations of pathology, important diseases that can result and their clinical presentations, treatments and prognoses are summarised in Table 2.55.

Table 2.55 Recent understanding of important glomerulonephritides

Location of pathology	Important diseases	Clinical presentation	Treatment and prognosis
Epithelial cell Epithelial cells, in conjunction with the basement membrane, allow filtration of plasma solutes but not proteins and cells. Diseases are typified by flattening or effacement of the foot processes (podocytes) that engage the basement membrane (minimal change disease) and subepithelial/basement membrane immune deposition with spikes and thickening (membranous nephropathy) resulting in disruption of the filtration barrier and proteinuria.	**Minimal change disease** Occasionally associated with Hodgkin's lymphoma or other diseases	Selective proteinuria or nephrotic syndrome, usually in children	Oral prednisolone 0.5–1 mg/kg daily for 6 weeks then tapered Steroid resistance and relapse more common in adults (cyclophosphamide or ciclosporin)
	Membranous nephropathy Secondary to malignancy (non-Hodgkin's lymphoma, paraneoplasia, carcinoma), drugs (e.g. gold, penicillamine), diabetes, autoimmune disease (lupus, rheumatoid), amyloid or infection (malaria, hepatitis, HIV)	Non-selective proteinuria or nephrotic syndrome	Oral cyclophosphamide and prednisolone achieves 50% remission rate 30% progress to end-stage over 10 years
	Focal and segmental glomerulosclerosis (FSGS)	Variably selective proteinuria or nephrotic syndrome	Nephrotic syndrome or ↓ GFR warrant immunosuppression – prednisolone 0.5–1 mg/kg daily for a few months 50% of steroid-resistant cases respond to cyclophosphamide Response reduces progression to end stage by 50% Common reason for renal replacement therapy
	Class V lupus nephritis Probably identical to membranous nephropathy	Nephrotic syndrome	
	Diabetic nephropathy	Nephrotic syndrome	Vigorous control of glycaemia, blood pressure (ACE inhibitor/ARB) and dyslipidaemia
Mesangial cell Mesangial cells are directly exposed to the circulation and deposition of immune complexes is typically seen in diseases such as IgA nephropathy (polymeric IgA deposits) that involve mesangial cells. This results in proliferation (increase in cell number) leading to haematuria, proteinuria and renal impairment.	**IgA nephropathy** Also known as mesangial proliferative GN Identical renal lesions are seen in Henoch–Schönlein purpura, of which IgAN may be the renal-limited form	Asymptomatic urinary abnormalities, notably macroscopic haematuria, often synpharyngitic (concurrent) with upper respiratory tract infection or nephritic syndrome	No satisfactory treatment Strict blood pressure control Combined ACE inhibitors and ARBs Steroids occasionally helpful Prognosis variable, a substantial proportion progressing to end-stage but asymptomatic prevalence unknown
	Class II lupus nephritis	Nephritic syndrome	
	Diabetic nephropathy Nodular and global sclerosis		Treatment not always indicated as prognosis good

Endothelial cell

Diseases can result from immune complex deposition, as in infection-associated GN and mesangiocapillary GN, antibody attachment to the basement membrane as in Goodpasture's disease, or trauma and activation of coagulation as in haemolytic–uraemic syndrome.

Endothelial cell proliferation and necrosis are accompanied by leucocyte accumulation, and rupture of the basement membrane, crescent formation and disruption of glomerular architecture can develop with nephritic syndrome or rapidly progressive GN.

Infection-associated GN Formerly known as diffuse proliferative and exudative endocapillary GN (endocapillary referring to endothelial and mesangial cells)	Nephritic syndrome, tending to be 7–10 days after infection, unlike IgAN. Hence its other names post-infectious GN (PIGN)/post-streptococcal GN (PSGN). It may be secondary to many other infections, including SBE.	Good prognosis if infection treated
Mesangiocapillary GN Also known as membranoproliferative GN Due to activation of complement Types 1 (classical pathway, often may be secondary to hepatitis C or cryoglobulinaemia) 2 (alternative pathway) and 3 (terminal pathway)	Nephritic syndrome	Anti-CD20 may be useful in cryoglobulin-associated disease Poor prognosis as tends to cause slowly progressive renal failure, predicted by rate of ↓ GFR and degree of proteinuria
Class III and IV lupus nephritis Proliferative lupus nephritis	Nephritic syndrome	Biopsy essential as type of lupus nephritis not clear clinically but determines therapy Pulsed methylprednisolone then monthly intravenous cyclophosphamide and oral steroid for 3–6 months (remission induction) Azathioprine or mycophenolate mofetil and reduced steroid (maintenance)
Vasculitis	Rapidly progressive GN	Pulsed methylprednisolone then oral cyclophosphamide and prednisolone
Antiglomerular basement membrane (Goodpasture's) disease	Rapidly progressive GN	Plasmapheresis, pulsed methylprednisolone followed by oral cyclophosphamide and prednisolone
Cryoglobulinaemia **Thrombotic microangiopathies** Thrombotic thrombocytopenic purpura/ haemolytic uremic syndrome		

ACE, angiotensin-converting enzyme; ARBs, angiotensin receptor blockers; GFR, glomerular filtration rate; GN, glomerulonephritis; IgA, immunoglobulin A.

What is Goodpasture's disease?

Goodpasture's disease is a pulmonary–renal syndrome that may cause renal failure, although it is not a vasculitis. Pathogenic antiglomerular basement membrane (GBM) antibodies target pulmonary and renal type IV collagen.

What is Alport's syndrome?

Mutations in the *COL4A5* (X-linked), *COL4A3* or *COL4A4* (both autosomal-recessive) genes cause defective synthesis of the α5-chain collagen type IV with dysfunction of the GBM and sensorineural deafness. Since donor kidneys contain the α5-chain, Alport's syndrome recipients may establish an immune response against them. This is a form of anti-GBM disease and can lead to graft failure.

What is thin basement membrane nephropathy?

This is one of numerous genetic disorders of GBM collagen, and a relatively common form of familial haematuria with a relatively good prognosis.

CASE 2.28

SYSTEMIC VASCULITIS

Candidate information

Role

You are a doctor in the emergency medical admissions unit. Please read the following letter from the patient's general practitioner. You may make notes on the paper provided. When the bell sounds, enter the examination room to begin the consultation.

Scenario

> Dear Doctor
>
> Re: Mr John Silver, aged 65 years
>
> Thank you for seeing this gentleman urgently. He has been breathless for the last two weeks and now has recurrent episodes of haemoptysis. His blood tests show a moderate leucocytosis with a neutrophilia, a moderate thrombocytosis, and normochromic normocytic anaemia. He has raised inflammatory markers with a C-reactive protein of 400. His urinalysis is strongly positive for blood and his serum creatinine is 350 µmol/l.
>
> Yours sincerely

Please take a history from the patient (you may continue to make notes if you wish on the paper provided). Your examiners will warn you when 12 minutes have elapsed. You have 14 minutes to take a history from the patient followed by 1 minute of reflection. There will then follow 5 minutes of discussion with the examiners. Be prepared to discuss solutions to the problems posed by the case and how you might reply to the GP's letter. You are not required to examine the patient.

Patient information

Mr John Silver is a 65-year-old gentleman who has been increasingly breathless for the last two weeks and over the last 48 hours has been coughing up blood. Over the last two months he has felt non-specifically unwell, with unintentional weight loss of around 8 kg and lethargy. His hearing became markedly reduced in his right ear over the course of a few days and he is awaiting an audiology appointment. For around 12 months he has noticed a little nasal stuffiness and on two occasions has been treated for sinusitis. Otherwise he has been a well man apart from mild hypertension, which is being monitored, and gout, for which he takes allopurinol 300 mg daily as prophylaxis. He takes no other medications. He does not have a history of asthma or lung disease. He has never smoked. He lives with his wife, who is wheelchair-dependent with multiple sclerosis but who is otherwise well. He has been told by his doctor that the diagnosis is uncertain, but Mr Silver feels that 'chronic' pneumonia is most likely.

How to approach the case

Data gathering in the interview and interpretation and use of information gathered

Presenting problem(s) and symptom exploration

He has a pulmonary–renal syndrome, possible causes of which are antineutrophil cytoplasmic antibody (ANCA)-associated systemic vasculitis (AASV), systemic lupus erythematosus (SLE), Goodpasture's disease and infection, e.g. pneumonia with acute tubular necrosis, bacterial endocarditis, post-streptococcal glomerulonephritis (GN). Although there is no agreed definition, the Chapel Hill Consensus Conference definitions provide a reasonable initial approach to AASV (Table 2.56).

There is considerable overlap between the AASVs in terms of symptoms:

- *Systemic* – Fever, night sweats, weight loss, myalgia and arthralgia are often present for two to three months before diagnosis.
- *Upper respiratory tract* – In Wegener's granulmatosis (WG), patients often present with limited upper airways disease – nasal stuffiness, mucosal discharge, crusting or septal perforation with a saddle nose deformity, sinusitis, epistaxis, otitis media or hoarseness. Sometimes symptoms may be chronic and insidious and predate systemic disease by months or many years before transforming. Subglottic stenosis affects many patients. Allergic rhinitis and nasal polyps often predate symptoms in Churg–Strauss syndrome (CSS) by many years.
- *Eyes* – Ocular inflammation may occur in all AASVs and includes conjunctivitis, episcleritis, scleritis, sight-threatening 'meltdown' keratitis and uveitis. Scleritis is typical, and untreated can lead to scleral perforation and blindness. Painful proptosis and

Table 2.56 Chapel Hill Consensus Conference criteria for antineutrophil cytoplasmic antibody (ANCA)-associated systemic vasculitis (AASV)

	Chapel Hill Consensus Conference criteria	Typical features
Wegener's granulomatosis (WG)	Granulomatous inflammation involving respiratory tract and necrotising vasculitis affecting small- to medium-sized vessels (capillaries, venules, arterioles) Necrotising glomerulonephritis (GN) common	Often presents with nasal and/or upper respiratory tract disease, e.g. nasal discharge, epistaxis, stridor Pulmonary granulomata and alveolitis may provoke lung haemorrhage Glomerulonephritis common Typically cANCA- and PR3-positive High relapse rate
Microscopic polyarteritis (MPA)	Necrotising vasculitis with few or no immune deposits, affecting small vessels (capillaries, venules, arterioles); necrotising arteritis of small and medium-sized arteries may occur Necrotising GN common Pulmonary capillaritis common	Pulmonary capillaritis leads to alveolitis, lung haemorrhage and fibrosis Focal necrotising GN most common manifestation Most pANCA- and MPO-positive but significant number PR3-positive Relapse less frequent with MPO positivity
Churg–Strauss syndrome (CSS)	Eosinophil-rich granulomatous inflammation involving respiratory tract and necrotising vasculitis affecting small to medium-sized vessels associated with asthma and eosinophilia	Nasal polyps and rhinitis Asthma and granulomatous inflammation Mononeuritis multiplex

diplopia may occur in WG with orbital granulomata. Optic nerve and retinal artery vasculitis are rare.

- *Lungs* – Both pulmonary nodules and diffuse alveolitis may occur. Acute haemorrhage is common in WG. Subsequent fibrosis is more common in microscopic polyangitis (MPA). Asthma and transient pulmonary infiltrates are common in CSS.
- *Renal* – Renal disease affects around 20% at presentation, but around 80% will develop GN, often rapidly progressive GN with significant (3 to 4+) blood and protein, variable renal impairment and necrotising GN on biopsy with inflammation surrounding the glomerulus (crescents) and negative (pauci-immune) immunofluorescence.
- *Skin* – Skin disease with purpura, ulcers or nodules occurs in a significant minority.
- *Neurological* – Sensorimotor neuropathy, typically mononeuritis multiplex, is most common in CSS.

Patient perspective

Vasculitis is not always easy to explain to patients, and further tests are needed. Explain that this could be infection but that other possibilities that require prompt treatment need to be considered.

Past medical history

The history of nasal stuffiness, and even more importantly the history of sudden hearing loss, is highly suggestive of Wegener's granulomatosis.

Drug and allergy history

Allopurinol is potentially nephrotoxic, and although only a small component of his problems, should at least be dose-adjusted.

Family history

Relevance here is unlikely.

Social history

Explore any difficulties that might arise for his wife if he is admitted to hospital.

SUMMARY – ASSESSMENT AND PLAN

- This is most likely an AASV with pulmonary haemorrhage and renal failure.
- Malignancy (primary lung cancer or metastatic to lungs) is possible given the weight loss, raised inflammatory markers and history of progressive symptoms over a few months; however, he is a non-smoker, the upper respiratory symptoms are highly suggestive of Wegener's granulomatosis and the active urine sediment with renal failure is typical of AASV.
- Chronic infection such as unresolving pneumonia with an underlying cause or tuberculosis should also be considered.
- His blood tests should be repeated with an urgent ANCA test. Urine should be analysed for casts and dysmorphic red cells. A chest X-ray in AASV may show nodules, reticulo-nodular shadowing, pneumonic changes, collapse, or pleural effusion. If AASV is likely and infection is not, immunosuppression with high-dose corticosteroids should be started promptly.
- If AASV is subsequently confirmed, other treatment considerations include osteoporosis prophylaxis and commencement of cyclophosphamide with monitoring for opportunistic infections and side effects, e.g. fungal infection, cyclophosphamide haemorrhagic cystitis, bladder tumours. Gout prophylaxis with allopurinol may not be possible if he subsequently takes azathioprine, although the combination may be used with caution if thiopurine methyltransferase levels are satisfactory. Regular monitoring of the white cell count is needed, e.g. twice weekly in the first month and alternate weeks in the second month and urgently if there are signs of infection or malignancy.

Discussion

What is vasculitis?

Vasculitis refers to fibrinoid necrosis and inflammation of blood vessels.

What types of vasculitis are there?

There is no indisputable classification. Vasculitides may be primary, the main damage being to blood vessels, or secondary to systemic, often connective tissue, disease such as SLE or rheumatoid. Vasculitides may be classified by vessel type (Table 2.57).

Despite the term 'systemic', vasculitis sometimes focuses on one organ as in a type of rapidly progressive glomerulonephritis caused by a type of renal-limited MPA and a form of WG limited to head and neck, usually granulomatous but with the potential to evolve into systemic vasculitis.

Why are vasculitides important to recognise?

Vasculitides are not common (but probably increasing in incidence), are easily missed and different vasculitides affect different age groups – Kawasaki disease only children, Henoch–Schönlein purpura usually children, WG/MPA only adults and giant cell arteritis older people. Overall, vasculitides are probably less easily recognised in older people but are equally common. They are medical emergencies – Kawasaki disease can cause myocardial infarction, WG/MPA can cause life-threatening renal failure and lung haemorrhage, and giant cell arteritis can cause blindness or stroke. Distinguishing the subsets is important because different vasculitides need different treatments.

How common is AASV?

WG and MPA have a prevalence of around 20 per million, an increasing incidence and are more common in white people with a peak age of onset of 55–70 years and no sex predilection. CSS is less common.

What are ANCAs?

AASVs are autoimmune and of unknown cause, although associations with certain drugs and nasal carriage of

Staphylococcus aureus (in WG relapse) have been identified. However, ANCAs, directed against neutrophil granules and monocyte/macrophage lysosomes and detected by immunofluorescence (more sensitive) and enzyme-linked immunosorbent assay (more specific), are sensitive (> 95%) and specific (> 99%) for active AASV.

Anticytoplasmic ANCA (cANCA)

This is directed against proteinase 3 (PR3) and is predominant in WG. α1-antitrypsin, the main inhibitor of PR3, is associated with WG in that patients with deficiency have more severe disease but deficiency is not sufficient to trigger WG.

Antiperinuclear ANCA (pANCA)

This is directed against myeloperoxidase (MPO) and is most common in MPA (70% of cases, although cANCA can also occur). In CSS 50% are pANCA-positive, 25% cANCA-positive and 25% ANCA-negative.

Positive ANCAs sometimes occur without obvious disease, and may be less relevant if subsequent testing for PR3 and MPO are negative.

What is the role of ANCAs in AASV?

ANCAs may be used to monitor disease activity and indicate risk of relapse. They correlate closely with disease activity in many, but not all, patients, and are thought to contribute to pathogenesis by binding to and activating primed neutrophils expressing PR3 or MPO (with release of proteolytic granules and pro-inflammatory cytokines) and impeding apoptosis, and so promoting highly inflammatory necrosis. This may cause endothelial damage and activation. Activated endothelium is prothrombotic and expresses adhesion molecules that attract neutrophils and a sustained proinflammatory response via monocytes and T cells, with ultimate scarring. The problem with ANCAs as markers of and contributors to disease is that in many patients correlation is poor and in some ANCAs are persistently negative.

How is a diagnosis of AASV confirmed?

Rapidly progressive renal failure with an active urine sediment or rapidly progressive haemorrhagic lung disease,

Table 2.57 Classification of vasculitis (Consensus Conference on the Nomenclature of Systemic Vasculitis 1994)		
Size of vessel	**Typical vessels affected**	**Diseases**
Small vessel vasculitis	Arterioles, capillaries and venules but may affect larger vessels	Wegener's granulomatosis (WG) Microscopic polyangiitis (microscopic polyarteritis) (MPA) Churg–Strauss syndrome (CSS) Henoch–Schönlein purpura Essential cryoglobulinaemic vasculitis Cutaneous leucocytoclastic vasculitis
Medium-sized vessel vasculitis	Main visceral arteries, e.g. renal, hepatic, coronary, mesenteric	Polyarteritis nodosa Kawasaki disease (children)
Large vessel vasculitis	Aorta and largest branches directed towards major body regions such as head and neck and extremities	Giant cell arteritis (GCA) Takayasu's arteritis

with a positive ANCA, are sufficient grounds to institute emergency immunosuppression. A renal biopsy for crescenteric GN is usually best for WG, because bronchoscopic biopsy may show granulomata but is often non-specific. C-reactive protein is increased in systemic vasculitis, but not in limited disease. Anaemia is common (haemoglobin 9–12 g/dl) and significant thrombocytosis (> 550 × 10⁹/l) is characteristic.

What is the treatment for AASV?

The prognosis for untreated AASV is very poor, with a one-year mortality of 80%. With treatment, survival is now 70–80% at five years (Table 2.58). Unsurprisingly, cytotoxic agents that improved survival were for many years used without being exposed to trials, but evidence has grown over the last few years, particularly with studies by the European Vasculitis Study Group.

What are indicators of relapse in AASV?

These include symptoms, rising inflammatory markers, recurrence of or a rising ANCA titre, active urinary sediment or deteriorating renal function.

What is polyarteritis nodosa?

This is a medium-vessel vasculitis that is ANCA-negative but which may share features with AASV.

What is Henoch–Schönlein purpura?

This is a syndrome with four variable features – immunoglobulin A nephropathy (which appears to be a renal limited form of Henoch–Schönlein purpura occurring in around 50%), vasculitic rash in children classically affecting the buttocks but in adults any distribution (100%), arthralgia (75%) and gastrointestinal disturbance (30–40%). In adults, unlike children, bowel wall oedema can be more likely.

What is Goodpasture's or anti-glomerular basement membrane (anti-GBM) disease?

This is an autoimmune pulmonary–renal syndrome, but not a vasculitis, characterised by anti-GBM antibodies that target renal and pulmonary type IV collagen. Histologically, there is linear GBM immunoglobulin G deposition. This causes rapidly progressive glomerulonephritis and pulmonary haemorrhage, although sometimes renal involvement is the overwhelming problem in isolation. Confusingly, the term Goodpasture's syndrome was used historically for what is now best termed Goodpasture's or anti-GBM disease, while Goodpasture's disease was often reserved for those patients with Alport's syndrome (in which type IV collagen is absent) in receipt of a kidney transplant who subsequently developed an anti-GBM response. Nowadays, Goodpasture's or anti-GBM disease refers to patients with anti-GBM antibodies and Goodpasture's syndrome is a rather vague term sometimes, but not ideally, used to denote any pulmonary–renal syndrome. Goodpasture's disease is treated as for AASV.

What is Behçet's diease?

Behçet's diease remains poorly understood. Pathologically, it is an inflammatory disease, mostly affecting blood vessels, although frank vascular injury is not always

Table 2.58 Treatment of antineutrophil cytoplasmic antibody (ANCA)-associated systemic vasculitis (AASV)	
Treatment stage	**Treatments**
Remission induction	Prednisolone 1 mg/kg reduced to 20 mg by week 5 and 10 mg by week 10 but tailored to response Oral cyclophosphamide 2 mg/kg daily (maximum 200 mg), 1.5 mg/kg in older people (pulsed treatment being evaluated) for 12 weeks or until remission achieved Weekly oral methotrexate an alternative to cyclophosphamide if not life-threatening disease and serum creatinine < 150 µmol/l (although relapse rate higher)
Adjuvant therapy for life-threatening disease	Plasma exchange considered if initial creatinine > 500 µmol/l (MEPEX), results better than methylprednisolone
Maintenance	Prednisolone 5–10 mg/day Azathioprine 2 mg/kg/day (maximum 200 mg) replacing cyclophosphamide at three months if initial creatinine < 500 µmol/l not associated with higher relapse rate; may reduce complications (CYCAZAREM) Cotrimoxazole prophylaxis considered in patients with Wegener's granulomatosis (recurrence may be linked with staphylococcal nasal carriage) Duration unclear; at least 18–24 months usual
Relapse (30–50% over 3–5 years) May occur at any time	3-monthly reviews with ANCA to detect early recurrence If major, return to initial induction If minor, increase steroid dosage
Rescue for relapsing and refractory disease	Standard induction fails in 10% Frequent relapse requiring recurrent cyclophosphamide also difficult
New therapies	Newer therapies include TNF blockade and polyclonal antithymocyte globulin (ATG)

apparent and it is not classified as a vasculitis. It probably has an infective or immunological basis in susceptible individuals, and its most constant geographical distribution is along the historical 'Silk Road', being most prevalent in Turkey. Clinical features are highly variable, and may include recurrent painful oral ulceration identical to aphthous ulceration, genital ulceration, gastrointestinal ulceration, skin lesions including pustules and erythema nodosum, uveitis or retinitis, arthritis, headaches or focal neurological symptoms. Venous thromboembolism occurs in around 20%; arterial occlusion is less common. The differential diagnosis includes sarcoidosis, inflammatory bowel disease and Reiter's syndrome and it is usually a diagnosis of exclusion. Corticosteroids may help in managing lesions.

CASE 2.29

HYPERCALCAEMIA

Candidate information

Role

You are a doctor in the emergency medical admissions unit. Please read the following letter from the patient's general practitioner. You may make notes on the paper provided. When the bell sounds, enter the examination room to begin the consultation.

Scenario

> Dear Doctor
>
> Re: Mr Jake Marley, aged 72 years
>
> Thank you for seeing Mr Marley, who has had back pain for a few months and whose blood tests show a corrected serum calcium of 2.9 mmol/l and a normochromic normocytic anaemia. He is previously well and I am concerned about the possibility of myeloma, although his protein electrophoresis shows a moderate polyclonal pattern without a monoclonal band. His renal function is normal. I would appreciate your urgent assessment.
>
> Yours sincerely

Please take a history from the patient (you may continue to make notes if you wish on the paper provided). Your examiners will warn you when 12 minutes have elapsed. You have 14 minutes to take a history from the patient followed by 1 minute of reflection. There will then follow 5 minutes of discussion with the examiners. Be prepared to discuss solutions to the problems posed by the case and how you might reply to the GP's letter. You are not required to examine the patient.

Patient information

Mr Jake Marley is a 72-year-old gentleman who has been losing weight for around four months, and in the last two months has developed a gnawing pain in his lower back that is now keeping him awake at night. More recently, he has had night sweats. His past medical history comprises a melanoma excision from his right shoulder area four years ago and prostate trouble. He has had a poor urinary stream for a couple of years and his GP told him it was probably the result of an enlarged prostate. He lives with his wife, who herself has osteoporosis and who has been struggling increasingly in the last few weeks to manage him at home. He does not have any lower limb weakness but is very disabled by the pain. He is a smoker of 10 cigarettes per day. He and his wife had thought his back pain might also be the result of osteoporosis.

How to approach the case

Data gathering in the interview and interpretation and use of information gathered

Presenting problem(s) and symptom exploration

■ **Explore symptoms of hypercalcaemia** These include polydipsia, polyuria and pain due to ureteric calculi. 'Moans, stones, bones and groans' (depression, ureteric calculi, bone pain, abdominal pain, dyspepsia) beloved of textbooks are not that common. Severe constipation, confusion or rigidity may occur with calcium levels over 3.0 mmol/l, where the cause is usually neoplastic.

■ **Explore the worrying symptoms** Weight loss, night sweats and the gnawing back pain are a significant worry and should alert you immediately to the possibility of cancer and prompt a full systematic enquiry. Back pain and urinary symptoms should raise the possibility of cord compression but the absence of lower limb symptoms is at least a little reassuring.

Patient perspective

There is a need to gently expose the possibility of an unwelcome diagnosis, without leaping to malignancy, given that it is not something he has considered. This may be done by expressing your concerns that things may not be as simple as they seem, that there is a wide range of possibilities but that you see a compelling need to investigate things urgently, keeping in mind the possibility of finding something that may not be nice. You could allude to the history of melanoma and say that sometimes there is a link with these sorts of symptoms and a history of melanoma.

Past medical history

The prostate symptoms and the history of melanoma are both potentially highly relevant.

Drug and allergy history

Not relevant here.

Family history

Hypercalcaemia only seldom has a familial basis and this is not a consideration here.

Social history

You should be concerned that he is becoming immobilised by pain and that his wife is struggling.

SUMMARY – ASSESSMENT AND PLAN

- Primary hyperparathyroidism (PHPT) and malignancy are the commonest causes of hypercalcaemia. Malignancy can cause hypercalcaemia by bone metastases or by release of parathyroid hormone (PTH)-related peptide (PTH-rp) by the tumour directly.
- PHPT is more common in outpatient settings and malignancy is more common in patients who have been admitted to hospital.
- Hypercalcaemia should usually be confirmed on two separate samples before further investigation.
- The next step is usually to perform a PTH assay. This is raised in PHPT, and often normal or suppressed in hypercalcaemia linked to malignancy. PTH-rp is not detected by the standard PTH assay and does not influence standard PTH levels. However, a PTH assay is not always needed in patients where hypercalcaemia is very likely to be a manifestation of malignancy.
- This patient very likely has malignancy, and bone metastases seem likely, either from prostate or melanoma. Bone metastases from melanoma can appear lytic, behaving not dissimilarly to myeloma. Examination should include prostate examination and further investigations should include a full screen of haematobiochemistry, inflammatory markers and prostate-specific antigen (PSA), chest X-ray, thoracolumbar spine X-ray and a bone scan. Urinary light chains should be sought for completeness if considering myeloma but the polyclonal electrophoresis and a more plausible sequence of pathological events make myeloma less likely. If these tests do not confirm a cause, a PTH assay and PTH-rp assay may be warranted, and a computed tomography scan of thorax, abdomen and pelvis might detect carcinoma or lymphoma.
- Hospital admission may be the most effective way of managing the overall situation – a need for urgent investigation, to manage his pain and to provide respite for his wife.

Discussion

What are the causes of hypercalcaemia?

These are listed in Box 2.66.

PHPT is usually due to a solitary adenoma but occasionally multiple adenomas or hyperplasia; carcinoma is exceptionally rare. It is occasionally associated with multiple endocrine neoplasia (MEN) syndromes (Case 1.43). In MEN1, PHPT is usual, often with pancreatic tumours and sometimes with pituitary adenomas. In MEN2 medullary thyroid cancer and phaeochromocytoma are more likely than PHPT.

What end-organ damage may be seen in PHPT?

Osteoporosis, osteitis fibrosa cystica, nephrolithiasis and nephrocalcinosis are common with uncorrected PHPT.

Box 2.66 Causes of hypercalcaemia

- Primary hyperparathyroidism (PHPT)
- Malignancy due to bone metastases or PTH-related peptide (PTHrp) produced by tumour
- Myeloma
- Tertiary hyperparathyroidism in kidney disease
- Thyrotoxicosis
- Addison's disease
- Excess calcium ingestion
- Milk-alkali syndrome
- Drugs, e.g. thiazides, lithium
- Paget's disease (if immobilisation)
- Familial hypocalciuric hypercalcaemia

Box 2.67 Indications for surgery in primary hyperparathyroidism

Indications for surgery for asymptomatic patients (generally evidence of end-organ damage):

- Serum calcium > 0.25 mmol/l above upper limit of normal
- 24-hour urinary calcium > 400 mg
- Creatinine clearance reduced by 30%
- Bone mineral density T score < −2.5
- Age < 50 years
- Medical surveillance not practical

What is familial hypocalciuric hypercalcaemia (FHH)?

This is a rare autosomal dominant condition with inactivating mutations in calcium-sensing receptor genes. Parathyroid cells are mildly resistant to calcium and there is reduced ability for the kidneys to up-regulate calcium excretion. Serum calcium is modestly elevated with an inappropriately normal PTH level and this can mimic PHPT. The calcium:creatinine clearance ratio can help distinguish FHH from PHPT, as can 24-hour urinary calcium levels.

What are the indications for surgery in primary hyperparathyroidism?

Indications for surgery in PHPT have been produced by the US National Institute of Health and their guidelines have been widely adopted. The indications are listed in Box 2.67.

What surveillance is needed for patients managed conservatively?

Serum calcium should be checked biannually and serum creatinine annually. Bone mineral density should be considered every two to three years. Baseline 24-hour urinary calcium and creatinine clearance, and a baseline renal ultrasound for stones are usual.

What is the surgical treatment of choice?

Minimally invasive surgery is often possible for patients where there is concordant nuclear medicine (SestaMIBI SPECT scan or thallium subtraction scan) and ultrasound evidence of an isolated adenoma. Otherwise, subtotal or total parathyroidectomy may be needed. Tests to establish disease extent may also include computed tomography or magnetic resonance imaging or selective venous sampling.

What are the potential complications of surgery?

These include hypoparathyroidism, which occurs in up to 70% of patients but which usually resolves quickly. Oral calcium and 1α hydroxyvitamin D are needed. More severe hypocalcaemia may result from 'hungry bones', often in patients with pre-existing bone disease, and may require intravenous calcium. Permanent hypoparathyroidism is rare.

What are the medical treatments for hypercalcaemia?

Adequate fluid replacement and bisphosphonate therapy may be needed. Steroids may be useful in malignancy. In PHPT, calcium tends to correct only with surgery.

What are the possible endocrine manifestations of malignancy?

Common hormones produced by tumours are listed in Table 2.59.

Rarer hormones produced by tumours include renin (renal cell cancer), insulin-like growth factors and vasoactive intestinal peptide (VIPoma).

How is serum calcium regulated?

Total serum calcium comprises the calcium that is bound to albumin and its ionised form. Calcium and phosphate homeostasis is maintained by PTH and 1,25-dihydroxyvitamin D (1,25(OH)$_2$D), also known as 1,25-dihydroxycholecalciferol.

PTH

This acts in the kidney, enhancing tubular resorption of calcium and excretion of phosphate, and converting 1,25(OH)D to 1,25(OH)$_2$D. It also acts on bone, promoting osteoclastic resorption, thereby increasing serum calcium and phosphate. PTH is normally suppressed by hypercalcaemia, and activated by hypocalcaemia. Calcitonin (from thyroid C cells) essentially opposes the actions of PTH.

1,25(OH)$_2$D

This is synthesised in the kidney from 25OHD, which is itself synthesised in the liver from vitamin D. Vitamin D is ingested or produced by the action of ultraviolet light on 7-dehydrocholesterol in the skin. 1,25(OH)$_2$D enhances tubular resorption of calcium and excretion of phosphate, increases gut absorption of calcium and phosphate and increases bone mineralisation.

What are secondary and tertiary hyperparathyroidism?

Primary hyperparathyroidism is discussed above. Secondary hyperparathyroidism corrects the tendency to hypocalcaemia in chronic kidney disease, causing calcium and phosphate release from bone. Phosphate cannot be cleared and so accumulates, creating a vicious cycle. In tertiary hyperparathyroidism the PTH rise is inappropriately large, overshooting its original purpose because the parathyroids have been chronically stimulated and have become autonomous secretors, leading to hypercalcaemia.

What happens to serum levels of alkaline phosphatase in hyperparathyroidism?

These increase, because bone turnover is increased.

What are the causes of hypocalcaemia?

These are outlined in Table 2.60.

Calcium may also be removed from the circulation in hyperphosphataemia, and by some blood products. It may be diminished in hypomagnesaemia.

What are the clinical features of hypocalcaemia?

These are outlined in Table 2.61. Chronic hypocalcaemia may be asymptomatic.

Table 2.59 Hormones produced by tumours	
Hormone	**Tumours**
Parathyroid hormone-related peptide (PTH-rp)	Breast cancer Squamous cell cancer, e.g. lung, head and neck, oesophagus Adenocarcinoma of lung Other solid tumours, e.g. ovary, bladder Lymphoma Phaeochromocytoma Myeloma
Antidiuretic hormone (ADH; in SIADH)	Small cell lung cancer Cancer of duodenum, pancreas, colon, genitourinary tract Squamous cell cancer of head and neck Lymphoma Carcinoid tumour
Adrenocorticotropic hormone (ACTH)	Lung cancer, especially small cell Pancreatic cancer Thymus cancer Bronchial carcinoid Many others less commonly

Table 2.60 Causes of hypocalcaemia	
Vitamin D deficiency states	Sunlight deficiency Dietary deficiency or impaired gut absorption Liver disease Kidney disease
Hypoparathyroid states	Post-parathyroidectomy Parathyroid infiltration (haemochromatosis, Wilson's disease, metastases) Inherited hypoparathyroidism Pseudohypoparathyroidism

What is 'simple' vitamin D deficiency and how does it differ from vitamin D deficiency with secondary hyperparathyroidism?

Biochemical changes in various types of vitamin D deficiency are outlined in Table 2.62.

What are the clinical manifestations of vitamin D deficiency?

The overall result is osteomalacia. This causes bone demineralisation and can cause myopathy and impaired balance.

What is hypoparathyroidism?

This causes hypocalcaemia and hypophosphataemia. It is most commonly the result of parathyroidectomy. Inherited hypoparathyroidism is rare and has numerous genetic causes. Autosomal dominant hypocalcaemia is caused by mutations in the *CasR* gene, which normally negatively regulates PTH secretion from the parathyroids and calcium resorption in the kidney. The mutation actually lowers the threshold for the action of *CasR*, so that PTH is more readily suppressed and calcium is more readily excreted by the kidney.

What is pseudohypoparathyroidism?

This refers to end-organ resistance to PTH, resulting in biochemical changes mirroring hypoparathyroidism, with hypocalcaemia and hyperphosphataemia, but PTH levels are raised. There are various forms of inheritance, one of these the result of mutations in the *GNAS* gene, which encodes a signalling effector on PTH action; the clinical features may include short stature, obesity, short fourth and fifth metacarpals, learning difficulties and basal ganglia calcification, a syndrome known as Albright's hereditary osteodystrophy.

What is pseudopseudohypoparathyroidism?

This refers to the phenotype of pseudohypoparathyroidism, but with normal biochemistry. PTH action on the kidney is normal but because of impaired PTH action on bone there are features of Albright's hereditary osteodystrophy.

Can hypomagnesaemia impair serum calcium?

Hypomagnesaemia can impair PTH secretion or cause PTH resistance and if hypocalcamia results, should if possible be corrected first.

How is acute, symptomatic hypocalcaemia treated?

Intravenous calcium is usually needed for levels under 1.9 mmol/l or with symptoms. Calcium gluconate is less irritating to veins than calcium chloride and is given slowly to avoid arrhythmias, e.g. 10% calcium gluconate 10–20 ml in 50–100 ml 5% dextrose over 10 minutes, repeated as needed. Magnesium may need concurrent correction. Oral calcium and vitamin should also be started.

How is chronic hypocalcaemia treated?

Oral calcium and vitamin D, either 25(OH)D or 1,25(OH)$_2$D, are usually suitable (e.g. alfacalcidol), with magnesium correction if needed.

How is vitamin D deficiency treated?

Dietary deficiency or deficient sunlight exposure may be treated with intramuscular ergocalciferol every few months. 1,25(OH)$_2$D deficiency is the result of chronic kidney disease and results in secondary hyperparathyroidism releasing calcium and phosphate from bone, correcting the hypocalcaemic tendency but at the expense of bone disease and phosphate accumulation, because the latter cannot be cleared in kidney disease. Treatment comprises oral phosphate binders, calcium and 1,25(OH)$_2$D. Newer agents, such as the calcimimetic Mimipara, can reduce PTH secretion (Case 2.26). Hypercalcaemia secondary to vitamin D

Table 2.61 Clinical features of hypocalcaemia	
Paraesthesia	Extremities and circumorally
Chvostek's sign	Twitching of circumoral muscles on gentle tapping of facial nerve just in front of the ear
Trousseau's sign	Carpal spasm on inflation of the blood pressure cuff, which can be very painful
Muscle cramps	Often of legs Carpopedal spasm (tetany) Most threateningly respiratory muscle spasm
Neurological	Altered behaviour Seizures
Cardiac	Prolonged QT interval and risk of ventricular arrhythmias

Table 2.62 Biochemical changes in vitamin D deficiency			
Vitamin D deficiency state	Vitamin D level	Serum calcium	PTH level
'Simple' vitamin D deficiency	Low	Normal	Normal
Vitamin D deficiency with secondary hyperparathyroidism	Low	Low	Raised (secondary, compensatory hyperparathyroidism)
Primary hyperparathyroidism masked by coexistent vitamin D deficiency	Low	Normal	Raised
PTH, parathyroid hormone.			

replacement is sometimes caused by unrecognised, coexistent primary hyperparathyroidism.

Is hypophosphataemia a problem?

This is under-recognised. It can be linked to decreased intake or absorption, vitamin D deficiency, liver disease or hyperparathyroidism. It causes organ dysfunction and along with potassium, magnesium and calcium disturbance should be corrected when low, as in, for example, re-feeding syndrome. It is available as oral phosphate or together with magnesium in magnesium glycerophosphate.

CASE 2.30

HYPONATRAEMIA

Candidate information

Role

You are a doctor in the emergency medical admissions unit. Please read the following letter from the patient's general practitioner. You may make notes on the paper provided. When the bell sounds, enter the examination room to begin the consultation.

Scenario

Dear Doctor

Re: Mr James Blonde, aged 58 years

Thank you for admitting Mr Blonde, who has had a week of diarrhoea and vomiting. He is now hypotensive (blood pressure 70/40), relatively bradycardic (heart rate 55) and tachypnoeic (respiratory rate 20). Examination is otherwise unremarkable. I obtained some blood tests yesterday and the results are appended. Blood tests taken a month ago were normal. His past medical history comprises hypertension, type 2 diabetes, Crohn's disease and a longstanding restrictive lung defect.

Yours sincerely

Test results

Sodium 117 mmol/l, potassium 2.9 mmol/l, creatinine 800 µmol/l, urea 35 mmol/l, calcium 1.80 mmol/l, phosphate 3.11 mmol/l, magnesium 0.50 mmol/l, albumin 28 g/dl, INR 1.8, C-reactive protein 140, haemoglobin 13.2 g/dl, mean cell volume normal, white cell count 11.5×10^9/l, platelets 300×10^9/l (venous blood gases show a marked acidosis – pH 7.05, pCO_2 4.7, pO_2 3.2, bicarbonate 7.3, base excess − 19.0, saturations 97%)

Please take a history from the patient (you may continue to make notes if you wish on the paper provided). Your examiners will warn you when 12 minutes have elapsed. You have 14 minutes to take a history from the patient followed by 1 minute of reflection. There will then follow 5 minutes of discussion with the examiners. Be prepared to discuss solutions to the problems posed by the case and how you might reply to the GP's letter. You are not required to examine the patient.

Patient information

Mr James Blonde is a 58-year-old gentleman who has been unwell for a week with diarrhoea and vomiting. His stools are watery; there is no blood or mucus. He has had some cramping abdominal pains. He now feels exhausted and weak, and has been admitted to hospital because he has developed 'kidney failure'. He is a widower living alone in a bungalow and usually manages well. He mobilises in a wheelchair because of peripheral vascular disease and neuropathy from type 2 diabetes, but has a good degree of assistance with meals and washing from relatives and friends. He also has hypertension, a minor longstanding chronic lung condition which causes minimal breathlessness and Crohn's disease, the latter poorly controlled over the last few years. He carries his list of medications with him and concordance with treatment is excellent. His medications are – metformin, gliclazide, insulin, bendroflumethiazide, atenolol, ramipril, azathioprine and mesalazine. He is not really sure why his GP is so concerned; he feels that once he gets better and starts drinking again things will be alright.

How to approach the case

Data gathering in the interview and interpretation and use of information gathered

Presenting problem(s) and symptom exploration

This is a complicated case, but the presentation of multiple acute problems on a background of multiple chronic diseases is now very common. The way forward is to take a standard history-taking approach to symptoms, with a full past medical history and drug history, and not to feel immediately swamped by the array of biochemical abnormalities. As you compile the information, consider potential triggers to each biochemical abnormality in turn.

Patient perspective

Explain that his GP was concerned that his current gastroenteritis illness has not just made him dehydrated but that his system may have become very sensitive to his medications while very dehydrated and unwell.

Past medical history

Take a list of each condition – type 2 diabetes, hypertension, Crohn's disease and a chronic respiratory condition – and explore the duration, complications and current symptoms of each; try to determine whether each is actively problematic or under control.

Drug and allergy history

The list of drugs is imperative because there are multiple iatrogenic contributors to his metabolic state.

Family history

Relevance here is unlikely.

Social history

Enquire fully into his home circumstances, his level of mobility and the degree of external support.

Table 2.63 Predominant ion composition of fluids		
	Extracellular fluid	**Intracellular fluid**
Cations	Sodium	Potassium Magnesium
Anions	Bicarbonate Chloride	Phosphate Proteins Organic acids

SUMMARY – ASSESSMENT AND PLAN

- Possible contributors to hyponatraemia include bendroflumethiazide, ramipril, diarrhoea and vomiting (with salt loss overriding the hypernatraemia seen in dehydration), hypoadrenalism, and pseudohyponatraemia (his blood glucose is unknown).
- Possible contributors to hypokalaemia include bendroflumethiazide and diarrhoea and vomiting. Hypomagnesaemia tends to have similar causes.
- Possible contributors to acute renal failure include dehydration and ramipril on the background of diabetic nephropathy and renovascular disease. The raised C-reactive protein also suggests sepsis, and immunosuppression and diabetes lower the threshold for this.
- Possible contributors to hypocalcaemia include acute renal failure (failure of conversion of inactive to active vitamin D) and malabsorption of vitamin D due to Crohn's disease.
- Possible contributors to the high INR include malabsorption of vitamin K and sepsis.
- The acidosis is probably caused by acute renal failure but diabetic ketoacidosis should be excluded.
- Immediate management includes fluid resuscitation and correction of life-threatening metabolic abnormalities. All drugs should be stopped and an insulin sliding-scale regimen started. Empiric antimicrobials might be considered.
- Calcium should be corrected first, before the acidosis, otherwise there is a risk of tetany.
- Hypokalaemia should also be corrected before acidosis, and can be given intravenously with magnesium.

Discussion

How is fluid distributed throughout the body and how does oedema arise?

The volume of total body water is approximately 45 litres. One-third of this is extracellular fluid (ECF) comprising plasma (3.5 l) and interstitial or tissue fluid (8.5 l) and two-thirds is intracellular fluid (ICF). The predominant ion composition of fluids is given in Table 2.63. Fluid flow between plasma and interstitium depends on the balance between outward pressures (capillary hydrostatic pressure, tissue oncotic pressure) and inward pressures (interstitial fluid pressure, plasma oncotic pressure). Oedema results when interstitial fluid increases because of a pressure gradient or excess capillary permeability.

What is osmolality?

Osmolality refers to the number of particles (osmoles) dissolved in 1 kg of solution (osmolarity refers to 1 litre rather than 1 kg). The main determinant of ECF osmolality is sodium and that of ICF osmolality is potassium. Normal plasma osmolality is 280–295 mOsmol/kg. Normal urine osmolality is 50–1400 mOsmol/kg (extremes, but commonly 500–800 mOsmol/kg).

How is sodium regulated?

Sodium is the prime ECF cation, the prime determinant of ECF osmolality and thus the prime determinant of ECF/ICF water distribution. The major sodium regulators are the kidney, aldosterone [Cases 2.31 (metabolic acidosis) and 2.14 (hypertension)] and antidiuretic hormone (ADH), otherwise known as vasopressin. ADH is the great evolutionary stress hormone – when sabre tooth tigers munched the limbs of our ancestors, ADH retained fluid by enhancing permeability at the collecting duct and made platelets sticky. Other contributors include atrial natriuretic peptide, angiotensin II (which may increase sodium reabsorption in the proximal tubule as well as promoting aldosterone), sympathetic nervous system activity (which also acts on the proximal tubule) and local paracrine factors such as endothelin-1, bradykinin and nitric oxide (which may inhibit sodium reabsorption in the collecting duct as well as altering vascular tone).

What happens to serum osmolality in dehydration?

Reduced body water leads to a rise in plasma osmolality, which is detected by osmotically sensitive neurons in the circumventricular organ of the hypothalamus which stimulate thirst and stimulate the paraventricular nucleus and supraoptic nucleus, the sites of ADH or 'sabre tooth tiger hormone'. These mechanisms increase total body water and return plasma osmolality to the normal range. At around 284 mOsm/kg ADH thirst is switched off to prevent over-hydration.

What are the causes of hyponatraemia?

Hyponatraemia is the commonest electrolyte disturbance. Mild hyponatraemia (126–135 mmol/l) is very common. Hyponatraemia is usually caused by relative water gain or sodium loss but is far more often the result of excess water relative to sodium. It may be spurious or true.

Pseudohyponatraemia

Spurious (laboratory assay) hyponatraemia occurs when protein (paraproteinaemias), lipid (hyperlipidaemias) or glucose (diabetic ketoacidosis) is high and plasma is hypertonic or isotonic. Parameters must be severely deranged to provoke significant pseudohyponatraemia – severe myeloma, hereditary dyslipidaemia or severe keto-acidosis (a 5 mmol/l glucose rise leads to an approximate 1.5 mmol/l drop in sodium).

True hyponatraemia

True hyponatraemia is always dilutional, with a low plasma osmolality (hypo-osmolar) indicating that water intake exceeds renal capacity to excrete it. Since normal kidneys can excrete up to 30 litres of dilute urine (< 100 mOsm/kg) daily, hyponatraemia usually occurs when the kidneys fail to generate and excrete enough solute-free water to balance intake. True hyponatraemia occurs in four groups of settings (Table 2.64).

What is cerebral salt wasting?

Hyponatraemia in the setting of traumatic brain injury or cranial surgery is often assumed to be the result of syndrome of inappropriate ADH (SIADH). It may be, but it is thought that the natriuretic peptides released in cerebral insults (mechanism unclear) also cause natriuresis and diuresis, leading to hyponatraemia and hypovolaemia.

What are the consequences of hyponatraemia?

When exposed to a hypotonic environment, cells tend to swell. The symptoms and signs of hyponatraemia depend both on its severity and the rapidity of the fall. Cerebral oedema is more likely the faster the fall. The body hates cell swelling, particularly the brain in its closed cavity where it can cause seizures and ultimately death. ADH levels are therefore normally low. Relative ADH excess plays a role in most causes of hyponatraemia because the body sees sodium as the instigator of cell swelling and water as the innocently seduced bystander. Hypernatraemia is therefore rare.

What is central pontine myelinosis (CPM)?

Cells adapt to the threat of cell swelling by limiting production of intracellular solutes to balance extracellular hypo-osmolality and maintain cell volume. Rapid correction of hyponatraemia, especially if chronic and adaptive (> 48 hours), may cause rapid cell shrinkage and the risk of osmotic demyelination syndrome, or CPM, e.g. spastic quadriparesis and pseudobulbar palsy. Extrapontine myelinosis occurs in 10% of cases, e.g. ataxia. Symptoms start two to three days after correction. A formula for sodium correction rates is available but in general correction should be limited to a few mmol/l over 24 hours (less than 12 mmol/l correction over 24 hours or less than 0.5 mmol/l per hour).

How should acute symptomatic hyponatraemia be treated?

Seizures and altered consciousness are an emergency and pose a high risk of cerebral herniation and death. Prompt treatment to prevent cerebral oedema may include hypertonic saline in an intensive-care environment to strictly monitor sodium rise, although some would say the risks of this therapy are never warranted. The risk of CPM is less in reversal of acute hyponatraemia but treatment should be stopped when asymptomatic, regardless of sodium concentration.

What are the causes of hypernatraemia?

Hypernatraemia is rare and usually the result of a failure to drink water (limited availability or blunted thirst mechanism). Even when the kidneys cannot excrete urine of low volume and high osmolality (> 1000 mOsm/kg) as in diabetes insipidus, hypernatraemia is rare. Some cell shrinkage occurs in hypernatraemia, but is minimised by other osmolytes. Rapid fluid replacement is dangerous because adapted cells may swell in the hypotonic environment.

What is the daily sodium requirement and how much sodium is there in normal saline?

60–100 mmol and 154 mmol/l, respectively.

Do the above figures influence sodium and fluid management of a patient with systemic inflammatory response syndrome?

A healthy person might ingest 100 mmol of sodium and 2500 ml of water daily and produce 2000 ml of urine and maintain a serum osmolality of 285 and normal urine osmolality. A dehydrated person might ingest only a litre of water and produce a litre of urine (minimum daily output is 500–750 ml) but maintain the same serum and urine osmolalities. An excessive water drinker might ingest 5000 ml of water daily, produce 5000 ml of urine and maintain the same serum and urine osmolalities.

The systemic inflammatory response involves inflammation (with increased vascular permeability and leakage of water, electrolytes and albumin), activation of the catecholamine and renin–angiotensin–aldosterone systems to retain salt and water, and metabolic effects such as cytokines that increase catabolism and raise urea and nitrogen loads and hence a need for increased urine output. Such patients frequently receive normal saline, but because of multi-organ failure and poor urine output they may rapidly become salt and water overloaded. Fluid restriction then

Table 2.64 The four settings of true hyponatraemia

	Causes	Volume status	Clinical signs	Biochemical changes	Treatment
Psychogenic polydipsia	Excess water drinking	Euvolaemic	Excess drinking High urine output	Hyponatraemia Urine sodium < 20 mmol/l	Water restriction
Unavoidable sodium loss	Renal loss due to tubular dysfunction or diuretics Hypoadrenalism Gastrointestinal loss Pancreatitis or skin loss in burns	Hypovolaemic/dehydrated	Tachycardia Hypotension Low jugular venous pulse (JVP) Decreased skin turgor Dry mucous membranes	Raised urea Natriuresis (urine sodium > 20 mmol/l) suggests renal sodium losses (thiazides the commonest cause of hypovolaemic hyponatraemia), or less commonly hypoadrenalism or cerebral salt wasting; some authorities use a threshold of 30 mmol rather than 20 mmol.	Rehydration Treat cause
Appropriate antidiuretic hormone (ADH) excess (body perceives volume depletion)	Cardiac failure Cirrhosis Nephrotic syndrome	Hypervolaemic/oedematous	Peripheral, sacral and pulmonary oedema Ascites Raised JVP (excess sodium and water but water gain proportionately greater)		Diuretics Fluid restriction treat cause
Syndrome of inappropriate ADH excess (SIADH)	Tumours, e.g. lung, mesothelioma, ureteric, pancreatic, duodenal, lymphoma, endometrial, leukaemia Lung disease, e.g. abscess, empyema pneumonia Central nervous system disease, e.g. tumour, abscess, hydrocephalus, haemorrhage, meningitis, encephalitis, acute intermittent porphyria Drugs, e.g. phenothiazines, tricyclics, ecstasy, carbamazepine, cyclophosphamide, selective serotonin reuptake inhibitors (SSRIs)	Euvolaemic	Signs of underlying cause	Urine is inappropriately concentrated in the setting of hyponatraemia Essential diagnostic criteria are: • Plasma osmolality < 270 mOsm/kg • Inappropriate urinary concentration (UOsm > 100 mOsm/kg) • Elevated urinary sodium (> 40 mmol/l) in presence of normal salt and water intake • Normal extracellular volume • Exclusion of hypothyroidism and glucocorticoid deficiency	Water restriction to 800–1200 ml/day Demeclocycline (inhibits ADH at the distal tubule, inducing nephrogenic diabetes insipidus) and may take a few days to work

Box 2.68 Diabetes insipidus

This is the result of antidiuretic hormone (ADH) deficiency or resistance to its action.

Cranial diabetes insipidus (CDI)

This is uncommon, because 80% of ADH-secreting neurons must be destroyed. It may be primary (possibly autoimmune) or secondary to trauma, tumours, craniopharyngioma, radiotherapy, infiltration (granulomatous, haemochromatosis), infection, human immunodeficiency virus, pregnancy (placental vasopressinase) or vascular compromise (Sheehan's syndrome, post-coronary artery bypass grafting).

Nephrogenic (NDI)

This may be primary, or secondary to chronic kidney disease, metabolic disturbance (hypokalaemia, hypercalcaemia), drugs (lithium is the commonest cause, accounting for 15% of NDI, demeclocycline), osmotic diuresis (glycosuria, poorly controlled diabetes) or systemic disease with tubular damage (amyloid, sickle cell disease, myeloma).

increases serum osmolality, with metabolic acidosis, and stimulates further water-retaining mechanisms including ADH release. Such patients often remain very unwell with the added complication of oedema. Ideal fluid replacement would provide maximum volume replacement with minimum salt and water loading. It does not exist, but normal saline is far from physiological and colloids may be preferable. This is, however, contentious because some colloids carry the potential for anaphylaxis, but newer albumin and starch solutions may be preferable.

What are the causes of polyuria?

Polyuria occurs because of excess thirst, which is rare (e.g. compulsive water drinking, hypothalamic infiltration, drugs such as anticholinergics) or diabetes insipidus (Box 2.68).

What is the water deprivation test?

This is a two-step test.

1. Dehydration step: 8-hour water deprivation

Normally a rise in osmolality stimulates osmoreceptors to promote ADH release and urine output falls, with a healthy rise in urine osmolality to > 700 mOsm/kg. Theoretically, primary thirst disorders have normal physiology and should respond to dehydration with appropriate urine concentration, whereas diabetes insipidus [cranial (CDI) or nephrogenic (NDI)] is unable to respond and urine remains dilute.

2. Desmopressin step

If DI is suspected, desmopressin is administered subcutaneously or intramuscularly. CDI responds with a rise in urine osmolality, while NDI does not. Desmopressin is thus a suitable treatment for CDI.

POISONING AND METABOLIC DISTURBANCE

Candidate information

Role

You are a doctor in the emergency medical admissions unit. Please read the following letter from the patient's general practitioner. You may make notes on the paper provided. When the bell sounds, enter the examination room to begin the consultation.

Scenario

Dear Doctor

Re: Ms Anita Radcliff, aged 24 years

Thank you for admitting this young lady who has taken an overdose of paracetamol following an argument with her boyfriend. She took the overdose yesterday evening and came to the surgery today to tell somebody. Please do the needful.

Yours sincerely

Please take a history from the patient (you may continue to make notes if you wish on the paper provided). Your examiners will warn you when 12 minutes have elapsed. You have 14 minutes to take a history from the patient followed by 1 minute of reflection. There will then follow 5 minutes of discussion with the examiners. Be prepared to discuss solutions to the problems posed by the case and how you might reply to the GP's letter. You are not required to examine the patient.

Patient information

Ms Anita Radcliff is a 24-year-old lady who took thirty 500-mg paracetamol tablets last night, around 12 hours ago. She also took 28 aspirin tablets. She subsequently feels a little anxious and breathless. She has no medical history of note, with no history of psychiatric disease or suicide attempts. She has now been admitted to hospital, having seen her GP. She did not want to die but took the overdose on impulse following an argument with her boyfriend. She subsequently told a friend what had happened who told her that paracetamol could cause liver damage and persuaded her to see her doctor. She is unaware that aspirin is also dangerous and will not volunteer this information to a doctor unless asked about other tablets. She also thinks she might be pregnant as she has missed her period and has not got around to telling her boyfriend this. She is now keen to go home if a blood test is normal.

How to approach the case

Data gathering in the interview and interpretation and use of information gathered

Presenting problem(s) and symptom exploration

▪ **Establish facts about the overdose**   Establish exactly what was taken, and when. Through a careful, empathetic approach, assuring her of confidentiality and that you are here to help, she will be likely to tell you exactly what she took, but ask specifically about other tablets as well as paracetamol. Explain that the first, urgent thing to do is to take blood for paracetamol and salicylate levels. The fact that she is breathless could represent anxiety, but acid–base disturbance from salicylate poisoning must go through your mind.

▪ **Establish events around the overdose**   Ask about events preceding the act, reasons for the act, suicide intent and support networks.

▪ **Assess suicide risk**   Ask if she took the overdose alone, about precautions to avoid discovery, whether with active preparation or on impulse, and why she alerted her friend and agreed to see her GP. Ask how she feels now about life.

Patient perspective

Show empathy. She is probably frightened. Assure her that you will firstly ascertain whether her overdose needs treatment, and that you can also establish whether or not she is pregnant, as this could have a bearing on monitoring and treatment.

Past medical history

Establish that there is no past history of psychiatric disease.

Drug and allergy history

Ask about all drugs including non-prescription ones.

Family history

Establish if there is any family history of psychiatric disease.

Social history

Ask about alcohol and drugs.

SUMMARY – ASSESSMENT AND PLAN

- Urgent blood tests include routine haematobiochemistry with liver function (INR especially important), paracetamol and salicylate levels, arterial blood gases and a pregnancy test (urine or blood β human chorionic gonadotrophin).
- She should be treated with *N*-acetyl cysteine (Parvolex) according to the nomogram.
- If she is pregnant then her case should be discussed with your consultant and potentially the poisons information service and an obstetrician.
- She should stay in hospital until it can be established that she is well and her blood tests are satisfactory, and until she has seen a psychiatrist.

Discussion

How is acid–base balance regulated?

Acids are hydrogen ion (H^+) donors and bases are H^+ acceptors. The main source of H^+ is oxidation of carbon compounds ($CO_2 + H_2O \rightleftharpoons HCO_3^- + H^+$). Buffers minimise changes in pH either by binding H^+ or by dissociating to release H^+. Buffers include intracellular fluid (50%) and plasma bicarbonate, phosphate, proteins and red cells.

What acid–base balance disturbances do you know of?

These are listed in Table 2.65.

pH reflects H^+ concentration on a logarithmic scale such that a small change in H^+ concentration causes a large change in pH. It may not therefore take very long in acute illness with lactic acid accumulation to fall from a normal pH of 7.4 to, for example, 7.1. However, CO_2 has a direct relationship with ventilation; if breathing at 5 l/minute were to give a pCO_2 of 5 kPa, then breathing at 2.5 l/minute would give an increased pCO_2 of 10 kPa and if hyperventilating at 10 l/minute the pCO_2 would fall to 2.5 kPa. Metabolic disturbances might be analysed by the bicarbonate or the base excess or deficit, the latter simply implying the amount of base needed to return the pH to normal.

Note that the pH gives the primary disturbance (acidaemia or alkalaemia), and this is useful to remember when interpreting arterial blood gases where there is compensation. For example, a patient with a high pH, hypocapnia, a low bicarbonate and appreciably negative base excess has primary respiratory alkalosis with metabolic compensation – the pH may correct with metabolic compensation but will not overshoot and overcorrect, i.e. this example could not be primary metabolic acidosis with respiratory compensation, although there is one exception in this example and that is salicylate poisoning because salicylates both stimulate the respiratory centre and cause metabolic acidosis to provoke a mixed picture. A patient with chronic obstructive pulmonary disease and primary respiratory acidosis may have a raised bicarbonate but this metabolic compensation will not overcorrect the pH to produce alkalosis. A patient with primary metabolic acidosis may hyperventilate with respiratory compensation but the hyperventilation will not tend to overcorrect the pH and produce alkalosis.

Table 2.65 Types of acid–base disturbance

Principal disturbance	Primary change	Secondary compensation
Metabolic acidosis	↓ HCO_3	↓ pCO_2
Metabolic alkalosis	↑ HCO_3	↑ pCO_2
Respiratory acidosis	↑ pCO_2	↑ HCO_3
Respiratory alkalosis	↓ pCO_2	↓ HCO_3

Table 2.66 Causes of increased anion gap metabolic acidosis

	Anions	Features
Ketoacidosis	Ketotic pathway	Diabetic ketoacidosis
Uraemia	Organic acids	Renal failure
Salicylate poisoning	Salicylic acid	Also respiratory alkalosis
Methanol poisoning	Formic acid	Visual disturbance
Alcohol/starvation	Ketotic pathway	
Lactic acidosis	Lactic acid	Ischaemia/infarction/sepsis
Ethylene glycol	Glycolate/oxalate	Oxalate crystals/renal failure

What are the causes of metabolic acidosis?

These can be associated with an increased or a normal anion gap.

Anion gap = plasma (sodium + potassium) − (chloride + bicarbonate)

i.e. normal anion gap = $(146 + 4) - (110 + 24)$

The normal value is 16 ± 2 mmol/l. The 'gap' comprises unmeasured anions such as albumin, phosphate and sulphate.

Increased anion gap metabolic acidosis

This is usually the result of the addition of endogenous or exogenous organic acid. A mnemonic for remembering its causes is KUSMALE – think of Kussmaul breathing in diabetic ketoacidosis (Table 2.66).

Normal anion gap metabolic acidosis

This is usually the result of loss of bicarbonate. Compensatory chloride retention maintains a normal gap and hence this is sometimes described as hyperchloraemic (and often hypokalaemic) metabolic acidosis. Causes include:

- Diarrhoea (loss of bicarbonate)
- Ureterosigmoidostomy (loss of bicarbonate)
- Renal tubular acidosis (RTA) (loss of bicarbonate in proximal RTA, impaired H^+ excretion in distal RTA)
- Ammonium chloride
- Acetazolamide

What are the causes of metabolic alkalosis?

Metabolic alkalosis is caused by a loss of H^+ or the addition of bicarbonate. Gastrointestinal H^+ losses include vomiting and intestinal secretions. Renal losses include diuretics, hyperaldosteronism, Cushing's syndrome and liquorice ingestion.

What are the causes of respiratory acidosis?

Respiratory acidosis is caused by hypoventilation.

What are the causes of respiratory alkalosis?

Respiratory alkalosis is caused by hyperventilation, e.g. anxiety, salicylate overdose, hypoxia (e.g. pulmonary embolism), fever, thyrotoxicosis.

Do you know anything about ethylene glycol and methanol poisoning?

Ethylene glycol is a constituent of antifreeze and screen wash. Toxicity is characterised by a severe high anion gap metabolic acidosis and calcium oxalate crystals in the urine. Following ingestion, peak serum concentration is reached in 1–4 hours and the sequence of clinical events is as follows:

- Stage 1 (30 min–12 hours): central nervous system disturbances
- Stage 2 (12–24 hours): metabolic acidosis and cardiopulmonary effects
- Stage 3 (24–72 hours): acute renal failure

Symptoms of methanol toxicity include weakness, nausea and headache. Eye effects include reduced vision, mydriasis and hyperaemia of the optic disc. Optic atrophy secondary to optic nerve anoxia can lead to blindness.

Treatments for ethylene glycol or methanol intoxication include fomepizole (first line), ethanol and haemodialysis.

What is the role of the proximal tubule and what disorders can occur here?

Exchange of H^+–Na^+ occurs in the proximal tubule, providing luminal H^+ for reclaiming most filtered bicarbonate. Two-thirds of filtered Na^+ (the prime determinant of extracellular fluid volume) and 80% of filtered water is reabsorbed here. Glucose and amino acids are reabsorbed completely here via a carrier protein. Also reabsorbed are phosphate (80%), urate (90%), potassium, chloride, calcium, urea (each approximately 50%) and a small amount of magnesium.

Glycosuria occurs when the 'renal threshold' for reabsorption (plasma glucose 10 mmol/l) is exceeded as in diabetes mellitus or in a genetic defect in the sodium–glucose transporter. Various aminoacidurias (e.g. Hartnup's disease, homocystinuria, cystinuria) result from defective amino acid transporters. In cystinuria there is excess secretion of cystine, ornithine, arginine and lysine (COAL), causing high urinary cystine levels and calculi. This is not the same disease as cystinosis, in which intracellular accumulation of the amino acid cystine disrupts tubular transport and can lead to renal Fanconi syndrome (failure of proximal tubule function) and renal failure. Renal tubular acidosis can also affect the proximal tubule.

What is the role of the loop of Henle, and how do loop diuretics work?

The loop of Henle comprises a proximal straight tubule, a thin descending limb, and thin and thick ascending limbs. It reabsorbs important additional sodium, water, potassium, chloride, calcium and magnesium. A Na^+/K^+-ATPase pump in the basolateral (non-luminal) membrane exchanges these two ions to maintain a baseline low intracellular sodium concentration, but this encourages sodium influx via the apical (luminal) membrane from the lumen, and this is coupled with one potassium and two chloride ions in a unique 'triple cotransporter' (sodium, potassium, chloride) carrier molecule.

Loop diuretics bind to the chloride site of this carrier molecule and inhibit triple cotransport and water transport. A potassium channel normally redirects some intracellular potassium back into the lumen but loop diuretics inhibit this too and encourage a gradient for calcium and magnesium to efflux into the lumen. Traditional thinking was that diuretics prompted compensatory aldosterone action on an H^+–Na^+ pump and that the resultant loss of H^+ caused alkalosis. However, loop diuretics seem to also enhance local bicarbonate uptake as the H^+–Na^+ pump operates faster to compensate for the diuretic action. Therefore, loop diuretics cause a hyponatraemic, hypokalaemic, hypomagnesaemic, hypocalcaemic, hypercalciuric (predisposing to calculi) metabolic alkalosis.

What is Bartter's syndrome?

Bartter's syndrome is a genetic defect of the triple cotransporter and numerous mutations have been described. It is a genetic loop diuretic.

How do thiazide diuretics work?

Fluid entering the distal tubule is hypo-osmotic. Here an apical sodium chloride cotransporter promotes sodium (and chloride) reabsorption (such that final excretion is < 1% of what is filtered) and calcium efflux into the lumen. Thiazide diuretics block the cotransporter and cause similar biochemical changes to loop diuretics, except that they may cause hypercalcaemia.

What is Gitelman's syndrome?

Gitelman's syndrome is a genetic defect of the above cotransporter. It is a 'genetic' thiazide.

What is the role of the terminal distal tubule and what is the effect of aldosterone here?

Aldosterone is secreted by the zona glomerulosa of the adrenal cortex in response to raised angiotensin II and high plasma potassium. It stimulates the absorption of Na^+ ions (via an H^+–Na^+ pump and apical Na^+ channel), exchanging these for K^+ and H^+. Some potassium-sparing diuretics inhibit aldosterone. Aldosterone disorders are discussed in Case 2.14 and the role of aldosterone in potassium disorders is discussed in Case 2.25.

What is the role of the collecting duct and antidiuretic hormone (ADH)?

The final common regulator of volume is ADH, which binds to the vasopressin-2 receptor (AVPR-2) on the basolateral membrane of the collecting duct. An intracellular cascade promotes insertion of the water-permeable channel aquaporin-2 into the apical membrane. A defective AVPR-2 or aquaporin-2 causing end-organ resistance

to ADH gives rise to nephrogenic diabetes insipidus (Case 2.30).

What is renal tubular acidosis (RTA)?

Various abnormalities of tubule mechanisms give rise to the normal anion gap hyperchloraemic metabolic acidosis of the various types of RTA. Type 1 RTA and type 2 RTA cause hypokalaemia; type 4 RTA causes hyperkalaemia. Renal function is usually normal.

Type 1 or distal RTA

The cells of the distal nephron normally acidify urine. Because of a defective apical H^+-ATPase in the distal tubule, the tubule cannot excrete H^+ or reabsorb sodium. This stimulates aldosterone, causing hypokalaemia. Bicarbonate buffering decreases serum bicarbonate levels (and reclamation of bicarbonate is functionally linked to H^+ secretion by H^+ ATPase) and bone buffering leads to release of calcium. Causes include autoimmune diseases such as systemic lupus erythematosus, hypergammaglobulinaemia, nephrocalcinosis (primary hyperparathyroidism, vitamin D excess, medullary sponge kidney), tubulointerstitial damage from drugs such as non-steroidal anti-inflammatory drugs and tubule pressure damage in obstructive uropathy. Patients may present with hypokalaemic complications, renal calculi or bone pain (late). Diagnosis is by serum biochemistry and is confirmed by alkaline urine, which fails to acidify to pH < 5.2 following an ammonium chloride acid load.

An autosomal recessive form of distal RTA is caused by a mutation in the apical H^+-ATPase. Some patients develop sensorineural hearing loss, probably because of a defective cochlear H^+-ATPase. An autosomal dominant form of distal RTA is recognised because of mutations in *AE1*, a basolateral chloride–bicarbonate anion exchanger which must be fully operational if bicarbonate reclaimed from lumen to tubule cell is to progress onwards from tubule cell to bloodstream.

Type 2 or proximal RTA

The H^+-sodium pump in the proximal tubule (above) operates but only slowly, so that bicarbonate recovery is slow. Causes include paraproteinaemias (amyloid), cystinosis and Wilson's disease, which may also induce wider proximal tubule damage resulting in Fanconi syndrome (failure to reabsorb glucose, phosphate and organic amino acids). Diagnosis is by serum biochemistry and detection of alkaline urine (bicarbonaturia). The urine can acidify because there is slowing rather than complete inhibition of normal function.

Type 4 RTA (associated aldosterone deficiency or resistance)

Aldosterone deficiency may be primary (Addison's disease) or secondary (to hyporeninaemia). Aldosterone resistance may be congenital (pseudohypoaldosteronism) or acquired (ACE inhibitors, potassium-sparing diurectics, systemic lupus erythematosus, amyloid, obstructive uropathy, diabetes). Aldosterone disorders are discussed in Case 2.14.

HAEMATOLOGICAL PROBLEMS

CASE 2.32

ANAEMIA

Candidate information

Role

You are a doctor in the medical outpatient clinic. Please read the following letter from the patient's general practitioner. You may make notes on the paper provided. When the bell sounds, enter the examination room to begin the consultation.

Scenario

Dear Doctor

Re: Mr Jim Case, aged 68 years

Thank you for seeing this gentleman with a haemoglobin of 8.2 g/dl. He has complained of several episodes of feeling tired and light-headed over the past six months and his haemoglobin a year ago was 11.5 g/dl. His current renal function is normal. His blood pressure is satisfactory. He had a sigmoid resection four years ago for colorectal cancer and no longer appears to be under surveillance for this and I wonder if he requires repeat colonoscopy and exclusion of other causes of anaemia.

Yours sincerely

Please take a history from the patient (you may continue to make notes if you wish on the paper provided). Your examiners will warn you when 12 minutes have elapsed. You have 14 minutes to take a history from the patient followed by 1 minute of reflection. There will then follow 5 minutes of discussion with the examiners. Be prepared to discuss solutions to the problems posed by the case and how you might reply to the GP's letter. You are not required to examine the patient.

Patient information

Mr Jim Case is a 68-year-old gentleman who for the last 12 months has felt increasingly tired and weak, and on occasion dizzy, although he has never passed out. His wife died a year ago, and since then he has been eating very little. He never cooks, and manages for the most part on 'cereal and toast'. He and his wife used to enjoy an active social life, and half a bottle of wine daily each was typical. Now he drinks closer to a bottle. He has hitherto been a generally well and active man. Four years ago he had an operation to remove part of the bowel for a malignant polyp but was subsequently given 'the all clear'. He has had no bleeding

per rectum (the mode of presentation of his bowel problem four years ago) and no other gastrointestinal symptoms. He has lost around 5 kg in weight. He takes aspirin (some years ago he was told it might be protective against bowel cancer) but no other drugs. He misses his wife dreadfully and sees life without her as bleak. He is now not too concerned about recurrence of bowel cancer; he would consider investigation for causes of anaemia, but only because his grandchildren make life tolerable.

How to approach the case

Data gathering in the interview and interpretation and use of information gathered

Presenting problem/s and symptom exploration

▪ **Consider possible causes**   Ask about possible sources of blood loss, especially rectal bleeding, dyspepsia and alarm symptoms. In females you would always ask about menorrhagia or vaginal bleeding.

▪ **Ask about symptoms**
- Ask about fatigue, presyncope or breathlessness.
- Very severe anaemia (not the case here) of any cause may cause high output cardiac failure.
- Megaloblastosis may occur outside the bloodstream; overt subacute combined degeneration of the cord (SACDC) is rare, but there may be paraesthesia and impaired vibration sense.
- Marrow infiltration of any cause can cause leucopenia (sepsis) and thrombocytopenia (petechiae).

Patient perspective

Try to establish why he has presented now, his thoughts about what his symptoms and anaemia might represent, and his keenness or otherwise for investigation. Here, keep closely in mind that bereavement and depression are likely to be playing a key role.

Past medical history

The history of colorectal cancer may be relevant. Ask about possible malabsorption symptoms such as diarrhoea or steatorrhoea (Crohn's disease, coeliac disease) and any history of autoimmune disease or gastrectomy (vitamin B12 deficiency).

Drug and allergy history

Ask about drugs that can provoke gastrointestinal bleeding, e.g. aspirin, non-steroidal anti-inflammatory drugs (NSAIDs), warfarin.

Family history

Relevance here is unlikely.

Social history

Dwell considerably on this. Discover why he has been drinking more and eating less and the impact of his bereavement on his feelings of social isolation and loneliness. Find out what, if any, support structures he currently has (family, friends, neighbours) and whether or not he goes out any more.

- Possible causes of anaemia include recurrence of colorectal cancer, aspirin-induced gastritis or ulcers, and dietary deficiency.
- He should have a full examination, including digital rectal examination.
- Investigations should include estimation of his red cell parameters, haematinics (ferritin, folate, vitamin B_{12}), and a biochemical profile including liver function. Ferritin might be raised in malignancy, hiding iron deficiency. Faecal occult blood testing is generally of no value in population screening.
- Colonoscopy and oesophagogastroduodenoscopy with duodenal biopsy should almost certainly be offered to him. The British Society of Gastroenterologists recommends that all iron deficiency requires oesophagogastroduodenoscopy and colonoscopy or barium enema (a computed tomography scan in frail elderly may be a reasonable substitute); sigmoidoscopy is insufficient. Occasionally small-bowel-related iron deficiency (e.g. some cases of coeliac disease or covert Crohn's) is to blame.
- Transfusion (not least because of its known and unknown potential risks, e.g. West Nile virus, new variant Creutzfeldt–Jakob disease, Simian foamy virus) is now only considered if patients are markedly symptomatic or the haemoglobin is around 8 g/dl or less; it should not be considered in megaloblastosis.
- Other possible contributors to anaemia could include myelodysplasia, anaemia of chronic disease (although no suggestion here) or non-gastrointestinal malignancy, notably renal cell carcinoma.
- His bereavement and depression warrant specific, specialist help.

Discussion

What are the general signs of anaemia?

There is pallor of conjunctival membranes, buccal membranes, palmar creases and nail beds. Iron deficiency anaemia may produce ridged brittle nails, koilonychia or spoon-shaped nails, angular stomatitis and dysphagia. Megaloblastic anaemia may produce atrophic glossitis. Haemolytic anaemia can lead to jaundice.

What is anaemia?

This refers to low haemoglobin concentration, which may occur if haemoglobin synthesis fails or if red blood cells are prematurely destroyed.

What do you know about iron uptake, transport and storage?

An average diet contains 15 mg of daily iron, of which 1 mg is absorbed from the duodenum and jejunum, increasing to a maximum of 3–4 mg in deficiency. The *HFE* gene product (abnormal in genetic haemochromatosis) is one protein responsible for its uptake. Iron is transported in plasma bound to transferrin, and cells requiring iron express receptors to which transferrin delivers its iron. In iron deficiency, the number of transferrin receptors, and hence total iron-binding capacity (TIBC), increases. Iron is stored in the liver and reticuloendothelial system (RES), and incorporated into haemoglobin in the bone marrow.

How might you confirm reduced iron status?

Serum iron status markers, peripheral blood film and bone marrow aspirate findings are shown in Table 2.67.

List some causes of microcytic anaemia

- Iron deficiency anaemia
- Thalassaemia
- Sideroblastic anaemia (failure of iron incorporation in cells leading to defective erythropoiesis)

How is sideroblastic anaemia treated?

If there is no reversible cause (e.g. myelodysplasia), folic acid 5 mg daily may counteract ineffective erythropoiesis. Transfusion is often required, and desferrioxamine may be needed in iron overload.

What is anaemia of chronic disease?

This occurs in a wide variety of inflammatory, infectious and neoplastic disorders but the severity of the anaemia does not correlate with the severity of the underlying systemic disease. Anaemia is initially normochromic and normocytic but tends to become hypochromic and microcytic with time, when small molecules like hepcidin involved in the pathogenesis inhibit iron absorption and inhibit iron release from macrophages. Since ferritin tends to be raised in inflammatory disease, the transferrin receptor assay is useful in identifying iron deficiency. Recombinant human erythropoietin, commonly used in CKD, is probably underused in malignancy – related anaemia and could reduce blood transfusion.

List some causes of normochromic normocytic anaemia

- Chronic disease
- Chronic kidney disease (anaemia of chronic disease as well as reduced erythropoietin) – irregular, spiky red blood cells called echinocytes or Burr cells sometimes seen
- Pregnancy
- Bone marrow failure

What is megaloblastic anaemia?

Megaloblastic anaemia is characterised by macrocytosis and megaloblastic erythropoiesis. The common denominator is faulty DNA synthesis resulting from deficiency of vitamin B12 or folate. It is occasionally the result of drugs inhibiting metabolism, e.g. azathioprine, aciclovir, hydroxyurea.

List some conditions which can cause macrocytosis

- Megaloblastosis (B12 or folate deficiency)
- Haemolysis or acute blood loss (abundant reticulocytes of larger diameter)
- Liver disease, especially alcohol, which alters red cell membrane lipids

Table 2.67 Differentiating microcytic anaemias and anaemias with altered iron status

	Iron deficiency	Thalassaemia trait	Sideroblastic anaemia	Anaemia of chronic disease
Causes	Blood loss Dietary deficiency	Genetic	Acquired, e.g. myelodysplasia, lead poisoning Congenital	Systemic inflammatory disease
Peripheral blood film				
MCV (normal 78–100 fl) and MCH	Microcytic and hypochromic (defective haemoglobinisation)	Marked microcytosis	Typically dimorphic with small population of microcytic, hypochromic red cells Mild macrocytosis usual in elderly Anaemia may be severe	Normochromic and normocytic initially Microcytic and hypochromic later
Other	Sometimes elongated pencil cells Occasional target cells (ring of pallor due to defective haemoglobinisation) ↑ red cell distribution width (RDW) – a measure of MCV uniformity	Basophilic stippling (RNA remains in cells with defective Hb) sometimes seen in thalassaemias and lead poisoning	Pancytopenia confers poor prognosis in myelodysplasia – high risk of transformation to acute myeloid leukaemia	Other anaemias often coexist altering the picture, e.g. iron deficiency
Serum iron status markers				
Serum iron	↓	Normal/↑	↑	↓
Transferrin/total iron binding capacity	↑	Normal	Normal	↓
Transferrin saturation	↓	Normal/↑	↑	↓
Ferritin	↓ (may be ↑ if concurrent inflammation)	Normal/↑	↑	Normal/↑
Soluble transferrin receptor assay	↑	Normal	Normal	Normal
Bone marrow				
Bone marrow erythroblast iron stores (Perl's stain)	↓ or absent stores and absent siderotic granules with normal cellularity	Normal/↑	↓	Normal/↑
Sideroblasts	↓/Absent	Present	Ring sideroblasts due to failure to incorporate iron into haemoglobin	Absent

Hb, haemoglobin; MCH, mean corpuscular haemoglobin; MCV, mean corpuscular volume.

- Hypothyroidism
- Pregnancy
- Myelodysplasia (dyserythropoiesis)

List some causes of vitamin B12 or folate deficiency

These are listed in Table 2.68.

What abnormalities may appear on a megaloblastic peripheral blood film?

Oval macrocytes and hypersegmented neutrophils (more than five lobes to the nucleus) are common. Bone marrow examination is seldom necessary with vitamin B12 and folate assays but would show increased cellularity, loss of fat spaces and accumulation of precursor cells – erythroid precursors, 'giant' metamyelocytes and megaloblasts. At all stages nuclei are primitive with an open 'lacy' chromatin pattern.

What is 'pernicious' anaemia?

This is the most common cause of vitamin B12 deficiency, caused by autoimmune gastritis with parietal cell destruction and intrinsic factor antibodies.

What are the complications of B12 deficiency?

Megaloblastosis can cause multisystem effects, notably cardiomyopathy and neurological disease, e.g. subacute combined degeneration of cord, peripheral neuropathy, dementia.

Table 2.68 Causes of B12 and folate deficiency	
Vitamin B12 deficiency	**Folate deficiency**
Inadequate intake Vegan	**Inadequate intake** Elderly Alcohol
Intrinsic factor deficiency Pernicious anaemia (autoimmune) Gastrectomy	**Malabsorption** Coeliac disease Tropical sprue

Small intestinal disease
Bacterial overgrowth (blind or
  'stagnant' loops)
Crohn's disease/terminal
  ileum resection
Coeliac disease
Tropical sprue
Miscellaneous (HIV, drugs –
  metformin, PPIs)
	Small bowel disease
	
	Increased utilisation or loss
	Pregnancy
	Haemolysis
	Myelofibrosis
	Malignancy
	Severe inflammation (exfoliative skin
	  disease, Crohn's disease)
	Liver failure, heart failure
	Homocystinuria

Pancreatic deficiency	**Drugs** Methotrexate (inhibits dihydrofolate reductase) Antiepileptics – valproate, phenytoin Trimethoprim

How would you treat B12 deficiency?

Hydroxycobalamin 1 mg intramuscularly on alternate days for two weeks, then three-monthly.

Is there a risk in administering a blood transfusion in the setting of B12 deficiency?

Severe vitamin B12 deficiency with megaloblastosis and a high lactate dehydrogenase (cells lyse easily) is dangerous. Transfusion is not necessary in pure B12 deficiency. In mixed anaemia with severe B12 deficiency, B12 should always be replaced before transfusion because transfusion can precipitate heart failure (megaloblastic cardiomyopathy) or provoke an aplastic crisis.

Are there risks in giving folate in the setting of B12 deficiency?

Giving folate in severe vitamin B12 deficiency can precipitate neurological problems. Vitamin B12 and folate (and ferritin because stores are often used up in B12 deficiency) may be given together, but B12 replacement should never be 'second'.

Is red cell folate a better marker of body folate status than serum folate?

Yes.

If both folate and iron levels are low, what condition would you screen for?

Coeliac disease. Indeed, coeliac disease is now one of the commonest causes of isolated iron deficiency.

What is haemolytic anaemia?

Haemolysis refers to destruction of peripheral red cells earlier than their normal life span of 120 days. Anaemia occurs if the marrow response fails to compensate. Most causes of haemolysis are extravascular (cells destroyed in the reticuloendothelial system, e.g. spleen), an accentuation of the normal destruction process. Some causes are intravascular, leading to red cell fragmentation being observed on the blood film.

What are the laboratory findings in haemolytic anaemia?

- Unconjugated hyperbilirubinaemia (jaundice is common)
- Increased urinary urobilinogen
- Reduced or absent serum haptoglobins
- Increased serum lactate dehydrogenase
- Reticulocytosis
- Bone marrow erythroid hyperplasia
- Polychromasia

What is reticulocytosis?

Young red cells, normally comprising < 1% of cells in the periphery, are 'churned out' when erythropoiesis is increased to compensate for peripheral destruction (acute blood loss or haemolysis). A blue tinge to the blood film, polychromasia, is seen in reticulocytosis because the ratio of nuclear remnant material to haemoglobin is high.

When might you suspect a haemolysed blood sample?

If there is raised potassium, lactate dehydrogenase and phosphate in a patient in whom you do not suspect cell lysis for any reason, e.g. post chemotherapy.

What are the causes of haemolytic anaemia?

These are listed in Table 2.69.

How is autoimmune haemolytic anaemia (AIHA) detected?

The direct antiglobulin test (DAT), detecting antibodies on the red cell surface, is usually positive. In this test, the autoantibody coating the surface of red blood cells is detected directly by application of an antiglobulin.

What types of AIHA are there?

Warm AIHA, in which the autoantibody reacts best at 37°C, may be idiopathic or secondary, e.g. systemic lupus erythematosus, lymphoproliferative disorders. There is often marked spherocytosis. Cold AIHA, in which the autoantibody reacts best at < 37°C, may occur in infections such as *Mycoplasma* and infectious mononucleosis.

How would you treat AIHA?

If there is no identifiable cause in warm AIHA, prednisolone 1 mg/kg is given for four weeks or until haemoglobin is 12 g/dl, then reduced slowly. Splenectomy may be needed

Table 2.69 Causes of haemolytic anaemia

Extrinsic RBC abnormality (acquired)	Intrinsic RBC abnormality (inherited)
Antibody-mediated Blood group incompatibility Autoimmune haemolytic anaemia (AIHA)	**Membrane abnormality** Hereditary spherocytosis/elliptocytosis
Non-antibody-mediated (tend to be intravascular) *RBC fragmentation (DIC/TTP/HUS, severe hypertension or renal failure, prosthetic valve) Infection (*Mycoplasma pneumoniae*, Epstein–Barr virus, *Clostridium welchii*, *Plasmodium falciparum*) Drugs Paroxysmal nocturnal haemoglobinuria March haemoglobinuria	**Metabolic abnormality** Glucose-6-phosphate dehydrogenase (G-6-PD) deficiency – by far most common Pyruvate kinase deficiency **Haemoglobin abnormality** Abnormal Hb structure (HbS – sickle cell disease, HbC, HbE) Abnormal Hb rate of synthesis (thalassaemias)

DIC/TTP/HUS, disseminated intravascular coagulation, thrombotic thrombocytopenic purpura, haemolytic uremic syndrome; Hb, haemoglobin; RBC, red blood cell.
*Microangiopathic haemolytic anaemia (MAHA) arises in these conditions, due to splicing of red cells into fragments (or schistocytes, referred to as 'helmets' if cut in half) as a result of clumping of platelets in small vessels in DIC/TTP/HUS, endothelial damage in severe hypertension and physical attack from prosthetic valves.

if there is no remission because red cells coated with immunoglobulin G are preferentially destroyed in the spleen (if complement-coated then mostly in the liver, and testing for this may predict the value of splenectomy). Plasma exchange may help. Other immune suppression may be considered if refractory, e.g. azathioprine or the newer experimental treatments rituximab (anti-CD20) and Campath-1H (anti-CD52). AIHA patients should avoid cold, and folic acid, transfusion, chlorambucil, steroids and splenectomy may be considered.

What are Howell–Jolly bodies?

These are nuclear remnants normally removed by the spleen, hence present post-splenectomy and in hyposplenic states such as coeliac and sickle cell disease.

List some other autoimmune cytopenias

- Autoimmune neutropenia
- Autoimmune thrombocytopenia (immune thrombocytopenic purpura)
- Autoimmune pancytopenia

What is schistocytosis?

This refers to the presence of fragmented red cells, seen in intravascular haemolysis, often as part of microangiopathic haemolytic anaemia. Strands of fibrin are laid down in small vessels and red cells are chopped into half (helmet cells) or multiple irregular fragments as they gush through.

What is paroxysmal nocturnal haemoglobinuria?

This is a rare condition in which the red blood cell membrane is abnormally sensitive to complement lysis because of aberrant membrane-anchored proteins which normally inhibit lysis. It can cause mesenteric thrombosis. Transfusion and anticoagulation may be needed.

What is aplastic anaemia?

This is pancytopenia due to marrow hypoplasia, which may be idiopathic or a consequence of drugs (e.g. chlor-

amphenicol, gold), chemicals or infection, e.g. parvovirus B19.

What is myelodysplasia?

The myelodysplastic syndromes are discussed in Case 1.45.

How might you manage pancytopenia of any cause?

As well as identifying and correcting any correctable cause, supportive care with blood and platelet transfusion and granulocyte colony-stimulating factor is often needed. Broad-spectrum antimicrobial therapy (e.g. tazocin, gentamicin) is needed in possible neutropenic sepsis.

CASE 2.33

SICKLE CELL DISEASE AND THALASSAEMIA

Candidate information

Role

You are a doctor in the emergency medical admissions unit. Please read the following letter from the patient's general practitioner. You may make notes on the paper provided. When the bell sounds, enter the examination room to begin the consultation.

Scenario

Dear Doctor
Re: Mr James Beech, aged 22 years
Thank you for admitting Mr Beech who has sickle cell disease and new abdominal pain. He frequently requires admission with his symptoms.
Yours sincerely

Please take a history from the patient (you may continue to make notes if you wish on the paper provided). Your examiners will warn you when 12 minutes have elapsed. You have 14 minutes to take a history from the patient followed by 1 minute of reflection. There will then follow 5 minutes of discussion with the examiners. Be prepared to discuss solutions to the problems posed by the case and how you might reply to the GP's letter. You are not required to examine the patient.

Patient information

Mr James Beech is a 22-year-old medical student with sickle cell anaemia. He has been admitted to the emergency ward again with abdominal pain. He was only here a month ago and is frustrated because his fourth year exams are pending. Past problems have included mild growth problems, recurrent abdominal pain, painful fingers (now with some deformities that limit his ability to write) and priapism. He does not smoke but does drink alcohol in binges close to exam time, not least because he feels annoyed that he has to work harder than his colleagues due to his condition; he knows that alcohol can precipitate sickling crises but is determined to lead as normal a life as possible and drinks plenty of water to try to compensate for his alcohol intake.

How to approach the case

Data gathering in the interview and interpretation and use of information gathered

Presenting problem(s) and symptom exploration

▪ **Evaluate symptoms** Take a thorough history of possible symptoms in sickle cell disease (SCD) (Box 2.69).

Patient perspective

Dwell considerably on this. Discover how he has been managing at medical school so far and what support structures he currently has (family, friends, mentors). Establish the difficulties posed by the unpredictability of symptoms, not least on his study and examinations.

Past medical history

Establish the range of hospital admissions he has endured before.

Drug and allergy history

Ask about prescription and non-prescription drugs.

Family history

This is very relevant.

Social history

Establish details about his drinking and its effects on symptoms.

Box 2.69 Clinical consequences of severe sickle cell disease (SCD)

Haemolysis

This can occur because red cells fail to negotiate tight capillaries resulting in anaemia, jaundice and a predisposition to pigment gallstones.

Vaso-occlusive or sequestration crises

These are caused by sickle cells impeding blood flow. Precipitating factors include infection and dehydration. Complications of occlusion can include:

- Abdominal pain
- Painful bone crises and dactylitis (digits of various lengths and/or deformed and there may be active finger swelling)
- Skin ulcers
- Splenic infarcts and tendency to sepsis from encapsulated organisms; severe SCD causes autosplenectomy but milder forms may cause splenic sequestration without infarction and the spleen may be palpable because of 'congestion' (the liver may be similarly enlarged) – where there is hyposplenism, there may also be an elevated white cell and platelet count
- Retinal infarcts
- Impaired renal tubule concentrating ability
- Renal papillary necrosis and chronic kidney disease
- *Salmonella* osteomyelitis
- Aseptic necrosis of the humeral and femoral heads
- Priapism
- Strokes
- Hepatic infarcts
- Growth impairment
- Pregnancy complications
- Pulmonary emboli

Aplastic crises

These are often the result of *parvovirus B19 infection*.

SUMMARY – ASSESSMENT AND PLAN

- The diagnosis is probably not really in doubt, but remember that other causes of abdominal pain such as appendicitis are of course possible.
- The peripheral blood film in sickle cell anaemia is likely to reveal anaemia (Hb 6–10 g/dl), reticulocytosis, target cells, and Howell–Jolly bodies due to autosplenectomy; definitive diagnosis requires haemoglobin electrophoresis.
- Treatment of a sickling crisis includes oxygen, hydration, analgesia and antibiotics. Numerous therapies are being evaluated which may reduce polymerisation.
- Appropriate psychological support may need to be sought in the longer term.
- Asplenic individuals should be vaccinated against *Pneumococcus*, *Meningococcus* and *Haemophilus*.

Discussion

How might abnormalities in red cell components give rise to inherited anaemia?

Red cells are approximately 8 μm wide and biconcave with an area of central pallor. Their size and shape enable them to squeeze through capillaries, with normally only minimal anisocytosis (variation in size) and poikilocytosis (variation in shape). Any of the three components of a red cell – membrane, enzymes and haemoglobin – may lead to anaemia if at fault.

Hereditary spherocytosis and abnormalities of the red cell membrane

The membrane bears blood group antigens and comprises a lipid bilayer and underlying protein skeleton. Alterations in its lipid can cause macrocytosis without anaemia. Alterations in cytoskeletal molecules (e.g. spectrin) can cause haemolysis. In hereditary spherocytosis abnormal membrane proteins render the red cell excessively permeable to sodium influx. Some of the membrane is spliced in the spleen to leave small spherical cells without central pallor (spherocytes). Ultimately, spherocytes are haemolysed in the reticuloendothelial system. Osmotic fragility tests reveal increased susceptibility to lysis compared to normal red blood cells. Splenectomy is often needed.

Enzymopathies

The metabolic energy-creating pathways are the Embden–Meyerhof pathway and the hexose monophosphate shunt. Energy is used to maintain osmotic stability by membrane pumps. Enzymopathies within these metabolic pathways cause haemolytic anaemia. Heinz bodies are inclusions of oxidised haemoglobin seen in glucose-6-phosphate-dehydrogenase deficiency.

Haemoglobinopthies – sickle cell disease and thalassaemias

Normal haemoglobin (Hb) comprises four haem groups (as a tetramer) and globin. Each haem group is an oxygen-binding site. Normal adult haemoglobin (HbA) comprises two α and two β globin polypeptide chains, with a trace of HbA2 (α2, δ2) and sometimes a trace of fetal Hb (α2, γ2). In the haemoglobinopathies, abnormal polypeptide chains are produced (sickle cell disease) or normal polypeptide chains are produced in decreased amounts (thalassaemias).

What is the underlying abnormality in sickle cell disease (SCD)?

SCD is caused by a structural abnormality in haemoglobin. Valine is substituted for glutamine at position 6 on the β globin chain, giving rise to the haemoglobin S gene. Sickle cell haemoglobin (HbS) molecules derived from this gene

tend to polymerise. The rate of polymerisation is accelerated by hypoxia, an increased concentration of intracellular haemoglobin or a decreased concentration of fetal haemoglobin (HbF). Polymerisation renders the red blood cell less pliable and it deforms into its characteristic sickle shape. Ischaemic damage from vaso-occlusion is self-evident, but haemolysis may contribute to some complications by free haemoglobin's binding to nitric oxide, promoting pulmonary hypertension, leg ulcers and priaprism.

The HbS gene occurs widely throughout Africa and in countries with African immigrant populations and also in parts of the Mediterranean, Middle East and India.

What types of SCD are there?

The spectrum of SCD is shown in Table 2.70.

How do thalassaemias arise?

Thalassaemias are caused by an inefficient rate of synthesis of one or more globin chains (compare with SCD in which normal globin chains are not produced).

This leads to underproduction of haemoglobin and imbalance in globin chain synthesis. The chains that are produced in excess precipitate, and formation of rigid inclusions (Heinz bodies) leads to premature cell destruction.

Depending upon which pair of globin chains, α or β, has inefficient production, α-thalassaemias or β-thalassaemias result. The α-thalassaemias are more common than β-thalassaemias. Thalassaemias are most common in people of Far and Middle Eastern origin.

What types of α-thalassaemia are there?

There are two α genes on each chromosome such that normal individuals have four copies of the α gene (unlike just two copies of the β gene). There are four possible genetic abnormalities (Box 2.70).

What types of β-thalassaemia are there?

β-thalassaemias are common in people of Mediterranean, Middle and Far Eastern origin, and over 180 different mutations of the gene have been described which decrease the output of β globin chains, either completely or partially. There is just one β gene on each chromosome such that normal individuals have only two copies of the β gene (unlike four copies of the α gene). There are two common genetic abnormalities (Box 2.71).

Table 2.70 The sickling spectrum	
Heterozygote (AS) sickle cell trait	Inheritance of the HbS gene from one parent and a normal β globin gene from the other results in this harmless carrier state.
Homozygous (SS) sickle cell anaemia	This occurs when HbS is inherited from both parents, and it tends to be severe.
Sickle cell/haemoglobin C (SC) disease	This occurs if HbS is inherited from one parent and HbC from the other. The HbC gene is the second commonest haemoglobin gene abnormality in West Africa. HbSC disease tends to be mild but important microvascular complications can occur.
Sickle cell/thalassaemia	This is designated β+ if 20–30% of HbA (normal adult haemoblobin) is present and β° if no HbA is present. β+ tends to be mild clinically but β° is severe.

- Deletion of one gene, resulting in an *asymptomatic carrier state* with a normal blood film
- Deletion of two genes (-α/-α or –/αα), resulting in the *thalassaemia trait* with mild hypochromic, microcytic anaemia
- Deletion of three genes (*HbH disease*) in which there is anaemia (Hb 7–10 g/dl), splenomegaly and the presence of 'golf ball cells' on the blood film due to precipitation of β globin chains in the red cell. The reduced rate of α chain synthesis generally leads to an excess of β and γ chains
- Deletion of all four genes (*Hb Bart's disease*) causing hydrops fetalis and stillbirth

---

Box 2.71 Types of β-thalassaemia

Thalassaemia major

Homozygotes (inheriting the same or different β-thalassaemia genes from each parent) develop thalassaemia major. This is characterised by:

- Severe anaemia (Hb 2–8 g/dl; much being HbF) resulting from deficiency of β chains
- Compensatory excess of α chains, which damage red cells
- Hypertrophy of ineffective marrow leading to bone expansion and skeletal abnormalities
- Extramedullary haemopoiesis and hepatosplenomegaly
- Failure to thrive, almost inevitable
- A blood film showing severe hypochromia and microcytosis, target cells and reticulocytosis
- A need for repeated blood transfusions which downregulate marrow dyserythropoiesis but lead to secondary haemochromatosis

Thalassaemia minor

Heterozygotes have the thalassaemia trait (thalassaemia minor). Individuals may be mildly anaemic during times of stress but otherwise have merely a hypochromic, microcytic blood film.

How are thalassaemias managed?

Haemoglobinopathies including severe thalassaemia may require blood transfusion and subcutaneous desferrioxamine. Both SCD and thalassaemia may develop pancytopenia and hypersplenism, and splenectomy has a role in both. Bone marrow transplantation may be considered in the most difficult cases and haematopoietic stem cell transplantation is the only curative treatment for β-thalassaemia.

Iron overload may occur; hepcidin, a small molecule that inhibits iron absorption in the small bowel, is inappropriately low in thalassaemia major. Accurate measurement of iron stores is important in gauging transfusion and desferrioxamine (or the newer deferiprone) chelation treatment.

Thrombotic problems, endocrinopathies (e.g. hypogonadism) and bone disease are common in β-thalassaemias and require specialised management.

CASE 2.34

PURPURA

Candidate information

Role

You are a doctor in the emergency medical admissions unit. Please read the following letter from the patient's general practitioner. You may make notes on the paper provided. When the bell sounds, enter the examination room to begin the consultation.

Scenario

> Dear Doctor
>
> Re: Mrs Megan May, aged 35 years
>
> Thank you for admitting Mrs May with a five-day history of an evolving purpuric rash. She does not appear to have any bleeding from anywhere. Her blood count is as follows: haemoglobin 11.5 g/dl, white cell count 8.0×10^9/l with a normal differential and platelets 15×10^9/l. She is usually very well and takes no medications.
>
> Yours sincerely

Please take a history from the patient (you may continue to make notes if you wish on the paper provided). Your examiners will warn you when 12 minutes have elapsed. You have 14 minutes to take a history from the patient followed by 1 minute of reflection. There will then follow 5 minutes of discussion with the examiners. Be prepared to discuss solutions to the problems posed by the case and how you might reply to the GP's letter. You are not required to examine the patient.

Patient information

Mrs Megan May is a 35-year-old lady who works as a writer for a national magazine. For the last few days she has noticed a gradually increasing purpuric, non-blanching rash which started in her hands but which now involves her arms, legs and trunk. The spots are flat, and many of them are tiny dots. She feels otherwise well. She has not experienced epistaxis, bleeding gums or bleeding from any other site. She has no headache or fever. There is no lymphadenopathy. There is no history of any recent viral illness. There are no unwell contacts. She lives with her husband and two children. Her last menstrual period was a week ago and a little heavier than usual. She does not smoke or drink alcohol. She has mild asthma for which she has an occasional ventolin inhaler. She does not take any regular medications other than the contraceptive pill and has not recently taken any tablets such as antibiotics or corticosteroids. She is clearly concerned about the rash.

How to approach the case

Data gathering in the interview and interpretation and use of information gathered

Presenting problem(s) and symptom exploration

▪ **Establish purpura details** Establish the duration of symptoms, the distribution of the rash, and its features (Table 2.71).

▪ **Ask specific questions** Ask specifically about:

- Fever
- Joint pains (Henoch–Schönlein purpura)
- Lymphadenopathy
- Recent viral symptoms

Patient perspective

Address her understandable concerns by sharing the possibilities. It is probably not wise to mention malignancy at this stage as a possibility unless she asks, but if so then to share that it seems unlikely with a severe but isolated drop in the platelet count.

Past medical history

Ask about any history of lymphoproliferative disease.

Drug and allergy history

Ask about prescription and non-prescription drugs. Drugs notorious for causing thrombocytopenia include sulphonamides and chloramphenicol and corticosteroids can cause purpura.

Family history

Ensure there are no unwell contacts.

Social history

Ask about alcohol intake. Human immunodeficiency virus (HIV) risk factors are important to exclude/establish.

SUMMARY – ASSESSMENT AND PLAN

- This is a typical presentation of idiopathic thrombocytopenic purpura (ITP). Other possibilities are drug-induced thrombocytopenia, infection (e.g. toxoplasmosis, cytomegalovirus, Epstein–Barr virus), bone marrow failure (e.g. leukaemia, metastatic malignancy or infiltration) or a coagulopathy.
- In ITP the blood count reveals isolated thrombocytopenia. Serology for infectious causes (including HIV if risk factors) should be requested, together with an autoimmune profile although in ITP platelet autoantibodies are generally unreliable. Bone marrow examination is often important to exclude other causes.
- Treatment of ITP is with corticosteroids (with concomitant bone protection) but in rare, serious cases intravenous immunoglobulin may have a role.
- Splenectomy is usually reserved for cases that are refractory to other measures.

Discussion

How is haemostasis regulated?

A tightly regulated homeostatic mechanism involving the endothelium, platelets, coagulation and fibrinolysis maintains physiological blood flow but permits rapid, localised thrombus formation at sites of tissue damage.

How does the endothelium contribute to haemostatic homeostasis? (Fig. 2.12A)

The endothelial surface normally inhibits thrombus formation. A negative charge repels platelets, ectoenzymes degrade platelet agonists such as adenosine diphosphate (ADP), the vasodilators nitric oxide and prostacyclin inhibit platelet adhesion and aggregation, and surface expression of thrombomodulin and heparan sulphate enhance anticoagulation.

With tissue damage, blood vessels constrict and the subendothelial extracellular matrix is exposed. Exposed collagen (types I and III), von Willebrand factor (VWF) and fibronectin promote platelet adhesion. Cytokines (interleukin-1, tumour necrosis factor, interferon-γ) or endotoxin render damaged endothelium prothrombotic. Tissue factor (TF) is expressed which initiates the coagula-

---

Table 2.71 Features of purpura (bruising) that help distinguish a platelet problem from a coagulopathy		
	Platelet problem	**Coagulopathy**
Sites of bleeding	Mucosal – epistaxis, genitourinary, gastrointestinal	Muscle and joint Visceral and intracranial bleeds potentially life threatening
Precipitating factor	Spontaneously or with minimal trauma	Spontaneously or with minimal trauma
Characteristic signs	Petechiae (representing small endothelial lesions that have failed to heal)	Haemarthroses Joint deformity ultimately Excessive bleeding from small cuts not typical because platelet activation, adhesion and aggregation are sufficient to seal small endothelial lesions; haemostasis of larger wounds requires fibrin reinforcement relying on effective coagulation

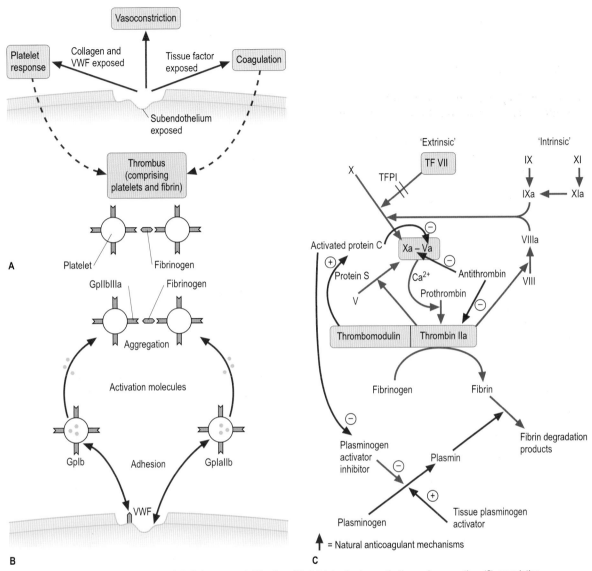

Fig. 2.12 Haemostatic homeostasis: (A) endothelial response to bleeding, (B) platelet adhesion, activation and aggregation, (C) coagulation.

tion pathway, plasminogen activator inhibitor (PAI) is secreted to impair fibrinolysis and thrombomodulin expression is reduced.

The endothelium is not just dynamic but is heterogeneous, leading to the modern concept of vascular-bed-specific haemostasis. Discrete thrombotic episodes are typical, and the ability of a vascular bed to compensate depends upon the local antithrombotic–prothrombotic seesaw.

List some vascular disorders that cause purpura

These are listed in Box 2.72.

Box 2.72 Vascular disorders that cause purpura

- Age-related purpura
- Corticosteroid-induced purpura
- Vasculitis
- Henoch–Schönlein purpura (an immunoglobulin A vasculitis affecting skin, joints and gastrointestinal tract, with immunoglobulin A nephropathy)
- Scurvy
- Infection (viral, bacterial, e.g. meningococcal septicaemia)
- Hereditary causes (hereditary haemorrhagic telangiectasia, Ehlers–Danlos syndrome, osteogenesis imperfecta, Marfan's syndrome)

How do platelets contribute to thrombus formation? (see Fig. 2.12B)

Platelets normally circulate in close contact with the endothelium, but adhesion is prevented by local nitric oxide and prostacyclin.

Platelet adhesion

With endothelial damage, platelet adhesion occurs rapidly between platelets and exposed subendothelium. Blood flow is faster at the centre of vessels than close to the endothelium, creating shear effects between adjacent layers of blood that are highest nearer the endothelium. In high flow conditions, platelets adhere to the subendothelium by the interaction of their glycoprotein (Gp) 1b receptors to VWF and in low-flow conditions platelets adhere to the subendothelium by the interaction of their GpIaIIb receptors to collagen, fibronectin and fibrinogen.

VWF is a large, multimeric protein synthesised by the endothelium and secreted into the subendothelium. After endothelial damage it binds to extracellular collagen, primarily through its A3 binding site. The Gp1b–IX-V complex binds to the A1 binding site of VWF despite high flow because of a high association rate. However, a concurrent high dissociation rate allows platelets to roll slowly along the endothelium.

Platelet activation

Platelet activation occurs during the rolling phase and is the result of the binding of various agonists (e.g. thrombin, thromboxane A2, ADP, collagen, arachidonic acid) to specific receptors leading to intracellular changes including reduced adenylate cyclase activity and cAMP, calcium mobilisation and secretion of platelet granules. These have many roles, including the release of receptors for activated factor V.

Platelet aggregation

During activation the platelet GpIIbIIIa receptor undergoes a conformational change, allowing it to bind to the dimeric fibrinogen molecule, and irreversible platelet aggregation occurs.

Which drugs interfere with platelet function?

Aspirin inhibits thromboxane A2 and other molecules, dipyridamole and clopidogrel exert effects on ADP-induced platelet activation and GPIIbIIIa inhibitors affect the final common denominator of platelet aggregation.

List some platelet disorders that cause a bleeding tendency

These are listed in Table 2.72.

What is idiopathic thrombocytopenic purpura (ITP)?

This commonly affects women between 20 and 40 years of age. It may present acutely with an abrupt fall in platelet count, or can be a chronic, relapsing condition. There is often a history of easy bruising or menorrhagia. Auto-antibodies directed against platelet glycoproteins lead to autoantibody–platelet complexes that are then sequestered in the spleen, but the trigger to this autoimmunity is usually unclear.

What is thrombotic thrombocytopenic purpura (TTP)?

TTP is characterised by microangiopathic haemolytic anaemia, thrombocytopenia, acute renal failure and microvascular neurological effects (usually causing confusion). Haemolytic uraemic syndrome, a similar condition, is more likely to present in children and with renal failure while in TTP neurological events including confusion often dominate. In sporadic TTP a metalloproteinase (VWF-cleavage protein ADAMTS-13) that normally degrades ultra-large multimers of VWF to smaller VWF proteins is dysfunctional; this leads to enhanced platelet–VWF adhesion, enhanced platelet aggregation and microangiopathic haemolysis. A familial form of TTP involves antibody dysfunction. LDH is high in TTP. Treatment is with plasma exchange.

What is disseminated intravascular coagulation (DIC)?

DIC is the enhanced and abnormally sustained generation of thrombin triggered by inflammatory mediators, usually in severe sepsis. Therapeutic activated protein C has had a limited role in treating DIC.

Table 2.72 Platelet disorders that cause a bleeding tendency	
Decreased bone marrow production	Myelodysplasia Aplasia, e.g. drugs, chemicals, radiation or infection, e.g. Parvovirus B19 Bone marrow infiltration, e.g. leukaemia, metastatic disease, tuberculosis Myelofibrosis Drugs, including alcohol Congenital disorders, e.g. May–Hegglin anomaly, Bernard–Soulier syndrome, Wiskott–Aldrich syndrome, Fanconi's anaemia, thrombocytopenia-absent radii syndrome
Increased peripheral destruction	Immune causes, e.g. drugs, infections, human immunodeficiency virus, idiopathic thrombocytopenic purpura, systemic lupus erythematosus or other autoimmune disorders, post transfusion Disseminated intravascular coagulation Thrombotic thrombocytopenic purpura Hypersplenism
Platelet dysfunction	Renal failure Congenital, e.g. Glanzmann's disease with GpIIbIIIa receptor deficiency (rare)

At what level of thrombocytopenia does purpura start to appear?

Purpura (petechial) is unusual spontaneously if normally functioning platelets are above 10×10^9 to 20×10^9/l, but may occur after injury at higher levels.

Do you know of any recent advances in the understanding of blood coagulation (see Fig. 2.12C)?

The coagulation 'jigsaw'

The traditional concept of intrinsic and extrinsic pathways failed to explain why factor XII deficiency does not cause bleeding despite its supposed role in initiating the intrinsic pathway, why factor IX deficiency causes only a mild bleeding tendency, why factor VIII and IX deficiencies cause severe bleeding but theoretically should be bypassed by factor VII activity and why thrombus generation in vitro has a lag phase. The two-pathway concept is being superseded with recognition of the tissue factor–factor VII complex (TF.VII) as central to coagulation.

The puzzle is less of a sequence and more of a jigsaw.

The central role of tissue factor and factor VIIa

TF is expressed on fibroblasts but may be induced by endotoxin, interleukin-1 and tumour necrosis factor in other cells, including endothelial cells. TF is only fully active in a damaged environment and subendothelial exposure causes factor VII or activated factor VII (VIIa) to bind to TF. Activation of VII to VIIa may be by autoactivation of the TF.VII complex, but trace amounts of Xa may aid activation and small amounts of basal VIIa are present (which are reduced in factor IX deficiency).

Why factor Xa is so important

Activated factor Xa is generated by TF.VII and stimulates sufficient amounts of factor IIa (thrombin) to induce local platelet aggregation and activation of the critical cofactors V and VIII. This is insufficient to sustain haemostasis because of rapid Xa inactivation by TF pathway inhibitor (TFPI). Instead, marked amplification of Xa is facilitated by factors IXa and VIIIa. Factor XIa may be needed to generate additional factor IXa if fibrinolysis is especially active, explaining why factor IX deficiency seldom causes spontaneous bleeds but can be problematic following trauma or surgery. Factor XI activation may involve thrombin. Much about coagulation remains unknown but the remaining pieces of the intrinsic jigsaw seem not to be important in haemostasis and relevant only in vitro.

Not forgetting factor Va and the prothrombinase complex

The prothrombinase or tenase complex (factor Xa–Va), incorporating Va that is crucial to Xa's activity, rapidly converts prothrombin (II) to thrombin (IIa).

And finally, the importance of thrombin

Thrombin converts soluble fibrinogen to insoluble fibrin, activates factor XIII, which stabilises the fibrin clot, and has positive feedback on coagulation by activating factors in the intrinsic pathway (including factor XI) and factor V.

Table 2.73 Coagulation disorders that cause a bleeding tendency	
Congenital disorders	Haemophilia A and B von Willebrand disease Factor XI deficiency Deficiencies of all other coagulation factors described but rare
Acquired disorders	Anticoagulant drugs Vitamin K deficiency Liver disease Disseminated intravascular coagulation Acquired factor inhibitors

Natural anticoagulation mechanisms

Procoagulation is itself regulated, to prevent unhindered thrombosis, by mechanisms that include:

* Thrombin binding to endothelial *thrombomodulin* (which on binding to thrombin activates *protein C* in the presence of its *cofactor protein S* rendering *activated protein C able to cleave and inactivate factor V* and the other cofactors)
* *Antithrombin* binding to and inactivation of thrombin and Xa; antithrombin is one of several 'serpins' that inhibit clotting proteases, including the recently discovered protein Z-dependent protease inhibitor
* *Tissue plasminogen activator* (tPA) secretion by endothelial cells.

List some coagulation disorders that cause a bleeding tendency

These are listed in Table 2.73.

CASE 2.35

HAEMOPHILIA

Candidate information

Role

You are a doctor in the emergency medical admissions unit. Please read the following letter from the patient's general practitioner. You may make notes on the paper provided. When the bell sounds, enter the examination room to begin the consultation.

Scenario

Dear Doctor

Re: Mr Nick Adler, aged 39 years

Thank you for seeing this gentleman with haemophilia who has had some bleeding today following a fall onto his knee. Although mild there is a steady leak from a laceration to his leg and the knee joint looks a little swollen to me.

Yours sincerely

Please take a history from the patient (you may continue to make notes if you wish on the paper provided). Your examiners will warn you when 12 minutes have elapsed. You have 14 minutes to take a history from the patient followed by 1 minute of reflection. There will then follow 5 minutes of discussion with the examiners. Be prepared to discuss solutions to the problems posed by the case and how you might reply to the GP's letter. You are not required to examine the patient.

Patient information

Mr Nick Adler is a 39-year-old gentleman with haemophilia A and a usual factor VIII level of around 10% of normal. This tends to result in continuous bleeding after mild to moderate trauma. Today he fell off his bicycle onto his left knee and sustained a laceration to it that is continuing to ooze after six hours of pressure. He has therefore been admitted to hospital. His knee joint is swollen but he has had multiple previous haemathroses of both knees and the left is usually a little more deformed and swollen than the right. He does not have pain. He has no history of intracranial bleeding and did not bang his head on this occasion. He is otherwise well but does carry the hepatitis C virus due to blood transfusions many years ago. He does not have human immunodeficiency virus infection. He is married, without children. He has come to terms with his condition very well, and sees a liver specialist six-monthly for monitoring of what is currently inactive hepatitis C. He works as a computer graphics designer. He is well informed about haemophilia and feels he will need factor VIII replacement on this occasion.

How to approach the case

Data gathering in the interview and interpretation and use of information gathered

Presenting problem(s) and symptom exploration

▪ **Evaluate symptoms** Haemophilia typically causes joint and muscle bleeding and symptom severity depends significantly on the factor level (Table 2.74).

▪ **Explore risks and complications** As well as blood transfusion risks, the significant problems of haemophilia relate to joint damage and comprehensive assessments often involve a haematologist, rheumatologist, orthopaedic surgeon and physiotherapist. Intracranial haemorrhage and visceral bleeds can occur with minimal trauma and are an important source of morbidity and mortality.

Patient perspective

Discover what he knows about his condition. He is probably more likely to know if he has sustained a haemarthrosis and what will be needed on this occasion to stem the bleeding than most doctors.

Table 2.74 Severity of haemophilia

Factor level	Clinical defect
> 50%	Normal
20–50%	Abnormal bleeding after severe trauma
5–20%	Abnormal bleeding after mild trauma
2–5%	Abnormal bleeding after trivial trauma/occasional spontaneous bleeding
< 2%	Spontaneous bleeding into joints, muscles and soft tissues

Past medical history

Explore the risk consequences of previous blood transfusions.

Drug and allergy history

He is likely to know which drugs to avoid in haemophilia.

Family history

The mode of haemophilia A and B inheritance is X-linked, such that all males carrying the affected X chromosome will have haemophilia and all females are carriers (unless, rarely, she is the daughter of a haemophilia male and carrier female). Carrier females may exhibit mild disease if factor production is sufficiently impaired. Around half of sons of carriers have haemophilia and half of daughters are carriers. The severity of disease tends to be similar between generations.

Social history

Establish if he is doing all that he can (within the limits of his wishes) to minimise injuries. Presumably the cycling was not competitive racing?

SUMMARY – ASSESSMENT AND PLAN

- You would arrange for baseline blood tests including an urgent haemoglobin and ensure that blood is available in the event that transfusion were absolutely necessary.
- You would liaise with his haematology team and arrange treatment, probably in the form of recombinant factor VIII.
- You would consult the orthopaedic team if you felt he had a significant haemarthrosis.

Discussion

What are the commonest haemophilias?

Haemophilia A and B are the commonest inherited coagulopathies but are rare (1 : 10 000). Haemophilia A (deficiency of factor VIII:C) is about five times more common than haemophilia B (deficiency of factor IX). Rarer deficiencies have been described for all clotting factors.

How might laboratory investigations be useful in haemophilia?

The activated partial thromboplastin time (APTT) is usually prolonged ('intrinsic' pathway) but the prothrombin time (tissue factor or 'extrinsic' pathway) is normal.

APTT corrects with the addition of normal plasma in a 50:50 mix in inherited haemophilia but not in the less common acquired factor VIII disease, where there is an inhibitor (autoantibody) against factor VIII. Specific assays demonstrate reduced factor VIII:C or IX levels.

How is bleeding in haemophilia managed?

A normal bleeding time is less than 10 minutes. In haemophilia, continuous bleeding often occurs, or becomes apparent hours or days after injury. Replacement of the missing factor is the key to therapy, freeze-dried factors from large donor pools were historically used but are gradually being replaced by recombinant factors. A formula for dosage is:

$$\text{Factor replacement} = \% \text{ increase in factor required} \times \text{body weight (kg)}/K$$

where $K = 2$ in factor VIII deficiency and 1 in factor XI deficiency.

Factors have only a short half-life (8–12 hours for factor VIII and 12–24 hours for factor IX) in vivo.

Desmopressin (DDAVP/synthetic ADH) combined with an antifibrinolytic agent increases factor VIII levels in patients with mild haemophilia A. Antifibrinolytic agents have been combined with factor concentrates for external bleeding but not usually with factor IX because of the risk of thrombosis or in haematuria because of risks of clot retention.

What is von Willebrand disease (VWD)?

This is caused by mutations in the von Willebrand factor (VWF) gene on chromosome 12, resulting in quantitative or qualitative abnormalities in VWF. The factor is synthesised in endothelial cells (to an extent bone marrow) and acts as a subendothelial binding protein for platelets via GP1b and as a carrier molecule for factor VIII in the bloodstream to sites of vascular injury. There are three types of VWD:

1. Type 1 (70% of cases, autosomal dominant) is a partial quantitative deficiency of VWF, with a propensity to mucocutaneous bleeding (epistaxis, menorrhagia). Laboratory findings are reduced levels of VWF antigen (protein) and activity (by ristocetin cofactor or RCo assay) with normal or increased ristocetin-induced platelet aggregation (RIPA), which measures sensitivity of ristocetin-induced interaction of the patient's VWF with their own platelets.
2. Type 2 has four subtypes:
   - Type 2A mutations result in a failure of VWF multimer assembly (group 1) or increased sensitivity to degradation by the VWF cleavage protease ADAMTS13 (group 2), resulting in loss of circulating high- and medium-molecular-weight multimers, with a corresponding low VWF antigen level and disproportionately lower RCo level.
   - Type 2B is a mutation of the platelet GP1b binding site that results in higher affinity of VWF for GP1b, so that VWF binds spontaneously to platelets in the circulation, causing loss of high-molecular-weight circulating multimers, with a corresponding low VWF antigen level and disproportionately lower RCo level.
   - Type 2M results in decreased affinity for the GP1b receptor. There is a corresponding low VWF antigen level and disproportionately lower RCo, and markedly reduced RIPA activity. Multimer analysis reveals a full set of multimers.
   - Type 2N (autosomal recessive) results in decreased affinity for the factor VIII binding site. Factor VIII levels in homozygotes may be in single figures; VWF antigen and activity levels, RIPA and multimer studies are normal.
3. Type 3 (5% of cases) is caused by two null VWF genes, with no detectable VWF antigen or activity levels, absent RIPA activity and no detectable multimers; Factor VIII levels are also low (prolonged APTT) and bleeding is of haemophilia and mucocutaneous type.

Treatment for all types may be with factor VIII concentrate containing VWF, or in types 1, 2A and 2B desmopressin.

CASE 2.36

DEEP VEIN THROMBOSIS

Candidate information

Role

You are a doctor in the emergency medical admissions unit. Please read the following letter from the patient's general practitioner. You may make notes on the paper provided. When the bell sounds, enter the examination room to begin the consultation.

Scenario

Dear Doctor

Re: Mrs Esther Summers, aged 60 years

Thank you for seeing this lady with a short history of leg swelling and breathlessness. She had a mastectomy for breast cancer two years ago and a perioperative DVT and I am concerned that this is further venous thromboembolism.

Yours sincerely

Please take a history from the patient (you may continue to make notes if you wish on the paper provided). Your examiners will warn you when 12 minutes have elapsed. You have 14 minutes to take a history from the patient followed by 1 minute of reflection. There will then follow 5 minutes of discussion with the examiners. Be prepared to discuss solutions to the problems posed by the case and how you might reply to the GP's letter. You are not required to examine the patient.

Patient information

Mrs Esther Summers is a 60-year-old lady with right-sided calf and leg swelling for the last three days. She usually has mild swelling of both legs but this does not unduly trouble her and she has been talking a small dose of frusemide for a couple of years on an occasional basis. She has also been more breathless in the last week. She does not have chest pain or other cardiorespiratory symptoms. She has a history of breast cancer with a mastectomy and axillary clearance two years ago and takes tamoxifen. She is not taking any other medications. She does not smoke. She recently visited her sister in the United States, returning two weeks ago. She is a widow, and is currently caring for one of her grandchildren. She is not particularly concerned about the possibility of another deep vein thrombosis (DVT).

How to approach the case

Data gathering in the interview and interpretation and use of information gathered

Presenting problem(s) and symptom exploration

■ **Evaluate symptoms** Unilateral leg swelling represents a DVT until proven otherwise, unless an alternative such as cellulitis is very evident. Bilateral leg swelling may be the result of heart failure, nephrotic syndrome and other low protein states, hypothyroidism or a saddle thrombosis (the latter usually in the setting of malignancy).

■ **Consider risk factors for venous thromboembolism** Risk factors include:

- Acute phase of illness
- Trauma, surgery
- Immobility/inactivity including long-haul flights
- Dehydration
- Pregnancy (oral contraceptive pill/hormone replacement therapy slightly increase risk)
- Obesity
- Malignancy, e.g. pancreas, prostate
- Myeloproliferative disorders and hyperviscosity syndromes

- Nephrotic syndrome
- Heart failure
- Antiphospholipid syndrome and hereditary thrombophilias
- Hyperhomocysteinaemia

■ **Clinical model** Post-test probability in venous thromboembolism (VTE) relates to pre-test clinical probability and the nature of the test, e.g. V/Q, CTPA. Accurate diagnosis of DVT can be a challenge, and various clinical scoring systems are used including the (maximum) nine-point version of the Canadian Wells score for predicting pre-test probability for DVT (Table 2.75). Note that this differs from the Wells score used in diagnosing pulmonary embolus. Clinical intuition has a strong place for experienced physicians.

The Wells DVT score probably performs differently in different clinical settings, but clinical judgement still has final veto.

Patient perspective

It is probably best to advise her that a DVT is likely but that you will need to confirm this with an ultrasound scan, and, if confirmed, consider whether or not the long-haul flight is enough to explain it but that you think it would also be sensible to recheck things from the point of the breast cancer to make absolutely certain things are still all clear.

Past medical history

The history of breast cancer and DVT is highly relevant.

Drug and allergy history

Tamoxifen is not a contributor.

Family history

Establish any family history of blood clots.

Social history

Establish who will look after her grandchild while she is in hospital.

Table 2.75 Wells scoring system for predicting pretest probability for deep vein thrombosis (DVT)	
Clinical feature	**Score**
Active cancer (treatment ongoing or within previous 6 months or palliative)	1
Paralysis, paresis or recent plaster immobilisation of legs	1
Recent bed rest for > 3 days or major surgery within 4 weeks	1
Localised tenderness along distribution of deep vein system	1
Entire leg swollen	1
Calf swelling by > 3 cm compared to asymptomatic leg (measured 10 cm below tibial tuberosity)	1
Pitting oedema (greater in symptomatic leg)	1
Collateral superficial veins (non-varicose)	1
Previous documented DVT	1
Alternative diagnosis as or more likely than that of DVT	−2
	Low probability 0 or less Moderate probability 1–2 High probability 3 or more

---

SUMMARY – ASSESSMENT AND PLAN

- Her risk factors for DVT include previous DVT and previous malignancy, and a recent long-haul flight.
- The diagnosis should be established by ultrasound scan; it might be suggested by a D-Dimer although here a negative D-Dimer is not likely to dissuade you from further testing (Table 2.76).
- Low-molecular-weight heparin (LMWH) is the initial treatment of choice for DVT and pulmonary embolism, with subsequent warfarinisation and if this proves to be recurrence of DVT then indefinite anticoagulation with warfarin is indicated.
- The possibility of recurrent malignancy should be explored.

Discussion

What do you know about the role of D-dimer testing in suspected VTE? (Table 2.76)

Plasma D-dimers are specific cross-linked derivatives of fibrin (fibrin degradation products). They are not specific for VTE but arise in many other situations including sepsis, trauma, surgery, pregnancy and post-partum. The usefulness also varies with age and co-morbidity.

Does the absolute level of a positive D-dimer correlate with the likelihood or severity of the VTE?

No. There is no evidence that any value above the cut-off correlates with the likelihood of VTE. It may correlate with the size of the DVT, age or likelihood of malignancy.

What treatment is advised for VTE in pregnancy?

LMWH is safe and effective in the treatment and prophylaxis of VTE in pregnancy.

How does heparin work?

Heparin forms a high-affinity complex with antithrombin and accelerates its action. Antithrombin inactivates both thrombin (IIa) and Xa when it binds to these (Fig. 2.12C, Case 2.34), but the rate of inactivation is relatively low. Heparin strongly catalyses the action of antithrombin by inducing a conformational change in antithrombin within the heparin–antithrombin–thrombin complex leading to irreversible binding of antithrombin to thrombin. Unfractionated heparin is a long molecule which complexes with antithrombin, causing it to bind with and accelerate the

action of both coagulation factors. Unfractionated heparin's anti-Xa:anti-IIa antithrombin binding ratio is 1:1. LMWH complexes with and accelerates mostly that region of antithrombin binding to Xa. In other words, LMWH exerts more effect on the proximal part of the coagulation pathway. This results in higher bioavailability, a longer half-life, and lower propensity to thrombocytopenia. There may also be a lower osteoporosis risk. Monitoring partial thromboplastin time is not required with LMWH. LMWHs are administered subcutaneously in the treatment and prophylaxis of DVTs, pulmonary emboli and acute coronary syndromes. Heparin can interfere with diagnostic testing for antithrombin deficiency.

How does warfarin work?

Warfarin inhibits the procoagulant factors II, VII, IX and X but also the anticoagulant protein C. Since the half-life of protein C is short, a procoagulant state may precede warfarin's anticoagulant effect. This is seldom clinically significant but may cause problems in patients with underlying protein C under-activity and is responsible for the phenomenon of warfarin-induced skin necrosis. It is also the reason that heparin should be continued at least until and probably for some days after the INR is therapeutic in those starting warfarin for VTE. Warfarin can interfere with diagnostic testing for protein C and S deficiency.

For how long should warfarin be administered after a first DVT or pulmonary embolism?

After a first DVT or pulmonary embolism without ongoing risk factors, three months is advised. There is no evidence supporting six months of treatment.

How may anticoagulation be reversed?

Heparin can be reversed if absolutely necessary with protamine, although LMWH reversal is incomplete. Over-anticoagulation with warfarin may need no treatment (INR < 10 and no bleeding) or vitamin K; it can be reversed rapidly with a prothrombin complex concentrate (Beriplex) in a life-threatening bleed, the dose being proportional to the INR and administered with vitamin K.

Do you know of any new antithrombotic agents?

New antithrombotic agents offer effective anticoagulation with less need for monitoring and may supersede warfarin

Pre-test probability of DVT/VTE	Likelihood of VTE on venography (gold standard)	Likelihood of VTE with negative D-dimer	Implications of D-dimer testing
High	75%	21%	D-dimer unhelpful because still need to ultrasound scan a 21% probability
Intermediate	17%	1.8%	Physicians might accept a 1.8% probability as sufficiently low to not test further, but the 1.8% figure relies on the more sensitive D-dimer assays
Low	3%	0.3%	D-dimer converts low to very low probability, i.e. no further testing needed

Table 2.76 The role of D-dimer testing in suspected venous thromboembolism (VTE)

in future. They include fondaparinux (a synthetic penta-saccharide that exclusively inhibits factor Xa by causing a conformational change in antithrombin promoting Xa binding) and direct thrombin inhibitors (DTIs).

What is the current state of play of DTIs?

DTIs are a new class of anticoagulant that bind directly to thrombin and block its interactions by binding to one of its three domains – the active or catalytic site or two exosites. Exosite 1 is a dock for fibrin. Exosite 2 is the heparin-binding domain. As well as heparin's ability to act in the heparin–antithrombin–thrombin complex, heparin can bind to both exosite 2 and fibrin. Because both thrombin exosites are occupied within this fibrin–heparin–thrombin complex, thrombin's activity is relatively protected from inactivation by the heparin–antithrombin complex. Thus, heparins have less capacity to inhibit fibrin-bound thrombin, which appears detri-mental. DTIs act independently of antithrombin, and can inhibit thrombin bound to fibrin or fibrin-degradation products. Bivalent DTIs (e.g. hirudin, bivalirudin) block the active site and exosite 1, and dissociate from thrombin, leaving a small amount of free active thrombin. Univalent DTIs (e.g. argatroban, melagatran and its oral precursor ximelagatran, dibigatran) block only the active site and inactivate fibrin-bound thrombin. DTIs, by reducing thrombin-mediated activation of platelets, also have an antiplatelet effect.

Evidence had been accumulating for the use of DTIs in atrial fibrillation and VTE treatment and prophylaxis, although their role in acute coronary syndromes and percutaneous coronary intervention had been less compelling. However, all uses of DTIs have now been put on hold because of concerns about liver toxicity and ximelagatran has been withdrawn.

Do you know of any roles of therapeutic activated protein C?

Intravenous infusion of activated protein C is administered in selected patients with severe sepsis and multi-organ failure.

CASE 2.37

THROMBOPHILIC TENDENCY

Candidate information

Role

You are a doctor in the medical outpatient clinic. Please read the following letter from the patient's general practitioner. You may make notes on the paper provided. When the bell sounds, enter the examination room to begin the consultation.

Scenario

> Dear Doctor
>
> Re: Mr Edward Ferrars, aged 28 years
>
> Thank you for seeing this gentleman who appears to have a family history of venous thromboembolism. He himself had an axillary deep vein thrombosis two years ago diagnosed in South East Asia but this was thought to be due to prolonged carriage of a rucksack. He was warfarinised for six months. He is a new patient to my surgery and at a routine medical examination he mentioned that a brother has just been diagnosed with a deep vein thrombosis. I wonder if you would consider thrombophilia testing and/or long-term anticoagulation.
>
> Yours sincerely

Please take a history from the patient (you may continue to make notes if you wish on the paper provided). Your examiners will warn you when 12 minutes have elapsed. You have 14 minutes to take a history from the patient followed by 1 minute of reflection. There will then follow 5 minutes of discussion with the examiners. Be prepared to discuss solutions to the problems posed by the case and how you might reply to the GP's letter. You are not required to examine the patient.

Patient information

Mr Edward Ferrars is a healthy 28-year-old who two years ago had an axillary vein thrombosis while backpacking in Thailand. This was thought to have been caused by prolonged axillary pressure of the backpack in combination with severe dehydration. He has two siblings, one of whom has just had a deep vein thrombosis (DVT) diagnosed at a slightly older age than he, but without any obvious cause. His mother had a DVT during pregnancy. To his knowledge his grandparents died of strokes and heart attacks at reasonable ages although he thinks a grandmother might have had a DVT when she sustained a hip fracture. There is no family history of recurrent miscarriage. He takes no medications, and does not drink or smoke. He is concerned that there appears to be a family history of blood clots and wonders if there is anything he might do to reduce his risk, especially as he is a professional wind-surfer and takes frequent long-haul flights.

How to approach the case

Data gathering in the interview and interpretation and use of information gathered

Presenting problem(s) and symptom exploration

Ask about:

- The circumstances and robustness of the diagnosis of the axillary vein thrombosis (diagnosis likely because he was taking warfarin)
- Family history (below)
- His general health now with a full systematic enquiry

The inherited thrombophilias are summarised in Box 2.73.

Patient perspective

His concerns are entirely understandable.

Past medical history

The history of an axillary vein thrombosis is highly relevant because this is unusual without a lesion obstructing axillary flow.

Drug and allergy history

Ask about prescription and non-prescription drugs, including anabolic steroids.

Box 2.73 Inherited thrombophilias

The natural anticoagulants, some of which are shown in Fig. 2.12C (Case 2.34), are impaired in inherited thrombophilias.

Protein C and S deficiencies and activated protein C resistance

Protein C is activated by thrombomodulin, an endothelial molecule that complexes with thrombin in homeostatic response to coagulation. Activated protein C cleaves factors Va and Vlla to prevent untamed clotting. Protein C deficiency may be autosomal dominant or recessive, the latter causing problems at birth. Protein S is a cofactor for protein C and protein S deficiency may cause similar disturbance. Factor V Leiden is a mutated form of factor V that is resistant to the effects of protein C. This is the commonest inherited thrombophilia and is also known as activated protein C resistance.

Antithrombin deficiency

Antithrombin deficiency is autosomal dominant and similarly common.

Prothrombin gene variant

G to A transposition at position 20210 in the 3′ untranslated region leads to elevated levels of prothrombin.

Dysfibrinogenaemia

This is rare and associated with low plasma fibrinogen levels.

Hyperhomocysteinaemia

This is discussed below.

Family history

The family history of at least two first-degree relatives with venous thromboembolism (VTE) is significant, and almost certainly warrants further assessment (see Case 2.36). Particular features to elicit are the age of family members when they developed symptoms and whether or not there were any clear provocative factors.

Social history

His active lifestyle may be protective although long-term anticoagulation could carry particular risks.

SUMMARY – ASSESSMENT AND PLAN

- There is probably an inherited thrombophilia exerting a modestly increased risk of venous thromboembolism.
- His active lifestyle may be protective against blood clots except for the long-haul flights, which merit advice about adequate hydration and mobility.
- Long-term anticoagulation might be considered pending the results of a thrombophilia screen (below).

Discussion

What do you understand by the term thrombophilia?

This refers to an inherited or acquired disorder of coagulation, with the potential for thromboembolism. The most important risk factors for VTE are a personal or family history, with an approximate 10-fold increased relative risk if there is a first-degree relative with a history of VTE. It has been difficult to quantify risk attributable to inherited thrombophilias, largely because these do not act alone but conspire with other factors. Thrombotic risk in factor V Leiden heterozygotes, for example, is increased dramatically by smoking and the oral contraceptive pill. Estimated increases in relative risk are given in Table 2.77.

How does hyperhomocysteinaemia lead to a prothrombotic tendency?

There are strong links between hyperhomocysteinaemia and occlusive vascular disease. The reasons are speculative, but homocysteine is atherogenic and causes oxidative damage to low-density lipoprotein. It may modify

---

Table 2.77 Risk of VTE attributable to inherited thrombophilia

	Approximate increased risk of VTE	Prevalence in patients with VTE (%)	Prevalence in normal population (%)
Protein C deficiency	10–15 ×	3	0.3
Protein S deficiency	10 ×	3	2
Antithrombin deficiency	25–50 ×	1	0.2
Heterozygous factor V Leiden (FVL) mutation	5 × (homozygous 10–80 ×)	25–50	5
Heterozygous prothrombin G20210A	4 × (homozygous unknown)	6	2
Heterozygous combined FVL and Prothrombin G20210a	20 ×		

apolipoproteins, and is hypertensive, interfering with endothelium-derived relaxation factor. It also seems to down-regulate anticoagulation, including protein C and thrombomodulin expression, and activate coagulants such as factor V.

How does hyperhomocysteinaemia arise?

The conversion of 5,10-methylenetetrahydrofolate (5,10-MTHF) to 5-methyltetrahydrofolate (5-MTHF) through methylene-tetrahydrofolate reductase (MTHFR) is a crucial starting point for normal homocysteine metabolism and DNA synthesis. The 5-MTHF is converted to tetrahydrofolate (THF) by MTHF : homocysteine methyltransferase, generating a methyl group that is transferred to homocysteine, converting homocysteine to methionine. It is the THF that is crucial to DNA synthesis. This series of reactions, known as the remethylation pathway of homocysteine metabolism, is folate dependent.

The mutated C677T MTHFR, known as the thermolabile variant, in its heterozygous form, is associated with a moderate (20%) increase in serum homocysteine and a modestly increased risk of arterial and venous thrombosis. The prevalence varies between populations but in many Western countries may be around 15%. Homozygous polymorphism is rare, but promotes markedly elevated homocysteine levels and vascular risk.

Homocysteine is not metabolised exclusively to methionine. In the alternative transulphuration alternative pathway it is metabolised to cysteine by the action of cystathione β-synthase. Mutations in cystathione β-synthase give rise to homocystinuria, in which homocysteine levels and thrombotic risk are very high.

Why is folate important?

The B vitamins, especially folate, may protect against vascular disease, birth defects (neural tube defects), recurrent pregnancy loss and cancer by lowering homocysteine or by epigenetic mechanisms (several mechanisms pivotal to genomic machinery are sensitive to B vitamin status).

Dietary methionine cannot provide all the methyl groups needed for cellular methylation reactions and so de novo production of methionine is important. Folate stabilises the *C677T* variant gene by preventing release of its flavin cofactor and as MTHFR is a flavin protein, riboflavin (B2) supplements may also lower homocysteine.

Precursors to DNA are dependent upon a healthy MTHFR pathway with adequate folate. If folate is low, uracil misincorporation occurs, leading to breaks in DNA and a predisposition to cancer.

Is there a role for folic acid in cardiovascular disease prevention?

High homocysteine levels contribute to arterial and venous thrombosis. Some evidence (not without some contradictions) suggests that lowering homocysteine levels by 3 µmol/l from current levels (achievable with folic acid 0.8 mg daily) reduces the risk of ischaemic heart disease by 16%, of stroke by 24% and of VTE by 25%, and that folate should be considered for primary or secondary prophylaxis in people at risk. Testing homocysteine levels may not be necessary to institute therapy because of the high rate of occurrence of hyperhomocysteinaemia in people with vascular disease.

Is folate supplementation a good idea for the general population?

Folate used in food fortification is not a natural coenzyme and the long-term effects of unmodified synthetic folate are unknown. Furthermore, there is an increasing tendency for clinicians to recommend 5 mg of folate daily, which is more than 10 times that needed to give maximal methylfolate concentrations.

What is antiphospholipid syndrome (APS)?

APS causes venous or arterial thrombosis (e.g. VTE, stroke), recurrent fetal loss and sometimes thrombocytopenia and is associated with persistent antiphospholipid antibodies, a group of autoantibodies directed against cell membrane phospholipids.

The antiphospholipid antibodies routinely tested for are lupus anticoagulant (LAC), which causes prolongation of phospholipid-dependent assays such as activated partial thromboplastin time (APTT) and anticardiolipin antibodies (ACL) of immunoglobulin G or M subclass.

The mechanism for thrombosis is not yet clear, but phospholipid-associated β_2-glycoprotein-1 (β_2-GP1) has an antithrombotic role and in APS the β_2-GP1 antibodies appear to activate endothelial cells and platelets and reduce activated protein C activity. Anti-β_2-GP1 detection is now an important part of assessment of APS.

APS may be primary or secondary, associated with chronic inflammatory diseases such as systemic lupus erythematosus and other connective tissue diseases, infections such as human immunodeficiency virus, hepatitis C and varicella viruses, lymphoproliferative diseases and certain drugs.

Diagnosis requires at least one of two clinical criteria (thrombotic event or recurrent pregnancy loss) and at least one of three laboratory criteria (LAC or ACL or β_2-GP1 positivity on two occasions at least 12 weeks apart).

Heparin is used in pregnancy to prevent pregnancy loss but evidence is insubstantial on anticoagulation versus antiplatelet therapy for treating and preventing other thrombotic manifestations of APS (see also Case 5.18).

Who should be considered for thrombophilia screening?

A normal thrombophilia screen does not exclude prothrombotic defects that may be yet to be discovered and cannot be assumed to imply 'normal' or 'no increased risk' in the future or in other family members. There is no evidence that identifying an abnormality influences the type of anticoagulant treatment, its intensity or its duration. Therefore, identifying a thrombophilia will not influence a patient's immediate treatment. Whether it may be of value in preventing further thrombosis and in counselling other family members, notably any family members contemplating pregnancy, is an area of uncertainty and possible indications for thrombophilia testing include:

- Patients with apparently spontaneous thrombosis, particularly if young or if pregnant, e.g. stroke at a young age without risk factors
- Patients with thrombosis at an unusual site, e.g. sagittal sinus thrombosis
- Patients with recurrent thrombosis
- Patients with VTE and a history of VTE in a first-degree relative
- Recurrent pregnancy loss
- Pre-pregnancy counselling

CASE 2.38

MYELOMA

Candidate information

Role

You are a doctor in the medical outpatient clinic. Please read the following letter from the patient's general practitioner. You may make notes on the paper provided. When the bell sounds, enter the examination room to begin the consultation.

Scenario

Dear Doctor

Re: Mr Frank Boyd, aged 66 years

Thank you for seeing this man, who 12 months ago was found to have a monoclonal paraprotein band on protein electrophoresis but was well at the time. He has no past medical history of note other than hypertension and stable chronic kidney disease with a creatinine of 150 μmol/l. For the last six months he has had intermittent watery diarrhoea, initially worse after new antihypertensive treatment was started but this has now been stopped and his blood pressure is now normal and without any postural drop. Coeliac antibodies are negative. However, repeat protein electrophoresis now shows two monoclonal bands, his plasma viscosity is 2.6 and his creatinine is 370 μmol/l. His serum potassium is 2.3 mmol/l with normal serum sodium. A skeletal survey is normal. I would appreciate your advice.

Yours sincerely

Please take a history from the patient (you may continue to make notes if you wish on the paper provided). Your examiners will warn you when 12 minutes have elapsed. You have 14 minutes to take a history from the patient followed by 1 minute of reflection. There will then follow 5 minutes of discussion with the examiners. Be prepared to discuss solutions to the problems posed by the case and how you might reply to the GP's letter. You are not required to examine the patient.

Patient information

Mr Frank Boyd is a 66-year-old with a six-month history of intermittent watery diarrhoea. Episodes last for a few days, although he may be well for weeks in between. He thinks it all started after a blood pressure tablet was started, but this was stopped soon afterwards and the diarrhoea has continued. He has a history of high blood pressure going back some years and takes amlodipine and ramipril, although his GP has recently stopped the ramipril because of worsening kidney tests. Mr Boyd is aware that his GP also obtained an abnormal blood test 12 months ago that can sometimes indicate a blood disease called myeloma. He refused referral to a hospital specialist at the time because he was afraid of a diagnosis of 'cancer'. However, the more recent tests indicate a worsening of that abnormality. He is a retired aircraft mechanic, lives happily with his wife and has smoked heavily since teenage years. He has not been overseas for 30 years and his wife is well.

How to approach the case

Data gathering in the interview and interpretation and use of information gathered

Presenting problem(s) and symptom exploration

Where confronted with a single problem you can delve deeply into its nuances. Here, you do not know which of the paraproteinaemia and hyperviscosity, the renal failure or the diarrhoea are more significant, whether they are equally important, whether they represent separate underlying pathologies or whether there is a unifying diagnosis. This case illustrates the importance of steering close to a standard history-taking framework. Ask particularly about:

- Symptoms of myeloma (Table 2.78)
- The nature of the diarrhoea
- Causes of renal failure (dehydration, symptoms of heart failure, renovascular risk factors, drugs, prostatic symptoms)

Patient perspective

Acknowledge and explore his earlier concerns about investigation.

Case 2.38 Myeloma

Table 2.78 Clinical features of myeloma			
Problem	**Prevalence**	**How it arises**	**Symptoms**
Bone disease	The most common presenting symptom (60% of patients)	Myeloma cells migrate from vessels and adhere to marrow stromal cells under the influence of cytokines. This causes stromal cells to produce IL-6, an important growth and survival factor for myeloma cells IL-1, IL-6 and TNF-α, all increased, mediate osteoclastic resorption through RANK-L while osteoprotegerin, a RANK-L inhibitor, is reduced Adhesion also causes myeloma cells to secrete vascular endothelial growth factor leading to new vessel formation, which may be important in tumour growth Alkaline phosphatase levels are normal, reflecting the normal or reduced osteoblast activity	Bone pain, especially back Osteoporosis and pathological fractures, especially vertebral Hypercalcaemia
Renal failure	25–30% 5% severe	Dehydration (unwell, pain, hypercalcaemia) Hypercalcaemia Hyperuricaemia Sepsis Direct proximal tubule damage from BJP Amyloid deposition	
Anaemia	Common presenting feature	Bone marrow infiltration Anaemia of chronic disease Cytokines such as IL-1 impair red cell production, iron incorporation and metabolism	Fatigue
Infection	Common	Myeloma impairs B-cell immunity with suppression of other normal immunoglobulins ('immune paresis') and also suppresses T cells A large quantity of immunoglobulin is around but is monoclonal and usually non-functional and suppresses residual normal polyclonal B cells	Lower respiratory tract infections common
Amyloidosis	10% of myeloma		Primary amyloidosis Kidney usually affected (nephrotic syndrome) Heart failure Peripheral neuropathy
Constitutional symptoms	Common	Cytokines produced by myeloma cells, e.g. TNF-α	Fatigue Fever
Hyperviscosity	More common with hyper IgM disease (Waldenstrom's)	Ig M load	Headache Blurred vision Dilated retinal veins and haemorrhages
Neurological	Less common		
Bleeding	Less common		
Asymptomatic	Common		Patients are increasingly diagnosed by way of raised inflammatory markers (plasma viscosity, ESR)

BJP, Bence Jones protein; IgM, immunoglobulin M; IL-6, interleukin-6; RANK-L, receptor activator of nuclear factor-κB ligand; TNF-α, tumour necrosis factor-α.

Past medical history

His background kidney disease renders his kidneys more susceptible to threat from any new insult.

Drug and allergy history

The angiotensin-converting enzyme (ACE) inhibitor might have been an important contributor to the renal failure.

Family history

Relevance here is unlikely.

Social history

This could be relevant, especially with respect to chronic infectious diarrhoea (overseas travel, unwell family members).

SUMMARY – ASSESSMENT AND PLAN

There are three highly plausible explanations for his symptoms and investigation results:

- *Myeloma with secondary renal failure*, although the normal haemoglobin and skeletal survey are a little unusual with this degree of renal failure. This would not explain the diarrhoea, and even although myeloma is immunosuppressive, infective gastroenteritis of this duration seems unlikely (*Giardia* can be notoriously recurrent and indolent with watery diarrhoea, but is not a typical infectious complication of myeloma).
- *Amyloid* causing the raised paraprotein level, renal failure and gastrointestinal involvement. This would be a unifying diagnosis.
- *Monoclonal gammopathy of undetermined significance* (MGUS) and a separate cause for the diarrhoea. The hypokalaemia might simply be secondary to chronic diarrhoea but is rather low, especially considering that he has renal failure. A potassium-secreting bowel tumour should certainly be considered. Renal failure is similarly not explained by MGUS (which by definition does not cause organ damage) but this could simply be pre-renal impairment consequent upon dehydration. An ex-heavy smoker, he may also have a precarious cardio-renal balance with incipient heart failure from ischaemia; furthermore, renovascular disease from previous hypertension and smoking may have taken their toll on his renal reserve, with a lower threshold for damage by dehydration. The ACE inhibitor would have been contributory.

Important next steps include:

- Referral to a haematologist and bone marrow examination
- Sigmoidoscopy and biopsy with Congo Red stain for amyloid
- Colonoscopy
- A renal opinion

Discussion

What is myeloma?

Myeloma refers to a malignant clone of B-cell-derived plasma cells in the bone marrow producing high concentrations of one particular (monoclonal) immunoglobulin. In 80% of patients there is a paraprotein in the serum, usually immunoglobulin G (IgG) or IgA class, but the abnormal cells may also produce free light chains small enough for excursion through glomeruli and tubules and appear in the urine as Bence Jones proteins (BJPs). In 20% of patients free light chains are present only without paraprotein in serum but with BJPs in the urine. Rarely, the cell clone does not secrete immunoglobulin or light chains (non-secretory myeloma).

What is the spectrum of plasma cell dyscrasias?

There is a range of plasma cell disorders (Box 2.74).

How common is myeloma?

The UK incidence is around 60 per million (around 3000 new cases per year), and it comprises 10% of haematological malignancies and 1% of all malignancies. The incidence increases with age, median age of presentation 60–65, peaking at 65–85. Under 2% are under 40 years of age. It is more common in males, and Afro-Caribbean people.

Box 2.74 Plasma cell disorders

- (Multiple) myeloma
- Monoclonal gammopathy of uncertain significance (MGUS)
- Plasmacytoma
- Plasma cell leukaemia
- Non-secretory myeloma
- POEMS syndrome (osteosclerotic myeloma with peripheral neuropathy, organomegaly, endocrinopathies and skin manifestations)
- Amyloidosis
- Hyper immunoglobulin M (Waldenström's macroglobulinaemia) – a lymphoplasmacytic disorder, with hyperviscosity, perhaps better classified with non-Hodgkin's lymphoma
- Heavy chain disorders

What causes myeloma?

This is unknown, but there are associations with ionising radiation, occupation (railroad workers and agriculture), rheumatoid arthritis and viruses such as human immunodeficiency virus and human herpes virus 8, together with familial clustering.

How is myeloma diagnosed?

The Duric and Salmon criteria published in 1975 are still widely used. These comprise three major criteria (plasmacytoma on biopsy, bone marrow plasma cells > 30%, monoclonal band – IgG > 35 g/l, IgA > 20 g/l, BJP > 1 g/24 hours) and four minor criteria (bone marrow plasma cells 10–30%, paraprotein present but less than above, lytic bone lesions, low immunoglobulins – immune paresis); diagnosis requires one major criterion plus one minor criterion, two major criteria or three minor criteria. New diagnostic criteria for myeloma were published in British Haematology Society guidelines in 2005 (Table 2.79).

There should be an index of suspicion. Test results warranting consideration of myeloma include unexplained anaemia with rouleaux on the blood film, raised inflammatory markers, renal impairment, hypercalcaemia and radiological lytic lesions. Baseline diagnostic tests include immunoglobulin levels and serum and urine electrophoresis for paraprotein. Diagnostic confirmation is by bone marrow examination, traditionally aspiration but increasingly with biopsy and staining for CD138 antibody to detect plasma cells. Plasma cells in myeloma may be morphologically different as well as abundant.

What is the place of radiology in myeloma?

A skeletal survey to demonstrate lytic lesions including the classic 'pepperpot skull' has low sensitivity and is less frequently performed. Computed tomography improves sensitivity but is not routine. Magnetic resonance imaging is good for detecting soft tissue masses, spinal cord compression and the pattern of bone marrow involvement, which has as yet postulated prognostic implications. Positron emission tomography scanning may be used in the future.

Table 2.79 Diagnostic criteria for myeloma

	MGUS (common; 1% per year progress to myeloma)	Asymptomatic myeloma (12–32% per year progress to symptomatic myeloma)	Symptomatic myeloma
M protein (g/l)	< 30	> 30	> 30
Bone marrow plasma cell percentage	< 10%	> 10%	> 10%, commonly > 30%
Organ or tissue involvement	No	No	Anaemia Renal disease Bone lesions Other

MGUS, monoclonal gammopathy of undetermined significance.

Table 2.80 Prognosis in myeloma

Stage	Features
I	Serum β_2-microglobulin < 3.5 mg/l (and albumin > 35 g/l)
II	Neither I nor III
III	Serum β_2-microglobulin > 5.5 mg/l

Other prognostic factors
Raised C-reactive protein
Atypical plasma cells
Cytogenetic abnormalities, e.g. trisomy 3, 7, 9, 11 or loss of 13q.

What treatments are there for myeloma?

Myeloma is incurable except possibly by allogeneic bone marrow transplantation (BMT), and even then cure rates are very small (around 5%). Median survival is 3–4 years.

Initial treatment achieves a response (decreased symptoms and tumour burden) in around two-thirds of patients but the paraprotein is seldom completely dispelled and tends to plateau at a low level after a few months of treatment, which is then stopped. Melphalan remains the most effective chemotherapy, usually given in combination with prednisolone for a few days each month. Interferon-α as maintenance treatment can prolong the plateau by a few months but has no significant survival effect and frequent side effects.

When paraprotein levels start to rise again, indicating relapse, further treatment, often with a different drug or combination, may achieve a further response although remission is usually sustained for a shorter time and ultimately the disease becomes refractory. Thalidomide achieves a response in up to 30% of patients with refractory disease, and improves survival in combination with melphalan and response rates in combination with prednisolone but with increased thromboembolic risk. Thalidomide analogues have been developed. Burtezemib, a proteosome inhibitor, has been used but remains low in the hierarchy of treatment.

Haematopoietic stem cell transplantation (HSCT) may be autologous or allogeneic. Cyclophosphamide is effective, and vincristine and adriamycin by four-day infusion into a Hickman line combined with dexamethasone (VAD) achieves rapid response in over 75% of patients and is used in younger patients before autologous transplantation. High-dose intensive chemotherapy with autologous stem cell support prolongs remission and survival but does not cure. Allogeneic transplantation, suitable for patients up to 55 years of age with a matched sibling donor, is potentially curative. It carries high transplant mortality but lower relapse rates because of graft versus myeloma effect. Reduced intensity conditioning regimens may extend the use of allogeneic transplantation to older patients.

Other standard treatments now include vaccination, bisphosphonate therapy and hydration for bone disease and analgesia.

What prognostic factors are there in myeloma?

A prognosis staging system (2003) is outlined in Table 2.80, as are other prognostic factors in symptomatic myeloma.

How would you manage suspected MGUS?

MGUS is common, and 10% of older people have a small detectable paraprotein. If anaemia, renal impairment, hypercalcaemia and evidence of organ involvement are excluded people can be observed. The combination of anaemia and a raised erythrocyte sedimentation rate or plasma viscosity should always prompt a paraprotein search. Referral to a haematologist is indicated if there is a high paraprotein, immune paresis or evidence of organ or tissue effects.

What is a plasmacytoma?

This is a localised cluster of myeloma cells which may produce any of the usual symptoms or pressure effects such as spinal cord compression (may also occur from vertebral collapse).

What is amyloidosis?

Amyloidosis is a spectrum of conditions resulting from amyloid fibril deposition and is classified according to the amyloidogenic protein that forms the fibrillary deposits:

- In *primary (AL) amyloidosis* the protein is an immunoglobulin light chain or fragment produced by a clone of plasma cells, although in most AL amyloidosis the plasma cell burden is typically low and only about 10% of AL amyloidosis is the result of myeloma.
- *Secondary (AA) amyloidosis* occurs in longstanding inflammation. Serum amyloid A protein, an acute-phase reactant produced in the liver, is the amyloidogenic protein.
- In the *familial amyloidosis* an amino acid substitution in a plasma protein, often transthyretin, renders it amyloidogenic.
- *Senile systemic amyloidosis* is also caused by transthyretin and tends to affect the heart.

The kidney is the most common site of damage in AL and AA amyloidoses, usually manifested as nephrotic syndrome, often with massive proteinuria and oedema resistant to diuretics. Renal failure is inevitable unless amyloid

Table 2.81 Clinical features of amyloidosis

Organ	Disorder
Kidney	Nephrotic syndrome Renal failure (an unusual combination which should always prompt consideration of amyloidosis)
Heart	Restrictive cardiomyopathy Cardiac arrhythmias Valvular heart disease
Gut and liver	Ischaemic colitis Hepatosplenomegaly and altered liver enzymes
Lung	Parenchymal infiltration Pleural effusions
Nervous system	Autonomic neuropathy Peripheral neuropathy
Other	Macroglossia (specific to AL amyloidosis, occurring in around 20%)

formation can be halted and is rare without marked proteinuria unless the amlyoid is predominantly confined to the tubulointerstitium and blood vessels, sparing the glomeruli. Amyloidosis (with the exeption of AA amyloidosis) also causes concentric left ventricular hypertrophy and a restrictive cardiomyopathy results from restriction to dilatation and filling that reduces cardiac output despite a relatively preserved ejection fraction. Clinical features of amyloidosis are given in Table 2.81. Diagnosing amyloidosis relies on demonstrating binding of Congo red dye to tissue deposits and birefringence when viewed with polarised light microscopy.

INFECTIOUS DISEASE PROBLEMS

CASE 2.39

HUMAN IMMUNODEFICIENCY VIRUS INFECTION

Candidate information

Role

You are a doctor in the emergency medical admissions unit. Please read the following letter from the patient's general practitioner. You may make notes on the paper provided. When the bell sounds, enter the examination room to begin the consultation.

Scenario

Dear Doctor

Re: Mr Jason Moriarty, aged 35 years

Thank you for admitting this gentleman with human immunodeficiency virus who has become breathless over a few days. He is slightly tachypnoeic, his temperature is 38°C, and he looks sweaty and unwell. I am concerned about pneumonia.

Yours sincerely

Please take a history from the patient (you may continue to make notes if you wish on the paper provided). Your examiners will warn you when 12 minutes have elapsed. You have 14 minutes to take a history from the patient followed by 1 minute of reflection. There will then follow 5 minutes of discussion with the examiners. Be prepared to discuss solutions to the problems posed by the case and how you might reply to the GP's letter. You are not required to examine the patient.

Patient information

Mr Jason Moriarty is a 35-year-old gentleman who is human immunodeficiency virus (HIV)-positive, infection acquired 12 years ago through homosexual intercourse. He has taken highly active antiretroviral treatment (HAART) for the past few years, although concordance with treatment has recently been problematic because of life stresses and side effects of treatment, and he has missed a number of follow-up appointments with his specialist. His last documented CD4 count was 250/μl, measured around four months ago. He now presents with a short respiratory illness comprising a dry cough, breathlessness and fever. He is worried about the possibility of *Pneumocystis jirovecii* pneumonia. His past medical history other than HIV is uneventful. In terms of HIV he has had problems with recurrent herpes zoster, recurrent candidiasis and white oral plaques. He has recently separated from his long-term partner and lives alone and describes himself as very depressed. He has given up work as a store designer. He is not infected with the hepatitis C virus.

How to approach the case

Data gathering in the interview and interpretation and use of information gathered

Presenting problem(s) and symptom exploration

▪ **Consider HIV-associated respiratory disease (but also the usual causes of breathlessness)** HIV-associated respiratory disease is common, affecting more than 50% of patients. Typical respiratory infections that affect non-HIV-infected people are common in early disease, but may be more severe. These include upper respiratory tract infections, sinusitis, bronchitis and bacterial pneumonia. With CD4 counts under 200/μl *P. jirovecii* is a problem (Box 2.75). Tuberculosis can occur at any stage. Non-infectious respiratory diseases in HIV include Kaposi's sarcoma, lymphoma, lung cancer and non-specific interstitial pneumonitis, the latter possible when the CD4 count is normal.

Patient perspective

Explore his reasons for stopping treatment, not least his depression.

Past medical history

Explore the duration of his diagnosis, how it came to be diagnosed and the likely mode of transmission and explore his list of symptoms and opportunistic infections to date and what treatments he has received for these.

Drug and allergy history

He has been taking HAART, but his poor concordance recently will have exposed him to a high risk of vigorous mutation of HIV with a further fall in the CD4 count and opportunistic infections, notably *P. jirovecii*. Enquire about side effects of HAART that might have contributed to his stopping treatment, rather than assuming it was exclusively depression.

Family history

Relevance here is unlikely.

Box 2.75 *Pneumocystis jirovecii* pneumonia

Formerly known as *Pneumocystis carinii*, this is a fungal infection that remains a common AIDS-defining disease. Most patients develop the disease without HAART. It is common in patients who cannot tolerate or who are non-compliant with HAART and probably arises as new infection, rather than reactivation as was once thought.

It causes a non-productive cough and breathlessness over two to three weeks, often with severe hypoxia, and minimal chest signs.

Social history

Explore what risk modification behaviour he has used to reduce the risk of transmission.

SUMMARY – ASSESSMENT AND PLAN

- He should have all the usual investigations first – a full screen of haematobiochemisty, a chest X-ray and arterial blood gases. The chest X-ray appearances in *P. jirovecii* range from mild, bilateral, perihilar interstitial infiltrates to confluent, diffuse alveolar opacification which can progress over a few days. Other appearances are possible, including upper zone infiltrates, pulmonary nodules or lobar consolidation.
- While the differential diagnosis in patients not known to be infected with HIV includes atypical pneumonia, a careful history in HIV usually reveals other signs of immune compromise such as oral candidiasis. Lymphopenia is common. *Pneumocystis jirovecii* may be confirmed by Giemsa staining or polymerase chain reaction of induced sputum or bronchoalveolar lavage fluid.
- Treatment is usually started empirically in patients with a presumptive diagnosis of *P. jirovecii* pneumonia and a CD4 count below 200/μl. First-line is co-trimoxazole, initially intravenously except in mild disease without hypoxia. Alternatives include clindamycin with primaquine, dapsone with trimethoprim or atovaquone. Pentamidine is now seldom used. Corticosteroids are given for moderate to severe disease.
- Prophylaxis uses co-trimoxazole first-line. Primary prophylaxis is indicated for a CD4 count below 200/μl, HIV-associated constitutional features or a history of any acquired immunodeficiency syndrome (AIDS) defining diagnosis. Secondary prophylaxis is indicated for all patients. Prophylaxis may be discontinued if patients on HAART exhibit sustained increases in CD4 counts greater than 200/μl and suppression of viral load below the limits of detection.

Discussion

What do you know about the epidemiology of HIV infection?

HIV affects 40 million adults worldwide. The major route of transmission is heterosexual (> 75%). About 5–10% of new infections are in children, usually acquired during pregnancy, birth or breastfeeding. Injecting drug users represent a smaller proportion of the mode of acquisition.

What types of HIV are there?

HIV-1 has multiple groups and genetic subtypes, and mutation of strains is part of its ability to survive. HIV-1 is derived from the simian immunodeficiency virus of chimpanzees. HIV-2 is quite dissimilar, common in parts of Africa and genetically closer to the sooty mangabey virus. It is inherently resistant to non-nucleoside reverse transcriptase inhibitors. Related viruses causing immunodeficiency infect other animals including cats, sheep, goats and horses.

Describe the structure of the HIV virion

HIV is a retrovirus comprising two RNA copies of the genes *env*, *gag* and *pol*; *env* encodes glycoprotein gp160, which is cleaved to form the gp120 surface molecule and the gp41 transmembrane molecule; *gag* encodes the precursor to the capsid molecules p24, p17, p9 and p6, the latter enabling budding of the virus; *pol* encodes the enzymes reverse transcriptase, protease and integrase. There are also regulatory genes – *tat*, which regulates transcription, *rev*, which aids translation and *nef*, which down-regulates expression of CD4, major histocompatibility complex (MHC) class 1 proteins and interleukin-2 (IL-2), and recruits lymphocytes to infected macrophages to aid spread.

How does the virus replicate?

Gp120 binds to CD4 surface antigens on T lymphocytes and macrophages. Entry of the HIV virion into host cells also requires the interaction of gp120 with chemokine co-receptor CCR5, found predominantly on macrophages, and with chemokine co-receptor CXCR4, found predominantly on lymphocytes. Binding leads to a conformational change in the envelope molecule such that a hydrophobic sharp tip of the transmembrane protein gp41 is exposed which can penetrate the host cell. Viral capsid is then released into the cytoplasm of the host cell. Reverse transcriptase converts the RNA genome into double-stranded DNA. DNA is then integrated into the host genome under the control of viral integrase. The integrated gene is treated by the host as a normal gene, transcribed and translated into a new virion aided by the regulatory genes, before budding out of the cell. Replication is rapid, with perhaps 10^{10} viruses produced daily and 10^8 host cells destroyed, especially at lymph node sites.

What is the pathogenesis of HIV infection and why do some people appear to be 'immune' to HIV?

The virus transmitted sexually across mucous membranes is almost exclusively macrophage tropic, and on infecting the macrophages it is transported to draining lymph nodes. People homozygous for CCR5 mutations appear to be protected from acquiring HIV by this route, and heterozygotes progress slowly. Macrophage-tropic HIV can infect central nervous system microganglia and probably accounts for HIV brain disease. Lymphocyte-tropic HIV may be acquired directly from contaminated blood but in most patients appears later in the course of infection as the macrophage-tropic virus evolves to use the CXCR4 receptor.

What is the immune response to HIV infection?

Innate immune responses are activated immediately but cannot stop the virus. Acquired, adaptive immune responses involve clonal expansion of B cells to produce antibodies and T-cell responses. Acute infection with HIV leads to rapid replication and within weeks several million copies of the HIV genome are found in the plasma, the peak level being determined by host immunity. However, this number rapidly declines to a steady state, because initial numbers comprise a wide variety of genetically different viruses because reverse transcriptase allows significant mutations as an in-built survival mechanism. Ultimately, the mutation potential of HIV is an important factor in the failure of host immunity to contain it.

Antibody responses

Antibodies against *gag* p24 and p17 tend to appear first within a few weeks, but are non-neutralising and non-sustained. Antibodies against envelope proteins needed for cell entry appear later – against a variable region, V3 loop, of gp120, the transmembrane protein gp41 and the binding sites for CD4 and the chemokine co-receptors CCR5 and CXCR4. However, these later antibodies tend to be directed against less crucial sites of these envelope proteins and even when neutralisation occurs, HIV can simply mutate.

Cellular responses

CD8 (cytotoxic) lymphocytes interact via their T-cell receptor (TCR) with MHC class I molecules of infected cells presenting HIV peptides. CD8 cells lyse infected cells directly and produce cytokines such as interferon-γ and tumour necrosis factor-α and chemokines such as macrophage inflammatory proteins 1α and 1β and RANTES (Regulated on Activation Normal T-Cell Expressed and Secreted) that suppress replication or block entry of HIV into CD4 cells. CD4 (T helper) lymphocytes interact via their TCR with the MHC class II molecules of specialised antigen-presenting cells presenting shed protein particles of the HIV virus. CD4 cells produce cytokines that perpetuate the T-helper response and collaborate with B cells in the production of specific antibodies (Case 2.46).

Why does the immune system not usually contain HIV?

Progressive CD4 cell depletion and development of immunodeficiency occur at a median of 10 years. There are numerous factors for this. Latent infection of CD4 cells means they are not visible for CD8 cytotoxicity. Envelope proteins tend to resist antibody neutralisation; numerous non-immunogenic proteins tend to coat more crucial envelope proteins; the V3 loop exhibits many mutations but antibodies to the V3 loop tend to be specific to a particular strain; although the CD4 binding domain is highly conserved between strains, antibodies to it tend to exhibit poor neutralising ability. Minimal mutations in the virus are enough to thwart MHC binding or for HIV particles to escape TCR recognition.

What is meant by the term 'long-term non-progressors' (LTNPs)

This refers to the small proportion (2%) of HIV-infected individuals who remain symptom-free and with low viral loads and stable CD4 counts for up to 20 years. Many have strong neutralising antibody responses. Many have mutant chemokine co-receptors.

Why are the symptoms of opportunistic disease in HIV often atypical?

The eloquent workings of the immune system are illustrated best when at fault. HIV, which parasitises the immune system, affirms that it is ravished defence rather than microbiological attack that causes the clinical manifestations of HIV disease and AIDS. Just as it is the powerful proinflammatory response causing fever, pharyngitis and pain in a common cold and not the furtive adenovirus, so impoverished inflammatory potential limits symptoms. Whilst meningococcal meningitis in immunocompetent individuals rapidly results in severe headache with a life-threatening acute-phase response, cryptococcal meningitis in HIV-infected individuals may be insidious with minimal signs despite a cerebrospinal fluid overrun with organisms.

What is the natural history of HIV infection?

The stages of HIV infection are illustrated in Table 2.82.

Other than *Pneumocystis jirovecii*, what other fungal infections can cause lung disease in HIV?

Cryptococcus neoforms, *Histoplasma capsulatum* and *Coccidioides immitis* are uncommon in the UK but occur in Africa and the USA. Treatment is with fluconazole or amphotericin.

What do you know about mycobacterial infection in HIV?

Tuberculosis may occur at any stage in HIV infection. There is a higher risk of tuberculosis latent reactivation, new acquisition, developing primary progressive disease or miliary, extrapulmonary or disseminated disease. More than two-thirds with tuberculosis present with pulmonary tuberculosis.

In early disease with near normal CD4 counts its behaviour is similar to that in non-HIV-infected adults with post-primary disease – i.e. cough, haemoptysis, dyspnoea, fever, night sweats or weight loss. The chest X-ray may show upper-zone opacification, the tuberculin test is positive and expectorated sputum or bronchoalveolar fluid analysis is often smear-positive.

More advanced HIV can cause atypical tuberculosis presentation, often with weight loss or fever that may be mistaken for HIV 'constitutional' disease. The chest X-ray may resemble primary tuberculosis with hilar lymphadenopathy, diffuse shadowing or even pleural effusion, or may be normal, the tuberculin test is usually negative and sputum or bronchoalveolar fluid analysis is often smear negative but culture positive.

Extrapulmonary tuberculosis is common with CD4 counts under 150/μl and often affects the lymph nodes, bone marrow, liver or pericardium.

Treatment for tuberculosis in HIV uses the standard four-drug regimens for six months used in non-HIV-

Table 2.82 Stages of HIV infection

Stage	When it occurs	Clinical manifestations		Management implications
Seroconversion	6–12 weeks	Seroconverson illness lasting 7–10 days in 40–90% with fever, malaise, arthralgia, maculopapular rash, myalgia, mouth ulcers and pharyngitis in decreasing likelihood Opportunistic infection if CD4 drops transiently below 200/µl Neurological problems occasionally, e.g. Guillain–Barré syndrome, facial nerve palsy, transverse myelitis, aseptic meningitis		Establish diagnosis
Centers for Disease Control (CDC) category A disease	Asymptomatic disease CD4 count usually 350–800/µl	Usually asymptomatic slow decline in CD4 count over 6–8 years Rapid progression usually implies virus using CXCR4 co-receptor Long-term non-progressors (up to 5–10%) Persistent generalised lymphadenopathy (PGL) may be the presenting feature of HIV infection; it persists for over three months in at least two extra-inguinal sites, usually symmetrically		Minor opportunistic infections
CDC category B disease	CD4 count 200–350/µl	Herpes zoster Pulmonary tuberculosis Streptococcal pneumonia (often recurrent and severe) Recurrent oropharyngeal or vaginal candidiasis (especially as approach 200/µl) Oral hairy leucoplakia Salmonellosis Kaposi's sarcoma Cervical intra-epithelial neoplasia II–III Lymphoid interstitial pneumonitis HIV-associated idiopathic thrombocytopenic purpura	**AIDS-defining conditions** *Pneumocystis jirovecii* pneumonia Miliary or extrapulmonary tuberculosis Disseminated *Mycobacterium avium intracellulare* Oesophageal candidiasis Chronic mucocutaneous herpes simplex Chronic cryptosporidial diarrhoea Recurrent non-*typhi* salmonella septicaemia Cryptococcal meningitis Cytomegalovirus retinitis HIV-associated wasting HIV-associated dementia Progressive multifocal leucoencephalopathy Cerebral toxoplasmosis Primary cerebral lymphoma Non-Hodgkin's lymphoma Kaposi's sarcoma	Start HAART
CDC category C disease	CD4 count < 200/µl	*Pneumocystis jirovecii* (formerly *carinii*) pneumonia Miliary or extrapulmonary tuberculosis Mucocutaneous herpes simplex Oesophageal candidiasis *Cryptosporidium* infection *Microsporidium* infection HIV-associated wasting Peripheral neuropathy		Opportunistic infections and neoplasms much more likely
CDC category D disease	CD4 count < 100/µl	Disseminated *Mycobacterium avium intracellulare* Cerebral toxoplasmosis Cryptococcal meningitis (occasionally pneumonia or skin lesions) Cytomegalovirus retinitis/colitis Primary central nervous system lymphoma Non-Hodgkin's lymphoma HIV encephalopathy leading to HIV-associated dementia Progressive multifocal leucoencephalopathy		Potentially fatal complications

infected individuals, but side effects are higher and HAART should be started.

Multi-drug-resistant (MDR) tuberculosis occurs in up to 2% of cases, often as a result of poor concordance with therapy.

Prophylaxis against tuberculosis in HIV-infected individuals is without consensus.

Tuberculosis is a potent stimulator of cell-mediated immunity and there have long been concerns that it may accelerate HIV replication in infected cells; this is also a concern with some other HIV opportunistic infections such as syphilis.

Other mycobacterial diseases occur in HIV. Disseminated *Mycobacterium avium intracellulare* causes fevers, weight loss and anaemia, and may cause diarrhoea. It is a late manifestation of HIV with CD4 counts less than 50/µl. Treatment is with azalide antibiotics such as azithromycin.

What HIV-related oral diseases do you know of?

Oral candidiasis and oral herpes simplex are common. Oral hairy leucoplakia refers to asymptomatic white corrugations on the side of the tongue and is the result of Epstein–Barr virus infection; it is highly suggestive of HIV infection, whereas oral candidiasis is common in many hospitalised and unwell patients.

What HIV-related oesophageal diseases do you know of?

Oesophageal candidiasis is the most common cause of oesophageal symptoms in HIV and an AIDS-defining condition, although it does occur not infrequently outside the setting of HIV. It causes pain on swallowing and dysphagia. It usually responds to single-dose fluconazole and, if that fails, itraconazole. Relapses are uncommon after HAART.

Oesophageal ulceration may be the result of cytomegalovirus or herpes simplex virus infections. Cytomegalovirus produces discrete ulcers of the lower oesophagus or haemorrhagic oesophagitis. Treatments include ganciclovir or foscarnet, and relapses are uncommon after HAART. Herpes simplex virus produces discrete, vesicular lesions and is treated with aciclovir.

What HIV-related diarrhoeal diseases do you know of?

Diarrhoea can occur at any stage of HIV disease and may be caused by various pathogens. It occurs in almost all patients at some point and is a presenting feature of AIDS in a considerable proportion.

Bacterial infections are common and include *Salmonella* and *Campylobacter* spp.

Cryptosporidium parvum is a zoonotic intestinal parasite. Cryptosporidiosis causes self-limiting diarrhoea in HIV-negative people and those with CD4 counts > 200/µl. Chronic diarrhoea with weight loss and malabsorption occur in immunodeficiency. It is identified on stool culture. *Microsporidium* causes less severe but similar symptoms. Treatment is with HAART aiming for a CD4 count over 200/µl.

Cytomegalovirus may affect the entire bowel, including the oesophagus, but most commonly causes inflammatory colitis with bloody diarrhoea in highly immunosuppressed patients.

What is HIV-associated wasting?

Loss of body weight by more than 10% without an obvious cause is an AIDS-defining condition but is now uncommon in the developed world. A pathogen should therefore generally be sought.

What is the range of HIV-related neurological disease?

Seroconversion may be associated with aseptic meningitis, ataxia, or cranial or peripheral neuropathy. Neurological manifestations of more advanced disease have been reduced with HAART and include HIV-associated wasting, cerebral toxoplasmosis, cryptococcal meningitis, cytomegalovirus retinitis or radiculopathy, primary central nervous system lymphoma, HIV encephalopathy leading to AIDS-related dementia and progressive multifocal leu-

coencephalopathy. Peripheral neuropathy is more common with HAART drugs.

What do you know about cerebral toxoplasmosis?

In more than 90% of cases this is the result of a reactivation of latent infection. There is usually a two- to three-week history of fever, headaches or seizures with localising signs. Multiple ring-enhancing lesions are seen on brain imaging. The absence of immunoglobulin G antibodies suggests an alternative cause. First-line treatment is with sulfadiazine and pyrimethamine. Prophylaxis is with cotrimoxazole and seronegative patients should not handle cat-litter or eat undercooked meat. The main differential diagnosis is cerebral lymphoma.

What do you know about cryptococcal meningitis?

Cryptocous neoformans is a fungus that is ubiquitous, especially in bird droppings. Cryptococcal meningitis tends to present insidiously with fever, headache and malaise. The fungus can be demonstrated by India ink staining of cerebrospinal fluid and antigen testing of cerebrospinal fluid or serum is almost always positive. Treatment is with amphotericin, usually with flucytosine, followed by fluconazole.

What are HIV encephalopathy and AIDS-related dementia?

This is a direct result of central nervous system infection and especially affects the central white matter, brainstem and spinal cord. Without HAART, up to 50% of patients develop HIV encephalopathy. Cytomegalovirus and herpes simplex virus encephalitis are in the differential diagnosis but they progress rapidly whereas HIV encephalopathy develops over months and may progress to severe dementia. It can be prevented, but not reversed, with HAART.

What is progressive multifocal leucoencephalopathy?

This is caused by reactivation of the Polyomavirus JC virus. It produces progressive, unrelenting neurological damage that may present in a wide variety of ways including localised hemiparesis, aphasia or ataxia over weeks to months. The JC virus can usually be detected by polymerase chain reaction on cerebrospinal fluid.

What is Kaposi's sarcoma?

This is the most common malignancy associated with HIV-1 and is caused by human herpes virus 8. It is probably derived from lymphovascular endothelium. Most patients present with mucocutaneous disease with discrete, non-itchy, non-tender, purple papules that are often arranged symmetrically on the limbs, trunk, face or hard palate. These may turn brown over time. Oedema from lymphatic involvement can precede lesions. Disease may be indolent or rapidly progressive with visceral as well as cutaneous involvement, especially of the lungs or gastrointestinal tract. HAART and local radiotherapy or intralesional chemotherapy are used for cutaneous disease and systemic chemotherapy, with liposomal doxorubicin or paclitaxel, may be needed in systemic disease.

What other AIDS-related cancers do you know of?

As HAART has reduced infectious disease complications and improved survival in HIV, longer-term malignant complications have become more prevalent. High-grade B-cell non-Hodgkin's lymphoma is 100 times more common in HIV-infected individuals. Systemic non-Hodgkin's lymphoma accounts for about 30% of malignancy-related death in HIV-positive individuals. HAART has not led to a dramatic decrease in the incidence. Primary central nervous system lymphoma is rare in the general population but was common in HIV before HAART. It is strongly associated with Epstein–Barr virus, occurs with CD4 counts less than 50/µl and may be difficult to distinguish from cerebral toxoplasmosis. Seropositivity for *Toxoplasma* antibodies favours toxoplasmosis and detection of Epstein–Barr virus DNA in cerebrospinal fluid suggests primary cerebral lymphoma, but diagnosis may be confirmed by open or stereotactic biopsy. Survival is usually only a few months. Human papillomavirus infection and cervical intraepithelial neoplasia are common in HIV.

What is HIV lipodystrophy?

Up to 30–50% of HIV-infected patients develop a form of lipodystrophy. This may be loss of subcutaneous fat (lipoatrophy) from the face and limbs, and increased central obesity. It is multifactorial, and may be the result of the virus, genetic factors, hypertriglyceridaemia, hypercholesterolaemia or anti-HIV drugs, protease inhibitors especially. Mitochondrial toxicity is mostly nucleoside reverse transcriptase inhibitor-related and insulin resistance is linked to protease inhibitors.

How would you test for HIV?

An antibody test in an HIV-infected individual is usually positive within 6–12 weeks after exposure. Antibody tests may be to various core or envelope proteins. Plasma HIV-1 load testing assesses disease progression and response to antiretroviral therapy; various assays include reverse transcriptase polymerase chain reaction. Specific genotypes can be detected by nucleic acid sequencing.

What do you know about antiretroviral treatment?

This is specialised treatment. The two broad categories of drug are reverse transcriptase inhibitors and protease inhibitors.

Reverse transcriptase inhibitors (RTIs)

These prevent conversion of viral RNA to DNA. Only DNA can be incorporated into the host genome.

- *Nucleoside RTIs* inhibit reverse transcriptase and act as DNA chain terminators. They include zidovudine, didanosine, zalcitabine, lamivudine, stavadine and abacavir.
- *Non-nucleoside RTIs* bind to reverse transcriptase at a site distant to the active site but lead to conformational changes in the reverse transcriptase that render it inactive. They include nevirapine and efavirenz.

Protease inhibitors

These bind competitively to the substrate site of viral protease. They include saquinavir, ritinavir, nelfinavir and amprenavir.

Highly active antiretroviral therapy (HAART)

The optimum time to start antiretroviral therapy is still not known but HAART, using combinations of at least three drugs for advanced HIV-1 disease, has dramatically improved life expectancy, maintaining viral RNA load at undetectable levels. There are concerns about cardiovascular mortality as HAART can induce endothelial dysfunction, increase plasma cholesterol and insulin resistance and possibly cause hypertension. HAART, using three antiviral agents, can suppress viraemia and restore normal CD4 counts and when critical 'cut-off' levels have been exceeded, prophylaxis against opportunistic infections may be stopped (although cellular specific immunity against HIV cannot be adequately restored). The lower limit for starting HAART is considered a CD4 count 200/µl because below this the chances of developing an AIDS-defining illness increase dramatically. Potentially, a considerable time span between counts of 350 µ/l and 200 µ/l exists, around two to five years given an average viral load.

Effects of HAART on survival

HAART has reduced the incidence of AIDS and AIDS-related mortality by over 40% in the 10-year period 1996 to 2006, with an 80% reduction in mortality in industrialised nations.

Treatment failure and emerging treatments

This is not uncommon and is indicated by an increase in plasma viral load. Failure is more likely with successive regimens. Drug-resistant viruses emerge when susceptibility of the virus to one or more drugs is reduced, and HIV's capacity to mutate vigorously means that stopping HAART even for a short time (often poor concordance) is very bad news. This problem is lessened with once-daily combined drug pills. Novel drugs on the horizon include integrase inhibitors (raltegravir and elvitegravir), R5 inhibitors which bind to CCR5 (although as disease advances patients are more likely to harbour viruses that utilise CXCR4 and there is also the potential for R5 inhibitors to promote switching to CXCR4 utilisation), and second-generation non-nucleoside RTIs (etravirine).

Table 2.83 Immune deficiency disorders

	Type of immune deficiency	Examples
Primary innate	Complement deficiency Neutrophil deficiency	Many complement deficiencies
Primary adaptive	Severe combined immune deficiency (SCID) MHC class 1 or 2 deficiencies X-linked agammaglobulinaemia Hyper-IgM syndrome Common variable immune deficiency	See Case 2.46 'Bald lymphocytes' (very rare) B lymphocytes unable to produce immunoglobulin Failure of class switching from IgM-producing B cells IgA deficiency commonest
Secondary immunodeficiency	Complement deficiency	Systemic lupus erythematosus Post-infectious glomerulonephritis Bacterial endocarditis
	Immunoglobulin deficiency	B-lymphocyte lymphoproliferative diseases Splenectomy Nephrotic syndrome
	Hypergammaglobulinaemia	Monoclonal lymphoproliferative disease (single B-lymphocyte clone 'crowds out' normal B lymphocytes) Polyclonal hypergammaglobulinaemia (chronic infection/inflammation)
	T-lymphocyte deficiency	T-lymphocyte lymphoproliferative diseases Immunosuppressant drugs HIV infection

Why is the profile of opportunistic infection and malignancy similar in patients with HIV to that of patients with renal transplants?

Impaired T-cell and B-cell immunity occurs in HIV, because T helper lymphocytes are affected. The profile of opportunistic organisms reflects those that normally require T helper lymphocytes for elimination such as *Mycobacterium*, viruses such as cytomegalovirus and fungi such as *Candida* and cryptococci. Neutrophil-mediated bacterial elimination is still largely intact. Many post-transplant immunosuppressive anti-rejection therapies inhibit IL-2, which is central to T helper lymphocyte proliferation.

Is an HIV vaccine likely?

This is difficult because of the terrific mutation potential of HIV. Neutralising antibodies, passively transferred or stimulated by immunisation with envelope protein, protect chimpanzees against a challenge with a homologous strain of HIV, but not humans.

Is post-exposure prophylaxis important?

Overall it appears to confer significant reduction in rates of seroconverison, but evidence varies.

How might immunodeficiency arise other than through HIV infection?

Immune deficiency disorders are outlined in Table 2.83.

OTHER GENERAL MEDICAL AND ELDERLY CARE PROBLEMS

CASE 2.40

FALLS AND REHABILITATION

Candidate information

Role

You are a doctor in the medical outpatient clinic. Please read the following letter from the patient's general practitioner. You may make notes on the paper provided. When the bell sounds, enter the examination room to begin the consultation.

Scenario

Dear Doctor

Re: Mrs Marianne Wood, aged 54 years

Thank you for seeing this lady who is having an increasing number of falls. She has sustained numerous injuries as a result. Last year she sustained a fractured ankle and humerus. She has no other medical history of note. She denies any loss of consciousness but I wonder if she merits investigation to search for possible causes.

Yours sincerely

Please take a history from the patient (you may continue to make notes if you wish on the paper provided). Your examiners will warn you when 12 minutes have elapsed. You have 14 minutes to take a history from the patient followed by 1 minute of reflection. There will then follow 5 minutes of discussion with the examiners. Be prepared to discuss solutions to the problems posed by the case and how you might reply to the GP's letter. You are not required to examine the patient.

Patient information

Mrs Marianne Wood is a 54-year-old primary school teacher with a lifelong history of falls. She describes herself as a 'clumsy child who always had a tendency to fall', but in adulthood these have become more frequent. She now falls approximately monthly. Her husband has adjusted to keeping close to her when walking, ready to break any fall. Last year she fractured her humerus and ankle, required intensive physiotherapy and was unable to write for two months or drive for six months. She also has a history of a vertebral compression fracture following a fall down stairs. She does not think she loses consciousness when she falls, but does not seem to be able to co-ordinate her legs, which seem to be clumsy. She has no apparent difficulty with sensation in the feet and legs, is able to sense pain,

hot and cold and joint position, and has no apparent difficulty with muscle strength. She has no other medical history of note, and takes no medications. She is extremely worried about having to give up work, which she loves.

How to approach the case

Data gathering in the interview and interpretation and use of information gathered

Presenting problem(s) and symptom exploration

▪ **Explore the frequency and time course of falls**   Ask the following:

- When did falls start?
- How often do they occur (how many in the last 12 months)?
- Are they becoming more frequent?
- Is there a circadian pattern?

▪ **Explore the characteristics of falls**   Patients often report one of light headedness, a sense of the room spinning, or feeling unsteady on their feet (Table 2.84).

Falls may occur:

- *with loss of consciousness* (usually syncope or seizure – Cases 2.41 and 2.42)
- *without loss of consciousness*, when they may be associated with neuromusculoskeletal instability or disequilibrium (Box 2.76) or be purely accidental ('the cat or the carpet'). Vertigo seldom provokes loss of consciousness. Most falls are in fact non-syncopal, and in older people are the result of poor mobility and frailty, or acute illness (intrinsic factors), often combined with extrinsic (environmental) factors.

Assessment in patients who are admitted must include cognitive assessment, an ECG and lying and standing blood pressure if relevant (although most falls on standing are caused by weakness).

- Ask about warning symptoms, whether there is recollection of falling or hitting the floor and whether protective responses to injury are used. Patients may lose consciousness so transiently as to be unaware of having done so. Associated symptoms, such as chest pain, palpitations or breathlessness should be elicited.
- Ask about direction of fall (in diffuse cerebrovascular disease, for example, gait tends to be upright or even

Table 2.84 Characteristics of the causes of falls	
Question	**Interpretation**
Do you feel lightheaded?	Pre-syncope or syncope
Is it a sense of the room spinning?	Vertigo
Do you feel unsteady on your feet (or wobbly on your legs)?	Disequilibrium

Box 2.76 Postural equilibrium and disequilibrium

The body has a small base compared to height and must constantly take automatic corrective actions to overcome destabilising gravitational forces and maintain postural stability. These actions can produce body sway and limits of sway are known as limits of stability. When the centre of mass is displaced beyond the limits a fall occurs unless there is rapid corrective action, e.g. moving the foot.

Neuromuscular mechanism for postural equilibrium

Balance is a complex sensorimotor process integrated centrally in the brainstem, cerebral cortex, cerebellum and extrapyramidal system, with stabilising sensory information from the vestibular system, vision and somatosensory afferents (e.g. joint position receptors in the lower limbs and spine and touch and pressure receptors in the sole). Somatosensory afferents are most important in postural stability when standing on a hard surface, and vision is important on unstable ground. The vestibular system largely detects head movement and is less perceptive for body sway. Much of this sensory information converges centrally and is used to produce corrective responses at the joints to keep the centre of mass within the limits of body sway, i.e. stabilisation of gaze during head movements and control of posture and equilibrium during movement. Effector pathways include the vestibulo-ocular reflex (stabilises retinal images with head movement) and vestibulospinal pathways to neck and trunk muscles and muscles in the lower limbs.

Postural disequilibrium

Postural unsteadiness or disequilibrium occurs when one of the sensory inputs is perturbed. Normally minor slips or trips provoke rapid motor responses to restore postural equilibrium. Some adaptation can occur to compensate for sensory perturbation, e.g. impaired proprioception compensated for by vision. When sensory compensation is inadequate, motor responses are inadequately evoked and this results in a fall.

Ageing and disequilibrium

Visual acuity, vestibulo-ocular reflexes, vestibular systems, proprioception and cutaneous sensation tend to decline with age or with disuse. These, combined with reduced cerebellar and cerebral processing and increased muscle stiffness, can all contribute to increased body sway over 60 years of age and an increased risk of falls.

Disease and disequilibrium

Many diseases contribute to disequilibrium, e.g. diabetic neuropathy, osteoporosis, stroke, postural hypotension, cataracts, glaucoma, macular degeneration.

Drugs and disequilibrium

Polypharmacy may contribute to disequilibrium.

Box 2.77 Falls risk assessment tool

- History of falling in past year
- Four or more medications
- Stroke or Parkinson's disease
- Balance problems
- Unable to rise from chair or knee height without using arms

---

stairs, lack of edge of step demarcations, lack of rails, slippery floors, loose rugs, pets, grandchildren's toys and cords of telephones and appliances. Outdoor hazards include uneven pavements, streets or paths, lack of safety equipment, snow and ice, traffic and public transportation. A description of footwear should always be elicited.

Assess falls risk The falls risk assessment tool predicts a high risk of falls if three or more of the five risks are present (Box 2.77).

People with syncope, recurrent falls in the past year, unexplained high-risk features or disturbance of gait or balance should be offered a specialist multifactorial falls risk assessment with a view to individualised multifactorial intervention.

Assessment should take account of number and description of falls, environmental and functional assessment, balance and gait assessment, confidence, cognition, medical disorders, past history, medications and osteoporosis risk.

Falls are often multifactorial. Chronic disorders causing problems with posture, balance and gait (e.g. peripheral neuropathy, joint disease, stroke, Parkinson's disease) may conspire with acute illness (e.g. pneumonia, urinary tract infection, acute confusion or dehydration), drug side effects (e.g. hypotension, sedation or electrolyte disturbances) and environmental hazards. In other words, if a cause of falls is found, assessment should continue to exclude yet more.

Patient perspective

Explore her ideas, concerns and expectations about her falls, especially her concerns about stopping work.

Past medical history

Establish the list of injuries sustained.

Drug and allergy history

Important medications contributing to falls risk include benzodiazepines, tricyclic antidepressants, antihypertensives, diuretics, levodopa and alcohol.

Family history

There is occasionally a familial neurodegenerative disorder.

Social history

Enquire about type of accommodation (stairs etc.), environmental hazards, hazardous tasks (e.g. climbing, reaching), functional abilities (mobility, transfer, activities of daily living, e.g. shopping, driving), support services and work.

---

tottering backwards a little, resulting in backward falls).

- Ask how long she is usually on the floor, and how she gets back up.
- Ask about vision and hearing.
- Ask about sensory symptoms.
- Ask about muscle weakness.
- Ask about joint symptoms (pain or swelling).
- Ask if there is vertigo (Table 2.85).

Explore environmental factors Environmental factors can contribute to falls risk, especially in the setting of disequilibrium. Indoor hazards include bad lighting, steep

Table 2.85 Vertigo (=the illusion of movement)

Type	Disease	Cause	Vertigo description	Other features	Natural history
Peripheral (three classic causes + local infective causes e.g. otitis media or cholesteatoma)	Vestibular neuronitis (acute labyrinthitis)	Common in younger people following upper respiratory tract infection ?Vestibular nerve degeneration	Often on waking Often marked	Nausea and vomiting Horizontal or rotatory nystagmus Hearing loss unusual	Usually resolves within days with vestibular compensation, which precedes nerve regeneration Milder symptoms may recur but over subsequent weeks
	Benign paroxysmal positional vertigo	Common in later life Probably caused by debris in inner canals May be triggered by infection, vasculitis or trauma	Recurrent vertigo provoked by change in head position, typically turning in bed, bending, straightening or looking upwards but provoked only by one direction of movement Short latent period (few seconds) after changing position before onset Short-lived and self-limiting Rapidly fatigues with repeated testing	Nausea common but seldom vomiting No associated hearing loss or tinnitus	Responds to Epley manoeuvre if Dix–Hallpike test positive (with head rotated at 45° to one side, patient lain back rapidly until head dependent over edge of bed; this induces self-limiting rotational nystagmus within 30 seconds – not always immediate because fluid viscous and it takes time for debris to move; procedure repeated on opposite side; direction of nystagmus – may be bilateral – indicates side of lesion)*
	Ménière's disease	Unknown	Vertigo at any time	Tinnitus Hearing loss	Tends to persist
Central	Disease of vestibular connections in brainstem (vertigo is never due to isolated cerebellar disease and causes should not be lumped with those of nystagmus)	Ischaemia (vertebrobasilar) Demyelination (may mimic peripheral vertigo) Space-occupying lesion (e.g. acoustic neuroma)	Vertigo immediate, persists and does not recover unless underlying cause can be treated May occur in all directions	Nausea less common Imbalance severe	

*Epley manoeuvre should follow positive test and involves tilting head contralateral to side of debris (to left if Dix–Hallpike test positive with manoeuvre to right indicating right-sided debris), followed by rolling the patient onto the contralateral (left) side, followed by sitting the patient forward with head still looking over the left shoulder and then turning and flexing the neck onto the chest, watching for rotational nystagmus and reproduction of symptoms (that would normally prevent the patient from moving into such positions) and waiting for resolution of these with each movement in the sequence.

SUMMARY – ASSESSMENT AND PLAN

- There is no apparent loss of consciousness, and the history suggests a problem with neuromusculoskeletal instability, or disequilibrium. She may have a progressive neurological disorder but the long history suggests a longstanding abnormality and impaired neuronal 'reserve'. New factors increasing her tendency to fall including syncope should still be considered.
- Osteoporosis risk should be assessed.
- A full examination, including blood pressure lying and standing, cardiovascular examination (notably for murmurs, and possibly carotid sinus massage with monitoring if no bruits) and neuromusculoskeletal

examination (notably cerebellar, peripheral nerve and joint examination) is the next step.
- Investigations should include routine haematobiochemisty, an ECG, magnetic resonance brain imaging and an osteoporosis dual energy X-ray absorptiometry scan. Further tests for syncope, including tilt-table testing, may be important later.
- Multifactorial intervention may include strength and balance re-training (e.g. Tai Chi), physiotherapy and occupational therapy assessment. Ear, nose and throat specialists have a role if vestibular disease is suspected. Bone protection should be started.

Discussion

Why is falls assessment important?

Falls may be the manifestation of an underlying cardiac or neurological disorder. The consequences of falls can be serious. Between 3% and 5% of all falls may result in a fracture and 10–15% of falls in people over 65 result in serious injury. Only around 10% of falls are reported, yet falls are very common; 30% of patients aged over 65 will have at least one fall in a year, and 50% over 80. Older people should be asked routinely if they have fallen in the last year and about the frequency, characteristics and context of the fall. Dedicated falls assessment and intervention clinics screen for medically treatable causes, assess using a clear and comprehensive pathway and reduce falls risk, even where there are multifactorial causes, by organised exercise programmes and occupational environmental adjustments. Falls assessment and management are all about identifying causes for and managing falls risk and reducing fracture risk with appropriate osteoporosis management.

Why are older people at increased risk of falls?

Older people are at increased risk of the features in Box 2.78, and when assessing older people with any condition it is useful to consider the special considerations highlighted by the mnemonic 'RAMPS'.

List some interventions that reduce falls

- Diagnosing and managing specific causes and risk factors (e.g. cardiac pacing)
- Strength and balance training (physiotherapist)
- Home hazard assessment and intervention (occupational therapist)
- Vision assessment and correction of visual impairment as part of multifactorial intervention
- Footwear assessment
- Medication review and modification/withdrawal

List some interventions that cannot be recommended because of insufficient evidence

- Low-intensity exercise combined with incontinence programmes in older people in extended-care settings
- Group exercise (not a reason to discourage, but little evidence for non-individualised programmes in older people)
- Cognitive/behavioural interventions

- Referral for correction of visual impairment as a single intervention
- Hip protectors in fracture prevention

Does vitamin D reduce falls risk in older people?

Vitamin D deficiency is common in older people and there is evidence that it impairs muscle strength and possibly neuromuscular function. However, evidence that replacement reduces falls risk is not yet strong. Vitamin D and calcium correction does reduce fracture risk in older people in care.

How might a patient's falls risk, balance and strength be assessed?

Overall falls risk

Perhaps the easiest initial assessment of falls risk is the *Get up and go* test. The patient is asked to get up from a chair without using their arms, walk a few paces, turn around and return to the chair. If this is normal falls risk is low. Walking can also be combined with distraction techniques that involve multi-tasking such as *walking and talking*.

Specific balance tests

Methods of assessing balance include:

- Functional reach (how far a patient can reach out without falling, a measure of the range of stability correlating with falls which improves with rehabilitation)
- Body sway (affected mostly by leg strength, peripheral sensation, visual acuity and reaction times and tested by swayometers)
- Step tests
- FICSITT 4 testing (to determine if a patient can stand with feet together side by side, semi-tandem, tandem or stand on one foot)

Balance assessment tools include the Berg balance scale and Tinetti balance assessment tool.

Strength

Strength may be assessed by dominant knee extension or hand dynamometry, standing from a chair without hands, gait speed or climbing stairs. Muscle force (strength × speed of contraction) reduces by 20% after a week spent in bed!

Which patients might be safely discharged following admission with a fall, and which patients admitted?

Discharge may be considered for patients who are continent, ambulant, rational, able to dress unaided and with safe social circumstances. Patients with injury, an abnormal ECG or a family history of sudden death should be admitted.

Box 2.78 Considerations in assessing older people

- **R**educed body reserve
- **A**typical presentation
- **M**ultiple medical problems
- **P**olypharmacy
- **S**ocial adversity

What is rehabilitation?

This is the process of actively restoring function. It is focused and purposeful and aims to improve quality, engagement and participation in life and decrease morbidity and mortality. It is not the same as convalescence, which implies spontaneous recovery. Conditions suitable for rehabilitation are wide ranging and include stroke, fractured neck of femur, heart failure and chronic obstructive disease. Rehabilitation generally starts on acute medical wards and may continue in community hospitals, care settings, outpatient units or at home with the community rehabilitation team.

List some challenges to rehabilitation

- Diagnostic uncertainty (the most important and, surprisingly, common, e.g. confusion in the setting of lung cancer when, for example, brain metastases should first be excluded)
- Constipation
- Incontinence
- Pain
- Sedation
- Pressure sores
- Parietal lobe neglect/inattention
- Cognitive impairment
- Communication problems (including hearing impairment)
- Depression

Which patients should not ideally be referred for rehabilitation?

- Those without a diagnosis
- Those needing complex further investigation
- Those who are medically unstable
- Those awaiting placement

Who should be referred?

Those with a diagnosis and forward plan and who are medically stable. The referral should not include the phrases 'acopia', 'convalescence' or 'awaiting placement'!

Is posture an important element of rehabilitation?

Muscle imbalance (due to neuromusculoskeletal problems, cognitive impairment or reduced activity) leads to disordered posture and sustained segmental (pelvis, hips, knees, feet, ankles, spine) malalignment. Physiotherapists assess posture by examining daily routines, the factors limiting stable posture and inhibiting neutral posture and the effects of posture (e.g. on function, comfort, contracture risk and pressure sore risk). Physiotherapy aims to limit deformity and discomfort and optimise function by, for example, moving all muscles and joints regularly and determining individually optimal bed and seating types.

CASE 2.41

SYNCOPE

Candidate information

Role

You are a doctor in the medical outpatient clinic. Please read the following letter from the patient's general practitioner. You may make notes on the paper provided. When the bell sounds, enter the examination room to begin the consultation.

Scenario

Dear Doctor

Re: Mr Walter Connelly, aged 74 years

Thank you for seeing Mr Connelly, who collapsed last week. He got up from his chair in the public library and promptly lost consciousness. He recovered rapidly but tells me this has happened before. He has a past medical history of hypertension and takes bendroflumethiazide and losartan. Examination is unremarkable except for an ejection systolic murmur. I would appreciate advice on further management.

Yours sincerely

Please take a history from the patient (you may continue to make notes if you wish on the paper provided). Your examiners will warn you when 12 minutes have elapsed. You have 14 minutes to take a history from the patient followed by 1 minute of reflection. There will then follow 5 minutes of discussion with the examiners. Be prepared to discuss solutions to the problems posed by the case and how you might reply to the GP's letter. You are not required to examine the patient.

Patient information

Mr Walter Connelly is a usually well 74-year-old gentleman who last week lost consciousness in the public library. He got up from his chair and with very little warning fell to the floor. He thinks his chest hit the back of the chair as he fell, as he had some discomfort on recovery. He recovered within minutes. He has had two or three similar episodes in the last year. He takes bendroflumethiazide and losartan for hypertension. He has no other past medical history of note, has never smoked, seldom drinks alcohol and lives with his wife in a house with stairs. He drives a car and is keen to continue doing so.

How to approach the case

Data gathering in the interview and interpretation and use of information gathered

Presenting problem(s) and symptom exploration

▪ **Establish the problem** Patients are often referred to out-patient clinics or admitted to hospital with 'dizziness', 'giddiness', 'faintness', 'blackouts' or 'collapse', or attacks of 'altered awareness'. It usually means one of the following:

- Pre-syncope (a sensation of impending loss of consciousness, which may lead to syncope) or syncope (Box 2.79)
- Vertigo (Case 2.40)
- Disequilibrium or some form of neuromusculoskeletal instability (Case 2.40)

If a patient has not lost consciousness, but has experienced altered awareness (best corroborated by a witness), then seizure activity seems more likely.

▪ **Try to differentiate between the two main causes of loss of consciousness – syncope or seizure ('faint or fit')** The term transient loss of consciousness (T-LOC) is gaining popularity, usually referring to syncope or seizure activity. The value of a description of episodes (patient or witness) cannot be overstated. Valuable discriminators are given in Table 2.86 but the key is to build up a picture rather than relying on one fact to make the diagnosis. Further, the differentiation can be more difficult in older people.

Other causes of loss of consciousness include metabolic disturbances (hypoglycaemia, hypoxia, hyperventilation), intoxication and vertebrobasilar transient ischaemic attacks but the latter, contrary to the belief of many doctors, almost never cause loss of consciousness.

▪ **If syncope is likely, try to differentiate between the various causes** These are outlined in Fig. 2.13. Increasingly, it is appreciated that the majority of loss of consciousness is the result of syncope and not seizures, and attempts should be made to try to demonstrate sinus pauses or asystole; 7- to 14-day Novacor recordings are useful for patients who lose consciousness without warning, and loop and non-loop event recorders for patients with warning. Implantable loop recorder or reveal devices are the gold standard, and can be implanted for over 12 months.

The term drop attack is unhelpful, but refers to a sudden fall with the legs giving way without loss of consciousness. Vertebrobasilar insufficiency is mooted as common but is

---

Box 2.79 Definition of syncope

Syncope is a symptom, and the defining characteristics are:

- Transient, self-limited loss of consciousness, usually leading to falling
- A relatively rapid onset
- Spontaneous, complete and usually prompt recovery

The underlying mechanism is transient global cerebral hypoperfusion. This occurs if cerebral blood flow ceases for 6–8 seconds or if systolic blood pressure falls to < 60 mmHg.

Table 2.86 Differentiating syncope and seizures

	Syncope	Seizure
Prodrome/warning symptoms	Minutes (often 1–10 minutes)	A brief (often 10–30 seconds, and sometimes only 3–4 seconds) aura is typical of a complex partial seizure
Duration of loss of consciousness	Usually < 1 minute (often 30 seconds to 2 minutes) May be longer if recovery thwarted by bystanders propping patient up!	Several minutes (usually 2–5 minutes)
Recovery/ first memory	Rapid recovery (wakes at scene) Retrograde amnesia more frequent than previously thought, especially in older people	More prolonged recovery (wakes in ambulance at around 20 minutes)
Skin colour (witness account)	Often 'deathly' pale	Red or blue (cyanosed) in tonic–clonic seizure
Abnormal movements (witness account)	Shaking or jerking can occur with syncope in the form of asynchronous myoclonic jerks or small, brief twitching movements ('syncopal seizure') but seldom last more than seconds. Automatisms, commonly ascribed to seizures, can also occur during syncope, and include lip smacking, chewing, head movements, fumbling movements and grunting	Limb jerks are common for 1–2 minutes Automatisms are common
Tongue biting	Biting the tip of the tongue can occur in both syncope and seizures	Biting the side of the tongue, if it occurs, is a robust sign of a generalised tonic–clonic seizure
Incontinence	Can occur	Can occur
Eyes	May be open or closed	May be open or closed
Injury	Less likely	More likely

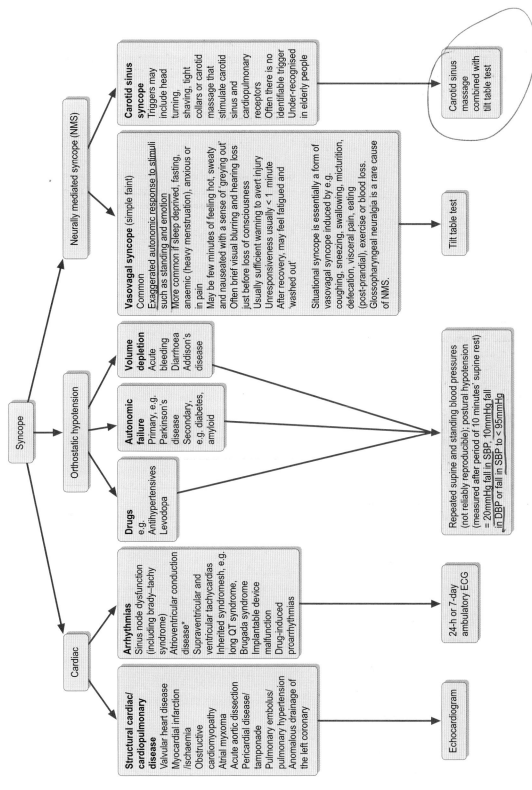

*Long sinus pauses (3 seconds is of definite significance and an indication for pacing, and shorter pauses with symptoms may be significant during daytime hours) tend to cause presyncope or syncope, and syncope may be so brief that patients do not admit to losing consciousness – they may genuinely not believe they did, but equally may not have an adequate explanation for what happened.

(Cerebrovascular syncope, due to vertebrobasilar insufficiency or vascular steal syndromes, is a different but very rare cause of syncope).

Fig. 2.13 Causes of syncope.

probably rare, much less common than carotid sinus disease. Vascular steal syndromes very rarely seduce blood away from the brainstem. Exceedingly rarely, syncope can occur due to intracranial lesions, such as space-occupying lesions causing effective 'coning' in certain head positions.

Patient perspective

Explore his ideas, concerns and expectations, especially about driving.

Past medical history

Establish the list of injuries sustained. A past medical history of anterior myocardial infarction should alert you to possible ventricular arrhythmias.

Drug and allergy history

Diuretics and angiotensin modulators can provoke syncope by postural hypotension, and can derange electrolytes.

Family history

Relevance here is unlikely, but ask about sudden cardiac death.

Social history

Ask about driving.

Discussion

List some ECG abnormalities that may suggest arrhythmic syncope

- Bifascicular block (left or right bundle branch block with left anterior or posterior fascicular block)
- Other intraventicular conduction abnormalities (QRS duration ≥ 0.12 seconds)

SUMMARY – ASSESSMENT AND PLAN

- Symptoms are consistent with neurally mediated syncope, although orthostatic hypotension may be a cause, and is a much more common cause than aortic stenosis, which has to be very severe to cause syncope and then often associated with other symptoms. However, the gradient across the valve in aortic stenosis is exacerbated by angiotensin receptor blockers.
- Echocardiography is important on account of the murmur, as is ambulatory ECG monitoring. The limitations of diagnostic tests such as ECG monitoring are that capturing a spontaneous event is unusual and a causal relationship between a diagnostic abnormality and syncope is often presumptive. The cause of syncope remains unknown in a substantial proportion of patients.
- An exercise tolerance test might be helpful because it is unclear whether his chest pain was secondary to trauma.
- A tilt table test will be helpful.
- If postural recordings confirm orthostatic hypotension, his antihypertensives should be weaned.
- The evidence base for investigations in syncope is limited, without gold standards (the diagnostic yield of tests being measured indirectly by the reduction of recurrence of events after administration of therapy as indicated by the test). Further, the evidence basis for many treatments is also limited.

- Mobitz 1-second degree atrioventricular block
- Asymptomatic sinus bradycardia (< 50 beats/minute), sinoatrial block or sinus pause ≥ 3 seconds in the absence of negatively chronotropic drugs
- Pre-excitation QRS complexes
- Prolonged QT interval
- Right bundle branch block pattern with ST elevation in leads V1–3 (Brugada syndrome)
- Negative T waves in right precordial leads, epsilon waves and ventricular late potentials suggesting arrhythmogenic right ventricular dysplasia
- Q waves as legacy of myocardial infarction

How would you approach and manage orthostatic hypotension?

This is confirmed by a systolic drop of 20 mmHg or a diastolic drop of 10 mmHg, or any drop with symptoms. Orthostatic hypotension may be worse after getting out of bed and not present in clinic. It may be delayed and only occur after a period of standing, diagnosed by a head-up tilt table test.

Thorough assessment to identify possible causes should consider volume status, drugs and diseases that can affect the autonomic nervous system.

Dehydrated patients should always be considered to have hypoadrenalism until a short synacthen test proves otherwise, particularly if there is hypoglycaemia or hyponatraemia, although these are late disturbances.

Euvolaemic patients may be on antihypertensives or other hypotension-inducing agents, or they may have long-standing diabetes or primary autonomic failure as in Parkinson's disease, multisystem atrophy or primary autonomic failure. Orthostatic hypotension with tachycardia suggests hypovolaemia, but failure to produce heart rate compensation suggests autonomic dysfunction.

Non-drug treatments include head-up bed tilting (thought to help maintain autonomic tone), compression stockings and salt. Drug treatments include fludrocortisone (25–50 µg increments generally up to a maximum of 300), slow sodium tablets and midodrine (2.5 mg twice daily up to 20 mg thrice daily – usually dangerous adrenaline-like side effects including tachycardia and supine hypertension). Midodrine is an α-agonist and so caution is needed with prostatism.

How would you manage orthostatic hypotension in heart failure?

More challenging are patients with heart failure or fluid overload and postural hypotension. This may be the result of heart failure drugs or simply a failing heart. Here, the above drug therapies are contraindicated (other than cautiously withdrawing antihypertensive heart failure drugs because of balance of risk) and it is counterintuitive to prescribe frusemide and fludrocortisone. Salt tablets and midodrine should also be used with extreme caution in patients with supine hypertension or a history of stroke.

How would you manage orthostatic hypotension with supine hypertension?

Some patients have supine hypertension and postural hypotension; theoretically it may be possible to re-sensitise cerebral autoregulation such that antihypertensives can be used without postural hypotension but in practice it may be necessary to accept hypertension and reduce falls risk by withdrawing drugs.

What is the mechanism of neurally mediated (also known as neurocardiogenic) syncope?

The basic problem is afferent pathways feeding to brainstem cardioinhibitory and vasodepressor centres leading to syncope by hypotension (vasodepressor) and variable bradycardia or asystole (cardioinhibitory).

Stimulation of the brainstem medullary vasodepressor region may follow activation of cardiac C-fibre mechanoreceptors (hypovolaemia causing reduced preload, Valsalva manoeuvre), cardiopulmonary baroreceptors (coughing, sneezing, carotid massage), cranial nerves (glossopharyngeal neuralgia), the cerebral cortex (anxiety, panic, pain) or gastrointestinal or genitourinary mechanoreceptors (defecation, micturition). In hypovolaemia and emotional states such as pain and anxiety the starting point may be increased sympathetic tone, leading to hypercontractility (increased ionotropy and chronotropy) of the volume-depleted left ventricle and subsequent stimulation of C fibres.

In all cases the common endpoint of receptor activation is compensatory parasympathetic (vagal) enhancement with bradycardia or transient asystole and decreased sympathetic tone with peripheral vasodilatation, reduced venous return, reduced cardiac filling, decreased cardiac output and cerebral hypoperfusion.

Which types of syncope generally have a good prognosis?

These include:

- Syncope in young, healthy people with a normal ECG
- Neurally mediated syncope
- Orthostatic hypotension with a correctable cause

Which types of syncope generally have a poorer prognosis?

Structural heart disease, independent of the cause of syncope, carries a poorer prognosis (Box 2.80). Syncope that has a probable structural cause, that is caused by arrhythmias or occurs on exertion or that has a family history of sudden cardiac death should be managed as an in-patient.

What is carotid sinus syncope or hypersensitivity (CSH)?

This is an exaggerated reflex response to carotid sinus stimulation. This reflex response has two components:

Box 2.80 Prognostic stratification in syncope

Risk stratification

- Age > 45 years
- History of heart failure
- History of ventricular arrhythmias
- Abnormal ECG

Arrhythmias or death within one year: 4–7% of patients with 0 factors, 58–80% in patients with three factors.

- A *cardioinhibitory* component due to parasympathetic over-activity causing sinus bradycardia or atrioventricular block
- A *vasodepressor* component due to sympathetic under-activity causing loss of vascular tone and hypotension independent of heart rate changes

CSH is much more common than vertebrobasilar insufficiency, the latter often being diagnosed as a cause of syncope on looking or reaching up but its existence is really very dubious and CSH more likely. CSH is more common in people with carotid or cerebrovascular disease, but the relationship is by no means reliable.

How is CSH diagnosed?

Carotid sinus massage (CSM) is performed in both supine and upright positions, firstly on the right for 5–10 seconds at the anterior margin of the sternocleidomastoid muscle at the level of the cricoid cartilage (angle of jaw where carotid pulse is maximally felt and massaged longitudinally), and repeated on the other side after a minute or so. CSM should be quite vigorous. Reproduction of spontaneous symptoms is required. CSM upright (during tilt test) better evaluates the vasodepressor component. Highly sensitive patients may be symptomatic with minimal provocation (even listening for bruits!).

Is CSM dangerous?

Neurological complications are reported with an incidence of 0.17–0.45%, and CSM should be avoided in patients with a carotid bruit, previous stroke, myocardial infarction in the past three months or a history of sustained VT. It should always be performed with recorded monitoring to avoid unnecessary repeat testing if positive to prove bradycardia or asystole and persuade the cardiology team to consider a pacemaker! A carotid ultrasound is safe practice prior to CSM where there is concern about possible carotid atheroma.

What is tilt table testing (TTT)?

Tilt table testing is an orthostatic stress test used when neurally mediated syncope is suspected. It should ideally be performed with beat-to-beat monitoring of blood pressure – the basic problem with vasovagal syncope is a drop in blood pressure, chased very quickly, within seconds, by a dramatic drop in heart rate.

Table 2.87 Tilt table testing responses and treatments – neurocardiogenic syncope

Type	Response	Definition	Treatment
Type 1	Mixed cardioinhibitory and vasodepressor	Heart rate falls but not to < 40 beats/minute	Cardiac pacing (less effective in mixed with important vasodepressor component)
Type 2A	Cardioinhibitory without asystole	Heart rate < 40 beats/minute for > 10 seconds	Cardiac pacing (considered for CSH more than vasovagal syncope)
Type 2B	Cardioinhibitory with asystole	Asystole > 3 seconds with symptoms	Cardiac pacing (considered for CSH more than vasovagal syncope)
Type 3	Vasodepressor	Fall in SBP of > 50 mmHg with symptoms. Heart rate does not fall by more than 10% of its peak at the time of syncope	More difficult to treat and evidence for treatments lacking. Compression hosiery. Salt tablets. Fludrocortisone. Beta blockers (apparently paradoxical but decreased contractility thought to decrease the cardioinhibitory response and peripheral vasoconstriction thought to prevent the vasodepressor activity that can then be chased by bradycardia). Selective serotonin reuptake inhibitors

CSH, carotid sinus hypersensitivity; SBP, systolic blood pressure.

Prolonged standing is estimated to lead to an effective 700-ml drop in plasma volume in healthy adults. This may cause a slight compensatory rise in heart rate, but ultimately this paradoxically slows in patients with vasovagal attacks.

A modern tilting protocol comprises 20 minutes of passive 70° head-up tilt followed by glyceryl trinitrate (GTN) spray. Exaggerated responses with progressive hypotension without bradycardia are an effect of GTN and more common in older people. Patients are supine for five minutes before the tilt and fast for two hours before the tilt. Tilts are best performed in the morning, in a quiet, darkened room to reduce sympathetic drive.

Upright tilting in people without neurally mediated syncope reduces venous return, but subsequent baroreceptor stimulation and increased α- and β-adrenergic tone averts syncope. In neurally mediated syncope there is decreased venous return, but sympathetic tone increases with the stimulation of C fibres leading to stimulation of the medullary vasodepressor region, sudden reduction in sympathetic tone (vasodilatation) and concurrent increase in vagal tone (bradycardia) causing syncope. In other words, a blood pressure drop may be chased rapidly by an inappropriate heart rate drop. The prodromal phase occurs at a systolic blood pressure (SBP) of around 90 mmHg then SBP rapidly falls and precedes a decrease in heart rate. Approximately 50% of patients with a positive baseline test become negative on repeat testing.

Tilt testing is considered positive (with 94% specificity) if there is reproduction of symptoms in conjunction with a sudden drop in blood pressure, heart rate, or both (Table 2.87).

A drop in blood pressure of > 20 mmg with no change or a rise in heart rate suggests orthostatic hypotension rather than neurocardiogenic syncope. A heart rate rise of > 30 mmHg with only a slight drop in blood pressure

(< 20/10 mmHg) suggests postural orthostatic hypotension syndrome, a form of autonomic dysfunction in younger people.

Is syncope a contraindication to driving?

It may not be (the rationale being that attacks are unlikely sitting down), although those waiting for a pacemaker are not permitted to drive. Frequently syncope versus other diagnoses has not been established without doubt and patients should be advised to inform the DVLA. A single simple faint with associated prodromal symptoms, clear provocation and of postural type (prodrome, provocation, posture), need not impose driving restrictions. Loss of consciousness likely to be unexplained syncope with a low risk of recurrence with no abnormal cardiac or neurological findings and a normal ECG imposes a four-week restriction. High risk of recurrence (abnormal ECG, evidence of structural heart disease, injury sustained, more than one episode in six months) imposes a four-week restriction if the cause is identified and treated and a six-month restriction otherwise. Strong suspicion of epilepsy within the differential diagnosis imposes a 12-month restriction. These rules apply to Group 1 entitlement (car, motorcycle) users, Group 2 entitlement users having steeper restrictions.

CASE 2.42

SEIZURES

Candidate information

Role

You are a doctor in the medical outpatient clinic. Please read the following letter from the patient's general practitioner. You may make notes on the paper provided. When the bell sounds, enter the examination room to begin the consultation.

Scenario

Dear Doctor

Re: Mr Julian Green, aged 40 years

Thank you for seeing Mr Green who had an episode of collapse last week. He was found confused in the kitchen by his wife, and had cut his head on a kitchen unit. She called the ambulance but he was recovering by the time it arrived. He had bitten his tongue but there was no incontinence. He was discharged from the emergency department following a normal computed tomography brain scan. He remembers going into the kitchen but then nothing until the ambulance arrived.

Yours sincerely

Please take a history from the patient (you may continue to make notes if you wish on the paper provided). Your examiners will warn you when 12 minutes have elapsed. You have 14 minutes to take a history from the patient followed by 1 minute of reflection. There will then follow 5 minutes of discussion with the examiners. Be prepared to discuss solutions to the problems posed by the case and how you might reply to the GP's letter. You are not required to examine the patient.

Patient information

Mr Julian Green is a usually well 40-year-old taxi driver who recently had an episode of collapse at home. He remembers walking into the kitchen at around 14.00 h but then has no recollection of events until an hour later, waking up in an ambulance. He sustained a laceration on the side of his head from a kitchen unit, together with a bite to the side of his tongue. He was taken to the emergency department where he received five sutures and underwent a computed tomography (CT) brain scan that he was told was normal. He felt slightly drowsy for the remainder of the day. He lives with his wife and does not drink or smoke or take illicit drugs. He had an episode three months previously of collapsing in the garden, but without injury. He had been at home alone, had spent five hours gardening on a hot day and felt a rubbery taste in his mouth before falling to the ground; he had come to after what seemed like minutes and attributed the episode to 'heat-stroke'.

How to approach the case

Data gathering in the interview and interpretation and use of information gathered

Presenting problem(s) and symptom exploration

▪ **Recognise the three phases of a seizure** There are, broadly, three phases to a seizure, details of which you should try to elicit (Table 2.88).

Patient perspective

Explore his concerns about driving, explaining that unexplained loss of consciousness poses a risk to himself and other road users.

Past medical history

Ask about predisposing and precipitating factors (Table 2.89).

Drug and allergy history

Some drugs can alter seizure threshold.

Family history

Relevance here is unlikely.

Social history

This is mandatory, not least with respect to occupation (operating machinery or working at heights), sport (e.g. diving, swimming alone) and driving.

SUMMARY – ASSESSMENT AND PLAN

- Partial complex seizures seem likely.
- An EEG and magnetic resonance imaging scan are warranted.
- He should be advised not to drive and to inform the DVLA.
- An anti-epileptic drug should be started after further assessment.

Discussion

How would you define a seizure?

A seizure is a clinically apparent episode of aberrant, paroxysmal electrical activity within the brain.

What is the risk of having a seizure?

The lifetime risk of having a seizure is around 5%, and around 30–50% of such people will have a recurrence.

How would you define epilepsy?

Epilepsy refers to recurrent seizures.

How are seizures classified?

Seizures may be partial or generalised (Table 2.90). Epilepsy is classified separately in terms of focal or generalised syndromes.

Table 2.88 Three phases of a seizure

Phase	Characteristics	Seizure type
Initial phase or aura	Aura can take almost any form. **Somatosensory** Olfactory/gustatory, e.g. tastes Auditory hallucinations, e.g. foreign voices, peculiar noises Visual, e.g. alterations in shape, size or distance of objects Vertigo (very rare) **Psychic** Déjà vu (sense of familiarity with the situation) Jamais vu (failure to recognise surroundings) Depersonalisation (sense of being detached from self) Derealisation (sense of the surroundings feeling unreal) Autoscopy (sense of seeing the body from the outside) **Autonomic auras** Include changes in heart rate, piloerection, sweats, nausea and strange rising epigastric sensation	**Primary generalised** Aura may be very brief **Absence and atonic drop attack** No warning Atonic drop attack can cause serious injury **Complex partial** Aura common (notably in temporal lobe epilepsy) May be protracted, sometimes even for days Occasionally spouses see changes days beforehand, and dogs sense something amiss! May be no warning at all
Loss of (or altered) awareness or consciousness	Patient inaccessible, failing to respond to other people	**Generalised** Usually lasts minutes Eyes may roll up, pupils dilate and 'wide-eyed stare' Period of rigidity (tonic phase) with or without cyanosis followed by generalised jerking (clonic phase) during which may be tongue biting, incontinence and vomiting **Absence** Brief (5–10 seconds) absence in which patient appears to be daydreaming; eyelids may flutter Rapid recovery Abnormal jerks, e.g. jerk of one arm resulting from abnormal discharge in contralateral motor gyrus **Complex partial** Abnormal behaviour and automatisms (repetitive stereotyped semi-purposeful movements), e.g. lip smacking and chewing May last seconds, minutes, hours or rarely days!
Post-ictal	Patient may be aware something has happened, but be confused afterwards	**Generalised** May remain confused for some hours afterwards Amnesia for its events Aphasia may be possible **Complex partial** Sometimes recollection of bizarre alterations of perception, e.g. visuospatial experiences such as micropsia or macropsia (a sense of the world shrinking or enlarging), altered time perception and 'magical thinking' Variety of experiences almost endless, and may culminate in psychiatric referral but: symptoms in complex partial seizures reflect the lobe involved; symptoms are much less common than psychiatric disorders with psychotic symptoms; violent behaviour rare in seizures and invariably non-directional

Table 2.89 Predisposing and precipitating factors for seizures

Predisposing factors	Precipitating or trigger factors
Birth injury	Sleep deprivation
Head injury	Alcohol or drug use
Stroke	Flashing lights
Space-occupying lesions	Stress
Meningitis/encephalitis	Menstruation

What causes epilepsy?

There may be a genetic contribution to idiopathic epilepsy. Mesial temporal/hippocampal sclerosis/calcification is increasingly detected on magnetic resonance images in patients with complex partial seizures and it is increasingly recognised that complex partial seizures are common, perhaps being the primary problem in up to 50% of all

Table 2.90 Partial and generalised seizures

Seizures may be simple (no loss of consciousness or awareness) or complex (loss of consciousness or awareness).	
Partial seizures (arising from a focal brain lesion, frequently the temporal lobe)	**Generalised seizures** (bilateral cortical discharges resulting in convulsive or non-convulsive seizures)
Partial evolving to secondary generalisation (very common)	Clonic (jerky), tonic (rigid) or tonic-clonic ('grand mal')
Myoclonic (single or multiple limb jerks, e.g. normal pre-sleep hypnic jerks)	Absence ('petit-mal')
	Atonic (drop attack with sudden loss of posture)

seizures, often with secondary generalisation. There are two peaks, in the young and the elderly.

New onset acute symptomatic seizures should always prompt a search for important causes. These include infection (cerebral abscess, meningitis, encephalitis, cerebral malaria), trauma, stroke, cerebral vasculitis, cerebral venous thrombosis, hypertensive encephalopathy, alcohol and drugs, neoplasm, porphyria, hypoglycaemia, hypocalcaemia, hyponatraemia and hypoxia.

What is juvenile myoclonic epilepsy?

This is a common, autosomal dominant generalised syndrome causing myoclonic jerks (patients may describe being 'jumpy' during the day and often wake up having bitten their tongue) and generalised seizures with a characteristic EEG. It may be triggered by sleep deprivation, common in students. Carbamazepine may make it worse but it responds to sodium valproate and lamotrigine.

How does a pseudoseizure differ from a seizure?

There is often a trigger (stress), the prodrome is often prolonged with anxiety a feature, the seizure is often of long duration (1–60 minutes), jerking is prolonged, erratic and variable, eyes are often closed with resistance to opening, tongue biting occurs occasionally but usually just the tip with additional cheek and lip biting, incontinence is uncommon, injury is uncommon (or trivial) and afterwards patients may be orientated and tearful. Fifty per cent of 'status epilepsy' presenting to emergency departments is 'functional'.

What is transient global amnesia?

This is often in the differential diagnosis of a seizure. During an attack, patients function almost normally but have no recollection of what has happened. They might go to the shops, or the golf course, or wander around town, and then drive home without recollection of their activities over the past few hours. An attack generally lasts under 24 hours, and seldom recurs. The cause is uncertain, but it does not seem to be due to seizure activity or a cerebrovascular disturbance.

Which investigations may help in diagnosing epilepsy?

A normal EEG does not exclude epilepsy and around 50% of patients with epilepsy have a normal EEG. The EEG

Box 2.81 Red flags warranting urgent investigation

- New focal neurology
- Persistent altered mental state
- Fever (but note that temperature and white cell count may rise after a seizure)
- Persistent headache (but many patients have a mild headache)
- Recent head injury
- History of malignancy
- Human immunodeficiency virus
- Anticoagulated patients or patients with a bleeding tendency
- Age > 40 years (NICE guidelines suggest all patients aged > 20 should have a CT or MRI)

waveforms include alpha (normal, 8–12 Hz), beta (fast normal or abnormal, > 12 Hz), theta (slow, usually abnormal, 5–7 Hz) and delta (very slow, abnormal, < 4 Hz). Common abnormalities include sharp/spiked complexes that may indicate epilepsy, focal abnormalities and diffuse slow-wave activity seen in encephalitis and diffuse cerebrovascular disease with dementia. Magnetic resonance imaging is increasingly used to investigate seizures because it is most likely to detect covert structural abnormalities and will detect hippocampal sclerosis. Functional magnetic resonance imaging can be used while a patient is performing a task.

Following a first seizure, when would you consider immediate or inpatient neuroimaging and management?

'Red flags' warranting rapid investigation, that may include neuroimaging and lumbar puncture as well as relevant blood tests, are listed in Box 2.81.

When would you consider anti-epileptic drug treatment?

Anti-epileptic drug (AED) treatment is usually indicated after more than one seizure. Many neurologists would not institute an AED after a single seizure. However, decisions should be reached with patients and AEDS may be considered after a first generalised tonic clonic seizure if:

- There is a birth abnormality
- There is a progressive neurological disorder or other underlying lesion identified
- There is a history of previous partial, absence or myoclonic seizures

- The EEG shows unequivocal epileptiform discharges
- The patient considers the risk of recurrence unacceptable

What are the choices for AED monotherapy?

Treatments are given in Box 2.82.

For seizures resistant to monotherapy, what are the choices?

Up to 60% of patients may be successfully treated with monotherapy and careful dose titration. If the first AED does not work then an alternative monotherapy is considered. Up to 40% of such patients may continue to fail to respond, often because of underlying damage such as hippocampal sclerosis.

Treatment resistance should prompt review of the diagnosis and concordance with treatment, but trial and error is needed to find the optimal regimen – make change, wait and see, make change, wait and see . . .

> **Box 2.82 Anti-epileptic drug (AED) monotherapy**
>
> Most AEDs inhibit excitatory neurotransmitters such as γ-aminobutyric acid (GABA).
>
> **Indications**
>
> - For partial and secondary generalised seizures, sodium valproate, carbamazepine (and oxcarbazepine), and lamotrigine are suitable.
> - For primary generalised seizures, sodium valproate is most effective, lamotrigine is effective in 30–40% and topiramate and levetiracetam are often effective. Phenytoin is no longer first-line because of side effects.
> - For uncertain seizure types, sodium valproate or lamotrigine are suitable. Some AEDs, notably carbamazepine, may worsen absences and myoclonic jerks.
>
> **Important side effects and interactions**
>
> - Phenytoin, sodium valproate and carbamazepine are older AEDs. Phenytoin can cause gum hypertrophy, hirsutism, ataxia and Stevens–Johnson syndrome. Valproate can cause tremor, hair loss and thrombocytopenia. Carbamazepine can cause ataxia, SIADH and neutropenia.
> - Lamotrigine is a newer AED that may act synergistically with valproate when either AED alone is ineffective. Rash is a major side effect of lamotrigine but can be limited by a slow initiation regimen.
> - Vigabatrin was the first of the newer generation AEDs but causes visual field constriction, and may cause psychosis and depression.
> - Gabapentin, also used to treat neuropathic pain, may be used for partial seizures but can cause ataxia and nightmares.
> - Topiramate can cause reversible cognitive slowing and weight loss.
> - Tiagabine is a newer AED and experience of it is still limited.
> - Levetiracetam is a novel, effective AED with a unique mode of action, fewer side effects or interactions, and is used as add-on treatment by many neurologists.
>
> **Pregnancy**
>
> Polypharmacy is more teratogenetic than monotherapy but sodium valproate is the most teratogenic AED, more so than lamotrigine and carbamazepine. It may also affect IQ in offspring and should be avoided in females of reproductive age (unless under supervision by a neurologist).

Combination therapy is considered when treatment with two first-line AEDs has failed or when the first well-tolerated drug improves control but fails to produce seizure freedom at maximum dosage. Sodium valproate and lamotrigine are suitable together. The choice should be matched to seizure type and limited if possible to two or at most three AEDs.

Vagal nerve stimulation (to reduce seizure frequency) and surgery may have a role in selected patients.

Is treatment different for provoked seizures?

Provocative metabolic or drug causes should be corrected or withdrawn. Benzodiazepines are indicated for alcohol withdrawal seizures and once withdrawn from alcohol and liberated from chlordiazepoxide other drugs are seldom needed. AEDs are not indicated for acute brain insults or for concussive convulsions.

List some treatments you would consider for status epilepticus

- Airway security, oxygen and early discussion with the intensive-care team
- Treatment of hypoglycaemia
- Thiamine if alcohol related
- Lorazepam 4 mg intravenously, repeated if no response
- Phenytoin 18 mg/kg intravenously with ECG monitoring

When would you consider AED withdrawal?

After at least two years of seizure freedom this might be considered. Factors to discuss include risks and fears of seizure recurrence, driving, employment and concerns about long-term treatment. Withdrawal should be gradual, usually over a few months.

What risk advice is important in epilepsy?

Risk advice is essential with respect to driving, occupation, sport and use of hot water at home (e.g. turning on the cold tap first as burns units frequently admit patients with epilepsy). Special considerations include preconception advice, pregnancy and lactation.

CASE 2.43

ACUTE CONFUSION

Candidate information

Role

You are a doctor on the ward. Please read the following scenario. You may make notes on the paper provided. When the bell sounds, enter the examination room to begin the consultation.

Scenario

> Re: Mrs Henrietta Smyth, aged 79 years
>
> Mrs Smyth was admitted to your ward last week with confusion and a possible urinary tract infection on the basis of blood and protein on urinalysis. Her sodium was 109 mmol/l on admission and is self-correcting slowly following withdrawal of bendroflumethiazide. Her abbreviated mental test score remains 4/10. Her daughter is present with her, and would like to report the presentation and background to you. Please take a history from the daughter.

Please take a history from the daughter (you may continue to make notes if you wish on the paper provided). Your examiners will warn you when 12 minutes have elapsed. You have 14 minutes to take a history followed by 1 minute of reflection. There will then follow 5 minutes of discussion with the examiners. Be prepared to discuss solutions to the problems posed by the case. You are not required to examine the patient.

Patient information

Mrs Henrietta Smyth, your mother, is a 79-year-old lady who has been admitted to hospital with confusion and a possible urinary tract infection. There have been numerous previous episodes of confusion, and this is her third admission to hospital in the last year. Mrs Smyth has lived alone in her three-bedroom house since being widowed two years ago but your major concern is that she appears to have hallucinations at home. She often talks about children behind the curtains in her bedroom at twilight. When challenged about this, her response is not denial but more matter of fact – that they can be a nuisance and often refuse to leave when she wants to go to sleep. The hallucinations seem to settle each time she comes into hospital when she simply reports that 'that is not happening any more'. Mrs Smyth has a history of hypertension, for which she was on treatment, but no other significant past medical history. She also takes diazepam at night to improve sleep. You are very concerned that when well enough for discharge the hallucinations will return and that her safety is increasingly challenged and precarious.

How to approach the case

Data gathering in the interview and interpretation and use of information gathered

Presenting problem(s) and symptom exploration

▪ **Recognise that the patient might be acutely confused**   Acute confusion or delirium is a common reason for admission to hospital and a common occurrence in patients admitted to hospital for another reason. Patients may present as 'confused', 'vague', 'a poor historian', 'uncooperative', 'rambling', 'incoherent', 'anxious' or 'tearful'. A witness account is essential.

The abbreviated mental test score (AMTS, Box 2.83) is a rudimentary test of cognition, a score of < 8/10 implying cognitive impairment. It does not diagnose acute confusion or dementia but can alert physicians to a need for further assessment.

▪ **Apply the Confusion Assessment Method (CAM)**   Acute confusion is characterised by its *sudden onset* and *fluctuating course*, *reduced attention*, *altered cognition* (memory deficit, disorientation, perceptual disturbance or language change) and *disturbance of consciousness* (reduced clarity of awareness of the environment). The *Confusion Assessment Method* (Table 2.91) is a validated screening tool that uses four features (a diagnosis of delirium requiring the presence of 1 and 2 and either 3 or 4).

▪ **Establish possible causes**   Often disturbance is multifactorial. AEIOUTHRIPS (Table 2.92) is a useful mnemonic for causes of confusion.

Patient perspective

It is important, when talking with relatives, to involve patients where appropriate to do so. Here, of course, you should elicit her daughter's concerns about safety.

Past medical history

This may reveal predisposing and precipitating risk factors (Table 2.93).

Drug and allergy history

Thiazide diuretics are a common cause of hyponatraemia. Benzodiazepines are a common cause of confusion.

Box 2.83 AMTS (abbreviated 10-item Roth–Hopkins – or later Hodkinson – test)

- Age
- Time (hour)
- Year
- Name of place
- Recognition of two people, e.g. relative and doctor
- Date of birth
- Date of World War I (or II)
- Monarch
- Counting 20→1
- Five-minute recall – 42 West Street

Table 2.91 Confusion Assessment Method for diagnosing delirium

1. Sudden onset and fluctuating course	Acute confusion develops over hours to days. Ask relatives about changes from the patient's normal baseline and whether behaviour fluctuates during the day.
2. Inattention	There is reduced ability to focus, sustain or shift attention. Establish if the patient is distractible, and has difficulty keeping track of what is said or following commands.
3. Disorganised thinking	Establish if the patient's thinking is muddled or incoherent, such as rambling or irrelevant conversation, unclear or illogical flow of ideas or unpredictable switching from subject to subject.
4. Altered level of consciousness (clouding, with reduced clarity of awareness of environment)	Patients may be *hyperactive* or agitated, with considerable psychomotor activity such as plucking bedclothes or non-directed aggression or *hypoactive*, quiet, apathetic and withdrawn, and this can easily be missed or diagnosed as depression. Establish if the patient is alert (normal), vigilant (hyperalert), lethargic (drowsy, easily aroused), stuporose (difficult to arouse) or comatose (unrousable). Reversal of the normal wake–sleep cycle is common.

Table 2.92 Causes of acute confusion

	Cause	Possible investigation
A	Alcohol (especially withdrawal)	History
E	Epilepsy/seizure	History, neuroimaging, EEG
I	Insulin – hypo/hyperglycaemia	Blood glucose
O	Oxygen – hypoxia/hypercapnia	Arterial blood gases
U	Urea and electrolytes and metabolic disturbance	Urea and electrolytes, creatinine, liver function tests and calcium
T	Trauma (e.g. subdural haematoma) Tumour Temperature (hypothermia/fever) Thyroid function Thiamine deficiency Thrombotic thrombocytopenic purpura (very rare)	Neuroimaging Temperature Thyroid function tests Blood film
H	Heart (acute coronary syndrome, heart failure, arrhythmia)	ECG, troponin, chest X-ray
R	Retention	Bladder scan, per rectal examination, abdominal X-ray
I	Infection	Urinalysis/MSSU, chest X-ray, blood cultures ± other tests directed by assessment, e.g. lumbar puncture, ultrasound for biliary obstruction/sepsis
P	Poisoning (usually iatrogenic from prescription drugs; occasionally withdrawal from psychotropic drugs)	Check prescription and other over-the-counter drugs Rare causes include toxic chemicals, e.g. bismuth in surgical dressings, lead, carbon monoxide from leaking gas fires (improves on admission to hospital)
S	SLE, autoimmune disease and vasculitides	Autoantibody screening

MSSU, mid-stream specimen of urine; SLE, systemic lupus erythematosus.

Table 2.93 Predisposing and precipitating risk factors for acute confusion

Predisposing factors	Precipitating factors (minimal provocation is all that is needed in vulnerable people with significant co-morbidity)
Multiple chronic diseases, e.g. chronic kidney disease, heart failure, stroke, fractures, metastatic malignancy Polypharmacy Alcohol Older age (over 65 years) Functional impairment/decreased mobility Poor nutrition Sensory impairment Dementia Depression	Acute illness Drugs Hospitalisation Surgery Physical restraints Bladder catheter Dehydration Constipation Pain Sleep disturbance

Family history

Relevance here is unlikely.

Social history

It is essential to establish the extent of involvement from the daughter and other relatives or carers.

SUMMARY – ASSESSMENT AND PLAN

- Hyponatraemia is a likely acute cause (beware of diagnosing urinary tract infection with only blood and protein on urinalysis).
- First steps are to stop bendroflumethiazide and diazepam and treat possible infection.
- Further investigations for hyponatraemia depend upon whether it corrects.
- The visual hallucinations are worrying, and suggest a possible background dementia such as Lewy body dementia. A 'dementia' screen including brain imaging is probably warranted.
- Although delirium is traditionally seen as transient, 30–60% of patients have clinically significant new cognitive impairment several weeks later, and there is an increased risk of dementia, functional decline and need for care placement. It is not clear if delirium is a marker of reduced cognitive reserve or a trigger for brain damage; it may be both.
- Assuming subsequent investigations are normal, involving the community psychiatric team at discharge would be sensible, and of course the daughter's concerns are perfectly legitimate and may prompt psychiatric review whilst her mother is an in-patient.

Discussion

What is the basic pathophysiology of delirium?

There is diffuse, reversible impairment of cerebral oxidative metabolism and neurotransmission and, theoretically, relative cholinergic deficiency and dopaminergic excess.

Which drugs may cause confusion?

Any drug! Common offenders are sedatives, opioids, corticosteroids, anticholinergics, dopaminergic drugs, antidepressants, anti-epileptic drugs and digoxin.

List some diffuse or focal encephalopathies that can cause acute or subacute confusion

These are listed in Table 2.94.

List some treatment principles in acute confusion

- Early diagnosis and treatment of causes
- Removal of precipitating factors
- Regular orientation to time and place (clocks)
- Familiar faces with continuity of staff where possible and presence of family and personal objects
- Reassurance of safety and reality (not colluding with perceptual disturbances!)
- Provision of usual visual and hearing aids
- Management of sensory inputs (noise, lighting)
- Avoidance of bedrails – which convert delirium into delirium with a hip fracture!
- Judicious use (if at all) of psychotropic drugs

Table 2.94 Encephalopathies

Pathology	Causes
Inflammation	Acute disseminated encephalomyelitis Cerebral lupus Cerebral sarcoid Behçet's disease Demyelination
Infection	Viral, e.g. Herpes simplex Bacterial, e.g. Lyme disease Abscesses Creutzfeldt–Jakob disease
Neoplasm	Primary tumour or metastases Paraneoplastic, e.g. limbic encephalitis
Vascular	Cerebral venous thrombosis Cerebral vasculitis Subdural haematoma Multifocal vascular damage, e.g. CADASIL
Structural	Hydrocephalus
Metabolic/toxic	Alcohol and drugs Hepatic encephalopathy Carbon monoxide poisoning Hashimoto's hypothyroidism Mitochondrial cytopathy

Do you envisage any potential problems of drug treatment for acute confusion?

Potential problems include:

- Treating without searching for causes
- Not tailoring treatment to age/weight/degree of agitation
- Not increasing the scheduled dose if patient requires large number of extra doses
- Overusing psychotropics or benzodiazepines
- Starting treatment too late
- A poisonous pot pourri

When necessary, what drug choices are there?

These are listed in Table 2.95.

CASE 2.44

MILD COGNITIVE IMPAIRMENT AND DEMENTIA

Candidate information

Role

You are a doctor in the medical outpatient clinic. Please read the following letter from the patient's general practitioner. You may make notes on the paper provided. When the bell sounds, enter the examination room to begin the consultation.

Table 2.95 Drugs for emergency sedation and treating confusion

Drug	Indications	When not to use	Side effects	Administration
Haloperidol	Emergency sedation	Withdrawal Anticholinergic toxicity Liver failure Dementia with Lewy bodies	Extrapyramidal Anticholinergic Hypotensive Prolonged QTc (Torsades de pointes)	p.o. peak effect 4–6 hours 0.5–1 mg twice daily and as required i.m. peak effect at 20–40 minutes useful for severe agitation 0.5–1 mg, repeated if needed at 30–60 minutes Maximum 5 mg in 24 hours
Lorazepam	Emergency sedation Alcohol withdrawal Parkinson's disease Adjunct to haloperidol to limit extrapyramidal effects	Respiratory depression	Respiratory depression Paradoxical excitement	p.o. 0.5–1 mg 4-hourly as required i.v. (emergency) 0.5 mg Maximum 2 mg in 24 hours
Atypical antipsychotics Risperidone R Olanzepine O Quetiapine Q	Longer-term sedation (O > Q > R) but potency R > O > Q	Limited evidence of increased cerebrovascular risk in dementia	Fewer interactions and fewer extrapyramidal side effects (safety Q > O > R) than haloperidol	Starting doses R 0.5 mg twice daily Q 25–50 mg once daily O 2.5–5 mg once daily
Valproate	Background cognitive impairment (sometimes useful if 'hyperactive')			

i.m., intramuscularly; i.v., intravenously; p.o. orally.

Scenario

> Dear Doctor
>
> Re: Mrs Elizabeth Russell, aged 82 years
>
> Thank you for seeing this lady who has become progressively confused and forgetful over the past year with a MMSE now of around 20/30. She lives alone and her past medical history includes a stroke three years ago for which she takes aspirin and simvastatin. Her blood pressure is well controlled. Her daughter is concerned that her mother is developing Alzheimer's disease.
>
> Yours sincerely

Please take a history from the patient (you may continue to make notes if you wish on the paper provided). Your examiners will warn you when 12 minutes have elapsed. You have 14 minutes to take a history from the patient followed by 1 minute of reflection. There will then follow 5 minutes of discussion with the examiners. Be prepared to discuss solutions to the problems posed by the case and how you might reply to the GP's letter. You are not required to examine the patient.

Patient information

Mrs Elizabeth Russell is an 82-year-old retired schoolmistress who has been increasingly confused and forgetful over the past year. Her daughter, who lives nearby, accompanies her. She reports that her mother has been increasingly frail since her stroke three years ago, but she has been managing alone with the aid of her daughter and son-in-law, having made a good physical recovery. She has had difficulties remembering days and months for a long time, but now worryingly has left the gas cooker switched on by mistake on at least two occasions. More rapid deterioration in short-term memory has been apparent in the last six months. Mrs Russell walks with a stick, and has a tendency to lean backwards with short, shuffling steps. There is no history of hallucinations. She has a history of hypertension. She takes aspirin, simvastatin and a sedative at night. She has never smoked and does not take alcohol. She herself does not believe there to be any cause for concern. Mrs Russell's daughter is concerned that her mother might have Alzheimer's disease.

How to approach the case

Data gathering in the interview and interpretation and use of information gathered

Presenting problem(s) and symptom exploration

▪ **Recognise that the patient may have dementia**   There are many definitions of dementia but those based on Diagnostic and Statistical Manual of Mental Disorders, 4th edition (DSM-IV) criteria are now standard (Box 2.84).

Folstein's mini-mental state examination (MMSE; Fig. 3.25), of which there are numerous versions, is the most widely used brief measure of cognitive function.

Box 2.84 Definition of dementia

1. _Memory impairment_ (problems with learning new information often precede problems with recall of previously learned information).
2. At least one of _another cognitive disturbance_:
   - _Aphasia_ (language disturbance)
   - _Apraxia_ (problems with motor activities despite intact motor function)
   - _Agnosia_ (problems recognising or identifying objects despite intact sensory function)
   - Disturbance in _executive functioning_ (planning, organising, sequencing, abstracting).
- The deficits in 1 and 2 _significantly impair social or occupational functioning_ and are a significant decline from before.
- The deficits are not part of delirium or better accounted for by another disorder, e.g. depression.

A score of < 23/30 usually indicates cognitive impairment and an MMSE of 22 with 0–1/3 on recall is likely to be dementia but no cognitive test alone should be used to diagnose dementia. Asking a patient to draw a clock face and set the hands to 11.10 is a useful addition to the MMSE. More specialist neuropsychological testing is useful in borderline or difficult cases, and mild cognitive impairment or early dementia is possible with a 'normal' MMSE, especially in those with premorbid high-level cognition; the MMSE, notably, may not detect vascular dementia where memory may be preserved until disease is advanced.

The features of dementia depend, crucially, on the lobes involved. The three common dementias, Alzheimer's dementia, vascular dementia and dementia with Lewy bodies tend to cause global cognitive impairment, but, for example, Alzheimer's pathology tends to progress from back to front, so that memory impairment occurs early and behavioural disturbance (frontal lobe) occurs late, in contrast to vascular dementia and the rare pure frontal lobe dementia which cause early and rapid behavioural change. As dementia progressively involves all parts of the brain recognisable features of other diseases may appear such as Parkinsonian features as the extrapyrmidal system degenerates; in such a case, the benefits of dopaminergic drugs are almost certainly outweighed by the risk of worsening confusion and postural instability.

■ **Establish possible causes of dementia**

- _Alzheimer's dementia (AD)_ is the commonest dementia in all age groups, accounting for 50–60% of all dementia in people aged > 65 years. Onset is gradual with continuing decline and in practice is diagnosed when other causes have been excluded as far as possible.
- _Vascular dementia (VaD)_ is the second commonest dementia, but may be the commonest in people aged > 85 years (Table 2.96).
- _Dementia with Lewy bodies (DLB)_ is probably the third commonest dementia and is under-recognised. It is suggested if one of the three features in Box 2.85 is present and probable if two are present.

Box 2.85 Dementia with Lewy bodies

This should be suspected when any of the following are present, particularly if exacerbated by antipsychotics which are absolutely contraindicated in DLB.

1. Fluctuating cognition

This is with marked variation in attention and alertness. Patients might typically be admitted to hospital with recurrent 'urinary tract infections and confusion'.

2. Recurrent visual hallucinations, often of people or animals

Typical hallucinations are of small children, cats and dogs, and exotic wildlife such as leopards, lions and elephants. In the author's experience, monkeys are inexplicably common. Sometimes there may be richly detailed panoramic visions of landscapes, rivers or armies of people. Typically hallucinations come at certain times of the day then dissipate, and may build over time. For example, a lady living alone might experience strangers coming to the house for tea in the late afternoon, who may subsequently visit each day and become more demanding, expecting meals and then settling in to watch television, ultimately staying very late. Her family might visit in the morning to find cups of tea and uneaten meals on the table and the television still on. Hallucinations tend to be more of a nuisance to patients than frightening. They may settle in hospital, where the distractions of light and noise suppress the twilight visits of children or cats that creep through curtains at home (sun-downing symptoms). These colourful, detailed hallucinations are quite unlike the disturbance of acute confusion, which tends to be a general agitation without such formed experiences and which often worsens in hospital.

3. Parkinsonian features

Lewy bodies may be restricted to the extrapyramidal system when they are associated with pure Parkinson's disease, scattered through the cortices to cause dementia with Lewy bodies or present in both areas, often causing dementia in the later stages of Parkinson's disease.

■ **Exclude reversible causes of cognitive decline** This requires investigation, but treatable causes of progressive cognitive decline include:

- Vitamin deficiency (B12, folate or B1) – ask about risk factors
- Hypothyroidism and hyperthyroidism (occasionally other endocrine diseases such as Cushing's disease, hypopituitarism or hypoadrenalism) – ask about thyroid disease
- Subdural haematoma – a history of trauma is not invariable
- Tumours – ask about recent headaches
- Normal pressure hydrocephalus – ask about gait disturbance and incontinence
- Drugs and alcohol and toxins (heavy metals) – ask about drugs and alcohol
- Depression
- Syphilis
- Acquired immunodeficiency syndrome dementia

Patient perspective

Insight into the safety issues appears to be blunted.

Table 2.96 Vascular dementia (VaD)

Risk factors	Morphological type			Clinical features
Age Hypertension Hyperlipidaemia Smoking Diabetes Heart disease Coronary artery bypass surgery (embolic showers, hypotension) Prothrombotic disorders	Classic multi-infarct dementia	Multiple infarcts in the territories of large cerebral arteries		Memory loss not always prominent
	Microangiopathic (small vessel) disease	Multiple lacunar infarcts in basal ganglia, white matter, cortex or hippocampus due to hypertensive microangiopathy or cerebral microembolism Various types according to location	Strategic infarct dementia	Infarcts in strategically important regions, e.g. thalamus, mesial temporal area, hippocampus	Executive dysfunction pronounced (mental slowing and impaired goal formation, planning, initiation, organisation, sequencing, executing and abstract thought) leading to difficulty with activities, e.g. driving, financial affairs
			Subcortical arteriosclerotic leucoencephalopathy or Binswanger's disease	Multiple small lacunar infarcts in basal ganglia often with diffuse white matter lesions Caused by hypertensive microangiopathy, reduced perfusion, cerebral autosomal dominant arteriopathy with subcortical infarcts and leucoencephalopthy (CADASIL) or amyloid angiopathy	Cortical VaD often causes abrupt sensorimotor signs, and stepwise progression with executive dysfunction
			Multilacunar state	Lacunae in basal ganglia, white matter or brainstem due to lipohyalinosis, arteriosclerosis or leakage of blood from abnormal vessels	Strategic VaD depends on the location but memory loss may be pronounced Subcortical VaD affects the prefrontal cortex with pronounced executive dysfunction
			Mixed cortical and subcortical disease	Multiple cortical and subcortical infarcts	
			Granular cortical atrophy	Multiple small infarcts in border-zone of anterior and middle cerebral arteries due to hypoperfusion from carotid stenosis or cerebral embolism	
	Post ischaemic encephalopathies Cerebral haemorrhages	Cortical laminar necrosis, multiple post ischaemic lesions or hippocampal sclerosis related to cardiac arrest or hypotension		
	Cerebrovascular changes with AD pathology – mixed dementia	Very common, pure AD and pure VaD increasingly seen as two extremes of a continuum		

VaD is a heterogeneous problem, both morphologically and clinically.
AD, Alzheimer's disease.

Past medical history

Hypertension and the previous stroke suggest that vascular dementia is rather likely. It is important to elicit any previous history of depression, as this can mimic dementia.

Drug and allergy history

Any drugs that can promote confusion such as sedatives can push patients more quickly down the slippery slope of cognitive decline.

Family history

Dementia is very rarely familial, e.g. Huntington's disease.

Social history

Patients and their relatives often mistake early signs of dementia for normal ageing, but the expected cognitive changes in normal ageing, such as slower information processing, generally do not impede independent function. Dementia often comes to light only when behaviour or function is impeded to a disabling extent and there are fears from relatives for safety.

Behavioural problems in dementia tend to occur late, and the order of prevalence is listed in Box 2.86.

Assessment of daily function (Table 2.97) is important in diagnosis, assessing response to treatment and planning future provision of care.

Box 2.86 Behavioural problems in dementia

- Verbal aggression/threats/mood swings (said to be more common in vascular dementia but a contentious supposition)
- Physical aggression/agitation
- Restlessness
- Wandering
- Apathy/withdrawal

Table 2.97 Activities of daily living

Basic activities	More complex activities
Eating	Shopping
Toileting	Telephone use
Washing/grooming	Cooking
Walking	Housekeeping
Dressing	Self-medication
	Handling finances
	Use of transport

SUMMARY – ASSESSMENT AND PLAN

- The risk factors and upright shuffling gait suggest vascular dementia is the most likely dementia.
- Investigations ('dementia screen') should include full blood count, urea, electrolytes and creatinine, liver function tests, calcium, glucose, B12 and folate, thyroid function tests, urinalysis and neuroimaging (evidence of small vessel disease, exclusion of hydrocephalus and subdural haematoma).
- Testing for neurosyphilis (cerebrospinal fluid for active disease) is occasionally indicated.
- Old age psychiatrists and clinical psychologists have an important role in the diagnosis, treatment, support and monitoring of patients with dementia, as does interception by the multidisciplinary team, e.g. occupational therapist.
- Cognitive enhancer therapy may be indicated if Alzheimer's dementia seems likely after more detailed assessment.
- Knowing the background level of physical agility and cognitive ability will aid explanation to patient and family of what is likely to be achieved; this patient would not be expected to be leaping like a gazelle on the African plains following treatment.

Discussion

What is the prevalence of dementia?

Up to 20% of people over 80 years have some form of dementia, and prevalence almost doubles every five years from age 60 to 94.

What causes Alzheimer's dementia?

Apolipoprotein E (ApoE) is a cholesterol transporter lipoprotein made in the liver with three isomers. The ApoE4 allele in its heterozygous and homozygous forms is associated with an increased risk of late onset Alzheimer's disease, while rarer early onset Alzheimer's disease may be attributable to rarer mutations in genes for presenilin and β-amyloid precursor protein. Alzheimer's disease is a neurodegenerative condition with progressive cerebral atrophy characterised histopathologically by neurofibrillary tangles containing the protein tau, and β-amyloid plaques.

Do similar changes occur in other neurodegenerative diseases?

The pathogenesis of many neurodegenerative disorders is associated with the accumulation of protein deposits in brain parenchyma. A normal soluble cellular protein is converted into an abnormal, insoluble, toxic, aggregated protein rich in β sheets, as in β-amyloid in Alzheimer's disease. Many neurodegenerative disorders are associated with amyloid accumulation and many are associated with trinucleotide CAG repeat sequences, which may cause protein aggregation. Research into treatments that inhibit or breakdown insoluble protein aggregates is ongoing.

Is vascular dementia easy to distinguish from Alzheimer's dementia?

No, and increasingly appreciated is the overlap. Indeed, it may be that vasculopathy is the trigger to the latent explosives that are neurofibrillary tangles and tau.

What do you know about Parkinson's disease dementia (PDD) and is it the same as DLB?

Up to 90% of PD patients develop cognitive impairment, and 20–40% frank dementia, associated with cholinergic deficiency. PDD is generally defined as dementia fulfilling dementia criteria (Box 2.84 Definition of dementia) in the setting of PD motor symptoms of at least a year's duration, DLB dementia that which arises earlier or without PD; they are both synucleinopathies (alpha-synuclein the protein that aggregates to form Lewy bodies) and distinguishable from AD by the features in Box 2.85 (Dementia with Lewy bodies), early sparing of short-term memory, a tendency to autonomic dysfunction and falls and sensitivity to neuroleptics, which should be avoided. Rivastigmine may be used in mild to moderate PDD and DLB.

Does neuroimaging aid dementia diagnosis?

Not usually. Atrophy is often seen first in the hippocampus and medial temporal lobe in AD. Evidence of small vessel disease and silent periventricular white matter lacunar infarcts is common on scans in people with and without dementia; the differential diagnosis of bright white matter lesions includes demyelination and inflammatory conditions but if the clinical context does not support these then testing for them is unnecessary. Single photon emission computed tomography (SPECT) scans with radionuclides sometimes help to enhance areas of pathology.

What are prions and Creutzfeld–Jakob disease?

The term prion disease is often used interchangeably with Creutzfeldt–Jakob disease (CJD) or transmissible spongiform encephalopathy (TSE). These diseases are caused by proteinaceous infectious agents (which are not organisms) called prions; these are proteins derived from simple genes on chromosome 20, coding for the prion protein (PrP). PrP is ubiquitous. We all have PrP, and its natural function is uncertain. When PrP is mutated it causes disease by aggregating into amyloid-like plaques. Prion diseases may be:

- Inherited (familial, autosomal dominant CJD)
- Acquired (iatrogenic CJD, such as that acquired from cadaver-derived growth hormone or from ingestion of brain tissue as in 'kuru')
- Sporadic (more than 85% of all CJD)

How does sporadic CJD present?

This is characterised by rapidly progressive dementia, myoclonus and ataxia resulting from neuron loss in a spongiform (vacuolated) brain with gliosis. Most patients have periodic sharp complexes on EEG.

What do you understand by the term new variant CJD?

The new variant CJD (nvCJD) or bovine spongiform encephalopathy (BSE) tends to affect a younger age group, and presents with early neuropsychiatric symptoms and ataxia. The EEG is not typical.

What is Charles Bonnet syndrome?

This is a syndrome of new visual hallucinations in the absence of delirium, dementia or neuropsychiatric disorder. Mean age of onset is 57 years. Hallucinations are often complex, and may be of animals or people or landscapes, often with distorted or magical shapes such as small people wearing bright clothes and silly hats. Patients usually have insight and may be visually impaired with age-related macular degeneration or cataracts. It seems that visual deprivation may lead to compensation by the brain to find patterns to explain the external world based on previous visual experiences, an extension of the vivid imagination that may lead us to see shapes in clouds or faces in flames, and is in a sense similar to phantom limbs in amputees or tinnitus in sensorineural hearing loss in that the cortex still searches for meaning with absent peripheral sensation. The differential diagnosis of course includes seizures, delirium and dementia, not least DLB, but in the latter cognitive impairment exists with hallucinations generally unleashed by sun-downing; in Charles Bonnet syndrome they appear in broad daylight.

What is normal pressure hydrocephalus (NPH)?

Cerebrospinal fluid (CSF) is produced by the choroid plexus and normally flows from the lateral ventricles, through the foramen of Monroe to the third ventricle, via the aqueduct of Sylvius to the fourth ventricle, and then via the foramina of Magendie and Luschka into the subarachnoid space where it is absorbed by the villi. In NPH there is no obstruction, the hydrocephalus communicating, and a CSF absorptive defect seems the most likely cause of CSF accumulation, the arachnoid villi seeming to take long tea breaks! This gives rise to the triad of:

- Gait change (there is no classical pattern but gait apraxia or an ataxic, wide-based gait are the commonest problems; a magnet gait, being glued to the spot, postural instability and a tendency to fall

backwards are also common and upper limb and mouth apraxia can occur)
- Dementia (this is a late sign, and usually mild to moderate; severe dementia is a bad prognostic sign unlikely to respond to shunting)
- Urinary incontinence (this is the result of frontal indifference, giving rise to frequency and urgency)

Psychological morbidity is high even without dementia – apathy, bradyphrenia, somnolence and asthenic emotional disorder. NPH can sometimes mimic Parkinson's disease – the frontal lobe connections to basal ganglia are involved in sequence learning.

CT scanning reveals ventricular dilatation out of proportion to sulcal enlargement because the problem is not atrophy. Frontal periventricular lucencies 'due to probable small vessel disease' are not a reason to dismiss possible NPH. Magnetic resonance imaging (MRI) may reveal an absence of gross hippocampal atrophy or marked subcortical white matter changes, periventricular high signal on T2 weighted images, upward bowing of the corpus callosum, flattening of gyri against the inner table or increased aqueductal flow, all strongly correlated with a response to shunting. MR may be important in confirming CT suspicions and in excluding non-communicating (obstructive) hydrocephalus – a colloid cyst, for example, may be difficult to see on CT but potentially lethal if it suddenly swings to obstruct flow (classically on fairground rides or with shifts in CSF pressure at lumbar puncture!).

Assessment for shunting can involve clinical tests such as walking tests pre and post therapeutic lumbar puncture, with physiotherapy assessment if gait disturbance is the most troublesome feature, reaction time tests such as pressing a mouse in response to auditory or visual stimulation and memory tests such as an MMSE if cognition is impaired. An improvement of 5% after CSF removal is often taken as a positive result. The best test might be if the patient or a spouse sees a difference.

Generally around 30 ml of CSF is appropriate to take off initially. An alternative lumbar infusion test (in specialised centres) is positive if CSF plateau pressure is over 22 mmHg or if it does not plateau but keeps rising to over 40 mmHg. Fifty millilitres CSF is then removed over 20 minutes and walking and reaction tests are repeated two weeks later.

NPH is a misnomer – there must be increased pressure at times, although when CSF is removed pressure is invariably normal and NPH might more accurately be called 'intermittently normal pressure hydrocephalus'. If diagnosed and managed early with a shunt, NPH is fully reversible, and a standard management pathway if NPH is suspected on CT is MR imaging, therapeutic lumbar puncture and if improvement is seen (sometimes early, sometimes after a week or two), referral to a neurosurgeon.

Can dementia be prevented?

Ageing involves two factors – programmed death and random damage.

Programmed mechanisms have genetic links, for example the *APOE4* genotype and a tendency to Alzheimer's dementia and *APOE2* and longevity. Cell senescence is linked with chromosome integrity. Chromosomes have non-sense, telomere sequences of DNA at their ends; these shorten with the number of cell replications and with age. Telomere shortening or damage is associated with senescence arrest (and essentially, the 'stuff of old age' such as osteoarthritis, atherosclerosis and skin fragility), apoptosis and attempts to repair; telomerases (which add DNA sequence repeats) prevent telomere shortening but at the price of increased mutation and susceptibility to cancer. Approximately 70% of genes are associated with repair rather than other functions, a reason why we share such genetic similarity to species as remote as bananas.

Random damage occurs in response to exogenous factors such as diet, infection and environmental toxins (essentially, the 'stuff of life') and, as common denominators, creation of oxygen free radicals, mitochondrial dysfunction (notable in dementia and cataracts) and telomere shortening. Protein and glucose, essential for life, produce protein glycosylation or advanced glycation end products (AGEPs) and these, along with oxygen species, are life's two notorious ageing substances. AGEPs, for example, produce browning of teeth, corneal staining and skin wrinkling and can associate with low-density lipoprotein-cholesterol to promote atherosclerosis, renal dysfunction and bone fragility, and are also linked with Alzheimer's disease. They are unavoidable, and irreversible.

Longevity elixirs, for which there is some evidence, include low-calorie diets and exercise. Low-energy diets with normal protein, fat and vitamins may postpone the disease of ageing, but at the price of a more miserable existence, growth reduction, decreased fertility and poor thermogenesis. Cardiovascular disease is associated with decreased physical activity at any age. Exercise improves blood pressure, insulin sensitivity, lipid profiles and even brainstem cell differentiation and learning, notably attention and reaction times. There is emerging evidence that 'thinking' affords us significant protection from dementia, and even where pathological changes of dementia are present clinical expression can be markedly tamed. Exercise and thinking appear to preserve telomere length, enhance growth factor expression and lower lipid peroxidase stress in the hippocampus, and increase brain capillary density, insulin-like growth factor-1 levels and antioxidant glutathione peroxidase levels.

What is the current place of cognitive enhancer drugs in dementia?

Reduced cholinergic activity is associated with Alzheimer's and other forms of dementia. The acetylcholinesterase inhibitors donepezil (Aricept), rivastigmine (Exelon) and galantamine (Reminyl) increase levels of acetylcholine, one of the depleted neurotransmitters in Alzheimer's disease, and are used in early disease. Vascular dementia is also associated with reduced cho-linergic function.

Selected patients with more advanced disease may benefit from the *N*-methyl-D-aspartate (NMDE) receptor antagonist memantine. The evidence for benefit is contentious, NICE guidelines taking a more restrictive stance than many clinicians. Six-monthly follow-up and stopping drugs if the MMSE falls below 10 is recommended. NICE supports use of the MMSE (with treatment between scores of 20 and 10 and six-monthly checks, stopping if < 10), but also the Addenbrooke's 100-point test battery to improve assessment. The MMSE may be less reliable in people with hearing or visual problems or without good English. The problem is that people with scores over 20 may derive significant benefit and a score of 27 or 28 may belie considerable global cognitive impairment, often compensated for if background intelligence is high, and unmasked only by behavioural psychology assessment. Acetylcholinesterase inhibitors are thus often used with scores above 20, not least by geriatricians. They are also sometimes used in non-cognitive (behavioural) disturbance in DLD (e.g. rivastigmine). Antipsychotics are generally not recommended for dementia except in severe non-cognitive behavioural disturbance or agitation, and not at all in DLB.

May patients with dementia drive?

Surveys of drivers aged more than 80 with normal cognition consistently show prudent driving behaviours. Further, many patients continue to drive safely after dementia has been diagnosed, and withdrawal of their licence should not be undertaken lightly since stopping driving can limit social interaction and is an independent risk factor for entry to a care home. However, people with dementia eventually lose the ability to drive safely and at that point Driver and Vehicle Licensing Agency (DVLA) regulations demand that driving stops. The risk of crashes in patients with dementia is significantly increased but generally seems acceptably low for up to three years after onset, by which time most patients have already surrendered their licence.

The DVLA is legally responsible for deciding medical fitness to drive, but for several conditions including dementia, doctors should advise patients of the possibility of stopping driving and take steps to ensure that the relevant statutory authorities are informed of breaches of regulations if there is concern about public safety. Any patient with dementia who is driving should be advised to inform the DVLA and their insurance company. If considered immediately unsafe by the doctor, the patient should be advised not to drive. If the patient fails to inform the DVLA, the advice should be reiterated, and then in writing, and if the patient still fails to notify then the doctor may disclose information to the DVLA, advising the patient of their intention to do so. The DVLA, informed by patient or notified by doctor, request a medical report with or without an on-road assessment and make a decision to issue an annual licence or revoke it.

The DVLA accepts the difficulty assessing driving ability in Alzheimer's disease. Clinicians can perform various clinical, cognitive and behavioural tests, and activities of daily living tests, to complete a DVLA report, but evidence suggests that no cognitive tests (e.g. MMSE, clock drawing or trails tests) are robust enough to distinguish between patients with early Alzheimer's disease with capacity to drive safely and only assist in determining the need for further evaluation of driving.

The DVLA states that anyone holding a driving licence must, by law, inform the DVLA when given a diagnosis of any medical condition that might affect safe driving (Box 2.87).

CASE 2.45

INCONTINENCE

Candidate information

Role

You are a doctor on the ward. Please read the following scenario. You may make notes on the paper provided. When the bell sounds, enter the examination room to begin the consultation.

Scenario

Re: Mrs Isabella Lincoln, aged 62 years

Mrs Lincoln is recovering from pneumonia on your ward. On your ward round, she mentions that she has been troubled by 'leakage of urine' for some years but that it is has become more troublesome in the past few months. She mentioned it to the admitting doctor but nothing appears to have been done and she wonders if this could be assessed before she is discharged.

Please take a history from the patient (you may continue to make notes if you wish on the paper provided). Your examiners will warn you when 12 minutes have elapsed. You have 14 minutes to take a history from the patient followed by 1 minute of reflection. There will then follow 5 minutes of discussion with the examiners. Be prepared to discuss solutions to the problems posed by the case. You are not required to examine the patient.

Patient information

Mrs Isabella Lincoln is a 62-year-old lady recovering in hospital from pneumonia. She has been troubled by urinary incontinence for years, and is now afraid to go out because of it. She finds her bladder will empty large volumes without provocation and she has to wear significant padding to prevent a 'flood'. She has no bowel symptoms. She is usually well, although her doctor commenced frusemide 20 mg some 10 years ago for ankle swelling around the time of the menopause, which she still takes. She has some vaginal irritation. She is a widow, and lives alone with two cats. She has plucked up the courage to ask the ward doctor if there are any treatments for incontinence.

How to approach the case

Data gathering in the interview and interpretation and use of information gathered

Presenting problem(s) and symptom exploration

Incontinence is a clinical diagnosis and a little knowledge about what to ask, investigation and treatment can make a large difference to a significant majority of patients.

■ **Explore symptoms of possible causes**   There are various types of urinary incontinence (Table 2.98).

An alternative way of categorising causes is as a *storage problem* (e.g. detrusor instability, stress incontinence, small bladder) or an *evacuation problem* (e.g. outflow obstruction, neuropathic bladder).

■ **Exclude aggravating factors**   These include:

- Urinary tract infections (most common cause)
- Mobility problems
- Dexterity problems
- Visual problems
- Cognitive impairment
- Drugs, e.g. sedatives, anticholinergics leading to a dry mouth, or a drink before bedtime

Table 2.98 Types of urinary incontinence

Type	Causes	Frequency	Symptoms	Management
Unstable, 'irritable' or overactive bladder ('detrusor instability')	Abnormal bladder contractions (can occur in anyone at any time, not always provoking incontinence) Some patients have non-sustained contractions because of a 'myopathic' ageing bladder with big residual volumes	Most common cause	Urgency and frequency May be triggered by coughing or sudden movements Large volumes of urine (a flood)	Bladder retraining Anticholinergics Botulinum toxin A Surgery, e.g. clam ileocystoplasty, ileal conduit
Bladder neck (sphincter)/pelvic floor weakness ('stress incontinence')		Common	Small volumes of urine (a leak) Triggered by coughing or sudden movements/activity *A rule of thumb is that stress incontinence occurs when getting out of a chair, whereas detrusor instability causes the urge to get out of the chair!* ± vaginal dryness/soreness or prolapse	Pelvic floor muscle exercises Oestrogen, topically or systemically (transdermal), in lower doses than used for HRT, suitable in post-menopausal patients with vaginal atrophy Surgery for prolapse
Outflow obstruction	Benign prostatic hypertrophy Urethral stricture Constipation	Common	Urinary retention ± overflow incontinence Small volumes of urine	Examination (constipation, large prostate, palpable bladder) 5α-reductase inhibition (finasteride) reduces prostatic bulk but takes months to work Alpha blockers improve flow but not urgency Surgery
Neuropathic bladder	**Frontal bladder** Dementia Normal pressure hydrocephalus	Less common	Voiding of large volumes with residual urine	
	Spinal bladder Multiple sclerosis Trauma	Less common	Urinary retention ± overflow incontinence Later bladder automatically contracts and voids small volumes but with incomplete emptying Associated constipation ± reflex priapism	Long-term 12–14 G indwelling catheter changed every 3–6 months Leakage or bypassing does not necessarily mean a blocked catheter but may indicate bladder contractions forcing more urine out than can enter the catheter; anticholinergics may help Infections only treated when symptomatic, and little place for antibiotic prophylaxis because of resistance
	Peripheral neurogenic (non-contracting 'atonic') bladder Cauda equina lesions, e.g. central lumbar disc protrusion Peripheral nerve lesions, e.g. diabetes	Least common	Painless distension of flaccid bladder with overflow incontinence and large residual volumes (i.e. continuous dribbling from large bladder whose fullness is not appreciated) Associated faecal incontinence, reduced anal tone and saddle anaesthesia	Intermittent self-catheterisation Long-term 12–14 G indwelling catheter changed every 3–6 months

- High urine output (diuretics or high solute load, e.g. diabetes)
- Surgical problems
- Hormonal (oestrogen deficiency, a leading factor)

A common scenario is an elderly patient in a hospital or nursing home with an overactive bladder who cannot mobilise easily, may not be able to navigate a new environment and may have difficulty undressing appropriately on finding a toilet.

Patient perspective

Incontinence is a common clinical problem, and is under-reported. It is more common in females, and more common in the elderly, although a number of studies (including one on college students in the United States) report that unstable bladder incontinence sometimes occurs in young healthy people. It can be psychologically disastrous.

Past medical history

The ankle swelling may not have justified diuretic treatment.

Drug and allergy history

The diuretic is likely to be contributory but not the full reason for incontinence.

Family history

It is unlikely that this is relevant in this case.

Social history

Incontinence can be the cause of huge embarrassment and social isolation.

SUMMARY – ASSESSMENT AND PLAN

- Assessment should include a full examination, e.g. bladder volume, atrophic vaginitis
- Investigations should include urinalysis and culture, ultrasound and urodynamics
- Frusemide should be stopped
- This is likely to be an overactive bladder and treatment could be with an anticholinergic, e.g. oxybutinin, imipramine, propiverine, tolterodine, trospium. Some anticholinergics are more likely to provoke confusion (trospium said to be less likely), and all can make outflow obstruction worse; they take weeks to months to work

---

Discussion

What are the neurological inputs to bladder control?

Bladder control has three main inputs:

- Parasympathetic, prompting detrusor contraction and sphincter relaxation hence promoting micturition
- Sympathetic, which does the opposite

- Voluntary, allowing contraction of a striated muscle sphincter

What are the principles of urodynamic studies?

Urodynamics involves catheterising the bladder (to obtain vesical pressure) and the rectum or vaginal fornix (to obtain abdominal pressure). Vesical pressure minus abdominal pressure gives a value for detrusor pressure. The bladder is filled at a non-physiological rate with a large volume of warm saline, which creates high pressures and flow rates can be recorded as a patient micturates. Pre- and post-micturition volumes, determined by ultrasound, aid urodynamics in determining a cause. For example in obstruction, there may be a very large residual of 800 ml on ultrasound with a low flow rate of 10 ml/second on urodynamics. Some normal values are:

- Normal bladder capacity 400–450 ml. Tolerance of this capacity decreases with age, so that an older person may have a tolerance capacity of only 100 ml, for example. Older people tend to get to know the locations of toilets because the time from urge to go to getting to a toilet without incontinence decreases.
- Normal residual volume < 50 ml (up to 100 ml in elderly).
- Physiologically the bladder fills at around 2 ml/minute.
- Normal flow rates ≥ 14 ml/minute (usually significantly higher). Urodynamic studies employ a fast flow rate such as 50 ml/minute (100 ml/minute would provoke instability in a healthy bladder).

What do you know about prostate-specific antigen (PSA) testing?

PSA levels vary with prostate size, and normal prostate cells contain PSA. Indeed, prostate cancer cells do not produce much PSA. It is possible to have advanced prostate cancer with metastases and a normal PSA, but usually the PSA that prostate cells contain leaks out easily and the PSA rises. Finasteride can reduce PSA levels with a danger of unwarranted reassurance. PSA is usually very high in prostate cancer with soft tissue metastases.

What treatment options are there for prostate cancer?

These include:

- Watchful waiting
- Radical prostatectomy with radical radiotherapy (can cure, or 'buy' 10 years of life if not curative); contemplated in fit patients with a normal rectal examination and a near normal PSA and diagnosis confirmed by transurethral ultrasound and biopsy
- Hormonal treatment if PSA high or metastases, e.g. Casodex, Zoladex
- Intermittent androgen blockade, combined androgen blockage or stilboestrol

CASE 2.46

RAISED INFLAMMATORY MARKERS

Candidate information

Role

You are a doctor in the medical outpatient clinic. Please read the following letter from the patient's general practitioner. You may make notes on the paper provided. When the bell sounds, enter the examination room to begin the consultation.

Scenario

Dear Doctor

Re: Ms Clarissa Dillon, aged 43 years

Thank you for seeing this lady who has a raised plasma viscosity of uncertain cause. She has felt tired and unwell for around four months, and routine blood tests showed the following: haemoglobin 11.0 g/dl, white cell count and platelet count normal, plasma viscosity 2.3 (normal < 1.65), erythrocyte sedimentation rate 40 mm/hour, C-reactive protein 28, liver and renal function normal.

Yours sincerely

Please take a history from the patient (you may continue to make notes if you wish on the paper provided). Your examiners will warn you when 12 minutes have elapsed. You have 14 minutes to take a history from the patient followed by 1 minute of reflection. There will then follow 5 minutes of discussion with the examiners. Be prepared to discuss solutions to the problems posed by the case and how you might reply to the GP's letter. You are not required to examine the patient.

Patient information

Ms Clarissa Dillon is a 43-year-old lady who for the last few months has felt lethargic and unwell to the extent that she has been unable to pursue a full day's work as a primary school teacher. She is a sensible lady who insists she is not 'making her symptoms up'. She has also had slightly more loose stools over this time period, on one or two occasions mixed with blood. She is usually well although she does have a heart murmur (mitral valve prolapse with mild regurgitation) for which she attends the cardiac clinic every two years. She does not smoke or drink alcohol. Six months ago she was in a road traffic accident in which she hurt her wrist but she made a full recovery. She lives alone, and reports no stress at work. She is understandably concerned that her blood tests have been abnormal.

How to approach the case

Data gathering in the interview and interpretation and use of information gathered

Presenting problem(s) and symptom exploration

The differential diagnosis of raised inflammatory markers is wide and essentially similar to those of pyrexia (Case 2.48). A full systematic enquiry here is essential.

Patient perspective

She is sensible and her concerns are entirely reasonable. The raised inflammatory markers and slightly low haemoglobin would dissuade from considering this to be chronic fatigue syndrome.

Past medical history

The history of a heart valve lesion cannot be ignored.

Drug and allergy history

Not relevant here.

Family history

A family history of colorectal cancer should be explored.

Social history

Her occupational history is unlikely to be relevant aetiologically and while sources of stress should be explored these are not likely to explain her new symptoms.

SUMMARY – ASSESSMENT AND PLAN

Further investigation is warranted. The two possibilities that immediately need to be considered are inflammatory bowel disease and infective endocarditis, the latter perhaps less likely given that her open injury was six months ago. Investigations that might be considered for any patient with raised inflammatory markers are listed below:

- Full blood picture
- Urea, creatinine and electrolytes, glucose
- Liver function tests
- Bone chemistry
- Thyroid function tests
- Plasma viscosity, erythrocyte sedimentation rate, C-reactive protein
- Immunoglobulin profile
- Serum electrophoresis for monoclonal band ± paraproteinaemia
- Urine for light chains
- Anti-nuclear antibodies/rheumatoid factor/extractable nuclear antigens/anti-neutrophil cytoplasmic antibodies (ANCA)
- Serum angiotensin-converting enzyme (ACE)
- Chest X-ray
- Abdominal ultrasound
- Chest, abdominal and pelvic computed tomography scan (?intra-abdominal solid tumour, lymphoma)
- Skeletal survey and bone marrow aspiration (if monoclonal band)
- Isotope bone scan (if bone pain or abnormal bone chemistry)
- Oesophageal-gastro-duodenoscopy (if dyspepsia, upper gastrointestinal alarm symptoms or iron deficiency anaemia)
- Colonoscopy (note that a significant proportion of patients with iron deficiency anaemia and an upper gastrointestinal cause will have a concomitant colorectal lesion)

Discussion

Does the immune system just respond to infection?

It evolved to combat traditional threats, notably infection and natural surveillance against tumours (especially of oncogenic virus origin). It may respond to self-antigens (tolerance versus autoimmunity).

What types of immunity do you know of?

The immune system can elicit *innate* responses involving neutrophils, natural killer cells and complement and *acquired specific or adaptive* responses involving T and B lymphocytes. The concepts of cell-mediated and humoral (antibody-mediated) immunity are now better replaced with appreciation of T helper lymphocyte differentiation and T-cell and B-cell collaboration. Primary lymphoid organs are the thymus and bone marrow. Stem cells destined to become T and B lymphocytes arise in bone marrow. T lymphocytes migrate to the thymus and B lymphocytes remain in the bone marrow and both undergo maturation at these primary lymphoid sites. Secondary lymphoid organs are the lymph nodes and spleen and mucosa-associated lymphoid tissue (MALT). Lymphocytes in the lymph nodes respond to tissue antigens, the spleen to blood antigens and MALT to mucosal antigens.

How does the immune system first respond to antigens?

Antigens may be exogenous (microorganisms) or endogenous (tumour proteins, transplant grafts, autoantigens). When an antigen invades a host cell it is processed such that some antigenic peptide is expressed on the host cell surface. Natural killer cells, which are large granular lymphocytes, may kill such a cell, but tend to leave damage in their wake (Fig. 2.14A). They will not seek out and destroy every last antigen and have no memory. For reliable elimination of infection a more eloquent and specific response is required.

Why is the major histocompatibility complex (MHC) important?

Also termed the human leucocyte antigen (HLA) complex, this is a segment of genes on chromosome 6 that encode MHC (HLA) molecules that are expressed on the surface of cells. Their four-subunit structure forms a cradle or peptide-binding groove in which antigenic peptide derived from infection may be presented to a cytotoxic T lymphocyte or a T helper lymphocyte. Each MHC molecule presents a specific antigenic peptide and an immune response is only triggered in the presence of the MHC molecule – such immune responses are said to be antigen-specific and MHC-restricted. Some diseases are associated with certain HLA variants such as B27 with seronegative arthropathies, DR2 with narcolepsy, DR4 with rheuma-

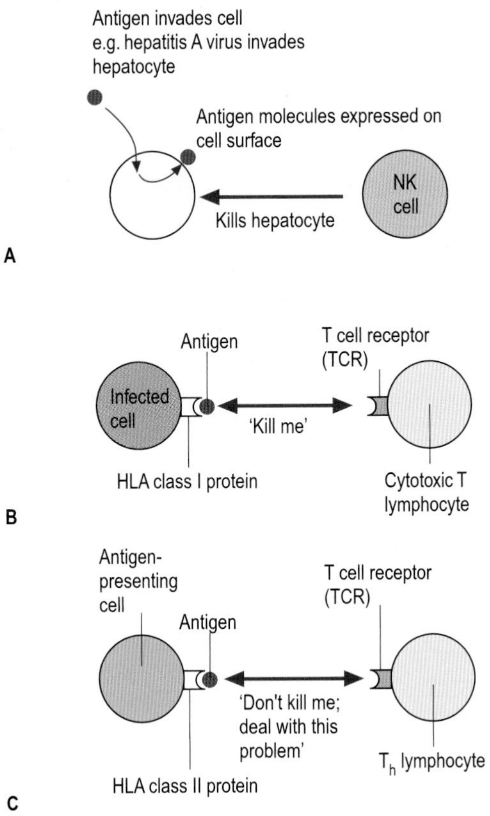

Fig. 2.14 Responses to antigen: (A) natural killer cell killing, (B) cytotoxic T lymphocyte response, (C) T helper lymphocyte response.

toid and B8, DR3 with many organ-specific autoimmune diseases. The HLA complex is highly polymorphic between individuals, resulting in a unique HLA or tissue type.

How does the MHC–peptide complex initiate a specific (adaptive) immune response by cytotoxic and T helper (Th) lymphocytes?

The MHC–peptide complex acts as a distress signal to either cytotoxic or Th lymphocytes.

MHC class I–peptide complex distress signal

MHC A, B and C genes encode MHC class I molecules (containing β_2-microglobulin) that are present on virtually all cells in the body. The *MHC class I–peptide complex on an infected cell is engaged by the T-cell receptor of a cytotoxic T lymphocyte* (also known as a CD8 cell), an interaction that *leads to killing of the infected cell by the cytotoxic T lymphocyte*. The MHC class I distress signal, capable of being elicited by most cells in the body, essentially says *'kill me'* (Fig. 2.14B).

MHC class II–peptide complex distress signal

MHC DP, DR and DQ genes encode MHC class II molecules that are present only on antigen-presenting cells

(APCs), which are mostly macrophages. MHC class II molecules are inducible, their genes up-regulated in response to antigen. The *MHC class II–peptide complex on the APC is engaged by the T-cell receptor of a Th lymphocyte* (also known as a CD4 cell), an interaction that *leads to Th lymphocyte activation and differentiation*. The MHC class II distress signal essentially says *'don't kill me, but deal with this problem'* (Fig. 2.14C).

MHC class I cytotoxic responses are very good at dealing with intracellular antigens. But MHC class II driven Th responses are better for eliminating extracellular organisms. Helminths, for example, are too big to be phagocytosed and so APCs take a snippet of worm and present it as antigen to Th cells which then decide what to do with it. This said, many bacteria, fungi and intracellular organisms also require a Th response.

How are T helper cells activated?

Two signals are needed for activation (Fig. 2.15), the first between the MHC class II–peptide complex and the T-cell receptor (TCR; CD3) of the Th cell (the almost infinite permutations of TCR gene rearrangement allowing the TCR to respond to an almost infinite variety of antigens) and a second *co-stimulatory signal*. Without the latter, the Th lymphocyte remains inactive or naive, a state known as anergy. There are many co-stimulatory signals, but that between APCs and TCRs is the B7–CD28 interaction.

There must also be immunological 'brakes' to Th activation otherwise lymphoproliferation would continue unchecked. One brake is cytotoxic T-lymphocyte antigen-4 (CTLA4), induced simultaneously with CD28 but with inhibitory rather than stimulatory activity. It may be aberrant in some lymphoproliferative disorders.

What do we mean by Th1 and Th2 pathways? (Fig. 2.16)

Cytokines produced by APCs during the activation process of Th lymphocytes direct whether naive (Th0) lymphocytes differentiate into Th1 or Th2 lymphocytes and thus down a Th1 or Th2 pathway. The cytokine interleukin-12 (IL-12) stimulates a Th1 response and IL-4 stimulates a Th2 response. The elected pathway depends upon numerous factors, including the nature of the antigen. Th1 and Th2 lymphocytes in turn secrete characteristic groups of cytokines that induce proliferation of Th lymphocytes along the designated Th1 or Th2 pathway. Th1 lymphocytes secrete IL-2 and interferon-γ (IFN-γ) and Th2 lymphocytes secrete interleukins 3,4, 5,10 and 13. An effective immune system that does not result in 'friendly-fire' relies on a well-balanced Th1–Th2 environment. Homeostasis is achieved by switch-off mechanisms and self-perpetuation mechanisms by cross-inhibition – IFN-γ inhibits the Th2 pathway and IL-10 inhibits the Th1 pathway.

What are cytokines?

Cytokines are molecules secreted by cells telling other cells what to do. There is a huge array of cytokines, and groups include interleukins (secreted by leucocytes and acting on leucocytes), interferons (IFNs), tumour necrosis factors (TNFs), chemokines (chemotactic) and colony-stimulating factors, promoting haematopoiesis. Most cytokines have multiple roles or effects. If one cytokine is absent, another may take its place. Cytokines are only produced by activated cells and are secreted locally. They bind with cytokine receptors on cells nearby. Cytokine receptors comprise polypeptide subunits with intra- and extracellular domains. One subunit, the common γ chain, is common to receptors for several interleukins. While cytokines will stand in for absent colleagues, cytokine receptors have no back-up. Mutations of the γ chain occur in *X*-linked severe combined immunodeficiency (SCID), with loss of function of several cytokine receptors; 'combined' implies that both T-cell and B-cell receptors are affected.

Just as there is a huge array of cytokines and cytokine receptors, there is a huge array of intracellular pathways. One such is the Jak (Janus kinase) and STAT (signal transducers and activators of transcription) pathway. Jaks are tyrosine kinases. After cytokine binding, a phosphorylation cascade of Jaks and STATs enables STATs to translocate to the nucleus, bind to DNA and act as transcription factors. Thus, mutations of Jak are another cause of SCID.

What is the role of the Th1 response?

This is proinflammatory. Th1 lymphocytes secrete cytokines that powerfully propagate the Th1 pathway (IL-2 induces Th1 cell proliferation and IFN-γ inhibits the rival Th2 pathway) and stimulate macrophages, which in turn synthesise and secrete the inflammatory cytokines IL-1, IL-6 and TNF-α (Fig. 2.16) that mediate the acute-phase response. If unchecked, chronic inflammation can ensue, and ultimately healing with fibrosis mediated by fibroblast-stimulating cytokines such as transforming growth factor-β. This immune response typifies many bacterial, viral and fungal infections, antitumour activity and many immune-mediated inflammatory disorders.

What is the acute-phase response?

Many systemic changes associated with proinflammatory cytokines are recognised. These changes, collectively termed the acute-phase response, include hepatic synthesis

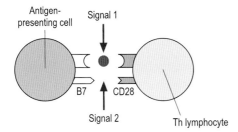

Fig. 2.15 Th lymphocyte activation.

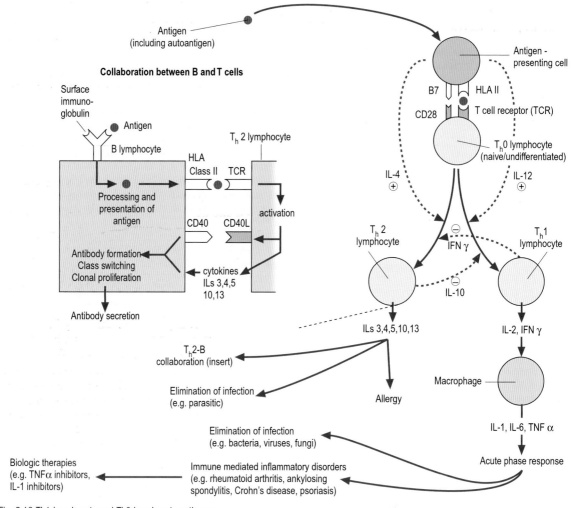

Fig. 2.16 Th1 lymphocyte and Th2 lymphocyte pathways.

and release of acute-phase proteins – complement proteins, coagulation proteins (including activated protein C), transport proteins and C-reactive protein (CRP). Some acute-phase proteins such as albumin decrease in concentration. Other acute-phase phenomena include fever, tachycardia, anorexia, rising concentrations of 'stress' hormones such as cortisol and catecholamines, decreased insulin-like growth factor 1 (IGF-1) levels, anaemia of chronic disease, leucocytosis, thrombocytosis, catabolism and cachexia.

How do you decide which inflammatory marker test to use – C-reactive protein (CRP), erythrocyte sedimentation rate (ESR) or plasma viscosity (PV)?

The ESR is a time-honoured test for red cell rouleaux formation that can alert clinicians to certain diagnoses such as polymyalgia rheumatica, giant cell arteritis or myeloma. An extremely elevated ESR is strongly associated with serious disease, most often infection, autoimmune disease or metastatic malignancy, but when moderately elevated

without clinical explanation, interval testing rather than indiscriminate investigation (other than perhaps a myeloma screen) may be preferable. Furthermore, the ESR can be very unreliable, being influenced by many factors (Table 2.99).

The advantages of CRP or plasma viscosity measurement over the ESR are outlined in Table 2.100.

What are immune-mediated inflammatory disorders?

These are diseases driven by a Th1 response, e.g. rheumatoid arthritis, ankylosing spondylitis, Crohn's disease, psoriasis.

What are 'biological' therapies?

These are therapies for immune-mediated inflammatory disorders which inhibit the Th1 response by cytokine manipulation, e.g. TNF-α inhibitors, IL-1 inhibitors. Non-Th1-cytokine molecular therapies such as growth factor receptor blockers in malignancy are also deemed 'biologics'.

Table 2.99 Factors that influence the erythrocyte sedimentation rate (ESR)

Factors that increase the ESR	Factors that decrease the ESR
Older age (traditionally cited, although this probably reflects a higher disease prevalence in older people!) Female (very slight) Pregnancy Anaemia, e.g. anaemia of chronic kidney disease Red blood cell abnormalities, e.g. macrocytosis Elevated fibrinogen (infection, inflammation, malignancy) Myeloma	Extreme leucocytosis Polycythaemia Red blood cell abnormalities, e.g. microcytosis, spherocytosis Protein abnormalities (hypofibrinogenaemia, hypogammaglobulinaemia)

Table 2.100 The advantages of C-reactive protein or plasma viscosity measurements

Test	Advantages
Erythrocyte sedimentation rate (ESR)	Inexpensive, but many limitations
C-reactive protein	More direct test of and more rapid response to proinflammatory activity Not influenced by those factors influencing the ESR
Plasma viscosity	Similar to ESR, but unaffected by anaemia or red cell abnormalities A non-specific 'red flag' for inflammation

What is the role of the Th2 response?

The Th2 response regulates the intensity of Th1 responses, dampening down the tendency to inflammation through the negative stimulus of IL-10. In this non-inflammatory respect, the Th2 pathway is 'anergic', although it is not anergic in the true sense of the word in that considerable activity is afoot!

Another major role of Th2 lymphocytes is collaborating with B cells in the production of specific antibodies (which are good at eliminating extracellular antigens such as encapsulated bacteria). While B lymphocytes can produce antibodies by direct stimulation from an antigen, Th2–B-lymphocytes collaboration is the more usual, optimal and efficient means of antibody production.

When an antigen stimulates a B lymphocyte, that B lymphocyte has the capacity to act as an antigen-presenting cell to Th2 lymphocytes via an MHC class II–peptide complex expressed on its surface (exactly analogous to a macrophage antigen-presenting cell presenting an MHC class II peptide to a Th lymphocyte). Again, a co-stimulatory signal is required, in this case CD40–CD40 ligand. The interaction leads to release of Th2 effector cytokines (interleukins 3, 4, 5, 10, 13) that feed back to the B lymphocyte (Fig. 2.16) and promote class switching, clonal proliferation, differentiation to plasma cells and antibody production.

Only some B cells become antibody-secreting plasma cells dedicated to the current threat. Others undergo identical specific somatic rearrangement of their immunoglobulin genes and then sit back as memory cells, armed and ready for any future secondary attack. T cells can similarly survive as memory cells.

IL-3 is also notorious for causing release of histamine from mast cells, IL-4 for stimulating immunoglobulin E production and IL-5 for stimulating eosinophils. These are of course central to parasite elimination, and the Th2 pathway is active in parasite infection. These are also central to atopy and allergy, which are characterised by an excessive Th2 response.

Do you know of any diseases that may have two presentations, depending upon which of the Th1 or Th2 pathways predominates?

There are many. Examples are leprosy (tuberculoid – Th1 response causes intense granulomatous inflammation, overt symptoms and effective organism elimination; lepromatous – Th2 response leads to persistence of organism), neurocysticercosis and sarcoidosis (erythema nodosum highly inflammatory and lupus pernio more anergic).

What are chemokines?

Chemokines (chemotactic cytokines) are cytokines that direct or attract leucocytes to sites of inflammation or injury. They are essential in evoking an adequate immune inflammatory response, but may also contribute to disease pathogenesis and are now potential targets for disease modification, such as chemokine receptor antagonists (Table 2.101 – for reference only!). Chemokines work with adhesion molecules called selectins and integrins in seducing leucocytes down extravasation pathways from blood to tissues.

Why are chemokines potentially important to clinicians?

A huge investment of research time and energy is currently being made in producing chemokine receptor antagonists to attempt to modify these disease processes.

What is haemophagocytic syndrome?

The term haemophagocytosis refers to the unusual problem in which activated macrophages engulf red cells, white cells, and platelets and their precursors. Haemophagocytic lymphohistiocytosis (HLH), the prototype haemophagocytic syndrome, is a condition of uncontrolled activation of the cellular immune system, mediated by numerous cytokines including IL-1, IL-2, soluble IL-2 receptor,

Table 2.101 Chemokines, their roles, and disease associations

Chemokine family	Broad role of that family of chemokines	Chemokine receptors	Examples of chemokines attracting cells bearing those chemokoine receptors	Examples of cells bearing chemokine receptors	Disease associations
CC First two of four cysteine residues adjacent	Attract mononuclear cells to sites of chronic inflammation, e.g. trauma, bacterial infection, ischaemia, chronic inflammatory disease	CCRI	Macrophage inhibitory protein MIP1α (CCL3) RANTES (CCL5)	T cells Monocytes	Rheumatoid arthritis Multiple sclerosis
		CCR2	Monocoyte chemoattractant proteins 1–4 (CCL2, 8, 7, 13)	Monocytes Macrophage antigen-presenting cells Memory T cells	Atherosclerosis Rheumaotid arthritis Multiple sclerosis Type 2 diabetes
		CCR3	Eotaxins (CCL11,13) MCP2 to 4 RANTES	Eosinophils Mast cells Th2 cells	Asthma and allergy
		CCR4	Thymus and activation regulated chemokine or TARC (CCL17) Macrophage-derived chemokine or MDC (CCL22)	Th2 cells	Parasite infection Graft rejection T lymphocyte attraction to skin
		CCR5	MIP-1α MIP-1β (CCL4) RANTES	T cells Monocytes	HIV requires CD4 and co-receptor CCR5 recognition to enter macrophages
		CCR6	CCL20	T cells B cells APCs	Mucosal humoral immunity T lymphocyte attraction to intestine
		CCR7	CCL19 CCL21	CCR7 on APCs and T cells CCL19 and CCL21 on endothelium and inside lymph nodes attract peptide-bound APCs and T cells for subsequent APC–T-cell engagement B cells also upregulate CCR7 expression to interact with Th cells After immune response subsides, CCR7 memory T cells continuously patrol tissues and lymph nodes via the bloodstream, some specialised for defending the skin or gastrointestinal tract	Exuberant chronic inflammation
		CCR8	CCL1	Th2 cells Monocytes Macrophage APCs	Granuloma formation
		CCR9	CCL25	T cells	Inflammatory bowel disease
		CCR10	CCL27	T cells	

Table 2.101 Chemokines, their roles, and disease associations—cont'd

Chemokine family	Broad role of that family of chemokines	Chemokine receptors	Examples of chemokines attracting cells bearing those chemokoine receptors	Examples of cells bearing chemokine receptors	Disease associations
CXC Single amino acid residue between first two cysteines	A subgroup of CXC chemokines with a glutamate–leucine–arginine motif (designated ELR+ chemokines) Notably attract neutrophils to sites of acute inflammation, induce granulocyte exocytosis and contribute to wound repair, e.g. interleukin 8 (CXCL8) attracts neutrophils to areas of acute inflammation and binds neutrophil receptors CXCR1 and CXCR2 to each other Inflammatory mediators such as IL-1, TNF-α and bacterial lipopolysaccharides elicit production of CXC chemokines	CXCR1	Interleukin-8 (CXCL8)	Neutrophils Monocytes	Inflammatory lung disease COPD
		CXCR2	Interleukin-8 CXCL1–3,5,6	Neutrophils Monocytes Endothelial cells	Inflammatory lung disease COPD Angiogenic factor for tumour growth
		CXCR3-A	CXCL4, 9, 10, 11	Th1 cells Mast cells Mesangial cells	Inflammatory skin disease Multiple sclerosis Transplant rejection
		CXCR3-B	CXCL4, 9–11	Endothelial cells Neoplastic cells	Angiostatic for tumour growth
		CXCR4	CXCL12	Wide expression	HIV requires CD4 and co-receptor CXCR4 recognition to enter T lymphocytes
		CXCR5	CXCL13	B cells	
		CXCR6	CXCR16	Mediates interaction between APCs and T cells Scavenger–receptor activity for oxidised lipids	Inflammatory liver disease May participate in atherosclerosis
CX₃C	CX₃CL1 arrests cells under normal physiological flow and may be cleaved from endothelium to act as soluble chemokine		CX₃CL1 (fractalcine)	Macrophages Endothelial cells Smooth muscle cells	Atherosclerosis
XC Single cysteine residue			XCL1 (lymphotaxin)	T cells Natural killer cells	Rheumaotid arthritis IgA nephropathy

APC, antigen-presenting cell; COPD, chronic obstructive pulmonary disease; HIV, human immunodeficiency virus; IgA, immunoglobulin A; IL-1, interleukin-1; TNF-α, tumour necrosis factor-α.

plasminogen activator and prostaglandins. The cause is usually infection (viral, bacterial, fungal or protozoal) or autoimmunity including the connective tissue disorders, but may be malignancy or familial. Still's disease may provoke macrophage activation syndrome, associated with very high inflammatory markers including ferritin. Clinical features include fever, splenomegaly, cytopenias, hypofibrinogen-aemia and rash, in the presence of haemophagocytosis.

What do immunoglobulins do?

During development in the bone marrow, virginal B cells contain 'unmutated' immunoglobulin V region genes. These genes undergo appropriate somatic mutation in response to antigen encounters in peripheral lymphoid sites, and B cells subsequently survive as memory cells in the lymph nodes or circulation, or undergo isotype class switching to become antibody-producing plasma cells.

Immunoglobulins (or antibodies) precipitate antigens and activate complement proteins, the role of complement being to eliminate precipitated antigens and immune complexes.

What are cryoglobulins?

A cryoglobulin is simply any antibody that precipitates in the cold (at < 4°C). It dissolves when warmed to 37°C. Cryoglobulins may be immunoglobulin G (IgG), IgM or IgA, and may be *monoclonal* IgM or IgG, tending to form precipitates (cryoprecipitation), *mixed* (usually monoclonal IgM directed against *polyclonal* IgG) or polyclonal (mixtures of polyclonal IgM and IgG). Mixed and polyclonal cryoglobulins tend to form immune complexes with antigens. Cryoglobulins, especially monoclonal, are often associated with lymphoproliferative disease and polyclonal with autoimmune disease such as systemic lupus erythematosus and infections such as hepatitis C. Cryoglobulinaemia may result in vasculitis, occlusive vascular disease and Raynaud's phenomenon.

What are cold agglutinins?

These are IgM antibodies that cause red blood cells to aggregate at < 37°C. They may be found in *Mycoplasma*, coxsackievirus and malarial infections and in lymphoproliferative disease. It is not surprising (given that both cryoglobulins and cold agglutinins are merely immunoglobulins secreted from plasma cells) that cryoglobulinaemia and cold agglutination are much more common in diseases of plasma cell proliferation. They merely represent a proportion of the immunoglobulin production in these diseases. They may also be found in otherwise healthy people, especially older people.

What are complement proteins?

The complement system is a cascade of plasma proteins, synthesised in the liver, whose role is to remove antigen precipitates and immune complexes (antigen–immunoglobulin complexes). The complement system may be activated by one of two routes, the classical pathway or the alternative pathway. The common result of both pathways is cleavage of the complement protein C3.

What is C1 (esterase) inhibitor deficiency?

This causes hereditary angio-oedema, in which attacks of non-inflammatory oedema are triggered by an excess of the complement protein C2.

What do you understand by the term hypersensitivity?

This refers to excessive immune responses (Table 2.102).

How does allergy arise?

It is suggested that we are born with a Th2-weighted imbalance (to fight worms!) with IL-4 in natural domination, but that in the first few months of life exposure to diseases like tuberculosis allows the emergence of Th1 to level the see-saw. Atopic predisposition seems to start in early life, with impaired IFN-γ production. Exposure to bacteria in early life may increase IFN-γ levels and lends weight to the 'hygiene' hypothesis, in which reduced exposure to bacteria, antibiotics and certain infant diets results in the persistence of a dominant Th2 pathway. Mycobacterial species are known to stimulate powerful IFN-γ production and research has examined vaccines to promote switching from Th2 to Th1 pathways.

How does tolerance give way to autoimmunity?

Immune responses to antigens and autoimmune responses to auto (self) antigens involve the same mechanisms. What is remarkable is how the immune system determines what is foreign and what is self. It does not normally respond to self-antigens, and this state of affairs is called tolerance. Tolerance is not fully understood. It begins in embryonic life, when lymphocytes 'learn' to react to antigens during their production in the thymus, bone marrow and lym-

Table 2.102 Hypersensitivity reactions

Type	Problem	What happens	Examples
I	Anaphylaxis	Antigens react with IgE on mast cells leading to release of vasoactive substances including histamine and leukotrienes. Reaction within minutes of exposure in previously sensitised individuals	Anaphylaxis
II	Antibody-dependent cytotoxicity	Cell surface antigens react with circulating antibody triggering complement activation	Transfusion reactions; Hyperacute transplant rejection
III	Immune complex-mediated	Circulating antigens react with circulating antibodies	Extrinsic allergic alveolitis; Serum sickness; Post-infectious glomerulonephritis
IV	Cell-mediated immunity: delayed hypersensitivity	Antigens, in association with HLA class II molecules on APCs, are presented to already sensitised (memory) Th lymphocytes	Tuberculin reaction; Contact dermatitis; Graft versus host disease (GvHD); Graft rejection

APC, antigen-presenting cell; HLA, human leucocyte antigen; IgE, immunoglobulin E.

phoid organs. Their developing cell receptors undergo random gene rearrangement in preparation for the diverse array of exogenous antigens in postembryonic life, and every T cell has a specific TCR encoded by a specific T-cell gene rearrangement. Understandably, during development, TCRs will encounter self-antigens. At this stage, any strong interactions between TCR and self-antigen will lead to de-selection – lymphocytes with a tendency to 'friendly-fire' are destroyed by apoptosis, or programmed cell death. However efficient this process, it is never enough to prevent some self-reacting lymphocytes from 'qualifying'. These dangerous cells, and their clonal offspring, must be kept in check by the immune system for the rest of an individual's life. One safeguard is called anergy. Anergy ensures the lack of response to a self-antigen by an autoimmune T lymphocyte unless a co-stimulatory signal is present. Most cells in the body are not competent to deliver such a signal. Another protective mechanism is ignorance. Frequently, autoimmune lymphocytes never encounter their respective self-antigens because the latter are 'hidden' behind cellular or vascular barriers. Equally, apoptosis ensures that, unlike necrotic cell death, antigenic intracellular contents do not spill out into the face of danger. Even these stealthy safeguards may fail, and the result is autoimmune disease.

CASE 2.47

POLYMYALGIA AND GIANT CELL ARTERITIS

Candidate information

Role

You are a doctor in the medical outpatient clinic. Please read the following letter from the patient's general practitioner. You may make notes on the paper provided. When the bell sounds, enter the examination room to begin the consultation.

Scenario

> Dear Doctor
>
> Re: Mrs Muriel Gray, aged 82 years
>
> Thank you for slotting this lady in urgently. She has had a right temporal and occipital headache for the past two weeks and this is out of character for her. She is a usually fit and active lady whom I seldom see at the surgery. I am concerned about the possibility of temporal arteritis. Her erythrocyte sedimentation rate was 45. I have started 60 mg of prednisolone.
>
> Yours sincerely

Please take a history from the patient (you may continue to make notes if you wish on the paper provided). Your examiners will warn you when 12 minutes have elapsed. You have 14 minutes to take a history from the patient followed by 1 minute of reflection. There will then follow 5 minutes of discussion with the examiners. Be prepared to discuss solutions to the problems posed by the case and how you might reply to the GP's letter. You are not required to examine the patient.

Patient information

Mrs Muriel Gray is an 82-year-old lady who for the past two weeks has had intermittent severe headaches over the right temporal area extending to the back of the neck. These have no diurnal pattern, are not related to posture or activity, and can be present at any time of the day or night. Her scalp is a little tender but not enough to stop her from washing or brushing her hair. She has not noticed any pain with chewing. She has no other symptoms. She has a past medical history of breast cancer with a mastectomy four years ago and remains on tamoxifen. She does not take any other medications. She feels a little better on prednisolone, which she has been taking for three days, but is very concerned about being on corticosteroids because her brother was on these for Crohn's disease and developed terrible osteoporosis. She is also concerned because her mother started to develop headaches at a similar age and turned out to have brain metastases from breast cancer. She lives with her husband and their dogs.

How to approach the case

Data gathering in the interview and interpretation and use of information gathered

Presenting problem(s) and symptom exploration

▪ **Explore possible symptoms of giant cell arteritis** The headache in giant cell arteritis (GCA) is classically temporal but potentially anywhere, relating to the diverse facial artery distributions. Up to 15% of GCA presents occipitally. Symptoms of GCA are outlined in Table 2.103 and you should explore these.

GCA occasionally presents with vascular occlusive disease elsewhere, e.g. chest pain, or as acute confusion with raised inflammatory markers in an elderly person.

▪ **Consider other conditions** Disorders that can mimic GCA are outlined in Box 2.88.

Patient perspective

Her fears of steroids are not unfounded and should be respected by outlining that:

• You will seek to establish the diagnosis quickly and the need or otherwise for these to continue

Table 2.103 Symptoms of giant cell arteritis

Typical symptoms	Diagnostic criteria	
Age > 60 years (less commonly 50–60) Headache – new or change in pattern Scalp tenderness Jaw claudication Visual disturbance, e.g. diplopia, blurring (may be transient and recurrent) Temporal artery tenderness, e.g. combing or washing hair Temporal artery thickening, redness or loss of pulsatility Systemic symptoms	Without visual symptoms	Three or more of: Age > 50 years New onset headache Temporal artery tenderness/ decreased pulsation ESR > 50 mm/hour Positive temporal artery biopsy
	With visual symptoms	Urgent ophthalmology review

ESR, erythrocyte sedimentation rate.

Box 2.88 Disorders which can mimic giant cell arteritis

Infective
- Viral illness
- Tuberculosis
- Infective endocarditis

Neoplastic
- Cancer
- Lymphoma
- Myeloma

SUMMARY – ASSESSMENT AND PLAN

- The two important differential diagnoses are giant cell arteritis and metastatic breast cancer.
- Urgent investigations should include routine haematobiochemistry and a computed tomography (CT) brain scan with contrast enhancement.
- If the CT scan does not reveal a structural lesion she should be considered for a temporal artery biopsy.
- If it is positive or if symptoms are persuasive corticosteroids should continue, a suggested regimen in Table 2.104. Bone protection is essential.

- You would recommend that she remains on these until then because GCA responds very well to steroid treatment but is potentially sight-threatening and stroke-provoking without
- You would start medication to protect the bones if it becomes necessary to recommend continuing steroids after further tests
- Steroids are gradually weaned in GCA

Past medical history

The history of breast cancer brings brain metastases into the differential diagnosis of her headaches.

Drug and allergy history

This is less relevant in this case.

Family history

There are no suggestions of a familial illness other than possible breast cancer, although this patient was only diagnosed with breast cancer in recent years.

Social history

Explore her active lifestyle, what her symptoms limit her from doing and whether the steroids have helped with some of these activities.

Discussion

Which tests might help confirm a diagnosis of GCA?

Ninety-five per cent of patients with GCA have raised inflammatory markers, notably an erythrocyte sedimentation rate (ESR) > 40 or plasma viscosity > 1.8 or C-reactive protein (CRP) > 10; the CRP is less likely to be raised because GCA does not involve a vigorous Th1-mediated immune acute-phase reaction. Thrombocytosis, normochromic normocytic anaemia and hypoalbuminaemia are common in GCA.

Temporal artery biopsy is positive in around 70–80% of GCA (especially if biopsies more than 2 cm long are taken to avoid missing skip lesions, or bilateral biopsies are undertaken) but there is uncertainty about for how long after starting corticosteroids a biopsy might be useful. The most popular view is that changes might disappear within three days, but some experts feel that histopathological legacies of GCA can remain for long time afterwards.

When would you consider a temporal artery biopsy?

There are no clear criteria for considering a biopsy but a pragmatic approach to biopsy is that it should be considered in all patients in whom there is diagnostic doubt. It is most useful before treatment or in the first 24 hours after starting treatment but treatment should not be delayed to get it. A negative biopsy does not exclude GCA. A positive

Table 2.104 Corticosteroid regimen in GCA	
Induction	40 mg + bone protection for one month (60–80 mg if visual disturbance)
Initial reduction	Reduce by 5 mg every 2 weeks until a dose of 5–7 mg is reached
Maintenance	Maintain 5–7.5 mg for around 12 months
Final reduction	Reduce by 1 mg every 6–8 weeks, more slowly below 3 mg, aiming for full weaning at 2–3 years

Table 2.105 Corticosteroid regimen in PMR	
Induction	15 mg + bone protection
Initial reduction	Aim for 12.5 mg at 2 weeks Aim for 10 mg at 4 weeks Reduce by 1 mg every 4–6 weeks until a dose of 5–7 mg is reached
Maintenance	Maintain 5–7 mg for around 12 months
Final reduction	Reduce by 1 mg every 6–8 weeks, more slowly below 3 mg

result prevents later diagnostic doubt, especially if there are treatment complications.

When should corticosteroids be started in suspected GCA?

Treatment should not be delayed if GCA is strongly suspected, and it should be immediate if there is visual disturbance, but patients with visual disturbance should also be seen by an ophthalmologist to look for evidence of ischaemic optic neuropathy or other causes of visual disturbance.

What might be a suitable corticosteroid regimen for GCA?

There is no evidence-based starting dose or regimen, but a suitable regimen is given in Table 2.104.

What is the place of steroid-sparing agents in GCA?

Azathioprine or methotrexate may be used if corticosteroids are contraindicated, or if it is not possible to wean successfully from steroids. They are sometimes used as steroid-sparing agents. They take three or four months to reach full effect and should never be used acutely. Methotrexate is started at 2.5 mg once weekly, increased to 5 mg, then at 7.5–10 mg once weekly long term. However, many patients following GCA or polymyalgia rheumatica (PMR) feel less well when off steroids and this is often not because of reactivation of GCA or PMR; hypoadrenalism from adrenal suppression may be the culprit.

In which patients is azathioprine dangerous?

Azathioprine can cause bone marrow suppression, more likely in those with genetically lower levels of thiopurine methyltransferase (TMPT), which should be checked before initiating treatment.

How does PMR present? (Box 2.89)

Like GCA, PMR has a mean age at presentation of 70 years, with the majority of cases presenting between 60 and 75 years. It is characterised by symmetrical pain and notably stiffness in the shoulders – especially deltoids and upper arms – or pelvis, and systemic symptoms may be present. Tenderness is not present in PMR, more likely in a myositis. Early morning symptoms are common. A

Box 2.89 Diagnostic criteria for polymyalgic rheumatica (PMR)
• Bilateral shoulder pain ± stiffness • Onset duration < 2 weeks • ESR > 40 mm/hour • Stiffness duration > 1 hour • Age > 65 years • Depression ± weight loss • Bilateral upper arm tenderness (not classic) Diagnosis if three or more of the above.

common differential diagnosis is rotator cuff pathology, or back pain radiating to the legs.

How is a diagnosis of PMR confirmed?

There is no diagnostic test. Inflammatory markers are raised but muscle enzymes, electromyographic studies and routine muscle biopsy are normal. The pathology of PMR is still unclear, unlike GCA with which PMR can be associated, but there are increased concentrations of T helper type 1 (interleukin-1 and interleukin-6) and type 2 (interleukin-10)-driven cytokines in affected tissues.

How is PMR treated?

Prednisolone at 15 mg is the right starting dose. This is sufficient to melt symptoms away within two or three days. A higher dose of prednisolone will 'treat' symptoms of a diverse array of pathology. If symptoms settle quickly, a reasonable reducing regimen is outlined in Table 2.105.

Corticosteroid-sparing agents such as azathioprine 1–2 mg/kg daily or methotrexate 7.5–15 mg once weekly may be considered.

CASE 2.48

PYREXIA AND SEPSIS

Candidate information

Role

You are a doctor in the emergency medical admissions unit. Please read the following letter from the patient's general practitioner. You may make notes on the paper provided. When the bell sounds, enter the examination room to begin the consultation.

Scenario

Dear Doctor

Re: Dr John Watson, aged 60 years

Thank you for admitting this 60-year-old ex-hospital ophthalmologist who is now engaged in regular overseas aid work. He presents with pyrexia of unknown origin. He has had night sweats and fever for the past few months. He has a documented temperature of 38°C. He has lost 2 kg in weight. He is usually well, although was briefly an inpatient in your hospital three months ago for incision and drainage of a staphylococcal abscess in his groin, when he was incidentally noted to have microcytic anaemia, with a haemoglobin of 10.5 g/dl. A subsequent ferritin was borderline low but his other haematinics were normal. He is awaiting outpatient endoscopies. I wondered if he had a soft systolic murmur, not previously documented, but examination is currently unremarkable. His blood tests reveal a C-reactive protein (CRP) of 156 and his white cell count is mildly elevated.

Yours sincerely

Please take a history from the patient (you may continue to make notes if you wish on the paper provided). Your examiners will warn you when 12 minutes have elapsed. You have 14 minutes to take a history from the patient followed by 1 minute of reflection. There will then follow 5 minutes of discussion with the examiners. Be prepared to discuss solutions to the problems posed by the case and how you might reply to the GP's letter. You are not required to examine the patient.

Patient information

Dr John Watson is a 60-year-old ex-hospital ophthalmologist with a month or so of fever, drenching night sweats and weight loss of around 2–3 kg. He has had occasional blood in his urine for around two months. He is usually well but three months ago developed an abscess in his groin, which required a short hospital admission to the surgical wards for incision and drainage. While in hospital he was found to be anaemic, and is awaiting outpatient endoscopies to exclude a source of covert bleeding. He has no symptoms of indigestion, change in bowel habit or family history of colorectal cancer. He has had a cough for the last few months, but it is mild and he had not thought much of it. His other past history is removal of a skin melanoma five years ago, thought to be completely excised. He does not take any medications. He is now semi-retired but does intermittent overseas medical work, largely cataract surgery. Six months ago he was in Africa, where he did not take adequate anti-malarial prophylaxis because

the tablets made him feel sick, but was well on return. Nevertheless, he feels he could still be at risk from malaria, and is a little concerned about the possibility of human immunodeficiency virus (HIV) having sustained occasional minor needlestick injuries overseas. He has never smoked. He is married with two children, and all are well at home although there has been a 'throat bug' in the family.

How to approach the case

Data gathering in the interview and interpretation and use of information gathered

Presenting problem(s) and symptom exploration

■ **Consider the causes of pyrexia**   Pyrexia of unknown origin (PUO) refers to a temperature > 38.3°C for at least 14 days or fever for three weeks and failure to reach a diagnosis within a week of tests. He therefore may have PUO, although strictly his temperature has not been documented and there are numerous potential causes that could be rapidly confirmed or excluded by tests. A full history of the nature of symptoms and their chronology, thinking of potential causes (Table 2.106) should be elicited, together with the pattern of fever (sustained, intermittent, remittent, relapsing).

Infections in immunocompromised patients (transplant recipients, HIV-infected patients, neutropenic patients) can present in an atypical fashion, as can infections in patients taking antipyretics, corticosteroids or antibiotics. The profile of causes of PUO in older people differs – infection is less common while lymphoproliferative disease, malignancy, giant cell arteritis, pulmonary emboli and drugs are much more common causes.

Patient perspective

His thoughts are entirely reasonable.

Past medical history

The recent staphylococcal abscess must be considered as a potential source of sepsis, perhaps with secondary sub-acute bacterial endocarditis, although staphylococcal endocarditis is invariably acute and aggressive. The history of melanoma cannot be ignored.

Drug and allergy history

It is unlikely that this is relevant in this case.

Family history

A family history of colorectal or renal cancer should be explored.

Social history

His occupational history with overseas travel is potentially highly relevant, exposing him to malaria and needlestick injuries. A history of exposure to animals including household pets and farm animals is part of routine enquiry for

Table 2.106 Causes of pyrexia of unknown origin (PUO)

Category	Causes		Clues in history
Infection	Localised pyogenic	Intra-abdominal: Subphrenic, diverticular, hepatic abscess	Abdominal pain
		Biliary sepsis	
		Osteomyelitis	Prostheses
		Septic arthritis	Exquisitely tender joint
		Soft tissue infection	History of oedema or eczema
		Dental abscess	Facial pain
		Sinusitis	Facial pain, worse coughing, bending and supine
		Chronic otitis media	Otalgia
			Conductive hearing loss
		Unresolving pneumonia	Chest symptoms
		Unresolving urinary tract infection	Frequency
			Dysuria
			Loin pain
		Genitourinary infection	Vaginal or urethral discharge
			Dysuria
			Dyspareunia
			Pelvic pain
	Systemic bacterial	Infective endocarditis	Prosthetic valve or native valve disease
			Invasive (including dental) procedures
		Salmonellosis	Gastroenteritis
		Atypical pneumonia	Usually very unwell
		Brucellosis	Unpasteurised milk
		Leptospirosis	Occupational history (sewers)
		Listeriosis	Dairy products, soft cheeses, etc
		Lyme disease	Tick bite
		Mycobacterial infection	Cough
			Night sweats
			Weight loss
	Viral	Human immunodeficiency virus	Lymphadenopathy
			Recurrent fungal/viral infections
		Hepatitis B or C virus	Risk factors
		Epstein–Barr virus	Sore throat
	Systemic fungal	Systemic candidiasis	Usually immunocompromised
	Protozoal	Malaria	Travel to malaria zone
		Giardiasis	Common
			Asymptomatic or watery diarrhoea/malabsorption
		Amoebiasis	Swimming in infected water
		Toxoplasmosis	Pet cat
	Worm	Toxocariasis	Pet dog
Neoplasm	Lymphoproliferative disease		Night sweats
			Lymphadenopathy
	Renal cell carcinoma		Lack of early warning symptoms
			Classic triad of flank pain (40%), haematuria (40%) and flank mass (25%) rare; 25–30% discovered as incidental finding
			Weight loss and night sweats
			Hypertension
			Varicocoele
			Paraneoplastic – hypercalcaemia (PTHrp), polycythaemia (EPO), iron deficiency anaemia, non-metastatic liver dysfunction, neuromyopathy
	Hepatocellular carcinoma		Complication of cirrhosis
	Colorectal cancer		Especially elderly
	Metastatic disease		Symptoms of primary, e.g. gastrointestinal, lung, breast, prostate, skin
	Atrial myxoma		Very high ESR

Table 2.106 Causes of pyrexia of unknown origin (PUO)—cont'd

Category	Causes	Clues in history
Inflammatory disease	Systemic vasculitides	Renal failure Haemoptysis or respiratory symptoms
	Systemic lupus erythematosus	Skin rashes Arthralgia
	Polymyositis	Muscle tenderness
	Adult Still's disease	Arthralgia
	Giant cell arteritis	Headache
Other	Pulmonary embolus	Tachypnoea
	Drugs	Antibiotics, NSAIDs, AEDs

AED, anti-epileptic drug; EPO, erythropoietin; ESR, erythrocyte sedimentation rate; NSAIDs, non-steroidal anti-inflammatory drugs; PTHrp, parathyroid hormone-related peptide.

PUO, as is a history of insect bites, including tick bites, a food history (poorly cooked meat, etc.), a history of unwell contacts, a sexual history and enquiry about intravenous drug taking.

SUMMARY – ASSESSMENT AND PLAN

- The differential diagnosis remains wide without further tests but possible infectious causes include staphylococcal bacteraemia (with endocarditis essential to exclude after his recent abscess and a possible new heart murmur), malaria and tuberculosis. Malignant causes include renal cell carcinoma and metastatic melanoma.
- Routine blood tests include full blood count, urea, electrolytes and creatinine, liver function tests, calcium, erythrocyte sedimentation rate (ESR), CRP and multiple blood cultures from separate sites. Blood film examination for malarial parasites should be performed.
- Urinalysis for blood is essential, and if present should be analysed for casts and dysmorphic red cells.
- A chest X-ray and echocardiogram are important early tests.
- Further tests are almost inevitable, but dictated by the preliminary information. A contrast enhanced computed tomography (CT) scan of chest, abdomen and pelvis would be important to look for metastatic disease or renal cell carcinoma, and differentiates between cystic and solid masses and determines lymph node and renal vein or inferior vena cava extension. Magnetic resonance imaging is excellent for further analysing the inferior vena cava and differentiates alternative diagnoses such as benign angiomyolipomata.

Discussion

What causes pyrexia?

The release of certain cytokines and acute-phase reactants involved in the immune response.

What is sepsis?

This refers to systemic illness caused by microbial invasion of parts of the body that are normally sterile. The term septicaemia is old-fashioned and encompasses the better terms sepsis (inflammation with evidence or suspicion of microbial cause), severe sepsis (sepsis with organ dysfunction) and septic shock (sepsis with hypotension despite volume replacement). Severe sepsis and septic shock have mortality rates of 25–30% and 40–70% respectively, partly because early phases may not be recognised as sepsis or sufficiently vigorously treated.

How do bacteria induce sepsis and septic shock?

Lipopolysaccharide-binding protein on host cells binds to lipopolysaccharide on Gram-negative bacteria and transfers it to CD14, which resides on the host cell membrane and as a soluble protein capable of transferring lipopolysaccharide to CD14-negative cells. Cellular activation requires CD14 and a co-receptor known as a Toll-like receptor (TLR-4 for lipopolysaccharide). Gram-positive bacteria may induce similar pathways via TLR-2 but more typically produce exotoxins that act as superantigens or directly stimulate immune cells via their proteins. Superantigens are molecules that bind to major histocompatibility complex class II molecules of antigen-presenting cells and T-cell receptors, activating large numbers of T cells and a powerful proinflammatory response. All cases of septic shock involve overt proinflammatory responses with vasodilatation and a tendency to intravascular coagulation disturbance.

What are some important clinical and laboratory markers of sepsis and its associated inflammation?

Important clinical markers may include fever (or hypothermia), tachycardia, tachypnoea, hypotension, confusion, oliguria, positive fluid balance and hypoxia.

Easily accessible laboratory markers may include leucocytosis, elevated C-reactive protein, hyperglycaemia, elevated creatinine, elevated plasma bilirubin, thrombocytopenia and elevated INR. Lactate is invariably elevated.

The pro-inflammatory response provoked after the initial recognition of lipopolysaccharides is complex, and it is increasingly understood that genetic factors often determine susceptibility or protection by the severity of this response. Many markers of this response are recognised, but few yet clinically available. These include:

- Leucocyte surface markers such as intracellular adhesion molecule (ICAM-1) and CD63, 64 and 66b
- Interleukins 1, 6, 8, 10, 15 and 18 and other monocyte/macrophage-released peptides such as macrophage migration inhibitory factor (MIF), soluble triggering receptor expressed on myeloid cells (sTREM-1) and high mobility group box protein 1 (HMGB-1)
- Leucocyte peptide products such as soluble L- and P-selectins (= CD62L and CD 62P)
- Endothelial peptide products such as soluble vascular cell adhesion molecule (sVCAM-1 = CD106) and soluble E-selectin (= CD62E)
- Other peptides produced by an array of cells including soluble TNF receptors and soluble ICAM-1
- Acute-phase reactants other than C-reactive protein including ferritin, procalcitonin, serum amyloid A, lactoferrin and neopterin
- Microbial products themselves including endotoxin

Staphylococcus is commonly detected in blood cultures. Which factors alert you to it reflecting true bacteraemia rather than being a 'contaminant'?

These include the presence of local or systemic signs of infection, detection of bacteria in both culture bottles, early detection (< 14 hours), coagulase-negative staphylococcus (although not always the case!) and previous colonisation with staphylococci.

What is the rate of nasal carriage of S. aureus?

This varies between around 10% and 40%.

What is 'MRSA'?

This is methicillin-resistant (but more appropriately multi-resistant) S. aureus because of its multi-resistant cassette gene. β-lactamase production was one of the traditional modes of antibiotic resistance, followed by production of antibiotics which inhibited β-lactamase. MRSA simply changed its target to become resistant again. In the early 1990s MRSA was a rare problem; now all doctors must be conscious of MRSA.

What are the risk factors for MRSA colonisation?

These include recent hospitalisation, recent (three to six months) antimicrobial use, invasive lines (intravenous, urinary catheters), recent surgery, nursing home residence, advanced age, underlying severe disease, exposure to a colonised or infected patient, morbid obesity and orthopaedic implant surgery.

What are the common sources of S. aureus bacteraemia?

About 20% of bacteraemia has an unidentified source. In hospital, wound infection and invasive lines are the biggest source, but other sources include skin and soft tissue infection, endocarditis, osteomyelitis, septic arthritis or prosthetic joint infections, and pneumonia. These should all be considered in patients with positive blood cultures.

What are the treatments for MRSA infection?

These are outlined in Table 2.107. Combination treatments are often best.

Who should receive MRSA eradication treatment?

Clinical indications are stronger than treatment for those with colonisation. Isolated nasal carriage has a reasonable chance of clearance but skin carriage and colonisation of indwelling catheters cannot be cleared.

Should NHS staff be screened for MRSA?

This was popular, but it is increasingly realised that many staff can have negative skin carriage at the start of a shift and be positive by the end of a shift.

Should screening be performed to detect hospital patient carriers?

Eighty-five per cent of carriage of MRSA is asymptomatic, but these people have a much higher risk of clinical infection when unwell; 15% of people have clinical infection. Same-day polymerase chain reaction testing has improved detection, and is being seen increasingly in at-risk patients such as those embarking on prosthetic surgery.

How can the MRSA prevalence be controlled?

Handwashing and prudent use of antibiotics (e.g. avoidance of quinolones which select MRSA) are imperative.

Can S. aureus affect healthy people in the community?

Previously well children and young healthy adults such as athletes are beginning to develop skin and soft tissue infections (SSTIs), pneumonia, empyema and invasive

Table 2.107 Treatments for methicillin-resistant *Staphylococcus aureus* (MRSA)	
Treatment	**Comment**
Glycopeptides – vancomycin, teicoplanin	Vancomycin is a little overrated, but so is its toxicity (nephrotoxicity and ototoxicity) Glycopeptide-resistant SA (GRSA) has occurred, the gene jumping form enteroccoccus
Rifampicin	
Fusidic acid	Causes jaundice
Linezolid	A novel antibiotic, an oxazolidinone Inhibits MRSA toxicity Useful for MRSA and vancomycin-resistant enterococcus (VRE) Usually reserved for pneumonia or complicated soft tissue infection May cause bone marrow suppression or peripheral and optic neuropathy
Clindamycin	Very effective for staphylococcal and streptococcal skin and soft tissue infections (SSTIs) Resistance occurs rapidly during treatment Often provokes *Clostridium difficile* infection
Tetracyclines – minocycline, doxycycline	For mild urinary or soft tissue infections
New agents, e.g. daptomycin, tigecycline	Daptomycin useful for SSTIs but not respiratory infections as inhibited by secretions

infections with particularly severe staphylococcal infection such as that produced by the Panton–Valentine Leucocidin (*PVL*) gene. *PVL* is a staphylococcal gene present in common, non-MRSA staphylococcous that may be switched on, promoting production of a toxin which attracts white cells and kills them; patients with PVL infections become very unwell with high inflammatory markers but low white cell counts. They can develop haemorrhagic purpura, sometimes resembling meningococcal septicaemia, with severe SSTI, pneumonia with heavy haemoptysis and cavitation and high fever. The myocardium may turn to pus. The CURB-65 score can underestimate severity. Neither flucloxacillin nor vancomycin will stop toxin production, and clindamycin and linezolid are often used, although it is the toxin, rather than ongoing infection, which gives rise to the high mortality.

How common is renal cell carcinoma?

This constitutes 2–3% of all adult malignancies, is twice as common in men, and usually presents in the fourth to sixth decades.

What causes renal cell carcinoma?

This is usually unknown. Smoking doubles the risk, and it is associated with obesity, unopposed oestrogen, hypertension, petroleum products, heavy metals, tuberose sclerosis and acquired cystic kidney disease of chronic renal failure, dialysis and immunosuppression (relative risk × 80). It also occurs in rare hereditary syndromes such as von Hippel–Lindau (autosomal dominant, 3p deletion, multiple cancers). Renal cell carcinoma usually arises in the proximal tubule epithelium and histologically may be clear cell 75% (proximal tubule origin, 3p deletion), chromophobic, chromophilic, oncocytic or of collecting duct type.

What are the symptoms of renal cell carcinoma?

Renal cell carcinoma is often an incidental finding. Haematuria, a flank mass or loin tenderness may occur, but symptoms may equally be the result of cytokines such as erythropoietin or interleukin-6 (IL-6). Renal cell carcinoma is a great mimicker. It can produce a raised haemoglobin or iron deficiency anaemia (a cytokine inhibits iron incorporation into the haem synthetic pathway), thrombocytosis or leucocytosis including eosinophilia (the tumour releases IL-5).

Thirty per cent of renal cell carcinoma presents with metastases, most commonly lung, but sometimes soft tissue, bone, liver, skin or central nervous system. Symptoms often improve after resection of the primary tumour.

How is renal cell carcinoma treated?

The mode of treatment depends upon staging because the disease may be confined to the kidney or extend to perinephric fat, the renal vein and inferior vena cava, regional nodes, adjacent viscera including adrenals, or more distantly with distant metastases. Surgery is the only potentially curative treatment for localised tumour, by radical nephrectomy. Palliative nephrectomy may alleviate symptoms such as pain, hypercalcaemia and polycythaemia. Regression of metastases has been reported after nephrectomy but nephrectomy cannot be considered adjuvant treatment. The disease is relatively resistant to radiotherapy or chemotherapy but the former may palliate bone or cerebral involvement. Immunotherapy shows promise. Mutation in the tumour suppressor gene at 3p drives renal cell cancer, upregulating growth factors (GF) including vascular endothelial GF (VEGF) and expression of receptors including epidermal GF receptor (EGFR) and Herceptin (cerbB-2). Therapies include neutralising VEGF antibodies, such as bevacizumab, and tyrosine kinase inhibitors, such as erlatinib which blocks EGFR, lapatinib which blocks cerbB-2 and sunitinib and sorefenib which block multiple receptors. Treatments may be combined with cytokines such as interferon.

CASE 2.49

WEIGHT LOSS

Candidate information

Role

You are a doctor in the medical outpatient clinic. Please read the following letter from the patient's general practitioner. You may make notes on the paper provided. When the bell sounds, enter the examination room to begin the consultation.

Scenario

Dear Doctor

Re: Mr George Ross, aged 86 years

Thank you for reviewing this gentleman, who was admitted to hospital last year with anaemia while staying with relatives. He was apparently transfused and on his return I referred him to the hospital here for further investigation. Unfortunately his appointment was superseded by a family bereavement and he missed it. He did, however, see a rheumatologist on account of joint pains and shoulder discomfort who felt the overall position to be anaemia of chronic autoimmune disease. He has been on steroids, with some improvement initially, for six months. But he has now become more unwell again, tired and, significantly, losing weight. On examination I did wonder about a mass in the right iliac fossa. He has type 2 diabetes and his blood glucose has risen to around 20. I wonder if you have any further advice on diagnosis and management.

Yours sincerely

Please take a history from the patient (you may continue to make notes if you wish on the paper provided). Your examiners will warn you when 12 minutes have elapsed. You have 14 minutes to take a history from the patient followed by 1 minute of reflection. There will then follow 5 minutes of discussion with the examiners. Be prepared to discuss solutions to the problems posed by the case and how you might reply to the GP's letter. You are not required to examine the patient.

Patient information

Mr George Ross is an 86-year-old gentleman who has become tired and has lost around 10 kg in weight over the last six months. His clothes have become extremely loose. He and his wife went to stay with their daughter and son-in-law in Scotland last year when Mr Ross became 'unwell' (a little light-headed and confused) and was admitted to hospital. There he was treated for a urinary tract infection and noted to be anaemic and was transfused with blood. Referral for investigation of his anaemia was interrupted when his brother died in London and family support was needed there. Mr Ross did see a rheumatologist, having also been troubled with joint pains, who felt he might have 'rheumatoid or polymyalgia'. He denies any history of proximal girdle pain or morning stiffness. Mr Ross also has type 2 diabetes and takes metformin and simvastatin, but is on no other medications. He has no other symptoms. He was a very active and well-maintained man until last year, playing golf most days.

How to approach the case

Data gathering in the interview and interpretation and use of information gathered

Presenting problem(s) and symptom exploration

▦ **Select the important presenting symptoms** This case very typically highlights the sort of presentation seen in elderly care. There is more than one thing going on, and it is important to keep an open mind about previous opinions and focus on what are important and potentially threatening symptoms now. These are undoubtedly tiredness (likely the result of anaemia) and weight loss.

▦ **Take a thorough systematic enquiry for causes of weight loss** (Box 2.90) Take a full systematic enquiry but pay particular attention to:

- Gastrointestinal symptoms – abdominal pain, nausea and vomiting, altered bowel habit (diarrhoea, constipation), gastrointestinal bleeding

---

Box 2.90 Causes of weight loss
• Malignancy – gastrointestinal or non-gastrointestinal
• Chronic disease, e.g. heart failure, chronic obstructive pulmonary disease
• Chronic infection
• Non-infectious inflammatory disease, e.g. vasculitis
• Neurodegenerative conditions
• Thyrotoxicosis
• Late onset type 1 diabetes
• Under-nutrition
• Depression

- Steatorrhoea – type 2 diabetes is occasionally the result of pancreatic infiltration
- Prostatic symptoms – difficulty getting started, thin stream, nocturia, incomplete emptying, frequency
- Adrenal insufficiency symptoms – dizziness, nausea and vomiting

■ **Decide what to do with less urgent symptoms and problems**   The joint symptoms might be less pressing than the abdominal mass and weight loss.

Patient perspective

Establish if he has had any thoughts about what his symptoms might represent.

Past medical history

There are no clues here.

Drug and allergy history

High-dose corticosteroids can mask symptoms of a wide range of diseases including cancer. Metformin is of course anorexogenic.

Family history

Ask about a family history of colorectal cancer.

Social history

As well as checking his alcohol and smoking history, aim to discover how his life has changed in the last few months, what he cannot do now that he could, any difficulties that might be posed by investigation (given recent family circumstances) and how he and his wife are currently managing.

SUMMARY – ASSESSMENT AND PLAN

- The anaemia warrants further investigation to exclude malignancy. The weight loss is the most worrying feature. The right iliac fossa mass could represent constipation, but a full examination including per rectal examination is imperative.
- The history of autoimmune disease is uncertain and needs clarification from the case notes, but polymyalgia does not seem likely.
- Repeat full haematobiochemistry is warranted, including blood count, haematinics and inflammatory markers, and a chest X-ray.
- Urgent investigation of the lower gastrointestinal tract is warranted first, either with colonoscopy or computed tomography scanning. The latter may be preferable and faster to organise in patients who are frail and may show disseminated disease.
- Metformin should be stopped in this anorexogenic situation, and perhaps substituted with a sulphonylurea.
- Bone protection should be instituted early for patients taking long-term corticosteroids (but is a lesser issue immediately and the aim here is likely to wean the steroids).

Discussion

Is there usually a C-reactive protein rise in cancer?

Inflammatory markers are often normal, and if elevated seldom very high (often under 50).

What is your differential diagnosis for weight loss?

Refer to Box 2.90.

CASE 2.50

TIREDNESS

Candidate information

Role

You are a doctor in the medical outpatient clinic. Please read the following letter from the patient's general practitioner. You may make notes on the paper provided. When the bell sounds, enter the examination room to begin the consultation.

Scenario

Dear Doctor

Re: Mr Christopher Brandon, aged 68 years

Thank you for seeing this gentleman with a history of tiredness and overall loss of energy for the last year. He has also been losing weight and feeling nauseated. He takes levothyroxine and his thyroid-stimulating hormone (TSH) and free thyroxine (T4) suggest adequate replacement. Examination is unremarkable save for a slightly tanned complexion but he says he has always had this. His wife agrees. His full blood count, urea, creatinine, liver function tests and inflammatory markers are normal. His serum sodium is 121 mmol/l and his potassium is 5 mmol/l. His random blood glucose is on the low side at 3.5 mmol/l. Please see and advise on further management.

Yours sincerely

Please take a history from the patient (you may continue to make notes if you wish on the paper provided). Your examiners will warn you when 12 minutes have elapsed. You have 14 minutes to take a history from the patient followed by 1 minute of reflection. There will then follow 5 minutes of discussion with the examiners. Be prepared to discuss solutions to the problems posed by the case and how you might reply to the GP's letter. You are not required to examine the patient.

Patient information

Mr Christopher Brandon is a 68-year old gentleman who has been feeling tired for around a year. He used to be very active, but since retiring from teaching a few years ago has found he has less energy, with a considerable decline in the last year. He now feels marked waning of energy and some dizziness on standing. He has lost a little weight but attributes this to nausea. He lives with his wife, is a lifelong non-smoker and seldom drinks alcohol. He has always tanned quickly, and is not sure if this has changed over the last year. He takes levothyroxine for an underactive thyroid but his tests indicate adequate dosage. He had a large operation for a maxillary sinus tumour 15 years ago followed by cranial radiotherapy, but was later told he was cured. Recently, his GP thought he might be depressed but he does not feel it. He and his wife would simply like to get back to 'doing things' again.

How to approach the case

Data gathering in the interview and interpretation and use of information gathered

Presenting problem(s) and symptom exploration

Patients may complain of feeling 'tired all the time', having 'no energy' or feeling 'exhausted'. It is important to try to establish:

- What is meant by tiredness (e.g. a general feeling of fatigue after minimal activity, or weakness in specific muscle groups)
- Whether symptoms are present all the time or are episodic. If episodic, do they occur at specific times of the day (e.g. rheumatoid arthritis causes morning stiffness which improves with activity while mechanical back pain may be worse towards the end of a working day) or after specific activities (e.g. myasthenia gravis causes fatiguable weakness in specific muscle groups)?
- The duration of symptoms
- The mode of onset of symptoms (insidious or sudden, following a specific illness?)
- Symptoms that might suggest a specific cause (Table 2.108)

Patient perspective

Establish if he has had any thoughts about what his symptoms might represent.

Past medical history

The history of pituitary radiation is potentially highly relevant.

Drug and allergy history

Levothyroxine is probably blameless here.

Table 2.108 Symptoms which might suggest a cause of tiredness

Cause	Symptoms and clinical clues
Anaemia	Pallor Per rectal or vaginal bleeding Diet
Hypothyroidism	Preference for warmth Weight gain Dry skin and hair thinning
Obstructive sleep apnoea –hypopnoea syndrome	Snoring Obesity
Heart failure	Dyspnoea, orthopnoea, paroxysmal nocturnal dyspnoea Ankle swelling
Chronic lung disease	Dyspnoea
Inflammatory bowel disease	Altered bowel habit with blood, mucus or pus
Diabetes mellitus	Polyuria and polydipsia Recurrent fungal infections
Addison's disease	Postural dizziness Nausea Pigmented skin creases Vitiligo
Chronic kidney disease	Nocturia Oliguria
Colorectal cancer	Altered bowel habit Per rectal bleeding Weight loss
Lung cancer	Cough Haemoptysis Weight loss Smoking history
Myopathy/polymyalgia rheumatica	Persistent proximal muscle weakness
Myasthenia gravis	Fatiguable weakness in certain muscle groups
Periodic paralysis (very rare)	Episodic marked generalised weakness
Depression	Depressed mood Loss of enjoyment, interest or pleasure in activities Diminished concentration Change in weight or appetite Sleep disturbance Suicidal ideation/attempts/specific plans Agitated behaviour or reduced activity
Chronic fatigue syndrome	Fatigue after minimal activity Antecedent viral illness
Iatrogenic, e.g. beta blockers	

Family history

Relevance here is unlikely.

Social history

As well as checking his alcohol and smoking history aim to discover how his life has changed due to his symptoms, notably what he cannot do now that he could.

SUMMARY – ASSESSMENT AND PLAN

- The history and biochemistry suggests hypocortisolism.
- The question is whether this is primary hypoadrenalism or secondary to hypopituitarism.
- Primary hypoadrenalism, most commonly the result of Addison's disease, may result in a tanned complexion and hyperpigmentation of palmar creases and the buccal mucosa [adrenocorticotrophic hormone (ACTH) excess]. It tends to be insidious but the history is usually months to a year or two before presentation. It may present as a crisis, or, frequently, with chronic symptoms without a crisis. Other causes of hypoadrenalism that should be considered include adrenal infiltration.
- Hypopituitarism is a common consequence of cranial irradiation. It can be much more insidious than Addison's disease, presenting many years, even decades, after initial damage to and subsequent atrophy of the pituitary gland. There may be pallor (loss of ACTH).
- He should have a synacthen test to confirm hypoadrenalism and if positive receive cortisol replacement (e.g. oral hydrocortisone). Large doses are unnecessary except in a patient presenting in an adrenal crisis. Imaging of the adrenal glands might identify a non-Addisonian cause. Pituitary disease may give rise to a positive synacthen test because of years of adrenal atrophy.

- ACTH levels can differentiate between primary hypoadrenalism (high) and hypopituitarism (low).
- Other tests to consider include a pituitary profile (TSH, prolactin, insulin-like growth factor 1, follicle-stimulating hormone, testosterone) and magnetic resonance image scanning (non-urgently).

Discussion

What is chronic fatigue syndrome?

This typically follows an upper respiratory tract infection with incomplete recovery. Many viruses have been implicated as possible causes. There are many possible symptoms, but profound fatigue, worsened by minimal physical or mental exertion, is central. Chronic fatigue syndrome is more common in females but there is no clear link with occupation or social class. Investigations are usually non-specific, although altered lymphocyte function, hypocortisolism and other altered blood parameters have been described in some patients. There may be full recovery, but symptoms may relapse and remit or persist as a chronic illness.

List some causes of hypoglycaemia

- Diabetic drugs
- Starvation
- Addison's disease
- Insulinoma

References and further reading

History-taking skills
Coderre S, Mandin H, Harasym PH et al. Diagnostic reasoning strategies and diagnostic success. Med Educ 2003; 37:695–703
Kurtz S, Silverman J, Benson J. Marrying content and process in clinical method teaching: enhancing the Calgary–Cambridge guides. Acad Med 2003; 78:802–809
Kurtz SM, Silverman JD, Draper J. Teaching and learning communication skills in medicine. Oxford: Radcliffe Medical Press; 1998
Neighbour R. The inner consultation. Lancaster: MTP Press; 1987
Norman GR, Eva KW. Doggie diagnosis, diagnostic success and diagnostic reasoning strategies: an alternative view. Med Educ 2003; 37:676–677
Silverman JD, Kurtz SM, Draper J. Skills for communicating with patients. Oxford: Radcliffe Medical Press; 1998
Tate P. The doctor's communication handbook. Oxford: Radcliffe Press; 1984

Respiratory problems
Asthma
The British Thoracic Society. Scottish Intercollegiate Guidelines Network. British Guidelines on the Management of Asthma. January 2003. Online. Available: www.brit-thoracic.org.uk; www.sign.ac.uk
The BTS/SIGN British guidelines on the management of asthma. April 2004 update. Thorax 2003; 58 (Suppl. I)
The BTS/SIGN British guideline on the management of asthma. The BTS/SIGN guideline on asthma management. November 2005 update. www.brit-thoracic.org.uk

Abdominal problems
Dyspepsia
Blatchford O, Murray WR, Blatchford M. A risk score to predict need for treatment for upper gastrointestinal haemorrhage. Lancet 2000; 356:1319

British Society of Gastroenterology (guidelines on dyspepsia management). Online. Available: www.bsg.org.uk
Fox M, Forgas I. Gastro-oesophageal reflux disease. BMJ 2006; 332:88–93
Harris A, Misiewicz JJ. Management of *Helicobacter pylori* infection. ABC of the upper gastrointestinal tract. BMJ 2001; 323:1047–1050
Jairith V, Langmead L. Acute gastroenterology. Clin Med 2007; 7:262–266
Logan RPH, Walker MM. Epidemiology and diagnosis of *Helicobacter pylori* infection. ABC of the upper gastrointestinal tract. BMJ 2001; 323:920–922
Rockall TA, Logan RF, Devlin HB et al. Risk assessment after acute upper gastrointestinal haemorrhage. Gut 1996; 38:316–321
Thompson I, Dixon J. Bradycardia in acute haemorrhage. BMJ 2004; 328:451–453
Wong T. The management of upper gastrointestinal haemorrhage. Clin Med 2006; 6:460–466

Abdominal pain
Lafferty K. Understanding abdominal pain. Practitioner 2001; 245:156–161
Sreenarasimhaiah J. Diagnosis and management of intestinal ischaemic disorders. BMJ 2003; 326:1372–1376

Altered bowel habit
Cairns S, Scholefield JH. Guidelines for colorectal cancer screening in high risk groups. Gut 2002; 51(Suppl. 5):1–28. www.bsg.org.uk
Hagee BH, Chung-Faye G. Colorectal cancer screening. Clin Med 2006; 6:453–456
Primary Care Society for Gastroenterology. Follow up care of adult celiac disease. 2001. Online. Available: www.pcsg.org.uk
Van de Wal Y, Kooy Y, van Veelen P et al. Selective deamidation by tissue transglutaminase strongly enhances gliaden-specific T cell reactivity. J Immunol 1998; 161:1585–1588

Cardiovascular problems

Cardiovascular disease prevention and weight gain
Antithrombotic therapy in cardiovascular disease
Antithrombotic Trialists Collaboration. Collaborative meta-analysis of randomised trials of antiplatelet therapy for prevention of death, myocardial infarction, and stroke in high-risk patients. Br Med J 2002; 324:71–86
CAPRIE Steering Committee. A randomised, blinded, trial of clopidogrel versus aspirin in patients at risk of ischaemic events (CAPRIE). Lancet 1996; 348:1329–1339

Lifestyle measures in cardiovascular disease and obesity
Bartsch P. Platelet activation with exercise and risk of cardiac events. Lancet 1999; 354:1747–1748
British Heart Foundation. Physical activity and the heart: an update. BHF Factfile 4/2001. London: British Heart Foundation
Brunner E. Oily fish and omega 3 fat supplements. BMJ 2006; 332:739–740
Din JN, Newby DE, Flapan AD. Omega 3 fatty acids and cardiovascular risk – fishing for a natural treatment. BMJ 2004; 328:30–35
Franco OH, Banneux L, de Leat C. The polymeal: a more natural, safer and probably tastier (than the polypill) strategy to reduce cardiovascular disease by more than 75%. BMJ 2004; 729:1147–1150
Hooper L, Thompson RL, Harrison RA et al. Risks and benefits of omega 3 fats for mortality, cardiovascular disease and cancer: systematic review. BMJ 2006; 332:752–755
Joint British Societies' guidelines on prevention of cardiovascular disease in clinical practice. Heart 2005; vol 91 suppl V
Lean MEJ. Prognosis in obesity. We all need to move a little more, eat a little less. BMJ 2005; 330:1339–1340
Little P, Byrne CD. Abdominal obesity and the 'hypertriglyceridaemic waist' phenotype. BMJ 2001; 322:687–689
Sundström J, Risérus U, Byberg L. Clinical value of the metabolic syndrome for long term prediction of total and cardiovascular mortality: prospective, population based cohort study. BMJ 2006; 332:878–882
Trichopoulou A, for members of the EPIC – elderly prospective study group. Modified Mediterranean diet and survival: EPIC – elderly prospective cohort study. BMJ 2005; 330:991–995
Wahrenberg H, Hertel K, Leijonhufvud BM et al. Use of waist circumference to predict insulin resistance: retrospective study. BMJ 2005; 330:1363–1364
Wald DS. The future of cornary heart disease prevention. Clin Med 2007; 7:392–396

Preventing diabetes
Chiasson JL, Josse RG, Gomis R et al. Acarbose for prevention of type 2 diabetes mellitus: the STOP-NIDDM randomised trial. Lancet 2002; 359:2072–2077
Knowler WC, Barrett-Connor E, Fowler SE et al. Reduction in the incidence of type 2 diabetes with lifestyle intervention or metformin. N Engl J Med 2002; 346:393–403
Pan XR, Li GW, Hu YH et al. Effects of diet and exercise in preventing NIDDM in people with impaired glucose tolerance. The Da Qing IGT and diabetes study. Diabetes Care 1997; 20:537–544
Tagerson JS, Hauptman J, Boldrin MN et al. Xenical in the prevention of diabetes in obese subjects (XENDOS) study: a randomised study of orlistat as an adjunct to lifestyle changes for the prevention of type 2 diabetes in obese people. Diabetes Care 2004; 27:155–161
Tuomilehto J, Lindstrom J, Eriksson JG et al. prevention of type 2 diabetes mellitus by changes in lifestyle among subjects with impaired glucose tolerance. N Engl J Med 2001; 344:1343–1350

Angiotensin-converting enzyme inhibitors (high cardiovascular disease risk and coronary artery disease)
EUROPA Investigators. European trial on reduction of cardiac events with Perindopril in stable coronary artery disease. Efficacy of perindopril in reduction of cardiovascular events among patients with stable coronary artery disease: randomised, double blind, placebo controlled, multicentre trial (the EUROPA study). Lancet 2003; 362:782–788
Mindlen F, Nordaby R, Ruiz M et al. The HOPE (Heart Outcomes Prevention Evaluation) Study Investigators. Effects of an angiotensin converting enzyme inhibitor, ramipril, on cardiovascular events in high risk patients. N Engl J Med 2000; 342:145–153

Angiotensin receptor blockers and risk modification in cardiovascular disease
Dahlof B, Devereux RB, Kjeldsen SE et al. LIFE Study Group. Cardiovascualr morbidity and mortality in the losartan intervention for endpoint reduction in hypertensive study (LIFE): a randomised trial against atenolol. Lancet 2002; 359:995–1003
Dickstein K, Kjekshus J; OPTIMAAL Steering Committee of the OPTIMAAL Study Group. Effects of losartan and captopril on

mortality and morbidity in-high risk patients after acute myocardial infarction: the OPTIMAAL randomised trial. Optimal Trial in Myocardial Infarction with Angiotensin II Antagonist Losartan. Lancet 2002; 360:752–760
Julius S, Kjeldsen SE, Weber M et al. VALUE Trial Group. Outcomes in hypertensive patients at high cardiovascular risk treated with regimens based on valsartan or amlodipine: the VALUE randomised trial. Lancet 2004; 363:2022–2031
Lithell H, Hansson L, Skoog I et al. The study on cognition and prognosis in the elderly (SCOPE): principal results of a randomised double-blind intervention trial. J Hypertens 2003; 21:875–876
McDonald MA, Simpson SH, Ezekowitz JA et al. Angiotensin receptor blockers and risk of myocardial infarction: systematic review. BMJ 2005; 331:873–876
Teo P, Yusuf S, Anderson C et al. Rationale, design and baseline characteristics of 2 large, simple randomised trials evaluating telmisartan, ramipril and their combination in high-risk patients: ongoing telmisartan alone and in combination with ramipril global endpoint trial/telmisartan randomised assessment study on Ace intolerant subjects with cardiovascular disease (ONTARGET/ TRANSCEND) trials. Am Heart J 2004; 148:52–61
The ONTARGET Investigators. Telmisartan, ramipril, or both in patients at high risk for vascular events. N Engl J Med [published online 31 Mar 2008]
Verma S, Strauss M. Angiotensin receptor blockers and myocardial infarction. BMJ 2005; 329:1248–1249

Chest pain
Pathophysiology of coronary heart disease
Hansonm GK. Inflammation, atherosclerosis and coronary artery disease. N Engl J Med 2005; 352:1685–1695
Keaney PM, Buigent C, Godwin J. Do selective cyclo-oxygenase inhibitors and traditional non-steroidal anti-inflammatory drugs increase the risk of atherosclerosis? Meta-analysis of randomised trials. BMJ 2006; 332:1302–1305

Diagnosis and treatment of chronic stable angina
Bucher HC, Hengstler P, Schindler C et al. Percutaneous transluminal coronary angioplasty versus medical treatment for non-acute coronary heart disease: meta-analysis of randomised controlled trials. BMJ 2000; 321:73–77
O'Toole L, Grech ED. Chronic stable angina: treatment options (ABC of interventional cardiology). BMJ 2003; 326:1185–1188
Tardiff JC, Ford I, Tendera M et al. for the INITIATIVE investigators, Efficacy of ivadrabine, a new selective I_f inhibitor, compared with atenolol in patients with chronic stable angina. Eur Heart J 205; 26:2529–2536
The IONA Study Group. Effect of nicorandil on coronary events in patients with stable angina: The Impact Of Nicorandil in Angina randomised trial. Lancet 2002; 359:1269–1275

Acute coronary syndrome
Fox KA, Poole-Wilson PA, Henderson RA et al. Interventional versus conservative treatment for patients with unstable angina or non-ST-elevation myocardial infarction: the British Heart Foundation RITA 3 randomised trial. Lancet 2002; 360:743–751
Fox KA, Dabbous OH, Goldberg RJ et al. Prediction of risk of death and myocardial infarction in the six months after presentation with acute coronary syndrome: prospective multinational observational study (GRACE): BMJ 2006; 333:1091–1094
Galasko GIW, Baker CSR. Acute cardiovascular emergencies. Clin Med 2007; 7:257–261
Hogg KJ, Docherty A. Acute coronary syndrome. J R Coll Physicians Edinb 2006; 36:132–135
National Institute for Health and Clinical Excellence. Clinical Guideline 48: MI: secondary prevention in primary and secondary care for patients following a myocardial infarction. London: NICE, 2007. Available: www.nice.org.uk/CG48
Peters RJS, Mehta S, Yusuf S. Acute coronary syndromes without ST elevation. BMJ 2007; 334:1265–1269
The Task Force on the management of acute coronary syndromes of the European Society of Cardiology. Management of acute coronary syndromes in patients presenting without persistent ST elevation. Eur Heart J 2002; 23:1809–1840
Van de Werf F, Ardissino D, Betriu A et al. Management of acute myocardial infarction in patients presenting with ST-segment elevation. The Task Force on the Management of Acute Myocardial Infarction of the European Society of Cardiology. Eur Heart J 2003; 24:28–66

Antithrombotic therapy
Bhatt DL, Fox KAA, Hacke W et al., for the CHARISMA investigators. Clopidogrel and aspirin versus aspirin alone for the prevention of atherothrombotic events. N Engl J Med 2006; 354:1706–1717
Chen ZM, Jiang LX, Chen YP et al. COMMIT (clopidogrel and metoprolol in myocardial infarction trial) collaborative group.

Addition of clopidogrel to aspirin in 45,852 patients with acute myocardial infarction: randomised placebo controlled trial. Lancet 2005; 366:1607–1621

Fox KA. Low molecular weight heparin (enoxaparin) in the management of unstable angina: the ESSENCE study. Efficacy and Safety of Subcutaneous Enoxaparin in Non-Q wave Coronary Events. Heart 1999; 82(Suppl. 1):I12–I14

Invasive compared with non-invasive treatment in unstable coronary-artery disease: FRISC II prospective randomised multicentre study. FRagmin and Fast Revascularisation during InStability in Coronary artery disease Investigators. Lancet 1999; 354:708–715

Mehta SR, Yusuf S, Peters RJ et al. Effects of pretreatment with clopidogrel and aspirin followed by long-term therapy in patients undergoing percutaneous coronary intervention: the PCI-CURE study. Lancet 2001; 358:527–533

Natarajan A, Tarique A, Zaman AG. Antiplatlet therapy in acute coronary syndromes. Clin Med 2007; 7:388–391

National Institute for Health and Clinical Excellence. TA080: acute coronary syndromes – clopidogel. London: NICE, 2004. Available: www.nice.org.uk

Sabatine MS, Cannon CP, Gibson CM et al. CLARITY_TIMI 28 Investigators. Addition of clopidogrel to aspirin and fibrinolytic therapy for myocardial infarction with ST elevation. N Engl J Med 2005; 352:1179–1189

Yusuf S, Zhao F, Mehta SR et al. Clopidogrel in Unstable Angina to Prevent Recurrent Events (CURE) Trial Investigators. Effects of clopidogrel in addition to aspirin in patients with acute coronary syndromes without ST-segment elevation. N Engl J Med 2001; 345:494–502

Thrombolysis

Fibrinolytic Therapy Trialists' (FTT) Collaborative Group. Indications for fibrinolytic therapy in suspected acute myocardial infarction: collaborative overview of early mortality and major morbidity results from all randomised trials of more than 1000 patients. Review. Lancet 1994; 343:311–322

ISIS-2 (Second International Study of Infarct Survival) Collaborative Group. Randomised trial of intravenous streptokinase, oral aspirin, both, or neither among 17187 cases of suspected acute myocardial infarction. Lancet 1988; 2:349–360

The GUSTO Angiographic Investigators. The effects of tissue plasminogen activator, streptokinase, or both on coronary-artery patency, ventricular function, and survival after myocardial infarction. N Engl J Med 1993; 329:1615–1622

Percutaneous coronary intervention

Andersen HR, Nielsen TT, Rasmussen K et al, and the DANAMI-2 investigators. A comparison of coronary angioplasty with fibrinolytic therapy in acute myocardial infarction. N Engl J Med 2003; 349:733–742

De Luca G, Suryapranata H, Ottervanger JP et al. Time delay to treatment and mortality in primary angioplasty for acute myocardial infarction: every minute of delay counts. Circulation 2004; 109:1223–1225

Dieker HJ, Brouwer Ma, Verheugt FW. ESC guidelines for percutaneous coronary interventions. Eur Heart J 2005; 26:2475

Fox KA, Poole-Wilson P, Clayton TC et al. 5-year outcome of an interventional strategy in non-ST elevation acute coronary syndrome: the British Heart foundation RITA 3 randomised trial. Lancet 2005; 366:914–920

Hochman JS, Sleeper LA, Webb JG et al., and the SHOCK investigators. Early revascularization in acute myocardial infarction complicated by cardiogenic shock. N Engl J Med 1999; 341:625–634

Lipid-lowering therapy

Cannon CP, Braunwald E, McCabe CH et al. Intensive versus moderate lipid lowering with statins after acute coronary syndromes. N Engl J Med 2004; 350:1495–1504

The Scandinavian Simvastatin Survival Study Group. Randomised trial of cholesterol lowering in 4444 people with coronary heart disease: the Scandinavian simvastatin survival study (4S). Lancet 1994; 344:1383–1389

Sacks FM, Pfeffer MA, Moye LA et al. Cholesterol and Recurrent Events (CARE) Trial investigators. N Engl J Med 1996; 335:1001–1009

Other

Freemantle N, Cleland J, Young P et al. Beta blockade after myocardial infarction: systematic review and meta regression analysis. BMJ 1999; 318:1730–1737

Malmberg K, Ryden L, Efendic S et al. Randomized trial of insulin-glucose infusion followed by subcutaneous insulin treatment diabetic patients with acute myocardial infarction (DIGAMI study): effects on mortality at 1 year. J Am Coll Cardiol 1996; 26:57–65

Wang K, Asinger RW, Marriot HJL. ST-segment elevation in conditions other than acute myocardial infarction. N Engl J Med 2003; 349:2128–2135

Heart failure

National Institute for Clinical Excellence. Chronic Heart Failure. Management of chronic heart failure in adults in primary and secondary care. NICE guideline July 2003. Available: www.nice.org.uk

National Institute for Health and Clinical Excellence. Clinical Guideline: Heart failure: Cardiac resynchronisation. London: NICE, 2007. Available: www.nice.org.uk

Padfield GJ, McMuray JJV. Current treatment of heart failure. J R Coll Physicians Edinb 2006; 36:141–146

Remme WJ, Swedberg K. Task Force for the Diagnosis and Treatment of Chronic Heart Failure. Guidelines for the diagnosis and treatment of chronic heart failure. Eur Heart J 2001; 22:1527–1560

Angiotensin-converting enzyme inhibitors (symptomatic LVSD)

Cohn JN, Johnson G, Ziesche S et al. A comparison of enalapril with hydralazine-isosorbide dinitrate in the treatment of chronic congestive heart failure. N Engl J Med 1991; 325:303–310 (VHeFT II)

Cohn JN, Archibald DG, Zeische S et al. Effect of vasodilator therapy on mortality in chronic congestive heart failure. N Engl J Med 1986; 314:1547–1552 (VHeFT)

The CONSENSUS Trial Study Group. Effects of enalapril on mortality in severe congestive heart failure. Results of the Cooperative North Scandinavian Enalapril Survival Study (CONSENSUS). N Engl J Med 1987; 316:1429–1435

Angiotensin-converting enzyme inhibitors (asymptomatic reduced LVEF)

The SOLVD Investigators. Effect of enalapril on survival in patients with reduced left ventricular ejection fractions and congestive heart failure. N Engl J Med 1991; 325:293–302

Angiotensin-converting enzyme inhibitors (LVSD post myocardial infarction)

The AIRE Study Investigators. Effect of ramipril on mortality and morbidity of survivors of acute myocardial infarction with clinical evidence of heart failure. The Acute Infarction Ramipril Efficacy (AIRE) Study Investigators. Lancet 1993; 342:821–828

Flather MD, Yusuf S, Kober L et al. Long-term ACE inhibitor therapy in patients with heart failure or left ventricular dysfunction: systematic overview of data from individual patients. Lancet 2000; 355:1575–1581

Hall AS, Murray GD, Ball SG. Follow up study of patients randomly allocated ramipril or placebo for heart failure after acute myocardial infarction: AIRE Extension (AIREX) Study. Lancet 1997; 349:1493–1497

Kober L, Torp-Pederson C, Carlsen JE et al. A clinical trial of the angiotensin converting enzyme inhibitor trandalopril in patients with left ventricular dysfunction after myocardial infarction (TRACE). N Engl J Med 1995; 333:1670–1676

Pfeffer MA, Braunwald E, Moye LA et al. Effect of captopril on mortality and morbidity in patients with left ventricular dysfunction after myocardial infarction. Results of the survival and ventricular enlargement trial (SAVE). The SAVE Investigators. N Engl J Med 1992; 327:669–677

Angiotensin receptor blockers

Granger CB, McMurray JJ, Yusuf S et al. CHARM Investigators and Committees. Effects of candesartan in patients with chronic heart failure and reduced left ventricular systolic function intolerant to angiotensin converting enzyme inhibitors: the CHARM Alternative Trial. Lancet 2003; 362:772–776

McMurray JJ, Ostergren J, Swedberg K et al. Effects of candesartan in patients with chronic heart failure and reduced left ventricular systolic function taking angiotensin converting enzyme inhibitors: the CHARM Added Trial. Lancet 2003; 362:767–771

Pfeffer MA, Swedberg K, Granger CB et al. Effects of candesartan on mortality and morbidity in patients with chronic heart failure: the CHARM Overall programme. Lancet 2003; 362:759–766

Pitt B, Poole-Wilson P, Segal R et al. Effect of losartan compared with captopril on mortality in patients with symptomatic heart failure: randomised trial – the Losartan Heart Failure Survival Study ELITE II. Lancet 2000; 355:1582–1587

Yusuf S, Pfeffer MA, Swedberg K et al. CHARM Investigators and Committees. Effects of candesartan in patients with chronic heart failure and preserved left ventricular ejection fraction; the CHARM Preserved Trial. Lancet 2003; 362:777–781

Aldosterone antagonists

Pitt B, Remme W, Zannad F et al. Eplerenone, a selective aldosterone blocker, in patients with left ventricular dysfunction after myocardial infarction. N Engl J Med 2003; 348:1309–1321

Pitt B, Zannad F, Remme WJ et al. for the Randomised Aldactone Evaluation Study (RALES) Investigators. The effect of spironolactone on morbidity and mortality in patients with severe heart failure. N Engl J Med 1999; 341:709–717

Beta blockers

Dargie HJ. Effect of carvedilol on outcome after myocardial infarction in patients with left ventricular dysfunction: the CAPRICORN randomised trial. Lancet 2001; 357:1385–1390

Poole-Wilson PA, Swedberg K, Cleland JG et al. Comparison of carvedilol and metoprolol on clinical outcomes in patients with chronic heart failure in the Carvedilol Or Metoprolol European Trial (COMET): randomised controlled trial. Lancet 2003; 362:7–13

Other

Massie BM, Krol WF, Ammon SE et al. The Warfarin and Antiplatelet Therapy in Heart Failure trial (WATCH): rationale, design, and baseline patient characteristics. J Card Fail 2004; 10:101–112

Palpitations

Hohnloser SH, Kucj KH, Dorian P. Prophylactic use of an implantable cardioverter–defibrillator after acute myocardial infarction. N Engl J Med 2004; 351:2481–2488

Jennings K. Sudden cardiac death. J R Coll Physicians Edinb 2006; 36:117–119

McComb JM, Camm AJ. Primary prevention of sudden cardiac death using implantable cardioverter defibrillators. BMJ 2002; 325:1050–1051

Priori SG, Aliot E, Blomstrom-Lundqvist C et al. Task force on sudden cardiac death of the European Society of Cardiology. Eur Heart J 2001; 22:1374–1450

Atrial fibrillation

Albers GW, Diener HC, Frison L et al. SPORTIF Executive Steering Committee for SPORTIF V Investigators. Ximelagatran versus warfarin for stroke prevention in patients with non-valvular atrial fibrillation: a randomised trial. JAMA 2005; 293:690–698

Alboni P, Botto GL, Baldi N et al. Outpatient treatment of recent onset atrial fibrillation with the 'pill-in-pocket' approach. N Engl J Med 2004; 351:2348–2391

American College of Cardiology, American Heart Association, European Society of Cardiology. ACC/AHA/ESC 2006 guidelines for the management of patients with atrial fibrillation. Europace 2006; 8:651–745

Connolly S, Pogue J, Hart R et al., and the ACTIVE writing group on behalf of the ACTIVE investigators. Clopidogrel plus aspirin versus oral anticoagulation for atrial fibrillation in the Atrial fibrillation Clopidogrel Trial with Irbesartan for prevention of Vascular Events (ACTIVE): a randomised controlled trial. Lancet 2006; 367:1903–1912

Lip GYH, Boos C. Antithrombotic therapy in non-valvular atrial fibrillation. Heart 2006; 92:155–161

National Institute for Health and Clinical Excellence (NICE). Atrial fibrillation. NICE June 2006. Available: www.nice.org.uk

Savelieva I, Camm J. Atrial fibrillation – all change! Clin Med 2007; 7:374–379

Taylor FC, Cohn H, Ebrahim S. Systematic review of long term anticoagulation or antiplatelet treatment in patients with non-rheumatic atrial fibrillation. BMJ 2001; 322:321–326

Watson T, Shanistila E, Lip GYH. Modern management of atrial fibrillation. Clin Med 2007; 7:28–34

Wyse DG, Waldo AL, DiMarco JP et al. The Atrial Fibrillation Follow-up Investigation of Rhythm Management (AFFIRM) Investigators. A comparison of rate control and rhythm control in patients with atrial fibrillation. N Engl J Med 2002; 347:1825–1833

Dyslipidaemia

ALLHAT Officers and Coordinators for the ALLHAT Collaborative Research Group. The antihypertensives and lipid-lowering treatment to prevent heart attack trial. Major outcomes in moderately hypercholesterolaemic, hypertensive people randomised to pravastatin vs. usual care: the antihypertensives and lipid-lowering treatment to prevent heart attack trial (ALLHAT-LLT). JAMA 2002; 288:2998–3007

Athyros V, Papageorgiou A, Bodosakis M et al. Treatment with atorvastatin to the National Cholesterol Education Programme goal versus 'usual' care in secondary coronary heart disease prevention. The Greek atorvastatin and coronary heart disease evaluation (GREACE) study. Cur Med Res Opinion 2002; 18:220–228

Bucher HC, Griffith LE, Guyatt GH. Effect of HMGc0-A reductase inhibitors on stroke. A meta-analysis of randomised controlled trials. Ann Intern Med 1998; 128:89–95

Cannon CP, Braunwald E, McCabe CH et al. for the Pravastatin or Atorvastatin Evaluation and Infection Therapy–Thrombolysis in Myocardial Infarction 22 Investigators. Intensive versus moderate lipid lowering with statins after acute coronary syndromes (PROVEIT). N Engl J Med 2004; 350:494–504

Cholesterol Treatment Trialists' Collaboration. Efficacy and safety of cholesterol lowering treatment: prospective meta-analysis to date from 90,056 participants in 14 randomised trials of statins. Lancet 2005; 366:1267–1278

Colhoun HM, Betteridge DJ, Durrington P et al. on behalf of the CARDS investigators. Primary prevention of cardiovascular disease in type 2 diabetes in the Collaborative Atorvastatin Diabetes Study (CARDS); multicentre randomised placebo controlled trial. Lancet 2004; 364:685–696

De Lemos JA, Blazing Ma, Wiviott SD et al. for the A to Z Investigators. Early intensive vs a delayed conservative simvastatin strategy in people with acute coronary syndromes: phase Z of the A to Z trial. JAMA 2004; 292:1307–1316

Downs JR, Clearfield M, Weiss et al. Primary prevention of acute coronary events with lovastatin in men and women with average cholesterol levels: results of AFCAPS/TexCAPS. Airforce/Texas coronary atherosclerosis prevention study. JAMA 1998; 279:1615–1622

Durrington P. Dyslipidaemia. Lancet 2003; 362:717–731

Heart Protection Study Collaborative Group. MRC/BHF Heart Protection Study of cholesterol lowering with simvastatin in 20536 high-risk individuals: a randomised placebo controlled trial. Lancet 2002; 360:7–22

Heart Protection Study Collaborative Group. MRC/BHF Heart Protection Study of cholesterol lowering with simvastatin in 5,963 people with diabetes: a randomised placebo controlled trial. Lancet 2003; 361:1149–1158

Holdaas H, Fellstrom B, Holme I et al. for the ALERT Study Group. Assessment of Lescol in renal transplantation. Effects of fluvastatin in cardiac events in renal transplant people: ALERT (assessment of Lescol in renal transplantation) study design and baseline data. J Cardiovasc Risk 2000; 8:63–71

Joint British Societies' guidelines on prevention of cardiovascular disease in clinical practice. Heart 2005; vol. 91 suppl. V

La Rosa JC, Grundy SM, Waters DD et al. for the Treating to New Targets (TNT) Investigators. Intensive lipid lowering with atorvastatin in patients with stable coronary disease. N Engl J Med 2005; 352:1–11

La Rosa JC, He J, Vupputuri S et al. Effect of statins on risk of coronary disease: a meta-analysis of controlled trials. JAMA 1999; 82:2340–2346

Law MR, Wald, NJ, Rudnicka AR. Quantifying effect of statins on low density lipoprotein cholesterol, ischaemic heart disease and stroke: systematic review and meta-analysis. BMJ 2003; 326:1423–1429

Lee CH, de Feyter P, Serruys PW et al. Beneficial effects of fluvastatin following percutaneous coronary intervention in people with unstable and stable angina: results from the Lescol intervention prevention study (LIPS). Heart 2004; 90:1156–1161

Lewis SJ, Maye LA, Sacks FM et al. Effect of pravastatin on cardiovascular events in older people with myocardial infarction and cholesterol levels in the average range. Results of the cholesterol and recurrent events (CARE) trial. Ann Intern Med 1998; 129:681–689

Pederson TR, Faergeman O, Kastelein JJP et al. High dose atorvastatin vs usual dose simvastatin for secondary prevention after myocardial infarction. The IDEAL study: a randomised controlled trial. JAMA 2005; 294:2437–2445

Sever PS, Dahlof D, Poulter NR et al. Prevention of coronary and stroke events with atorvastatin in hypertensive people who have average or lower than average cholesterol concentrations, in the Anglo-Scandinavian cardiac outcomes trial – lipid lowering arm (ASCOT-LLA): a multicentre randomised controlled trial. Lancet 2003; 361:1149–1158

Shepherd J, Blauw GJ, Murphy M et al. Pravastatin in elderly individuals at risk of vascular disease (Prospective Study of Pravastatin in Elderly at Risk PROSPER): a randomised controlled trial. Lancet 2002; 360:1623–1630

Shepherd J, Cobbe SM, Ford I et al. Prevention of coronary heart disease with pravastatin in men with hypercholesterolaemia. West of Scotland Coronary Prevention Study group (WOSCOPS). N Engl J Med 1995; 333:1301–1307

The FIELD Study Investigators. Effects of long-term fenofibrate therapy on cardiovascular events in 9795 people with type 2 diabetes mellitus (the FIELD study): randomised controlled trial. Lancet 2005; 366:1849–1861

The Long-term Intervention with Pravastatin in Ischaemic Disease (LIPID) Study Group. Prevention of cardiovascular events and death with pravastatin in patients with coronary heart disease and a broad range of initial cholesterol levels. N Engl J Med 1998; 339:1349–1357

The Scandinavian Simvastatin Survival Study Group. Randomised trial of cholesterol lowering in 4444 people with coronary heart disease: the Scandinavian simvastatin survival study (4S). Lancet 1994; 344:1383–1389

Thompson GR. Is good cholesterol always good? BMJ 2004; 329:471–472

Waner C, Krane V, Winfried M et al. Atorvastatin in patients with type 2 diabetes undergoing haemodialysis. N Engl J Med 2005; 353:238–248

Waters DD, Guyton JR, Herrington DM et al. Treating to new targets (TNT) study: does lowering low density lipoprotein cholesterol levels below currently recommended guidelines yield incremental clinical benefit? Am J Cardiol 2004; 93:154–158

Hypertension

ALLHAT Collaborative Research Group. Major outcomes in high-risk hypertensive patients randomised to angiotensin converting enzyme inhibitor or calcium channel blocker versus diuretic. JAMA 2002; 2888:2981–2997

Blood Pressure Lowering Treatment Trialists' collaboration. Effects of different blood pressure lowering regimens on major cardiovascular events: results of prospectively designed overviews of randomised trials. Lancet 2003; 362:1527–1545

Brown MJ, Cruickshank JK, Dominiczak AF et al. Executive Committee, British Hypertension Society. Better blood pressure control: how to combine drugs. J Human Hypertens 2003; 17:81–86

Dahlof B, Devfereux RB, Kjeldsen SE et al. LIFE Study Group. Cardiovascular morbidity and mortality in the Losartan Intervention For Endpoint reduction in hypertension study (LIFE): A randomised trial against atenolol. Lancet 2002; 359:995–1003 (a subgroup of the LIFE study in patients with diabetes: 1004–1010)

Dahlof B, Sever PS, Poulter NR et al. ASCOT investigators. Prevention of cardiovascular events with an antihypertensive regimen of amlodipine adding perindopril as required versus atenolol adding bendroflumethazide as required, in the Anglo-Scandinavian Cardiac Outcomes Trial-Blood Pressure Lowering Arm (ASCOT-BPLA): a multicentre randomised controlled trial. Lancet 2005; 366:895–906

Goh KP, Subramaniam T. An update on biochemical evaluation, imaging and treatment of phaeocromocytoma. J R Coll Physicians Edinb 2006; 35:206–213

Hansson L, Zanchetti A, Carruthers SG et al. for the HOT Study Group. Effects of intensive blood pressure lowering and low-dose aspirin in patients with hypertension: principal results of the hypertension optimal treatment (HOT) randomised trial. Lancet 1998; 351:1755–1762

National Institute for Health and Clinical Excellence. Clinical Guideline 18 – management of hypertension in adults in primary care. London: NICE; 2004

Nisen SE, Tuzcu EM, Libby P et al. Effect of antihypertensive agents on cardiovascular events in patients with coronary disease and normal blood pressure. The CAMELOT Study: a randomised controlled trial. JAMA 2004; 292:2217–2226

PROGRESS Collaborative Group. Randomised trial of a perindopril based blood pressure lowering regimen among 6105 individuals with previous stroke or transient ischaemic attack. Lancet 2001; 358:1033–1041

Sacks FM, Svetky LP, Vollmer WM et al. DASH-sodium Collaborative Research Group. Effects on blood pressure of reduced dietary sodium and the dietary approaches to stop hypertension (DASH) diet. N Engl J Med 2001; 344:3–10

Sever PS, Dahlof B, Poulter NR et al. ASCOT investigators. Prevention of coronary and stroke events with atorvastatin in hypertensive patients who have average or lower than average cholesterol concentrations, in the Anglo Scandinavian Cardiac Outcomes Trial-Lipid Lowering Arm (ASCOT-LLA): a multicentre randomised controlled trial. Lancet 2003; 361:1149–1158

The Heart Outcomes Prevention Evaluation Study Investigators. Effects of an angiotensin converting enzyme inhibitor, ramipril, on cardiovascular events in high risk patients. New Engl J Med 2000; 342:145–153

Williams B, Poulter NR, Brown MJ et al. British Hypertension Society guidelines for hypertension management 2004 (BHS-IV): summary. BMJ 2004; 328:634–640

Williams B, Poulter NR, Brown MJ et al. Guidelines for management of hypertension: report of the fourth working party of the British Hypertension Society, 2004 – BHS-IV. J Human Hypertens 2004; 18:139–185

Neurological problems

Headache

van de Beek D, de Gans J, McIntyre P et al. Steroids in adults with acute bacterial meningitis: a systematic review. Lancet Infect Dis 2004; 4:139–143

van de Beek D, de Gans J, Tunkel AR et al. Community-acquired bacterial meningitis in adults. Review. N Engl J Med 2006; 354:44–53

Davenport R. Diagnosing acute headache. Clin Med 2004; 4:108–112

De Gans J, van de Beek D. European Dexamethasone in Adulthood Bacterial Meningitis Study Investigators. Dexamethasone in adults with bacterial meningitis. N Eng J Med 2002; 347:1549–1556

Fuller G, Kaye C. Headache. BMJ 2007; 334:254–256

Goadsby PJ. Recent advances in the diagnosis and management of migraine. BMJ 2006; 332:25–29

Headache Classification Committee of the International Headache Society. The international classification of headache disorders (second edition). Cephalgia 2004; 24(suppl. 1):1–160

Linn FH, Rinkel GJ, Algra A et al. Headache characteristics in subarachnoid haemorrhage and benign thunderclap headache. J Neurol Neurosurg Psychiatry 1998; 65:791–793

Peatfield R. A revised classification of headache disorders. BMJ 2004; 328:119–120

Raza MM, Heyderman RS. Acute fever and headache – is it meningitis? Royal College of Physicians of Edinburgh 2006

Tomlinson SE, Hanna MG. Acute neurology. Clin Med 2007; 7:272–277

Transient ischaemic attack

Diener HC, Bogousslavsky J, Brass LM. Aspirin and clopidogrel compared with clopidogrel alone after recent ischaemic stroke or transient ischaemic attack in high-risk patients (MATCH): randomised, double blind, placebo-controlled trial. Lancet 2004; 364:331–337

Hill MD, Yiannakoulias N, Jeerakathil T et al. The high risk of stroke immediately after transient ischaemic attack: a population-based study. Neurology 2004; 62:2015–2120

Johnston SC, Rothwell PM, Nguyen-Huynh MN et al. Validation and refinement of scores to predict very early stroke risk after transient ischaemic attack. Lancet 2007; 369:283–292

Knight R. The Poohsticks phenomenon. BMJ 2004; 329:1432–1434

Rothwell PM. Atherothrombosis and ischaemic stroke: unstable plaque is the main mechanism of stroke in patients with carotid stenosis. BMJ 2007; 334:379–380

The ESPRIT Study Group. Aspirin plus dipyridamole versus aspirin alone after cerebral ischaemia of arterial origin (ESPRIT): randomised controlled trial. Lancet 2006; 367:1665–1673

Weakness and wasting

Gutowski N. Neurological problems in cancer. Clin Med 2007; 7:159–164

Multiple sclerosis

McDonald WI, Compston A, Edan G et al. Recommended diagnostic criteria for multiple sclerosis: guidelines from the international panel on the diagnosis of multiple sclerosis. Ann Neurol 2001; 50:121–127

Murray TJ. Diagnosis and treatment of multiple sclerosis. BMJ 2006; 332:525–527

Multiple sclerosis. National clinical guideline for diagnosis and management in primary and secondary care. www.rcplonodn.ac.uk/pubs/books/ms/

Whiting P, Harbord R, Main C et al. Accuracy of magnetic resonance imaging for the diagnosis of multiple sclerosis: systematic review. BMJ 2006; 332:875–878

Tremor

Medcalfe P, Bhatia KP. Restless legs syndrome. BMJ 2006; 333:457–458

www.rls.org

Locomotor problems

Back pain and osteoporosis

Beral V, Banks E, Reeves G. Evidence from randomised trials on the long-term effects of hormone replacement therapy. Lancet 2002; 360:942–944

Black DM, Cummings SR, Karpf DB et al. Randomised trial of the effects of alendronate on risk of fracture in women with existing vertebral fracture. Fracture Intervention Trial Research Group. Lancet 1996; 348:1535–1541

Chapuy MC, Arlot ME, DuBoeuf F et al. Vitamin D3 and calcium to prevent hip fractures in elderly women. N Eng J Med 1992; 327:1637–1642

Compston JE, Rosen CJ. Osteoporosis, 4th edition. Oxford: Health Press; 2004

Ettinger B, Black DM, Mitlak BH et al. Reduction of vertebral risk in postmenopausal women with osteoporosis treated with raloxifene: results from a 3-year randomised clinical trial. Multiple Outcomes of Raloxifene Evaluation (MORE) Investigators. JAMA 1999; 282:637–645

Harris ST, Watts NB, Genant HK et al. Effects of risedronate treatment on vertebral and non-vertebral fractures in women with postmenopausal osteoporosis: a randomised controlled trial. Vertebral Efficacy with Risedronate Therapy (VERT) Study Group. JAMA 1999; 282:1344–1352

McClung MR, Geusens P, Miller PD et al. Effect of risedronate on the risk of hip fracture in elderly women. N Eng J Med 2001; 344:333–340

Meunier PJ, Roux C, Seeman E at al. The effects of strontium ranelate on the risk of vertebral fracture in women with postmenopausal osteoporosis. N Eng J Med 2004; 350:459–468

Meunier PJ, Slosman DO, Delmas PD et al. Strontium ranelate: dose-dependent effects in established postmenopausal vertebral osteoporosis – a 3 year randomised placebo controlled trial. J Clin Endocr Metab 2002; 87:2060–2066

Neer RM, Arnaud CD, Zanchetta JR et al. Effect of parathyroid hormone (1–34 on fractures and bone mineral density in postmenopausal women with osteoporosis. N Eng J Med 2001; 344:1434–1441

National Institute for Health and Clinical Excellence. Clinical Guideline: Primary and Secondary Prevention of Osteoporosis in Postmenopausal Women. NICE guideline, August 2007. Available: www.nice.org.uk

Poole KES, Compston JE. Osteoporosis and its management. BMJ 2006; 333:1251–1256

Reginster J-Y, Mine HW, Sorensen OH et al. Effect of risedronate on the risk of hip fracture in women with established osteoporosis. Vertebral Efficacy with Risedronate Therapy (VERT) Study Group. Osteoporosis Int 2000; 11:83–91

Royal College of Physicians and the Bone and Tooth Society. Osteoporosis: clinical guidelines for prevention and treatment. London: Royal College of Physicians; 2000

Zanchetta JR, Bogado CE, Ferreti JL et al. Effects of teriparatide (recombinant human parathyroid hormone 1–34) on cortical bone in postmenopausal women with osteoporosis. J Bone Miner Res 2003; 18:539–543

Endocrine problems

Type 1 diabetes

Atkinson MA, Eisenbarth GS. Type 1 diabetes: new perspectives in disease pathogenesis and treatment. Lancet 2001; 358:221–229

DCCT Research Group. The effect of intensive treatment of diabetes on the development and progression of long-term complications in insulin dependent diabetes mellitus. N Engl J Med 1993; 329:977–986

DCCT Research Group. Effect of intensive therapy on the development and progression of nephropathy in the DCCT. Kidney Int 1995; 47:1703–1720

DPT-1 Study Group. Effects of insulin in relatives of patients with type 1 diabetes. N Engl J Med 2002; 346:1685–1691

European Nicotinamide Diabetes Intervention Trial (ENDIT) Group. European Nicotinamide Diabetes Intervention Trial (ENDIT): randomised controlled trial of intervention before onset of type 1 diabetes. Lancet 2004; 363:925–931

MacLeod KM. Hypoglycaemia in diabetes. Clin Med 2004; 4:307–310

Wilkin TJ. The accelerator hypothesis: weight gain the missing link between type I and type II diabetes. Diabetologia 2001; 44:914–922

Type 2 diabetes

Pathophysiology

Fajans SS, Bell GI, Polonsky KS. Molecular mechanisms and clinical pathophysiology of maturity onset diabetes of the young. N Engl J Med 2001; 345:971–980

Polonsky KS, Sturis J, Bell GI. Non-insulin dependent diabetes mellitus – a genetically programmed failure of the beta cell to compensate for insulin resistance. N Eng J Med 1996; 334:777–783

General management

Bhattacharya A, Dornan T. Diabetes in hospital. Clin Med 2004; 4:314–317

Department of Health. National Service Framework Diabetes. Online. Available: www.doh.gov.uk/nsf/diabetes

Joint British Societies' guidelines on prevention of cardiovascular disease in clinical practice. Heart 2005; vol. 91 suppl. V

Diabetes and cardiovascular disease risk

Haffner SM, Lehto S, Ronnemaa T et al. Mortality from coronary heart disease in subjects with type 2 diabetes and in non-diabetic subjects with and without prior myocardial infarction. N Engl J Med 1998; 339:229–234

Harvey JN. Preventing cardiovascular disease in diabetes. Clin Med 2004; 4:311–314

Marshall SM, Flyvbjerg A. Prevention and early detection of vascular complications of diabetes. BMJ 2006; 333:475–480

Glycaemic control

Page S. Glycaemic management of type 2 diabetes. Clin Med 2004; 4:302–306

Dormandy JA, Charbonnel B, Eckland DJA et al. Secondary prevention of macrovascular events in patients with type 2 diabetes in the PROactive study (prospective pioglitazone clinical trial in macrovascular events): a randomised controlled trial. Lancet 2005; 366:1279–1289

Malmberg K. Prospective randomised study of intensive insulin treatment on long-term survival after acute myocardial infarction in patients with diabetes mellitus. DIGAMI (Diabetes Mellitus, Insulin Glucose Infusion in Acute Myocardial Infarction) Study Group. BMJ 1997; 314:1512–1515

Malmberg K, Ryden L, Wedel H et al. Intense metabolic control by means of insulin in patients with diabetes and myocardial infarction (DIGAMI 2): effects on mortality and morbidity. Eur Heart J 2005; 26:650–661

Stratton IM, Adler AI, Neil HA et al. Association of glycaemia with macrovascular and microvascular complications of type 2 diabetes (UKPDS 35): prospective observational study. BMJ 2000; 321:405–412

UKPDS Group. Intensive blood glucose control with sulphonylureas or insulin compared with conventional treatment and risk of complications in patients with Type 2 diabetes (UKPDS 33). Lancet 1998; 352:837–853

UKPDS Group. Effect of intensive blood glucose control with metformin on complications in overweight patients with Type 2 diabetes (UKPDS 34). Lancet 1998; 352:854–865

Diabetes and blood pressure

ALLHAT Officers and Coordinators for the ALLHAT Collaborative Research Group. Major outcomes in high-risk hypertensive patients randomised to angiotensin-converting enzyme inhibitor or calcium channel blocker vs diuretic. The antihypertensive and lipid-lowering treatment to prevent heart attack trial (ALLHAT). JAMA 2002; 288:2981–2997

Dahlof B, Severs PS, Poulter NR et al. for the ASCOT Investigators. Prevention of cardiovascular events with an antihypertensive regimen of amlodipine adding perindopril as required versus atenolol adding bendroflumethazide as required, in the Anglo-Scandinavian Cardiac Outcomes Trial-Blood Pressure Lowering Arm (ASCOT-BPLA): a multicentre randomised controlled trial. Lancet 2005; 366:895–906

Hansson L, Zanchetti A, Carruthers SG et al. for the HOT Study Group. Effects of intensive blood pressure lowering and low-dose aspirin in patients with hypertension: principal results of the hypertension optimal treatment (HOT) randomised trial. Lancet 1998; 351:1755–1762

Heart Outcomes Prevention Evaluation (HOPE) Study Investigators. Effects of ramipril on cardiovascular and microvascular outcomes in people with diabetes mellitus: results of the HOPE study and micro-HOPE sub-study. Lancet 2000; 355:253–259

Lindholm LH, Ibsen H, Dahlof B et al. Cardiovascular morbidity and mortality in patients with diabetes in the Losartan Intervention For endpoint reduction in hypertension study (LIFE): a randomised trial against atenolol. Lancet 2002; 359:1004–1010

UKPDS Group. Efficacy of atenolol and captopril in reducing risk of macrovascular and microvascular complications in type 2 diabetes (UKPDS 39). BMJ 1998; 317:713–720

UKPDS Group. Tight blood pressure control and risk of macrovascular and microvascular complications in type 2 diabetes (UKPDS 38). BMJ 1998; 317:703–713

Diabetes and lipids

Colhoun HM, Betteridge DJ, Durrington P et al. on behalf of the CARDS investigators. Primary prevention of cardiovascular disease in type 2 diabetes in the Collaborative Atorvastatin Diabetes Study (CARDS); multicentre randomised placebo controlled trial. Lancet 2004; 364:685–696

Costa J, Borges M, David C et al. Efficacy of lipid lowering drug treatment for diabetic and non-diabetic patients: meta-analysis of randomised controlled trials. BMJ 2006; 332:1115–1118

Heart Protection Study Collaborative Group. MRC/BHF Heart Protection Study of cholesterol lowering with simvastatin in 20536 high-risk individuals: a randomised placebo controlled trial. Lancet 2002; 360:7–22

Heart Protection Study Collaborative Group. MRC/BHF Heart Protection Study of cholesterol lowering with simvastatin in 5,963 people with diabetes: a randomised placebo controlled trial. Lancet 2003; 361:1149–1158

Lewis SJ, Maye LA, Sacks FM et al. Effect of pravastatin on cardiovascular events in older people with myocardial infarction and cholesterol levels in the average range. Results of the cholesterol and recurrent events (CARE) trial. Ann Intern Med 1998; 129:681–689

Sever PS, Dahlof D, Poulter NR et al. Prevention of coronary and stroke events with atorvastatin in hypertensive people who have average or lower than average cholesterol concentrations, in the Anglo-Scandinavian cardiac outcomes trial – lipid lowering arm (ASCOT-LLA): a multicentre randomised controlled trial. Lancet 2003; 361:1149–1158

Diabetic nephropathy

Brenner BM, Cooper ME, Zeeuw D et al. for the RENAAL Study Investigators. Effects of losartan on renal and cardiovascular outcomes in patients with type 2 diabetes and nephropathy. N Engl J Med 2001; 345:861–869

Lewis E, Hunsicker L, Bain R et al. The effect of angiotensin converting inhibition on diabetic nephropathy. N Engl J Med 1993; 329:1456–1462

Lewis EJ, Hunsicker LG, Clarke WR et al. for the Collaborative Study Group. Renoprotective effect of the angiotensin-receptor antagonist irbesartan in patients with nephropathy due to type 2 diabetes. N Engl J Med 2001; 345:851–860

Mogensen CE, Neldam I, Tikkanen I et al. Randomised controlled trial of dual blockade renin–angiotensin system in patients with hypertension, microalbuminuria and non-insulin dependent diabetes: the candesartan and lisinopril microalbuminuria (CALM) study. BMJ 2000; 321:1440–1444

Parving H-H, Lehnert H, Brochner-Mortensen J et al. for the Irbesartan in Patients with Type 2 Diabetes and Microalbuminuria Study Group. The effect of irbesartan on the development of diabetic nephropathy in patients with type 2 diabetes. N Engl J Med 2001; 345:870–878

Renal and metabolic problems

Acute renal failure

Australian and New Zealand Intensive Care Society (ANZICS) Clinical Trials Group. Low dose dopamine in patients with early renal dysfunction: A placebo-controlled randomised trial. Lancet 2000; 356:1239–1245

Genarri FJ. Hypokalaemia. N Engl J Med 1998; 339:451–458

Hilton R. Acute renal failure. BMJ 2006; 333:786–790

Chronic kidney disease

Coresh J, Astor BC, Greene T et al. Prevalence of chronic kidney disease and decreased kidney function in an adult US population: Third National Health and Nutrition Examination Survey. Am J Kidney Dis 2003; 41:1–12

GISEN Group. Randomised placebo-controlled trial of effect of ramipril on decline in glomerular filtration rate and risk terminal renal failure in proteinuric non-diabetic nephropathy. Lancet 1997; 349:1857–1863

GISEN Group. Renoprotective properties of ACE-inhibition in non-diabetic nephropathies with non-nephrotic proteinuria. Lancet 1999; 354:359–364

GISEN Group. ACE inhibitors to prevent end stage renal disease: When to start and why possibly to never stop: a post hoc analysis of the REIN trial results. J Am Soc Nephrol 2001; 12:2832–2837

Holdaas H, Fellstrom B, Jardine AG et al. Assessment of Lescol in Renal Transplantaton (ALERT) Study Investigators. Effect of fluvastatin on cardiac outcomes in renal transplant recipients: a multicentre, randomised, placebo-controlled trial. Lancet 2003; 361:2024–2031

Jafar TH, Schmid CH, Landa M et al. Angiotensin converting enzyme inhibitors and progression of non-diabetic renal disease. Ann Intern Med 2001; 135:73–87

Johnson S, Hewlins P. What's new in renal medicine. Medicine 2004; 32(Suppl. 10):1–4

Levey AS, Coresh J, Balk E et al. National Kidney Foundation practice guidelines for chronic kidney disease: evaluation, classification and stratification. Ann Intern Med 2003; 139:137–147

Murtagh et al. Dialysis or not? A comparative survival study of patients over 75 years with chronic kidney disease. *Nephrol Dial Transplant* 2007

Nakao N, Yoshimura A, Morita H et al. Combination treatment of angiotensin II receptor blocker and angiotensin converting enzyme inhibitor in non-diabetic renal disease (COOPERATE): a randomised controlled study. Lancet 2003; 361:117–124

National Institute for Health and Clinical Excellence Clinical Guideline 39. Anaemia management in people with chronic kidney disease. NICE; 2006

Pastan S, Soucie JM, McClellan WM. Vascular access and increased risk of death among haemodialysis patients. Kidney Int 2002; 62:620–626

Glomerulonephritis

Chadban SJ, Atkins RC. Glomerulonephritis. Lancet 2005; 365:1797–1806

Systemic vasculitis

Gaskin G et al. Adjunctive plasma exchange is superior to methylprednisolone in acute renal failure due to ANCA-associated glomerulonephritis (MEPEX). *J Am Soc Nephrol* 2002; 13:2A

Jayne D et al. Randomised trial of cyclophosphamide versus azathioprine during remission in ANCA associated vasculitis (CYCAZAREM). *J Am Soc Nephrol* 1999; 10:105A

Jennette JC, Falk RJ, Andrassy K et al. Nomenclature of systemic vasculitides: The Proposal of an International Consensus Conference. *Arthritis Rheum* 1994; 37:187–192

Kluth DC, Hughes J. ANCA-associated systemic vasculitis. J R Coll Phys Ed 2007; 37:128–134

Hyponatraemia

Adrogue H J, Madias NE. Hypernatraemia. N Engl J Med 2000; 342:1493–1499

Adrogue HJ, Madias NE. Hyponatraemia. N Engl J Med 2000; 342:1581–1589

Moore K, Thompson C, Trainer P. Disorders of water balance. Clin Med 2003; 3:28–33

Reynolds RM, Padfield PL, Seckl JR. Disorders of sodium balance. BMJ 2006; 332:702–705

Unwin R, Capasso G. Common fluid and electrolyte disorders. Medicine 2003; 5:11–17

Poisoning and metabolic disturbance

Adrogue J, Madias NE. Management of life-threatening acid-base disorders. First of Two Parts. N Engl J Med 1998; 338:26–34

Adrogue HJ, Madias NE. Management of life-threatening acid-base disorders. Second of Two Parts. N Engl J Med 1998; 338:107–111

Karet F. Inherited distal renal tubular acidosis. J Am Soc Nephrol 2002; 13:2178–2184

Haematological problems

Anaemia

Bain BJ. Diagnosis from the blood smear. N Engl J Med 2005; 353:498–507

Thalassaemia

Rund D, Rachmilewitz E. β-Thalassaemia. N Engl J Med 2005; 353:1135–1146

Haemophilia

Wilde JT. von Willebrand disease. Clin Med 2007:629–632

Deep vein thrombosis

Di Nisio M, Middeldorp S, Buller HR. Direct thrombin inhibitors. N Engl J Med 2005; 353:1028–1040

Goodacre S, Sutton AJ, Sampson FC. Meta-Analysis: the value of clinical assessment in the diagnosis of deep venous thrombosis. Ann Intern Med 2005; 143:129–139

Oudega R, Hoes AW, Moons KGM. The Wells Rule does not adequately rule out deep venous thrombosis in primary care patients. Ann Intern Med 2005; 143:100–107

Wells PS, Hirsh J, Anderson DR et al. Accuracy of clinical assessment of deep-vein thrombosis. Lancet 1995; 345:1326–1330

Wells PS, Anderson DR, Bormanis J et al: Value of assessment of pretest probability of deep-vein thrombosis in clinical management. Lancet 1997; 350:1795–1798

Wells PS, Anderson DR, Rodger M, et al: Evaluation of D-dimer in the diagnosis of suspected deep-vein thrombosis. N Engl J Med 2003; 349:1227–1235

Thrombophilic tendency

Baglin T. Acquired bleeding disorders. Clin Med 2005; 5:326–328

International Consensus Statement on an update of the classification criteria for definite antiphospholipid syndrome (APS). J Thromb Haemost 2006; 4:295–306

Lucock M. Is folic acid the ultimate functional food component for disease prevention? BMJ 2004; 328:211–214

Infectious disease problems

Deeks SG. Antiretroviral treatment of HIV infected adults. BMJ 2006; 332:1489–1493

Other general medical and elderly care problems

Falls and rehabilitation

National Institute for Clinical Excellence. Falls: the assessment and prevention of falls in older people. NICE Guideline 21

Syncope

Brignole M, Alboni P, Benditt D et al. Guidelines on management (diagnosis and treatment) of syncope. Eur Heart J 2001; 22:1256–1306

European Society of Cardiology – Task Force Report. Guidelines on Management (Diagnosis and Treatment) of Syncope – Update 2004. Europace 2004; 6:467–537

Chen-Scarabelli C, Scarabelli TM. Neurocardiogenic syncope. BMJ 2004; 329:336–341

Seizures

International League against Epilepsy (ILAE) (publishes the International Classification of Epileptic Seizures). Available: www.ilae-epilepsy.org

Scottish Intercollegiate Guidelines Network (SIGN) Guideline no. 70. Diagnosis and management of epilepsy in adults. Available: www.sign.ac.uk

Acute confusion

Hodkinson HM. Evaluation of a mental test score for assessment of mental impairment in the elderly. Age and Ageing 1972; 1:233–238

Inouye S. Delirium in older people. N Engl J Med 2006; 354:1157–1165

Nayeem K, O'Keefe ST. Delirium. Clin Med 2003; 3:412–415

Scolding N, Fuller G. Subacute neurological syndromes. Clin Med 2004; 4:122–124

Mild cognitive impairment and dementia

Breen DA, Breen DP, Moore JW et al. Driving and dementia. BMJ 2007; 334:1365–1369

Folstein MF, Folstein SE, McHugh PR. 'Mini-Mental State'. A practical method for grading the cognitive state of patients for the clinician. J Psychiatr Res 1975; 12:189–198

McKeith IG, Galasko D, Kosoka K et al. Consensus guidelines for the clinical and pathological diagnosis of dementia with Lewy bodies (DLB): a report of the consortium on DLB international workshop. Review. Neurology 1996; 47:1113–1124

McKhann G, Drachmann D, Folstein M et al. Clinical diagnosis of Alzheimer's disease. Report of the NINCDS-ADRDA Work Group under the auspices of the Department of Health and Human Services Task Force on Alzheimer's disease. Neurology 1984; 34:939–944

National Institute for Health and Clinical Excellence. Clinical Guideline: Demantia. NICE guideline, Autumn 2006. Available: www.nice.org.uk

Roman GC, Tatemichi TK, Erkinjuntli T et al. Vascular dementia: diagnostic criteria for research studies. Report of the NINDS-AIREN International Workshop. Neurology 1993; 43:250–260

Snowdon DA, Greiner LYH, Mortimer JA et al. Brain infarction and the clinical expression of Alzheimer's disease. The Nun Study. JAMA 1997; 277:813–817

Raised inflammatory markers

Charo IF, Ransohoff RM. The many roles of chemokines and chemokine receptors in inflammation. N Engl J Med 2006; 354:610–621

Polymyalgia and giant cell arteritis

Frearson R, Cassidy T, Newton J. Polymyalgia rheumatica and temporal arteritis: evidence and guidelines for diagnosis and management in older people. Age Ageing 2003; 32:370–374

Pyrexia and sepsis

Brugarolas J. Renal-cell carcinoma – molecular pathways and therapies. N Engl J Med 2007;356:185–187

Lever A, Mackenzie I. Sepsis: definition, epidemiology, and diagnosis. BMJ 2007; 335:879–883

Station 3
Cardiovascular and nervous system

CARDIOVASCULAR SYSTEM

Examination of the cardiovascular system 346

Cases

3.1 Mitral stenosis 355
3.2 Mitral regurgitation 357
3.3 Aortic stenosis 359
3.4 Aortic regurgitation 361
3.5 Tricuspid regurgitation and Ebstein's anomaly 363
3.6 Other right-sided heart murmurs 364
3.7 Mixed valve disease 365
3.8 Mitral valve prolapse 365
3.9 Prosthetic valves 367
3.10 Permanent pacemaker 368
3.11 Infective endocarditis 370
3.12 Congenital acyanotic heart disease 373
3.13 Cyanotic heart disease 375
3.14 Hypertrophic (obstructive) cardiomyopathy 375
3.15 Pericardial rub and pericardial disease 378

NERVOUS SYSTEM

Examination of the nervous system – overview 380

Examination of the cranial nerves 380

Examination of higher cortical function and specific lobes 387

Examination of speech and language 389

Examination of coordination 390

Examination of power and sensation – overview 392

Examination of the upper limbs 397

Examination of the lower limbs 402

Examination of gait 406

Cases

3.16 Visual field defects 406
3.17 Ocular nerve lesions 407
3.18 Internuclear ophthalmoplegia 409
3.19 Nystagmus 411
3.20 Ptosis 412
3.21 Large pupil 413
3.22 Small pupil 414
3.23 Horner's syndrome 415
3.24 Cerebellopontine angle syndrome 416
3.25 Facial nerve palsy 418
3.26 Bulbar palsy 420
3.27 Anterior circulation stroke syndromes 421
3.28 Dysphasia/dysarthria 431
3.29 Pseudobulbar palsy 431
3.30 Agnosias and apraxias 432
3.31 Posterior circulation stroke syndromes 435
3.32 Parkinson's disease 438
3.33 Cerebellar disease 442
3.34 Spastic paraparesis and Brown–Séquard syndrome 443
3.35 Syringomyelia 446
3.36 Absent ankle jerks and extensor plantars 447
3.37 Motor neurone disease 449
3.38 Cervical myeloradiculopathy 451
3.39 Cauda equina syndrome 452
3.40 Carpal tunnel syndrome (median nerve lesion) 454
3.41 Ulnar nerve lesion 455
3.42 Radial nerve lesion 457
3.43 Wasting of the small (intrinsic) muscles of the hand 459
3.44 Common peroneal nerve lesion 460
3.45 Peripheral neuropathy 461
3.46 Charcot–Marie–Tooth disease and hereditary neuropathies 468
3.47 Guillain–Barré syndrome 469
3.48 Myasthenia gravis 472
3.49 Myopathy and myositis 474
3.50 Myotonic dystrophy 479

References and further reading 482

CARDIOVASCULAR SYSTEM

Examination of the cardiovascular system

Inspection

Hands and arms

- Look for finger clubbing, characterised by fluctuant nail beds, loss of angle between the nail plate and posterior nail fold, and increased nail curvature. Cardiac causes include cyanotic heart disease and infective endocarditis.
- Look for cyanosis caused by right to left cardiac shunts.
- Look for palmar or tendon xanthomata.
- Look for peripheral stigmata of infective endocarditis (Table 3.1).

Face and neck

- Look for central cyanosis at the tongue.
- Note any pallor or abnormal skin markings, specifically a malar flush. A malar flush may be a sign of pulmonary hypertension and you should especially consider mitral stenosis as a cause.
- Look for corneal arcus, a creamy yellow discoloration at the boundary of the iris and cornea caused by cholesterol deposition; it can be normal. Look for xanthelasmata.

Jugular venous pulse (JVP)

There are no valves between the right atrium and the internal jugular vein, such that the degree of rise and distension of the JVP is dictated by right atrial pressure. The external jugular vein is superficial, prone to kinking in the fascial layers and thus not a guide to right atrial pressure. The right internal jugular vein is used in preference to the left. It runs a relatively straight course medial and deep to the sternomastoid, from between the sternal and clavicular heads to the angle of the jaw. It differs from the arterial pulse (Table 3.2) in numerous ways.

The JVP has a characteristic waveform (Table 3.3, Fig. 3.1).

Note that in relation to the ECG the 'a' wave thus corresponds to a P wave and the 'x' descent to the QRS complex.

- Examine the JVP by positioning the patient at 45° and estimate the vertical height in centimetres between the top of the venous pulsation and the sternal angle to give the venous pressure in cm (Fig. 3.2, Table 3.4). Normal is up to 3–4 cm.

Chest wall

- Look for a median sternotomy scar consistent with coronary artery bypass grafting, open mitral

Table 3.1 Peripheral signs of infective endocarditis

Sign	Appearance
Splinter haemorrhages	Multiple linear reddish-brown marks on linear axis of nails (one or two may occur in healthy people)
Osler's nodes	Small painful, purplish nodules at the finger pulps representing digital microinfarction
Janeway lesions	Pink palmar macules
Roth's spots	Flame-shaped retinal haemorrhages with a cotton wool centre

Table 3.2 Differences between jugular and carotid pulse

	Jugular	Carotid
Number of waveforms	Two – 'a' and 'v'	One
Upper level	Definite	Not defined
Shape of movement	Rapid inward	Rapid outward
Palpability	Impalpable	Palpable
Effect of respiration	Falls during inspiration (venous return increased by suction effect of lungs)	No effect
Effect of position	Varies	No effect
Effect of abdominal pressure	Rises	No effect

Table 3.3 Normal waveform of the jugular venous pulse (see Fig. 3.1)

Waveform	When it occurs	What it represents
'a'	Presystolic	Venous distension due to right atrial contraction – blood, as well as entering the right ventricle, passes back through the open channel between the right atrium entrance and the jugular vein
'c' (a flicker in the x descent)	Ventricular systole	Closure of tricuspid valve whose leaflets bulge back towards right atrium during ventricular systole
'x'	Synchronous with carotid pulse	Tricuspid valve drawing away from right atrium as right ventricle empties in systole (atrial relaxation also contributes to 'x')
'v'	*Not* synchronous with ventricular systole	Venous return to right atrium while tricuspid valve still closed
'y'	Precedes atrial contraction	Opening of tricuspid valve and blood rushing from right atrium into right ventricle just before 'kick' of atrial contraction

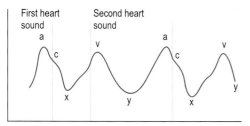

Fig. 3.1 Normal waveforms of the jugular venous pulse.

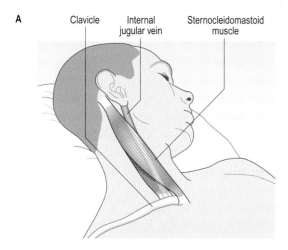

A

Clavicle   Internal   Sternocleidomastoid
            jugular vein   muscle

B

Sternocleidomastoid muscle

Top of jugular venous pulsation

Clavicle

Measure
vertical
height in
centimetres

Sternal angle

Patient lying at 45°

Fig. 3.2 Measuring the jugular venous pulse.

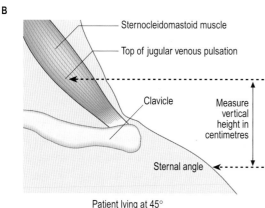

Box 3.1 Apex beat abnormalities

- A **double impulse** may be a sign of hypertrophic cardiomyopathy
- A **tapping apex** is the palpable equivalent of a loud first heart sound and should alert you to mitral stenosis
- A **hyperdynamic** or **thrusting apex** should alert you to aortic regurgitation
- A **sustained apex beat** should alert you to aortic stenosis
- A **heaving apex** is a sign of left ventricular hypertrophy

Apex beat abnormalities can be difficult. As a rule of thumb, try to determine if the apex beat is displaced or undisplaced and whether or not it is forceful.

Undisplaced apex

This is normal or implies pressure overload, as in aortic stenosis (raised left ventricular pressure with hypertrophy) and mitral stenosis (raised left atrial pressure with hypertrophy/dilatation).

Displaced apex

This implies volume overload, as in aortic regurgitation (left ventricular dilatation) and mitral regurgitation (left atrial and left ventricular dilatation).

Palpation

Arterial pulse

- Note the heart rate and rhythm.
- Palpate the radial or carotid pulse. Important abnormalities in arterial pulse character are shown in Table 3.5.

Blood pressure

- Take (or ask for) the blood pressure. Ensure you have the correct cuff size. Obese patients need a large cuff; a standard cuff will exert greater pressure to compress the artery and give falsely elevated readings. The point at which you hear the first Korotkoff sound is the systolic pressure and the point at which sound disappears (fifth Korotkoff sound) is the diastolic pressure. The fourth Korotkoff sound (muffling) is acceptable in patients in whom sound does not disappear.

Be alert to a wide pulse pressure (aortic regurgitation) and a narrow pulse pressure (aortic stenosis). Be aware of the significance of differences in blood pressure between arms (leaking thoracic aneurysm) and greater than 15–20 mmHg between arms and legs, always palpating for radio-femoral delay otherwise silent aortic coarctation is missed.

Apex

- Aim to locate the apex beat with your middle finger, normally palpable in the fifth intercostal space at the midclavicular line, and determine if it is displaced (see Fig. 3.3). An absent apex beat may be a sign of obesity, emphysema, pericardial effusion or dextrocardia, but it may be best palpable in the left lateral position. Many terms have been used to describe abnormalities in apex beat character (Box 3.1).

---

valvotomy or valve replacement, aortic valve surgery or mediastinal surgery.
- Look for a left lateral/inframammary thoracotomy scar consistent with closed mitral valvotomy.
- Look for the scar of (and palpable) a permanent pacemaker or implantable cardiac defibrillator.

Table 3.4 Abnormal waveforms of the jugular venous pulse

Abnormality		Causes	What it represents
Loss of 'a' wave		Atrial fibrillation	Loss of effective atrial contraction
Systolic V wave		Tricuspid regurgitation	'x' descent lost and replaced by very prominent upright systolic wave representing blood shooting back up into neck as right ventricle contracts Synchronous with carotid pulse and called systolic 'V' wave (not to be confused with 'v' wave) Sometimes called 'cV' wave Frequently seen rising to the earlobes 'y' descent steep as a result
Prominent 'a' wave		Tricuspid stenosis Pulmonary hypertension of any cause resulting in right ventricular overload Pulmonary stenosis	Atrium contracting against resistance 'y' descent also slowed because ventricular filling impeded
Giant 'a' or cannon wave		Complete heart block	Atrium contracting against a closed ventricle
Kussmaul's sign		Pericardial constriction Also restrictive cardiomyopathy and severe right heart failure of any cause when venous pressures are high	Paradoxical rise in JVP on inspiration due to inability of right heart to accommodate blood volume of venous return without a marked rise in filling pressure 'x' and 'y' descents correspondingly deep between the steep upstrokes
Raised venous pressure (> 4cm)		Congestive biventricular cardiac failure Pericardial effusion Cardiac tamponade	In all of these arterial blood pressure may be low and in large effusions and tamponade apex beat absent In tamponade only the 'x' descent is prominent Raised JVP + hypotension + absent apex beat = Beck's triad.
Non-pulsatile (fixed) raised neck veins		Superior vena cava obstruction	Obstructed venous return at the level of the SVC

Right ventricular parasternal lift

- Also known as a right ventricular heave or a left parasternal heave, this is detected by placing your palm over the left lower parasternal edge (Fig. 3.3). It will palpably (and visibly) lift if there is right ventricular hypertrophy, itself usually a consequence of pulmonary hypertension of any cause.

Palpable heart sounds and murmurs ('thrills')

- Feel for any thrills. Thrills are palpable murmurs (like touching a purring lion cub) usually caused by blood being squeezed through a narrow aperture. They are the tactile manifestation of murmur energy. A systolic thrill at the apex suggests mitral regurgitation. An upper parasternal thrill suggests aortic stenosis (right

Table 3.5 Abnormalities in arterial pulse character

Pulse character	Causes	Description/What it represents
Normal		The percussion wave is the dominant wave transmitted along elastic arterial walls The dicrotic notch (difficult to detect) is a normal blip on the downstroke of the percussion wave representing aortic valve closure
Slow rising, plateau pulse ('anacrotic' pulse)	Aortic stenosis	Slow rising with delayed percussion wave and sometimes a palpable judder on the upstroke Characteristically associated with narrow pulse pressure (narrow difference between systolic and diastolic pressure) if severe
Collapsing pulse	Aortic regurgitation Arteriovenous fistula Patent ductus A large volume, hyperkinetic pulse may occur in any cause of high cardiac output, e.g. thyrotoxicosis, Paget's disease, severe anaemia; a small volume collapsing pulse (quickly rising but small percussion wave) is associated with ventricular run-off states, e.g. mitral regurgitation, ventricular septal defect	Very brisk upstroke followed by 'collapse' occurs when there is 'run-off' from the aorta Characteristically associated with wide pulse pressure (wide difference between systolic and diastolic blood pressure) if severe May be visible at brachials or carotids and best felt by raising patient's arm, feeling the radial pulse 'slap' against your fingertips or palm
Pulsus alternans	Aortic stenosis Left ventricular failure	Alternating large and small beats A sign of poor left ventricular function
Pulsus paradoxus	Cardiac tamponade Pericardial constriction Acute severe asthma compromising venous return	Excessive fall in pulse pressure (> 10 mmHg) during inspiration Not, in fact, a paradox, but an exaggeration of normal physiology Difficult to detect
Jerky pulse	Hypertrophic cardiomyopathy	Ventricular ejection in 'stops and starts'

Table 3.6 Predicting valve abnormalities before auscultation

Pulse character	Pulse pressure	Apex position	Diagnosis
Normal (may be atrial fibrillation)	Normal	Undisplaced	Mitral stenosis (or normal!)
Large volume	Wide	Displaced	Aortic regurgitation
Small volume	Narrow	Undisplaced	Aortic stenosis
Normal	Normal	Displaced	Mitral regurgitation

parasternal edge) or pulmonary hypertension (left parasternal edge).

Predicting valve abnormalities before auscultation

One of your aims in cardiovascular examination to this point should be to try to predict any valve abnormality before auscultation. Ideally, auscultation should confirm already aroused suspicions. Common examples are given in Table 3.6.

Percussion

Percussion of the cardiac border or cardiac dullness adds little to clinical assessment. Omit unless other signs suggest the presence of a pericardial effusion.

Auscultation

Auscultation sites

- Start at the apex with the diaphragm followed by the bell of your stethoscope, then move through the areas shown in Fig. 3.4 with the diaphragm. The bell is a resonating chamber that amplifies low-pitched sounds, such as the diastolic murmur of mitral stenosis or a third or fourth heart sound. If not applied lightly it becomes a diaphragm.
- Next listen at the *apex* with the patient in *the left lateral position* and at the *aortic and pulmonary areas* with the patient *sitting forward*. Which you do first depends upon where you think the pathology lies, but

be seen to do both. *In both positions listen in expiration ('breathe in, and out, and hold your breath . . . and breathe again') and in inspiration if you suspect a right-sided (pulmonary or tricuspid) murmur.* Inspiration increases the loudness of right-sided murmurs and expiration the loudness of left-sided murmurs.

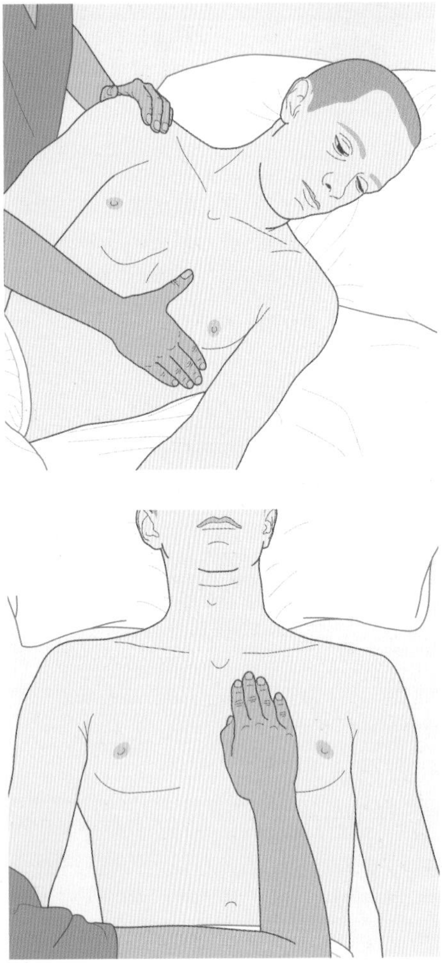

Heart sounds

Heart sounds are vibrations caused by the closure of heart valves combined with rapid changes in blood flow and tensing within cardiac structures.

- Listen for the first and second heart sounds, and any extra third or fourth heart sound.

■ **First heart sound (S1)**   S1 ('*lub*') represents mitral (and to a lesser extent tricuspid) valve closure at the onset of ventricular systole. Only one sound is audible. The intensity of S1 may be altered (Table 3.7) by the position of the

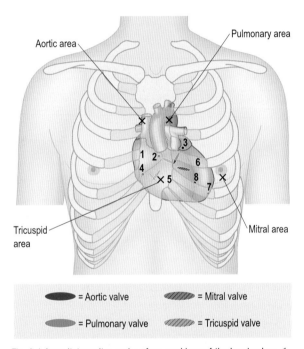

Fig. 3.4 Auscultatory sites and surface markings of the heart valves. 1, right atrium; 2, right atrial appendage; 3, left atrial appendage; 4, atrioventricular groove; 5, right ventricle; 6, left ventricle; 7, apex of the heart; 8, anterior interventricular groove. Note: areas refer to where sound best heard, not anatomical location of valve.

A

B

Fig. 3.3 Determining the position of the apex beat (A) and palpating for a right ventricular heave (B).

Table 3.7 Abnormalities of S1 intensity		
Loud S1	**Soft S1**	**Variable S1**
Tachycardia (shortened diastolic filling time and faster valve closure)	Bradycardia (prolonged diastolic filling time)	Atrial fibrillation Ventricular ectopic beats
Short PR interval (atrial contraction precedes ventricular contraction in an unusually short time, again with faster valve closure)	Long PR interval (first-degree heart block)	Complete heart block
Mitral stenosis with pliable valve (high left atrial pressure forces leaflets further apart during atrial systole so that they are very far apart by the end of ventricular diastole and come together again more forcefully) Tricuspid stenosis	Mitral stenosis with non-pliable valve (anterior leaflet immobile because of rigid calcification) Mitral regurgitation and left ventricular failure (imperfect closure or coaption of leaflets)	
Increased atrioventricular flow in high cardiac output states	Poor chest wall conduction	

Box 3.2 Abnormalities of S2 intensity

Loud S2

- Tachycardia
- Systemic hypertension – loud A2 (forceful aortic valve closure because of high aortic pressure)
- Pulmonary hypertension – loud P2 (high pulmonary pressure)
- Congenital aortic stenosis (mobile but narrowed valve closes suddenly at end of diastole)

Soft S2

- Severe aortic stenosis with calcified valve (reduced movement of leaflets)
- Aortic regurgitation (leaflets cannot coapt)

---

mitral valve leaflets at the onset of systole, the rate of rise of the left ventricular pressure pulse, the amount of tissue, fluid or air between valve and stethoscope, and mitral valve disease.

▪ **Second heart sound (S2)** S2 ('*dub*') comprises aortic valve closure (A2) followed by pulmonary valve closure (P2) at the onset of diastole. Diastole is normally longer than systole. S2 is of slightly lower intensity than S1. Normally A2–P2 is slightly split (< 0.05 seconds apart) and A2 comes first – think of the efficient left ventricle contracting swiftly, offloading its stroke volume compared to the lower pressure within the right side of the heart.

There are four types of S2 splitting (Table 3.8).

The intensity of S2 may be altered in disease (Box 3.2).

▪ **Third heart sound (S3)** This is described in Box 3.3.

▪ **Fourth heart sound (S4)** This is described in Box 3.3.

If the heart rate is very fast, S3 and S4 may be superimposed as one audible sound. It does not necessarily imply a heart under stress unless one or both sounds persist when the heart is slowed. If both S3 and S4 are present the situation is a quadruple rhythm, a sign of severe ventricular dysfunction.

Added sounds

- Listen for added sounds (Box 3.4).

Murmurs

Heart murmurs result from vibrations in the bloodstream and surrounding heart and great vessels due to turbulent flow.

- Try to determine the character, location and radiation of any murmur you hear (Box 3.5).
- Try to grade the intensity or loudness of any murmur you hear (Table 3.9).
- Try to determine the timing (with the carotid pulse) and duration of any murmur you hear (Table 3.10). While this is expected by examiners and is straightforward in theory, many candidates find timing difficult; what sounded like the typical whispering decrescendo murmur of aortic regurgitation suddenly becomes mitral regurgitation on the basis of dubious timing when all the evidence is with the former and against the latter. Keep in

---

Box 3.3 Extra heart sounds

Third heart sound (S3)

S3 is a low-pitched sound just after S2 (causing a gallop rhythm – 'Tennessee' or 'lub-dub-d' or 'd-d-d'). It is the result of rapid ventricular filling in early diastole from a very full or engorged left atrium such that blood crashes into the left ventricle with a 'boing'. A left-sided S3 is best heard with the bell at the apex in the left lateral position in expiration. A right-sided S3 is best heard at the left sternal edge in inspiration. S3 occurs normally in healthy children, young adults, athletes, pregnancy, fever and other hyperdynamic states, but usually signifies a heart under strain as in heart failure or mitral regurgitation. Some physicians describe a 'tic-tac' rhythm in which S1 and S2 appear to be in a hurry ('lub-dub'-'lub-dub'-'lub-dub' becomes 'dd'-'dd'-'dd'') just before a true gallop arises (the heart anticipating S3!) or coexisting with gallops.

Fourth heart sound (S4)

S4 is a low-pitched, presystolic sound occurring before S1 due to vigorous atrial contraction filling a stiff (less compliant) ventricle ('d-lub-dub'). As the mitral valve opens, the left atrium is 'looking down into a half-full ventricle'. S4 peaks in intensity at the left ventricular apex and is heard best with the bell in the left lateral position. There may be palpable or even visible presystolic distension of the left ventricle. S4 may be accentuated by isotonic and isometric exercise. It may occur in systemic hypertension, aortic stenosis, left ventricular hypertrophy, ischaemic heart disease and restrictive cardiomyopathies. Most typically, it occurs in heart failure and simply represents a 'tired heart'; it is also common in acute myocardial infarction. It is always pathological. It cannot occur in atrial fibrillation.

S3 and S4 are rarely detected by doctors but become easier to detect if you are expecting them, in heart failure for example. If S1 and S2 appear in a hurry (tic-tac rhythm or 'dd'), then S3 or S4 may become apparent ('dd'-'d'-'dd'-'d'-'dd'-'d', where 'd' is S3 if detected just after 'dd' or S4 if detected just before 'dd').

Box 3.4 Added sounds

Opening snap (OS)

This is a brief, high-pitched, early diastolic sound occurring as the mitral valve is forced open by high left atrial pressure in mitral stenosis. The S2–OS interval is shorter the higher the left atrial pressure.

Ejection click or sound

This is a sharp, high-pitched sound in early systole soon after S1. It may occur in non-calcified aortic stenosis or pulmonary stenosis with a pliable valve, the mechanism similar to an opening snap and the sound preceding the typical ejection systolic murmur.

Mid-systolic (non-ejection) click

This may occur in mitral valve prolapse as one or both leaflets prolapse into the left atrium. There may be an accompanying late systolic murmur of mitral regurgitation.

Metallic prosthetic sounds

These may be audible without auscultation.

Pericardial knock

This is a third heart sound equivalent heard in diastole in constrictive pericarditis.

Pericardial friction rub

This is a scratching presystolic, systolic or early diastolic sound heard best with the diaphragm. It is due to pericarditis.

Table 3.8 Types of S2 splitting

Type of splitting (all splitting best heard at left sternal edge with diaphragm)	Explanation	Causes
Inspiratory splitting	Reduced intrathoracic pressure on inspiration 'sucks' blood into the pulmonary vessels of the lungs. There is increased venous return and inflow to the right ventricle, which increases right ventricular stroke volume and right ventricular ejection time and so delays right ventricular emptying and thus P2. *In short, more blood is flowing through the right side of the heart in inspiration.* This is entirely logical because the lungs need more blood in inspiration for oxygenation purposes. Blood is 'held back' from entering the left side of the heart by the reduced intrathoracic pressure and this decreased blood flow out of the lungs into the left side of the heart gives rise to earlier left ventricular emptying and an earlier A2. The diminished cardiac output during inspiration also explains why blood pressure falls and heart rate rises in inspiration. The converse of these rules applies in expiration.	The normal physiological situation

Accentuated physiological splitting and expiratory splitting	Physiological splitting is accentuated by right ventricular volume overload. Splitting that persists in expiration is usually pathological, and occurs when right ventricular emptying is further delayed or when left ventricular emptying is fast.
	 Splitting may be accentuated, normal or diminished in pulmonary hypertension depending upon the cause, pulmonary vascular resistance and the degree of right ventricular decompensation.
		Delayed right ventricular emptying
		   Right bundle branch block (delayed activation)
		   Pulmonary embolism
		   Pulmonary stenosis (prolonged right ventricular contraction)
		   Right ventricular failure (right ventricular volume overload)
		 Fast left ventricular emptying
		   Mitral regurgitation (some ejection into left atrium)
		   Ventricular septal defect (if shunted to right)
		   Left ventricular ectopics and left ventricular pacing

Wide and fixed splitting	Equalisation of volume loads between the two atria occurs in an atrial septal defect producing a common chamber. The proportion of blood contributed to the right atrium by the left atrium and the vena cava varies reciprocally throughout the respiratory cycle such that right ventricular inflow (and thus volume and duration of right ventricular ejection) is constant or *fixed* throughout the respiratory cycle. Since the right side of the heart is maximally overloaded, systole is prolonged and cannot be further delayed *(wide and fixed).*	Atrial septal defect

Reversed (paradoxic) splitting	Left ventricular emptying is delayed or right ventricular emptying is fast.	Delayed left ventricular emptying
		   Left bundle branch block
		   Aortic stenosis
		   Hypertrophic obstructive cardiomyopathy
		   Systemic hypertension
		   Left ventricular failure
		 Fast right ventricular emptying
		   Right ventricular pacing

Table 3.9 Intensity of murmurs

Grade	Description
1	Very soft, heard only by experts
2	Heard by non-expert in optimum conditions
3	Easily heard but no thrill
4	Loud with thrill
5	Very loud with easily palpable thrill
6	Extremely loud and heard without stethoscope

Box 3.5 Character, location and radiation of murmurs

Specific murmurs are described in more detail in individual cases. The location and radiation help diagnostically. For example, aortic stenosis murmurs are usually loudest in the right second intercostal space and may radiate to the carotids; mitral regurgitation murmurs are often loudest at the apex and may radiate to the axilla (especially if the anterior leaflet is mostly affected) or the left sternal border and base of the heart (especially if the posterior leaflet is mostly affected). As a rule, aortic murmurs tend to radiate more than mitral murmurs. However, the *character or quality of a murmur is invariably more helpful than its location. You are the same person wherever you go – murmurs are no different.*

Table 3.10 Timing of murmurs

Timing		Mechanism	Causes
Systolic murmurs	Pansystolic murmur (PSM)	Flow between two chambers that have widely different pressure throughout systole	Mitral regurgitation Tricuspid regurgitation Ventricular septal defect Sometimes aorto-pulmonary shunt
	Mid- or ejection systolic murmur (ESM)	Crescendo–decrescendo in shape (the sound of a 'woodcutter sawing wood in a forest') as pressure rises and falls	Aortic stenosis Pulmonary stenosis HCM Pulmonary flow murmur of ASD
	Early systolic murmur (unusual)		Large VSD with pulmonary hypertension Very small VSD Triscuspid regurgitation without pulmonary hypertension
	Late systolic murmur	Mitral regurgitation after the valve has clicked open in mitral valve prolapse	Mitral valve prolapse Mitral regurgitation from papillary muscle dysfunction
Diastolic murmurs	Early diastolic murmur	Begins with or shortly after S2 as soon as ventricular pressure falls below pressure in the aorta or pulmonary artery High-pitched, whispering and decrescendo	Aortic regurgitation Pulmonary regurgitation
	Mid-diastolic murmur	Disproportion between valve orifice and flow rate	Mitral stenosis Tricuspid stenosis Atrial myxoma *Carey–Coombs* murmur of acute rheumatic fever attributed to mitral valve inflammation In severe aortic regurgitation, a mid-diastolic murmur (*Austin–Flint murmur*) may arise at the anterior mitral valve leaflet as jets of blood from the aortic root and left atrium collide
	Presystolic murmur or presystolic accentuation of murmurs	Typical of mitral stenosis when the pressure-overloaded left atrium forcefully contracts and the mid-diastolic murmur crescendos into S1; only occurs in sinus rhythm	Mitral stenosis Tricuspid stenosis Atrial myxoma
Continuous murmurs	Combined systolic and diastolic murmurs may appear to fill cardiac cycle but are not continuous murmurs, by definition	Starts in systole, peaks near S2 and continues through all or much of diastole	Patent ductus arteriosus Arteriovenous fistulae (coronary, pulmonary, systemic) Aortic coarctation Venous hum Mammary soufflé (late pregnancy/early postpartum)

ASD, atrial septal defect; HCM, hypertrophic cardiomyopathy; VSD, ventricular septal defect.

Table 3.11 Effect of dynamic auscultation on murmurs

Manoeuvre	Effect on murmur		
	Most murmurs, e.g. mitral regurgitation, aortic stenosis	Mitral valve prolapse	Hypertrophic cardiomyopathy
Valsalva strain phase During the strain phase (forceful expiratory pressure against a closed glottis) there is raised intrathoracic pressure leading to reduced right and left ventricular filling (reduced preload to both ventricles); this leads to reduced cardiac output and blood pressure falls and heart rate rises to compensate. *Note from Table 3.8 that reduced intrathoracic pressure in inspiration augments venous return, the opposite rule to the strain phase of Valsalva, but that both inspiration and the strain phase of Valsalva lead to a fall in blood pressure and cardiac output – in inspiration the negative pressure in the lungs 'sucks' blood from the right side of the heart and 'holds it back' from entering the left side of the heart (blood pools in the pulmonary vessels during inspiration for oxygenation purposes); in the strain phase of Valsalva, the positive intrathoracic pressure impedes venous return into the thorax, and reduced delivery of blood to the left side of the heart is the natural consequence. Thus, both in inspiration and the strain phase of Valsalva, cardiac output falls with a fall in blood pressure and rise in heart rate, although stretch receptor and baroreceptor autonomic responses contribute to these responses in inspiration and the strain phase of Valsalva respectively.* **Valsalva release phase** During the release phase there is a transient overshoot correction of blood pressure, which rises, and heart rate falls.	Softer and shorter because less blood is flowing in the heart	Louder and longer and follows earlier click because prolapse is enhanced when the heart is underfilled; this may be because a greater left ventricular end diastolic volume exerts tension on the valve that maintains it in normal position; furthermore, a left atrium filled with blood may counteract prolapse	Louder because reduced heart filling in diastole worsens the subsequent dynamic obstruction
Position **Standing** Reduces venous return and murmurs follow same rules as strain phase of Valsalva	Softer and shorter	Louder and longer and follows earlier click	Louder
Squatting or passive leg raising Enhance venous return and have the opposite effect on murmurs to strain phase of Valsalva and standing	Louder and longer	Softer and shorter and follows later click	Softer
Exercise **Isometric** (e.g. sustained hand grip for 20–30 seconds) Increases systemic blood pressure (afterload) and heart rate and generally opposite effect on murmurs to strain phase of Valsalva and standing, although aortic stenosis murmurs may be softer because of a decreased gradient across the valve. Compare this with isotonic exercise (e.g. jogging), which also increases blood flow through the heart	Aortic stenosis softer Most other murmurs louder	Softer and shorter and follows later click	Softer

mind that the character of a murmur is more compellingly helpful than anything else when you might otherwise 'hedge your bets'.

Murmurs and physiological manoeuvres

▪ **Murmurs and respiration** Right-sided heart murmurs are louder in inspiration because in inspiration blood flow increases through the right side of the heart. Left-sided heart murmurs are louder in expiration because in expiration blood flow increases through the left side of the heart.

▪ **Murmurs and dynamic auscultation** Subtle murmurs may be enhanced by certain manoeuvres (Table 3.11). Tell the examiners that you would consider them but never ask a patient to perform these unless directed to do so by examiners.

Additional examination

Complete cardiovascular system examination includes assessment of lower limb pulses and examining for pulmonary, sacral and lower limb oedema.

Summary

A summary of the cardiovascular examination sequence is in the Summary Box.

SUMMARY BOX – CARDIOVASCULAR SYSTEM EXAMINATION SEQUENCE

- Look at the hands and arms for clubbing, peripheral cyanosis, xanthomata or peripheral signs of endocarditis
- Look at the face for central cyanosis, pallor, a malar flush, corneal arcus or xanthelasmata
- Determine the height of the JVP and any abnormal waveform
- Determine pulse rate, rhythm and character
- Ask for the blood pressure
- Determine the position of the apex and any abnormalities in apex beat character
- Feel for a right ventricular heave
- Feel for thrills
- Ask yourself if pulse character, blood pressure and apex position predict any valve abnormality
- Listen for S1 and S2; note any abnormal intensity of S1 and any abnormal splitting of S2
- Listen for any S3 or S4
- Listen for added sounds
- Listen for murmurs
- Consider the character, location, radiation, intensity and timing of murmurs (but give greatest attention to character)
- Remember to listen in the left lateral position and with the patient sitting forward

---

CASE 3.1

MITRAL STENOSIS

Instruction

This 65-year-old lady is thought to have a heart murmur. She is short of breath on exercise. Please examine her pulse, and palpate and auscultate her heart. Tell the examiners the signs you elicit, and discuss your proposed management.

Recognition

Signs of mitral stenosis are shown in Fig. 3.5.

Interpretation

Confirm the diagnosis

Listen in the left lateral position and in expiration to accentuate the murmur. The differential diagnosis includes:

- Tricuspid stenosis (rare, louder in inspiration)
- Atrial myxoma (rare, fever, constitutional symptoms, raised inflammatory markers)
- Carey Coombs murmur (acute rheumatic fever)
- Austin Flint murmur (see Case 3.4)

Encountering a 'full-house' of signs is improbable and even when present they are difficult to elicit. Many physicians say they have never heard an opening snap. Atrial fibrillation renders a murmur difficult to time. But the rumbling murmur is characteristic, not unlike heavy rain on a tin roof, the rumble of a subway train or a buffalo stampede!

What to do next – consider causes

Tell the examiners that causes of mitral stenosis include:

- Rheumatic heart disease (the most common cause worldwide; in Australia, for example, where streptococcal infection is highly prevalent within the Aboriginal population, rheumatic heart disease is a major health burden)
- Congenital
- Left atrial myxoma
- Connective tissue disease

Two-thirds of patients are female.

Consider severity/decompensation/complications

Signs of severe mitral stenosis are listed in Box 3.6.
Tell the examiners that:

- Pulmonary hypertension may be irreversible.
- Thromboembolic disease, especially stroke, may result from systemic emboli originating in the left atrium
- Infective endocarditis may lead to valve decompensation.
- Ortner's phenomenon is rare and refers to hoarseness resulting from an enlarged left atrium exerting pressure on the left recurrent laryngeal nerve supplying the vocal cord.
- Any situation that increases heart rate, such as exercise, pregnancy or sepsis, further increases the trans-mitral pressure gradient and can provoke increased pulmonary pressure and pulmonary oedema.

Consider function

Tell the examiners you would establish the limitations provoked by exertional dyspnoea and consider fitness for surgery.

Box 3.6 Signs of severe mitral stenosis

- Signs of pulmonary hypertension (Case 1.18)
- Short interval between S2 and opening snap (the shorter the interval the higher the left atrial pressure)
- Long diastolic murmur

Case 3.1 Mitral stenosis

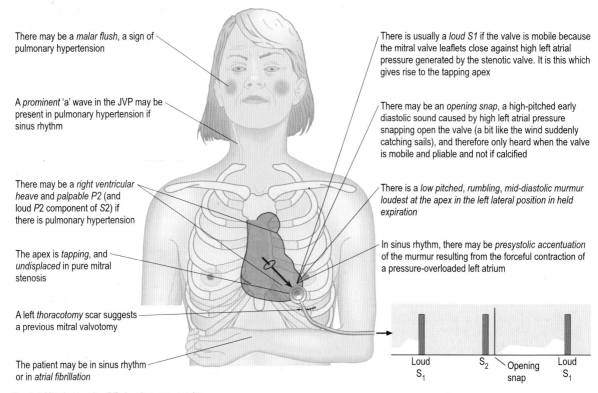

There may be a *malar flush*, a sign of pulmonary hypertension

A *prominent 'a' wave* in the JVP may be present in pulmonary hypertension if sinus rhythm

There may be a *right ventricular heave* and *palpable P2* (and loud *P2* component of *S2*) if there is pulmonary hypertension

The apex is *tapping*, and *undisplaced* in pure mitral stenosis

A left *thoracotomy* scar suggests a previous mitral valvotomy

The patient may be in sinus rhythm or in *atrial fibrillation*

There is usually a *loud S1* if the valve is mobile because the mitral valve leaflets close against high left atrial pressure generated by the stenotic valve. It is this which gives rise to the tapping apex

There may be an *opening snap*, a high-pitched early diastolic sound caused by high left atrial pressure snapping open the valve (a bit like the wind suddenly catching sails), and therefore only heard when the valve is mobile and pliable and not if calcified

There is a *low pitched, rumbling, mid-diastolic murmur* loudest at the apex in the left lateral position in held expiration

In sinus rhythm, there may be *presystolic accentuation* of the murmur resulting from the forceful contraction of a pressure-overloaded left atrium

Loud S₁   S₂   Opening snap   Loud S₁

Fig. 3.5 Mitral stenosis. JVP, jugular venous pulse.

Discussion

What happens to the valve pathologically?

The mitral valve is funnel shaped, dipping into the left ventricle. In mitral stenosis the valve leaflets are diffusely thickened by fibrosis and calcification. The commissures fuse, the chordae tendinae fuse and shorten, and the cusps become rigid. These narrow the apex of the funnel. The normal orifice is 4–6 cm². In significant obstruction the valve is < 2 cm² and blood can be propelled to the ventricle only by an abnormally elevated left atrial pressure.

What is the most common presenting symptom of mitral stenosis?

Exertional dyspnoea.

Why should patients experience exertional dyspnoea?

As blood flow increases with exercise across the mitral valve, the increased left atrial pressure needed to propel blood across the valve raises pulmonary venous and capillary pressures, which reduce pulmonary compliance, and pulmonary artery pressure increases.

Tachycardia also diminishes diastole disproportionately more than systole and thus the time for flow across the stenosed valve is reduced. Therefore at any given level of

cardiac output, tachycardia increases the transvalvular gradient and further elevates left atrial pressure.

When the valve orifice is reduced to 1 cm², a left atrial pressure of 25 mmHg is needed to maintain normal cardiac output. Pulmonary oedema may occur if there is a sudden surge of flow across a tight valve.

Eventually there is decreased cardiac output on exertion and at rest. The ability of the left atrium to generate sufficient pressure to maintain transvalvular flow is overcome.

What other symptoms may occur in mitral stenosis?

Symptoms may be the result of atrial arrhythmias, including premature atrial contractions, paroxysmal atrial tachycardia, atrial flutter and atrial fibrillation. Haemoptysis, due to the rupture of pulmonary–bronchial venous connections in pulmonary venous hypertension, is unusual but occurs in patients with raised left atrial pressure but without significantly increased pulmonary vascular resistance.

How does pulmonary hypertension arise?

Passive transmission backwards of raised left atrial pressure leads to raised pulmonary venous and capillary pressure, pulmonary arteriolar constriction triggered by pulmonary venous hypertension (reactive pulmonary

Box 3.7 Diagnostic criteria (Jones) for rheumatic fever

Major criteria

- Carditis
- Migratory polyarthritis
- Erythema marginatum
- Chorea
- Subcutaneous nodules

Minor criteria

- Fever
- Arthralgia
- Raised acute-phase reactants
- Prolonged PR interval

hypertension), interstitial oedema and pressure damage to and fibrosis or obliteration of the pulmonary vascular bed.

What are the diagnostic criteria for rheumatic fever?

Rheumatic fever (Box 3.7) and rheumatic heart disease remain common in the developing world, the latter a common usher for infective endocarditis. In the developed world the legacy of rheumatic fever remains, most commonly as mitral stenosis. Two major criteria *or* one major and two minor criteria *plus* evidence of antecedent group A streptococcal infection are required.

List some features the ECG might show in mitral stenosis

- p pulmonale if pulmonary hypertension (tall and peaked in II and upright in V1 if severe)
- Atrial fibrillation
- Right axis deviation
- Right ventricular hypertrophy in pulmonary hypertension

List some features the chest X-ray might show in mitral stenosis

- Enlarged left atrium
- Widened carinal angle
- Kerley B lines (indicating a left atrial pressure > 20 mmHg)
- Alveolar oedema
- Pulmonary haemosiderosis (haemosiderin containing macrophages in airways)

What might echocardiography be used to assess in mitral stenosis?

- Transvalvular gradient
- Orifice area (1.5–2.2 cm^2 mild stenosis, 1.0–1.5 cm^2 moderate stenosis, < 1 cm^2 severe stenosis)
- Rigidity and nature of valve disease
- Cardiac chamber dimensions
- Pulmonary artery pressure
- The presence of any associated mitral regurgitation

What is the place of cardiac catheterisation?

This may provide more accurate assessment of pulmonary artery and heart chamber pressures, and can be used to assess both pressure gradient and flow rate across the valve. Left ventricular end diastolic pressure (LVEDP) is normal in pure mitral stenosis. It is often raised, however, with co-existing impaired left ventricular function because of ischaemic heart disease, mitral regurgitation, aortic valve disease or systemic hypertension. The end diastolic gradient between left atrial pressure and LVEDP is a guide to severity and need for surgery, and surgery would not normally be performed for a gradient of < 5 mmHg. Note that mitral valve prostheses are slightly obstructive by their nature. Theoretically a gradient is a rate of change and the term pressure drop is sometimes used, although most argue that gradient is an appropriate term because the pressure changes continuously as blood crosses a valve.

How might you clinically detect if there is significant concomitant mitral regurgitation?

There would be significant diminution of S1 and the opening snap, together with a pansystolic murmur.

Which treatments may be considered for mitral stenosis?

Most asymptomatic patients with mild to moderate mitral stenosis can be reviewed annually with echocardiography.

The primary indication for intervention is relief of symptoms in patients with a valve area ≤ 1.5 cm^2. Mitral balloon valvuloplasty (percutaneous transmitral commissurotomy), rather than mitral valve replacement, is favoured if the valve is mobile and relatively undistorted, provided there is no/minimal mitral regurgitation and no left atrial thrombus. It can delay mitral valve replacement by around 10 years in suitable patients. Otherwise, a prosthetic mitral valve is needed. Minimally invasive valve replacement may become more prominent in future.

All patients should be considered for anticoagulation if there are no contraindications, and receive antibiotic prophylaxis during procedures.

CASE 3.2

MITRAL REGURGITATION

Instruction

This 66-year-old lady is thought to have a heart murmur. Please palpate and auscultate her praecordium and discuss your findings.

Recognition

Signs of mitral regurgitation are shown in Fig. 3.6.

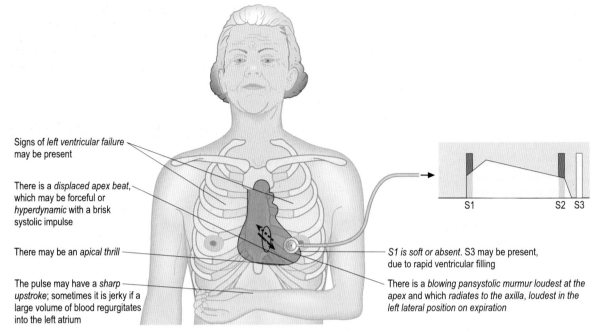

Signs of *left ventricular failure* may be present

There is a *displaced apex beat*, which may be forceful or *hyperdynamic* with a brisk systolic impulse

There may be an *apical thrill*

The pulse may have a *sharp upstroke*; sometimes it is jerky if a large volume of blood regurgitates into the left atrium

S1   S2 S3

S1 is soft or absent. S3 may be present, due to rapid ventricular filling

There is a *blowing pansystolic murmur loudest at the apex* and which *radiates to the axilla, loudest in the left lateral position on expiration*

Fig. 3.6 Mitral regurgitation.

Interpretation

Confirm the diagnosis

Listen in the left lateral position and in expiration to accentuate the murmur. The differential diagnosis includes:

- Tricuspid regurgitation (pansystolic murmur louder in inspiration, 'V' waves, pulsatile liver)
- Ventricular septal defect
- Other systolic murmurs, e.g. ejection systolic murmur of aortic stenosis radiating to carotids

What to do next – consider causes

Mitral regurgitation can result from malfunction of the valve leaflets, the valve annulus, the chords, the papillary muscles or the underlying myocardium. Tell the examiners that causes include:

- Degenerative mitral disease in which chordal elongation leads to systolic prolapse of one or both leaflets back into the left atrium
- Ischaemic heart disease with left ventricular dysfunction
- Rheumatic heart disease (this deforms and stiffens the valve, fusing the commissures, contracting and fusing the chordae tendinae and retracting the cusps; unlike

> **Box 3.8 Signs of severe mitral regurgitation**
>
> - Left ventricular failure is the most obvious feature of advanced mitral regurgitation
> - When the left atrium is markedly enlarged, it may be palpable at the left sternal edge and resemble a right ventricular heave
> - Combined retraction of the left ventricle and expansion of the left atrium during systole may create a characteristic chest wall rocking motion (rare)
> - Progressively rising pulmonary venous and capillary pressure may progress to raised pulmonary artery pressure with signs of right-sided heart failure.

rheumatic mitral stenosis, this is more common in men)
- Mitral valve prolapse

Acute mitral regurgitation may be the result of papillary muscle rupture (infarction) or infective endocarditis.

Consider severity/decompensation/complications

Signs of severe mitral regurgitation are listed in Box 3.8.

Consider function

Tell the examiners you would establish the limitations provoked by symptoms (fatigue, exertional dyspnoea, orthopnoea) and consider fitness for surgery (mitral regurgitation is seldom treated surgically).

Discussion

What is the pathophysiology of mitral regurgitation and does it tend to progress?

During systole there is ejection into both aorta and left atrium. This reduces left ventricular afterload and left ventricular tension but ultimately creates a volume overloaded left side of heart as the left ventricle becomes the recipient of its intended volume of blood plus that which it ejected aberrantly into the left atrium. Irrespective of cause, mitral regurgitation tends to progress, because the enlarging left atrium pulls the posterior mitral valve leaflet away from the orifice and the dilating left ventricle enhances the regurgitation.

List some features the ECG might show in mitral regurgitation

- Left atrial enlargement (P mitrale)
- Atrial fibrillation if left atrium enlarged
- Left ventricular hypertrophy (often coexists with dilatation)

List some features the chest X-ray might show in mitral regurgitation

- Left atrial and left ventricular enlargement
- Signs of left ventricular failure

What are the treatments for mitral regurgitation?

Asymptomatic patients should receive antibiotic prophylaxis during procedures and be followed up with serial echocardiography. Asymptomatic patients with moderate or worse mitral regurgitation should be followed at least annually with echocardiography. Vasodilators have no proven role in delaying progression. The aim is to operate before severe symptoms or left ventricular dysfunction occur.

CASE 3.3

AORTIC STENOSIS

Instruction

Please examine this 80-year-old lady's cardiovascular system and discuss your findings.

Recognition

Signs of aortic stenosis are shown in Fig. 3.7.

Interpretation

Confirm the diagnosis

Listen with the patient sitting forward and in expiration to accentuate the murmur. The differential diagnosis includes:

- Pulmonary stenosis (murmur louder on inspiration, radiates to left clavicle)

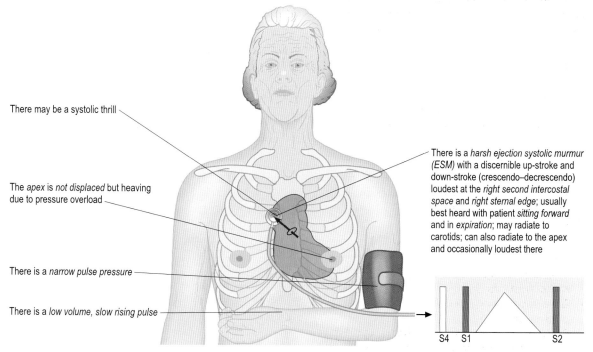

There may be a systolic thrill

The *apex* is *not displaced* but heaving due to pressure overload

There is a *narrow pulse pressure*

There is a *low volume, slow rising pulse*

There is a *harsh ejection systolic murmur (ESM)* with a discernible up-stroke and down-stroke (crescendo–decrescendo) loudest at the *right second intercostal space* and *right sternal edge*; usually best heard with patient *sitting forward* and in *expiration*; may radiate to carotids; can also radiate to the apex and occasionally loudest there

S4   S1   S2

Fig. 3.7 Aortic stenosis.

- Hypertrophic (obstructive) cardiomyopathy
- Other systolic murmurs, e.g. pansystolic murmur of mitral regurgitation, loudest at apex

What to do next – consider causes

Tell the examiners that causes include:

- Calcific degeneration (by far the commonest cause)
- Rheumatic heart disease, usually with associated mitral valve disease (now much less common)
- Congenital bicuspid valve (may affect 1–2% of people and tends to present in the fifth and sixth decades)

Consider severity/decompensation/complications

Signs of severe aortic stenosis are listed in Box 3.9. Additionally, an early peaking murmur may be associated with a less stenotic valve and a late peaking murmur more severe stenosis.

Average time to death with angina or syncope is 3 years, with dyspnoea 2 years and with heart failure 1.5 years. Asymptomatic patients even with severe stenosis have an excellent prognosis with surgery.

Consider function

Tell the examiners you would establish the limitations provoked by symptoms (gradually decreasing exercise tolerance is usually the presenting symptom) and consider fitness for surgery.

Discussion

How does the pathophysiology of aortic stenosis correlate with the pulse, pulse pressure and murmur?

This is described in Box 3.10.

Box 3.9 Signs of severe aortic stenosis

- Small volume pulse
- Narrow pulse pressure
- Soft S2 (the valve leaflets neither open nor close well rather than crisply opening and snapping shut)
- Reversed S2
- Thrill/heave
- Left ventricular failure with S4

Box 3.10 Pathophysiology of aortic stenosis

- Aortic stenosis is a condition of pressure overload in which reduced left ventricular outflow results in left ventricular hypertrophy; the left ventricle is essentially 'weight-lifting' against progressive weights, as it does with systemic hypertension. The ejection pressure rises and falls between a peak in mid-systole to produce the ejection systolic murmur.
- The stroke volume ejected from the left ventricle is limited, and results in a small volume pulse that is slow rising.
- Because the obstructed valve limits the amount of pressure the systemically ejected jet can achieve, the pulse pressure is narrow with a low systolic component.

Why might patients with aortic stenosis develop angina?

This might be due to:

- Outflow obstruction impairing coronary sinus filling
- Squeezing of coronary arteries by hypertrophied muscle
- Increased myocardial demand from hypertrophied muscle

However, aortic stenosis is usually asymptomatic and the majority of patients with aortic stenosis and angina will have typical coronary artery disease.

Is there a difference between aortic sclerosis and aortic stenosis?

Aortic sclerosis refers to thickening of the valve because of calcification without stenosis and can progress over years to aortic stenosis. Once thought to be different conditions, they are now viewed as part of the same spectrum. Aortic stenosis is the commonest adult valve lesion and aortic sclerosis affects 20–30% of people over 65 years and 48% of those over 85 years. The pulse volume tends to be normal and the murmur does not radiate to the carotids. Aortic sclerosis is not usually of haemodynamic significance, but can be.

How does calcific aortic stenosis arise?

Traditionally it is attributed to degeneration of an ageing valve. However, many people over 80 years have no calcification, and increasingly calcific aortic stenosis is viewed as a chronic inflammatory condition, not dissimilar pathophysiologically to those mechanisms described for atherosclerosis in coronary artery disease. There is, not surprisingly, emerging evidence for the role for statin therapy in modifying this process. While non-specific thickening of the valve tips is very common in anyone over 80 years of age, calcific thickening characteristically results in irregular nodules on the aortic surfaces of the leaflets. Furthermore, the risk factors for calcific aortic stenosis are similar to those for coronary artery disease – age, male sex, smoking, dyslipidaemia, hypertension, diabetes, coronary heart disease, chronic kidney disease, hypercalcaemia.

Do you know of any unusual anaemia associations with aortic stenosis?

These include angiodysplasia and microangiopathic haemolytic anaemia.

List some other forms of left ventricular outflow obstruction

- Hypertrophic (obstructive) cardiomyopathy
- Discrete congenital subvalvular aortic stenosis
- Supravalvular aortic stenosis (uncommon, congenital)

Table 3.12 Echocardiographic measurement of severity of aortic stenosis

	Normal	Mild	Moderate	Severe
Aortic valve area (cm^2)	2.0–3.5	> 1.5	1.0–1.5	< 1.0
Aortic jet velocity (m/s)	0.9–2.5	< 3.0	3.0–4.0	> 4.0
Mean gradient (mmHg)	< 25	< 25	25–40	> 40

List some features the ECG might show in aortic stenosis

- Left ventricular hypertrophy
- ST segment depression and T wave inversion (left ventricular strain) in leads I and aVL and in anterolateral precordial leads

What might the chest X-ray show in aortic stenosis?

This is normal unless a calcified valve is visible.

How is aortic stenosis severity determined by echocardiography?

The current gold standard for assessing severity is two-dimensional and Doppler echocardiography, although magnetic resonance imaging and computed tomographic scanning have been evaluated. Narrowing of the valve results in acceleration of blood flow across the valve and larger pre–post valve peak and mean pressure differences or gradients (Table 3.12). The peak pressure gradient across the aortic valve has a simple relationship with the aortic jet velocity and is described as four times the square of that velocity (modified Bernoulli equation). A peak velocity of 4 m/s, for example, gives a peak pressure gradient of $4 \times 4^2 = 64$ mmHg with a mean gradient of 40 mmHg.

What is the rate of progression of aortic stenosis?

In people with aortic sclerosis, progression to stenosis (arbitrarily defined as a peak post-valve velocity ≥ 2.5 m/s or peak gradient ≥ 25 mmHg) is relatively slow, with mean increases per year in peak post-valve velocity and peak gradient of 0.07 m/s and 1.4 mmHg, respectively. However, once stenotic, severity rates accelerate with average yearly increases of 0.3 m/s and 7–8 mmHg, corresponding to a decrease in valve area of 0.1 cm^2 per year.

Which drugs may be used for symptomatic aortic stenosis and which drugs should be used with caution or avoided?

Symptomatic aortic stenosis might require treatment with diuretics, vasodilators or digoxin. Excessive diuretic use should be avoided in severe aortic stenosis because diastolic dysfunction is common and an adequate preload is needed to maintain cardiac output. Although the evidence for so doing is limited, drugs that reduce afterload or preload, notably angiotensin-converting enzyme inhibitors, angiotensin II receptor blockers and nitrates, should be avoided with advancing severity (although increasing evidence supports a beneficial role for angiotensin inhibition). A reduction in afterload will increase the gradient across the valve. The heart responds by increasing cardiac output but cannot do so if preload is compromised. In practice, any antihypertensives should be used with caution but further evidence is needed to establish the dangers or possible benefits. In angina, beta blockers and even nitrates may be used with caution.

What are the indications for surgery in aortic stenosis?

No therapy can currently slow or reverse disease progression in calcific aortic stenosis, although statins are being evaluated and early evidence is promising. Current management involves monitoring progression, ensuring antibiotic prophylaxis during procedures and, for those with severe symptoms, conventional medical therapy or aortic valve replacement. The optimum timing for aortic valve replacement remains contentious. It is universally accepted that surgery is indicated as soon as symptoms start. Although often intuitively worrying to see patients with severe asymptomatic stenosis not proceed to surgery, annual mortality figures in this latter group are low, less than 1% per year, pitched against a combined risk of aortic valve replacement mortality (2–10% per year) and prosthesis-related complications (2–3% per year). Patients requiring bypass grafting with aortic stenosis should also undergo valve replacement.

What surgical options are there for aortic stenosis?

Balloon valvotomy has largely been abandoned in adults and most patients receive a bioprosthetic or metallic valve. Minimally invasive percutaneous transfemoral valve replacement may assume a greater role in future in selected cases.

CASE 3.4

AORTIC REGURGITATION

Instruction

Please examine this 70-year-old gentleman's cardiovascular system and discuss your findings.

Recognition

Signs of aortic regurgitation are shown in Fig. 3.8.

Some eponymous signs of the hyperdynamic circulation in aortic regurgitation are given in Box 3.11.

Interpretation

Confirm the diagnosis

Listen with the patient sitting forward and in expiration to accentuate the murmur. The differential diagnosis includes:

Case 3.4   Aortic regurgitation

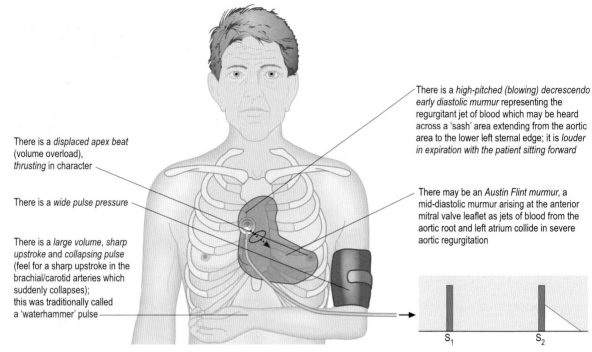

There is a *displaced apex beat* (volume overload), *thrusting* in character

There is a *wide pulse pressure*

There is a *large volume, sharp upstroke* and *collapsing pulse* (feel for a sharp upstroke in the brachial/carotid arteries which suddenly collapses); this was traditionally called a 'waterhammer' pulse

There is a *high-pitched (blowing) decrescendo early diastolic murmur* representing the regurgitant jet of blood which may be heard across a 'sash' area extending from the aortic area to the lower left sternal edge; it is *louder in expiration with the patient sitting forward*

There may be an *Austin Flint murmur*, a mid-diastolic murmur arising at the anterior mitral valve leaflet as jets of blood from the aortic root and left atrium collide in severe aortic regurgitation

S_1 S_2

Fig. 3.8 Aortic regurgitation.

Box 3.11 Eponymous signs in aortic regurgitation (some are hard to believe!)

- *Corrigan's sign* – visible rise and fall of pulsation; often vigorous or 'dancing' brachial or carotid arteries
- *De Musset's sign* – head nodding with each pulsation (Abraham Lincoln probably had this)
- *Quincke's sign* – alternate flushing and paling of the skin at the nail bed while pressure is applied to tip of nail (may occur at mucous membranes)
- *Lighthouse sign* – flushing and paling of the forehead
- *Traube's sign* – pistol shot systolic and diastolic sounds heard at the femoral arteries
- *Duzroziez's sign* – a systolic sound heard at the femoral artery when compressed proximally and a diastolic sound if compressed distally; essentially a to-and-fro sound at the femoral artery
- *Muller's sign* – uvula pulsation
- *Rosenbach's sign* – hepatic pulsation
- *Gerhardt's sign* – splenic pulsation (if enlarged)
- *Landolfi's sign* – change in pupil size synchronous with cardiac cycle

---

Box 3.12 Signs of severe aortic regurgitation

- Wide pulse pressure
- Soft S2
- Short early diastolic murmur (earlier equalisation of aortic and ventricular pressures)
- S3/left ventricular failure
- Austin–Flint murmur
- Hill's sign (popliteal cuff exceeding brachial cuff systolic pressure by ≥ 20 mmHg; 20–39 mild, 40–59 moderate, > 60 severe)

- Pulmonary regurgitation, which is a similar murmur but loudest at the pulmonary area and louder in inspiration.

What to do next – consider causes

Tell the examiners that causes include:

- Infective endocarditis
- Prosthetic valve paravalvular leak – acute or chronic
- Rheumatic heart disease

- Ankylosing spondylitis (kyphosis, question mark posture)
- Marfan syndrome (tall, long extremities with arm span > height, arachnodactyly, high arched palate)
- Rheumatoid arthritis (rheumatoid hands)
- Syphilitic aortitis (rare)

Aortic regurgitation is more common in males, and usually due simply to an ageing degenerative valve.

Consider severity/decompensation/complications

Signs of severe aortic regurgitation are listed in Box 3.12.

Consider function

Tell the examiners you would establish the limitations provoked by symptoms (although often asymptomatic until too late) and consider fitness for surgery.

> **Box 3.13 Pathophysiology of aortic regurgitation**
>
> - The left ventricle dilates to accommodate the increased blood volume that results from a reverse pressure gradient and regurgitation from aorta to left ventricle. This pressure gradient falls during diastole to produce the decrescendo of the early diastolic murmur.
> - The total stroke volume ejected from the left ventricle (effective forward stroke volume plus regurgitated volume) is increased, resulting in a large volume pulse with a sharp upstroke. This collapses when arterial pressure falls rapidly in late systole and diastole.
> - Because there is high systolic outflow but aortic run-off back into the ventricle in diastole, the pulse pressure is wide, with increased systolic and decreased diastolic components; ultimately, of course, the stretching, floppy sack that is the left ventricle decompensates (heart failure) with decreased output.

Discussion

How does the pathophysiology of aortic regurgitation correlate with the pulse, pulse pressure and murmur?

This is described in Box 3.13.

What might the ECG show in aortic regurgitation?

Left ventricular strain is common.

List some features the chest X-ray might show in aortic regurgitation

- Left ventricular enlargement
- Prominent aorta

What are the indications for surgery in aortic regurgitation?

Surgery is the definitive treatment to halt volume overload. The aim is to replace the valve before significant left ventricular dysfunction occurs, the current criteria for defining the onset of left ventricular systolic dysfunction in chronic aortic regurgitation being a left ventricular end-systolic dimension > 55 mm or an ejection fraction < 55%. Nifedipine may delay the need for surgery in asymptomatic patients with severe aortic regurgitation but long-term vasodilator treatment is not recommended for patients with significant systolic dysfunction.

CASE 3.5

TRICUSPID REGURGITATION AND EBSTEIN'S ANOMALY

Instruction

Please examine this 48-year-old lady's cardiovascular system and discuss your findings.

Recognition

Signs of tricuspid regurgitation are shown in Fig. 3.9.

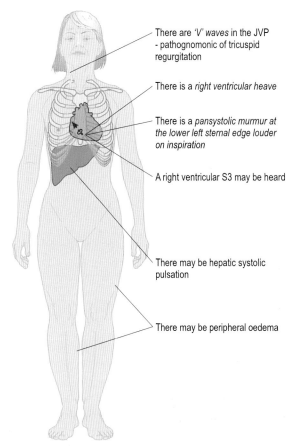

- There are 'V' waves in the JVP - pathognomonic of tricuspid regurgitation
- There is a *right ventricular heave*
- There is a *pansystolic murmur at the lower left sternal edge louder on inspiration*
- A right ventricular S3 may be heard
- There may be hepatic systolic pulsation
- There may be peripheral oedema

Fig. 3.9 Tricuspid regurgitation. JVP, jugular venous pulse.

Interpretation

Confirm the diagnosis

Listen in inspiration to accentuate the murmur. The differential diagnosis includes:

- Mitral regurgitation (murmur at apex radiating to axilla, louder in expiration)
- Other systolic murmurs, e.g. ejection systolic murmur of aortic stenosis

What to do next – consider causes

Tell the examiners that tricuspid regurgitation is usually functional, secondary to dilatation of the annulus. It may occur in:

- Heart failure
- Right ventricular infarction
- Pulmonary hypertension of any cause (cor pulmonale, mitral stenosis, primary pulmonary hypertension)
- Eisenmenger's syndrome

Primary causes include:

- Rheumatic heart disease
- Right-sided endocarditis
- Carcinoid syndrome

Consider severity/decompensation/complications

Signs of severe tricuspid regurgitation are:

- Hepatic pulsation
- Peripheral oedema

Consider function

Tell the examiners you would establish the limitations provoked by symptoms (although often asymptomatic until too late) and consider fitness for surgery.

Discussion

What other right-sided valve abnormalities do you know of?

- Tricuspid stenosis (rare; generally part of rheumatic heart disease)
- Pulmonary regurgitation (usually the result of dilatation of the pulmonary valve ring in pulmonary hypertension – Graham–Steel murmur)
- Pulmonary stenosis (rare; may be congenital or due to carcinoid syndrome)

What do you know about Ebstein's anomaly?

This is congenital, isolated tricuspid regurgitation (without signs of pulmonary hypertension), which leads to cardiomegaly and right-sided heart failure. Ebstein's anomaly is characterised by downward displacement of the tricuspid valve into the right ventricle due to anomalous attachment of the tricuspid leaflets. The abnormally situated tricuspid orifice produces an 'atrialised' portion of right ventricle, which lies between the atrioventricular ring and origin of the valve. The right ventricle is often hypoplastic. Cyanosis results because of right to left shunting at the atrial level (through a patent foramen ovale or an atrial septal defect).

CASE 3.6

OTHER RIGHT-SIDED HEART MURMURS

Instruction

Please examine this 28-year-old lady's cardiovascular system and discuss your findings.

Recognition

Signs of pulmonary regurgitation are shown in Fig. 3.10.

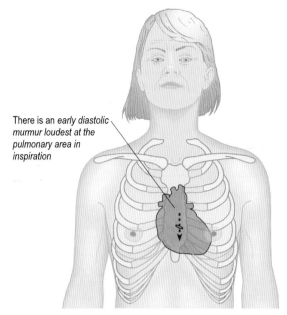

There is an *early diastolic murmur loudest at the pulmonary area in inspiration*

Fig. 3.10 Pulmonary regurgitation.

Interpretation

Confirm the diagnosis

Listen in inspiration to accentuate the murmur. The differential diagnosis of right-sided heart murmurs includes:

- Tricuspid regurgitation
- Tricuspid stenosis (rare; generally part of rheumatic heart disease)
- Pulmonary stenosis (rare; may be congenital, e.g. Noonan's syndrome, or due to carcinoid syndrome)

What to do next – consider causes

Pulmonary regurgitation is usually the result of dilatation of the pulmonary valve ring in pulmonary hypertension causing the classic Graham–Steel murmur. Tell the examiners that other important causes include:

- Infective endocarditis from intravenous drug use
- Carcinoid syndrome

Consider severity/decompensation/complications

Valve decompensation is common in infective endocarditis.

Consider function

Tell the examiners you would establish the limitations provoked by symptoms (although often asymptomatic until too late) and consider fitness for surgery.

Table 3.13 Determination of predominant mitral valve abnormality

	Mitral stenosis	Mitral regurgitation
Pulse	Small volume	Normal volume or hyperdynamic
Blood pressure	Usually unhelpful	Usually unhelpful
Apex	Not displaced Tapping	Displaced Thrusting
Heart sounds	Loud S1	Soft or absent S1 ± S3
Murmur	Rumbling mid-diastolic	Blowing pansystolic

Discussion

Which valve is most commonly affected in infective endocarditis secondary to intravenous drug use?

Tricuspid valve endocarditis is common.

CASE 3.7

MIXED VALVE DISEASE

Instruction

This patient has a mixture of heart valve abnormalities. Please decide which valve abnormality is dominant.

Recognition

Aortic stenosis with mitral regurgitation is the most common combination of valve abnormalities. Mixed mitral and mixed aortic valve disease is also common.

Mixed mitral valve disease

Pulse character, apex, S1 examination and the character of the murmur may help to determine which is dominant (Table 3.13). Further, the presence of an S3 would imply the absence of significant stenosis.

Mixed aortic valve disease

Pulse, blood pressure, apex examination and the character of the murmur may be used to determine which is dominant (Table 3.14). Consider also the possibility of a prosthetic aortic valve with an ejection systolic flow murmur and an early diastolic murmur suggesting a paravalvular leak.

Interpretation

Confirm the diagnosis

Use Tables 3.13 and 3.14 to determine the likely dominant lesions but tell the examiners that echocardiography is needed to resolve the issue.

Table 3.14 Determination of predominant aortic valve abnormality

	Aortic stenosis	Aortic regurgitation
Pulse	Slow rising	Collapsing
Blood pressure	Narrow pulse pressure with low systolic pressure	Wide pulse pressure with high systolic pressure
Apex	Not displaced Heaving	Displaced Thrusting
Heart sounds	Soft/absent S2	Quiet S1 Normal/soft S2
Murmur	Harsh 'sawing wood' ejection systolic Thrill	Whispering early diastolic

What to do next – consider causes

Causes of mitral stenosis, mitral regurgitation, aortic stenosis and aortic regurgitation are described in Cases 3.1–3.4.

Consider severity/decompensation/complications

Signs of severe mitral stenosis, mitral regurgitation, aortic stenosis and aortic regurgitation are described in Cases 3.1–3.4.

Consider function

Tell the examiners you would establish the limitations provoked by symptoms (although often asymptomatic until too late) and consider fitness for surgery.

Discussion

Questions about valve lesions are answered in cases on specific valve lesions.

CASE 3.8

MITRAL VALVE PROLAPSE

Instruction

This 30-year-old lady is thought to have a heart murmur. Please examine her cardiovascular system and report your findings.

Recognition

Signs of mitral valve prolapse are shown in Fig. 3.11.

Interpretation

Confirm the diagnosis

Tell the examiners that you would like to perform dynamic auscultation (Table 3.15).

Case 3.8   Mitral valve prolapse

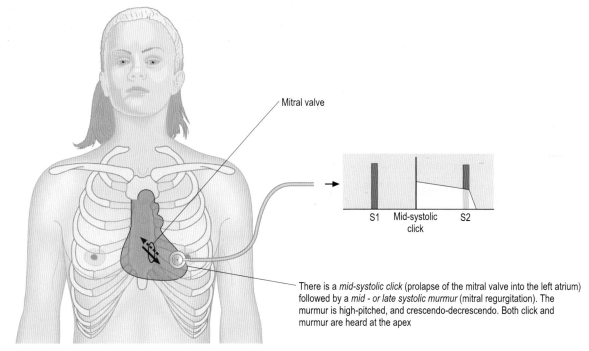

Mitral valve

S1   Mid-systolic   S2
      click

There is a *mid-systolic click* (prolapse of the mitral valve into the left atrium) followed by a *mid - or late systolic murmur* (mitral regurgitation). The murmur is high-pitched, and crescendo-decrescendo. Both click and murmur are heard at the apex

Fig. 3.11 Mitral valve prolapse.

Table 3.15 Effect of dynamic manoeuvres on mitral valve prolapse murmur		
Manoeuvre		**Effect**
Valsalva Reduces venous return		Longer and louder and follows earlier click because prolapse enhanced when heart under-filled
Position	**Standing** Reduces venous return	Longer and louder and follows earlier click
	Squatting or passive leg raising Enhances venous return	Softer and shorter and follows later click
Exercise	**Isometric** (hand grip) Enhances venous return	Softer and shorter and follows later click

What to do next – consider causes

Mitral valve prolapse is common, affecting between 2% and 10% of the population. Tell the examiners that occasionally it may be associated with:

- Marfan syndrome (tall, long extremities with arm span > height, arachnodactyly, high arched palate)
- Rheumatic heart disease
- An ostium secundum atrial septal defect
- Ehlers–Danlos syndrome
- Ebstein's anomaly
- Systemic lupus erythematosus

Consider severity/decompensation/complications

Complications of mitral valve prolapse include:

- Severe mitral regurgitation
- Arrhythmias
- Atypical chest pain
- Transient ischaemic attacks or strokes
- Infective endocarditis (usually only if associated with mitral regurgitation)
- Sudden cardiac death

Consider function

Tell the examiners you would establish the limitations provoked by symptoms (although often asymptomatic) and consider the need for surgery.

Discussion

What is the pathophysiology of mitral valve prolapse?

Mitral valve prolapse encompasses a spectrum of severities. Some patients have 'floppy' but non-prolapsing mitral valves. In cases of prolapse, the posterior leaflet is usually more affected, but both can prolapse. The mid-systolic click may be produced by the sudden tensing of the slack, elongated chordae tendinae or by the prolapsed leaflet at maximum excursion. Ruptured chordae tendinae and progressive annular dilatation may contribute to the subsequent regurgitation and eventually mitral valve prolapse may be extinguished by the signs of severe mitral regurgitation. Some patients have a click and no murmur and some patients have a murmur and no click.

CASE 3.9

PROSTHETIC VALVES

Instruction

Please examine this lady's cardiovascular system and discuss your findings.

Recognition

Mitral valve prosthesis

There is a *midline sternotomy scar*. There is a *metallic S1 click* representing closure of the prosthesis, *a metallic opening snap* in diastole and a *normal S2*. Systolic murmurs are common and do not necessarily indicate valve dysfunction.

Aortic valve prosthesis

There is a *midline sternotomy scar*. *S1 is normal* and is followed by an *ejection click* (often synchronous with S1) representing opening of the prosthesis, an *ejection systolic murmur* and an *S2 click* representing closure of the prosthesis. An early diastolic murmur and collapsing pulse imply a leaking prosthetic aortic valve.

Mitral and aortic valve prostheses

Both mitral and aortic valves may be prosthetic.

Interpretation

Confirm the diagnosis

The click of a mechanical valve is unmistakeable.

What to do next – consider causes

The most common reason for valve replacement is valve degeneration. Other causes include congenital heart disease and infective endocarditis.

Box 3.14 Complications of valve replacement

- Thromboembolic sequelae
- Infective endocarditis
- Valve regurgitation
- Ball thrombus/valve obstruction
- Haemolysis

Consider severity/decompensation/complications

Look for splinter haemorrhages or other signs of infective endocarditis. Listen for regurgitation. List some complications of valve replacement to the examiners (Box 3.14).

Consider function

Tell the examiners that a normal functioning valve should not give rise to symptoms.

Discussion

What types of prosthetic valve are available, and what are the pros and cons?

Mechanical valves

These are more durable than bioprosthetic valves, but more thrombogenic and require anticoagulation. Three designs are available. *Caged-ball valves* (e.g. Starr–Edwards) were the first and are highly durable but have significant problems with haemolysis, thrombogenesis and regurgitation. *Titling disc valves* (e.g. retired Björk–Shiley) improved the haemodynamic profile with reduced thrombogenic potential in the aortic position. *Bileaflet valves* (e.g. St Jude) are now invariably used, with a leaflet hinge mechanism. These valves enable 'washing' of the leaflets by allowing haemodynamically insignificant regurgitation across the valve during diastole. Most modern mechanical valves have 98% freedom from degeneration at 10 years.

Bio-prosthetic valve

These are less durable but are preferred in some circumstances (e.g. the elderly) because anticoagulation is not needed. Three types of bio-prosthesis are available. *Xenografts* are the most common, porcine or bovine with or without a wire or polyacetal stent. They are prone to degeneration, affecting around 5% of valves in the aortic position at 5 years and 30% at 10 years, due to calcification. *Homografts (allografts)* and *autografts* are less commonly used, the latter sometimes used to replace a diseased pulmonary valve with an aortic valve, which lasts longer in the pulmonary position because of lower pressure; but double valve surgery is needed for single valve pathology.

Which factors help to determine the choice of valve?

Aortic valve

Generally patients over 75 years of age receive a xenograft. These close against the lower diastolic pressure of the aorta and are more durable than in the mitral position. In patients under 50 years of age a homograft or autograft might sometimes be considered because they are more durable than xenografts and avoid the need for anticoagulation. Other patients usually receive a mechanical valve, unless there are contraindications to anticoagulation such as liver disease, haemorrhagic stroke, frequent falls or pregnancy.

Mitral valve

Preservation and repair of native valves is generally preferable to mitral valve replacement. Xenografts are avoided except in very elderly patients with limited life expectancy because of the need for durability.

Why might prosthetic valves become regurgitant?

Degeneration and endocarditis are the usual suspects. A trivial paravalvular leak is invariable with any prosthetic valve.

CASE 3.10

PERMANENT PACEMAKER

Instruction

Please examine this gentleman's cardiovascular system and discuss your findings.

Recognition

There is a permanent pacemaker in situ (Fig. 3.12).

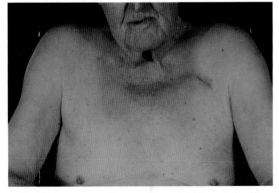

Fig. 3.12 Permanent pacemaker.

Interpretation

Confirm the diagnosis

There will usually be an additional cardiovascular finding.

What to do next – consider causes

The indications for a permanent pacemaker and other implantable cardiac devices are described below. Permanent pacemakers are most commonly inserted when ischaemic or degenerative conducting pathways give rise to sinus pauses causing presyncope or syncope.

Consider severity/decompensation/complications

Tell the examiners that regular pacemaker interrogation is necessary to ensure optimal function.

Consider function

This depends on the underlying cause. Pacemaker syndrome, now less common, arises when retrograde conduction produces atrial contraction against a closed atrioventricular valve; this leads to decreased ventricular filling and decreased cardiac output with presyncopal symptoms.

Discussion

What kinds of pacing do you know about?

Traditionally there has been a code to pacing with three letters: the first implies the paced chamber (atrium A, ventricle V or dual D), the second the sensed chamber (A, V or D) and the third the mode of pacing (inhibited I, triggered T or dual D). All modes may include R. R implies rate responsive – movement is sensed and the pacing rate increases if the pacer 'thinks' the patient is exercising.

VVI pacing via a temporary pacing wire placed into the right ventricle after inferior myocardial infarction is common. A single electrode senses QRS, a single electrode paces QRS and pacing is inhibited if QRS is sensed. In other words, this is on-demand pacing only. The operator may adjust the rate at which pacing is triggered. If the heart rate falls from 60 to 59 and the pacer is set to trigger at < 60, V will take over; thus a small change in intrinsic heart rate can result in a large change physiologically – if the patient's intrinsic heart rate happens to be around 60, continual switching in and out of pacing can be very uncomfortable and VVI pacing can produce cannon waves. AAI pacing is similar but paces the right atrium and is inhibited if P waves are sensed. It is used in sick sinus syndrome and requires normal conducting pathways distal to the atrioventricular node. The advantage is that it provides the physiological atrial 'kick' or systole. DDD dual chamber pacing is more physiological and in patients with heart block and P wave activity it has largely superseded single chamber pacing.

What do you understand by the terms underdrive and overdrive pacing for tachyarrhythmias?

Underdrive pacing was used in early pacemakers to treat supraventricular tachycardia (SVT) and ventricular tachycardia (VT). Extra stimuli are introduced at a constant interval but a slower rate than the tachycardia, until one arises during the critical period to terminate it. Because of a lack of sensing of the underlying tachycardia, there is a risk of a paced beat falling on the T wave, producing VT or ventricular fibrillation (VF) or converting atrial tachycardias into atrial fibrillation. It is not especially successful and has been superseded by *overdrive pacing*. Radiofrequency ablation has reduced some need for implantable devices to terminate arrhythmias, although pacing is increasingly used for atrial as well as ventricular arrhythmias, including selected patients with paroxysmal atrial fibrillation. Any device capable of pace termination of VT must also have defibrillatory capacity.

What drug treatments are there for ventricular arrhythmias?

Drug therapy for ventricular arrhythmias is limited by the pro-arrhythmic potential of anti-arrhythmic drugs. Agents known to safely reduce the risk of sudden cardiac death in patients with ischaemic heart disease and cardiomyopathies are beta blockers (CIBIS-II). Amiodarone can reduce risk in patients who have already had a ventricular arrhythmia but it has wide ranging side effects and primary prevention benefit after myocardial infarction has not been established.

What implantable devices are there for treating tachyarrhythmias?

These are overdrive pacing devices and implantable cardiac defibrillators.

What is an implantable cardioverter–defibrillator (ICD)?

Since the 1990s transvenous ICD systems have been implanted like a permanent pacemaker, under sedation without anaesthesia. The ICD lead is placed in the right ventricle and has one or two shock coils. It delivers a shock between the coils and the casing of the device. Devices not only defibrillate but also can recognise and treat VT by overdrive pacing and have all the functions of a bradycardia pacemaker. Dual-chamber devices are suitable for patients with atrioventricular block and have enhanced ability to discriminate between ventricular and supraventricular arrhythmias by sensing both atrial and ventricular rhythm. Ventricular fibrillation is induced at implantation to ensure function and the device is programmed with several rate zones to respond to patient's individual arrhythmia rates. Modern devices can incorporate QRS analysis and analyse to minimise the risks of inappropriate shocks in patients with rapidly conducted supraventricular arrhythmias.

What is the evidence base for ICDs?

Evidence is based on primary and secondary prevention trials:

- AVID for survivors of VT or ventricular fibrillation
- MADIT for primary prevention (at risk patients after myocardial infarction who had not had an arrhythmia which involved electrophysiological testing in patients with impaired left ventricular ejection fraction (LVEF) and ambulatory ECG monitoring)
- MADIT-2 for patients after myocardial infarction with LVEF < 30% (no need for electrophysiological testing)
- DINAMIT for timing after myocardial infarction (at least one month after)
- CABG-PATCH for inherited cardiac conditions
- SCD-HeFt for NYHA class III heart failure due to left ventricular systolic dysfunction

Should patients with non-ischaemic cardiomyopathy be considered for an ICD?

The situation is unclear, although the DEFINITE trial found significant reduction in arrhythmias but not all-cause mortality with an ICD in dilated cardiomyopathy. An ICD should probably be offered to patients with a history of syncope or documented ventricular arrhythmias.

What are the indications for ICD placement?

NICE guidance (Box 3.15) covers ICD placement in ischaemic cardiomyopathy.

Box 3.15 Recommendations for implantable cardioverter–defibrillators (ICDs) in ischaemic cardiomyopathy

Secondary prevention (one of the following in the absence of a treatable cause)

- Survival from cardiac arrest caused by ventricular tachycardia (VT) or ventricular fibrillation
- Spontaneous sustained VT causing syncope or significant haemodynamic compromise
- Sustained VT without syncope or cardiac arrest and left ventricular ejection fraction (LVEF) < 35% (no worse than NYHA class III heart failure)

Primary prevention

- History of previous (more than four weeks) myocardial infarction
  and
  either
  LVEF < 35% (no worse than NYHA class III heart failure) *and* non-sustained VT on 24-hour ECG *and* inducible VT on electrophysiological testing
  or
  LVEF < 30% (no worse than NYHA class III heart failure) *and* QRS duration ≥ 120 milliseconds
- A familial cardiac condition with high risk of sudden cardiac death, e.g. long QT, hypertrophic cardiomyopathy, Brugada syndrome, arrhythmogenic right ventricular dysplasia, surgical repair of congenital heart disease

What is cardiac resynchronisation therapy (CRT)?

Around 20% of patients with heart failure have left bundle branch block (LBBB). This can result in desynchronisation of left ventricular systolic contraction by causing delayed contraction of the posterior left ventricle relative to the septum, a phenomenon known as left ventricular dyssynchrony with significant effects on cardiac haemodynamics and symptoms. CRT partially corrects this by simultaneously pacing the septum and left ventricular free wall. The device is similar to a conventional dual-chamber pacemaker but has an additional ventricular lead, which is introduced via a guiding catheter into the coronary venous system via the coronary sinus, which drains into the right atrium. CRT works by sensing sinus node activity via the atrial lead and simultaneously pacing both ventricles in response to each sensed sinus beat. For this reason, it has not been evaluated extensively in atrial fibrillation. Evidence for CRT has evolved from the MIRACLE, COMPANION and CARE-HF trials. CRT indications are evolving but CRT significantly improves symptoms, exercise tolerance and quality of life in patients in sinus rhythm with moderate to severe heart failure and reduces mortality. Further, combined CRT and ICD device therapies may confer incremental risk reduction.

CASE 3.11

INFECTIVE ENDOCARDITIS

Instruction

Please examine this lady's hands and then auscultate the heart. Discuss your proposed further assessment and management.

Recognition

Peripheral signs include *anaemia, clubbing, Janeway lesions* (non-tender red palmar or plantar haemorrhagic macules or pustules), *Osler's nodes* (tender nodules of the finger and toe pulps), *splinter haemorrhages* and areas of *digital infarction*. A *murmur* is present (state location and describe).

Janeway lesions and Osler's nodes are the result of immunological activity or septic embolisation and are less common peripheral stigmata these days because infective endocarditis tends to present at an earlier stage. Vasculitic phenomena, such as splinter haemorrhages are more common; splinter haemorrhages appear as red lines for the first two or three days and are brown thereafter (Fig. 3.13).

Interpretation

Confirm the diagnosis

Tell the examiners that diagnosis is supported by high inflammatory markers and confirmed by positive blood

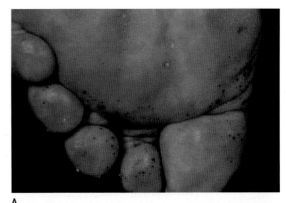

A

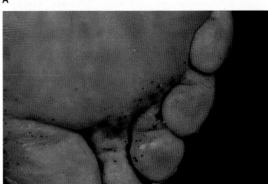

B

Fig. 3.13 (A,B) Vasculitic rash.

cultures (multiple, from different sites) and transthoracic or transoesophageal echocardiographic evidence of vegetations. Blood cultures are positive in over 90% of patients cultured from two sites, provided an antibiotic has not been administered. Serological assays and polymerase chain reaction testing may aid diagnosis when organisms are difficult to culture. Criteria for diagnosing infective endocarditis are outlined below.

What to do next – consider causes/assess other systems

Tell the examiners you would ask about:

* Valvular or congenital heart disease
* Recent surgery or dental procedures

Tell the examiners you would look for:

* Fever, and a history of rigors and night sweats
* Roth's spots
* Splenomegaly – because of the generalised activation of the reticuloendothelial system in subacute bacterial endocarditis
* Haematuria

Note that in right-sided endocarditis, peripheral stigmata will not occur.

Box 3.16 Complications of infective endocarditis

- Disseminated sepsis and multi-organ failure
- Embolic complications: these affect around 30% of patients and are often the presenting feature – up to two-thirds are neurological complications (e.g. stroke, cerebral metastatic abscess formation, mycotic aneurysms – septic embolisation of vegetations to a vessel wall, more common in delayed presentation) but other sites of embolic spread include the lungs, spleen, kidneys, gut and liver
- Valve destruction and heart failure; changing murmurs are common, indicating change in size of a vegetation or embolisation of part thereof, or worsening valve destruction
- Intracardiac abscess formation, e.g. aortic root abscess
- Pulmonary emboli (common in intravenous drug users, seeding from tricuspid vegetations)
- Circulating immune complexes causing glomerulonephritis

Consider severity/decompensation/complications

Tell the examiners of possible complications (Box 3.16).

Consider function

This is dependent on symptoms and the underlying cause.

Discussion

How does infective endocarditis arise?

Infective endocarditis arises when trauma or ulceration to the valvular endothelial surface promotes bacterial adherence by one of two mechanisms. Firstly, it could induce a valve thrombus when subendothelial components are in direct contact with blood; pathogens arising in transient bacteraemia bind avidly to this potential culture medium and subsequent cytokine activation by monocytes progressively enlarges the subsequent vegetation. Secondly, local inflammation promotes the cellular expression of transmembrane proteins that bind fibronectin; pathogens such as *Staphylococcus aureus* carry fibronectin-binding protein on their surface and so can adhere to the inflammatory focus. Staphylococcal endocarditis often occurs on previously normal valves, probably induced by microulcerations.

Valve trauma is more likely in the presence of a structurally abnormal valve or where there is turbulent blood flow. High shear stress is more likely in the region of the mitral and aortic valves, the tricuspid and pulmonary valves being colonised with decreased frequency, respectively. Once seeded with infection, 'vegetations' tend to appear downstream of the jet of blood flow on the low-pressure side of the valve (e.g. the ventricular side of the aortic valve) normally close to the closure line of the leaflet.

What is a vegetation?

A vegetation is a collection of platelets, fibrin, microorganisms and inflammatory cells.

How does the bacteraemia that causes infective endocarditis arise?

Bacteraemia is usually part of a nosocomial or iatrogenic infection. Areas more heavily colonised with bacteria (mouth, gastrointestinal tract) are more likely to predispose to bacteraemia. Bacteraemia can occur with very mild trauma, dental interventions being a notable, although hitherto overemphasised, source, whilst cumulative risks from routine tooth-brushing may be underestimated. Intravenous drug users are at particularly high risk. NICE guidelines do not advocate prophylaxis for gastrointestinal, genitourinary, respiratory or gynaecological procedures.

Which valve lesions are susceptible to infective endocarditis?

These are any valve disease (commonly degenerative, mitral valve prolapse with regurgitation, prostheses or damage from previous endocarditis, but historically rheumatic), hypertrophic cardiomyopathy or congenital heart disease. ASD endocarditis is rare.

Which organisms cause endocarditis?

The profile of organisms varies geographically and changes over time.

Native valve endocarditis

This has tended to be the caused by viridans streptococci, which colonise the oral cavity, lower gastrointestinal tract and genitourinary tract, but may also be the result of staphylococci, Gram-negative bacilli (e.g. enterococcus via bowel pathology or urinary tract infection) or organisms that are notoriously culture negative, such as the HACEK group of organisms (*Haemophilus* species, *Actinobacillus actinomycetemcomitans*, *Cadiobacterium hominis*, *Eikenella corrodens*, *Kingella* species), *Coxiella burnetti*, *Brucella*, *Bartonella*, *Chlamydia*, and fungi and yeasts (*Candida*, *Aspergillus*, *Histoplasma*, *Cryptococcus*). Antibiotic use remains the most common cause for culture negativity, however. Staphylococci, especially *S. aureus*, are now surpassing viridans streptococci as the most common cause of endocarditis. *Staphylococcus lugdunensis* is a less common but particularly destructive cause of endocarditis, surviving patients usually needing valve replacement. The most common streptococci continue to be *Strep. sanguis*, *Strep. bovis*, *Strep. mutans* and *Strep. mitis*. *Streptococcus bovis* is especially common in older people with colonic lesions. Native valve endocarditis is more common in men, with an increasing incidence in older people as valves degenerate and nosocomial infection becomes more likely.

Prosthetic valve endocarditis

This accounts for around 10–15% of infective endocarditis. It may occur early, mostly caused by coagulase-negative staphylococci, including *S. aureus* and *S. epidermidis*, or late with a similar organism profile to native valve disease.

Table 3.16 Modified Duke Criteria for diagnosing infective endocarditis

Major	Microbiological If infective endocarditis likely and haemodynamic compromise, treatment should start immediately after three sets of blood cultures at separate sites; otherwise, diagnostic work-up should pre-empt treatment		Typical microorganism isolated from two separate blood cultures: viridans streptococci, *Streptococcus bovis*, HACEK group, *Staphylococcus aureus* or community-acquired enterococcal bacteraemia without a primary focus
			Microorganism consistent with but less specific for infective endocarditis isolated from persistently positive blood cultures
			Single positive blood culture for *Coxiella burnetii* or appropriate serology for *Coxiella burnetii*, *Bartonella* species or *Chlamydia psittici*
			Positive molecular assays for specific gene targets
	Evidence of endocardial involvement		Positive echocardiogram showing oscillating structures, abscess formation, new valvular regurgitation, or dehiscence of prosthetic valves
Minor	Predisposition (includes predisposing heart disease and injection drug-use)	High risk	Previous infective endocarditis Aortic valve disease Rheumatic heart disease Prosthetic valve Aortic coarctation Acyanotic congenital heart disease
		Moderate risk	Mitral valve prolapse with mitral regurgitation or leaflet thickening Isolated mitral stenosis Tricuspid valve disease Pulmonary stenosis Hypertrophic cardiomyopathy
		Low or no risk	Secundum atrial septal defect Ischaemic heart disease Previous coronary artery bypass grafting Mitral valve prolapse with thin leaflets in absence of mitral regurgitation
	Fever	> 38°C	
	Vascular phenomena	e.g. major emboli, splenomegaly, clubbing, splinter haemorrhages, petechiae or purpura	
	Immunological phenomena	e.g. glomerulonephritis, Osler's nodes, Roth's spots, positive rheumatoid factor	
	Microbiological findings	Positive blood cultures that do not meet major criteria	
	Elevated C-reactive protein or erythrocyte sedimentation rate		
Pathological	Positive histology or microbiology of autopsy or cardiac surgery material		

Definite infective endocarditis is diagnosed by positive pathological criteria OR two major criteria OR one major and two minor criteria OR five minor criteria.

How do subacute bacterial endocariditis (SBE) and acute bacterial endocarditis differ?

The term infective endocarditis is generally replacing these two terms. Viridans streptococci grow slowly and have tended to be associated with SBE, presenting with fevers and weight loss. *Staphylococcus aureus* tends to cause acute bacterial endocarditis and is common in patients with prosthetic heart valves and in intravenous drug users; acute fever is more likely, as are abscess formation, valve destruction and metastatic infection causing brain abscesses and intracerebral haemorrhage. Fungi and *S. aureus* carry the highest mortality.

Do you know of any criteria that can aid diagnosis?

The Duke criteria were initially proposed in 1994 to standardise diagnostic criteria and have been modified recently (Table 3.16).

What is the most common valve lesion predisposing to infective endocarditis?

Mitral valve prolapse is the most common valve lesion.

List some indications for urgent surgery in infective endocarditis

- Haemodynamic compromise due to valve destruction
- Persistent infection or fever despite appropriate antimicrobial therapy
- Development of abscesses or fistulas because of perivalvular spread of infection
- Involvement of highly resistant organisms
- Prosthetic valve endocarditis, especially when early postoperative
- Large vegetations with high embolic potential (> 10 mm or on mitral valve)

CASE 3.12

CONGENITAL ACYANOTIC HEART DISEASE – VENTRICULAR SEPTAL DEFECT, ATRIAL SEPTAL DEFECT, PATENT DUCTUS ARTERIOSUS, AORTIC COARCTATION

Instruction

This gentleman has a congenital heart murmur. Please examine his cardiovascular system and report your findings.

Recognition

At birth, pulmonary vascular resistance falls as the lungs inflate and more blood flows through them. Left atrial blood flow increases causing closure of the foramen ovale (a connection between the atria). The ductus arteriosus usually closes within 24 hours of birth. Congenital heart disease is common and often multiple abnormalities occur. It may be acyanotic or cyanotic (Table 3.17).

Ventricular septal defect (VSD)

There is a *pansystolic murmur* and often a *thrill* at the *left sternal edge*. This represents blood flowing from the high-pressure left ventricle to the low-pressure right ventricle. There may be a *mid-diastolic flow murmur* at the apex and a *right ventricular heave* due to right ventricular volume overload.

Atrial septal defect (ASD)

Ostium secundum atrial septal defect (OS ASD)

This is the commonest ASD, presenting in childhood or adulthood. There is a *right ventricular heave*, reflecting right ventricular overload with hypertrophy. Left to right shunting causes increased flow across the pulmonary valve and results in an *ejection systolic murmur* in the *pulmonary area* (left second/third intercostal space). *S2* (A2–P2) is *widely split*, because of delayed pulmonary valve closure (Table 3.8), and *fixed*. ASDs are often large and under low pressure with little turbulence, and it is a common misconception that the murmur is the result of the ASD itself. There may also be a *mid-diastolic flow murmur* across the *tricuspid valve* (heard best at the left fourth intercostal space).

Ostium primum ASD (OP ASD)

This is less common and usually presents in childhood with associated mitral regurgitation.

Patent ductus arteriosus (PDA)

Small defect

There is a *loud continuous 'machinery' murmur*. This is caused by the increased blood flow through the lungs (pulmonary arteriovenous fistulae also sound like this). The continuous murmur is *pansystolic/early diastolic* and heard best over *the left upper sternal edge and clavicle*. There may be an associated *thrill*.

Large defect

There is a *collapsing pulse* (aortic diastolic run-off), and a *mid-diastolic tricuspid flow murmur* because of right-sided heart overload.

Aortic coarctation

There are *large volume radial pulses* (left may be weaker) and there is vigorous *carotid pulsation* (although aortic regurgitation is a much more common cause). Blood pressure would be lower in the legs than arms and there is *radiofemoral delay* – the femoral pulse is delayed and of small volume. There is an *ejection systolic murmur* (which may be loud posteriorly but not audible anteriorly). There are *bruits* over the *scapulae, anterior axillary areas and left sternal edge* (internal mammary artery). *Collateral* blood vessels may be visible when the patient sits forward.

Table 3.17 Congenital heart disease			
Acyanotic (majority of congenital heart disease)			Cyanotic
With left to right shunt (high to low pressure unless shunt reversal occurs)	Without shunt		Always right to left shunt
Ventricular septal defect Atrial septal defect Patent ductus arteriosus and other aorto-pulmonary shunts Aortic root to right heart shunts Multilevel shunts	Aortic coarctation (narrowing just below the origin of the left subclavian artery) Congenital left heart inflow abnormalities, e.g. pulmonary vein stenosis Congenital mitral stenosis Congenital mitral regurgitation Congenital aortic stenosis Ebstein's anomaly Congenital pulmonary stenosis Congenital pulmonary regurgitation		Fallot's tetralogy Transposition of the great arteries (TGA), which presents at birth Eisenmenger's syndrome

Interpretation

Confirm the diagnosis

Tell the examiners that further investigations include ECG, chest X-ray, echocardiography and cardiac catheterisation (Table 3.18).

What to do next – consider causes/assess other systems

Tell the examiners likely causes and associations (Table 3.19).

Consider severity/decompensation/complications

Tell the examiners of important potential complications (Table 3.20).

Consider function

The patient might look well or chronically unwell (e.g. underweight, cyanosed, clubbed).

Discussion

Where do types of VSD occur?

There are four common sites for VSDs:

- *Membranous septum* ('infracristal') – the most common site, just behind the medial papillary muscle of the tricuspid valve which may oppose it and help it to close spontaneously
- *Muscular septum* – variable site and may be multiple (acquired VSD after septal infarction is usually the 'Swiss cheese' type)
- *Infundibular* ('supracristal') – a high VSD just beneath the pulmonary valve and below the right coronary cusp of the aortic valve; the latter may be inadequately supported and prolapse, causing aortic regurgitation; an infundibular VSD may also be associated with malalignment of the infundibular septum, e.g. with shift of the septum to the right as in

Table 3.18 Diagnosing acyanotic congenital heart disease

Ventricular septal defect	Atrial septal defect (ASD)	Patent ductus arteriosus	Aortic coarctation
ECG may show signs of right or left ventricular hypertrophy Chest X-ray may show enlarged pulmonary arteries Echocardiography and cardiac catheterisation would confirm anatomical abnormalities, pressures and oxygen saturations	ECG differentiates between ostium secundum (OS) and ostium primum (OP) ASDs – OS ASDs tend to cause right bundle branch block and right axis deviation and OP ASDs cause right bundle branch block and left axis deviation Echocardiography confirms suspicions	Diagnosed by echocardiography	ECG may show left ventricular hypertrophy Chest X-ray may show rib notching on the inferior surfaces of ribs due to tortuous arterial collaterals and there may be a 'figure 3' pattern resulting from an upper bulge (the left subclavian artery, a notch (representing coarctation) and a lower bulge (poststenotic dilatation) Thoracic imaging confirms suspicions

Table 3.19 Causes and associations in acyanotic congenital heart disease

Ventricular septal defect	Atrial septal defect (ASD)	Patent ductus arteriosus	Aortic coarctation
Usually congenital Occasionally post myocardial infarction	Holt–Oram syndrome: Ostium secundum ASD + hypoplastic thumbs Lutembacher syndrome: ASD + rheumatic mitral stenosis Usually isolated	Congenital	Usually idiopathic (males, commonly, sometimes asymptomatic until adulthood and presenting at around the third decade with hypertension) Turner's syndrome

Table 3.20 Complications in acyanotic congenital heart disease

Ventricular septal defect (VSD)	Atrial septal defect	Patent ductus arteriosus	Aortic coarctation
Infective endocarditis Aortic regurgitation due to prolapse of right coronary cusp (5% of VSDs) Infundibular stenosis – right-sided heart failure Reversal of shunt and Eisenmenger's syndrome (cyanosis)	Infective endocarditis Atrial fibrillation Eisenmenger's syndrome (cyanosis)	Infective endocarditis Pulmonary hypertension Eisenmenger's syndrome (cyanosis)	Infective endocarditis Hypertension (may persist post surgery) Bicuspid aortic valve Cerebral aneurysms

Fallot's tetralogy or shift of the septum to the left with a double outlet left ventricle and subaortic stenosis.

- *Posterior* (atrioventricular defect) – a paratricuspid defect

How are VSDs treated?

Small defects often close spontaneously in childhood, especially membranous VSDs. Infundibular VSDs do not close spontaneously. VSDs should be assessed regularly for complications and closed before the onset of Eisenmenger's syndrome. Indications for surgery include recurrent endocarditis, aortic regurgitation or volume overload, and acute septal rupture.

When should surgery be contemplated for an ASD?

The OS ASDs have traditionally been closed in or before the third decade, but recent thinking is that there may be less gained from surgery in asymptomatic adults.

CASE 3.13

CYANOTIC HEART DISEASE – EISENMENGER'S SYNDROME, FALLOT'S TETRALOGY

Instruction

This young lady has a congenital heart murmur. Please examine her cardiovascular system and report your findings.

Recognition

There is *cyanosis*, *clubbing*, a *right ventricular heave* and an *intense pulmonary ejection systolic murmur* at the *left sternal edge* with an associated *thrill*.

Interpretation

Confirm the diagnosis

Tell the examiners that further investigations include ECG, chest X-ray, echocardiography and cardiac catheterisation. In Fallot's tetralogy the ECG usually shows sinus rhythm, right axis deviation and right ventricular hypertrophy with right bundle branch block and the chest X-ray shows a classic *coeur en sabot* (heart in a boot) shape.

What to do next – consider causes

Cyanotic congenital heart disease may be the result of Eisenmenger's syndrome or primary cyanotic congenital heart disease. Transposition of the great arteries is managed at birth but Fallot's tetralogy is, occasionally, not detected until the second or third decade, especially in people from

countries with poorly resourced health care. The complete syndrome comprises:

- Ventricular septal defect with right to left shunt
- Aorta overriding septal defect
- Pulmonary stenosis (resulting in diversion of right ventricular blood straight into the aorta)
- Right ventricular hypertrophy

Consider severity/decompensation/complications

Eisenmenger's syndrome or primary cyanotic congenital heart disease represents a decompensated situation. Other complications of Fallot's tetralogy include poor growth, infective endocarditis and cerebral abscesses (absence of lung filter with left to right shunt).

Consider function

The patient might look well or chronically unwell (e.g. underweight, cyanosed, clubbed).

Discussion

What is Eisenmenger's syndrome?

Longstanding right-sided heart overload leads to pulmonary hypertension and reversal of the left to right shunt (Eisenmenger's syndrome). It leads to clubbing and central cyanosis and the progressive backward pressure consequences of pulmonary hypertension.

How is Fallot's tetralogy treated?

Treatments include total correction or Blalock–Taussig shunting, in which the left subclavian artery is anastomosed to the left pulmonary artery to increase pulmonary blood flow.

CASE 3.14

HYPERTROPHIC (OBSTRUCTIVE) CARDIOMYOPATHY

Instruction

This 35-year-old gentleman is thought to have a heart murmur. Please examine his cardiovascular system and report your findings.

Recognition

The arterial *pulse* is *jerky*. A sharp early rise of rapid ejection is followed by a late systolic phase as the dynamic obstruction supervenes (Fig. 3.14). Contrast this with the slow rising plateau pulse of aortic stenosis in which there is obstruction from the outset of systole (Table 3.22). There may be an '*a*' wave in the jugular venous pulse reflecting forceful atrial contraction of a hypertrophied atrium. There is a *double impulse at the apex*; this represents presystolic ventricular expansion from forceful atrial systole followed by a systolic left ventricular heave.

There may be a *fourth heart sound* due to atrial systole. A *late systolic ejection murmur at the left sternal edge* is caused by dynamic obstruction (Fig. 3.14). This may be associated with a *systolic thrill at the left sternal edge*, from turbulence. There may be an associated *pansystolic murmur at the apex* because mitral regurgitation is commonly associated. These findings suggest classic hypertrophic (obstructive) cardiomyopathy.

Interpretation

Confirm the diagnosis

Tell the examiners that you would ask about presenting symptoms, which may include any of the features in Box 3.17.

Tell the examiners that you would perform dynamic auscultation (Table 3.21).

What to do next – consider causes

Differentiate clinically between an ejection systolic murmur due to hypertrophic (obstructive) cardiomyopathy and one due to aortic stenosis, the latter in a young person often being the result of a congenital biscuspid valve (Table 3.22).

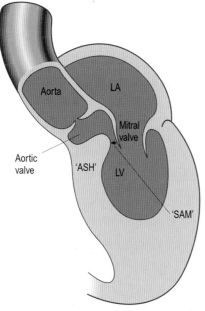

Fig. 3.14 Asymmetrical septal hypertrophy (ASH) and systolic anterior motion (SAM) during systole. LA, left atrium, LV, left ventricle.

Box 3.17 Symptoms of hypertrophic cardiomyopathy

- Asymptomatic
- Dyspnoea on exertion and symptoms of heart failure (diastolic dysfunction)
- Syncope or presyncope
- Palpitations (ventricular arrhythmias or atrial fibrillation common)
- Chest pain (in the absence of coronary atherosclerosis possibly microvascular dysfunction)
- Family history of syncope or sudden cardiac death
- Sudden cardiac death

Table 3.21 Effect of dynamic manoeuvres on murmur of hypertrophic (obstructive) cardiomyopathy

Manoeuvre		Effect
Valsalva Reduces venous return		Louder because reduced heart filling in diastole worsens the subsequent dynamic obstruction
Position	**Standing** Reduces venous return	Louder
	Squatting or passive leg raising Enhances venous return	Softer
Exercise	**Isometric** (hand grip) Enhances venous return	Softer

---

Table 3.22 Aortic stenosis versus hypertrophic (obstructive) cardiomyopathy

	Aortic stenosis	Hypertrophic (obstructive) cardiomyopathy
Carotid character	Slow rising	Bifid, jerky
Thrill	Upper right parasternal area	Lower left parasternal area
Ejection murmur	Characteristic up and down stroke around mid-systole	Late systolic
Aortic early diastolic murmur	Often present	Rare
Effect of manoeuvres	Fixed murmur	Variable murmur

Table 3.23 Risk stratification of hypertrophic cardiomyopathy

Risk stratification	Features	Treatment
High	Family history of premature sudden death Extreme left ventricular hypertrophy (≥ 30 mm) in young patients Unexplained syncope in young patients Non-sustained ventricular tachycardia (NSVT) in patients aged ≤ 30 years Abnormal blood pressure response during exercise	Implantable cardioverter defibrillator for primary prevention if high-risk features or secondary prevention if sustained ventricular tachycardia or survived cardiac arrest
Low	Mild left ventricular hypertrophy (< 20 mm) and no risk factors	Medical therapy as required

Consider severity/decompensation/complications

Hypertrophic cardiomyopathy (HCM) is a heterogeneous disease with a wide spectrum of severity, and classic hypertrophic (obstructive) cardiomyopathy occupies only a small part (around 20%) of that spectrum. In HCM the myocardium is hypertrophied. Septal hypertrophy usually dominates and asymmetrical septal hypertrophy (ASH) is the characteristic pattern. There may, in addition to hypertrophy, be obstruction to the left ventricular outflow tract, which is dynamic, appearing in late systole – the hypertrophied septum distorts systolic movement of the left ventricle, and the most significant effect of this is systolic anterior movement of the anterior leaflet of the mitral valve (SAM); this results in mid-late systolic subaortic obstruction caused by mitral–septal contact and occurs at rest. There may also be diastolic dysfunction generated by stiffness of the hypertrophied ventricle.

Neither the severity of symptoms nor the left ventricular outflow gradient appear to correlate with prognosis as much as the underlying genetic mutation. However, outflow obstruction is associated with an increased risk of heart failure and sudden death. Features helpful in risk stratification are listed in Table 3.23.

Consider function

Tell the examiners you would establish the limitations provoked by symptoms (although often asymptomatic).

Discussion

What is meant by the term cardiomyopathy?

It generally refers to structural or functional myocardial disease in the absence of coronary disease, hypertension, valvular heart disease and congenital heart disease.

How common is HCM?

HCM is the most common familial genetic disease of the heart (from 1:500 to 1:1000) and the most common cause of sudden cardiac death in young people and athletes.

What is the cause of HCM?

The genetic basis is a mutation in one of the genes coding for one of the myocardial contractile proteins – β-myosin heavy chain, cardiac myosin binding protein C, cardiac troponin I, troponin T, troponin C, α-tropomyosin, essential myosin light chain, regulatory myosin light chain, cardiac actin, β myosin heavy chain, titin. A large number of mutations have been described, many with autosomal dominant inheritance, which share the basic histopathological consequence of myocardial fibre disarray. The major risk is arrhythmias resulting from the microarchitecture, such that the high proportion of people with hypertrophic cardiomyopathy without any obstructive features are at no less risk. Indeed, the greater determinant of risk is the underlying microarchitectural type. Some patients at risk even have no detectable hypertrophy.

Other causes of HCM with a systemic basis include glycogen and lycosomal storage diseases, diseases of fatty acid metabolism, mitochondrial cytopathies, athletic training, obesity, amyloidosis and genetic syndromes such as LEOPARD syndrome.

What might the ECG show in HCM?

The ECG might show left ventricular hypertrophy, deep Q waves and conduction defects. It may be normal.

What might the echocardiogram show in HCM?

The echocardiogram might confirm ASH and SAM in HCM, and there might be almost complete obliteration of the left ventricular cavity with a large outflow tract gradient.

Does magnetic resonance imaging have a place in evaluating hypertrophic cardiomyopathy?

Magnetic resonance imaging might detect hypertrophy that is confined to segments that are not identifiable on echocardiography.

How might the diagnosis be confirmed?

DNA analysis is now the definitive method for diagnosing many genetic diseases. However, hypertrophic cardiomyopathy is caused by mutations in any one of the genes encoding proteins of the cardiac sarcomere and DNA analysis for diagnostic and screening purposes is not currently routine.

What are the treatment options for HCM?

Because of the relative rarity of hypertrophic cardiomyopathy, randomised trials have not been conducted for treatment, and remain unlikely. Evidence is based on retrospective studies and clinical experience.

Medical treatment of heart failure

Dyspnoea on exertion in hypertrophic cardiomyopathy is usually the result of heart failure, and heart failure, to a great extent, reflects diastolic dysfunction because of the stiff left ventricle. Systolic function is usually well preserved. Medical treatment with beta blockers improves the exertional symptoms in patients with outflow obstruction but has not been shown to modify the clinical course. Diuretics are sometimes useful. Angiotensin-converting enzyme inhibitors must be used with caution because by reducing afterload they may favour the development or worsening of outflow obstruction. Atrial fibrillation develops in around 20% of patients with hypertrophic cardiomyopathy and is rate controlled with beta blockers or verapamil and anticoagulation is usually indicated for thromboembolic prophylaxis.

Surgery

Patients with marked outflow obstruction (≥ 50 mmHg at rest) and severe symptoms (NYHA class III or IV) that are unresponsive to medical therapy represent about 5% of patients with HCM and may be considered for surgical myectomy or alcohol septal ablation to relieve outflow obstruction.

Prevention of sudden cardiac death

A cardioverter defibrillator is the only effective treatment for prevention of sudden cardiac death. Indications include high-risk features (see Table 3.23).

Is prophylaxis against infective endocarditis needed in HCM?

It is only indicated if there is obstruction at rest.

Does HCM increase pregnancy risk?

It generally carries little additional risk.

What lifestyle consequences are there for people with HCM?

Competitive sports associated with intense exertion or other strenuous physical activities should be avoided. People with a favourable clinical profile – asymptomatic, normal or only mildly increased left atrial dimension (< 45 mm), mild left ventricular hypertrophy (< 20 mm), no outflow obstruction at rest, no risk factors for sudden death – may participate in sports associated with mild or moderate physical activity.

What is the current screening practice for HCM?

Genetic screening is complex, as alluded to. Clinical screening of first-degree relatives is based on ECG and echocardiographic evaluation and is recommended every two years in children (when disease can change rapidly with growth) and every five years in adults.

What is dilated cardiomyopathy?

This refers to a dilated ventricle in the absence of ischaemic heart disease or abnormal loading (hypertension or valvular heart disease) and causes systolic dysfunction. Causes include alcohol, genetic disorders (Duchenne muscular dystrophy, myotonic dystrophy), nutritional deficiencies (e.g. thiamine), inflammatory causes (infection, toxic, eosinophilic) and drugs (e.g. anthracyclines).

What is restrictive cardiomyopathy?

Myocardial infiltration generally results in a degree of restriction. Amyloidosis and sarcoidosis are important causes. Haemochromatosis can cause dilatation or restriction. Endomyocardial fibrosis is a chronic non-eosinophilic condition affecting young Africans and is difficult to treat. Loefler's endocarditis is an aggressive, eosinophilic cause of restriction. Diastolic dysfunction and conduction disturbances are the common manifestations of restrictive cardiomyopathy. Breathlessness, a positive Kussmaul's sign and other symptoms of heart failure without radiological evidence of cardiac enlargement should alert suspicion. The main differential diagnosis is constrictive pericarditis. Treatment is tricky.

What is myocarditis?

Myocarditis is relatively uncommon and caused by viruses (e.g. coxsackievirus), radiation, drugs, chemicals (e.g. lead) and Chagas' disease. It results in a dilated heart and heart failure, often in young adults. Sudden cardiac death is a possible complication and as well as treating heart failure, the cause should be identified where possible and, at least in the early stages of the insult when sudden death appears especially risky, excessive exertion should be avoided. Around one-third of patients die or proceed to cardiac transplant, one-third have residual symptoms and one-third return to a normal life.

CASE 3.15

PERICARDIAL RUB AND PERICARDIAL DISEASE

Instruction

This patient is thought to have pericardial disease. Please examine her and discuss your diagnosis.

Recognition

Pericarditis

There may be a *pericardial rub*. This is a scratching or creaking sound, like snow underfoot or sometimes a little more high-pitched like the creaking of timbers on an old ship. It is usually only apparent over an isolated area of cardiac auscultation and often changes or disappears with position, as does the patient's pain. It may be present at any stage in the cardiac cycle, but is often systolic.

Constrictive pericarditis

The signs of a constricted pericardium are similar to restrictive cardiomyopathy – both result in a *raised jugular venous pulse with prominent x and y descents*, and *non-pulsatile hepatomegaly*. There may be a *pericardial knock*, representing an abrupt halt to rapid ventricular filling. There is often ascites and peripheral oedema, although signs of pulmonary congestion are absent.

Pericardial effusion

There may be a raised jugular venous pulse with hypotension and quiet heart sounds.

Interpretation

Confirm the diagnosis

Tell the examiners that you would like to see an ECG (saddle-shaped ST segments in pericarditis – often in only some leads reflecting patchy inflammation, small complexes in pericardial effusion), a chest X-ray (large globular heart shadow in pericardial effusion) and an echocardiogram. Acute pericarditis typically presents with pleuritic central chest pain, worse lying flat and relieved sitting forwards. Raising the legs of the supine patient to increase venous return classically induces sudden pericardial pain in pericarditis, which then eases as the legs are again lowered.

What to do next – consider causes

Tell the examiners that common causes of pericarditis include viruses (e.g. coxsackievirus), tuberculosis, autoimmune-disease-associated serositis, malignancy, Dressler's syndrome (post-myocardial infarction with fever), drugs, hypothyroidism and uraemia. Constrictive pericarditis is classically the result of tuberculosis, but is more usually caused by viruses, and sometimes malignancy. All causes may lead to a pericardial effusion.

Consider severity/decompensation/complications

Pericarditis may lead to pericardial effusion and even tamponade (small volume pulse, hypotension, raised jugular venous pulse). An ECG might show small complexes. Echocardiography is essential to estimate the volume of

Table 3.24 Signs differentiating constrictive pericarditis from cardiac tamponade

Constrictive pericarditis	Tamponade
Prominent x and y descents	Prominent x descent
Kussmaul's sign positive	Kussmaul's sign negative
Pulsus paradoxus uncommon	Pulsus paradoxus present
Pericardial knock	No pericardial knock

fluid accumulated, assess cardiac contractility and guide diagnostic or therapeutic pericardiocentesis. Pericarditis may be part of a myopericarditis, in which the troponin is elevated. Constrictive pericarditis causes diastolic dysfunction.

Consider function

Tell the examiners you would establish the limitations provoked by any symptoms.

Discussion

What ECG changes may be seen in pericarditis?

There is classically concave, saddle-shaped ST elevation, typically more widespread than in STEMI, involving more than one coronary territory. But it may be normal. T wave inversion may occur before the ECG normalises. Atrial repolarisation is affected, leading to PR elevation in aVR (in association with ST depression) and PR depression elsewhere (in association with ST elevation). Q waves do not develop and reciprocal ST depression does not occur.

How is pericarditis managed?

This is symptomatic, with non-steroidal anti-inflammatory drugs. Anticoagulants should be discontinued and any underlying cause treated. Steroids may be given if it relapses.

Which signs help differentiate constrictive pericarditis from cardiac tamponade?

Differentiating signs are shown in Table 3.24.

How is constrictive pericarditis treated?

In addition to treating the underlying causes, pericardectomy is the definitive treatment to release constriction.

NERVOUS SYSTEM

Examination of the nervous system – overview

Context

Candidates (and examiners!) find neurological examination difficult. They find it difficult to know what to do, what they are looking for and how to interpret their findings.

The nervous system is complicated; the human brain comprises one hundred billion neurons, each neuron making thousands of synaptic connections with others, and it has been calculated that the number of possible permutations of brain activity or information exchange exceeds the number of elementary particles in the known universe. Not surprisingly, different neurologists and cognitive neuroscientists have different ways of approaching such a complex body system; more than any other specialty, there is often a sense of inaccessibility to those outside it. Lists of signs are somewhere in memory like fragments of jigsaw but form no real picture. 'Absent ankle jerks and extensor plantars' is a list learned by rote and raised to a mythical proportion of difficulty.

Although science is poised to understand a lot more about the human brain, to de-mystify this walnut-shaped piece of jelly that subserves all that humans think and do, neurologists and neuroscientists remain in the shallows. You may feel you have not set foot in the water, but remember that in this largely unexplored ocean your interpretations may be as valid as anyone's. To make some sense of the nervous system, it is necessary to oversimplify it, and there is nothing wrong with that. To get glimpses of how it really works, two things often help us. The first is to understand things from an evolutionary vantage; this often helps to explain why things might be so. The second is to understand neurological curiosities, anomalies and disease; these often help to explain how the normal brain works. More and more, the study of curious diseases is providing insights into the murky neuroscientific ocean, exchanging it for a giant aquarium as the windows slowly slot into place.

Neurological examination is best performed in context. Rather than trying to examine everything hurriedly and with little grasp of what you are looking for, it is better to be selective. Patients with different neurological problems need different types of examination.

Levels of the nervous system

A basic grasp of the different levels of the nervous system and the patterns of signs that arise from disease at these different levels helps candidates know what to do, what to look for and how to interpret their findings. Interpreting findings should be anatomical and pathological.

Box 3.18 Levels of the nervous system

- Cranial nerves (peripheral nerves of the head and neck)
- Cerebral hemispheres
- Brainstem
- Extrapyramidal system and cerebellum
- Spinal cord
- Nerve plexi
- Nerve roots
- Specific nerves
- Neuromuscular junction
- Muscles

Anatomical interpretation of findings

Attempt to identify if there is one or more than one lesion and the level or levels involved (Box 3.18). Findings may form a recognisable syndrome, such as Horner's syndrome or Parkinsonism, but diseases may also coexist. A combination of upper and lower motor neuron signs in an older patient is common with cervical myelopathy, multilevel radiculopathy and peripheral neuropathy. Remember that systems degenerate with age and as neuronal reserve declines so vision, hearing, balance, reflexes and gait can change. In general, signs are more likely to represent pathology if there are associated symptoms. If you think 'perhaps the left triceps jerk is a little less brisk than the right', it may well be normal.

Pathological interpretation of findings

Consider which diseases are consistent with the anatomical findings. History taking is the most important part of neurological assessment because it helps to localise the level and site of a lesion and determine its duration – intermittent unilateral headache for many years is likely to be migraine, abrupt hemiparesis and facial weakness is likely to be cerebral ischaemia; worsening sensory symptoms over a few months in the median nerve distribution is likely to be carpal tunnel syndrome and so forth. Since history taking is not possible in PACES, the examination schemes that follow are selective sequences appropriate for the cases that are likely to occur in PACES. With any examination, remember that neurology is a highly observational specialty. Much can be missed by stepping forward instantly to examine 'hands on'.

Examination of the cranial nerves

Introduction

Cranial nerves in context

When we examine the limbs we consider upper and lower neuron lesions. Cranial nerves are simply lower (motor, sensory or both) neurons. Examining them in order from I to XII detracts from the concept that these peripheral nerves connect proximally via their nuclei with central nerves and distally with neuromuscular junctions and muscles (Fig. 3.15). What we are really doing with so-called 'cranial nerve' examination is examining the head

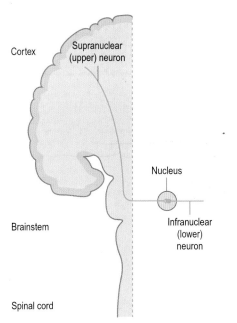

Fig. 3.15 Supranuclear, nuclear and infranuclear arrangement of the nervous system.

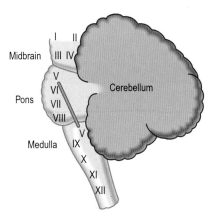

Fig. 3.16 Location of cranial nerve nuclei in the brainstem. I–XII nuclei present bilaterally.

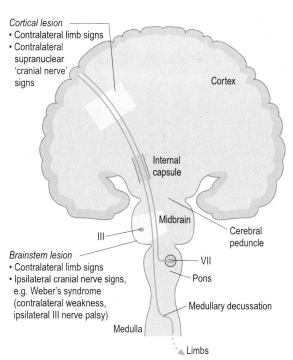

Fig. 3.17 Cortical versus brainstem lesions. Cerebellum not shown for simplification.

and neck and when examining head and neck neurology a functional approach is more logical than a numerical one – examining 'the eyes', 'visual fields', 'eye movements' and so on rather than 'the cranial nerves'.

The value of cranial nerve and long tract lesions in localisation

Cranial nerve nuclei are where cranial nerves synapse with their supranuclear pathways within the brainstem. Many brainstem lesions may, theoretically, be localised by cranial nerve lesions and long tract signs.

Cranial nerve lesions

Brainstem lesions can be localised in the vertical plane by cranial nerve lesions. The 12 nuclei broadly descend from

midbrain to medulla (Fig. 3.16). In reality, there are more than 12 nuclei, some nerves with a main nucleus and smaller satellite nuclei.

Long tracts

Brainstem lesions can be localised in the transverse plane by signs of damage to long motor and sensory tracts (motor being ventral to sensory).

Corticospinal tracts (Fig. 3.17) are long motor tracts that descend from the precentral gyrus of the frontal lobe, through the internal capsule, cerebral peduncle, midbrain and pons, and decussate at the medullary 'pyramids' to supply the contralateral limbs. They are sometimes called pyramidal tracts. Arm fibres lie medial to leg fibres. Fibres synapse at their destined ventral horn exit sites in the spinal cord. *Supranuclear pathways destined to innervate cranial nerves* descend with the corticospinal fibres as far as the brainstem where they decussate and synapse with and innervate their respective cranial nerve nuclei and cranial nerves, which may be pure motor, pure sensory, or both (see Fig. 3.17). Supranuclear fibres innervating the lower cranial nerves that mediate speech and swallowing are often called corticobulbar fibres.

The *dorsal columns* carrying sensory information for accurate localisation of touch, vibration and proprioception synapse and decussate in the medulla and project to the contralateral thalamus and parietal lobe (Fig. 3.18). The *spinothalamic tracts* carrying pain and temperature information have already synapsed and crossed lower in the spinal cord and also project to thalamus and parietal

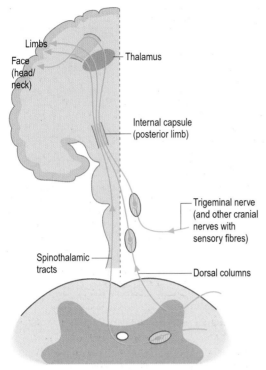

Fig. 3.18 Sensory pathways from the spinal cord to the parietal cortex via the brainstem.

Box 3.19 Brainstem versus cortical lesions and the value of cranial nerves in localisation

Cortical lesions

A cortical lesion such as an internal capsule stroke may cause *contralateral long tract signs* and *contralateral supranuclear cranial signs* (Fig. 3.17). If the tongue and face are affected on the same side as a hemiparesis the lesion must be supranuclear to the XIIth and VIIth nuclei respectively. However, some cranial nerves, indeed most, receive bilateral supranuclear innervation and function is unaffected. The trigeminal motor nucleus is one example, and facial nerve fibres supplying the upper face another; 'spare parachutes' for chewing and eye protection carry survival advantages. Spare parachutes for the bulbar cranial nerves (IX, X, XII) often exist but they often require recruitment before they become affected – it is not uncommon following a cortical stroke to develop speech and swallowing problems that improve with rehabilitation as the brain's plasticity declares itself.

Brainstem lesions

A brainstem lesion may cause *contralateral long tract signs* (if the lesion is above the medullary decussation of the corticospinal tracts and dorsal columns; the spinothalamic tracts have already crossed in the spine and any pain and temperature loss is contralateral to the side of a brainstem lesion) with *ipsilateral cranial nerve signs* because the cranial nerve nuclei or nerves are damaged directly (Fig. 3.17). This combination is sometimes referred to as crossed signs. A lesion is, for example, at the level of the midbrain if III is involved, the pons if VI or VII are involved and the medulla if IX, XI or XII are involved. A brainstem lesion may extend bilaterally (e.g. demyelination, space occupying lesion, basilar artery occlusion) causing bilateral motor or sensory long tract and cranial nerve signs.

Box 3.20 Cranial nerve syndromes

- Unilateral V, VII and VIII – cerebellopontine angle lesion
- Unilateral III, IV, V, and VI – cavernous sinus lesion
- Unilateral IX, X and XI – jugular foramen lesion
- IX, X and XII – bulbar palsy

---

lobe (see Fig. 3.18). *Supranuclear fibres from sensory cranial nerves* and their nuclei (e.g. the trigeminal sensory nucleus) project to the contralateral thalamus and parietal lobe (see Fig. 3.18). The exception is the corneal reflex, where evolution felt a rapid protective response would be best served by an involuntary relay between trigeminal-nerve-mediated sensation and facial-nerve-mediated eye closure within the brainstem. There is bilateral supranuclear innervation to the trigeminal motor nucleus, such that chewing persists in the face of hemianaesthesia. Chewing is more important to survival than facial sensation!

All of this information has localising value (Box 3.19).

Implications of multiple cranial nerve lesions

Multiple cranial nerve lesions may occur where nerves run close together (often resulting in the recognised syndromes in Box 3.20), in generalised disorders (e.g. myasthenia gravis) or due to multiple discrete lesions (e.g. basal meningitis, strokes).

Olfactory nerve (I)

Olfactory testing is seldom expected in PACES.

Eyes

Visual acuity (VA) – optic nerve (II)

VA testing is seldom expected in PACES. Problems with VA may arise from refractive errors, anterior eye disease such as cataracts or retinal disease, or disease of the optic nerve itself.

- Ask the patient to close each eye in turn and read the letters on a near vision chart at 30 cm. Vision should be corrected with glasses if the patient wears them, but a pinhole could also be used to correct refractive errors because it filters out angled rays of light entering the eye. A 6-m Snellen wall chart is more accurate. Normal distance VA is 6/6, meaning that the eye sees at 6 m what it should see at 6 m. 6/60 (the letters on the 6/60 line are 10 times larger) means it sees at 6 m what it should see at 60 m. If letters cannot be seen, bedside tests such as counting fingers, seeing hand movements and perception of light may be performed.
- Test colour vision using a red hatpin. Central vision is colour (cones) and especially sensitive for red. Red desaturation, an impaired ability to detect red, suggests an optic nerve lesion.

Visual fields (VFs) – optic nerve (II)

Different patterns of VF abnormality arise from lesions at different sites (Case 3.16). VFs are divided vertically into

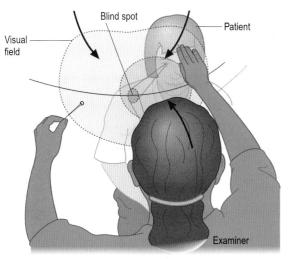

Box 3.21 The light and accommodation reflexes

Light reflex

Light impulses travel along the optic nerve and both optic tracts. Approximately 10% of fibres reaching the level of the lateral geniculate ganglion subserve the light reflex and connect with both Edinger–Westphal nuclei (and adjacent third nerve nuclei) in the periaqueductal matter of the midbrain. Parasympathetic fibres, entwined around both oculomotor nerves, are 'excited' by the light impulses, and stimulate the ciliary ganglion, ciliary nerves and ultimately the pupillary sphincter muscle of each pupil, causing bilateral pupillary constriction.

Accommodation reflex

A similar efferent mechanism subserves accommodation, although the afferent pathway is in the frontal lobe rather than the optic nerve. The third nerve nuclei also control the action of the medial rectus muscles and convergence. The ciliary nerves also supply the ciliary muscle, altering the lens's shape for focusing. Many more ciliary fibres are dedicated to the ciliary muscle than to the pupillary muscle and the accommodation reflex is often regarded as 'stronger' than the light reflex. This may be the reason why accommodation is preserved in otherwise unreactive Argyll Robertson pupils.

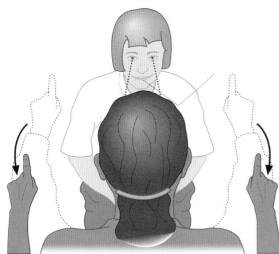

Fig. 3.19 Visual field testing: (A) confrontation method, (B) screening for large defects.

nasal and temporal fields such that an object on your right looking ahead is in the temporal field of your right eye and the nasal field of your left eye. VF defects are described according to the patient's perspective and are homonymous if the same part of the VF is affected in each eye.

- Sit just under one arm's length away from the patient and at the same level. Cover one of their eyes, close your opposing eye and ask the patient to look at you. Slowly introduce a finger or white hatpin in a plane halfway between you and the patient from each quadrant (Fig. 3.19A), ensuring that the pin cannot be seen when you start. A white pin is used because peripheral vision is monochrome. Major VF defects can be screened for using the method shown in Fig. 3.19B, asking the patient to tell you which index finger or hand is moving – right, left or both.

- Examine for a scotoma by moving the hatpin (a red one will detect more significant deficits) slowly at eye level in a temporal to nasal direction and asking the patient to tell you if it disappears or changes colour. In a central scotoma there will be loss of central vision. The blind spot 30° into the temporal field can be mapped in the same way. It corresponds to the optic disc.

Pupils – optic nerve (II), oculomotor nerve (III)

- Check that pupils are of equal size and shape. Ptosis on the side of a larger pupil should alert you to a third nerve palsy, and on the side of a smaller pupil to Horner's syndrome.
- Place your finger 10 cm in front of the patient's nose and check the accommodation response (Box 3.21). The eyes should constrict as they converge.
- Check the direct and consensual light reflexes by shining the light twice in each eye (Fig. 3.20, Box 3.21).
- Note any afferent pupillary defect by swinging the light repeatedly (the swinging light test) from eye to eye, dwelling for a second or two on each eye (Box 3.22). Observe paradoxical dilatation of the pupil of an affected eye, implying a damaged afferent pathway (optic nerve).

Eye movements – oculomotor nerve (III), trochlear nerve (IV), abducens nerve (VI)

- Observe the eyes in primary gaze. Misalignment may be the result of a latent strabismus (constant convergent or divergent strabismus in all directions of gaze), a third nerve palsy or skew deviation in which the eyes are aligned in different vertical planes (brainstem pathology).
- Observe slow, smooth pursuit movements used for fixation on a moving object (the lioness on the

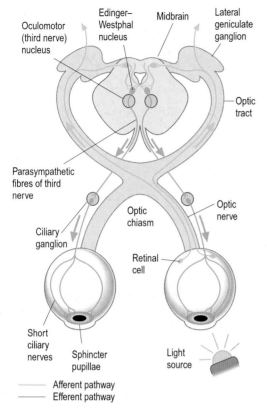

Fig. 3.20 The light reflex.

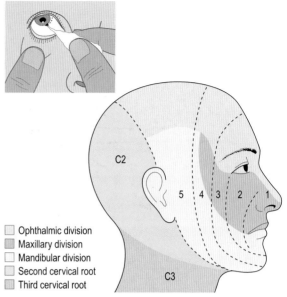

Ophthalmic division
Maxillary division
Mandibular division
Second cervical root
Third cervical root

Fig. 3.21 Facial sensation. Insert: Testing the corneal reflex. Areas 1–5 indicate distribution of sensory fibres from the Vth nerve's long nucleus that extends from the pons (1) to the upper cervical cord (5); the implication of this is that Vth nucleus lesions, unlike Vth nerve lesions, produce (bilateral if both nuclei affected) 'onion skin' patterns of facial sensory loss.

Box 3.22 How the swinging light test detects an afferent pupillary defect (APD)

This relies on the fact that the pupils receive dual innervation from the mid-brain.

A   Shining light into the affected eye causes absent or sluggish direct and consensual responses.
B   Shining light into the normal eye stimulates normal direct and consensual responses.
C   If there is complete damage to the afferent pathway of the affected eye, whatever lighting the normal eye (dominant response) is exposed to will determine the size of both pupils. When light is swung back into the affected eye the normal pupil dilates and so does the affected pupil. If there is partial damage to the afferent pathway recovery from B (the dominant response) is swifter and stronger than the sluggish response to A, so the affected eye still dilates. The latter is known as a relative afferent pupillary defect (RAPD). An APD is also known as a Marcus Gunn pupil.

Serengeti eyeing a roaming zebra or gazelle). Do this by gently fixing the patient's head with one hand and ask the patient to follow the index finger of your other hand using midline horizontal and vertical movements, not a letter H. Look for an ocular palsy due to a lesion of III, IV or VI. Be alert to more than one lesion. Ask about double vision. Also be alert to supranuclear disorders of eye movements that may

not result in double vision, such as lateral gaze palsy (frontal or parietal lesion when the patient looks away from the side of the lesion or pontine lesion when the patient cannot look away from the side of the lesion) or a vertical gaze palsy (upper brainstem lesion).

- Observe faster saccadic movements, the rapid movement from one point of fixation to another (the zebra catches sight of the lioness), asking the patient to look from side to side. This may elicit internuclear ophthalmoplegia.
- Note any nystagmus, normal at extremes of gaze.
- Note any ptosis.

Fundoscopy

Fundoscopy is discussed in Station 5.

Trigeminal nerve (V)

The trigeminal nerve is sensory to the face and motor for the muscles of mastication.

- Feel for any wasting of the masseters, the muscles of jaw closure.
- Ask the patient to clench their teeth (masseters) and open their mouth against the resistance of your hand on their chin (pterygoids).
- Test light touch and pinprick in the ophthalmic (V_1), maxillary (V_2) and mandibular (V_3) distributions (Fig. 3.21).

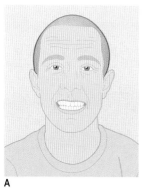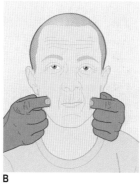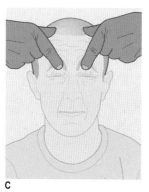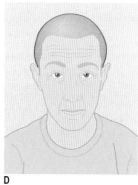

A　　　　　　　　B　　　　　　　　C　　　　　　　　D

Fig. 3.22 Facial nerve examination. Ask the patient to do the following: (A) show me your teeth, (B) puff your cheeks out, (C) close your eyes tightly and do not let me open them, and (D) raise your eyebrows.

- Tell the examiners that you would check the corneal reflex (Fig. 3.22) with a wisp of cotton wool (touching the cornea, not the white sclera), its absence often the first sign of a trigeminal lesion.
- Test the jaw jerk, which can be brisk with bilateral supranuclear lesions above the level of the pons (e.g. pseudobulbar palsy)

Facial nerve (VII)

This is motor to the face and provides taste to the anterior two-thirds of the tongue.

- Look at facial symmetry, noting the nasolabial folds and forehead wrinkles and watch spontaneous movements such as smiling and blinking.
- Ask the patient to show you their teeth, whistle or blow out their cheeks, close their eyes tightly and look up at the ceiling, again looking for symmetrical movement (Fig. 3.22). Bell's phenomenon (eye turns upwards on attempted closure) is the result of a lower motor neuron lesion.
- Compare power in the forehead and lower face. Since upper facial muscles receive bilateral supranuclear innervation, unilateral upper motor neuron lesions spare the forehead whereas facial nerve palsy (lower motor neuron) paralyses the upper and lower face (Case 3.25). Bilateral facial nerve lesions sometimes occur.

Ptosis is not the result of a facial nerve lesion.

Hearing

Hearing testing is seldom expected in PACES. Clinical tests can be unreliable, as demonstrated by formal audiometry.

Rinne's test

Rinne's test (Fig. 3.23A) compares sound from a vibrating 512-Hz tuning fork on the mastoid (bone conduction) with the external auditory canal (air conduction). Normally air conduction is better than bone conduction (bone, denser than air, is actually a better conductor of vibration but here 'conduction' refers to the unimpeded transmission of sound through the air and external canal to the middle ear and inner ear), by convention a Rinne positive test. If bone conduction is better, this implies conductive deafness (everything other than the sensorineural aspect of hearing is conductive), usually because of middle ear disease or wax.

Weber's test

In Weber's test (Fig. 3.23B), sound should be heard in both ears equally when the tuning fork is applied to the central forehead or vertex. In sensorineural deafness sound is not detected by the affected ear. In conductive deafness sound is louder in the affected ear although this phenomenon is difficult to explain. Certainly, when a tuning fork is placed directly on bone, there is no significant sound transmission through the air and all conduction is through bone to the inner ear. Any additional solid material in the ear (e.g. wax, tympanosclerosis, middle ear debris or even poking a finger into the ear!) probably attenuates the normal energy loss at a bone–air interface and enhances sound transmission to the inner ear from the vertex.

Bulbar function – speech and swallowing

The lower ('bulbar') cranial nerves IX, X and XII are integral to speech and swallowing. The proximity of these nerves implies that several combinations of lesion are possible, and that presenting symptoms may be similar whatever the diagnosis – loss of strength in speech and swallowing with hoarseness, nasal speech, nasal regurgitation of fluids or food particles with aspiration and attacks of choking – in other words, a bulbar palsy (Case 3.26).

Glossopharyngeal nerve (IX)

This is mostly sensory, relaying information from the palate, pharynx and posterior third of the tongue via the trigeminal nucleus to the sensory cortex. It is motor only to stylopharyngeus. A glossopharyngeal lesion is rare in isolation and invariably part of a wider bulbar palsy.

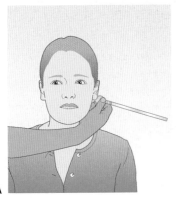
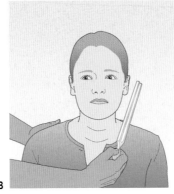
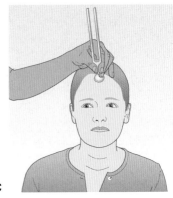

Fig. 3.23 Rinne's test. Bone conduction (A) and air conduction (B). (C) Weber's test; placing the tuning fork on the teeth is more sensitive but only to be done with care.

- Touch the palate each side with an orange stick or touch the pharyngeal wall each side with the patient saying 'Aah', asking the patient to compare right and left.
- Touching the posterior third of the tongue is of less value.
- The gag reflex (sensory via IX, motor to palate via X) is usually too gross to test and unreliable, not present in many people.

Vagus nerve (X)

This is motor to the palate, pharynx, larynx and vocal cords and sensory to the tympanic membrane, external auditory meatus and external ear.

- Watch the patient say 'Aah'. The palate and uvula normally move upwards. In a vagus lesion the paralysed side is immobile and tends to be pulled towards the intact side. The palate fails to elevate and the uvula is seen dragged across to the unaffected side. It may be completely immobile in bilateral vagus lesions. These problems lead to the bulbar palsy symptoms described above.
- Assessment should include voice and cough as well as palatal movements. A paralysed vocal cord lies limply abducted to the midline, giving rise to a hoarse voice and a bovine cough.

Since sensory fibres from X are conveyed in the auricular branch, malignant lesions of the throat may sometimes cause earache, as may the common cold.

Hypoglossal nerve (XII)

This is motor to the tongue.

- Observe the tongue at rest. It is paralysed on the side of a lesion and deviates to the side of that lesion. It may also be unilaterally wasted.
- On attempted tongue protrusion, the deviation can become more obvious.

- Tongue fasciculation is best observed with the tongue at rest inside the mouth because normal rippling movements can occur when the tongue exerts itself.

Coordination of cranial nerves in swallowing

Perhaps the best test of overall bulbar function is to ask the patient to drink a glass of water. Swallowing is a complex process involving many cranial nerves and comprises a voluntary phase, a reflex phase and an oesophageal phase. In the voluntary phase VII holds the mouth shut, IX relays information about food bolus position to the sensory cortex, V controls chewing, IX senses the arrival of the bolus at the palate and XII pushes the chewed bolus up and back against the palate. In the reflex phase XII pulls the hyoid upwards and forwards to bring the larynx beneath the back of the tongue, IX, via stylopharyngeus, assists the hyoid elevators and lifts the larynx forwards and X elevates the palate to occlude the nasopharynx (preventing nasal regurgitation), flips the epiglottis forwards over the top of the elevated and tilted larynx (preventing food falling into trachea), dilates the hypopharynx (allowing the bolus to fall into the oesophagus) and initiates oesophageal peristalsis.

Accessory nerve (XI)

This innervates the trapezius and sternocleidomastoid muscles.

- Test trapezius by asking the patient to shrug their shoulders against resistance (Fig. 3.24A).
- Test the sternocleidomastoids by asking the patient to turn their head against resistance (Fig. 3.24B). The right sternocleidomastoid turns the head to the left and vice versa.

Summary

A summary of the cranial nerve examination sequence is in the Summary Box.

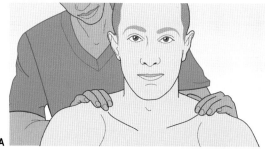

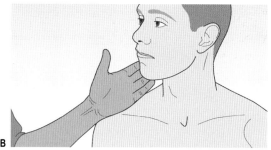

Fig. 3.24 Testing the accessory nerve: (A) trapezius, (B) left sternocleidomastoid.

SUMMARY BOX – CRANIAL NERVE EXAMINATION SEQUENCE

- Test visual acuity and then colour vision using a red hatpin
- Test visual fields (an initial screen detects major homonymous defects)
- Check pupil size and shape
- Test the accommodation reflex
- Test the direct and consensual light reflexes and check for an afferent pupillary defect
- Look at the eyes in primary gaze and then test eye movements
- Note any internuclear ophthalmoplegia
- Note any nystagmus
- Note any ptosis
- Test masseter strength
- Test touch in all the divisions of the trigeminal nerve and tell the examiners you would check for a corneal reflex
- Look at facial symmetry and test facial movements, noting any upper and lower facial discrepancy
- Tell the examiners you would formally assess hearing in the presence of symptoms or in the presence of cerebellopontine neuropathies
- Test palatal sensation
- Test uvula and palatal movement
- Look at the tongue at rest inside the mouth for deviation, wasting and fasciculation and then look for more obvious deviation of a protruded tongue
- Test the accessory nerve

Examination of higher cortical function and specific lobes

Higher cortical function

Examining higher cortical function adequately is complex and cannot be performed in PACES. A 30-point mini-mental state examination is frequently performed on the

---

Box 3.23 Functions of the frontal lobe

- Planning
- Initiation of movement
- Speech expression involving Broca's speech area (in the dominant hemisphere)
- Attention and concentration
- Voluntary control of micturition
- The more enigmatic aspects of thinking and behaviour, such as wisdom, intelligence, ambition, moral sense and judgement
- Acquired social behaviour

Box 3.24 Potential effects of frontal lobe disease

- Akinesia (difficulty with movement)
- Apathy (loss of initiative) and abulia (loss of spontaneity)
- Motor or expressive dysphasia (if dominant hemisphere)
- Distractibility, perseveration
- Incontinence
- Mood disturbance and disinhibition

Primitive reflexes

- Grasp – stroking the palm induces a grasp
- Palmomental – firmly stroking the thenar eminence induces an ipsilateral grimace
- Rooting – stroking the cheek induces a gnawing mouth movement
- Sucking – touching the lips promotes sucking
- Snout – tapping the upper lip makes it pucker upwards
- Glabellar – tapping the forehead stimulates eye closure

---

wards, and a 10-point abbreviated mental test score forms an initial clerking screen (Fig. 3.25 and Box 2.83, Case 2.43).

Lobe syndromes

The cranial nerves send sensory information to the brain and receive motor information from it. Likewise, the rest of the body, through peripheral nerves and nerve roots, sends sensory information to the central nervous system and receives motor information from it. Some of this information does not involve the hemispheres of the cerebral cortex – the corneal reflex, for example, and spinal reflexes. But for most information, the cortex is involved, perceiving everything in our world and initiating almost everything we do. Its different lobes have specific functions.

The frontal lobe

This is a motor lobe. It plans and initiates tasks. The precentral gyrus puts thoughts into action; it is here that the cascade of messages to move a body part begins. Functions of the frontal lobe are shown in Box 3.23. The posterior parts of the lobe are most important. Frontal lobe disease may result in those features in Box 3.24. The frontal lobes not only inhibit undesirable behaviour but also primitive reflexes that are present at birth. These may be disinhibited by frontal lobe disease.

Connections between different parts of the brain explain many neurological signs. Patients with Parkinson's disease

Mini-mental state examination (MMSE)

ONE POINT FOR EACH ANSWER

ORIENTATION		
	Year Month Day Date Time	/5
	Country Town District Hospital Ward	/5
REGISTRATION		
	Examiner names 3 objects (e.g. apple, table, penny) Patient asked to repeat (1 point for each correct) then patient to learn the 3 names repeating until correct	/3
ATTENTION AND CALCULATION		
	Subtract 7 from 100, then repeat from result Continue 5 times: 100 93 86 79 65 Alternative: spell 'WORLD' backwards – dlrow	/5
RECALL		
	Ask for names of 3 objects learned earlier	/3
LANGUAGE		
	Name a pencil and watch	/2
	Repeat 'No ifs, ands or buts'	/1
	Give a 3-stage command. Score 1 for each stage, e.g. 'Place index finger of right hand on your nose and then on your left ear'	/3
	Ask patient to read and obey a written command on a piece of paper stating 'Close your eyes'	/1
	Ask patient to write a sentence. Score if it is sensible and has a subject and a verb	/1
COPYING		
	Ask the patient to copy a pair of intersecting pentagons:	/1
		TOTAL /30

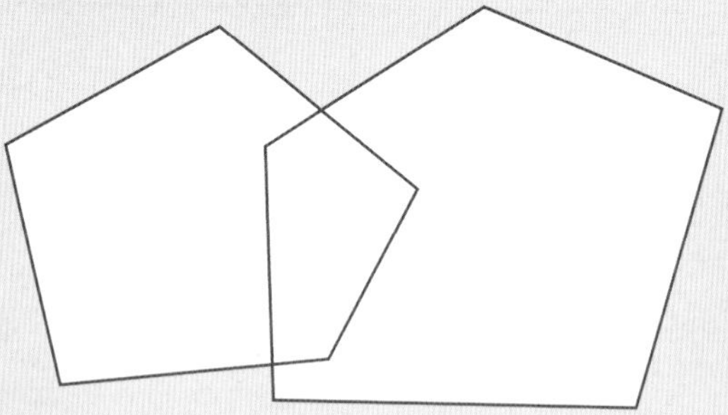

Fig. 3.25 Mini-mental state examination.

may have a positive glabellar tap because of disease in the frontal lobe's extrapyramidal connections.

The parietal lobe

The parietal lobe contains the sensory cortex or post-central gyrus. Unlike the frontal lobe, the parietal lobe very much senses, and is concerned with appreciating the world around us, creating a three-dimensional representation of the spatial layout of the external world, and also of your body within

that three-dimensional representation. Both the dominant and non-dominant parietal lobes are concerned with recognition and awareness. Both relay the parietal radiations of the visual pathways. Disease in a parietal lobe may manifest itself broadly in one of two ways (Box 3.25).

Lesions may cause a single problem or a recognised syndrome (Case 3.30). The dominant parietal lobe is usually left sided (even in left-handed people, whose 'dominant' hemisphere we often assume as being the right).

There is much overlap of dominant and non-dominant parietal lobe function.

The occipital lobe

The occipital lobe is the common endpoint of the visual nerve pathways. Lesions may result in cortical blindness, visual agnosia (parieto-occipital connections) or specific visual processing defects such as impaired perception of colour or movement.

The temporal lobe

The temporal lobe subserves memory (hippocampus and other areas) and emotion, certain aspects of perception, central representation of hearing, taste and smell, speech interpretation, transmission of visual impulses via the temporal visual radiations, and some aspect of behaviour via frontal lobe connections. Lesions may result in memory impairment, auditory agnosia (temporo-parietal connections), cortical deafness (if bilateral) and receptive dysphasia.

The limbic system

The cerebral hemispheres perceive and initiate. They make contact with the outside world through sensory and motor pathways. But what of the inside world? There is extreme complexity in the visual pathways relaying what we see, but we always see a particular object in the same way. A monkey always looks like a monkey, a giraffe always looks like a giraffe, and we would not mistake one for another. But the visual pathways are crude compared with the mechanisms of recognition, learning, thought and emotion. The limbic system is a part of the brain where science has more questions than answers. It has to do with memory. It is also thought to be a centre for smell. Have you noticed that some smells instantly evoke distant memories?

Examination of speech and language

Ensure that the patient can hear, then consider in turn if there is:

- Dysphasia
- Dysarthria
- Dysphonia

Dysphasia

Types of dysphasia

Dyphasia is a disorder of language and refers to the inability to understand or find words (Table 3.25) due to a lesion in the dominant (usually left) hemisphere.

Wernicke's area recognises sounds as language, but a higher concept area is required to convert sounds into meaning. This concept area then connects to Broca's area, where speech output is generated. A direct connection, the arcuate fasciculus, also exists between Wernicke's and Broca's areas. Transcortical sensory dysphasia is similar to receptive dysphasia but with preserved repetition and is caused by a lesion in the parietal-occipital concept area. Transcortical motor dysphasia is similar to expressive dysphasia but with preserved repetition and is the result of an incomplete lesion in Broca's area. Conductive dysphasia refers to preserved comprehension and output with loss of repetition and is the result of a lesion in the arcuate fasciculus. Difficulty naming objects, or nominal dysphasia, is the result of an angular gyrus lesion.

Examining for dysphasia

- Introduce yourself and ask a few simple questions, e.g. *Can you tell me your name and date of birth?*
- Is there receptive dysphasia? Give a simple command, e.g. *Close your eyes/With your right hand touch your*

Box 3.25 Two important manifestations of parietal lobe disease

Agnosias

There is *difficulty in recognising things*, despite intact sensory pathways peripheral to the parietal lobe. These problems with recognition are often termed agnosias.

Apraxias

There is *difficulty in performing tasks*, not because of any problem with motor nerves or muscles, which are all intact – but because the parietal lobe fails to process information about the environment. It would normally pass on this processed information to the frontal lobe, which in turn would normally initiate a course of action in response to it. These problems with performing tasks are often termed dyspraxias or apraxias.

Table 3.25 Receptive and expressive dysphasia

	Receptive dysphasia	Expressive dysphasia
Problem	Inability to understand	Inability to express, despite comprehension
Clinical findings	May be fluent, but words meaningless	Can cause immense frustration to patients, who know in their minds what they want to say but cannot get the words out (if less severe can answer questions and speak spontaneously but often struggle, making mistakes)
Location of lesion	Wernicke's area in the temporal lobe (may be a visual field defect)	Broca's area in the frontal lobe (connected to Wernicke's area by the arcuate fasciculus)

In reality it is less useful to distinguish expressive and receptive dysphasia, and the concept of two discrete language areas is somewhat artificial. Dysphasia usually involves both expressive and receptive components, and testing more complex sequence tasks or non-verbal language skills in a patient with obvious word-finding difficulty who appears to understand simple commands can reveal this to be so.

nose and then more complex, two-step or three-step commands.

- Is there expressive dysphasia? Get the patient talking further, e.g. *Tell me a little about where you live.*
- Is there global dysphasia? If the patient cannot perform either task, there is global dysphasia (the lesion affects both receptive and expressive areas).
- Is there nominal dysphasia? Ask the patient to name some objects, e.g. *What is this?* (show pen, tie and watch). If unable to name objects, ask *Is it a . . . ?*
- Assess word-finding ability, e.g. *Name as many animals as you can think of.*
- Assess repetition by asking the patient to repeat a sentence, e.g. *A giraffe is a tall, graceful animal.*
- Tell the examiners that you would assess reading and writing; similar categories of problem can occur with other aspects of language such as reading and writing (dyslexia and dysgraphia).

Dysarthria

Types of dysarthria

Dysarthria refers to impaired articulation and is the result of a lesion in any of the structures coordinating voice production:

- Upper motor neuron lesion (pseudobulbar palsy)
- Extrapyramidal lesion, e.g. Parkinson's disease
- Cerebellar lesion
- Lower motor/cranial nerve lesion (bulbar palsy)
- Neuromuscular junction lesion (myasthenia)
- Myopathy
- Local lesion of the palate, tongue or lips

Examining for dysarthria

- Ask the patient to say some simple and more difficult (*eleven benevolent elephants, baby hippopotamus*) phrases
- The sequence *ppp, lll, kkk* and a *cough* is a rapid screen for lip, tongue, palate and vocal cord function

Fig. 3.26 can be used to determine the type of dysarthria; Box 3.26 describes how to differentiate bulbar from pseudobulbar palsy.

Dysphonia

Types of dysphonia

Dysphonia refers to impaired voice production or phonation due to a lesion in the vocal cords or larynx (such as laryngitis) or vagal nerve supply. It is common when muscles are weak, as in Parkinson's disease.

Examining for dysphonia

- Determine if the patient coughs or produces a sustained *eee*. Dysphonia with a normal cough suggests a local (laryngeal) lesion. A bovine cough (without an explosive start) suggests vocal cord palsy.

> **Box 3.26 Bulbar and pseudobulbar palsy**
>
> **Bulbar palsy**
>
> Bulbar palsy refers to infranuclear or lower motor neurone disease, usually involving cranial nerves X (palate) or XII (tongue) with flaccid, nasal speech. Nasal speech/escape is the characteristic sign of bulbar palsy and nasal regurgitation of fluids and food with choking or aspiration may be prominent. Analogies are 'drowning' or 'choking' and a sense that 'everything is in the way'. The tongue seems too big for the mouth and seems to hang out with salivary pooling. Patients sometimes say it feels as if the mouth is numb like being at the dentist and cannot spit out toothpaste.
>
> **Pseudobulbar palsy**
>
> Pseudobulbar palsy refers to supranuclear or upper motor neurone disease with spastic speech. The tongue appears small and 'tight', and cannot be protruded, lying immobile on the floor of the mouth. Analogies include 'high pitched', 'Donald Duck', 'hot potato' or 'strained' speech. Bilateral supranuclear innervation of the lower (bulbar) cranial nerves necessary for speech and swallowing means that bilateral cortical or brainstem lesions are required to induce a pseudobulbar palsy. Causes include bilateral internal capsule strokes or demyelination. Dysarthria and swallowing problems in a cortical stroke are due to unilateral supranuclear disease, often a combination of facial and bulbar weakness, but the spare parachute afforded by bilateral innervation to the swallowing muscles means that it is a much attenuated form of pseudobulbar palsy.

Summary

A summary of the speech and language examination sequence is given in the Summary Box.

> **SUMMARY BOX – SPEECH AND LANGUAGE EXAMINATION SEQUENCE**
>
> - Introduce yourself and ask a few simple questions, e.g. *Can you tell me your name and date of birth?*
> - Test for receptive dysphasia with a simple command, e.g. *Close your eyes/With your right hand touch your nose* and then more complex, two- or three-step commands
> - Test for expressive dysphasia by getting the patient to talk more, e.g. *Can you tell me a little about where you live?*
> - Consider global dysphasia
> - Test for nominal dysphasia by asking the patient to name some objects. If unable to name, ask *Is it a . . . ?*
> - Assess word-finding ability, e.g. *Name as many animals as you can think of*
> - Assess repetition by asking the patient to repeat a sentence, e.g. *A giraffe is a tall, graceful animal*
> - Tell the examiners that you would assess reading and writing.
> - Use the sequence *ppp, lll, kkk* and a *cough* as a rapid screen for lip, tongue, palate and vocal cord function
> - Ask the patient to say some phrases, e.g. *eleven benevolent elephants, baby hippopotamus*

Examination of coordination

The motor cortex exerts voluntary or conscious control of movement via its descending motor pathways to cranial nerves and corticospinal tracts and conscious sensory information travels via the ascending dorsal columns, spinothalamic tracts and sensory pathways from cranial nerves to the thalamus and sensory cortex.

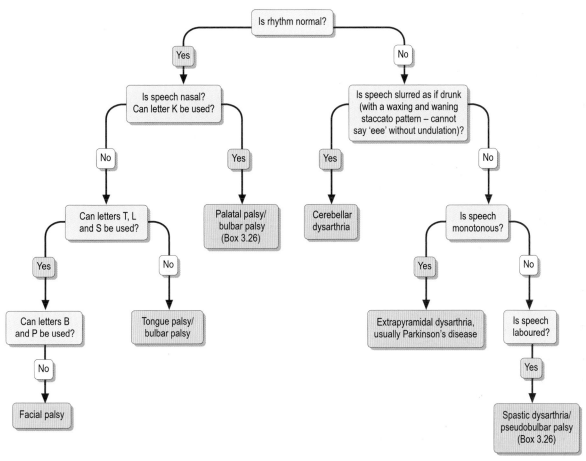

Fig. 3.26 Dysarthria.

That conscious motor pathways are not enough to control movement is evident from diseases of the extrapyramidal system. The extrapyramidal system adds unconscious fine-tuning to every move we make.

That conscious sensory pathways are not enough to appreciate the body's position in space is evident by diseases of the cerebellum. The cerebellum sends unconscious feedback to the cortex about every move we make.

There is, in essence, a loop (Fig. 3.27). The motor cortex initiates activity, movements are adjusted by the extrapyramidal system, and the cerebellum provides feedback information about the movements made.

When examining coordination, be aware that the dominant side may have a slight advantage.

- Look for nystagmus.
- Ask the patient to hold their arms outstretched and close their eyes. Look for any oscillation.
- Ask the patient to touch your finger, held out about an arm's length away. Look for an intention tremor or overshoot (past pointing). Then ask the patient to touch their nose. Repeat this movement at faster speeds, the patient touching your finger then their nose repetitively, but with your finger fixed, not as a moving target.

- Assess rapid movements by asking the patient to twist their hand, as when turning a doorknob, and to tap the back of their hand quickly (and then rapid alternating movements by turning it over and back again quickly). Look for dysdiachokinesis.
- Assess heel–shin coordination (Fig. 3.28).
- Gait, discussed separately, is crucial to the assessment of coordination.

Cerebellar disease

Incoordination in PACES is usually the result of cerebellar disease (Box 3.27).

Movement disorders

Types of movement disorder are listed in Table 3.26.

Dystonia

If there is focal pathology it tends to be found in the basal ganglia (putamen) or midbrain. The most common dystonia is primary torsion dystonia (PTD). Tests to exclude a secondary cause (e.g. Wilson's disease) should be considered in young patients, those with generalised dystonia and those with features not seen in PTD, such as additional neurological signs. Types of dystonia are listed

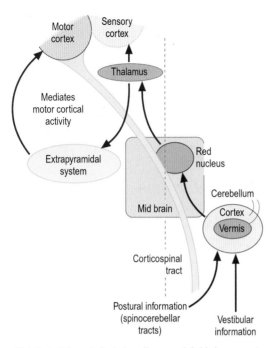

Note that a left cerebellar lesion will cause a *left* sided movement disturbance and vice versa

Fig. 3.27 The loop.

Box 3.27 Cerebellar signs

A mnemonic for the typical 'syndrome' of cerebellar signs is DASHING

- **D**ysdiadochokinesis with rapid alternating movements
- **A**taxia of limbs
- **S**lurred speech
- **H**eel–shin ataxia
- **I**nability to judge distance (dysmetria) with past pointing
- **N**ystagmus
- **G**ait wide based

Note in Fig. 3.27 how unilateral cerebellar disease causes ipsilateral signs. A cerebellar hemisphere feeds information to the contralateral cerebral hemisphere but then that cerebral hemisphere exerts control of movement back on the opposite side. Midline (vermis) lesions cause midline or truncal ataxia. Gait is broad-based and the patient is unable to tandem-walk or stand like a flamingo! They might even be unable to sit up without falling to one side. Cerebellar hemisphere lesions cause appendicular or limb ataxia. These principles may suggest whether cerebellar pathology is unilateral or bilateral, midline, hemispheric or pancerebellar. This should narrow the differential diagnosis to structural lesions or more generalised insults.

---

in Table 3.27. A rare group of genetic paroxysmal dyskinesias may be dystonic or choreic and include paroxysmal kinesigenic dyskinesia (PKD), paroxysmal non-kinesigenic dyskinesia (PKND), paroxysmal exercise-induced dyskinesia (PED) and paroxysmal hypnogenic dyskinesia (PHD), some linked to writer's cramp.

Drug-induced movement disorders

These are outlined in Box 3.28.

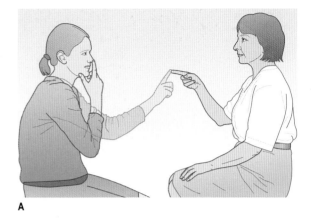

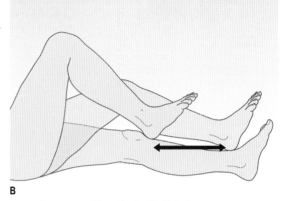

Fig. 3.28 Finger–nose (A) and heel–shin (B) testing.

Summary

A summary of the coordination examination sequence is given in the Summary Box.

SUMMARY – COORDINATION EXAMINATION SEQUENCE

- Look for nystagmus
- Ask the patient to hold their arms outstretched and close their eyes, looking for any oscillation.
- Ask the patient to touch your finger, held out about arm's length away. Look for an intention tremor or overshoot (past pointing)
- Assess rapid movements by asking the patient twist their hand, as when turning a doorknob, and to tap the back of their hand quickly (and then rapid alternating movements by turning it over and back again quickly)
- Look for dysdiachokinaesis
- Assess heel–shin coordination
- Assess gait

Examination of power and sensation – overview

The spinal cord

The spinal cord

The spinal cord extends from behind the C1 vertebral body to the lower end of the L1 vertebra. A cord level is thus

Table 3.26 Types of movement disorder

Type of movement disorder	Clinical features
Akinetic-rigid syndromes/ Parkinsonism	Clinical syndromes with bradykinaesia as the defining feature, almost always accompanied by rigidity and often by tremor. Parkinsonism is discussed in Case 3.32
Tremor	A rhythmic oscillation of a body part produced by alternating or synchronous contraction of antagonistic muscles All tremors are worse with performance, anxiety and tiredness and are subdivided into predominantly rest, action or postural tremors. While resting tremors can be due to many diseases, especially of the basal ganglia, action tremors usually imply cerebellar disease; a postural tremor characterises essential tremor. To see if the tremor is truly an action tremor, lie the patient on the bed with their arms fully supported to abolish any muscle activation; a cerebellar tremor disappears. A further way to assess subtle tremor is to observe writing or drawing, e.g. an Archimedes spiral. Tremors are further discussed in Case 2.19.
Dystonia (athetosis is an obsolete term for dystonia)	Sustained muscle contraction leading frequently to twisting and repetitive movements or abnormal postures
Chorea	Involuntary or semi-purposive abrupt, irregular and random movements Usually affect face, hands and feet, i.e. usually distal Large-amplitude movements (ballismus) are disabling but mild chorea is easy to miss
Myoclonus	Brief, sudden, shock-like jerks caused by active muscle contraction Sudden pauses are termed 'asterixis' Causes include epilepsy, anoxia, encephalitis, and prion disease
Tic	Rapid, brief jerk or sound Usually affects head or arms Suppressible at expense of tension and distress

Table 3.27 Types of dystonia

Type of dystonia	Features and causes
Focal	Focal involvement, e.g. cervical dystonia (spasmodic torticollis), blepharospasm (involuntary spasm of eye closure), oromandibular dystonia, laryngeal dystonia, brachial dystonia (writer's cramp) and foot dystonia
Segmental	Adjacent regions affected, e.g. cranial + oromandibular ± cervical dystonia
Generalised	Legs and other areas usually affected
Hemidystonia	Unilateral dystonia due to a lesion in the contralateral basal ganglia

Box 3.28 Drug-induced movement disorders

Dyskinesia

Dyskinesia strictly means disordered movement but the term is often used synonymously with drug-induced chorea and dystonia that occur, for example, in the later stages of Parkinson's disease.

Acute dystonia

Prochlorperazine, metaclopramide and antipsychotic drugs can produce sudden, severe dystonia, often of the head or neck. Oculogyric crises may occur. Treatment is with an intravenous anticholinergic drug (e.g. procyclidine).

Tardive dyskinesia

Continuous involuntary movements are common with long-term antipsychotics, and are difficult to treat.

above its designated vertebral root exit site (Fig. 3.76, Case 3.38). The cord is encased by the pia, subarachnoid space, arachnoid, potential dural space and dura, and is supplied by branches of the vertebral arteries.

Long tracts

Knowledge of the long tracts of the spinal cord (Fig. 3.29) is essential to knowing what you are looking for when examining power and sensation in the limbs and trunk.

■ **Motor (descending) tracts** The *corticospinal tracts* (CSTs) run downwards and throw off fibres to ventral horn cells. Arm fibres run medially to leg fibres. The CST supplying each side of the body in fact divides into a lateral CST, carrying at least 80% of fibres (decussating in the medulla), and an anterior or ventral CST, carrying less than 20% of fibres (not decussating until the spinal cord). For practical purposes, the CST is considered here as one lateral tract.

■ **Sensory (ascending) tracts** The *dorsal* or posterior columns (DCs) relay *proprioception* (joint position sense) and *vibration* sense from peripheral nerves, roots and dorsal horns, along their gracile (arm) and cuneate (leg) fibres. These fibres synapse in the brainstem then cross, or decussate, from the brainstem to the contralateral thalamus and sensory cortex. If a dog rubs its nose up your leg sequential segments of cortical representation or homunculus (Fig. 3.64, Case 3.27) will be stimulated and each will inform you exactly where its nose is. The *spinothalamic tracts (STTs)* rapidly convey *pain* and *temperature* (and some *light touch*) information to the contralateral sensory cortex but cross early, either immediately or within a few segments in the spinal cord. STTs are fast pathways. The differential crossing of DCs and STTs accounts for the signs in Brown–Séquard syndrome.

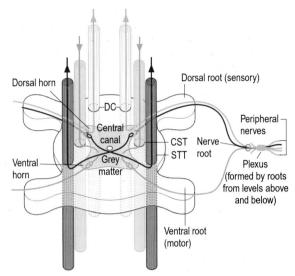

Fig. 3.29 The long tracts – cross-section of one level of the spinal cord, showing the major tracts running up and down it and fibres that connect with a nerve root at that level. DC, dorsal columns; STT, spinothalamic tracts; CST, corticospinal tracts.

Spinal cord lesions and radiculopathies

The level of a cord lesion or the presence of a radiculopathy (root lesion) can be determined by knowledge of root myotomes and dermatomes (Box 3.29). Power is most easily assessed in the limbs but sensation can be assessed in the limbs and trunk.

The limbs

Rapid examination screen

In the upper limbs, rapid inspection for wasting then testing for weakness of shoulder abduction, wrist extension and finger extension should detect subtle upper motor neuron (UMN) weakness, proximal weakness due to a proximal myopathy and distal weakness because of a lower motor neuron (LMN) lesion. In the lower limbs, hip flexion and ankle dorsiflexion are the most discriminatory tests of power. Sensation can be left until last when findings should be predictable from the pattern of weakness.

Examining power

While the above is a useful screen when you do not suspect neurological disease, a more complete examination is required in neurological cases. *The key to examining the limbs is in examining power.*

Box 3.29 Spinal cord lesions and radiculopathies

Spinal cord lesions

- In a complete spinal cord lesion there is spastic weakness of all muscle groups below the level of the lesion. There is sensory loss in all areas below the level of the lesion if sensory tracts are also involved.
- Sometimes only one half of the cord is damaged (hemisection, or Brown–Séquard syndrome) with ipsilateral weakness, and the sensory loss is said to be dissociated: ipsilateral loss of sensation carried by the dorsal columns and contralateral loss of sensation carried by the spinothalamic tracts.
- Furthermore, there may be detectable lower motor neuron myotomal weakness at the level of a lesion if there is damage to the ventral horn cell or ventral nerve root at that level.

In T2–L1 lesions all muscle groups in the lower limbs are spastic and testing power has no localising value. Seeking where trunk dermatomal sensory loss (below) starts is the most effective way of assessing the level of thoracic spine lesions. Abdominal reflexes are easy to understand when you think of a 'tummy tickle'. The tickly feeling is the result of stimulation of the lower thoracic sensory fibres T8–12 and is lost in lower thoracic lesions. In lumbar, sacral and cervical lesions identifying dermatomal loss helps to determine the level of the lesion. Early in disease there may be considerable pain at the level of a lesion. When limb dermatomes are painful, spinal cord and root disease are often considered; this is not so for thoracic cord or root disease; in these cases, heart, lung and abdominal diagnoses are often considered before dermatomal pain, and thoracic root shingles or vertebral collapse are easily ignored.

Radiculopathies

- In a radiculopathy there is discrete myotomal weakness and dermatomal sensory loss.
- The term myotome refers to the muscles supplied by a particular nerve root, no matter how the nerve fibres within that root are finally distributed via the limb plexuses and peripheral nerves. In root lesions, affected muscles are weak and flaccid, and any reflexes involving that root are lost.
- The term dermatome refers to the area of skin supplied by a nerve root (Fig. 3.30). Dermatomes vary between individuals and overlap in individuals.

Myotomes

Movements supplied by specific roots are:

- C5   shoulder abduction (+ biceps reflex)
- C6   elbow flexion (+ supinator reflex)
- C7   elbow extension (+ triceps reflex)
- C8   finger flexion and extension
- T1   movements of the small muscles of the hand
- L2   hip flexion/adduction
- L3   knee extension (+ knee reflex)
- L4   ankle inversion (+ knee reflex)
- L5   ankle dorsiflexion
- S1   ankle plantar flexion/eversion (+ ankle reflex)

Generally two, and sometimes more, roots contribute to a particular movement, but one (listed above) makes the major contribution. Reference sources vary in ascribing nerve roots to particular movements, and in reality there is considerable biological variation between individuals. There are eight cervical roots but seven vertebrae. Root C1 exits above the C1 vertebra and C8 below the C7 vertebra. All thoracic and lumbar roots exit below their designated vertebra and sacral roots from foramina in the coccyx. Lumbar and sacral roots travel a long distance from their cord segment of origin to their exit site.

Dermatomes

Dermatomes are shown in Fig. 3.30.

■ **Grading power** There are numerous ways of grading power (Table 3.28), but it is also useful to describe weakness in terms of functional loss.

■ **Five patterns of weakness** It is important diagnostically to consider *five patterns of weakness* (Table 3.29). Each has *characteristic signs*. Recognising the pattern offers a *clinical correlate*. The clinical correlate connects the site of the lesion, determined from the pattern of weakness, to *numerous possible pathologies* or *diagnoses*. Generally, reaching the clinical correlate is by clinical examination and determining the pathology by history and investigation. When examining limbs, aim to identify the clinical correlate before considering possible diagnoses. Sometimes multiple patterns of weakness occur, e.g. cervical myeloradiculopathy, cervical myelopathy with peripheral neuropathy, diabetic peripheral neuropathy with mononeuritis multiplex.

Examining tone

A little resistance is normal. Increased tone is the result of UMN lesions. Increased tone because of *spasticity* is best elicited by rapid movements and is present if resistance increases suddenly ('the catch' or clasp-knife), e.g. the heel flings up from the bed when the knee is lifted quickly. *Lead-pipe rigidity* is when tone is increased throughout movement. Extrapyramidal *cogwheel rigidity*, with regular intermittent breaks, is best elicited by slow movements. *Paratonia* or *Gegenhalten* refers to resistance due to frontal

Table 3.28 Medical research council grading of power

Grade	Definition
5	Normal
4	Active movement against gravity and resistance but not full strength
3	Active movement against gravity but not against resistance
2	Active movement with gravity eliminated
1	Flicker of movement on voluntary contraction
0	No visible or palpable movement

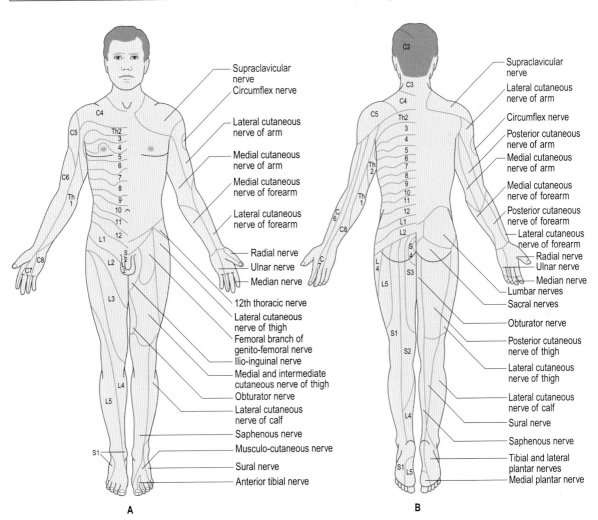

Fig. 3.30 Dermatomes.

Table 3.29 Five patterns of weakness

	Pattern of weakness	Characteristic signs	Clinical correlate	Possible pathologies or diagnoses
Upper motor neuron weakness	All muscle groups in the arm, leg or both (although arm flexors tend to be stronger than extensors and leg extensors stronger than leg flexors) But note that isolated bits of limb may be affected if only a small part of the homunculus is damaged (Fig. 3.64, Case 3.27); this may be especially so higher in the cortex where fibres travelling to and from their destined home on the homunculus map are more sparsely populated, whereas lower in the cortex they have all bunched together; it is analogous to rural living high in the cortex, before they head to work on the motorway that is ultimately the internal capsule	Increased tone or spasticity Enhanced reflexes Extensor (upgoing) plantar response	Monoparesis (one limb) Hemiparesis (arm and leg on one side)	Stroke Internal capsule stroke (e.g. + upper motor neuron facial weakness ipsilateral to hemiparesis) Brainstem stroke (e.g. + cranial neuropathies contrateral to hemiparesis)
			Tetra(quadri)paresis (all four limbs, e.g. high cervical cord lesion, bilateral brainstem or cerebral hemisphere lesions)	Cervical myelopathy
			Paraparesis (both legs due to spinal cord disease below the level of the arms)	Demyelination
Lower motor neuron weakness – focal	Weakness due to disease in spinal nerve (root), nerve plexus (web of neurons with fibres from different roots) or specific peripheral nerve. Site of weakness depends on the root, plexus or nerve affected. Specific myotomal patterns of weakness and dermatomal patterns of sensory loss are associated with root lesions (Box 3.29). Specific weakness and sensory loss occur in specific nerve lesions. Patchy signs may occur with multiple nerve lesions (mononeuritis multiplex)	Wasting (± fasciculation) Flaccid tone Attenuated reflexes (in affected muscle groups)	Radiculopathy Plexopathy Mononeuropathy Mononeuritis multiplex	Box 3.29 Brachial plexopathy in Pancoast's syndrome Carpal tunnel syndrome Ulnar nerve lesion Radial nerve lesion Common peroneal nerve lesion Diabetes Vasculitis
Lower motor neuron weakness – diffuse and distal	Symmetrical weakness in all muscle groups distally	Multiple nerve tips are involved and weakness, sensory loss and reflex loss start at the feet and ankles and ascend (fingertips starting to be affected by the time disease reaches knees)	Peripheral neuropathy	Many causes, some predominantly sensory, some motor and some both
Neuromuscular junction weakness	Muscular weakness	Muscle weakness – limbs, bulbar, ptosis Fatiguability (muscles becoming weaker with activity)	Myasthenia	Myasthenia
Muscle weakness	Symmetrical weakness in all muscle groups, (usually) proximally	No other neurological signs	Myopathy Dystrophy	Many causes

lobe damage and is common in cerebrovascular disease. Flaccid tone, with loss of resistance throughout movements, indicates LMN lesions. The heel does not lift off the bed when the knee is lifted quickly.

Examining reflexes

Reflexes are monosynaptic responses to the stretch of muscle fibres, mediated in the spinal cord. Reflexes and tone have a further inhibitory input from higher neurons in the muscles they supply. In LMN lesions, reflexes are reduced or absent. In UMN lesions there is disinhibition from higher neurons and reflexes are increased. Always use a long tendon hammer, and let it swing with its own weight onto the muscle. Patients should be relaxed, best achieved by not telling them to relax! Reflexes are graded as in Box 3.30.

Box 3.30 Grading reflexes	
–	Absent
+	Present only with reinforcement
+	Diminished
++	Normal
+++	Hyperactive
++++	Clonus

Increased reflexes occur in UMN lesions. Absent or reduced (more difficult to judge) reflexes occur in LMN lesions. The term 'inverted reflex' merely implies the absence of a reflex at one, or sometimes more, levels (e.g. C5 and C6) and brisk reflexes below, and indicates a spinal cord lesion at the level of the absent reflexes.

Examining sensation

Usually, examiners will stop you before you embark on sensory examination. The exceptions are with a radiculopathy, a specific mononeuropathy or peripheral neuropathy. For these, the modalities to test for are proprioception (joint position sense), vibration, temperature and pinprick.

■ **Proprioception** Grasping the sides of a finger or big toe, move it up and down, demonstrating to the patient, before asking them to close their eyes and report the direction of movement being applied (Fig. 3.31).

■ **Vibration** A 128-Hz tuning fork may be applied over the first metatarsophalangeal joints, medial malleoli, knee, greater trochanters, anterior superior iliac spines, ribs, sternum, wrists, elbows and shoulders) (Fig. 3.32).

■ **Temperature** A cold tuning fork tests the spinothalamic tracts.

■ **Light touch and pinprick** Using a disposable neurological pin, first confirm on the patient's sternum that the difference between sharp and blunt is appreciated. Light touch may also be assessed, with cotton wool, and not a stroking movement. 'Light' is the operative word – many candidates apply touch that pachyderms such as elephants or hippos would detect!

Pinprick and light touch loss are often the first to be noticed by patients but the other sensory modalities may be more discriminating. For all sensory modalities you can interpret patterns of sensory loss (Table 3.30).

Examination of the upper limbs

Inspection

Note any obvious wasting, fasciculation, tremor or unusual posture. The face may reveal asymmetry, wasting, a Parkinsonian expression, Horner's syndrome, nystagmus and so on.

Tone

Take the hand as if to shake it and hold the forearm. Pronate and supinate the forearm, then roll the hand at the wrist and finally flex and extend the elbow. Repeat movements at different speeds.

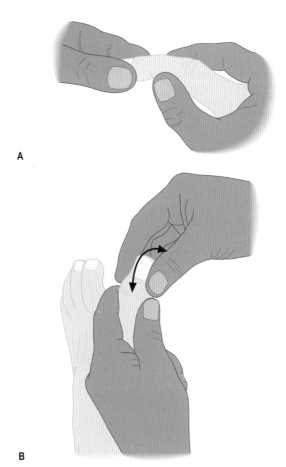

A

B

Fig. 3.31 Testing proprioception in finger (A) and toe (B).

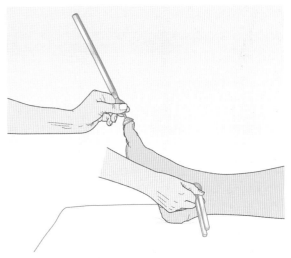

Fig. 3.32 Testing vibration sense.

Table 3.30 Patterns of sensory loss

Lesion	Pattern of sensory loss
Parietal lobe lesion	Sensory inattention or neglect Recognition of all types of sensation may be intact but poor localisation – two point discrimination lost
Thalamic lesion	Hemisensory loss of all modalities of sensation
Brainstem lesion	Loss of pain and temperature on face and opposite side of body in lateral medullary syndrome

Spinal cord lesions
  Complete transverse lesion
  Brown–Séquard hemisection
 	
  Central cord lesion, e.g. syringomyelia
 	
  Dorsal column lesion, e.g. tabes dorsalis
  Anterior spinal syndrome
	
	Complete loss of all sensory modalities below lesion
	Loss of pain and temperature sensation contralaterally and proprioception and vibration sense ipsilaterally below lesion
	Loss of pain and temperature sensation bilaterally below lesion with other modalities preserved (dissociated sensory loss)
	Loss of proprioception and vibration sense bilaterally below lesion
	Loss of pain and temperature sensation bilaterally below lesion with preserved proprioception and vibration sense

Radiculopathy	Dermatomal loss
Mononeuropathy	Sensory loss in distribution of nerve
Peripheral neuropathy	Peripheral symmetrical sensory loss

Power

Instruct the patient 'Hold your arms out in front of you and close your eyes' and look for:

- Upper motor neuron weakness (the arm falls)
- Drift (the arm wanders in the presence of a parietal lesion)
- Overshoot (when the arm is tapped with eyes closed it fails to rediscover its point of origin) and the action tremor of cerebellar disease.

If there is an obvious upper motor neuron weakness it is not necessary to examine every muscle group. Full examination would begin by asking the patient to shrug their shoulders adducting the scapulae (C3,4 roots and trapezius muscles), brace back their shoulders (C4,5 roots and rhomboids) and push forward against resistance (C5–7 roots and serratus anterior muscles) but these instructions are seldom necessary.

Examining shoulder movements

Refer to Fig. 3.33.

Examining elbow movements

Refer to Fig. 3.34.

Examining wrist movements

Refer to Fig. 3.35.

Examining finger movements (that do not involve small muscles of the hand)

Refer to Fig. 3.36.

Examining the small (intrinsic) muscles of the hand

Refer to Fig. 3.37. These muscles all originate within the hand and are supplied from the T1 nerve roots via the median and ulnar nerves. The median nerve supplies just four small muscles (lateral two umbricals, opponens pollicis, abductor pollicis brevis, flexor pollicis brevis – 'LOAF', which are the thenar muscles) and the ulnar nerve supplies all other small muscles – hypothenar muscles, medial two lumbricals, interossei which abduct and adduct the fingers, and adductor pollicis.

Reflexes

With the patient's arms relaxed and rested lightly on the abdomen, test the upper limb reflexes (Fig. 3.38).

Coordination

A rapid finger–nose test should tell you whether or not to pursue cerebellar examination as outlined in 'Examining coordination'.

Sensation

Refer to 'Examining power and sensation – overview'.

Summary

A summary of the upper limb examination sequence is given in the Summary Box.

SUMMARY BOX – UPPER LIMB EXAMINATION SEQUENCE

- Look for wasting, fasciculation, tremor or unusual posture
- Assess tone
- Examine shoulder movements (Fig. 3.33)
- Examine elbow movements (Fig. 3.34)
- Examine wrist movements (Fig. 3.35)
- Examine finger movements (Fig. 3.36)
- Examine the small muscles of the hand (Fig. 3.37)
- Examine biceps, triceps and supinator reflexes
- Examine coordination with a rapid finger–nose test
- Examine sensation

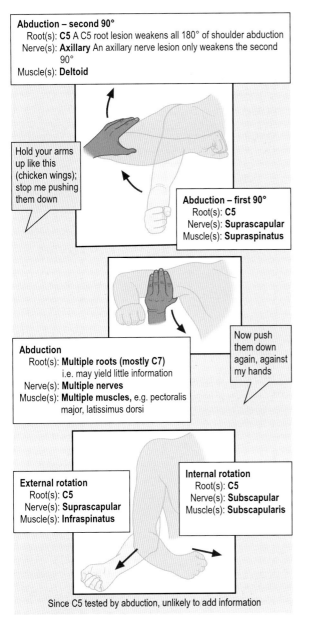

Fig. 3.33 Examining shoulder movements.

Abduction – second 90°
Root(s): **C5** A C5 root lesion weakens all 180° of shoulder abduction
Nerve(s): **Axillary** An axillary nerve lesion only weakens the second 90°
Muscle(s): **Deltoid**

Hold your arms up like this (chicken wings); stop me pushing them down

Abduction – first 90°
Root(s): **C5**
Nerve(s): **Suprascapular**
Muscle(s): **Supraspinatus**

Abduction
Root(s): **Multiple roots (mostly C7)**
i.e. may yield little information
Nerve(s): **Multiple nerves**
Muscle(s): **Multiple muscles**, e.g. pectoralis major, latissimus dorsi

Now push them down again, against my hands

External rotation
Root(s): **C5**
Nerve(s): **Suprascapular**
Muscle(s): **Infraspinatus**

Internal rotation
Root(s): **C5**
Nerve(s): **Subscapular**
Muscle(s): **Subscapularis**

Since C5 tested by abduction, unlikely to add information

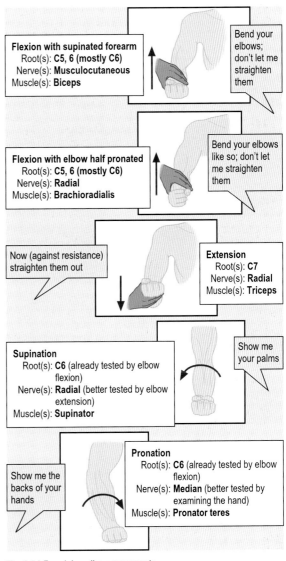

Fig. 3.34 Examining elbow movements.

Flexion with supinated forearm
Root(s): **C5, 6 (mostly C6)**
Nerve(s): **Musculocutaneous**
Muscle(s): **Biceps**

Bend your elbows; don't let me straighten them

Flexion with elbow half pronated
Root(s): **C5, 6 (mostly C6)**
Nerve(s): **Radial**
Muscle(s): **Brachioradialis**

Bend your elbows like so; don't let me straighten them

Now (against resistance) straighten them out

Extension
Root(s): **C7**
Nerve(s): **Radial**
Muscle(s): **Triceps**

Supination
Root(s): **C6** (already tested by elbow flexion)
Nerve(s): **Radial** (better tested by elbow extension)
Muscle(s): **Supinator**

Show me your palms

Show me the backs of your hands

Pronation
Root(s): **C6** (already tested by elbow flexion)
Nerve(s): **Median** (better tested by examining the hand)
Muscle(s): **Pronator teres**

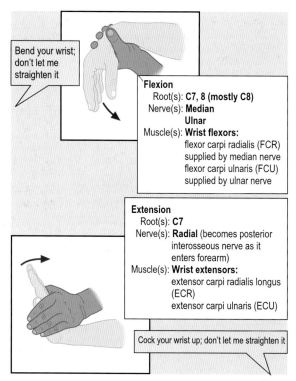

Bend your wrist; don't let me straighten it

Flexion
Root(s): **C7, 8 (mostly C8)**
Nerve(s): **Median**
Ulnar
Muscle(s): **Wrist flexors:**
flexor carpi radialis (FCR) supplied by median nerve
flexor carpi ulnaris (FCU) supplied by ulnar nerve

Extension
Root(s): **C7**
Nerve(s): **Radial** (becomes posterior interosseous nerve as it enters forearm)
Muscle(s): **Wrist extensors:**
extensor carpi radialis longus (ECR)
extensor carpi ulnaris (ECU)

Cock your wrist up; don't let me straighten it

Fig. 3.35 Examining wrist movements.

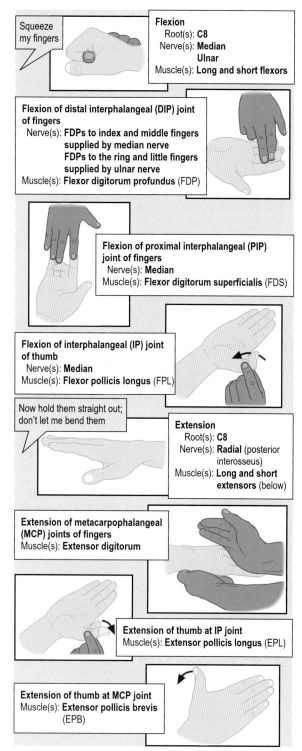

Squeeze my fingers

Flexion
Root(s): **C8**
Nerve(s): **Median**
Ulnar
Muscle(s): **Long and short flexors**

Flexion of distal interphalangeal (DIP) joint of fingers
Nerve(s): **FDPs to index and middle fingers supplied by median nerve**
FDPs to the ring and little fingers supplied by ulnar nerve
Muscle(s): **Flexor digitorum profundus (FDP)**

Flexion of proximal interphalangeal (PIP) joint of fingers
Nerve(s): **Median**
Muscle(s): **Flexor digitorum superficialis (FDS)**

Flexion of interphalangeal (IP) joint of thumb
Nerve(s): **Median**
Muscle(s): **Flexor pollicis longus (FPL)**

Now hold them straight out; don't let me bend them

Extension
Root(s): **C8**
Nerve(s): **Radial** (posterior interosseus)
Muscle(s): **Long and short extensors** (below)

Extension of metacarpophalangeal (MCP) joints of fingers
Muscle(s): **Extensor digitorum**

Extension of thumb at IP joint
Muscle(s): **Extensor pollicis longus (EPL)**

Extension of thumb at MCP joint
Muscle(s): **Extensor pollicis brevis (EPB)**

Fig. 3.36 Examining finger movements.

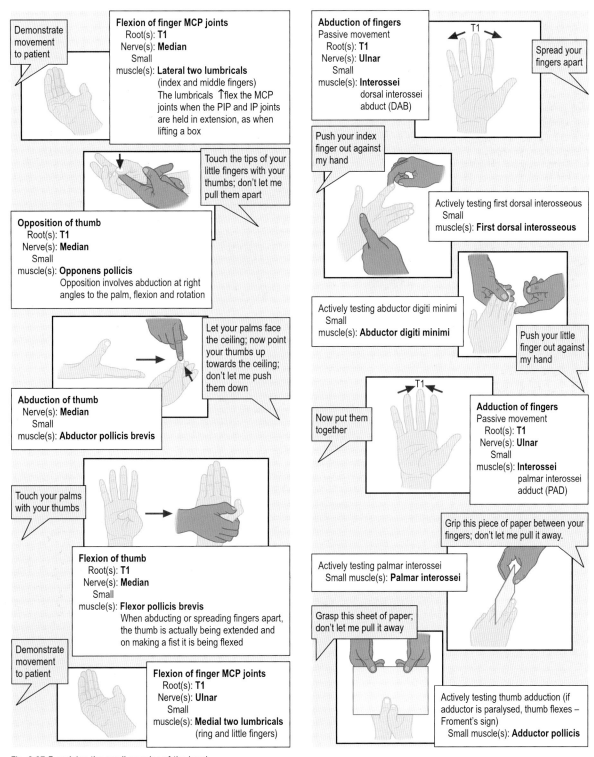

Flexion of finger MCP joints
Root(s): **T1**
Nerve(s): **Median**
Small
muscle(s): **Lateral two lumbricals**
(index and middle fingers)
The lumbricals ↑flex the MCP
joints when the PIP and IP joints
are held in extension, as when
lifting a box

Demonstrate movement to patient

Touch the tips of your little fingers with your thumbs; don't let me pull them apart

Opposition of thumb
Root(s): **T1**
Nerve(s): **Median**
Small
muscle(s): **Opponens pollicis**
Opposition involves abduction at right
angles to the palm, flexion and rotation

Let your palms face the ceiling; now point your thumbs up towards the ceiling; don't let me push them down

Abduction of thumb
Nerve(s): **Median**
Small
muscle(s): **Abductor pollicis brevis**

Touch your palms with your thumbs

Flexion of thumb
Root(s): **T1**
Nerve(s): **Median**
Small
muscle(s): **Flexor pollicis brevis**
When abducting or spreading fingers apart,
the thumb is actually being extended and
on making a fist it is being flexed

Demonstrate movement to patient

Flexion of finger MCP joints
Root(s): **T1**
Nerve(s): **Ulnar**
Small
muscle(s): **Medial two lumbricals**
(ring and little fingers)

Abduction of fingers
Passive movement
Root(s): **T1**
Nerve(s): **Ulnar**
Small
muscle(s): **Interossei**
dorsal interossei
abduct (DAB)

T1

Spread your fingers apart

Push your index finger out against my hand

Actively testing first dorsal interosseous
Small
muscle(s): **First dorsal interosseous**

Actively testing abductor digiti minimi
Small
muscle(s): **Abductor digiti minimi**

Push your little finger out against my hand

T1

Now put them together

Adduction of fingers
Passive movement
Root(s): **T1**
Nerve(s): **Ulnar**
Small
muscle(s): **Interossei**
palmar interossei
adduct (PAD)

Grip this piece of paper between your fingers; don't let me pull it away.

Actively testing palmar interossei
Small muscle(s): **Palmar interossei**

Grasp this sheet of paper; don't let me pull it away

Actively testing thumb adduction (if
adductor is paralysed, thumb flexes –
Froment's sign)
Small muscle(s): **Adductor pollicis**

Fig. 3.37 Examining the small muscles of the hand.

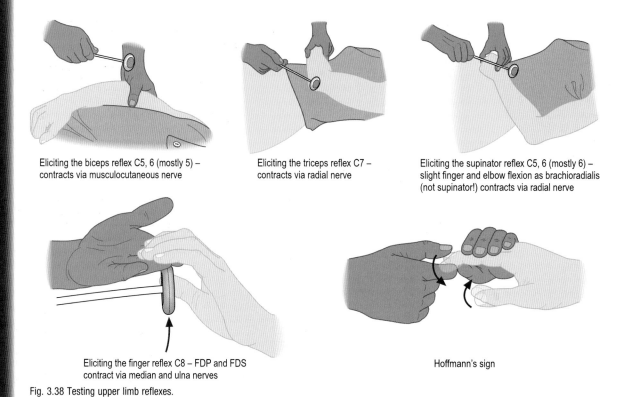

Eliciting the biceps reflex C5, 6 (mostly 5) – contracts via musculocutaneous nerve

Eliciting the triceps reflex C7 – contracts via radial nerve

Eliciting the supinator reflex C5, 6 (mostly 6) – slight finger and elbow flexion as brachioradialis (not supinator!) contracts via radial nerve

Eliciting the finger reflex C8 – FDP and FDS contract via median and ulna nerves

Hoffmann's sign

Fig. 3.38 Testing upper limb reflexes.

Examination of the lower limbs

Inspection

Note any deformity or positional abnormality. Look for wasting and fasciculation.

Tone

Roll the legs, externally and internally rotating the hips (Fig. 3.39A). Flick them up from behind the knees – the heel will 'fly' if there is spasticity and remain in contact with the bed at all times if the leg is flaccid. Normally there is only minimal departure of the heel from the bed. Check for ankle clonus. With the knee semiflexed and the foot relaxed, suddenly pull the foot dorsally and hold it, looking for sustained contractions at the ankle joint (Fig. 3.39). More than three beats is abnormal.

Power

The patient should be lying supine. Examine sections of the upper limbs as follows.

Examining hip movements

Refer to Fig. 3.40.

Examining knee movements

Refer to Fig. 3.41.

Examining ankle movements

Refer to Fig. 3.42. Note that the *sciatic nerve* has two divisions, the *common peroneal* (lateral popliteal) nerve and the *tibial* (medial popliteal) nerve. The *common peroneal nerve* has two subdivisions, the *deep* and *superficial* peroneal nerves.

Examining toe movements

Refer to Fig. 3.43.

Reflexes

With the patient's legs relaxed, test the lower limb reflexes (Fig. 3.44).

Coordination

Ask the patient to run their heel smoothly up and down the shin and watch for any tremor or difficulty coordinating this movement.

Sensation

Refer to 'Examining Power and Sensation – Overview'.

Summary

A summary of the lower limb examination sequence is given in the Summary Box.

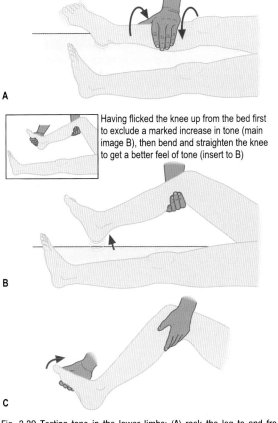

A

B

Having flicked the knee up from the bed first to exclude a marked increase in tone (main image B), then bend and straighten the knee to get a better feel of tone (insert to B)

C

Fig. 3.39 Testing tone in the lower limbs: (A) rock the leg to and fro, (B) flick the leg up from behind the knee, (C) test for ankle clonus.

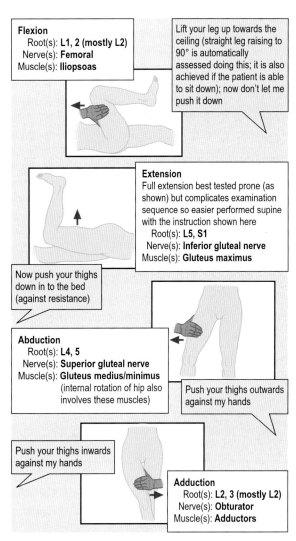

Flexion
Root(s): **L1, 2 (mostly L2)**
Nerve(s): **Femoral**
Muscle(s): **Iliopsoas**

Lift your leg up towards the ceiling (straight leg raising to 90° is automatically assessed doing this; it is also achieved if the patient is able to sit down); now don't let me push it down

Extension
Full extension best tested prone (as shown) but complicates examination sequence so easier performed supine with the instruction shown here
Root(s): **L5, S1**
Nerve(s): **Inferior gluteal nerve**
Muscle(s): **Gluteus maximus**

Now push your thighs down in to the bed (against resistance)

Abduction
Root(s): **L4, 5**
Nerve(s): **Superior gluteal nerve**
Muscle(s): **Gluteus medius/minimus**
(internal rotation of hip also involves these muscles)

Push your thighs outwards against my hands

Push your thighs inwards against my hands

Adduction
Root(s): **L2, 3 (mostly L2)**
Nerve(s): **Obturator**
Muscle(s): **Adductors**

Fig. 3.40 Examining hip movements.

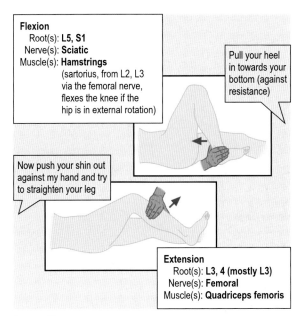

Flexion
Root(s): **L5, S1**
Nerve(s): **Sciatic**
Muscle(s): **Hamstrings**
(sartorius, from L2, L3 via the femoral nerve, flexes the knee if the hip is in external rotation)

Pull your heel in towards your bottom (against resistance)

Now push your shin out against my hand and try to straighten your leg

Extension
Root(s): **L3, 4 (mostly L3)**
Nerve(s): **Femoral**
Muscle(s): **Quadriceps femoris**

Fig. 3.41 Examining knee movements.

SUMMARY – LOWER LIMB EXAMINATION SEQUENCE

- Look for deformity or any positional abnormality, wasting and fasciculation
- Assess tone and examine for clonus
- Examine hip movements (Fig. 3.40)
- Examine knee movements (Fig. 3.41)
- Examine ankle movements (Fig. 3.42)
- Examine toe movements (Fig. 3.43)
- Examine knee and ankle reflexes
- Assess the plantar responses
- Examine coordination with a rapid heel–shin test
- Examine sensation

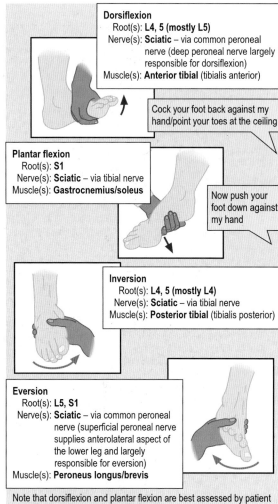

Dorsiflexion
  Root(s): **L4, 5 (mostly L5)**
  Nerve(s): **Sciatic** – via common peroneal nerve (deep peroneal nerve largely responsible for dorsiflexion)
  Muscle(s): **Anterior tibial** (tibialis anterior)

Cock your foot back against my hand/point your toes at the ceiling

Plantar flexion
  Root(s): **S1**
  Nerve(s): **Sciatic** – via tibial nerve
  Muscle(s): **Gastrocnemius/soleus**

Now push your foot down against my hand

Inversion
  Root(s): **L4, 5 (mostly L4)**
  Nerve(s): **Sciatic** – via tibial nerve
  Muscle(s): **Posterior tibial** (tibialis posterior)

Eversion
  Root(s): **L5, S1**
  Nerve(s): **Sciatic** – via common peroneal nerve (superficial peroneal nerve supplies anterolateral aspect of the lower leg and largely responsible for eversion)
  Muscle(s): **Peroneus longus/brevis**

Note that dorsiflexion and plantar flexion are best assessed by patient standing on heels and toes respectively

Fig. 3.42 Examining ankle movements.

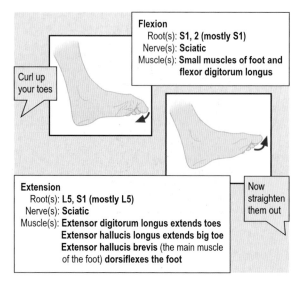

Flexion
  Root(s): **S1, 2 (mostly S1)**
  Nerve(s): **Sciatic**
  Muscle(s): **Small muscles of foot and flexor digitorum longus**

Curl up your toes

Now straighten them out

Extension
  Root(s): **L5, S1 (mostly L5)**
  Nerve(s): **Sciatic**
  Muscle(s): **Extensor digitorum longus extends toes**
  Extensor hallucis longus extends big toe
  Extensor hallucis brevis (the main muscle of the foot) **dorsiflexes the foot**

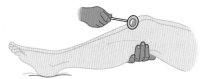

Eliciting the knee reflex L3, 4 – strike the quadriceps and watch it contract and the knee extend

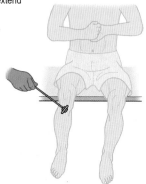

Reinforcement may be used to enhance reflexes which are difficult to elicit (ask patient to clasp hands tightly as shown or clench teeth)

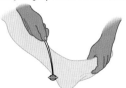

Eliciting the ankle reflex of recumbent patient (*Bend your knee slightly and let it flop to the side*) L5, S1 (mostly S1) – strike the Achilles tendon, having induced relaxed tone in the calf muscle by adjusting the amount of ankle flexion and watch for plantar flexion and calf contraction.

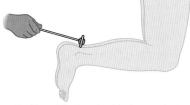

Alternative method is to strike the sole of the foot to stimulate sudden Achilles stretch

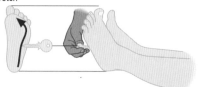

Plantar response – scrape the outer border of the foot from heel to toe and then across sole of the forefoot. Watch the toes curl (normal) or extend (positive Babinski's sign – upper motor neuron lesion, or withdrawal).

Alternative stimuli include stimulating the lateral aspect of the foot (Chaddock's sign) or running the thumb and index finger down the medial aspect of the tibia (Oppenheim's reflex) – both stimuli only of use if present

Fig. 3.44 Lower limb reflexes.

Fig. 3.43 Examining toe movements.

Table 3.31 Common abnormal types of gait

Gait		Signs	What to look for next	Possible causes
Spastic		Awkward, as if wading through mud, with foot turned inwards May be part of hemiplegia or paraplegia – in hemiplegia pelvis on affected side tilted upwards to raise spastic leg off the floor; in paraplegia gait is scissoring, as if the legs are trying to cross over each other	Upper motor neuron signs Hemiplegia Sensory level if paraplegia	Stroke Demyelination
Cerebellar		Wide based Lurching as if on the deck of a ship	Other cerebellar signs	Alcohol Cerebellar degeneration
Parkinsonian		Short, shuffling steps Lack of arm swing Stooped posture as though shuffling steps are hurrying to keep up with it—so called festinant gait	Other signs of Parkinson's disease, e.g. bradykinaesia, hypomimia, rigidity, asymmetrical resting tremor	Parkinson's disease
Marche à petit pas		Short steps Preserved arm swing Upright posture	Assess cerebrovascular risk factors	Diffuse small vessel disease
Sensory ataxic (stamping) gait		Foot seems to stamp down onto the floor Movements of leg(s) bear(s) no relation to its/their position in space Wide based and apprehensive, patient looking to floor to aid unsure steps	Positive Romberg's sign Impaired proprioception and vibration sense	Subacute combined degeneration of cord Tabes dorsalis Friedreich's ataxia Cervical myelopathy
High stepping		Foot drop Patient lifts leg or bends knee to avoid forefoot scraping ground	Signs of common peroneal nerve palsy	Common peroneal nerve palsy Hereditary motor and sensory neuropathy 1 Sciatic nerve lesion L4,5 radiculopathy
Waddling		Wide-based gait with weight shifting from side to side of pelvis as patient waddles forwards	Inspection for likely causes of proximal myopathy, e.g. Cushing's syndrome	Cushing's syndrome Thyrotoxicosis Polymyositis
Apraxic		Patient cannot walk Neuromuscular system works Sometimes visual aids compensate and override faulty brain processing of walking mechanism	Other apraxias Other frontal lobe signs	Normal pressure hydrocephalus Frontal lobe disease

Examination of gait

Gait abnormalities

Examining gait is an essential part of both lower limb and more generalised neurological examination. Common abnormal types of gait are illustrated in Table 3.31 and while these may become easy to recognise, a suggested sequence for their detection is given in the Summary Box.

Most gaits are symmetrical. Asymmetric gaits may be the result of hemiplegia, a foot drop or pain.

Summary

A summary of the gait examination sequence is given in the Summary Box.

SUMMARY BOX – GAIT EXAMINATION SEQUENCE

- Observe the patient walking
- Note any obvious inward turning of foot or scissoring *(spastic)*
- Observe the patient turning and note any loss of arm swing *(Parkinsonian)*; note posture
- Observe the patient standing (and then walking) on their heels and toes *(high stepping/foot drop)*
- Observe patient walking heel to toe or 'tandem' walking *(cerebellar)*
- Check Romberg's test *(sensory ataxia)*; this is only positive if the patient is more unsteady with eyes closed than open – 'pseudo-Rombergism' is common because without vision, unsteadiness is always a little worse – and a truly positive Romberg's test is associated with proprioceptive and vibration sense impairment occurring in dorsal column disease and some peripheral neuropathies
- Observe the patient squatting *(proximal myopathy)*

CASE 3.16

VISUAL FIELD DEFECTS

Instruction

Please examine this patient's eyes/visual fields and comment on your findings.

Recognition

There is (depending on the site of the lesion):

- A left/right *central scotoma*
- *Tunnel* (more correctly *funnel*) vision
- *Unilateral blindness*
- *Bitemporal hemianopia*
- *A left/right homonymous hemianopia*
- *A left/right homonymous quadrantanopia*
- *Loss of vision in the left/right eye with macular sparing*

Interpretation

Confirm the diagnosis

What to do next depends upon the defect (Fig. 3.45).

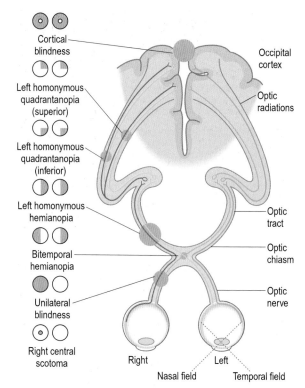

Fig. 3.45 Visual field defects (visual field testing and visual field defects).

Box 3.31 Five Signs of Optic Nerve Damage

1. Central scotoma
2. Decreased visual acuity
3. Decreased colour vision
4. Relative afferent papillary defect (the most sensitive and specific sign)
5. Optic atrophy

What to do next – consider causes/assess other systems

Central scotoma

This indicates disease of the macula or nerve fibres from the optic nerve head (optic disc) that supply it. Look for evidence of disease at the macula or disc such as diabetic maculopathy or optic atrophy. Five signs of optic nerve damage are listed in Box 3.31.

Unilateral blindness

This indicates that damage is to the eye itself.

Bitemporal hemianopia

This implies a lesion at the optic chiasm. A pituitary tumour may cause compression from below the optic chiasm. Look for signs of acromegaly (Fig. 3.46) or hypopituitarism. Rare causes include craniopharyngiomas, which compress the chiasm from above, meningiomas and aneurysms.

Homonymous hemianopia

This usually results from a total or partial anterior circulation stroke (TACS or PACS). A right TACS or PACS causes a left homonymous hemianopia – look then for a

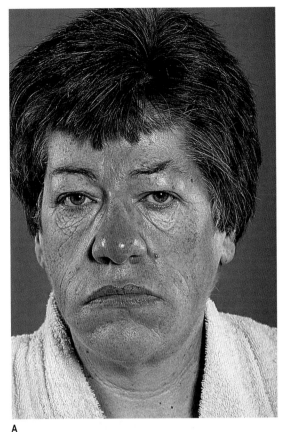

A

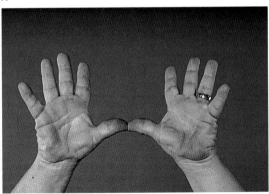

B

Fig. 3.46 (A,B) Acromegaly.

left supranuclear facial palsy and left upper motor neuron limb signs.

Homonymous quadrantanopia

Consider a lesion in the temporal radiations if there is a superior homonymous hemianopia and in the parietal radiations if there is an inferior homonymous quadrantanopia. The cause again is usually a contralateral TACs or PACS.

Cortical blindness

This is the result of bilateral posterior cerebral artery strokes. The macula is spared because the macular cortex

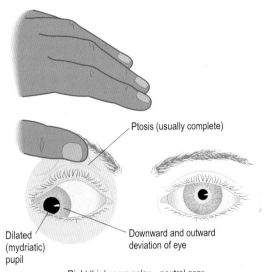

Ptosis (usually complete)

Dilated (mydriatic) pupil

Downward and outward deviation of eye

Right third nerve palsy – neutral gaze

Fig. 3.47 Right third nerve palsy.

is supplied by the middle cerebral artery. Structural lesions destroying a hemioccipital cortex can cause complete contralateral blindness and visual hallucinations.

Consider severity/decompensation/complications

This relates very much to the underlying diagnosis. A visual field defect that is part of a TACS or PACS might lead to a discussion about stroke (Case 3.27).

Consider function

Comment on the functional significance of visual loss.

Discussion

List some causes of a visual field defect in one eye

- Scotoma
- Altitudinal defect (lesion confined to the upper or lower half of the visual field but crossing the vertical meridian) – usually a retinal artery branch problem
- Funnel vision (e.g. retinitis pigmentosa)

CASE 3.17

OCULAR NERVE LESIONS (THIRD NERVE, SIXTH NERVE, FOURTH NERVE)

Instruction

Please examine this patient's eyes/eye movements and discuss your findings.

Recognition

Third nerve (oculomotor) lesion

The left/right eye adopts a *'down and out'* position because only the superior oblique and lateral rectus muscles are intact (Fig. 3.47). There is *ptosis* and the *pupil is dilated* if

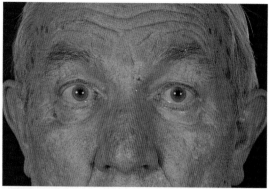

A

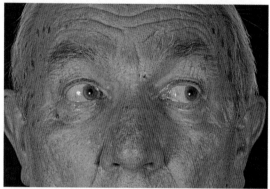

B

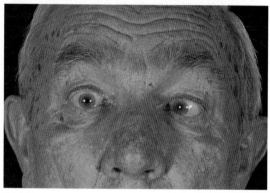

C

Fig. 3.48 Sixth nerve palsy: (A) primary position, (B) looking left, (C) looking right.

there is parasympathetic damage. Because the parasympathetic nerves destined for the pupillary sphincter are entwined around the third nerve, compressive lesions damage them while intrinsic (medical) causes like diabetes spare them. Medical causes tend to be painless.

Sixth nerve (abducens) lesion

There is a gaze palsy, the left/right eye *failing to abduct* (Fig. 3.48).

Fourth nerve (trochlear) lesion

Isolated fourth nerve palsies are rare. Unopposed external rotation of the affected eye may result in a compensatory head tilt.

Interpretation

Confirm the diagnosis

The type of ocular palsy is usually clear if a single lesion is present. If this is not the case, consider the possibility of a complex ophthalmoplegia.

What to do next – consider causes

Tell the examiners possible sites of lesions:

Brainstem

The lesion may be of the nerve or of its nucleus connecting with central pathways. Causes include vascular lesions (isolated sixth nerve palsies often with diabetes), demyelination and compressive lesions. Look for diabetic retinopathy and tell the examiners you would exclude diabetes.

Basal area

Causes include infection (bacterial, fungal or tuberculous infection), carcinomatous meningitis, basal infiltration from neurosarcoid or lymphoma, or infiltration from the nasopharynx or sinuses.

- Multiple lower cranial nerves are often involved, with a bulbar palsy.
- A posterior communicating artery aneurysm may compress the third nerve and is often painful.
- The third nerve may occasionally be stretched by a prolapsing temporal lobe (haemorrhage) and the sixth nerve may be stretched over the petrous tip by posterior fossa tumours. These ocular palsies are 'false localising' signs.

Cavernous sinus and orbit

Sepsis, tumours, intracavernous carotid aneurysms and infiltrative conditions like Wegener's granulomatosis may damage ocular nerves as they traverse the cavernous sinus.

Consider severity/decompensation/complications

This relates very much to the underlying diagnosis.

Consider function

Comment on the functional significance of diplopia.

Discussion

What are the actions of the muscles controlling eye movements?

These are shown in Fig. 3.49. The rectus muscles are straightforward. The medial rectus of one eye and the lateral rectus of the other work as a conjugate pair for

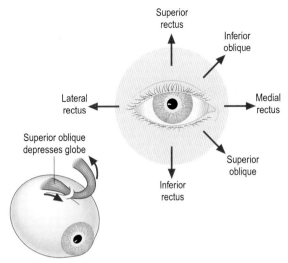

Fig. 3.49 Actions of the muscles controlling eye movements (insert: action of superior oblique).

horizontal conjugate gaze. The actions of the obliques are more difficult to remember:

- When abducting, the superior and inferior rectus muscles dominate vertical gaze.
- When adducting, the superior and inferior oblique muscles dominate vertical gaze.
- Superior oblique, unlike superior rectus, depresses the eye while inferior oblique, unlike inferior rectus, elevates the eye! This is because the oblique muscles swing through hooks of tissue then double back on the globe to exert traction on it in a line of pull contrary to their nomenclature (see Fig. 3.49: insert)
- As the oblique muscles sit slightly medially, they also attempt rotatory movements of the eyes, being unsuccessful in normal circumstances because of the opposing strength of other muscles. Acting alone, superior oblique would cause internal rotation or 'intorsion', and inferior oblique would cause external rotation or 'extorsion'.

By which ocular nerves are these muscles supplied?

- Oculomotor nerve – superior oblique, inferior rectus, medial rectus and inferior oblique
- Abducens nerve – lateral rectus
- Trochlear nerve – superior oblique

How does ophthalmoplegia cause diplopia?

When you take a romantic walk with your partner on a sunny day you may catch the sunlight in her or his eyes and see that it falls on exactly the same spot on each eye. Likewise, images from the world around us fall on corresponding spots of each retina. Slight displacement of either eye causes diplopia or double vision.

Which is the false image in diplopia?

The direction of gaze in which separation of images and corresponding diplopia is maximal is the direction of action of the paretic muscle. The false image (resulting from the paretic eye) falls progressively away from the macula and is always the outer or peripheral image seen. By covering the paretic eye this false image disappears.

What is meant by the term dysconjugate gaze?

This simply means that the eyes do not move together synchronously.

What is meant by the term strabismus or squint?

Strabismus or squint refers to misalignment – convergence (exotropia) or divergence (esotropia) – in the primary position (looking straight ahead), which remains constant in all directions of gaze. Cranial nerve ocular palsies and lateral and vertical gaze palsies arising from supranuclear disturbances should not be termed 'squints'.

What is meant by the term latent strabismus?

The visual axes are misaligned, even in the primary or neutral position, because of an imbalance of muscle tone rather than paresis. We all have a tendency to this, overcome by fusion mechanisms. It manifests in those with a history of a childhood squint, especially when tired. The squint does not settle in either eye. Rather, it is an angle that remains fixed between the eyes in any direction of gaze.

How might a latent strabismus be confirmed?

The cover test may be useful in eliciting a latent squint. To elicit the squint a hand covers one eye. The covered eye moves towards the squinting position, while the free eye fixes on an object. When the covered eye is uncovered, the squint is transiently observed.

Is ophthalmoplegia always due to a cranial nerve lesion?

No. It can arise from cranial nerve, neuromuscular junction or muscle abnormalities. Myasthenia gravis causes a complex ophthalmoplegia (multiple nerve lesions) and ptosis, and may be bilateral. A complex ophthalmopathy may also occur in thyroid eye disease due to compression from orbital infiltration or thyrotoxic myopathy, and vasculitis. Rare ocular myopathies include some mitochondrial cytopathies and oculopharyngeal muscular dystrophy.

CASE 3.18

INTERNUCLEAR OPHTHALMOPLEGIA

Instruction

Please examine this patient's eye movements and proceed as you think appropriate before discussing your findings.

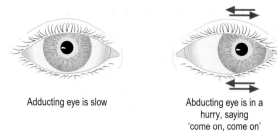

Adducting eye is slow

Abducting eye is in a hurry, saying 'come on, come on'

Fig. 3.50 Internuclear ophthalmoplegia.

Recognition

On horizontal gaze, the abducting eye appears impatient because the *adducting eye* is *slow*. There is *divergent gaze* and the *abducting eye* appears to be coaxing the slow adducting eye, saying to it 'come on, come on!' in the only way it knows – with coarse, jerky *nystagmus* (Fig. 3.50)!

Interpretation

Confirm the diagnosis

This combination of eye anomalies is specific to internuclear ophthalmoplegia. Be alert, however, to the possibility of bilateral internuclear ophthalmoplegia.

What to do next – consider causes

In internuclear ophthalmoplegia the medial longitudinal fasciculus is damaged, most commonly by demyelination in multiple sclerosis. Look for signs of optic nerve damage – central scotoma, decreased visual acuity, decreased colour vision, relative afferent pupillary defect and optic atrophy – and tell the examiners you would look for other signs of demyelination, e.g. cerebellar signs, spastic paraparesis, sensory disturbance or bladder catheterisation.

Consider severity/decompensation/complications

This relates very much to the underlying diagnosis, usually the severity of multiple sclerosis.

Consider function

Comment on the functional significance of diplopia.

Discussion

Explain the mechanism of horizontal voluntary conjugate gaze and therefore how internuclear ophthalmoplegia arises

The supranuclear or central processes governing eye movements are not well established but the following are thought to be true:

- Saccadic movements, under voluntary control, are initiated in the frontal cortex.
- Pursuit movements are initiated in the parieto-occipital cortex.

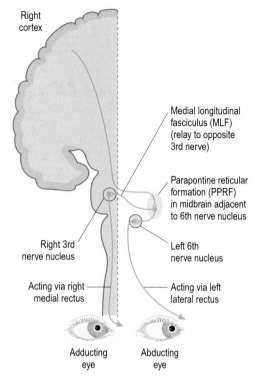

Fig. 3.51 The role of the medial longitudinal fasciculus in voluntary gaze, looking to the left.

Box 3.32 Horizontal voluntary gaze and how internuclear ophthalmoplegia arises

Higher initiating pathways descend from the *frontal cortex* to the level of the contralateral sixth nerve nucleus at the *parapontine reticular formation (PPRF)*. Some neurons from the PPRF stimulate the *adjacent sixth nerve nucleus*. Other neurons from the PPRF travel back upwards and decussate to stimulate the *opposite third nerve nucleus* via a pathway called the *medial longitudinal fasciculus (MLF)* (Fig. 3.51). The MLF allows the lateral rectus of one eye and the medial rectus of the other to contract synchronously. Each cerebral hemisphere controls horizontal gaze in the contralateral direction. The right hemisphere stimulates the ipsilateral third nerve and the contralateral sixth nerve and the eyes look to the left.

Damage to the MLF causes internuclear ophthalmoplegia (INO). Bilateral INO (BINO) is common because of the close midline proximity of the right and left MLF.

- The eyes must continuously adjust in relation to the position of the head in space, and this requires complex vestibular and proprioceptive inputs mediated through the brainstem.
- The eyes must move together, requiring synchronous contraction of ocular muscles in one eye and reciprocal muscles in the other. Monkeys relied on this evolution of binocular vision to judge swinging distances and evade death!
- Vertical gaze is mediated by the midbrain and is not well understood. Skew deviation refers to eyes that are misaligned at different vertical levels.

- Horizontal gaze is mediated by the pons; the best understood horizontal gaze mechanism is that of voluntary gaze (Box 3.32; Fig. 3.51).

CASE 3.19

NYSTAGMUS

Instruction

Please examine this patient's eyes/eye movements and discuss your findings.

Recognition

There is difficulty in maintaining conjugate deviation. The *abducting eye drifts slowly back to the central position* (slow, pathological phase) and *then flicks back to its correct position* (fast phase). The direction of nystagmus, by convention, is the direction of the fast phase. This is known as *jerk nystagmus*.

Interpretation

Confirm the diagnosis

Jerk nystagmus should be distinguished from two other types of nystagmus:

- *Optokinetic* (physiological or end point) nystagmus, which refers to the few nystagmoid jerks at extremes of lateral gaze that are normal; this happens, for example, to a passenger in a car continuously watching the world go by.
- *Pendular nystagmus*, which is a congenital difficulty with fixation, due to, for example, retinal disease; nystagmus is pendular or symmetrical with no distinct slow and fast phases, the speed and amplitude being equal in all directions, and the eyes seem to be searching forever for an elusive resting place.

What to do next – consider causes/assess other systems

Nystagmus implies irregular, rhythmic oscillations of one or both eyes, and may be horizontal, vertical or rotatory. Since there is much mystery about the mechanism of conjugate gaze, the pathophysiology of nystagmus is obscure but:

- Vertical nystagmus is rare and indicates brainstem disease
- Horizontal nystagmus is common and includes internuclear ophthalmoplegia and jerk nystagmus caused by cerebral or peripheral disease (Fig. 3.52)

Jerk nystagmus occurs in diseases of the peripheral vestibular apparatus or central diseases involving brainstem vestibular connections or the cerebellum. Cerebellar disease is the commonest cause of nystagmus in PACES and you should look for other cerebellar signs.

Consider severity/decompensation/complications

This relates very much to the underlying diagnosis.

Consider function

Comment on the functional significance of nystagmus.

Discussion

What are the differences between peripherally and centrally provoked nystagmus?

These are listed in Table 3.32.

In a cerebellar lesion, the fast phase of nystagmus is towards the side of the lesion. In practice, the cerebellum and its brainstem connections are intimately associated and the pathophysiology of these abnormal eye movements probably involves brainstem nuclei. With progressive disease abnormal eye movements may also include: *ocular dysmetria*, an overshoot of target-directed fast eye 'saccadic' movements resembling limb past pointing and in which the eyes take a few moments to stabilise in the primary position after lateral gaze; *ocular flutter*, in which involuntary horizontal eye movements may occur in the

Table 3.32 Peripherally and centrally provoked nystagmus

	Peripheral	Central
Causes	Disease of the vestibular system, e.g. vestibular neuronitis	Brainstem or cerebellar disease, e.g. demyelination, ischaemia, structural lesion
Direction of fast phase of nystagmus	Away from side of lesion	May be multidirectional or towards lesion Vertical nystagmus suggests brainstem disease
Associated symptoms	Vertigo ± auditory symptoms common (vertigo is discussed in Case 2.40)	Vertigo and auditory symptoms rare. May be cerebellar symptoms
Nausea and vomiting	Common	Rare
Effect of lying still	Improves nystagmus and other symptoms	Does not improve symptoms
Recovery	Usually recover quickly (central adaptation)	Slow or no recovery

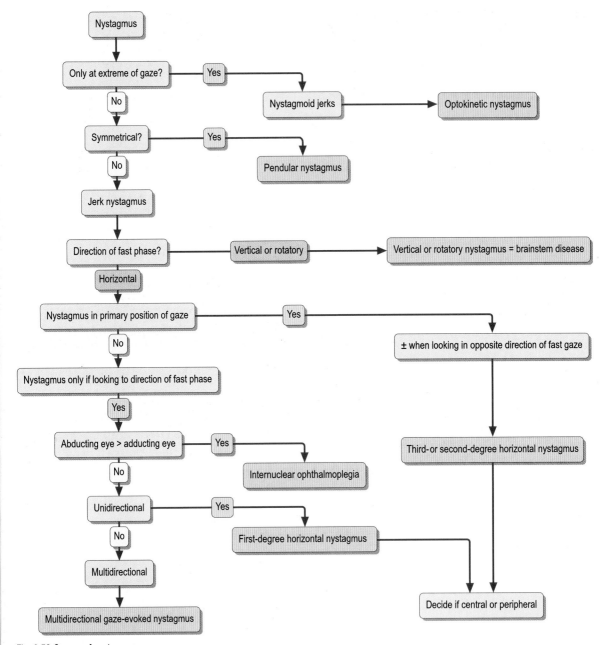

Fig. 3.52 Causes of nystagmus.

primary position; and *opsoclonus*, in which the eyes continuously oscillate in all directions.

CASE 3.20

PTOSIS

Instruction

Please examine this patient's eyes and discuss your findings.

Recognition

There is a *ptosis* (drooping upper eyelid) (Fig. 3.53).

Interpretation

Confirm the diagnosis

Ensure that the ptosis is not part of wider facial weakness.

What to do next – consider causes

Determine three things when you recognise ptosis (Box 3.33).

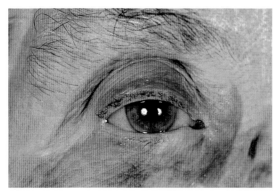

Fig. 3.53 Ptosis (due to Horner's syndrome).

Box 3.33 Determine three things when you recognise ptosis

1. Check for equal pupils
2. Check eye movements
3. Note if the ptosis is unilateral or bilateral

Third nerve palsy

There is a dilated pupil on the side of the ptosis and a 'down and out' eye. Ptosis is usually complete, so you may need to retract the lid to see these signs. The degree of ptosis alone should alert you to a third nerve palsy.

Horner's syndrome

There is a small pupil on the side of the ptosis. Ptosis is partial. Proceed as for Horner's syndrome (Case 3.23).

Myasthenia gravis

The pupils are normal. There is often a complex ophthalmoplegia and fatiguable weakness of eyelid closure (seventh nerve) and eyelid opening (third nerve). Ptosis may be unilateral or bilateral.

Myotonic dystrophy

Pupils and eye movements are normal. Cataracts may be present. Ptosis is bilateral. The face is typically myotonic (Case 3.50).

Other

Rarer causes, with normal pupils and eye movements, include congenital ptosis, oculopharyngeal muscular dystrophy and oedema.

Consider severity/decompensation/complications

This relates very much to the underlying diagnosis. A Horner's syndrome due to an apical lung tumour, for example, has a vastly different prognosis to a third nerve palsy in diabetes or myasthenia gravis.

Consider function

Comment on the functional significance of ptosis if it obscures the pupil; this is common in a third nerve palsy.

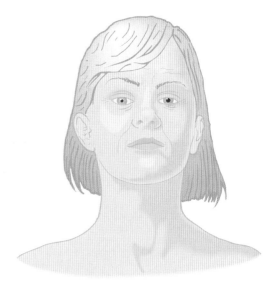

Fig. 3.54 Holmes–Adie pupil.

Discussion

What other causes of large/small pupils do you know?

These are discussed in Cases 3.21 and 3.22.

CASE 3.21

LARGE PUPIL

Instruction

Please examine this patient's pupils and eyes and discuss your findings.

Recognition

There may be difficulty in deciding whether one pupil is *too big* or if the other is too small. Fortunately, knowledge of causes helps you to determine the abnormality.

Interpretation

Confirm the diagnosis

The most straightforward way is to consider causes.

What to do next – consider causes

Third nerve palsy

Look for ptosis on the side of the larger pupil and a 'down and out' eye. Examine eye movements.

Holmes–Adie (tonic) pupil (Fig. 3.54)

This is likely to be the result of damage to the ciliary ganglion. It often affects young women. The dilated pupil may be present long before attention is drawn to it. Holmes–Adie pupils are often widely dilated, and react slowly to light but react to accommodation. They are usually unilateral, at least at first. Check ankle and knee reflexes. Absent reflexes suggest Holmes–Adie syndrome.

Traumatic iridoplegia

This is the result of damage to the ciliary pupilloconstrictor mechanism.

Drug causes

If both pupils are dilated, consider a drug-induced cause. If both eyes are blind for any reason in which light is prevented from reaching both optic nerves and triggering the light reflex response, there will also be bilateral mydriasis.

Consider severity/decompensation/complications

This relates very much to the underlying diagnosis. A third nerve palsy has many causes including stroke; a Holmes–Adie pupil is not a threat.

Consider function

Comment on the functional significance of any visual loss or diplopia.

Discussion

List some drugs which act as mydriatics

- Tropicamide
- Cocaine or amphetamines
- Atropine and other anticholinergics (gardeners may develop mydriasis after contact with plants which have anticholinergic properties, 'cause–effect' often elusive without a thorough history)

What governs pupil size?

Pupil size is balanced by the effect on the ciliary muscle of constricting parasympathetic fibres acting via the ciliary ganglion and dilating sympathetic fibres acting via the superior cervical ganglion.

CASE 3.22

SMALL PUPIL

Instruction

Please examine this patient's pupils and eyes and discuss your findings.

Recognition

There may be difficulty in deciding if one pupil is *too small* or the other too big. If there are *no obvious signs of a third nerve palsy* and the *larger pupil reacts quickly to light*, consider the causes of a small pupil.

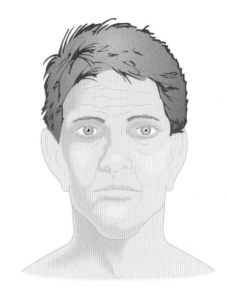

Fig. 3.55 Argyll Robertson pupils.

Interpretation

Confirm the diagnosis

The most straightforward way is to consider causes.

What to do next – consider causes

Horner's syndrome

A Horner's syndrome is usually unilateral and the pupil reacts to light. Look for partial ptosis.

Argyll Robertson pupils (ARPs) (Fig. 3.55)

These are bilaterally small, irregularly shaped pupils that accommodate but do not react to light. The accommodation reflex is subserved by more pupilloconstrictor fibres than the light reflex, and this may explain the dissociation. ARPs are classically attributed to neurosyphilis.

Anisocoria

Twenty per cent of people normally have pupil asymmetry.

Age-related miosis

Both pupils can become smaller with age, but still react to light and accommodation, and this probably represents autonomic degeneration.

Consider severity/decompensation/complications

This relates very much to the underlying diagnosis. A Horner's syndrome may be the result of an apical lung tumour, for example.

Consider function

Comment on the functional significance of any visual symptoms.

Discussion

List some common drugs causing miosis

- Pilocarpine
- Opiates

What causes of miosis might you consider in a patient with a depressed consciousness level?

Opiates and pontine lesions such as haemorrhage or encephalitis cause miosis.

What cause of miosis would you consider were the eye red and painful?

Iritis.

CASE 3.23

HORNER'S SYNDROME

Instruction

Please examine this patient's pupils and anything else you think appropriate, then discuss your findings.

Recognition (Fig. 3.56)

This is a syndrome with four potential features:

1. There is *miosis* (reduced pupillodilator activity) ipsilateral to the site of the lesion.
2. There is *partial ptosis* (because the levator palpebrae of the upper lid is partially supplied by the sympathetic nervous system as well as the parasympathetic supply that travels with the third nerve) ipsilateral to the site of the lesion.
3. There may be *anhydrosis* or absence of sweating (in preganglionic lesions only because sweat gland outflow is proximal to the superior cervical ganglion).
4. Apparent *enophthalmos* (because of paralysis of the upper and lower eyelid tarsus muscles) is seldom seen.

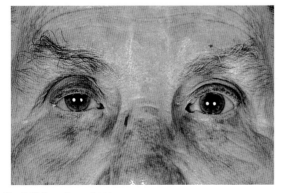

Fig. 3.56 Horner's syndrome.

Interpretation

Confirm the diagnosis

Unlike a third nerve palsy, ptosis is partial and the pupil is small.

What to do next – consider causes

Horner's syndrome is the result of an interruption of the sympathetic chain and may originate anywhere along this chain (Fig. 3.57). Lesions can occur within one of three general sites.

The first neuron

The sympathetic pathway starts in the hypothalamus and travels through the brainstem, terminating in the grey matter of the spinal cord at C8–T1. Lesions include:

- Brainstem strokes, e.g. lateral medullary syndrome
- Demyelination in the brainstem or spinal cord
- Syringomyelia/syringobulbia, resulting in a 'cape' distribution of dissociated sensory loss
- Spinal cord tumours or trauma

The second neuron

Sometimes referred to as the preganglionic neuron, referring to the superior cervical ganglion (SCG), the sympathetic pathway travels from C8–T1 via their nerve roots to

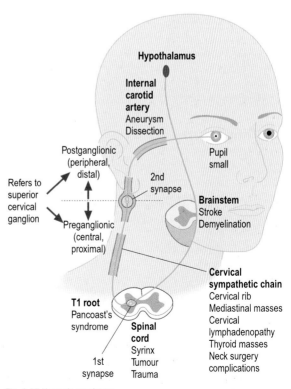

Fig. 3.57 Horner's syndrome.

the SCG. Preganglionic (also known as central or proximal) lesions are the most common causes of Horner's syndrome and include:

- Pancoast's syndrome, in which a tumour of the thoracic inlet infiltrates and causes pain in the distribution of T1 or C8; percuss and auscultate the supraclavicular area for signs of consolidation and look for ipsilateral wasting of the small muscles of the hand.
- A cervical rib, which may be confirmed by chest X-ray and may cause thoracic outlet syndrome
- A mediastinal mass; look for signs of superior vena cava obstruction
- Cervical lymphadenopathy
- Thyroid masses
- Complications of neck surgery

The third neuron

The postganglionic sympathetic pathway travels from the SCG in close proximity to the carotid artery and innervates the pupil (via long ciliary nerves which traverse around the eye), the blood vessels of the eye (via vasomotor fibres in the nasociliary branch of the trigeminal nerve) and the upper and lower lid tarsus muscles (which open the eye and oppose the action of orbicularis). Postganglionic (otherwise known as peripheral or distal) lesions include carotid aneurysms and carotid dissection.

Consider severity/decompensation/complications

Tell the examiners that a Pancoast's tumour implies invasive disease.

Consider function

This depends on the underlying cause.

Discussion

How might you determine the site of a Horner's syndrome lesion?

This is usually by identifying the cause. The use of chemical eye drops to determine if a lesion is central or peripheral is historical.

Can loss of pain and temperature sensation occur in Horner's syndrome?

The sympathetic pathway in the brainstem lies close to the spinothalamic tracts and contralateral body loss of pain and temperature sensation is frequent in Horner's syndrome arising from the brainstem.

What is thoracic outlet syndrome?

This is impingement of the subclavian arteries, which may occur with cervical ribs but which is often a variation of normal anatomy and dependent upon position (patients may experience paraesthesia and arterial symptoms in the arms on elevating the arms).

CEREBELLOPONTINE ANGLE SYNDROME

Instruction

Please examine this patient's cranial nerves and then discuss your findings.

Recognition

Any combination of *cranial neuropathies* involving the *trigeminal*, *facial* and *vestibulocochlear* nerve may occur. *Corneal reflex* loss is often the first sign, followed by facial sensory loss. Facial weakness can be a late sign. There may be *nystagmus*. There may be *sensorineural hearing loss*.

Interpretation

Confirm the diagnosis

A combination of pontine emanating cranial neuropathies without other neurological findings should alert you to this diagnosis. In practice, cerebellar signs and long tract involvement may occur depending upon the exact site of the lesion and the cause.

What to do next – consider causes

Cerebellopontine angle lesions, including acoustic neuromas and meningiomas, may cause slowly progressive hearing loss or tinnitus. Vertigo may occur. The next step is neuroimaging.

Consider severity/decompensation/complications

Tumours causing this syndrome are often benign but very awkwardly situated.

Consider function

Tell the examiners that hearing loss may be the first difficulty for patients.

Discussion

What is the cerebellopontine angle?

This is a triangle between the cerebellum, lateral pons and petrous bone (Fig. 3.58). Cranial nerves V–VIII emerge into it from the pons in craniocaudal sequence. The cerebellopontine angle stops just above IX, which emerges from the medulla.

What are the functions of the trigeminal nerve?

The trigeminal nerve divides into three from the trigeminal ganglion, which lies on the petrous tip. Each division conveys sensation (from many distal branches) from the face:

A

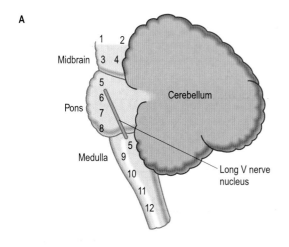

B

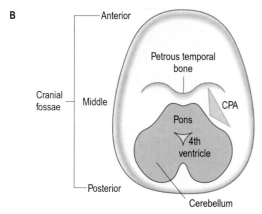

Fig. 3.58 The cerebellopontine angle (CPA).

Ophthalmic

This runs via the superior orbital fissure and cavernous sinus conveying sensation from the forehead and scalp. The nasociliary branch supplies the nostril and the tip and upper border of the nose, carries sympathetic fibres to the pupil and conveys the sensory limb of the corneal reflex.

Maxillary

This runs via the inferior orbital fissure and cavernous sinus conveying sensation from the cheek, much of the oral cavity and mid-face. One branch thickens into a special ganglion called the pterygopalatine ganglion. This receives preganglionic parasympathetic fibres from the nervus intermedius (a branch of the facial nerve), which supply the lacrimal gland.

Mandibular

This exits at the foramen ovale and supplies the jaw and lower face. It also carries motor branches to the muscles of mastication, the masseter, which is very strong (jaw closure), and the pterygoids, which are weak (jaw opening). Alligators and crocodiles demonstrate how powerful masseters and weak pterygoids confer evolutionary advantage.

What trigeminal neuropathies do you know of?

Trigeminal neuropathies may be part of a wider cerebellopontine angle syndrome, with loss of the corneal reflex often the first clinical sign. Other clinical conditions affecting the trigeminal nerve include herpes zoster ophthalmicus and trigeminal neuralgia.

What is trigeminal neuralgia?

This is a rare but characteristic pain syndrome with sudden and severe lancing pain lasting from seconds to minutes within the trigeminal nerve distribution, typically the maxillary or mandibular branches, often evoked by trivial stimulation in 'trigger zones'. Atypical symptoms with altered sensation may occur. It is a variable condition, and some patients only have one episode.

Most cases are still referred to as idiopathic, although vascular compression of the trigeminal nerve by an aberrant loop of artery or vein at its exit site from the brainstem is increasingly appreciated. A minority of cases are the result of nerve compression by a tumour, or occur in multiple sclerosis. Accordingly, the threshold for magnetic resonance imaging that includes the brainstem should be low.

The differential diagnosis includes dental disease, temporomandibular joint pain, persistent idiopathic facial pain ('atypical facial pain'), migraine and temporal arteritis.

Treatment is usually effective. Carbamazepine is first-line treatment. Surgical treatments are possible if carbamazepine is ineffective or not tolerated. Ablative surgery is seldom associated with severe complications but may cause facial sensory loss and there is a high rate of pain recurrence; microvascular decompression has a lower relapse rate but a higher risk of serious complications.

What do you know about sensorineural hearing loss (SNHL)?

Sensorineural hearing loss is popularly attributable to an acoustic neuroma in the cerebellopontine angle. These are overall rarer than perceived as a cause of SNHL and often slowly progressive. Other central causes, which may present abruptly, include demyelination and stroke, each described, but unusual causes of isolated SNHL. The commonest form of SNHL occurs insidiously with age. Sometimes, SNHL is 'idiopathic' (ISNHL) and abrupt, postulated as viral, autoimmune or ischaemic and prompting a standard battery of haematobiochemistry, inflammatory markers, autoimmune screening and a syphilis test. MR imaging is mandatory. ISNHL is usually unilateral, occasionally bilateral if autoimmune, and has a variable prognosis. Adjacent cranial nerves are not affected. Treatment is with high-dose steroids and, where available, hyperbaric oxygen; acyclovir is recommended if herpes simplex or zoster are even remote possibilities.

As well as hearing loss, unilateral ISNHL produces problems with localisation of sound as stereosound is lost, a problem that the brain may slowly adjust to.

SNHL is vital to distinguish from conductive hearing loss such as wax in the external ear or fluid in the middle ear, conductive hearing loss being much more amenable to treatment. Abrupt SNHL is an emergency.

What might the audiogram show in SNHL?

An audiogram has two axes, the *x*-axis on the top representing increasing frequency from 0 and 250 Hz (very low rumbles) on the left to 8000 Hz, the point at which humans start to stop hearing but beyond which dogs can still detect even higher frequencies or pitches, on the right. Little useful hearing in adults occurs beyond 6000 Hz and in age-related SNHL it is these higher frequencies that are impaired first of all. On the *y*-axis downwards is the intensity of sound, in decibels (dB), a logarithmic scale going from 0 at the top to around 100 at the bottom.

An audiologist in a silent room will produce sound at various frequencies and decibels to determine the minimum threshold in decibels that a sound is heard at a particular frequency. Gradually an average map is built up for each ear. As a very general rule, normal hearing detects most frequencies at around 0 dB but it is common to see the threshold a bit higher, at say 5–10 dB, with a tendency for even higher thresholds at higher frequencies; in very good hearing even negative results such as −5 or −10 dB may be seen, especially at lower frequencies and in children.

With SNHL the trend is for a downward sloping line on the graph rather than a horizontal one. The descent may be very early and very steep in severe ISNHL.

As a general rule, sounds heard below 30 dB give rise to adequate hearing, sounds audible at 50–60 dB may be corrected to around 30 dB with a hearing aid, and sounds detected only below 50–60 dB are usually not amenable to treatment without significant sound distortion when sound is amplified.

The audiogram illustrates the amazing spectrum of frequency and loudness detected by the ear, even individual spoken words comprising a vast array of internal differences; hearing words is a function not just of the spectrum of capability of the hearing mechanism but also of an individual's learned interpretation of how these diverse sounds come together to form words.

Is vertigo a frequent association of SNHL?

It is, and in a sense represents a 'screaming', diseased nerve that settles when the nerve is more severely damaged and the brain adjusts. It is more likely continuous than paroxysmal when present.

What is tinnitus?

Tinnitus is often ascribed to Meniére's disease but in fact is a common feature of any severe SNHL or damage to the vestibulocochlear nerve. It may be a high-pitched whine or hiss or a washing machine whir. It can be alarmingly disabling, a fact often underappreciated since many benign noises in the ear such as awareness of the pulse are often inadvertently reported as tinnitus. Tinnitus may be due to the brain detecting background noise previously blotted out by normal hearing from ear structures; other theories suggest it is due to the hearing compartment in the brain still being receptive whilst its sensory nerve has dwindled, analogous to the sensory experiences of a phantom limb. Rehabilitation training can overcome tinnitus, just as ticking clocks can become inaudible with time, and hearing aid technologies can help.

What is jugular foramen syndrome?

The final four cranial nerves, IX, X, XI and XII, occupy an area around the jugular foramen. Lesions in this area may extend from the cerebellopontine angle, or arise as localised or diffuse basal skull lesions as in tuberculosis or meningeal malignancy. Lesions may provoke a bulbar palsy.

CASE 3.25

FACIAL NERVE PALSY

Instruction

Please examine this patient's face. Discuss your differential diagnosis.

Recognition

There is *paralysis of one side of the face* (Fig. 3.59). In the *upper face*, the *eye does not close fully* (the eyeball may roll up on attempted closure – Bell's phenomenon). Muscles that do not work include the orbicularis oculi (closes eye), the frontalis (raises eyebrow) and the corrugator superficialis (frowns). In the *lower face*, the *mouth droops* and the *nasolabial fold* is *smooth*.

Interpretation

Confirm the diagnosis

A facial nerve palsy is just that! There is paralysis of the upper and lower parts of the face because of a lesion in the facial nerve (see Fig. 3.60). Candidates often talk of 'lower motor neuron facial nerve weakness'. By definition, facial nerve lesions are lower neuron lesions because the facial nerve is a cranial nerve innervating the face! Upper motor neuron facial weakness, due to a lesion in supranuclear neurons innervating the facial nerve, spares the upper face because there is bilateral supranuclear or upper motor neuron innervation selectively to those facial nerve fibres that supply the upper face. This said, bilateral innervation may not be even (e.g. 70:30 rather than 50:50), such that a little upper facial weakness may be seen.

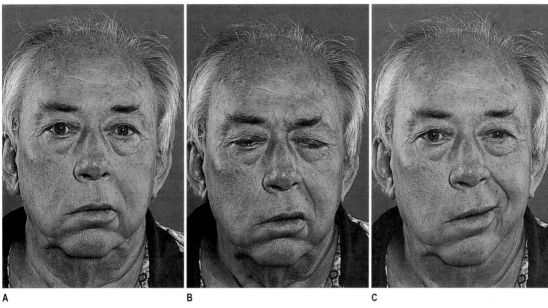

Fig. 3.59 Facial nerve palsy: (A) at rest, (B) closing eyes, (C) smiling.

What to do next – consider causes

Tell the examiners that you would consider whether loss of taste to the tongue with loss of salivation, hyperacusis or loss of lacrimation have occurred. These respectively, theoretically, help localise the lesion proximally (Fig. 3.60).

Knowing the possible causes of facial nerve palsy enables you to rapidly look for other relevant signs:

Bell's palsy

This is probably viral. Usually, but not always, the only sign is facial weakness, the presumed site of inflammation distal in the facial canal.

Ramsay Hunt syndrome

This is the result of re activation of herpes zoster virus in the geniculate ganglion. Taste tends to be affected and there may be vesicles over the external auditory meatus. Occasionally vesicles hide exclusively within the ear canal.

Parotid swellings

Look and feel for a swollen parotid gland, which may be the result of infection secondary to a duct calculus, or a parotid tumour.

Brainstem strokes or demyelination

These may involve the facial nerve nucleus and precipitate facial weakness.

Cerebellopontine lesions

These should always be considered, especially if there is loss of the corneal reflex or hearing.

Cholesteatoma

A rare cause, in which epithelial cells accumulate behind the tympanic membrane, sometimes leading to perforation. An ENT appraisal is mandatory.

Bilateral facial nerve weakness

Often missed, although weakness may not be symmetrical. Causes include bilateral Bell's palsy, Guillain–Barré syndrome, neurosarcoid and Lyme disease.

Consider severity/decompensation/complications

This very much relates to the underlying cause. Facial palsy as part of Guillain–Barré syndrome, for example, clearly has different implications to a Bell's palsy; the former might just as easily recover, but the condition is potentially much more serious. Most Bell's palsies will recover, but persistent weakness can occur.

Consider function

Tell the examiners you would wish to assess bulbar function. Tell the examiners you would wish to exclude exposure keratitis and consider corneal protection.

Discussion

Which viruses probably cause Bell's palsy?

Herpes simplex virus type 1 and herpes zoster virus are probably frequently to blame.

Would you treat Bell's palsy?

Combined treatment with oral aciclovir or valaciclovir or famciclovir for 7–10 days and prednisolone 60 mg reduced

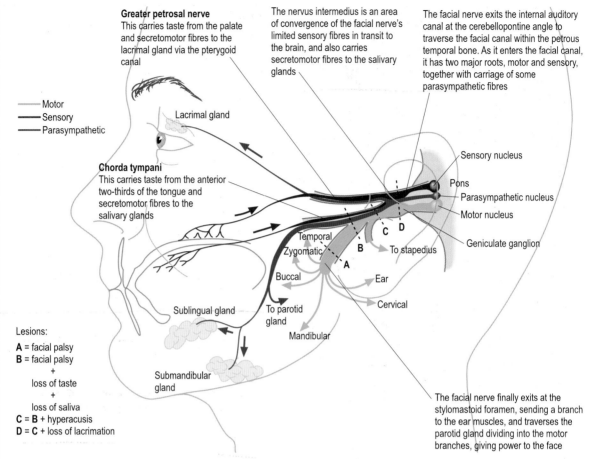

Motor
Sensory
Parasympathetic

Greater petrosal nerve
This carries taste from the palate and secretomotor fibres to the lacrimal gland via the pterygoid canal

The nervus intermedius is an area of convergence of the facial nerve's limited sensory fibres in transit to the brain, and also carries secretomotor fibres to the salivary glands

The facial nerve exits the internal auditory canal at the cerebellopontine angle to traverse the facial canal within the petrous temporal bone. As it enters the facial canal, it has two major roots, motor and sensory, together with carriage of some parasympathetic fibres

Lacrimal gland

Chorda tympani
This carries taste from the anterior two-thirds of the tongue and secretomotor fibres to the salivary glands

Sensory nucleus

Pons

Parasympathetic nucleus

Motor nucleus

Geniculate ganglion

Temporal
Zygomatic

C   D

B

A

To stapedius

Buccal

Ear

Sublingual gland

To parotid gland

Cervical

Mandibular

Submandibular gland

Lesions:

A = facial palsy
B = facial palsy
       +
   loss of taste
       +
   loss of saliva
C = **B** + hyperacusis
D = **C** + loss of lacrimation

The facial nerve finally exits at the stylomastoid foramen, sending a branch to the ear muscles, and traverses the parotid gland dividing into the motor branches, giving power to the face

Fig. 3.60 The facial nerve and localisation of damage.

to zero over three weeks is now recommended, although the evidence supporting this is equivocal. Treatment of partial Bell's palsy is controversial but a few patients do not recover if left untreated. Treatment is probably most effective before 72 hours and less effective after seven days.

CASE 3.26

BULBAR PALSY

Instruction

This lady has been in the intensive therapy unit recently. Please examine her speech.

Recognition

There is *dysarthria*. There is *nasal speech (nasal escape)*. Speech may have a 'drowning' or 'choking' quality and it often seems that 'everything is in the way'. There may be salivary pooling.

Interpretation

Confirm the diagnosis

Try to distinguish a bulbar from a pseudobulbar palsy, although this is not always so easy in practice. A bulbar palsy caused by unilateral cranial nerve insults should, in addition to the characteristic bulbar pattern of speech, produce:

• A uvula that is pulled away from the side of unilateral weakness – Xth nerve palsy (Fig. 3.61)
• A tongue that deviates to side of the lesion – XIIth nerve palsy (Fig. 3.62)

A bulbar palsy due to bilateral cranial nerve, neuromuscular or muscle disease may not produce asymmetry but the characteristic bulbar pattern of speech is present.

What to do next – consider causes/assess other symptoms

Causes of a bulbar palsy are listed in Box 3.34.

Tell the examiners that full assessment includes testing all cranial nerves, noting any ptosis and asking about

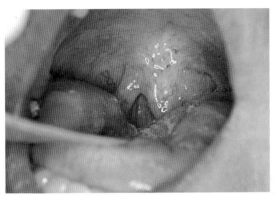

Fig. 3.61 Bulbar palsy. Xth nerve palsy – note asymmetric uvula.

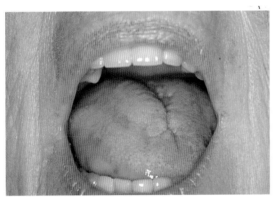

A

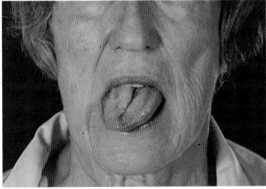

B

Fig. 3.62 Bulbar palsy. XIIth nerve palsy: (A) tongue at rest, (B) tongue protruded.

diplopia (myasthenia), testing power, testing reflexes (Guillain–Barré syndrome) and checking for fatiguability (myasthenia).

Consider severity/decompensation/complications

Tell the examiners that you would ask about nasal regurgitation of fluids or food particles with aspiration or attacks of choking and that you would wish to assess vital

---

> **Box 3.34 Causes of a bulbar palsy**
>
> - Motor neuron disease
> - Guillain–Barré syndrome
> - Myasthenia gravis
> - Lambert–Eaton myasthenic syndrome
> - Basal meningitis
> - Botulism (*Clostridium botulinum*)
> - Tetanus
> - Diphtheria
> - Lyme disease
> - HIV-related neuropathy
> - Malignancy

capacity (and ask about respiratory symptoms) and arrange a swallow assessment.

Consider function

Tell the examiners that you would ensure assessment by a speech and language therapist. Mention if there is a nasogastric tube or percutaneous gastrostomy tube in situ.

Discussion

Explain the difference between a bulbar palsy and a pseudobulbar palsy

This is explained in Box 3.26.

List some investigations you might consider for a patient with a rapidly progressive bulbar palsy

- Visualisation of the vocal cords by an ear, nose and throat specialist
- Brain/brainstem imaging
- Cerebrospinal fluid examination
- Tensilon (edrophonium) test/acetylcholine receptor antibodies
- Infection serology and testing for botulism, tetanus and diphtheria
- HIV testing

What would you regard as essential immediate management for a patient with a rapidly progressive bulbar palsy?

Assessment of respiratory rate and vital capacity and early liaison with the intensive-therapy unit and a neurologist.

CASE 3.27

ANTERIOR CIRCULATION STROKE SYNDROMES

Instruction

Please examine this patient's speech, face and limbs and discuss your findings.

Recognition

Circulation and cortical representation

Circulation

Each lobe does not have a discrete blood supply and so *stroke syndromes* are different to *lobe syndromes*. It is helpful to briefly revise brain vascular anatomy (Fig. 3.63).

Cortical representation

In terms of stroke, it is useful to remember that each cortical hemisphere represents the contralateral limbs and cranial nerves (homunculus). The left hemisphere has a major role in language. The right hemisphere has a major role in awareness of the left side of the body. This said, both hemispheres contribute to language and awareness (Fig. 3.64).

Total anterior circulation stroke (TACS), partial anterior circulation stroke (PACS), lacunar strokes (LACS) and posterior circulation stroke (POCS)

Bamford et al. devised and published this classification in Oxford in 1991 and it is now widely used because it is relatively straightforward, widely applicable and prognostic (Fig. 3.65). The suffix stroke may be substituted for infarct (I) or haemorrhage (H).

Total anterior circulation stroke (TACS) (see Fig. 3.17)

The anterior communicating artery is a protective anastomosis between the two anterior cerebral arteries and so middle cerebral artery territory strokes are much more common. Strokes arising in the proximal trunk of the middle cerebral artery or the internal carotid artery result in a *total anterior circulation syndrome* (Box 3.35). TACS account for around 20% of strokes.

Conjugate eye deviation (and sometimes head deviation), known as Prevost's sign, sometimes occurs in cortical strokes due to disturbance in cortical or subcortical pathways involved in control of voluntary eye movements. Deviation is towards the side of the lesion. For example, in a right cortical stroke, disrupted signals to the left eye with normal signals to the right eye cause an imbalance in neural tone that causes the right eye to tend to move to the right at rest because of the absence of counter pull to the left; the left eye follows in a yoking manner because

the pontine neural connections (e.g. the medial longitudinal fasciculus) to the left medial rectus are intact, leading to conjugate deviation of the eyes to the right.

Partial anterior circulation stroke (PACS) (see Fig. 3.17)

More common (around 35% of strokes) is a stroke arising in one of the middle cerebral artery's branches giving rise to a *partial anterior circulation syndrome* (Box 3.36).

Lacunar strokes (LACS) (see Fig. 3.17)

Small localised infarcts are often the result of lipohyalinosis of penetrating arteries (lenticulostriate arteries) and are referred to as LACS (Box 3.37). They are very common, and often silent. They often affect the internal capsule; the anterior limb of the internal capsule relays only motor fibres and so strokes are pure motor whereas the posterior limb of the internal capsule relays sensory fibres to the thalamus destined for the parietal lobe and strokes cause contralateral hemianaesthesia. LACS generally affect subcortical structures (e.g. basal ganglia, thalamus) and so do not exhibit higher cortical signs such as dysphasia or neglect. LACS occasionally stutter for a day or two as the occluding artery expands and contracts around its clot.

Strokes exemplify the eloquence of small parts of the brain, a minor fault evoking a clinical earthquake. The contemporary threat of atherosclerosis has taken evolution by surprise. As it is, the internal capsule, the main thoroughfare for nerve excursion from the cortex, has a disappointing blood supply ill-equipped for breakdown and an internal capsule LACS is a small area of damage with clinically large repercussions. The internal capsule is the motorway for all motor and sensory neurons whose

---

Box 3.36 Partial anterior circulation syndrome (PACS)

This requires two out of the three TACS criteria or restricted criteria:

- *Contralateral weakness of arm or leg or hand* or part thereof (corticospinal tract infarction referable to the appropriate area of homunculus) *or face* (supranuclear infarction of fibres supplying facial nerve). A monoparesis may be the sole manifestation of a PACS.
- Higher cortical dysfunction alone (*dysphasia or dyspraxia*), which may be the only manifestation of a PACS.

  Visual field defects are less common if the upper division of the middle cerebral artery is affected and motor and sensory deficits are uncommon if the lower division is affected.

Box 3.35 Total anterior circulation syndrome (TACS)

This requires all three of:

- *Contralateral* hemiparesis or *weakness* of at least *two out of three of face, arm or leg*, usually with increased tone and reflexes, with or without contralateral hemisensory loss
- *Contralateral homonymous hemianopia* (infarcted optic radiations in parietal and temporal lobes)
- A higher cortical function abnormality, usually *dysphasia* if left TACS or *dyspraxia (sensory inattention or neglect)* if right TACS

  If a patient is drowsy or has a decreased Glasgow Coma Score and 1, then 2 and 3 are assumed.

Box 3.37 Lacunar strokes (LACS)

These can affect the anterior or posterior circulation but are most common in the basal ganglia and pons. Possible LACS are:

- Pure motor (contralateral arm, leg and facial weakness, often with dysarthria)
- Pure sensory
- Sensorimotor
- Ataxic hemiparesis – contralateral hemiparesis and ipsilateral cerebellar signs due to small infarcts in basal ganglia or pons

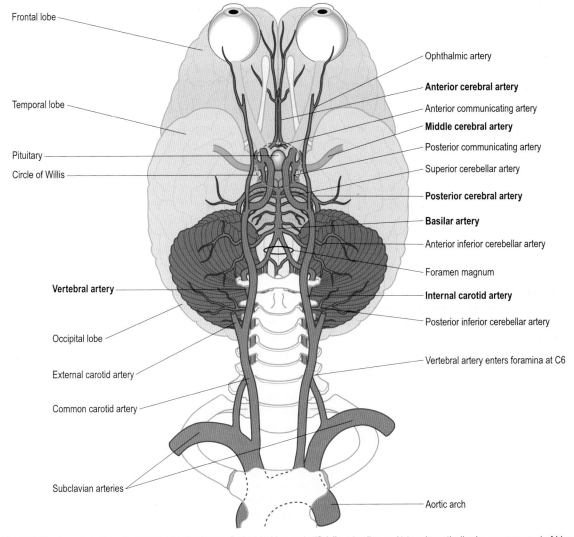

Fig. 3.63 Blood supply to the anterior and posterior fossae. Patient looking up (artificially extending neck) to schematically show arrangement of blood vessels.

Bilateral vertebral arteries fuse to form a single midline basilar artery, these arteries collectively supplying the brainstem (medulla, pons and midbrain) and cerebellum. The basilar artery runs midline along the ventral surface of the brainstem, feeding it with small, deep perforators, and then merges with the Circle of Willis, giving off the posterior cerebral arteries at the basilar bifurcation. The posterior cerebral arteries supply the upper brainstem, occipital lobes and visual cortex (via the terminal calcarine artery), posterior temporal lobes and thalamus (not visible here).

The anterior cerebral artery supplies the parasagittal cortex including the motor (predominantly frontal lobe) and sensory (predominantly parietal lobe) cortices for the leg. The middle cerebral artery supplies most of the lateral cortex, its main trunk dividing into three major branches; smaller lenticulostri- ate branches supply the anterior limb of the internal capsule and the basal ganglia. The main vessel terminates as a wisp in the occipital lobe supplying the macular cortex.

At the Circle of Willis, note how the internal carotid artery essentially trifurcates into the middle cerebral artery, the anterior cerebral artery and the pos- terior communicating artery, the last providing communication with the posterior circulation via connection with the posterior cerebral artery; this con- nection is seldom sufficient to nourish the brainstem via the anterior circulation, however, in the event of basilar occlusion.

Note, too, that the anterior communicating artery provides some exchange of blood between the right and left anterior cerebral arteries; in the event of internal carotid artery occlusion, the middle cerebral artery, is clearly compromised, and the anterior cerebral artery may or not be compromised depending upon the degree of compensation afforded by the anterior communicating artery. The anterior cerebral artery provides blood supply to leg fibres in the motor cortex, and so in internal carotid artery occlusions, leg weakness may be a little more spared than arm and facial weakness, arm and face fibres in the motor cortex being much more fully dependent on middle cerebral artery supply; occlusion of the anterior cerebral artery distal to the anterior communicating artery could give rise to a leg monoparesis, and occluded branches of the middle cerebral artery similarly may produce restricted monoparesis of arm or paresis of face (partial anterior circulation strokes).

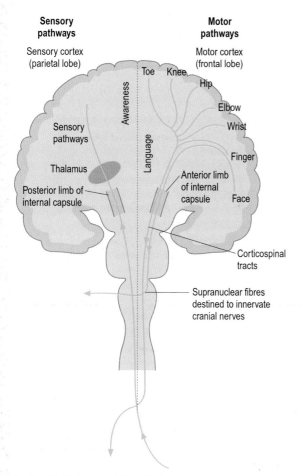

Fig. 3.64 Cortical representation of body structures.

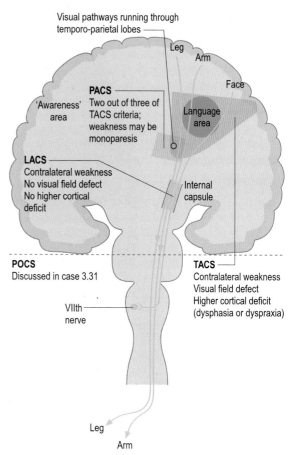

Fig. 3.65 Total or partial anterior circulation stroke (TACS, PACS), lacunar strokes (LACS) and posterior circulation stroke (POCS). Cerebellum not shown for simplification.

distant homes were dotted in the widely spaced uplands of the homunculus. Those heading to work (the motor tracts) will never make it if the motor lanes of the internal capsule are closed. Those coming home from work (the sensory tracts) will never make it if the sensory lanes of the internal capsule are closed.

None of this is to say, of course, that LACS are more devastating than the higher cortical PACS or TACS. PACS or TACS tend to involve larger (middle cerebral) artery occlusions and so although the traffic is more widely dispersed above the internal capsule the damage is also on a larger scale. Conceivably, however, a small distal branch of the middle cerebral artery could be affected in isolation, damaging merely a few neurons' far upland homes on the map that is the homunculus; this might then give rise to weakness that is isolated to a small part of the limb, and may be mistaken for a peripheral nerve lesion, when in fact it is a small PACS.

Posterior circulation stroke (POCS) (see Fig. 3.17)

POCS affect the brainstem, cerebellum and occipital lobes and are discussed in Case 3.31.

Interpretation

Confirm the diagnosis

Tell the examiners you would ask about onset. Strokes are abrupt (or stepwise) clinically. They cause focal weakness. Strokes are thus primarily clinical diagnoses; infarcts are sometimes invisible on early scans and the role of imaging is to exclude stroke mimics and determine whether infarct or haemorrhage.

If facial weakness is a prominent sign, confirm it is an upper motor neuron or supranuclear facial weakness (Box 3.38; Fig. 3.66).

Tell the examiners you would arrange neuroimaging to confirm and characterise stroke and exclude stroke mimics.

What to do next – consider causes

Occlusive stroke

Strokes are usually occlusive (embolic or atherosclerotic with thrombosis). LACS are commonly silent events seen on magnetic resonance imaging as deep white matter

List some stroke mimics

In order of frequency, these include:

- Seizure (far more likely than stroke if there is a history of epilepsy)
- Delirium
- Flare-up of old stroke (under-recognised, but not uncommon in new illness and logical because exact symptoms and signs of a previous stroke in that territory are unlikely to be replicated)
- Syncope (global rather than focal event but surprisingly common mistake)
- Tumour (contrary to traditional teaching, may present acutely – just as strokes can occasionally disobey the acute rule)
- Psychiatric disturbance
- Alcohol- or drug-related symptoms

Hypoglycaemia should always be excluded with acute neurological signs.

What key advances in stroke care have been made in recent years?

Three major advances in stroke care are:

- The introduction of rapid access stroke/transient ischaemic attack (TIA) clinics
- The increasing use of thrombolysis
- The introduction of dedicated stroke rehabilitation units as well as acute stroke units

Discuss the role of brain imaging in acute stroke

Imaging has hitherto used computed tomography (CT) to rapidly exclude intracerebral haemorrhage (ICH) and detect certain stroke mimics. CT is readily available and thus allows the exclusion of contraindications to thrombolysis, and practical, because some unwell patients cannot tolerate magnetic resonance (MR) imaging. However, improvements in MR imaging are leading to it superseding CT as the most favourable test because it can now give rapid positive diagnoses rather than simply exclude haemorrhage. Three areas of information may be useful in stroke imaging.

Imaging vascular occlusion

This is still not crucial until or unless direct angiographic intervention is possible. Traditional angiography is seldom performed. CT angiography shows occluded vessels as hyperdense or white; mimics include a raised haematocrit, microcalcification or hypodense parenchyma giving the appearance of hyperdense vessels, or indeed appearances may be normal, all vessels appearing whiter than usual. MR angiography is an alternative.

Imaging acute parenchymal infarction

CT shows loss of grey/white matter distinction before three hours in 50–70% of infarcts, together with obscuration of deep nuclei and loss of the insular 'ribbon'. The parenchyma is hypodense or dark. Very dark areas with encephalomalacia reflect old strokes. Gyral swelling occurs at 12–24 hours. Haemorrhagic transformation shows a variety of changes.

MR imaging is by a number of methods:

- T1 imaging shows loss of grey/white differentiation and early swelling.
- T2 imaging shows early swelling, hyperdense (reflecting water) change and 'fogging' at two to three weeks; T1 and T2 techniques differ in many subtle ways, and essentially cerebrospinal fluid is black in T1 and white in T2; infarcts are white in both, as are small vessel disease and lacunar infarcts.
- FLAIR images may be positive as early as six hours.
- Gadolinium-contrast-enhanced MR images show intravascular slowing or stasis immediately, pial collaterals at 24–48 hours resolving by three to four days and parenchymal changes at 24–48 hours, which may persist for a few weeks.

Thus, in terms of speed of detection, CT shows blood immediately but may miss smaller infarcts and may be difficult to interpret in the first few hours; T1, T2 and FLAIR imaging show infarcts at 6–12 hours. But modern treatment of stroke requires earlier detection and MR diffusion weighted imaging (DWI) has improved the detection of infarcts to within one hour and perfusion imaging by CT or MR can detect infarcts immediately. Diffusion imaging is based on water molecule movement; as cerebral blood flow slows, there is failure of sodium membrane pumps, leading to oedema. DWI is abnormal within 30–60 minutes of an infarct, abnormalities peaking at two to three days and normalising at around one month. The size of the infarct on DWI is proportional to outcome. Furthermore, DWI also detects many small infarcts previously attributable to transient ischaemic attacks.

Imaging reversible ischaemia

Cerebral blood flow is the gold standard method of detecting this. This may be by CT or MR imaging, either requiring rapid repeat slices for 40 seconds to detect perfusion defects or perfusion/diffusion mismatch. Thus, DWI detects infarction and perfusion weighted imaging (PWI) identifies what is potentially salvageable.

What pitfalls might there be when imaging in acute stroke?

Apart from the difficulties in early diagnosis, vascular territories are very variable, and odd variants include, for example, a dominant posterior cerebral artery arising from an internal carotid artery, leading to apparent middle cerebral artery occlusion. Watershed infarcts occur between rather than within territories. Less common causes of infarct outlined in Table 3.33 should also be considered.

List some causes of multiple small bleeds noted on MR imaging

These may be detected on MR imaging when not apparent on CT, and include diffuse small vessel disease, cerebral amyloid angiopathy (can produce larger bleeds), haemorrhagic metastases, septic emboli and multiple arteriovenous malformations.

Are infarcts easy to distinguish from tumours or inflammation with imaging?

Cytotoxic oedema of infarcts affects white and grey matter whereas vasogenic oedema of tumours and inflammation affects only white matter. Sometimes follow-up scanning is required to be certain.

When should imaging be performed urgently in stroke?

Situations in which imaging should be preformed rapidly in stroke are listed in Box 3.39.

How important are stroke units?

Stroke units save lives (number needed to treat [NNT] 33) and improve independence (NNT 20). They may be acute, rehabilitative or combined and evidence is that patients do much better than on mixed rehabilitation wards and undifferentiated medical wards. Mobile stroke units appear not to be as effective, and it seems that the combined beneficial features of a dedicated stroke unit cannot be reproduced outside it.

What are the benefits of thrombolysis in stroke?

The key is to identify the infarct early and institute treatment to limit its size by reperfusion of the ischaemic, threatened penumbra. 'Time is brain'. Penumbra gives way to cell death as oedema, lactate and perturbed neuro-electrical activity occur.

There have been numerous trials of thrombolysis, e.g. NINDs, ECASS I, ECASS II, and a meta-analysis with 'intention to treat analysis' of 2775 patients (a high number for stroke evidence-based medicine). Median age was 68 years and mean National Institute for Health Severity Score (NIH-SS) was 11; one-third of patients were treated within 180 minutes and two-thirds beyond 180 minutes. The tendency was for earlier treatment in the US NINDS study (before three hours) and later treatment in the European ECASS studies (up to six hours) explaining the overall benefit seen in the former and its lack in the latter. The risk of bleeding is increased with longer time frames, with significant overall benefit within three hours, uncer-tain benefit between three to four hours and beyond four hours benefit crossing confidence intervals. Thrombolysis can achieve a 45% overall decrease in death or dependence, the number needed to treat (NNT) 8, comparing well with many cardiac trials. The NNT approximately doubles with each hour, 2–3 in the first hour, 6 in the second and 25 in the third. Overall bleeding rates were 5.9% but there are so many exclusion criteria in considering thrombolysis and inadvertent protocol violations were probably not uncommon. In hospital, mortality was not prevented by thrombolysis but long-term disability was.

List some exclusion criteria to thrombolysis in stroke

Some important exclusion criteria are listed in Table 3.35. The NIH-SS is a means of scoring functional deficit, and should be incorporated into the weighing up of potential candidacy for thrombolysis; a very low score with minimal deficit is likely to improve without exposure to the bleeding risks of thrombolysis and a high score carries a high risk of bleeding because brain is 'mushier'; stroke suitable for thrombolysis is hence neither too mild nor too severe.

Scoring is from 0 to 42, < 10 being mild, 10–20 moderate and > 20 severe with thrombolysis advocated with extreme caution over 22. However, a score of 22 because of drowsiness might be considered more risky than a score of 22 with severe focal signs in an alert patient. Furthermore, a low score such as 6 or 7 might be considered worthy of thrombolysis in a PACI where extending damage might otherwise occur, but not in a LACI.

The NIH score may be aided by imaging findings in determining candidacy for thrombolysis, the Alberta Stroke Program Early CT Score (ASPECT) out of 10 – one point subtracted for each of a list of defined abnormalities – being considered more risky with a score of less than seven.

What are the major barriers to thrombolysis in stroke?

A major barrier to thrombolysis is time, which requires coordination across the NHS, e.g. public and primary-care provider awareness, ambulance response times, prioritisation on arrival to hospital, immediate imaging, immediate access to a physician trained in assessing the patient and obtaining consent. The early problems of awareness and ambulance response times have been improved with the 'FAST' tool, a simple screen with an 85% specificity and similar sensitivity for hemispheric stroke – facial weakness, arm weakness, speech problems, test all three.

Where thrombolysis is given, the NIH score is repeated at 2 hours, 24 hours and 7 days, and antiplatelet therapy is withheld for the first 24 hours.

What other drug treatments are important in acute stroke?

Aspirin should be given once imaging has excluded ICH, the optimum dose contentious but there is some evidence for 300 mg daily for two weeks and then 75–150 mg daily (enterally or rectally if dysphagic). The high initial dose

---

Box 3.39 Situations in which imaging should be performed rapidly in stroke

- Anticoagulant treatment or bleeding tendency
- Decreased Glasgow Coma Score
- Unexplained progressive or fluctuating symptoms
- Papilloedema, neck stiffness or fever
- Severe headache at onset
- Thrombolysis being considered

Table 3.35 Some important exclusion criteria to thrombolysis in stroke

From history	Initial assessment	Laboratory results	Imaging
Age < 18 years, > 80 years > 3 hours from onset (onset of sleep if woke with deficit) Generalised seizure at onset or within last six months Arterial puncture at non-compressible site or lumbar puncture in last week Major surgery in last 14 days Gastrointestinal or genitourinary haemorrhage in last 21 days Head injury, intracranial surgery or stroke in last three months Any history of intracranial haemorrhage, brain tumour, intracranial AVM or aneurysm (Antiplatelet treatment or anticoagulation with an INR or APTT are not exclusions)	Coma Hemiplegia plus fixed head/eye deviation Minor stroke symptoms, e.g. sensory loss only, dysarthria only, ataxia only, minimal weakness, partial visual field defect Rapidly improving symptoms or signs Presentation suggests SAH, even if CT normal Systolic blood pressure > 185 mmHg or diastolic blood pressure > 110 mmHg	Platelets < 100 INR > 1.7 APTT > 1.2 Plasma glucose < 2.8 or > 22.0	ICH Diffuse swelling of a cerebral hemisphere Brain swelling, sulcal effacement or parenchymal hypo-density involving more than one-third of MCA territory or entire ACA or PCA territory

ACA, anterior cerebral artery; APTT, activated partial thromboplastin time; AVM, arteriovenous malformation; ICH, intracerebral haemorrhage; INR, international normalised ratio; PCA, posterior cerebral artery; SAH, subarachnoid haemorrhage.

compensates for early prostaglandin handling. Dipyridamole modified release 200 mg twice daily is also given to patients able to swallow, but blocks nasogastric tubes. In future other antiplatelet agents may achieve greater significance, and testing for an individual's genetic resistance to various antiplatelet agents may allow more targeted treatment. Aspirin should be withheld for 24 hours after thrombolysis.

Routine anticoagulation therapeutically is of no benefit and increases the risk of bleeding (International Stroke Trial, Chinese Acute Stroke Trial). It is used for deep vein thrombosis prophylaxis in high-risk patients. Patients in AF should receive antiplatelet therapy for 14 days before anticoagulation is considered, as should those warfarinised for a prosthetic valve with a disabling stroke and high risk of haemorrhagic transformation. Therapeutic anticoagulation may be considered for patients with venous thromboembolism and stroke (even ICH) with careful balances of risk. Hyperglycaemia acutely may be associated with a less favourable outcome warranting an insulin regimen. Supplemental oxygen is not recommended without hypoxia.

General supportive measures, including fluids, make sense but are without an evidence base. The FOOD trials with three arms did not show overt evidence in favour of nutritional supplements in patients able to swallow, advocated early feeding where possible by nasogastric tube if swallowing was impaired (although evidence was not strong enough to provoke alarm if proving an initial challenge), and showed that gastrostomy feeding was more risky than beneficial early, within the first three weeks.

Do you know of any potential novel treatments in ischaemic stroke?

Endovascular techniques to 'fish' or 'suck' out the clot do not yet have a sturdy evidence base. Localised intra-arterial thrombolysis may develop further. Glutamate receptor antagonists may limit ischaemic penumbra.

Novel antiplatelet therapies include phosphodiesterase III inhibitors. For large middle cerebral artery strokes (NIHSS > 15 with decreased GCS, ≤ 60 years, > 50% territory on CT or > 145 cm^2 on DWI MR) with cerebral oedema, decompressive hemicraniotomy, perhaps in conjunction with osmotherapy (mannitol), may have a role; fears of poor long-term prognosis based on infarct size and consciousness level may not always be borne out, some studies suggest.

Should antihypertensive therapy be started in acute stroke?

Trials are ongoing to determine this. Physiological arguments for are that it may reduce oedema and the risk of haemorrhagic transformation and arguments against are that it may jeopardise cerebral perfusion. The traditional practice is to continue the antihypertensives that patients are already taking but not to escalate treatment for two weeks as blood pressure rises in the first few days post-stroke, reflecting the increased perfusion pressure needs. Exceptions might include hypertensive encephalopathy or nephropathy, heart failure, aortic dissection, pre-eclampsia or ICH with SPB > 200 mmHg. This may be particularly important in haemorrhagic stroke, either to treat possible accelerated hypertension or to limit damage from further bleeding. Possible treatments include an intravenous nitrate infusion or intravenous boluses of labetalol followed by a labetalol infusion.

What do you know about secondary prevention of stroke with angiotensin-converting enzyme (ACE) inhibition?

PROGRESS was a secondary prevention multi-centre randomised controlled trial of over 6000 patients with stroke or TIA in the previous five years. Active treatment comprised perindopril alone or in combination with indapamide (added at the clinician's discretion). Combination therapy achieved a relative stroke risk reduction of 28% after four years. The risk of fatal or disabling stroke was

429

reduced by 24%, ischaemic stroke by 24% and cerebral haemorrhage by 50%. A further study by the PROGRESS Collaborative Group found that treatment also substantially reduced adverse cardiac outcomes. PROGRESS showed a mild mean blood pressure reduction (12/5 mmHg) with combination treatment, perindopril alone 5/3 mmHg with no significant effect on stroke or other vascular events. PROGRESS suggested that the lower the blood pressure in stroke secondary prophylaxis the better and that there may be a benefit in treating normotensive patients.

The Heart Outcomes Prevention Evaluation study (HOPE) compared ramipril 10 mg with placebo in 9297 patients over 55 years of age with a wide range of vascular disease or risk factors, i.e. a high-risk population. At 4.5 years there were significant relative risk reductions in fatal and non-fatal stroke (0.68 or 32% risk reduction), cardiovascular events (0.8) and cardiovascular death (0.74) in patients randomised to ramipril. Blood pressure at entry was 139/79 mmHg in both groups and at the end it was 136/76 (ramipril) and 139/77 (placebo). The benefits were thus not only the result of blood pressure lowering, and possibly were irrespective of it. Furthermore, patients with left ventricular dysfunction (where ACE inhibitors already have proven benefits) had been excluded and most patients were already taking other drugs such as aspirin and beta blockers.

ACE inhibitors probably protect by many mechanisms, including reduction of oxidative stress, regulation of pro-inflammatory cytokines, decreased progression of atherosclerotic plaques and plaque stabilisation.

What other secondary prevention measures are there after a stroke?

All patients with ischaemic stroke in sinus rhythm should receive antiplatelet therapy – aspirin 75–300 mg daily, or clopidogrel (aspirin intolerance), or a combination of low-dose aspirin and modified release dipyridamole. Aspirin and clopidogrel as a combination appears to be less beneficial in ischaemic stroke than in coronary disease and the MATCH trial showed that benefits did not outweigh risks. Aspirin gives incomplete protection after a first episode of stroke or TIA and NICE guidelines recommend adding dipyridamole, but the evidence for this is not strong. Anticoagulation is indicated for all patients with persistent or paroxysmal atrial fibrillation. It should not be started until brain imaging has excluded haemorrhage and usually until 14 days have elapsed from the ischaemic event.

Early carotid endarterectomy should be considered if there is symptomatic carotid stenosis of 70–99% (ECST criteria) it should be performed as soon as possible, the risk of major stroke up to 30% in the first month, falling rapidly with time, as does the benefit of endarterectomy – the number needed to treat to prevent one major event is five in the first two weeks but 125 after 12 weeks. The benefit may be particularly great after a small stroke compared with a TIA; the evidence for treating asymptomatic stenosis is growing. Blood pressure targets (130/80) and treatments should follow blood pressure guidelines; a slightly higher target (SBP 150) may be warranted in severe bilateral carotid stenosis. Statins should be considered for all patients. Rehabilitation should not be underestimated because the brain has much plasticity and neuronal reserve needs encouragement. Lifestyle measures are essential.

What are the management principles for ICH?

Management is often supportive but neurosurgeons should be consulted unless the situation is hopeless or the ICH is clearly inaccessible, and the neurosurgical team may provide optimum supportive care even where surgery is inappropriate. Outcomes are best in patients who are awake before the intervention (Glasgow Coma Score > 8), younger and where the ICH is superficial. Any anticoagulation should be reversed. Early conservative management versus early surgery for supratentorial ICH was evaluated in the ISTITCH trial and this showed that ICH of any size or location was best managed conservatively, at least initially. The overall prognosis remains poor, with a 60–65% six-month survival. Previously fit people may be considered for surgery with lobar ICH and hydrocephalus or deteriorating neurology. Small deep ICHs, lobar ICH without hydrocephalus/rapidly deteriorating neurology, large ICHs in patients with significant comorbidity, or patients with a GCS < 8 seldom warrant surgery. Surgery is often undertaken for a cerebellar ICH > 3 cm or progressive because outcome is poor without surgery and the ICH is often accessible. Pontine ICHs are not indications for surgery. There is no evidence for blood pressure lowering, but it may be used empirically for very high pressures aiming for slow, smooth reduction. Vasodilators seem theoretically risky agents because of cerebral oedema. Anti-epileptic drugs are not routinely given for prophylaxis. There is no evidence of benefit for corticosteroids (role confined to tumour oedema), osmotic agents such as glycerol or mannitol, or hyperventilation. Recombinant factor VII for ICH may limit haematoma extension and improve functional outcomes. Larger studies are under way to identify optimum dose and patient selection, because thrombotic complications are common.

What is 'phantom limb syndrome' and what insights does it give us into brain plasticity?

This refers to the sensory appreciation of a limb that has been amputated. At first sight this seems illogical, and phantom limb 'pain' was once considered to be a psychological grief reaction. But take a closer look at Penfield's homunculus (see Fig. 3.64). The entire surface of the body is repeatedly mapped on the opposite hemisphere, one such map the post-central gyrus, like a little person draped on the surface of the brain. For the most part, it is continuous, but a discrepancy is that the face is next to the hand, rather than next to the neck. Nobody knows why, although it may relate to feeding. If a hand or arm is amputated, its cortical representation is not receiving signals, and open to alternative sensory input, and it seems that in phantom limb syndrome sensory input from adjacent cortical areas, in this case the face, invades the vacant territory corresponding to the missing hand or arm, and is then misinterpreted in higher centres – touching the cheek, for example, may feel like touch to the thumb. The broader implications of this phenomenon relate to rehabilitation, the brain's plasticity being increasingly understood.

Do you know of any predictors of poor outcome after stroke?

In the early phases of stroke, high temperature, low oxygen saturation and hyperglycaemia are all associated with worsening outcomes. These may, however, reflect stroke severity although it makes sense to correct these. Despite advances in acute care and rehabilitation, overall prognosis in stroke remains unsettlingly poor; 20–30% of patients die within a month and 13% of survivors are placed in care at discharge.

Functional status at 6 months, independent of age or type of stroke influences prognosis – median survival is 9.7 years if independent, 6 years if dependent. The key is early treatment to reduce dependency in the early days, weeks and months, a major contributor to which is stroke unit care, yet in 2006 only 62% of patients were admitted to a stroke unit, and only 54% spent more than half of their inpatient stay in one.

How might you investigate and manage suspected cerebral venous sinus thrombosis?

This is referred to in Case 2.15.

CASE 3.28

DYSPHASIA/DYSARTHRIA

Instruction

Please examine this patient's speech.

Recognition

There is *word-finding difficulty* and there appears to be an element of *receptive dysphasia*. Articulation appears to be mostly intact although speech is a little slurry at times.

Interpretation

Confirm the diagnosis

The findings suggest dysphasia, a cortical lesion, of language. An element of dysarthria is sometimes present due to facial weakness after a stroke.

What to do next – consider causes/assess other systems

Tell the examiners that the most common cause is a left cortical stroke and that you would like to assess visual fields and limb function.

Consider severity/decompensation/complications

Tell the examiners that you would wish to arrange a swallow assessment and be concerned about the risk of aspiration.

Consider function

Tell the examiners that you would ensure assessment by a speech and language therapist. Mention if there is a nasogastric tube or percutaneous gastrostomy tube in situ.

Discussion

What is dysphasia?

Dysphasia refers to the inability to understand or find words due to a lesion in the dominant (usually left) hemisphere. It is unusual for pure word-finding difficulty to exist without an element of receptive dysphasia, often unmasked by more complicated sequences of commands.

What is dysarthria?

Dysarthria refers to impaired articulation and is the result of a lesion in any of the structures coordinating voice production – upper motor neuron lesion (pseudobulbar palsy), extrapyramidal lesion, cerebellar lesion, lower motor neuron/cranial nerve lesion (bulbar palsy), neuromusuclar junction lesion (myasthenia), myopathy or local lesion of the palate, tongue or lips.

CASE 3.29

PSEUDOBULBAR PALSY

Instruction

This 65-year-old gentleman has some speech difficulties. Please examine his speech.

Recognition

There is *dysarthria*. The *tongue appears small and 'tight'*, and cannot be protruded, lying immobile on the floor of the mouth. There is *no word-finding difficulty* and comprehension appears to be fully intact with *no evidence of receptive dysphasia*. There might be a positive jaw jerk, but this is an unreliable sign (Fig. 3.67).

In some patients there may be more complete dysarthria or anarthria with difficulty even opening the mouth and drooling, and this can very much resemble a bulbar palsy.

Interpretation

Confirm the diagnosis

Try to distinguish a bulbar from a pseudobulbar palsy, although this is not always so easy in practice.

What to do next – consider causes/assess other symptoms

Common causes of a pseudobulbar palsy are listed in Box 3.40 (see also Box 3.26).

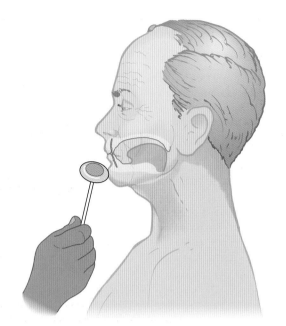

Fig. 3.67 Pseudobulbar palsy.

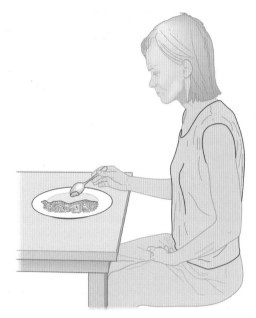

Fig. 3.68 Parietal neglect or inattention.

Box 3.40 Common causes of a pseudobulbar palsy

- Bilateral (usually disseminated in time) strokes – cortical or brainstem
- Demyelination

Consider severity/decompensation/complications

Tell the examiners that you would wish to arrange a swallow assessment and be concerned about the risk of aspiration.

Consider function

Tell the examiners that you would ensure assessment by a speech and language therapist. Mention if there is a nasogastric tube or percutaneous gastrostomy tube in situ.

Discussion

Explain the difference between a bulbar palsy and a pseudobulbar palsy

This is explained in Box 3.26.

CASE 3.30

AGNOSIAS AND APRAXIAS

Instruction

Please examine this lady's arms and visual fields and comment on any higher cortical disturbance.

Recognition

There is *left-sided upper motor neuron weakness*. There is a *left homonymous hemianopia*. There appears to be some

sensory inattention or neglect of the left side (Fig. 3.68) (this can make visual field testing difficult).

Interpretation

Confirm the diagnosis

Ask the patient to touch her left ear with her right hand (the tendency is to touch the right ear). Ask the patient to close her eyes and tell you which hand you are touching; stroking both hands, she is likely to report touch only to the right hand.

What to do next – consider causes

Parietal lobe signs are common after stroke but can also be caused by space-occupying lesions.

Consider severity/decompensation/complications

Tell the examiners that the combination of weakness, homonymous hemianopia and sensory inattention suggests a right total anterior circulation syndrome.

Consider function

Sensory inattention is a considerable challenge to rehabilitation.

Discussion

What is meant by the term agnosia?

This refers to difficulty recognising things, despite intact sensory pathways from periphery to parietal lobe, and results from parietal lobe damage, most commonly the non-dominant lobe. Some important agnosias are given in Table 3.36.

Table 3.36 Some important agnosias

Agnosia	Description
Sensory inattention or neglect	Neglect or unawareness of one side of body, invariably left side Lesion in dominant right parietal lobe *Autotopagnosia* refers to inability to identify parts of body *Anosagnosia* refers to unawareness of any disability

Tactile agnosia (astereognosis)	Inability to recognise an object placed in the hand with the eyes closed, e.g. a key; this despite intact sensory
	    pathways from hand to brain and motor pathways from the brain allowing adequate manipulation of the object;
	    opening the eyes or rattling the key may prompt recognition
	Lesion in contralateral parietal lobe
	Agraphaesthesia refers to inability to interpret numbers stroked on the palm of the hand

Visual agnosia	Inability to recognise familiar object by sight, despite intact visual pathways to occipital lobe; touching the object may prompt recognition Lesion in contralateral parieto-occipital area *Prosopagnosia* refers to inability to recognise a familiar face
Auditory agnosia	Inability to recognise familiar sounds, e.g. voices, music, telephone

What is prosopagnosia and does it give any insights into the mechanisms of visual processing?

Proposagnosia, or 'face blindness' illustrates a not uncommon agnosia. It is caused by damage to a structure called the fusiform gyrus in the temporo-parietal area. Patients are not 'blind' (they can still read), but simply cannot recognise people's faces. Much less common, but intriguing, is Capgrass syndrome, in which a patient can recognise faces but not make the association with familiarity. A patient might recognise his wife but say 'doctor, she looks like my wife but she is not; she is an impostor'. Capgrass syndrome explains the intricate steps in visual recognition well. Images are relayed via the optic nerve, optic tracts and optic radiations to around 30 visual areas at the back of the brain for analysis. After analysing all of the individual features, such as shapes, colours and textures, identification takes place in the fusiform gyrus – 'is it my wife, or somebody else, or a tiger or a wolf?' – the structure at fault in prosopagnosia. Once the image is recognised, a message is sent to the amygdala, the gateway to the limbic system, the brain's emotional core, which judges the emotional significance of the image – 'is it family, friend or foe, predator or prey, or something insignificant like a cloud in the sky?' Capgrass syndrome implies a disconnection between vision and emotion. Lending weight to the theory is that a separate pathway connects the auditory cortex in the superior temporal gyrus to the amygdala, so that if the patient hears his wife on the telephone, the auditory–emotional recognition mechanism kicks in immediately. The emotional response to visual images is fascinating because it represents the foothills in our understanding of how we, as humans, probably unlike other species, appreciate and respond to art, aesthetics and beauty.

Where is the visual external world perceived in the brain?

It is a fallacy that an image inside the eyeball excites photoreceptors on the retina and then that image is transmitted faithfully along the optic nerves, tracts and fibres and is displayed on a screen that is the visual cortex in the occipital lobe. Obviously, you would need a little person inside the brain to watch the image, and another to look inside his or her brain and so ad infinitum with an endless regress of little people watching images without really solving the problem. So we must think instead of representations of the external world. There is not just one visual area, the visual cortex; there are around 30 at the back of the brain that allow us to perceive the world and make sense of a bunch of green and yellow foliage and decipher whether or not the yellow pieces are lion fragments obscured by a bush. One area, called V4, is involved with colour processing and another, called the middle temporal (MT) area, in the parietal lobe, is involved with sensing movement. When V4 is damaged bilaterally, cortical colour blindness or achromatopsia results, in which only shades of grey are seen, but there is no difficulty in reading a book, recognising faces or sensing movement. Dogs and many animals are thought to only see shades of grey, because they lack V4. People with MT damage cannot sense movement and might be terrified to cross the street but can read books, recognise faces and see colour.

There are, in fact, two evolutionary visual centres. The old centre, the superior colliculus in the brainstem, is the ancient one, present when we were fish. The new one is what we understand as representing vision today, the visual cortex. The old pathway is involved in locating an object in the visual field, swivelling the eyeballs and head and directing the high acuity central foveal region of the retina towards it. The new, visual cortex is for identifying objects and generating appropriate responses.

Blindsight is an unusual condition in which there is damage to the visual cortex on one side leading to blindness in the contralateral visual field. Patients cannot 'see', or at least consciously see, but if asked to touch your finger in the 'blind' visual field, might do so accurately. It seems that the old pathway, also linked to the parietal lobe, allows identification without conscious awareness. In a sense, we all have blindsight. We might switch off awareness when watching a lion on television but were a real lion to enter the living room, the old visual pathway would rapidly alert us!

How do these processes explain sensory inattention or neglect?

Sensory inattention or neglect, in a sense, is the opposite of blindsight (if blindsight implies appreciation of the world without cortical vision, then neglect implies failure to appreciate part of that world even though it may be seen), but much more common. Cortical vision is intact, but when the right parietal lobe is damaged the left side of the body, as well as often paralysed, is ignored, not recognised as existing. It is a challenge to rehabilitation, and it is vital to continually encourage the brain's plasticity and stimulate the left side; visitors, for example, should be encouraged to sit at the left. We might postulate what might happen were a mirror held up to the patient's right side, so that the patient could see the reflection of their left. We might expect one of two reactions – sudden realisation of half a world hitherto ignored, or nonchalance that although the left is represented it does not exist in the patient's world and can be ignored. In fact, if asked to touch an object on the left with the aid of a mirror, neither happens. The patient reaches into the mirror and tries to capture it through it, something a young child or even a chimpanzee realises is futile. It has been termed 'mirror agnosia' or 'looking glass syndrome', since Alice walked into her world through a mirror; patients seem aware that it is a mirror, that they are seeing a reflection, and that the object is on their left, but because left does not exist in their world, all knowledge of laws of physics are disbanded to accommodate this strange new sensory world into which they have emerged.

Why is inattention not explained by a visual field defect?

Patients with sensory inattention often have a left homonymous hemianopia (especially if they have a right total anterior circulation syndrome), compounding their difficulties. In broad terms, if there is a problem with the eyes or the visual pathways then a patient is blind, either completely or partially, as in the case of left homonymous hemianopia. If there is a problem with the visual cortex then a patient is blind because of failure of visual processing (albeit potentially with 'blindsight' alluded to above). If there is a problem with the right parietal lobe, whilst visual pathways might be intact, these are over-ridden by the failure of awareness produced by the diseased right parietal lobe; this is illustrated by the fact that even with a right homonymous hemianopia, patients with left parietal lobe disease (the left parietal lobe not so crucially allied with visuospatial awareness) can still turn their heads to the right and are aware of their right side whereas this is not so with patients with a diseased right parietal lobe.

What is anosagnosia?

Sometimes patients with right parietal damage do not have neglect but do deny that their left side is paralysed. This is called anosagnosia. It may be that the left hemisphere's coping style is to ignore discrepancies, pretend they do not exist, and forge ahead while the right hemisphere is highly sensitive to discrepancies. So if the right parietal lobe is damaged, the left simply gets on with things as if nothing has happened, whereas if the left is damaged the right is very aware of what has happened. Even more interesting is the concept of mirror neurons. It is sometimes the case that patients with denial will deny the paralysis of other patients on the ward! Cognitive neuroscientists are learning that just as motor command neurons are stimulated by certain actions, they can also be stimulated in observers of those actions. This 'mirror neuron' activity probably has vital roles in learning, and in reading other people's expressions, intentions and actions.

How does the body perceive pain?

Pain sensation is a vital evolutionary mechanism for survival. That nerve fibres to the spinothalamic tracts carry pain sensation is what we all learnt at medical school. What happens beyond is interesting. Signals are first relayed, via the thalamus, to the insular cortex in the temporo-parietal area, and thence to the amygdala, and especially part of the amygdala called the anterior cingulate, where the emotional response to pain is seated, such that pain produces an appropriate response. One part of the brain signals danger, the other formulates a response.

What is meant by the term apraxia?

This refers to difficulty in performing tasks such as combing hair, brushing teeth or writing, not because of any damage to sensory pathways, motor pathways or adjustment pathways (cerebellum and extrapyramidal system), which all work normally, but due to the failure of the parietal lobe to process information about the environment. Some important apraxias are given in Table 3.37.

An important specific syndrome of the dominant parietal lobe is Gerstmann's syndrome (Box 3.41).

What is synaesthesia?

This is not a PACES question but it illustrates perfectly the heterogeneity of the brain. Synaesthesia literally means a mixing of senses. Colour and number mixing is not uncommon, such that numbers or sequences such as days of the week or months of the year appear to be coloured. The fusiform gyrus of the temporal lobe contains the colour area V4, which processes colour information, and it so happens that the number processing area is right next to it. It may be that 'cross-wiring' or lack of pruning of neurons in early life associates each number with a colour, and this is highly preserved, unchanging and indelible throughout one's life. It was once thought that such people should be locked away! Happily, science advances and so

Table 3.37 Some important apraxias

Apraxia	Description
Dressing apraxia	e.g. inability to put on pyjama top, especially if turned inside out
Gait apraxia	Inability to put one foot in front of the other, sensation of ground and motor mechanisms of walking and balance normal Problem may be in parietal lobe itself or in its connections with the frontal lobe or extrapyramidal system; may be overcome if other parts of brain compensate, e.g. the patient may be able to walk by looking at the ground – 'the cracks between paving slabs' provide assisted visual input
Topographic apraxia	Inability to appreciate geography, e.g. patient might not be able to find way back to bed
Constructional apraxia	Inability to construct shapes or patterns using, for example, matchsticks or wooden blocks, and inability to copy shapes such as a five-pointed star or fill in numbers on a clock face
Ideomotor apraxia	Inability to perform a task automatically but not on command
Ideational apraxia	Inability to perform a series of tasks

Box 3.41 Gerstmann's syndrome

- Agraphia (inability to write)
- Alexia (inability to read)
- Finger agnosia/acalculia (inability to name and count fingers)
- Right–left agnosia (inability to determine right from left)

Problems with numeracy (e.g. recounting serial 7s) more commonly seen as part of global cortical decline in dementia

---

Box 3.42 Common symptoms and signs in posterior circulation strokes

Symptoms

- Dizziness
- Vertigo
- Headache
- Diplopia
- Loss of vision
- Ataxia (often bilateral)
- Numbness (often bilateral)
- Weakness (often bilateral)

Signs

- Limb weakness
- Ataxia of gait or limbs
- Ocular palsies
- Oropharyngeal dysfunction

A key feature of brainstem pathology is a constellation of symptoms or signs. The presence of one symptom or sign alone occurs in less than 1% of brainstem strokes; vertigo, for example, with no other symptoms, is more likely to have a peripheral cause

---

does understanding. It is now appreciated that there are also 'higher' synaesthetes who probably have 'cross-wiring' higher up in the temporo-parietal-occipital (TPO) junction of the brain, in the vicinity of the angular gyrus, and this is the concept area of a number or day of the week or month of the year; in such people, rather than the appearance of numbers or words, it is the abstract concept or thought that provokes the sensation. Some people even perceive multi-colours and shapes and movements. Synaesthesia can involve much more elaborate mixtures such as hearing colour. What is fascinating is that people with synaesthesia tend to be more prone to using metaphors, thinking in abstract ways and lateral thinking; it is seven times more common in novelists and artists.

CASE 3.31

POSTERIOR CIRCULATION STROKE SYNDROMES

Instruction

Please examine this lady's eye movements and limbs and report your findings.

Recognition

There is a large range of brainstem and vertebrobasilar syndromes, many comprising a pot pourri of motor or sensory long tract, cranial nerve and cerebellar signs.

Common symptoms and signs of posterior circulation stroke syndromes are outlined in Box 3.42.

Broadly, syndromes may be midbrain, pontine or medullary. Two well-described syndromes are Weber syndrome and lateral medullary (or Wallenberg) syndrome, the latter classically the result of occlusion of the posterior inferior cerebellar artery, but it may represent a variety of occlusions, and even lateral medullary syndrome exhibits variations on a theme (Fig. 3.69). The corticospinal tracts are spared in a true lateral medullary syndrome because the lesion is isolated to the dorsolateral area of brainstem.

Interpretation

Confirm the diagnosis

Tell the examiners you would ask about onset. Strokes are abrupt. Tell the examiners you would arrange neuroimaging to confirm and characterise stroke and exclude stroke mimics.

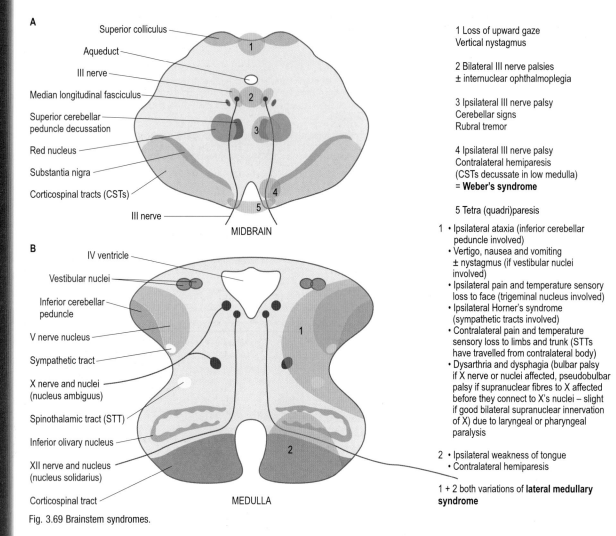

A

Superior colliculus
Aqueduct
III nerve
Median longitudinal fasciculus
Superior cerebellar peduncle decussation
Red nucleus
Substantia nigra
Corticospinal tracts (CSTs)
III nerve
MIDBRAIN

1 Loss of upward gaze
Vertical nystagmus

2 Bilateral III nerve palsies
± internuclear ophthalmoplegia

3 Ipsilateral III nerve palsy
Cerebellar signs
Rubral tremor

4 Ipsilateral III nerve palsy
Contralateral hemiparesis
(CSTs decussate in low medulla)
= **Weber's syndrome**

5 Tetra (quadri)paresis

B

IV ventricle
Vestibular nuclei
Inferior cerebellar peduncle
V nerve nucleus
Sympathetic tract
X nerve and nuclei (nucleus ambiguus)
Spinothalamic tract (STT)
Inferior olivary nucleus
XII nerve and nucleus (nucleus solidarius)
Corticospinal tract
MEDULLA

1 • Ipsilateral ataxia (inferior cerebellar peduncle involved)
• Vertigo, nausea and vomiting ± nystagmus (if vestibular nuclei involved)
• Ipsilateral pain and temperature sensory loss to face (trigeminal nucleus involved)
• Ipsilateral Horner's syndrome (sympathetic tracts involved)
• Contralateral pain and temperature sensory loss to limbs and trunk (STTs have travelled from contralateral body)
• Dysarthria and dysphagia (bulbar palsy if X nerve or nuclei affected, pseudobulbar palsy if supranuclear fibres to X affected before they connect to X's nuclei – slight if good bilateral supranuclear innervation of X) due to laryngeal or pharyngeal paralysis

2 • Ipsilateral weakness of tongue
• Contralateral hemiparesis

1 + 2 both variations of **lateral medullary syndrome**

Fig. 3.69 Brainstem syndromes.

What to do next – consider causes

Consider the causes and risk factors described in Case 3.27.

Consider severity/decompensation/complications

Tell the examiners you would listen for signs of aspiration pneumonia.

Consider function

Tell the examiners of the vital role of physiotherapists, occupational therapists and speech and language therapists in assessment and rehabilitation.

Discussion

What are some common patterns of presentation of posterior circulation strokes?

These are outlined in Table 3.38.

The following are not usually the result of posterior circulation disease:

• Isolated light-headedness, dizziness or vertigo, (usually pre-syncope or peripheral disturbance)
• Transient decrease in consciousness (usually due to syncope or seizure)
• Drop attacks (sudden loss of postural tone and falling without warning)

What do you know about vertebral artery dissection (VAD)?

VAD is an important cause of stroke in younger people. With the advent of modern magnetic resonance (MR) imaging, it is clearly much more prevalent than previously recognised, often detected in asymptomatic people, or often with relatively limited neurological sequalae such as vertigo or isolated cranial neuropathies, although sometimes effects can be much more serious. It is much less

Table 3.38 Common patterns of presentation of posterior strokes

Process	Vascular supply involved	Territory of infarct	Clinical features	
Embolic	Intracranial vertebral arteries	Cerebellar infarct	Dizziness Ataxia – veer to one side, need support to sit Vertigo Blurred vision Nausea and vomiting ± hypotonia, nystagmus and overshoot of arm with eyes closed No motor or sensory symptoms if pure cerebellar infarct	
	Distal basilar artery	Upper cerebellum Midbrain Thalamus Posterior cerebral artery territories ('top of the basilar' infarct)	Somnolence No new memory formation Small pupils Impaired vertical gaze	
	Single posterior cerebral artery	Upper brainstem (midbrain) Occipital lobe and visual cortex Posterior temporal lobe Thalamus	Hemianopia of contralateral visual field ± Motor or sensory disturbance in contralateral limbs Left-sided infarct may produce reading and naming colour difficulties Right-sided infarct may produce neglect	
	Bilateral posterior cerebral arteries		Bilateral visual field defects or cortical blindness	
Atherosclerosis (emboli from may cause any of the embolic phenomena here or above)	Near origin of vertebral arteries in neck	Vestibulocerebellar structures in medulla and cerebellum	Brief transient ischaemic attacks	When both vertebral arteries are affected, the most common pattern is brief spells of ataxia and blurred vision, often precipitated by prolonged standing or hypotension
	Intracranial vertebral arteries	Lateral medulla	Laterally medullary syndrome (Fig. 3.69)	
	Basilar artery	Midbrain Pons	Bilateral signs or crossed findings (ipsilateral face and contralateral limbs) Motor and oculomotor signs predominate Corticospinal tract involvement causes limb weakness (may be bilateral) with hypertonia and hyperreflexia Oculomotor features include diplopia, gaze palsies, nystagmus or internuclear ophthalmoplegia Corticobulbar involvement may occur with dysarthria, dysphagia and diminished gag reflex Facial weakness may occur Most severe form is 'locked-in syndrome' sometimes embolic (Case 4.35)	
Penetrating artery disease (lacunar infarcts)		Paramedian pons	Pure motor stroke with face, arm or leg weakness and ataxic hemiparesis	
		Thalamus	Pure sensory stroke with numbness or paraesthesia of face, arm or leg	
Dissection	Vertebral artery	Medulla Pons Cerebellum	Pain often a cardinal symptom, at back of neck and occiput Dizziness/vertigo Diplopia/other cranial nerve signs Motor or sensory symptoms Ataxia	

prevalent over 50 years of age as arteries stiffen. VAD is typically provoked by minor trauma, such as neck twisting in sport, tugging at roots whilst gardening, after a minor whiplash or after spinal manipulation; even sneezing is reported as provocative. Typically within a few days thrombus that has formed in the dissected crescent may dislodge or fragment and emboli cause a posterior circula-tion stroke, sometimes with progressive signs as a flurry of emboli are released over time. Clinical effects may also relate to the extent of the dissection, often modest when isolated to a small section of the vertebral artery but some-times extending into the basilar and causing luminal nar-rowing as well as embolic potential if the dissection is large. Carotid artery dissection may occur, but seems not to be as common as VAD. Diagnosis requires an index of suspicion, and whilst MR angiography may reveal the dissection, other MR techniques such as T1 fat subtraction imaging may reveal haematoma for months afterwards. Early anticoagulation to thwart progressive symptoms is often favoured, with a growing evidence base. Recurrence rates seem to be low.

CASE 3.32

PARKINSON'S DISEASE

Instruction

Please examine this patient's movements/upper limbs/gait and discuss your findings.

Recognition

The UK Parkinson's Disease Society brain bank clinical diagnostic criteria for diagnosing Parkinson's disease utilises a three-step approach:

Step 1 Diagnose a Parkinsonian syndrome

This requires the presence of bradykinesia + more than one of:

- *Rigidity*
- *Tremor*
- *Postural instability:*
  - *disorder of posture* (flexion of neck and trunk)
  - *disorder of balance* (loss of righting reflexes)
  - *disorder of gait* (short steps, shuffling, festination, freezing)

Bradykinesia

This is essential to diagnose Parkinson's disease (Box 3.43).

Rigidity

This is a '*lead pipe*' rather than 'clasp knife' resistance to passive movement with superimposed '*cogwheeling*'. The rigidity may increase if the patient is asked to perform a concurrent distracting manoeuvre in the opposite limb – *synkinesis* – such as drawing circles in the air or tapping the knee.

Tremor

This is a *low frequency (4–6 Hz) asymmetrical 'pill rolling'* tremor most pronounced at *rest* (Fig. 3.70). An action tremor is possible in Parkinson's disease but this tends to be re-emergent rather than immediate. A *jaw or tongue tremor* is common in Parkinson's disease but a head tremor is seldom if ever a feature of Parkinson's disease and should prompt alternative diagnoses.

Step 2 Apply exclusion criteria

Exclusion criteria are listed in Box 3.44.

Box 3.43 Bradykinesia

Bradykinesia refers to *slowness and progressive decrease in amplitude* of movement and is central to diagnosing Parkinson's disease. *Initiating*, rather than sustaining, movement, is the biggest problem.

Loss of spontaneous movement such as *diminished gesturing in conversation, reduced facial expression* and *reduced blinking* are often specific to Parkinson's disease, but tend to be preserved in cerebrovascular disease, a common differential diagnosis. Early signs can be subtle, and may predate diagnosis by many years.

Freezing (becoming 'glued to the spot') is a relatively late feature of Parkinson's disease.

Slowing of speech, and even *cognitive 'freezing'* are also features of Parkinson's disease.

Gait is usually affected, with *loss of arm swing*, a stooped or *forward flexed posture, difficulty initiating steps, short steps, shuffling* and *festination*, in which the patient appears to be chasing his or her centre of gravity. There is *difficulty turning* and *righting reflexes are reduced* (demonstrated by gently pushing your patient forwards or pulling your patient backwards, but best avoided in PACES).

Fatiguability of repeated movements is impaired; *rhythmic movements*, such as stirring tea, cutting food and heel taps, are difficult, as are *rapid alternating movements* such as touching each finger in turn with the thumb.

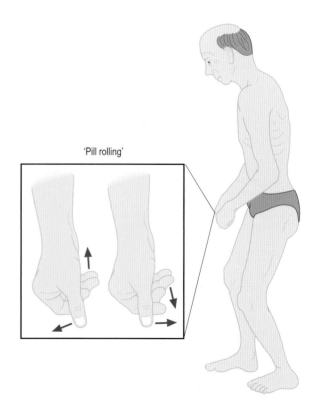

'Pill rolling'

Fig. 3.70 Parkinson posture and 'pill rolling'.

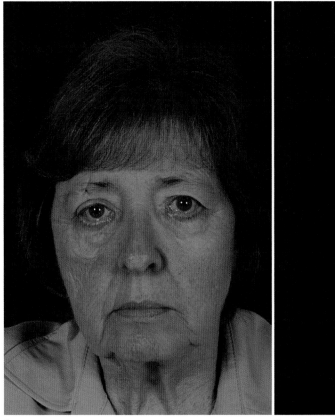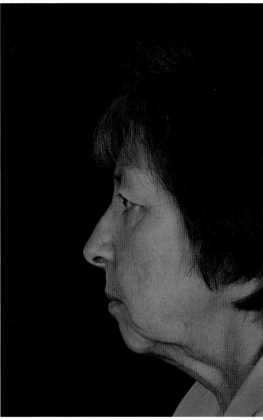

A   B

Fig. 3.71 (A,B) Parkinson's disease.

Box 3.44 Exclusion criteria

- Repeated strokes with stepwise progression
- Repeated head injury
- Antipsychotic and dopamine-depleting drugs
- Definite encephalitis and/or oculogyric crises on no drug treatment
- More than one affected relative
- Sustained remission
- Negative response to large doses of levodopa
- Strictly unilateral features after three years
- Other neurological features: supranuclear gaze palsy, cerebellar signs, early severe autonomic involvement, Babinski's sign, early severe dementia with disturbances of language, memory or praxis
- Exposure to known neurotoxin
- Presence of cerebral tumour or communicating hydrocephalus

Box 3.45 Supportive criteria

The presence of three or more of the following is required:

- Unilateral onset
- Persistent asymmetry
- Rest tremor
- Progressive symptoms
- Good response to levodopa
- Development of levodopa-induced chorea after 10 years
- Levodopa response for over 5 years
- Clinical course of over 10 years

Step 3 Elicit positive supportive criteria

Supportive criteria are listed in Box 3.45.

Fig. 3.71 illustrates Parkinson's disease.

Interpretation

Confirm the diagnosis

The diagnosis of Parkinson's disease is typically made at a mean age of 62–63 years, with a life expectancy of 16–17 years. Diagnosis typically takes 12–18 months, during which time various differential diagnoses of idiopathic Parkinson's disease may be considered. The overall diagnostic accuracy is around 80% in specialist clinics and 55% in general practice. Diagnosis remains clinical. 'Red flags' that should alert you to possible causes of symptoms other than Parkinson's disease are given in Box 3.46.

Parkinson's disease tends to fluctuate in severity (some days in a wheelchair, some days pushing it!) and be aware of the variable expression of Parkinson's disease. Tremor-predominant Parkinson's disease is often recognised. Postural instability is marked in some patients. Some patients have faster progression than expected, often with more intellectual impairment, and some have slower progression, with less intellectual impairment.

What to do next – consider causes

Parkinsonism has a number of differential diagnoses other than Parkinson's disease.

Parkinsonism secondary to other causes

Secondary causes include:

- Vascular Parkinsonism
- Drugs/toxicity
- Structural lesions
- Huntington's chorea
- Wilson's disease
- Neuroacanthocytosis

Some features that are more persuasive of a diagnosis of vascular Parkinsonism than idiopathic Parkinson's disease are listed in Box 3.47.

Parkinson-plus syndromes

These include multiple system atrophy (MSA), progressive supranuclear palsy (PSP) and corticobasal degeneration (CBD). These tend to progress more rapidly than Parkinson's disease, often leading to considerable disability within 18 months or so. Parkinsonism also occurs with other neurodegenerative disorders, e.g. dementia with Lewy bodies (Case 2.44), Alzheimer's dementia, normal pressure hydrocephalus with dementia and gait apraxia; this is not surprising because many dementias are diffuse processes and therefore disrupt extrapyramidal pathways.

■ **Multiple system atrophy (MSA)** This is the largest of the atypical group and embraces numerous diseases, often with overlap – a cerebellar syndrome (olivopontocerebellar), *Shy–Drager syndrome* (autonomic symptoms) and striatonigral syndrome (like Parkinson's disease but no response to levodopa).

■ **Progressive supranuclear palsy (PSP)** PSP is not rare, and is characterised by vertical supranuclear gaze palsy. Typically patients lose downward gaze, leading to falls. Other features are symmetrical bradykinaesia, axial rigidity, pseudobulbar dysarthria and mild dementia. The response to levodopa is poor.

■ **Corticobasal degeneration (CBD)** This is a less common degenerative asymmetric akinetic–rigid syndrome with cortical signs. An early clumsy limb, often a rigid arm, is characteristic, the rigidity very much more marked than that in Parkinson's disease. The arm later becomes useless, often with focal myoclonus. Cortical signs include dyspraxia, cortical sensory and sometimes the so-called 'alien limb syndrome' in which the limb appears to the patient to have a life of its own. The response to levodopa is poor.

Consider severity/decompensation/complications

There are various staging and rating scales for the ongoing assessment of Parkinson's disease, including UK Parkinson's Disease Rating Scale (UKPDRS), but this is more for use in specialist clinics. Rating scales examine both symptoms and function. The UKPDRS examines in detail:

- Mentation, mood and behaviour
- Activities of daily living (speech, salivation, swallowing, handwriting, cutting food and handling utensils, dressing, hygiene, turning in bed, falling, freezing, walking, tremor, sensory complaints)
- Motor function (speech, facial expression, tremor, rigidity, finger tapping, hand movements, rapid alternating hand movements, leg agility, arising from chair, posture, gait, postural stability, body bradykinesia)
- Complications of therapy (dyskinesias, clinical fluctuations – on/off)

It should be possible to determine if a patient has entered the stage of complex Parkinson's disease (below).

Consider function

There are many different scales to assess activities of daily living and function in Parkinson's disease. The Northwestern University disability scale, for example, assesses five areas – walking, dressing, hygiene, eating and speech.

Discussion

Do you know of any risk factors for Parkinson's disease?

Documented risk factors include age, a non-smoking status, low caffeine intake, reduced olfaction, major depression, decreased arm swing, more than one first-degree relative affected, anhedonia, low mood, novelty-seeking personality, mental inflexibility and alcoholism. However, some of these, such as reduced olfaction and reduced arm swing, are more likely early features of disease. Others are not convincingly associated.

What causes Parkinson's disease?

Parkinson's disease has a prevalence of 1% at > 65 years rising to 2% by > 80 years. The cause is unknown, apart from a very small proportion of patients with identified genetic predisposition (alpha-synuclein). In most, there is no family history, although the evidence for a genetic role is increasing. Many environmental causes have been postulated but most of these probably induce a Parkinsonian syndrome rather than being causative for Parkinson's disease.

What is the pathology in Parkinson's disease?

The pathology is degeneration of dopaminergic pathways with a depigmented substantia nigra, and the presence of cytoplasmic inclusions called Lewy bodies. Lewy bodies may also occur diffusely and give rise to dementia with Lewy bodies (DLB). Lewy bodies may also cause rapid eye movement (REM) sleep disturbance or autonomic disturbance. A few Lewy bodies can be a normal finding.

What is essential tremor?

This is a bilateral postural tremor (action, kinetic) but there can be a resting component. It is increasingly not viewed as a monosymptomatic disorder but as a neurodegenerative disorder that can produce cerebellar and gait problems. Half are alcohol responsive. It may be familial, but there is increasing evidence for environmental toxins, such as harmanes, which are products of burnt food. Essential tremor is discussed in Case 2.19.

Is there a role for neuroimaging in Parkinsonism?

Computed tomography (CT) can be useful in excluding other conditions, such as cerebrovascular disease, and normal pressure hydrocephalus in patients with an early gait disorder. Magnetic resonance (MR) imaging can sometimes be useful if MSA or PSP is suspected but there is poor sensitivity for the changes suggesting these conditions. Functional imaging with single photon emission tomography (SPECT) uses the tracer FP-Cit, otherwise known as a DaT scan. The tracer binds to dopamine transporters on pre-synaptic dopaminergic neurons and gives an indirect measure of dopaminergic function. It may be used to distinguish Parkinson's disease from essential tremor; the latter is normal but in Parkinson's disease loss of the 'tail of the comma' bilaterally is seen, representing putaminal degeneration. A DaT scan is capable of distinguishing these two conditions with 97–98% sensitivity and specificity. It cannot reliably distinguish Parkinson's disease from other Parkinsonian syndromes, although neuron loss is more likely to be asymmetrical in Parkinson's disease.

What do you know about non-motor symptoms in Parkinson's disease?

Many neurotransmitters are disrupted in Parkinson's disease, and the diverse array of structures involved, and therefore symptoms, is increasingly appreciated. These include early olfactory dysfunction, sleep disorders, restless legs and psychiatric disease.

What are the stages of Parkinson's disease?

Parkinson's disease is a progressive disease requiring a multidisciplinary team approach. It is helpful to consider the four management stages proposed by MacMahon and utilised in NICE guidelines:

- Diagnosis
- Maintenance treatment
- Complex disease
- Palliative care

Diagnosis is around 18 months, usually with observation. It is usually important not to plunge into treatment quickly before getting an idea of the individual pattern of disease.

Treatment should always be individualised. Once treatment is started, it is seldom stopped, and most patients receive maintenance treatment for around five years before entering the complex stage.

Complex may mean more than two drugs or more than four doses or frequent drug changes or side effects. Patients in the complex stage generally attend Parkinson's Disease or Movement Disorder clinics where they may benefit additionally from multidisciplinary care, e.g. physiotherapists to help with gait and postural instability and activities of daily living, speech and language therapists to assist with speech and swallowing and occupational therapists to assess the need for domiciliary adjuncts.

If a patient survives long enough, the priority may no longer be to increase drug doses but to maintain dignity. Important issues may include managing dementia, managing drug-induced psychiatric side effects and appropriate reduction in pharmacotherapy.

Box 3.48 Strategies for treating motor symptoms in Parkinson's disease

Aims of treatment

Currently there is not a cure for Parkinson's disease and the aim of drug treatment is to control symptoms and so improve function and quality of life. It is seldom possible to abolish symptoms, and treatment is often a trade-off between improving one symptom and potentially inducing a drug side effect. There is no evidence that any drug improves prognosis but the concepts of neuro-protection, which would ideally start before symptoms, and neuro-restoration remain unresolved.

Types of treatment

There are three strategies to treating motor symptoms, all the results of dopamine depletion – replacing dopamine with *levodopa*, enhancing the effects of dopamine with *dopamine agonists* or reducing dopamine breakdown with *enzyme inhibitors*. The ongoing PD Med trial aims to determine which drugs might be favourable as initial treatment and how best to escalate treatment. However, the best strategy is likely to remain individually determined.

Dopamine – levodopa (LD)

LD is the most potent drug for Parkinson's disease and is the mainstay of therapy. It is generally used as first-line in patients with co-morbidity or cognitive impairment. Essentially all new patients with Parkinson's disease respond. Preparations are Sinemet or Madapar in various doses; both contain a peripheral decarboxylase inhibitor. LD can reduce disability and prolong activities of daily living, but it does not stop disease progression.

The side effects of LD are postural hypotension, cognitive disturbance, dyskinesias and on–off phenomena (sudden, unpredictable fluctuations between bradykinesia or freezing and LD-induced dyskinesia). The problem with dyskinesias is progressively more likely with time and it seems preferable to limit LD dosage to a maximum of 500 mg daily. Dyskinesias generally do not develop for a few years.

Dopamine agonists (DAs)

A DA may be considered as initial therapy if there is no comorbidity and no cognitive impairment and the patient has a considerable life expectancy. DAs provide enhanced 'background' levels of dopamine, which may be sufficient to help patients with mild disease or, as add-in therapy, to help smoothen the effects of LD or spare high-LD doses. DAs may be *ergot-derived* (cabergoline, bromocriptine, lisuride, pergolide) but these carry a risk of pulmonary fibrosis, retroperitoneal fibrosis and pleural effusions; in practice, therefore, *non-ergot DAs* (ropinorole, pramipexole), which do not carry the same side effect profile (although there are concerns about gambling, punding and hypersexuality, collectively termed dopamine dysregulation syndrome), are now almost always prescribed in new patients.

Enzyme inhibitors reducing dopamine breakdown

Catechol-O-methyl transferase (COMT) inhibitors may be especially useful if there is a wearing-off effect before the next dose of LD is due. However, they may also have a place at any stage of the disease. Entacapone is the main COMT inhibitor, but tolcapone has recently been reintroduced after being withdrawn because of a small but important risk of serious liver disease. *Monoamine oxidase (MAO) inhibitors* (selegiline and rasagiline) are also used.

Current common treatment regimens

Primary treatment is usually with LD or a DA. Add-in treatment is then often as follows:

- DA + LD + COMT inhibitor or
- LD + COMT inhibitor + DA

Other treatments

Apomorphine is a potent DA that is used in advanced disease subcutaneously. *Anticholinergics* may be used for tremor, but side effects (confusion, constipation, blurred vision, dry mouth) are seldom worth the price. *Amantadine* was introduced historically as a treatment for Parkinson's disease but is relatively ineffective; it has, however, re-emerged as a treatment for LD-induced dyskinesias in some patients. Surgery is occasionally considered.

What are the treatments in Parkinson's disease?

Broadly, the treatments for the motor symptoms centre on dopamine replacement and fall into three categories (Box 3.48).

CASE 3.33

CEREBELLAR DISEASE

Instruction

Please examine this patient's speech and upper limbs and discuss your findings.

Recognition

There is slurred speech dysarthria. There is *upper limb ataxia, inability to judge distance (dysmetria) with past pointing* and *dysdiadochokinesis*.

Interpretation

Confirm the diagnosis

Tell the examiners that you would examine for nystagmus and for heel–shin ataxia and for a wide-based gait.

What to do next – consider causes

Unilateral cerebellar disease causes ipsilateral signs. Midline (vermis) lesions cause midline or truncal ataxia. Cerebellar hemisphere lesions cause appendicular or limb ataxia. These principles may suggest whether cerebellar pathology is unilateral or bilateral, midline, hemispheric or pancerebellar. This should narrow the differential diagnosis to structural lesions or more generalised insults. Causes of cerebellar disturbance are shown in Fig. 3.72.

Consider severity/decompensation/complications

This depends upon the underlying cause.

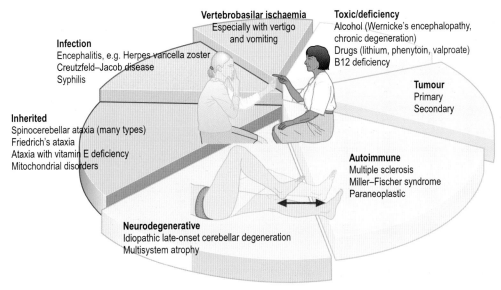

Vertebrobasilar ischaemia
Especially with vertigo and vomiting

Toxic/deficiency
Alcohol (Wernicke's encephalopathy, chronic degeneration)
Drugs (lithium, phenytoin, valproate)
B12 deficiency

Infection
Encephalitis, e.g. Herpes varicella zoster
Creutzfeld–Jacob disease
Syphilis

Tumour
Primary
Secondary

Inherited
Spinocerebellar ataxia (many types)
Friedrich's ataxia
Ataxia with vitamin E deficiency
Mitochondrial disorders

Autoimmune
Multiple sclerosis
Miller–Fischer syndrome
Paraneoplastic

Neurodegenerative
Idiopathic late-onset cerebellar degeneration
Multisystem atrophy

Fig. 3.72 Cerebellar ataxia.

Consider function

Tell the examiners that you would like to assess gait and falls risk.

Discussion

List some conditions that can give rise to cerebellar disturbance and limb weakness/sensory disturbance and state how you might investigate for these

- Multiple sclerosis (MR imaging, cerebrospinal fluid examination)
- Friedreich's ataxia (frataxin gene)
- Spinocerebellar ataxias (*SCA* genes – many and best to involve a neurogeneticist)
- Vitamin E deficiency (level)
- B12 deficiency (level)
- Hypothyroidism (thyroid function tests)
- Neurosyphilis (serology ± CSF examination)
- Adrenoleucodystrophy and other fatty acid disorders (long-chain fatty acids, pristanic acid, phytanic acid)
- Combined cerebellar disease and spastic paraparesis or peripheral neuropathy (brain imaging, spinal cord imaging, nerve conduction study)

CASE 3.34

SPASTIC PARAPARESIS AND BROWN–SÉQUARD SYNDROME

Instruction

Please examine this patient's lower limbs and discuss your findings.

Recognition (Fig. 3.73)

Spastic paraparesis

There is *weakness, increased tone and clonus in both legs* with *enhanced reflexes* and *extensor plantar responses* – an upper motor neuron pattern of weakness. There may be signs of radiculopathy at the level of the lesion.

Brown–Séquard syndrome

There is *spastic weakness* (monoplegia – one limb, or hemiplegia – arm and leg), with *enhanced reflexes* and *loss of proprioception and vibration sense* on one side (ipsilateral to the lesion), and *loss of pain and temperature sensation* on the other (contralateral to the lesion). There may also be ipsilateral root signs at the level of the lesion.

Interpretation

Confirm the diagnosis

Confirm spastic paraparesis (lower limbs only) and not tetraparesis (four limbs). Tetraparesis implies a lesion above C4. Try to seek a sensory level. True Brown–Séquard syndromes, with 50% hemisection, are rare; usually lesions are more or less than one wing of the butterfly that is spastic paraparesis, and a spastic paraparesis can be markedly asymmetrical.

What to do next – consider causes/assess other systems

An *anterior cord syndrome* refers to complete motor paralysis (corticospinal tracts) and sensory anaesthesia (spinothalamic tracts). *Brown–Séquard syndrome* is an *incomplete* cord syndrome. A *central cord syndrome* is typically the result of an extension injury to an osteoarthritic spine; the

Case 3.34   Spastic paraparesis and Brown–Séquard syndrome

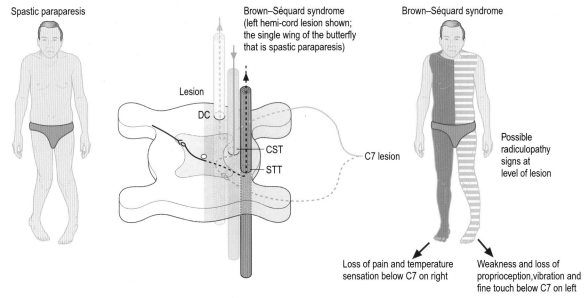

Fig. 3.73 Spastic paraparesis and Brown–Séquard syndrome. CST, corticospinal tracts; DC, dorsal columns; STT, spinothalamic tracts.

central grey matter is mostly affected and motor loss tends to be greater in the arms than the legs (fibres to the lower body are more peripheral) with variable sensory sparing. Cord lesions may be non-compressive (Table 3.39) or compressive.

Lesions that can appear to be spinal because of tetraplegia but are not include bilateral cortical lesions, parasagittal meningiomas and syringomyelia/bulbia.

Non-compressive spinal cord disorders

These are shown in Table 3.38.

Compressive spinal cord disorders

Extradural lesions include cervical spondylosis (myelopathy or radiculopathy), cervical/lumbar disc prolapse, tumours and trauma. Intradural lesions may be intramedullary such as meningiomas or neurofibromas or extramedullary such as astrocytomas.

Consider severity/decompensation/complications

Tell the examiners that you would ask about sphincter disturbance (bladder or bowel symptoms, urinary catheter) and initially exclude acute cord compression, a neurosurgical emergency.

Consider function

Tell the examiners you would determine the level of disability and, as well as identifying and correcting any correctable cause, would work closely with physiotherapy and occupational therapy colleagues to optimise function.

Discussion

How does the blood supply to the spinal cord influence clinical features of infarction?

The anterior cord is supplied by the anterior spinal artery, artery of Adamkiewicz, a radicular artery that contributes significantly to the lower thoracic and lumbar cord and multiple radicular arteries. The posterior cord is supplied by the posterior spinal arteries supplemented by posterior radicular arteries. Infarction may occur in watershed areas between the anterior and posterior systems, e.g. after cardiac arrest. The dorsal columns are invariably preserved, with normal proprioception and sensation of vibration and light touch.

What is the prognosis for recovery in spinal cord infarction?

This is generally poor if there is no improvement in the first 48 hours.

Where do spinal arteriovenous malformations (AVMs) tend to occur?

Dural AVMs are mostly thoracolumbar, and lie in the spinal dura and nerve roots, supplied by branches of the intercostal and lumbar arteries.

What is spinal muscular atrophy?

This is the second commonest hereditary neuromuscular disorder after Duchenne muscular atrophy (1 in 25 000 live births). It has many forms, localised to the SMN gene on chromosome 5, which has a role in RNA processing. SMA is classified according to age (childhood or adult), distribu-

Table 3.39 Non-compressive spinal cord disorders

	Causes	Clinical clues

Acute transverse myelopathy
Acute weakness
Sensory level
Bilateral
Sometimes asymmetrical
	Multiple sclerosis (Case 2.18)
	Viral
	
	Autoimmune
		Transverse myelitis or partial cord syndrome
		Radicular pain at onset
		  (can also occur in compressive lesions)
		Plateau phase for several months
		Partial recovery
		Residual disability 30%
		  e.g. systemic lupus erythematosus

Vascular	Infarction Haemorrhage Arteriovenous malformation	Sudden painful flaccid paraparesis Urinary retention Later spasticity and hyperreflexia Normal proprioception, vibration and light touch Similar to infarction Slowly evolving mixed upper and lower motor neuron signs Sensory disturbance Sometimes sphincter disturbance

Hereditary/degenerative	Friedreich's ataxia
	Spinal muscular atrophy
	
	Hereditary spastic paraparesis
	
	Rare causes, e.g. Abetalipoproteinaemia,
	  X-linked adrenoleukodystrophy
		Absent ankle jerks and extensor plantars
		Progressive weakness and wasting and hypotonia due to degeneration of
		  anterior horn cells or bulbar motor nuclei
		Differential diagnosis of motor neurone disease
		Spasticity
		Hyperreflexia and extensor plantars
		Weakness less striking
		Mild sensory symptoms
		Mild pes cavus possible

Infective	HIV Syphilis Lyme disease West Nile virus	Slowly progressive spastic paraparesis and sensory ataxia in late disease Acute seroconversion myelitis Absent ankle jerks and extensor plantars Radiculoneuromyelitis involving lower and upper motor neurons Resembles amyotrophic lateral sclerosis Acute, asymmetrical flaccid weakness due to anterior horn cell involvement
Motor neuron disease	Amyotrophic lateral sclerosis	Refer to Case 3.37
Nutritional	Subacute combined degeneration of cord Vitamin E deficiency	Absent ankle jerks and extensor plantars
Toxic	e.g. lathyrism, konzo, tropical ataxic neuropathy	Endemic in some parts of the world

tion (proximal, distal, bulbar) and mode of inheritance (dominant, recessive, X-linked).

What is hereditary spastic paraparesis?

This is a typically, but not exclusively, an X-linked recessive disease developing at any age with difficulty walking. Paradoxically, the earlier the presentation the milder the disease. The spastin gene is one of numerous genes that can be at fault.

Is myelopathy common in human immunodeficiency virus (HIV)?

It occurs clinically in 7% of patients and at post-mortem in 50%, and may be vacuolar or multinucleate giant cell, the former being more common and a marker of late disease (CD4 count < 200/μl). The mechanism is uncertain and may involve microglial neurotoxicity, gp120 protein myelin toxicity or vitamin B12 deficiency. There is no treatment. Myelitis may occur at seroconversion. Human T-cell lymphotropic virus type 1 (HTLV-1), endemic in parts of the world, is transmitted similarly to HIV and may cause insidious spastic paraparesis, peripheral neuropathy, ataxia or optic atrophy.

What investigations might you consider when investigating a spinal cord syndrome?

These include MR imaging, cerebrospinal fluid examination (for microscopy and culture, protein, glucose, oligoclonal bands and polymerase chain reaction testing for viruses), electrophysiology, erythrocyte sedimentation rate and autoimmune profile, vitamin B12, viral serology and syphilis serology (if suspicion).

Box 3.49 Treatments for myelopathy

- Surgical decompression
- Intravenous acyclovir 10 mg/kg eight-hourly for suspected or confirmed herpes simplex myelitis
- Pulsed methylprednisolone 0.5–1 mg daily for three days for suspected multiple sclerosis
- Vitamin B12 replacement as hydroxycobalamin 1000 µg daily for five days then monthly
- Antiretroviral therapy to prevent vacuolar myelopathy
- Symptom control, e.g. pain
- Rehabilitation

How might MR imaging further the diagnosis?

It can exclude cord compression and sometimes identify signal change consistent with myelitis. Cord atrophy is possible in neurodegenerative and nutritional causes, and signal change may occur in subacute combined degeneration of the cord. Cord infarction or inflammation may appear as a high signal on T2-weighted scans, sometimes associated with focal cord swelling.

What treatments are there for myelopathy?

Treatments are outlined in Box 3.49.

CASE 3.35

SYRINGOMYELIA

Instruction

Please examine this patient's arms neurologically. He has a history of altered pain sensation.

Recognition

The slowly expanding central canal of syringomyelia results in those signs in Fig. 3.74.

- The spinothalamic tracts (STTs) are always affected because their fibres cross near the centre of the cord leading to *loss of hot/cold discrimination and pain sensation in a 'cape' distribution*. This is often the earliest sign.
- There is bilateral *wasting and weakness of the small muscles of the hands* caused by bilateral compression of T1 ventral nerve roots. The syrinx generally originates in the cervical cord. Other anterior horn cells and nerve roots are affected as it elongates, resulting in *loss of upper limb reflexes and flaccid tone*.
- The dorsal columns (DCs) are spared because they are too far from the site of disease. Because vibration, joint position and fine touch sense are preserved but

pain and temperature sense are lost, the sensory loss is referred to as *dissociated sensory loss.*
- The corticospinal tracts (CSTs) may rarely be affected in late disease, resulting in spastic paraparesis or tetraparesis.

Interpretation

Confirm the diagnosis

Diabetes (foot and ankle joints) and tabes dorsalis (knee joints) can also cause Charcot's joints. The clue to syringomyelia should be the dissociated sensory loss.

What to do next – assess other systems

Other features that may be present are Horner's syndrome, Charcot's joints and other skeletal abnormalities:

- Horner's syndrome is common because the syrinx disrupts the sympathetic nerve fibres, especially at C8, T1.
- In longstanding disease loss of pain sensation causes Charcot's joints.
- Other skeletal abnormalities include kyphoscoliosis and cervical ribs. *La main succulemente* is the term given to the cold, swollen, dystrophic hands that may occur in syringomyelia due to autonomic vasomotor disturbance.

Consider severity/decompensation/complications

In syringobulbia the syrinx originates in the brainstem or extends upwards into it. There may be:

- Facial dissociated sensory loss (the decussating pain and temperature fibres from the descending trigeminal nucleus are affected)
- Wasting and weakness in the bulbar muscles giving rise to a bulbar palsy
- Nystagmus and cerebellar ataxia

Consider function

Tell the examiners you would determine the level of disability and as well as identifying and correcting any correctable cause work closely with physiotherapy and occupational therapy colleagues to optimise function.

Discussion

What is the differential diagnosis of syringomyelia?

Syringomyelia is rare and has an equal sex incidence and an age of onset in early middle age. Intramedullary tumours of the spinal cord may cause a similar clinical picture to syringomyelia.

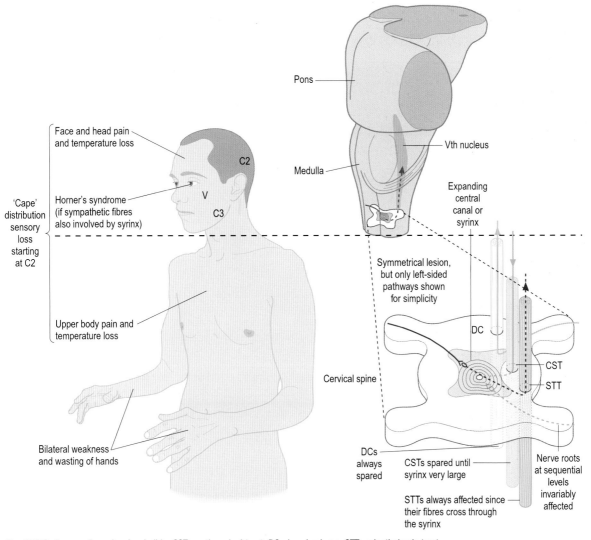

Fig. 3.74 Syringomyelia and syringobulbia. CST, corticospinal tract; DC, dorsal column; STT, spinothalamic tract.

ABSENT ANKLE JERKS AND EXTENSOR PLANTARS (SUBACUTE COMBINED DEGENERATION OF THE CORD, TABES, FRIEDREICH'S ATAXIA)

Instruction

Please examine this patient's legs (you may be asked specifically to examine reflexes and sensation) and discuss your findings.

Recognition

This implies no more than a combination of lower and upper motor neurone disease, described classically in:

- Subacute combined degeneration of the cord
- Taboparesis
- Friedreich's ataxia

But most commonly these signs are visible when two common conditions occur together, e.g. cervical myelopathy causing extensor plantar responses and diabetes causing peripheral neuropathy with loss of ankle reflexes. Motor neuron disease and lesions at the conus medullaris may also cause a combination of upper and lower motor neuron signs.

Table 3.40 Differentiating clinical signs of causes of absent ankle jerks and extensor plantars

	Subacute combined degeneration of cord (SACDC)	Tabes	Friedreich's ataxia
	DC, CST, STT, DC and CST degeneration, Peripheral nerve degeneration	DC, CST, STT, DCs and dorsal roots degenerate, CSTs not affected unless taboparesis	DC, CST, STT, DC and CST degeneration. Note that the spinocerebellar tracts also degenerate in Friedreich's ataxia, Peripheral nerve degeneration
Dorsal columns (DCs)	Degenerate. Loss of vibration and proprioception over feet (± legs and hands). +ve Romberg's sign	Degenerate. Signs as for SACDC. Without CST involvement = tabes dorsalis	Degenerate. Signs as for SACDC
Corticospinal tracts (CSTs)	Weakness. Extensor plantars. Possible brisk knee reflexes (i.e. spastic paraparesis). Ankle reflexes absent because full-blown upper motor neuron picture prevented by peripheral nerve damage (loss of dorsal root ganglion cells)	If CSTs involved signs as for SACDC = taboparesis	Signs as for SACDC
Spinothalamic tracts (STTs)	Spared or involved as part of peripheral neuropathy	Spared	Spared
Other possible differentiating features	Optic atrophy with centrocaecal scotoma. Dementia. Autoimmune disease (if due to pernicious anaemia)	Ultimately neuropathic joint destruction – Charcot's joints, and trophic ulceration. Argyll Robertson pupils. Autonomic degeneration with neuropathic bladder and constipation. Optic atrophy (rare)	Skeletal deformity – pes cavus, kyphoscoliosis. Cerebellar signs e.g. ataxia with wide-based gait, dysarthria. Cardiomyopathy. Diabetes

Interpretation

Confirm the diagnosis

A positive Romberg's sign (unsteadiness with the eyes closed or sensory ataxia) confirms dorsal column disease.

What to do next – consider causes

The three classic causes are differentiated by the clinical signs in Table 3.40. Though classic, they are not inevitable. It is perfectly possible, for example, to have Friedreich's ataxia with flexor plantars and without dorsal column involvement.

Consider severity/decompensation/complications

The spectrum of severity in each of the conditions is highly variable. Note in the final row of Table 3.40 the additional complications that may occur.

Consider function

Tell the examiners you would determine the level of disability and as well as identifying and correcting any correctable cause work closely with physiotherapy and occupational therapy colleagues to optimise function.

Discussion

What causes subacute combined degeneration of cord (SACDC)?

Vitamin B12 is a co-enzyme for transmethylation in DNA and myelin protein synthesis. Vitamin B12 deficiency may cause an array of insidious neurological problems including SACDC, pure peripheral neuropathy (often precedes SACDC) and dementia.

What are the stages of syphilis?

These are outlined in Box 3.50.

Syphilis is caused by the spirochaete *Treponema pallidum*, which can reach the central nervous system early in the course of infection, even in the primary stage. In meningovascular syphilis, leptomeningeal exudates, granulomata and arteritis produce progressive spastic paraparesis and radicular pain is common. In tabes dorsalis, a cellular reaction in the dorsal roots causes retrograde sensory loss up to 20 years after infection; characterised by lancinating pain that may be viscerally sited, then hypoalgesia.

What do you know about Friedreich's ataxia?

This constitutes 50% of all inherited ataxias. It is an autosomal recessive spinocerebellar degeneration (referring not to spinocerebellar tracts in isolation, but to degeneration of multiple tracts within the spinal cord together with cerebellar degeneration) caused by an increased number of GAA trinucleotide repeat sequences at a gene encoding the protein frataxin on chromosome 9–9q13. Essential diagnostic criteria are listed in Box 3.51.

What are the spinocerebellar tracts?

These tracts convey unconscious proprioceptive information to the cerebellum. This is in contrast to the dorsal columns transmitting conscious sensation directly to the sensory cortex.

CASE 3.37

MOTOR NEURONE DISEASE

Instruction

Please examine this patient's arms and legs and then discuss your findings.

Recognition

There is *asymmetrical muscle wasting and weakness* in the *limbs* (e.g. foot drop, weakness of the small muscles of the hand) (Fig. 3.75).

Interpretation

Confirm the diagnosis

Motor neuron disease should be in the differential diagnosis of a patient with weight loss, muscle wasting or muscle weakness that is not otherwise easily explained. The hallmark of motor neurone disease is muscle weakness or wasting with preserved or brisk reflexes. Sensory disturbance is not present.

- Presentation is often in an arm or leg, with a mixture of lower and upper motor neuron signs. Brisk reflexes, fasciculation (commonly in the deltoid, first dorsal interosseous and thigh muscles), corticobulbar signs with a brisk jaw jerk, and extensor plantar reflexes are common.
- Progressive bulbar involvement (predominant in some patients, especially older women) causes drooling (sialorrhoea; because of impaired swallowing), dysarthria and risk of nasal regurgitation of liquids.

Differential diagnoses include benign cramp fasciculation, cervical myeloradiculopathy, dual pathology (e.g. cervical myelopathy and peripheral neuropathy), multifocal neuropathy with conduction block, and myopathy.

What to do next – assess other systems

Tell the examiners that you would assess respiratory function (spirometry) and swallowing (speech and language therapist).

Consider severity/decompensation/complications

Tell the examiners that:

- Muscle wasting leads to progressive weakness, ultimately of respiratory movements.
- A pure lower motor neuron form can be confined to the arms or legs for many years, with a better prognosis. More generalised lower motor neuron forms can be rapidly progressive.
- Primary lateral sclerosis, a pure upper motor neuron form characterised by ascending, relatively symmetrical spasticity including the face

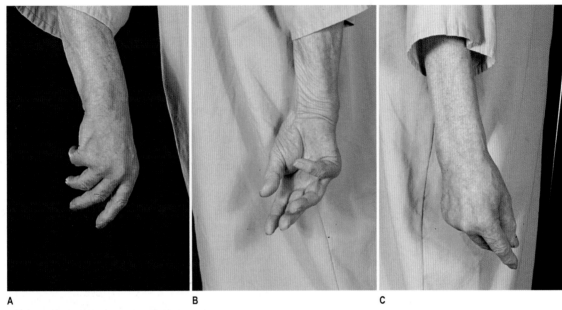

A   B   C

Fig. 3.75 (A–C) Radial and ulnar nerve palsy and wasting in motor neurone disease.

Box 3.52 Predictors of long-term survival in motor neurone disease

- Pure lower or upper motor neurone disease
- Absence of bulbar involvement
- Absence of respiratory involvement
- Confined to specific regions, e.g. arm or leg for long period
- Slow progression in first year

(corticobulbar dysarthria or pseudobulbar palsy) is often associated with long-term survival of beyond 15–20 years.

- Frontotemporal dementia is the presenting form in about 3–4% of patients, and may precede motor symptoms by years.

The prognosis in motor neurone disease is wide. Fifty per cent of patients with amyotrophic lateral sclerosis die from respiratory failure, almost always peacefully, at a mean of 40 months from symptom onset; 20% are alive at 5 years and 10% at 10 years. Predictors of long-term survival are shown in Box 3.52.

Consider function

About one-third of patients have mild executive dysfunction.

Discussion

What is motor neurone disease?

Motor neuron disease is an inexorably progressive neuro-degenerative disease, characterised by degeneration of spinal cord ventral horn motor neurons, cerebral motor pathways and brainstem motor nuclei. Amyotrophic lateral sclerosis is the typical form of motor neurone disease, presenting with mixed upper and lower motor neuron features, often focal at first (e.g. wasted, fasciculated biceps muscle with brisk reflex, foot drop) or with asymmetrical distal weakness and wasting of the small muscles of the hand, patients often dropping objects. Bulbar onset affects 20%. Respiratory onset may occur. Rarer variants include pure upper motor neuron involvement (e.g. primary lateral sclerosis) or pure lower motor neuron involvement (e.g. progressive muscular atrophy, which tends to be spared of any cognitive problems).

How common is motor neurone disease?

The incidence is around 2 per 100 000 and the prevalence 4–7 per 100 000 per year in the UK. The median age of onset is 60 years, but 5–10% of patients are under 40. The male:female ratio is 1.5:1.

What causes motor neurone disease?

Around 5–10% is caused by a dominantly inherited genetic mutation and tends to present earlier. Some have a mutation in the gene for Cu–Zn superoxide dismutase (*SOD1*), whose overexpression rather than loss of enzyme function in microglia (the main immune cells of the nervous system) may cause disease. TAR DNA-binding protein 43 is the main component of the pathological hallmark protein inclusions found in surviving motor neurons in sporadic motor neurone disease (also in frontotemporal dementia and progressive muscular atrophy). Selective suppression of mutant *SOD1* in microglia improves survival in mice; astrocytes, cells which support neuronal structure and function, are responsible for reuptake of excitotoxic neurotransmitters such as glutamate, receptors for which may be aberrant in motor neurone disease (the basis for riluzole therapy).

How is motor neurone disease diagnosed?

Imaging has a limited role. Electromyography shows diffuse anterior horn cell disease. However, these tests are usually undertaken to exclude structural lesions and provide further confirmation of the diagnosis. The mean time to diagnosis is 1–1.5 years because early symptoms and signs are often subtle and mistaken for minor musculoskeletal disease or a mononeuropathy.

Is there any treatment for motor neurone disease?

Riluzole is a glutamate antagonist with a modest survival benefit of 3–4 more months in some patients. Unhappily, there remains no cure and no adequate brake to the relentless progression of motor neurone disease. Information, psychological support and physiotherapy aids, such as mobile support arms, neck braces and foot splints, are important. Occupational therapy input is frequently valued. Gastrostomy feeding may be needed.

Symptom control is vital. Sleep disturbance with hypopnoea may be helped by non-invasive ventilation, which may prolong life. Cramps and spasms occasionally warrant baclofen. Sialorrhoea is difficult to treat but hyoscine or tricyclics, or botulinum toxin to salivary glands, are sometimes used. Emotionality (incongruous laughing or crying seen in patients with bulbar involvement, perhaps due to the loss of cortical inhibition of reflex emotional behaviours and which is not depression) is not uncommon but is difficult to treat.

Do you know of any other motor neurone diseases?

Many single gene disorders lead to progressive motor neuron degeneration. Spinal muscular atrophy (SMA) is a slowly progressive motor neurone disease of the spinal cord with many predisposing genes and taking many different forms. Kennedy's disease (spinobulbar muscular atrophy) is an X-linked disorder causing slowly progressive motor neurone disease and partial androgen insensitivity with gynaecomastia and is caused by mutations in the androgen receptor gene.

CASE 3.38

CERVICAL MYELORADICULOPATHY

Instruction

Please examine this patient's arms and legs and then discuss your findings.

Recognition

There is *weakness* and *increased tone in the lower limbs* with *enhanced reflexes* and *extensor plantar responses*. There may be sensory impairment (compression of dorsal columns). There may be inversion of the biceps and supinator reflexes. In middle-aged to older patients the most likely diagnosis is cervical spondylosis.

> **Box 3.53 Inverted reflexes**
>
> This is a phenomenon caused by combined spinal cord and root disease. It simply means absent reflexes at the segmental level of the lesion and enhanced reflexes below. With an inverted biceps reflex (C5/6 segment lesion), when the biceps tendon is tapped there is no biceps reflex but the triceps (C7) may be stimulated by the manoeuvre. In an inverted supinator reflex (C5/6) there is no supinator response but finger flexion (C8) may be seen to have been stimulated.

Interpretation

Confirm the diagnosis

The most common level of cervical spondylosis is C5,6. Always check for inversion of the biceps and supinator reflexes (Box 3.53). Upper motor neuron signs are present below the level of the lesion, giving rise to brisk triceps (C7) and finger (C8) reflexes.

What to do next – consider causes

If there is spastic paraparesis or tetraparesis, the numerous differential diagnoses are given in Case 3.34.

Consider severity/decompensation/complications

Tell the examiners that you would ask about sphincter disturbance (bladder or bowel symptoms, urinary catheter) and initially exclude acute cord compression, a neurosurgical emergency.

Consider function

Tell the examiners you would determine the level of disability and, as well as identifying and correcting any correctable cause, work closely with physiotherapy and occupational therapy colleagues to optimise function.

Discussion

What is cervical spondylosis? (Fig. 3.76)

Cervical spondylosis is the most common cause of cervical myeloradiculopathy, and the signs are frequently subtle. It is often painless and may be suspected with brisk lower limb reflexes but minimal or no other neurological signs. Sometimes it gives rise to Lhermitte's phenomenon, with a burning sensation on neck flexion. Commonly C5/6 is affected with signs of radiculopathy at that level and signs of myelopathy below. The lower cervical thoracic spine and roots are less susceptible because their vertebrae undergo less 'wear and tear' over a lifetime. The cervical and lumbar spine is subjected to most movement with greater propensity to degeneration.

What do you know about disc prolapse?

Cervical disc lesions may provoke cervical myeloradiculopathy. Disc prolapse is more common in young to middle-aged adults, and especially affects vertebral levels C5/C6 and C6/C7, with marked radicular pain. Lumbosacral disc prolapse is much more common and causes

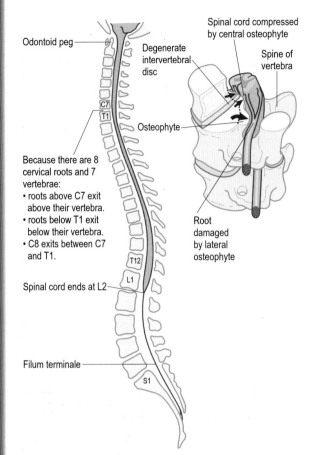

Fig. 3.76 Spinal cord, roots and compression.

Labels on figure:
- Odontoid peg
- Degenerate intervertebral disc
- Spinal cord compressed by central osteophyte
- Spine of vertebra
- C7
- T1
- Osteophyte
- Because there are 8 cervical roots and 7 vertebrae:
  - roots above C7 exit above their vertebra.
  - roots below T1 exit below their vertebra.
  - C8 exits between C7 and T1.
- Root damaged by lateral osteophyte
- Spinal cord ends at L2
- T12
- L1
- Filum terminale
- S1

radiculopathy but not myelopathy because the spinal cord has terminated at the lower level of the L1 vertebra.

CASE 3.39

CAUDA EQUINA SYNDROME

Instruction

Please examine this patient's legs and then discuss your findings.

Recognition

There is *flaccid weakness* in the lower limbs with *loss of the knee and ankle reflexes* and *normal plantar responses*. There is *dermatomal sensory loss below L1*. These findings suggest a complete cauda equina lesion.

Interpretation

Confirm the diagnosis

Flaccid weakness and areflexia in the lower limbs can be the result of Guillain–Barré syndrome. Tell the examiners

that you would take a history for ascending symptoms over a few days. Overt sensory loss is not a feature of Guillain–Barré syndrome.

What to do next – consider causes

Causes of cauda equina lesions and their clinical features are outlined in Table 3.41.

Consider severity/decompensation/complications

Tell the examiners that you would ask about sphincter disturbance (bladder or bowel symptoms, urinary catheter) and initially exclude acute cord compression, a neurosurgical emergency.

Consider function

Tell the examiners you would determine the level of disability and, as well as identifying and correcting any correctable cause, work closely with physiotherapy and occupational therapy colleagues to optimise function.

Discussion

What is the cauda equina?

The spinal cord is shorter than the vertebral column, its roots sloping inferiorly from their levels of origin to their designated intervertebral foraminae, especially further down the cord. Below the inferior end of the cord, the dural–arachnoid sac contains a leash of roots (T12–S5) and the filum terminale – a complex called the cauda equina ('horsetail').

What is the conus medullaris?

This refers to the terminal portion of the spinal cord, at vertebral level L1, and from it emerge the lower sacral roots.

What is cauda equina syndrome?

A lesion in the spinal canal below the conus medullaris can cause a cauda equina syndrome. Because the spinal cord ends at the lower end of the L1 vertebra, the lumbar and sacral roots pursue a long course (unlike cervical roots) within the lumbar canal and can be injured anywhere within it to their intervertebral foramina exit sites.

Can lumbar disc disease cause upper motor neuron signs?

Because the spinal cord ends at the L1 vertebral level, lumbar disc disease should never cause upper motor neuron signs.

How does cauda equina syndrome differ from lumbar disc disease?

Lumbar disc prolapse causing isolated radiculopathies is very common. For example, the highly prevalent L4/5 and L5/S1 disc prolapses compress the L5 or S1 roots at their exit foraminae (although these roots originated from their cord segment at a much higher level). The term cauda equina syndrome is usually reserved for more widespread damage arising within the canal and involving multiple nerve roots. Pain in the distribution of L4, L5 or S1 may

Table 3.41 Cauda equina lesions

	Type	Causes	Features
	Lateral	Neurofibroma	Anterior thigh pain Quadriceps wasting Ankle inversion (L4 lesion) Absent ankle reflex Enhanced ankle reflexes and extensor plantars if terminal cord impinged Sphincter disturbance (if cord compression)
	Midline intrinsic lesion	Terminal cord lesion, e.g. dermoid tumour, ependymoma, lipoma	Roots damaged from 'inside out', i.e. S5 → S4 → S3 and so on Rectal pain Genital pain Sphincter disturbance Loss of perianal/sacral sensation (saddle anaesthesia) Anal reflex/rectal tone loss Loss of ankle reflex and weakness as S1 and L5 affected
	Midline extrinsic lesion	Bilateral lumbar and sacral root lesions, e.g. lumbosacral disc lesions Sacral tumour Bone metastases	Any pattern of root disturbance

reasonably be attributed to lumbosacral disc disease, but root pain in unusual dermatomes or evidence of higher lumbar disc disease or lower sacral root damage is unusual, and should ring alarm bells to the possibility of cauda equina syndrome.

CASE 3.40

CARPAL TUNNEL SYNDROME (MEDIAN NERVE LESION)

Instruction

Please examine this patient's hands and discuss your findings.

Recognition

There is *thenar wasting*. There is *weakness of opposition, abduction and flexion of the thumb* and weakness of the index and middle finger lumbricals. *Sensation is impaired over the palmar aspect of the lateral side of the hand, thumb, index finger, middle finger and lateral (radial) border of the ring finger* (Fig. 3.77).

Interpretation

Confirm the diagnosis

Tell the examiners you would ask about symptoms, particularly nocturnal pain or tingling, which often radiates up the forearm. Percussing over the median nerve at the wrist may reproduce the tingling – Tinel's sign (Fig. 3.78). Flexing the wrist for one minute may do the same (Phalen's sign). Neither of these eponymous signs has been discriminating in clinical studies.

Clinical tests predictive of neurophysiological evidence of a median nerve lesion include:

*   Hyperalgesia in the median nerve territory
*   The classic Katz hand diagram (patient draws the area of sensory loss)
*   Weakness of abductor pollicus brevis

What to do next – consider causes

Causes of carpal tunnel syndrome are listed in Box 3.54.

Consider severity/decompensation/complications

Worsening weakness may be more of an imperative than sensory symptoms.

Consider function

Tell the examiners how you think it might affect the patient's life, especially the nocturnal discomfort.

Discussion

What is the nerve root supply to the median nerve?

See Table 3.42.

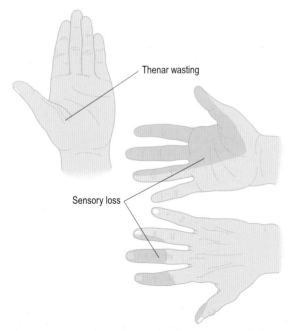

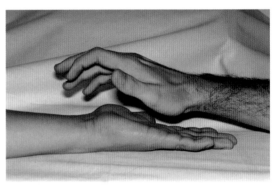

A

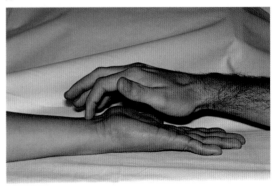

B

Fig. 3.77 Thenar wasting and sensory loss in a median nerve lesion.

Thenar wasting

Sensory loss

Fig. 3.78 (A,B) Eliciting Tinel's sign.

Table 3.42 The median nerve

Roots supplying the median nerve	Muscles supplied by these roots	Common sites of a median nerve lesion
C6	Forearm pronators	Carpal tunnel (carpal tunnel syndrome)
C7	Lateral wrist flexors – flexor carpi radialis	Wrist (lacerations, trauma)
C8	Long finger flexors (via anterior interosseous branch of median nerve) – FDPs to index and middle fingers, FDSs to index and middle fingers, flexor pollicis longus	Forearm (fractures) Elbow (fractures/dislocations)
T1	'LOAF' intrinsic muscles of the hand (Fig. 3.37)	

FDP, flexor digitorum profundus; FDS, flexor digitorum superficialis.

Box 3.54 Causes of carpal tunnel syndrome

- Often idiopathic entrapment
- Diabetes
- Connective tissue disease, e.g. rheumatoid arthritis
- Hypothyroidism
- Acromegaly
- Pregnancy
- Osteoarthritis
- Amyloid
- A family history of small carpal tunnels

Which muscles are supplied by the median nerve?

See Table 3.42.

Which common sites are affected in a median nerve palsy?

See Table 3.42.

Are the signs of a median nerve lesion different if the lesion is at or above the elbow?

There may be lateral forearm wasting and the index (± middle) finger is held in extension (Benediction attitude).

What is the investigation of choice?

A nerve conduction study is imperative before surgical decompression is contemplated.

How would you recognise an anterior interosseous nerve lesion?

An isolated lesion of the anterior interosseous nerve, albeit rare, causes isolated weakness of pincer grasp.

What is the treatment for carpal tunnel syndrome?

Steroids, splinting and yoga may have modest benefits. Surgical decompression is the treatment of choice but benefit in severe lesions is uncertain and where other causes will settle or are treatable, as in pregnancy or hypothyroidism, management is usually conservative.

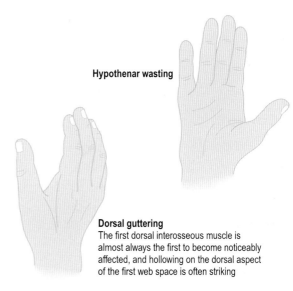

Hypothenar wasting

Dorsal guttering
The first dorsal interosseous muscle is almost always the first to become noticeably affected, and hollowing on the dorsal aspect of the first web space is often striking

Fig. 3.79 Wasting in an ulnar nerve lesion.

CASE 3.41

ULNAR NERVE LESION

Instruction

Please examine this patient's hands and discuss your findings.

Recognition

There is *generalised wasting* of the hand muscles (Fig. 3.79), *sparing only* the *thenar eminence*. Look especially for *dorsal guttering*; the first dorsal interosseus is invariably the first muscle to be noticeably affected, causing hollowing of the first web space.

In a low ulnar nerve lesion the hand is claw shaped – the metacarpophalangeal (MCP) joints of the ring and little fingers are hyperextended and the interphalangeal (IP) joints remain flexed. There is weakness in abduction and adduction of the fingers and thumb.

Sensation is impaired over the medial side of the hand, little finger and medial (ulnar) border of the ring finger (Fig. 3.80).

Ulnar nerve palsy is illustrated in Fig. 3.81.

Interpretation

Confirm the diagnosis

Consider other causes of wasting of the intrinsic muscles of the hand (Case 3.43).

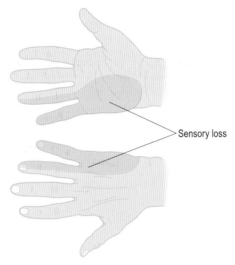

Fig. 3.80 Sensory loss in an ulnar nerve lesion.

What to do next – consider causes

Be sure that you can differentiate between a low and a high ulnar nerve lesion (Box 3.55; Fig. 3.82).

Consider severity/decompensation/complications

Worsening weakness may be more of an imperative than sensory symptoms.

Consider function

Tell the examiners how you think it might affect the patient's life – grip, and so forth. Check for *Froment's* sign – ask the patient to grip a piece of paper or a book between the index finger and thumb (Fig. 3.83). Because thumb adduction is weak, the IP joint must flex to perform this

---

Box 3.55 Differentiating low and high ulnar nerve lesions

Low lesion

The hand is clawed. The lumbricals of the ring and little fingers are paralysed causing hyperextension of the metacarpophalangeal joints but the flexor digitorum profundus (FDP) muscles are intact and flex the distal interphalangeal (DIP) joints. The paralysed interossei also make a contribution to proximal interphalangeal (PIP) flexion. Low lesions occur at the wrist.

High lesion (above the wrist)

The FDPs are also paralysed. The DIPs are hence not flexed and so clawing is less obvious. This has been termed the *ulnar paradox*. High lesions occur commonly at the elbow and include osteoarthritis and fractures/dislocations. The ulnar nerve is particularly vulnerable in the cubital tunnel or ulnar groove. Some people are particularly prone to pressure palsy of the ulnar nerves, provoked by prolonged leaning on desks. As with all mononeuropathies, consider diabetes, connective tissue disorders and vasculitides.

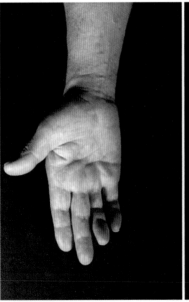

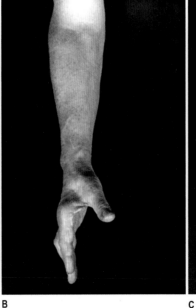

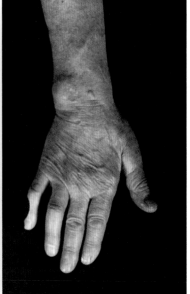

A   B   C

Fig. 3.81 (A–C) Ulnar nerve palsy.

task, possible because flexor pollicis longus is supplied by the median nerve.

Discussion

What is the nerve root supply to the ulnar nerve?

See Table 3.43.

Which muscles are supplied by the ulnar nerve?

See Table 3.43.

Which common sites are affected in an ulnar nerve palsy?

See Table 3.43.

What is the differential diagnosis of a 'claw hand'?

Two conditions should always be considered:

* Volkmann's ishaemic contracture, usually a consequence of brachial artery damage by a supracondylar fracture.

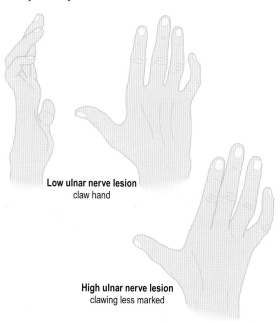

Low ulnar nerve lesion
claw hand

High ulnar nerve lesion
clawing less marked

Fig. 3.82 Claw hand.

* Diabetic cheiropathy, a complication of longstanding type 1 diabetes mellitus, in which there is skin tightening, joint restriction and sclerosis of tendon sheaths.

Is leprosy still common?

Worldwide, leprosy remains a common cause of peripheral nerve thickening and damage, notably the greater auricular nerve and the ulnar nerve (Fig. 3.84).

What is the treatment for an ulnar nerve lesion at the elbow?

Most patients would be offered decompression, with or without transposition, with significant signs and not improving having avoided repeated minor trauma.

CASE 3.42

RADIAL NERVE LESION

Instruction

Please examine this patient's hands and discuss your findings.

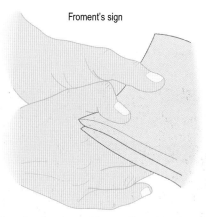

Froment's sign

Fig. 3.83 Normal and paralysed adductor pollicus giving rise to Froment's sign.

Table 3.43 The ulnar nerve		
Roots supplying the ulnar nerve	**Muscles supplied by these roots**	**Common sites of an ulnar nerve lesion**
C8	Medial wrist flexors – flexor carpi ulnaris Long finger flexors – FDP and FDS to ring and little fingers	Ulnar tunnel, where the nerve passes between the pisiform and hamate bones (trauma, ganglion) Wrist (Guyon's canal – ganglion, laceration, trauma – increasingly seen in mountain bikers)
T1	Intrinsic muscles of the hand other than the 'LOAF' muscles (Fig. 3.37)	Medial epicondyle (friction, pressure, stretching, osteoarthritis, trauma) Brachial plexus
FDP, flexor digitorum profundus; FDS, flexor digitorum superficialis.		

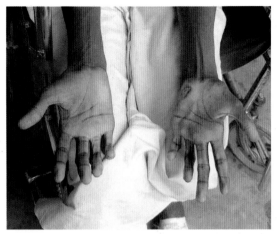

Fig. 3.84 Bilateral ulnar nerve palsy in leprosy.

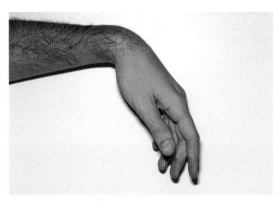

Fig. 3.85 Wrist drop.

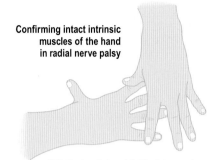

**Confirming intact intrinsic
muscles of the hand
in radial nerve palsy**

With the hand placed flat the interossei can use
their attachments to the long extensor tendons
effectively to abduct and adduct

Fig. 3.86 Radial nerve lesion.

Recognition

There is a *wrist drop* (Fig. 3.85) and *weakness of finger extension*. There is *sensory impairment over the first dorsal interosseous* ('anatomical snuffbox', considerable sensory overlap with the other nerves meaning the area is small). Straightening fingers at the interphalangeal (IP) joints is made possible if the wrist is passively straightened because the intrinsic muscles of the hand supplied by the ulnar nerve (interossei and lumbricals) permit some extension. No extension is possible at the metacarpophalangeal joints (MCPs).

Grip is impaired, not because any flexors are weak but because a degree of wrist extension facilitates good grip. Likewise, abduction and adduction of the fingers are unaffected but may appear to be with a flexed wrist. Testing movements with the palm placed on a flat surface demonstrates that they are nicely intact (Fig. 3.86).

Interpretation

Confirm the diagnosis

Check elbow extension and the triceps reflex. An intact triceps reflex indicates a lesion below the spiral groove. Triceps wasting and an absent reflex imply a high (axillary) radial nerve lesion or a C7 radiculopathy. A C7 root lesion causes weakness of shoulder adduction, elbow extension, wrist flexion and wrist extension because it makes a significant contribution to both the median and radial nerves. A radial nerve lesion cannot affect shoulder adduction or wrist flexion.

What to do next – consider causes

This is the most common acute mononeuropathy, presenting after deep sleep or coma.

Consider severity/decompensation/complications

Worsening weakness may be more of an imperative than sensory symptoms.

Consider function

Tell the examiners how you think it might affect the patient's life.

Discussion

What is the nerve root supply to the radial nerve?
See Table 3.44.

Which muscles are supplied by the radial nerve?
See Table 3.44.

Which common sites are affected in a radial nerve palsy?
See Table 3.44.

Table 3.44 The radial nerve

Roots supplying the radial nerve	Muscles supplied by these roots	Common sites of a radial nerve palsy
C6	Supinator Brachioradialis	At or below the elbow (fracture, dislocation, ganglion) Shaft of humerus (fracture) Axilla (crutches, overnight 'stupor' paralysis sleeping with arm slumped over chair)
C7	Elbow extensors – triceps Wrist extensors	
C8	Long finger extensors – extensor digitorum, extensor pollicis longus, extensor pollicis brevis	

How would you recognise an axillary nerve lesion?

This is usually the result of a traumatic lesion at the humeral head, and causes weakness of the deltoid and sensory loss over the lateral shoulder.

How would you recognise an isolated lesion of the posterior interosseous branch of the radial nerve?

This is rare, usually the result of compression as the nerve enters the supinator muscle. It causes weakness of finger extension without a wrist drop or sensory loss. The differential diagnosis is a radiculopathy of C7.

Box 3.56 Testing just two muscles can yield much information!

Abductor pollicis brevis (APB) – median nerve

Let your palm face the ceiling; now point your thumb up towards the ceiling; don't let me push it down.

First dorsal interosseous (1st DI) – ulnar nerve

Push your index finger out against my hand.
The little finger may be tested (abductor digitorum minimi) instead of the index finger (1st DI) to assess ulnar nerve integrity.

Interpretation

- APB weak + 1st DI weak = T1 radiculopathy
- APB weak + 1st DI spared = median nerve lesion
- APB spared + 1st DI weak = ulnar nerve lesion

CASE 3.43

WASTING OF THE SMALL (INTRINSIC) MUSCLES OF THE HAND

Instruction

Please examine this patient's hands and discuss your findings.

Recognition

There is *wasting and weakness of all the small or intrinsic muscles* (Fig. 3.87) of the hand.

Interpretation

Confirm the diagnosis

Signs may be similar to those of an ulnar nerve lesion but with additional thenar wasting.

What to do next – consider causes

Causes can be considered under the following headings:

- T1 radiculopathy or plexopathy involving T1
- Concurrent median **and** ulnar nerve lesions
- Polyneuropathy (if bilateral and with motor predominance)
- Disuse atrophy (bilateral/asymmetrical), e.g. longstanding rheumatoid arthritis

If wasting is unilateral it can be hard to know whether you are looking at a radiculopathy, an ulnar nerve lesion or even a median nerve lesion. A quick way of tackling this is to focus on testing the two muscles in Box 3.56.

Consider severity/decompensation/complications

This rather depends upon the cause. A diffuse cause, such as motor neurone disease, can be overlooked in the early stages, often dismissed as a minor mononeuropathy.

Consider function

Tell the examiners how you think it might affect the patient's life, with particular regard to fine tasks.

Discussion

List some causes of a C8/T1 root lesion

- Cervical spondylosis
- Syringomyelia (may be bilateral)
- Motor neuron disease
- Pancoast's tumour
- Cervical rib

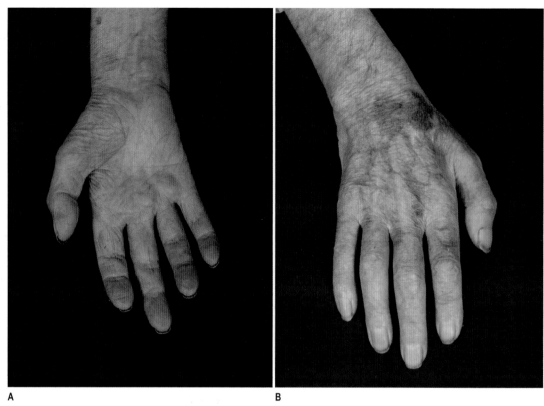

A   **B**

Fig. 3.87 (A,B) Wasting of the small muscles of the hand (in multifocal motor neuropathy).

COMMON PERONEAL NERVE LESION

Instruction

Please examine this patient's lower limbs and discuss your findings.

Recognition

There is *wasting of the lateral muscles of the lower leg*, and *weakness of dorsiflexion and eversion* of the ankle provoking a foot drop (Fig. 3.88) and weakness of toe extension. There may be sensory loss over the lateral calf and dorsum of the foot, but in practice it tends to be slight.

Interpretation

Confirm the diagnosis

Check the ankle reflex. It should be intact. The sciatic nerve has two branches – the common peroneal and tibial

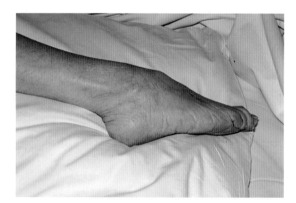

Fig. 3.88 Foot drop.

nerves. The ankle reflex is conveyed through the S1 root via the tibial nerve, and thus is spared in a peroneal nerve lesion. An absent ankle reflex indicates one of three possible lesions (Box 3.57).

What to do next – consider causes

Consider all causes of a foot drop (Box 3.58).

Table 3.45 The peroneal nerve		
Roots supplying the common peroneal nerve	**Muscles supplied by these roots**	**Common sites of a common peroneal nerve lesion**
L4,5 (mostly L5)	Dorsiflexors – tibialis anterior (deep peroneal branch of common peroneal nerve)	Most commonly compression (plaster casts, leg crossing) or trauma at the fibula neck – the nerve twines around this
L5, S1	Evertors – peroneus longus, peroneus brevis (superficial peroneal branch of common peroneal nerve)	Diffuse lesions, e.g. diabetes mellitus, vasculitis, leprosy

---

Box 3.57 Causes of an absent ankle reflex

- S1 radiculopathy (by far the most common cause)
- Complete sciatic nerve lesion
- Tibial nerve lesion (much rarer than lesions of the common peroneal nerve or its deep and superficial divisions)

Box 3.58 Causes of foot drop

- Common peroneal nerve lesion
- Sciatic nerve lesion
- L4/5 (especially 5) radiculopathy (prolapsed lumbar disc)
- Polyneuropathy, especially hereditary sensory and motor neuropathy/Charcot–Marie–Tooth disease
- Upper motor neuron lesion (spinal cord or cortex)

   Preserved inversion strongly suggests a common peroneal nerve lesion; any weakness of inversion indicates a more proximal lesion

---

Consider severity/decompensation/complications

This rather depends upon the cause (see Table 3.45).

Consider function

Observe gait. A common peroneal nerve lesion causes a foot drop, resulting in a high stepping gait. Correcting callipers may be at the bedside.

Discussion

What is the nerve root supply to the common peroneal nerve?

See Table 3.45.

Which muscles are supplied by the common peroneal nerve?

See Table 3.45.

Which common sites are affected in a common peroneal nerve palsy?

See Table 3.45.

How would you recognise a sciatic nerve lesion?

This is a less common mononeuropathy in the leg, the site of damage the pelvis, buttock or thigh and usually the result of trauma, buttock compression or tumour. It causes weakness in the hamstrings plus common peroneal and tibial nerve deficits and sensory loss over areas of the posterior cutaneous nerve of the thigh plus the common pero-neal and tibial nerves. The differential diagnosis is a radiculopathy of L5 or S1.

How would you recognise a femoral nerve lesion?

This is a less common mononeuropathy in the leg, usually the result of a psoas haematoma or trauma. It causes weakness of hip flexion and knee extension and sensory loss over the anterior thigh and medial calf. The differential diagnosis is a radiculopathy of L3 or L4, or diabetic amyotrophy.

What is diabetic amyotrophy?

This refers to pain, weakness and wasting in one or both quadriceps in diabetes mellitus, probably due to lumbosacral plexus microvasculitis.

How would you recognise an obturator nerve lesion?

This is a rare mononeuropathy, usually the result of a pelvic tumour or surgery. It causes weakness of hip adduction and sensory loss over the medial thigh. The differential diagnosis is a lumbosacral plexopathy.

How would you recognise a lesion of the lateral cutaneous nerve of the thigh or 'meralgia paraesthetica'?

This is a common mononeuropathy in the leg, the site of damage is often the inguinal ligament and it is commonly the result of obesity, pregnancy or surgery. It causes sensory disturbance, often pain or tingling, at the lateral mid-thigh, without weakness. The differential diagnosis is a radiculopathy of L2.

CASE 3.45

PERIPHERAL NEUROPATHY

Instruction

Please examine this patient's legs and discuss your findings.

Recognition

There may be *symmetrical impairment of sensation to all modalities in a stocking (and sometimes also glove)*

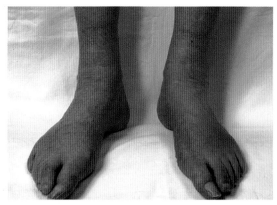

Fig. 3.89 Stocking distribution.

distribution (Fig. 3.89) There may be *distal wasting* and *weakness* and *distal areflexia*.

Interpretation

Confirm the diagnosis

The classic picture of stocking sensory loss and/or distal wasting, weakness and diminished reflexes due to a distal symmetrical polyneuropathy is likely (Box 3.62).

What to do next – consider causes/assess other systems

Look for punched-out foot ulcers suggesting diabetic neuropathy. Tell the examiners you would:

- Take a history for systemic disease (especially for diabetes, chronic kidney and liver disease), infection (tick bites for Lyme disease, HIV) and malignancy (Table 3.48)
- Take a drug and possible toxin exposure history (Table 3.48)
- Take a family history (inherited neuropathies, shared toxin exposure)

Diabetes is the most common cause in the developed world and globally, leprosy remains a common cause. Other common causes include metabolic disorders, infection, vasculitis, drugs and toxins. Dysimmune and inherited polyneuropathies are not uncommon chronic causes.

Tell the examiners you would ask about sensory and motor symptoms, and autonomic symptoms (Box 3.59). Autonomic symptoms occur mostly in generalised polyneuropathy, e.g. diabetes polyneuropathy, Guillain–Barré syndrome, porphyria and amyloid neuropathy; rarely, they occur as a pandysautonomia, presumably with a dysimmune basis.

Consider severity/decompensation/complications

If there is a predominant symmetrical motor neuropathy, tell the examiners you would immediately attempt to

---

Box 3.59 Autonomic symptoms

- Postural hypotension
- Atonic bladder
- Constipation
- Erectile dysfunction
- Dry eyes and mouth
- Anhidrosis
- Paroxysmal hypertension, tachycardia or bradycardia (rare)
- Hyperhidrosis (rare)
- Diarrhoea (rare)

Box 3.60 Definitions of sensory symptoms

- Paraesthesia – abnormal sensations evoked or spontaneous and not unduly painful or unpleasant
- Dysaesthesia – unpleasant paraesthesia
- Hyperaesthesia – increased sensitivity to a stimulus
- Allodynia – painful sensation resulting from a non-painful stimulus, e.g. light touch

---

exclude Guillain–Barré syndrome (Case 3.47), which can cause acute severe ascending paralysis involving the arms, chest, neck and cranial nerves (facial and bulbar weakness), and respiratory failure.

Consider function

Tell the examiners you would ask about sensory symptoms (Box 3.60) and the limitations posed by weakness and gait disturbance. Motor tasks requiring manual dexterity are often impaired.

Discussion

What is meant by the term peripheral neuropathy?

It is a general term for any disorder of the peripheral nervous system. The causes are disparate and the presentation is variable. Most can be categorised by subtype and cause through a logical and sequential approach using clinical findings, electrodiagnostic and laboratory tests, with implications for management and prognosis.

How common is peripheral neuropathy?

It is common, with an overall prevalence of 2.4% of the population rising to 8% over 55 years.

How would you further evaluate a peripheral neuropathy?

This requires clinical evaluation, electrodiagnostic studies and laboratory tests (see also Table 3.48).

Clinical evaluation and electrodiagnostic studies

The clinical manifestations of peripheral neuropathy vary widely, with varying presenting combinations of sensory symptoms, pain, muscle weakness or atrophy, and autonomic symptoms. Electrodiagnostic studies, including

Table 3.46 Important details to determine from clinical evaluation and electrophysiological tests

Rate of development and duration	Acute (up to 4 weeks) Subacute (4–8 weeks) Chronic (> 8 weeks)
Pattern of progression	Gradual progression Relapsing–remitting
Pattern of distribution	Mononeuropathy Mononeuropathy multiplex Plexopathy Polyneuropathy
Pattern of symptoms	Predominantly motor Predominantly sensory Both
Pattern of fibre involvement	Most polyneuropathies involve large and small fibres Weakness or wasting indicates large fibre involvement because all motor fibres except gamma efferents to muscle spindles are large Sensory ataxia or areflexia indicates large sensory fibre involvement because vibration, proprioception and reflex afferent fibres are large Positive sensory symptoms such as pain and burning dysaesthesias indicate small fibre involvement because pain and temperature sensitivity and peripheral autonomic functions rely on small fibres; causes include diabetes, amyloidosis and HIV
Electrophysiological type	Mainly demyelinating Mainly axonal

Table 3.47 Causes of a mononeuropathy

External insult Acute onset or insidious onset as in repeated minor external compression such as habitual leaning on the elbow (ulnar lesion) or kneeling (common peroneal lesion)	Direct trauma, including prolonged external compression, e.g. coma Repeated minor trauma Traction Injection Cold, burns, radiation
Internal entrapment or compression Usually insidious onset	Median nerve entrapment in carpal tunnel Ulnar nerve entrapment at elbow Rarely, compression by tumours or vascular malformations
Intrinsic lesion Usually acute onset	Infarct, usually a focal manifestation of a generalised process, e.g. vasculitis, conduction block in multifocal motor neuropathy
Increased susceptibility to injury Usually insidious onset	e.g. diabetes, alcohol, nutritional deficiency, hereditary liability to pressure palsies, combined with minor compression or entrapment

nerve conduction studies and needle electromyography, are sensitive, specific and validated measures of peripheral neuropathy and should be considered whenever peripheral neuropathy is suspected. A nerve conduction study involves electrical stimulation of a peripheral nerve and recording, further along that nerve, the latency and amplitude of the action potential. From the latency, a conduction velocity may be calculated; normal is 50–60 m/second in the arm and 40–50 m/second in the leg. Amplitude is normally small for small nerves and large for larger compound muscle action potentials. In demyelinating neuropathies, the velocity is slowed but the amplitude is preserved. The opposite is characteristic of axonal neuropathies. Although some recommend investigation for common causes before using electrophysiological tests, evidence does not support this and many neurologists consider it a mandatory exten-

sion of neurological examination. The most important details to determine are outlined in Table 3.46. An overview of evaluation of peripheral neuropathy is shown in Fig. 3.90.

What is meant by the term mononeuropathy?

This refers to a lesion of a single peripheral nerve. Typical causes are outlined in Table 3.47.

There are essentially three types of focal peripheral nerve lesion:

- Neuropraxia, focal or segmental demyelination with preservation of the axon and recovery in 2–12 weeks
- Axonotmesis, in which the axon is divided but the epineurium remains intact and regrowth occurs at 1 mm/day from the injured site

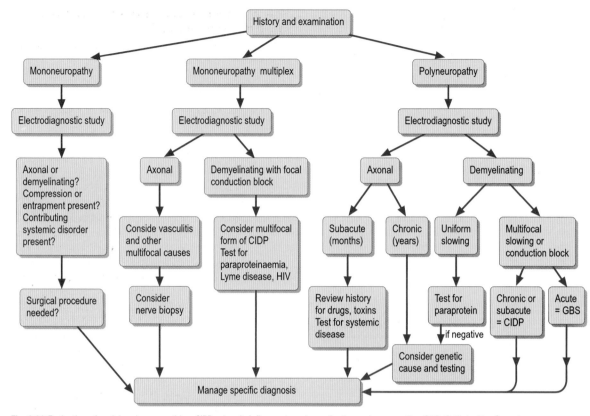

Fig. 3.90 Evaluation of peripheral neuropathies. CIPD, chronic inflammatory demyelinating polyneuropathy; GBS, Guillain–Barré syndrome.

- Neurotmesis, where the nerve is divided and no longer in continuity, with no recovery

These can occur together, appreciated clinically when relatively rapid neuropraxic recovery is followed by slower axonotmesis recovery. Appreciation of the likely mechanism of injury helps guide investigation.

What are the common mononeuropathies and how are they diagnosed?

Diagnosis of mononeuropathies depends on recognising that the neurological deficit involves the distribution of a single nerve. This requires knowledge of anatomy and of the motor and sensory territories of nerves, but fortunately relatively few nerves are prone to mononeuropathies, notably:

- Median nerve compression in carpal tunnel syndrome (the commonest)
- Ulnar nerve compression at the elbow (the next most common)
- Radial nerve lesion after acute compression ('Saturday night' palsy)
- Common peroneal nerve lesion

Peripheral nerves are arranged in fascicles so that a more proximal lesion may be mistaken for a more distal one, e.g.

a foot drop following hip replacement with weak eversion and preserved inversion and sensory loss in the common peroneal nerve distribution is almost certainly a sciatic nerve lesion involving the common peroneal fascicle rather than a more distal common peroneal nerve lesion. Electrodiagnostic studies help localise, determine severity and exclude unsuspected mononeuropathy multiplex. Multiple compression mononeuropathies are often part of the spectrum of hereditary neuropathy with liability to pressure palsies.

What is meant by the term mononeuropathy multiplex?

This refers to involvement of multiple separate non-contiguous peripheral nerves, either simultaneously or serially. The pattern of nerve involvement is random, multifocal and often evolves quickly, sometimes progressing to a summation of nerve lesions with confluent, symmetric deficits mimicking a distal symmetrical polyneuropathy. The early pattern of onset is important. Urgent assessment is important because vasculitis is a common cause, and usually systemic but may be confined to the peripheral nerves. Common causes of mononeuropathy multiplex are listed in Box 3.61.

Sural or superficial peroneal nerve biopsy may be helpful unless the diagnosis is clear, as in diabetic amyotrophy, or a systemic cause has been identified.

Box 3.61 Common causes of mononeuropathy multiplex

Axonal

- Vasculitis, e.g. Churg–Strauss syndrome, connective tissue disease, e.g. rheumatoid arthritis
- Diabetic amyotrophy (acute pain in thigh, probably due to vasculitis in lumbosacral plexus)
- Leprosy
- Lyme disease
- Human immunodeficiency virus
- Carcinoma
- Lymphoma
- Sarcoidosis
- Amyloidosis
- Cryoglobulinaemia

Demyelinating

- Chronic inflammatory demyelinating polyradiculopathy (CIDP) or variant, e.g. multifocal motor neuropathy
- Multifocal neuropathy with liability to pressure palsies (deletion in PMP22 gene)

Box 3.62 Typical progression of symptoms and signs in distal symmetrical polyneuropathy

- Distal, symmetrical sensory symptoms (numbness, burning, paraesthesia or dysaesthesia of toes or feet); weakness sometimes comes first, of toe and foot dorsiflexion
- Ascending sensory symptoms, weakness of toe and foot dorsiflexion (unable to stand on heels) and depression or loss of ankle reflexes
- Plantar flexion remains relatively strong (able to stand on toes)
- Shin and fingertip sensory symptoms
- Gait disorder – proprioceptive loss and extensor muscle weakness
- Mid-thigh, upper forearm and lower abdominal sensory symptoms – a triangular-shaped area of hypoaesthesia with its apex in the midline; may ascend as far as umbilicus or even manubriosternum (unlike a spinal cord lesion, with sensory loss at front and back)
- Advanced polyneuropathy with stocking-glove diffuse sensory loss, distal muscle wasting and weakness and absent reflexes

---

What types of polyneuropathy are there clinically?

The most common variety is distal symmetrical polyneuropathy; nerve fibres are affected in a length-dependent manner, length meaning distance from the parent nerve cell body (either the dorsal root ganglion sensory neuron or the anterior horn motor neuron), irrespective of root or nerve trunk distribution. The typical progression of symptoms and signs is outlined in Box 3.62.

What are the causes of distal symmetrical polyneuropathy?

This pattern is associated with many systemic diseases, metabolic disorders, infections, malignancies, drugs and toxins (Table 3.48), the main cause being the chronic sensory and motor polyneuropathy associated with diabetes.

How are polyneuropathies classified on the basis of nerve conduction studies?

Polyneuropathies are most practically subtyped as acute, chronic demyelinating or chronic axonal.

Acute polyneuropathy

Guillain–Barré syndrome and the differential diagnosis of acute neuropathy are discussed in Case 3.47.

Chronic polyneuropathy

Chronic symmetrical polyneuropathy is the commonest type of polyneuropathy, and differential diagnosis is usually narrowed down on the basis of history, examination and electrodiagnostic studies to a few possibilities. For example, a chronic, steadily progressive distal symmetrical sensorimotor polyneuropathy with predominantly axonal features is most likely to be the result of systemic or metabolic disease, or drugs or toxins; a longstanding chronic, predominantly motor distal symmetrical polyneuropathy with uniformly demyelinating features is most likely an inherited polyneuropathy, e.g. Charcot–Marie–Tooth type 1; acquired mimics, e.g. chronic inflammatory demyelinating poly(radiculo)neuropathy (CIDP) or paraproteinaemia are excluded by electrodiagnostic studies and electrophoresis.

Chronic demyelinating polyneuropathy   The causes are limited. Genetic causes include Charcot–Marie–Tooth disease type 1, 4 or X1, hereditary liability to pressure palsies, metachromatic leucodystrophy, globoid cell leucodystrophy and Refsum disease. Acquired causes include CIDP, multifocal motor neuropathy (MMN) and paraproteinaemic demyelinating polyneuropathy (associated with antibodies to myelin-associated glycoprotein), monoclonal gammopathy of uncertain significance and osteosclerotic myeloma. Acquired causes are mostly immunologically mediated. CIDP is the most common type, either gradually progressive or relapsing. It is usually, but not always, predominantly motor, causing proximal as well as distal weakness. Cerebrospinal protein concentration tends to be very high. MMN, related to CIDP, produces partial conduction block and is restricted to motor axons, usually producing weakness and atrophy in the hands and forearms. Around 10% of acquired causes are the result of paraproteinaemias, usually producing slowly evolving distal symmetrical sensory abnormalities in the feet.

Chronic axonal polyneuropathy   This is the commonest type of polyneuropathy and there are many causes (Table 3.48). Several varieties of hereditary neuropathy, especially axonal types of Charcot–Marie–Tooth disease (CMT2) present with this pattern. No cause is found in up to 25% of patients. Proof of diagnosis can be made on unmyelinated nerve fibre density in a skin biopsy, but this is not widely available. Most idiopathic distal symmetrical polyneuropathies progress slowly and seldom produce

Table 3.48 Causes of polyneuropathy

Causes		Sensory (S), motor (M), sensorimotor (SM)	Axonal (A) or demyelinating (D)	Notes
Systemic disease and metabolic	Diabetes mellitus	S, SM, rarely M	A and D	Commonest cause of chronic polyneuropathy Glucose intolerance can produce polyneuropathy
	Chronic kidney disease	SM	A	Controlled with dialysis Cured by transplant
	Chronic liver disease	S or SM	A and D	Mild
	Nutritional deficiency – B vitamins, thiamine, folic acid, often alcoholism	SM	A	
	B12 deficiency	S	A	Myelopathy may dominate
	Malabsorption, e.g. inflammatory bowel disease, coeliac disease	S or SM	A	Not necessarily vitamin deficiency ? Immune/autoimmune basis
	Porphyria (rare)	M or SM	A	Often acute, often proximal and upper limbs Differential diagnosis Guillain–Barré syndrome (GBS)
	Sarcoidosis	S or SM	A	Polyneuropathy or mononeuropathy multiplex Facial neuropathy common
	Primary systemic amyloidosis (rare)	SM	A	Most associated with paraproteinaemia (myeloma, Waldenstrom's macroglobulinaemia, lymphoproliferative disease)
	COPD (rare) Hypothyroidism (very rare)	S or SM	A	Severe chronic obstructive pulmonary disease
Infection	Leprosy	S > SM	A	Cutaneous nerves
	Lyme disease	S > M	A	Focal or multifocal radiculoneuropathy Facial neuropathy
	Human immunodeficiency virus	S > M	A	Chronic distal sensory polyneuropathy Other types in early infection
Malignancy	Carcinoma	SM Pure S (rare)	A	Lung cancer Paraneoplastic ganglionitis with small cell or breast cancer
	Lymphoma	SM	A > D	
	Myeloma	S, M or SM	A	Uncommon
	Osteosclerotic myeloma Plasmacytoma	SM	D	Association with POEMS syndrome – polyneuropathy, organomegaly, endocrinopathy, monoclonal gammopathy, skin changes
	Monoclonal gammopathy of uncertain significance (MGUS)	S or SM	A or D	IgM, G or A
Drugs	Amiodarone	SM	D > A	Dose related; may cause tremor, optic neuropathy
	Antibiotics, e.g. chloramphenicol, chloroquine, dapsone, ethambutol, isoniazid, metronidazole, nitrofurantoin, nucleoside anti-retrovirals	SM common	A D	Chloramphenicol reversible Myopathy more common with chloroquine Upper limb with dapsone Ethambutol mild Isoniazid slow acetylators, avoid with pyridoxine Metronidazole dose related Nitrofurantoin rapid, worse with renal failure Nucleoside painful, dose related
	Chemotherapeutic, e.g. platinum, taxol	S	A	May start abruptly
	Colchicine	S or SM	A	Myopathy more common
	Hydralazine	S > M	A	Pyridoxine antagonist
	Phenytoin	S > M	A	Rare, decades of use
	Pyridoxine (vitamin B6)	S	A	High doses
	Thalidomide	S > M	A	Pain insensitivity

Table 3.48 Causes of polyneuropathy—cont'd

Causes		Sensory (S), motor (M), sensorimotor (SM)	Axonal (A) or demyelinating (D)	Notes
Toxins	Arsenic	SM	A or D	Painful sensory symptoms then weakness, systemic illness, e.g. genitourinary symptoms, Mees lines on nails Differential diagnosis GBS
	Carbon disulphide (cellophane manufacturing)	S > M	A	Sensory then motor symptoms
	Diphtheria toxin	SM	D	Rare, 8–12 weeks after infection
	Hexacarbons (gasoline or glue)	SM	A and D	May be severe
	Lead	M	A	Wrist drop Differential diagnosis GBS
	Mercury	M > S	A	Differential diagnosis GBS
	Organophosphates (insecticides)	M > S	A	10–20 days after exposure
	Thallium (rodenticides)	S > M	A	Differential diagnosis GBS
Inherited neuropathies	Charcot–Marie–Tooth disease types 1,4 and X1	SM	D	
	Hereditary liability to pressure palsies	SM	D	

overt disability and treatment of sensory symptoms is paramount.

What laboratory and other tests would you consider in the investigation of peripheral neuropathy?

These are outlined in Table 3.49.

What is the role of a nerve biopsy in peripheral neuropathy?

Nerve biopsy is useful in documenting inflammatory disorders such as vasculitis, sarcoidosis, CIDP, infectious diseases such as leprosy, or infiltrative disorders such as amyloidosis or tumour. It is usually reserved for cases when diagnosis cannot be reached by other means.

What are the principles of treatment in peripheral neuropathy?

These can be divided into specific and general approaches.

Specific

Treatments specific to the subtype include removal of any exogenous cause or treatment of any medical cause. CIDP and MMN can respond to immunotherapy, both respond to intravenous immunoglobulin, but only CIDP responds to corticosteroids and plasma exchange; some patients with MMN have deteriorated with steroids.

General

Foot care, ankle supports and physiotherapy can be useful. Painful peripheral neuropathy is difficult to treat. The most useful agents are anticonvulsants (especially gabapentin and carbamazepine) and tricyclic antidepressants (especially amitriptyline).

How might you treat a patient with diabetic neuropathy with refractory burning sensations or dysaesthesia?

A stepwise approach might start with amitriptyline, sedating alternatives including imipramine or lofepramine. Gabapentin might be tried as first line, at a dose of 100–300 mg daily and incremented. Carbamazepine is an alternative but ataxia is a common side effect.

MR spinal imaging might be performed to exclude spinal stenosis or radiculopathy in patients with refractory symptoms and a not unequivocal diagnosis. The differential diagnosis of thigh pain, for example, might include femoral neuropathy, diabetic amyotrophy or meralgia paraesthetica.

Referral to a pain clinic for consideration of epidural analgesia might be a next step, or consideration of opioid analgesia such as morphine sulphate MST twice daily and oramorph for breakthrough pain; the combination of oxycontin, at a starting dose of 5 mg twice daily, and oxynorm for breakthrough pain may be preferable if confusion is a side effect. A 35 mg buprenorphine patch with antiemesis is an alternative. Topiramate at a dose of 25 mg once or twice daily has been used with some effect, but by this stage the law is generally that of diminishing returns and acupuncture is sometimes tried. Some patients are helped by clonazepam, but this is rather sedating.

Table 3.49 Laboratory and other tests in peripheral neuropathy

Initial tests	Haematology	Full blood count
		Erythrocyte sedimentation rate
		B12
		Folate
		?Homocysteine levels for B12 levels in low normal range
	Biochemistry	Fasting blood glucose or oral glucose tolerance test
		Renal function
		Liver function
		Calcium
		Thyroid function
		Protein electrophoresis and immunoglobulins
	Autoimmune profile	ANA and rheumatoid factor
		ENA for Sjögren's syndrome and systemic lupus erythematosus
		ANCA for vasculitis
		Cryoglobulins
	Urine	Glucose
		Protein
	Radiology	Chest X-ray
More specialised tests for specific causes	Systemic/metabolic	Serum (± cerebrospinal fluid) angiotensin-converting enzyme
		Coeliac disease antibodies
		Porphyrins in blood, urine or stool
	Infection	Lyme serology
		HIV testing
		Campylobacter jejuni, cytomegalovirus, hepatitis viruses B and C, and herpes virus serology
	Malignancy	Mammography
		Skeletal survey
		CT thorax, abdomen, pelvis (TAP)
		Antineuronal antibodies (anti-HU, anti-CV2)
	Drugs and toxins	Heavy metal toxicity from blood, urine, hair or nail analysis
	Dysimmune	Anti-ganglioside antibody profile (GM1 – MMN with conduction block, other – see Case 3.47
		Anti-myelin associated glycoprotein (MAG) antibodies (IgM paraproteinaemic neuropathy)
		Cerebrospinal fluid analysis including immunoglobulin oligoclonal bands
	Inherited	Tailored to clinical profile, e.g. chromosome 17 (duplication for Charcot–Marie–Tooth disease type 1a, deletion for hereditary neuropathy with liability to pressure palsies), familial amyloid polyneuropathy

ANA, antinuclear antibodies; ANCA, anti-neutrophil cytoplasmic antibody; CT, computed tomography scan; ENA, extractable nuclear antigens.

CASE 3.46

CHARCOT–MARIE–TOOTH DISEASE AND HEREDITARY NEUROPATHIES

Instruction

Please examine this patient's legs and discuss your findings.

Recognition

A severe, predominantly motor, peripheral neuropathy with marked wasting (causing distal narrowing or *inverted champagne bottle legs*) may be caused by *hereditary sensory and motor neuropathy (HSMN)* (Fig. 3.91). There may also be *clawing of the toes* and *pes cavus* with marked weakness of dorsiflexion. Thickened nerves and tremor are sometimes present.

Interpretation

Confirm the diagnosis

In pes cavus, the arch of the foot is high, the foot shortened with bunched up, clawed toes, and its lateral border does not contact the ground. Foot drop usually develops later.

What to do next – consider causes

Charcot–Marie–Tooth disease type 1 (CMT-1)

Of CMT-1 (HMSN type 1) cases, 70–80% are caused by a duplication in the *PMP22* gene (probably encoding myelin protein) on chromosome 17. The phenotype is highly variable, ranging from the classic picture with pes cavus and 'stork legs' (severe distal wasting or 'inverted champagne bottle legs') to minimal deficit with almost undetectable clawing of the toes. Different mutations can cause a similar phenotype, and classification relies on genetic testing, which is now widely available.

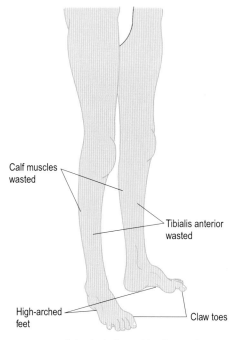

Calf muscles
wasted

Tibialis anterior
wasted

High-arched
feet

Claw toes

(Lateral sole does not touch ground)

Fig. 3.91 Hereditary sensory and motor neuropathy (HSMN) type 1.

CMT-2

CMT-2 (HSMN type 2) accounts for one-third of dominantly inherited neuropathies and is also clinically heterogeneous, but often only becomes detectable in later life.

Consider severity/decompensation/complications

The neuropathy often ascends relentlessly to cause wasting of the intrinsic muscles of the hands, while sensory impairment is usually minimal or absent.

Consider function

If you suspect HSMN a marked, bilateral high-stepping gait, caused by bilateral foot drop, is likely; this is predominantly the result of bilateral common peroneal nerve palsy, these nerves being especially vulnerable in this condition and often thickened.

Discussion

What hereditary neuropathies do you know?

The hereditary neuropathies are a complex and heterogeneous group of disorders with an estimated prevalence of 1–3/10 000. Many genes and linkage sites have been described. Most are extremely rare. The most common are dominantly inherited CMT, also known as HSMN, types 1 (demyelinating) and 2 (axonal), and X-linked CMT (CMT-X). Spontaneous mutations also occur. CMT was once known as 'peroneal muscle atrophy'. Other hereditary neuropathies, of chronic demyelinating polyneuro-

pathy type, are CMT type 4, hereditary liability to pressure palsies, metachromatic leucodystrophy, globoid cell leucodystrophy and Refsum's disease.

CASE 3.47

GUILLAIN–BARRÉ SYNDROME

Instruction

Please examine this patient's lower limbs and discuss your findings.

Recognition

There is *symmetrical weakness in an ascending distribution with areflexia.*

Interpretation

Confirm the diagnosis

Guillain–Barré syndrome is an acute, predominantly motor, distal but rapidly ascending, symmetrical polyneuropathy. It often starts with mild extremity weakness or distal paraesthesia, which is easy to dismiss. Areflexia is characteristic but may not occur in the first few hours. Contrary to what is often written, sensory symptoms do occur, although they are often mild. Diagnosis is often clinical, supported by examination of cerebrospinal fluid and neurophysiological studies.

What to do next – consider causes

Mention a differential diagnosis of acute flaccid paralysis to the examiners (Box 3.63).

Guillain–Barré syndrome has numerous subtypes (see Table 3.50) and is arbitrarily defined by an onset lasting up to four weeks. Subacute inflammatory demyelinating polyradiculoneuropathy and chronic inflammatory demyelinating polyradiculoneuropathy (CIDP) are defined by four to eight weeks and over eight weeks, respectively. Some patients with Guillain–Barré syndrome have recurrent peaks of symptoms within an apparent single but protracted episode of illness and then it may be difficult to distinguish from CIDP; indeed, the two conditions may overlap.

Consider severity/decompensation/complications

Progression is often swift and life-threatening respiratory muscle paralysis can occur. A quarter to a third of patients need ventilatory support. Tell the examiners that you would arrange regular spirometry.

Consider function

Patients have flaccid paralysis of the lower limbs especially and cannot walk. Complete or near-complete recovery, while likely, is not assured.

Box 3.63 Differential diagnosis of acute flaccid paralysis

Brainstem disease

- Brainstem stroke
- Brainstem encephalitis

Acute myelopathy

- Acute transverse myelitis
- Space-occupying lesion

Anterior horn cell disease

- Poliomyelitis or other neurotropic virus

Peripheral neuropathy

- Guillain–Barré syndrome
- Diphtheritic neuropathy
- Botulinum neuropathy
- Heavy metal, biological toxin or drug intoxication neuropathy
- Acute intermittent porphyria
- Vasculitis neuropathy
- Critical illness neuropathy
- Lymphomatous neuropathy
- Post rabies vaccine neuropathy

Neuromuscular junction disease

- Myasthenia gravis
- Toxins

Myopathy

- Hypokalaemia
- Hypophosphataemia
- Inflammatory myopathy
- Acute rhabdomyolysis
- Periodic paralysis

Discussion

How common is Guillain–Barré syndrome?

The incidence is reported as around 0.6–4 cases per 100 000, with relative uniformity between countries, although it may be more common where infectious causes are common.

What causes Guillain–Barré syndrome?

Guillain–Barré syndrome is not a single disease but has various subtypes. There is no single cause, and the cause is often unknown, but infections that are known to trigger forms of Guillain–Barré syndrome include *Campylobacter jejuni*, cytomegalovirus, Epstein–Barr virus and *Mycoplasma pneumoniae*.

What is the pathophysiology of Guillain–Barré syndrome?

Guillain–Barré syndrome comprises at least four subtypes of acute peripheral neuropathy.

Acute inflammatory demyelinating polyradiculoneuropathy (AIDP)

The AIDP subtype is mediated by T cells against peptides from myelin proteins PO, P2 and PMP22, although antibodies and complement are also involved.

Axonal subtypes of Guillain–Barré syndrome – acute motor axonal neuropathy (AMAN) and acute motor and sensory axonal neuropathy (AMSAN)

These are caused by antibodies to gangliosides on the axonomella that target macrophages to invade the axon at the node of Ranvier and cause damage and degeneration. Around 25% of patients with Guillain–Barré syndrome have had recent *Campylobacter jejuni* infection, and axonal subtypes are especially common in these people. The *Campylobacter* bacterial wall contains ganglioside-like structures and antibodies against it may similarly attack axons in AMAN, in which antibodies to GM1, GM1b, GD1a and Ga1Nac-GD1a are implicated, and ASMAN, in which all of the above, except Ga1Nac-GD1a, are implicated.

Fischer syndrome

This subtype is especially associated with antibodies to GQ1b, and similar cross-reactivity with ganglioside structures in *Campylobacter* has been observed.

What are the clinical manifestations of the different types of Guillain–Barré syndrome?

These are described in Table 3.50.

How is Guillain–Barré syndrome diagnosed?

Investigations in Guillain–Barré syndrome are listed in Table 3.51.

Electrodiagnostic studies are important in diagnosis, subtype classification and confirmation of peripheral neuropathy. Sufficient data are needed, as described in Table 3.50, and with these data one of three subtypes – AIDP, AMAN, AMSAN – can be identified. However, unlike for clinical criteria, there is no consensus on neurophysiological criteria. Sometimes an 'inexcitable' result is obtained, dCMAP absent in all nerves or present in only one nerve with dCMAP < 10%, and then it is not possible to determine if the absence of recordable action potentials is the result of complete conduction block from demyelinaton or of axonal degeneration or dysfunction. A common finding in Guillain–Barré syndrome is a normal sural sensory action potential (SAP) and abnormal median SAP, the 'normal sural–abnormal median pattern.'

Raised cerebrospinal fluid protein (higher the longer the evolution of the illness) with a normal white cell count is characteristic but not specific in Guillain–Barré syndrome.

Nerve biopsy can differentiate between demyelination and axonal disease but is seldom performed in Guillain–Barré syndrome.

How is Guillain–Barré syndrome treated?

Results of international trials have shown equivalent efficacy of intravenous immunoglobulin and plasma exchange, but not corticosteroids, and these treatments minimise worsening, hasten recovery and reduce long-term disability. Intravenous immunoglobulin is usually preferred

Table 3.50 Features of the different subtypes of Guillain–Barré syndrome

	Features	Antibodies	Neurophysiology
Acute inflammatory demyelinating polyradiculoneuropathy (AIDP)	Most common subtype by far Acute weakness of all four limbs with hyporeflexia or areflexia, reaching peak within four weeks Can involve cranial nerves Can cause respiratory muscle weakness Autonomic involvement common, especially if severe respiratory weakness	Unknown	At least one of the following in each of at least two nerves, or at least two of the following in one nerve if all others inexcitable and compound muscle action potential amplitude after distal stimulation (dCMAP) > 10% of lower limit of normal (LLN): Motor conduction velocity < 90% LLN (85% if dCMAP < 50%) Distal motor latency > 110% upper limit of normal (ULN) (> 120% if dCMAP < 100% LLN) Proximal CMAP (pCMAP)/dCMAP ratio < 0.5 and dCMAP > 20% ULN F-response latency > 120% ULN
Acute motor axonal neuropathy (AMAN)	Acute weakness of all four limbs with hyporeflexia or areflexia, reaching peak within four weeks Can involve cranial nerves Can cause respiratory muscle weakness Autonomic involvement less common	GM1, GM1b, GD1a, Ga1Nac-GD1a	No features of AIDP except one demyelinating feature allowed in one nerve if dCMAP < 10% LLN Sensory action amplitudes normal
Acute motor and sensory axonal neuropathy (AMSAN)	Acute weakness and sensory disturbance of all four limbs with hyporeflexia or areflexia, reaching peak within four weeks Can involve cranial nerves Can cause respiratory muscle weakness Autonomic involvement less common	GM1, GM1b, GD1a	No features of AIDP except one demyelinating feature allowed in one nerve if dCMAP < 10% LLN Sensory action amplitudes < LLN
Acute sensory neuropathy		GD1b	
Acute pandysautonomia/ regional variants	Fischer syndrome — Triad: Acute ophthalmoplegia, Ataxia, Areflexia May have facial and lower cranial nerve involvement Generally benign	GQ1b, GT1a	Sensory nerve demyelination with sensory nerve conduction slowing
	Oropharyngeal	GT1a	
Overlap – Fischer syndrome/Guillain–Barré syndrome overlap	Overlap forms of Fischer syndrome with limb weakness and respiratory involvement not uncommon	GQ1b, GM1, GM1b, GD1a, GalNac-GD1a	

Table 3.51 Investigations in Guillain–Barré syndrome

Aim	Investigations
To establish diagnosis	Electrodiagnostic studies – minimum study comprises three sensory nerves (conduction velocity and amplitude), three motor nerves (conduction velocity, amplitude and distal latency) with F waves and bilateral tibial H-reflexes Cerebrospinal fluid examination (raised protein)
To establish cause	Stool culture and serology for *Campylobacter jejuni* Stool culture for poliovirus in pure motor syndromes Acute and convalescent serology for cytomegalovirus, Epstein–Barr virus and *Mycoplasma pneumoniae* Antibodies to gangliosides GM1, GD1a and GQ1b
General monitoring	Urinalysis Haematobiochemistry Chest radiograph Spirometry
In certain circumstances	Antinuclear antibody Urine porphobilinogen and delta-aminolaevulinic acid Drug and toxin screen HIV test

because it is more convenient with fewer side effects, although potential side effects include anaphylactic reactions and venous thromboembolism. The earlier treatment is started, the better the outcome. Supportive and essential adjuncts to immunological therapies include thromboembolic prophylaxis, physiotherapy, speech and language therapy for swallow assessment and pain management.

CASE 3.48

MYASTHENIA GRAVIS

Instruction

Please examine this patient's eye movements/arms and discuss your findings.

Recognition

There is *weakness of the extraocular muscles* giving rise to a *complex ophthalmoplegia* and unilateral or bilateral *ptosis* (the pupil is never involved) and *weakness of proximal limb muscles* (weakness of elbow and finger flexion is not uncommon).

Weakness is induced or worsened by sustained activity – *fatiguability*. Ptosis and diplopia are worsened by two minutes of upward gaze (Fig. 3.92).

Bulbar muscle weakness may occur, with *dysarthria* (*nasal speech*) and *dysphagia*. Facial involvement may cause difficulty with eye closure and a snarling smile, and weakness of jaw closure may cause chewing difficulty. Trunk involvement may occur. Neck muscle weakness may cause head drooping.

Box 3.64 Features that differentiate myasthenia from alternative diagnoses

- Fatiguable weakness is absolutely characteristic of myasthenia
- Non-limb features of generalised myasthenia (ocular and bulbar dysfunction) are not features of most myopathies
- Muscle wasting may be a feature of neuropathies and myopathies but not myasthenia
- Tendon reflexes are normal or slightly brisk in myasthenia but reduced in peripheral neuropathies
- Chronic progressive external ophthalmoplegia (a mitochondrial disorder) can mimic the ocular symptoms of myasthenia but fatigue is not typical

Interpretation

Confirm the diagnosis

Features that can help differentiate myasthenia from alternative diagnoses are shown in Box 3.64.

What to do next – assess other systems

Look for overt signs of other autoimmune diseases, e.g. Graves' disease (3%).

Consider severity/decompensation/complications

Tell the examiners that:

- Respiratory muscle involvement can be life threatening; dyspnoea, particularly lying supine, is common because of diaphragmatic weakness. Forced vital capacity is monitored.
- Aspiration pneumonia is a potential complication with bulbar myasthenia

Consider function

Tell the examiners that limb weakness, diplopia and bulbar palsy can have devastating effects on physical and psychological health.

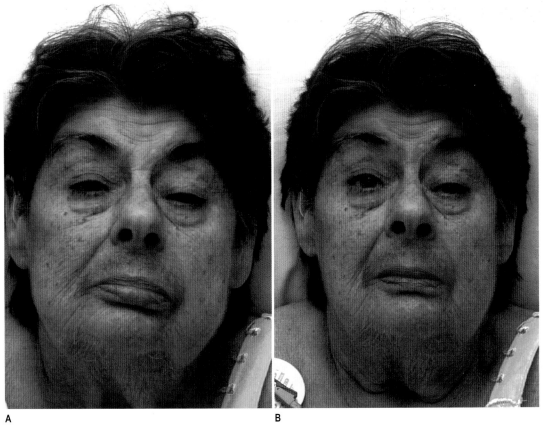

A   B

Fig. 3.92 Myasthenia gravis: (A) ptosis and facial weakness, (B) some improvement after Tensilon.

Discussion

What causes myasthenia gravis?

It is an autoimmune disease of the neuromuscular junction in which autoantibodies directed against the postsynaptic acetylcholine receptor (AChR) of the neuromuscular junction cause functional blockade and destruction of receptors. About 85% of patients with generalised myasthenia are seropositive and 55% with isolated ocular myasthenia are seropositive. About 40% of patients with seronegative generalised myasthenia have autoantibodies to the postsynaptic protein muscle-specific kinase (MuSK). Antibody titre does not correlate with disease activity or progression. The thymus is important in pathogenesis, the normal thymus a source of AChR; expression may be upregulated in patients with thymoma. The thymus may also have a role in deleting autoreactive T cells specific for self-antigens, and thus any disturbance of function allowing escape of such cells. The hyperplastic thymus may also be a site of anti-AChR production.

> **Box 3.65 Subtypes of myasthenia gravis**
>
> - Early-onset (age < 40 years) myasthenia with thymic hyperplasia, *HLA B8DR3* association and a 4 : 1 female : male ratio
> - Late-onset myasthenia with thymic atrophy, *HLA B7, DR2* association and a 1 : 2 female : male ratio (most common subtype)
> - Thymoma without HLA association and a 1 : 1 female : male ratio
> - Ocular myasthenia (20% of patients have pure ocular myasthenia)
> - A MuSK antibody-positive group that overlaps with late-onset seronegative patients

Who tends to be affected?

It affects all races and ages and has a prevalence of around 1/7000 and an incidence of 1/100 000. There are five subtypes with useful treatment implications (Box 3.65).

How useful are AChR antibodies diagnostically?

AChR antibodies are detectable in most patients; a negative test does not exclude but a positive test is highly specific.

What is the role of anticholinesterase testing?

A positive response to anticholinesterases (e.g. oral pyridostigmine) is common, and pyridostigmine is also the first-line treatment. The *Tensilon* test with intravenous edrophonium (Tensilon) assesses immediate and short-acting effects of anticholinesterase, but there is a risk of bradycardia and other cholinergic side effects. With antibody testing and electromyography, Tensilon testing is now less common.

Does electromyography (EMG) help diagnostically?

It shows decreasing muscle action potentials with repetitive stimulation. Increased jitter and blocking are found on single-fibre EMG and the diagnosis is questioned when single-fibre studies in weak muscle are normal. Abnormal single-fibre EMG can be found in motor neurone disease and some myopathies.

Should all patients have mediastinal imaging?

This is good practice, to characterise thymic pathology.

How is myasthenia gravis treated?

Treatments are outlined in Box 3.66.

What is the prognosis in myasthenia gravis?

Treatment is usually needed life-long and mortality is slightly increased.

List some causes of a myasthenic crisis

- Tiredness
- Infection
- Drugs (many)

What is Lambert–Eaton myasthenic syndrome (LEMS)?

LEMS is much less common than myasthenia, and more common after the fifth decade. Sixty per cent of cases are associated with small cell lung cancer, as a paraneoplastic syndrome. LEMS also has an autoimmune basis with antibodies to P/Q-type voltage-gated calcium channels in most patients. Autoantibodies to these channels on malignant cells are thought to cross-react with those at the pre-synaptic membrane of the neuromuscular junction. LEMS may precede cancer by up to five years, and even be associated with tumour suppression. It causes fatiguability but does not affect ocular or bulbar muscles, nor cause ptosis. Reflexes are absent but return with exercise, unlike myasthenia gravis, and the EMG shows improved amplitude with repetitive stimulation. LEMS can be treated with 3,4-diaminopyridine in specialist centres. Anticholinesterases tend to be less effective.

Box 3.66 Treatments for myasthenia gravis

Anticholinesterase

First-line treatment is usually pyridostigmine, a long-acting cholinesterase inhibitor, slowly titrated up to 60 mg three to four times daily. Cholinergic side effects include abdominal cramps and diarrhoea and can be controlled with anticholinergic drugs such as propantheline bromide 15 mg thrice daily. High doses of anticholinesterase can precipitate a cholinergic crisis causing worsening weakness or pulmonary oedema. A need for more than 90 mg four times daily indicates a need for immunosuppression.

Immunosuppression

Prednisolone alone, or with azathioprine as a steroid-sparing agent, is first-line immunosuppression. Treatment should be started in hospital in all but the mildest cases because steroids can initially exacerbate symptoms and impair ventilatory capacity. Slowly introducing prednisolone reduces the risk with a target of 1.5 mg/kg. Azathioprine should be prescribed only after exclusion of low thiopurine methyltransferase activity, which would cause slow metabolism of azathioprine and is a contraindication. There is no evidence for teratogenicity of prednisolone or azathioprine. Other immunosuppressants are seldom used.

Remission

Anticholinesterase should be withdrawn, and, if still free of symptoms, prednisolone is withdrawn slowly to the lowest dose that maintains remission.

Ocular myasthenia

This is relatively benign, with seldom a need for more than anticholinesterases and low-dose steroid.

Surgery

The benefits of thymectomy are not conclusively established, but it is generally recommended in patients with onset before 40 years of age, and generally soon after diagnosis.

Non-response

Misdiagnosis or rare, congenital myasthenic syndromes are reasons for a failed response to immunotherapies.

CASE 3.49

MYOPATHY AND MYOSITIS

Instruction

Please examine this patient's arms and legs and discuss your findings.

Recognition

There is *symmetrical weakness* (and possibly wasting) in the *proximal muscles*. There is *inability to rise from a squatting position or to raise the arms above the head*. There are no other neurological signs (Fig. 3.93).

Interpretation

Confirm the diagnosis

Features than can help differentiate myopathy from myasthenia or neuropathy are shown in Box 3.67. Tell the

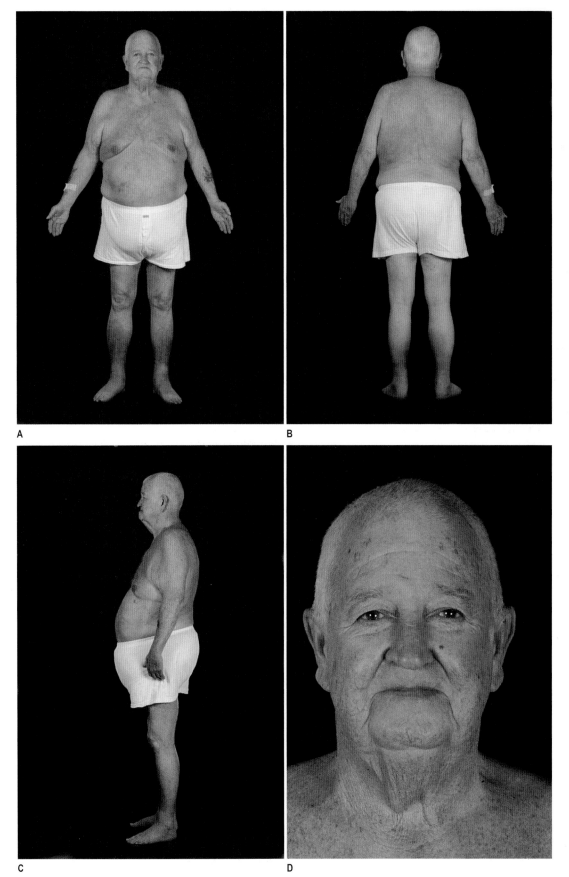

A

B

C

D

Fig. 3.93 (A–D) Cushing's syndrome.

examiners that the diagnosis of the type of myopathy may be based on history and clinical features, and biopsy.

What to do next – consider causes

The more common of many potential causes with potential diagnostic clues are listed in Table 3.52 (Fig. 3.94).

Consider severity/decompensation/complications

This depends on the underlying cause (Table 3.52).

Consider function

Tell the examiners that life would be very restricted, obvious problems being lifting objects overhead, combing and washing hair, climbing stairs and rising from a chair.

Box 3.67 Features than differentiate myopathy from myasthenia or neuropathy

- Proximal muscle weakness is usually due to myopathy
- Distal muscle weakness is sometimes due to myopathy but much more commonly due to peripheral neuropathy
- Myasthenia gravis is unusual without ophthalmoplegia or ptosis or bulbar symptoms, and characteristically fatiguable

---

Discussion

What is myositis and what types of myositis are there?

Myositis is inflammation of skeletal muscle and has many causes (Box 3.68).

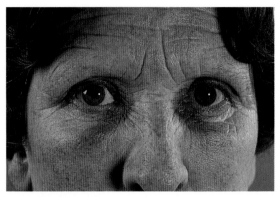

Fig. 3.94 Dermatomyositis.

Table 3.52 Causes of myopathy and potential clues

	Causes		Diagnostic clues
Acquired myopathies	Inflammatory myopathies (myositis)	Polymyositis	May be painful and tender
		Dermatomyositis	Rash
		Inclusion body myositis	Marked distal atrophy
		Other, e.g. drugs	History
	Metabolic/endocrine myopathies	Cushing's syndrome	Cushingoid morphology
		Thyrotoxicosis or hypothyroidism	Hypothyroid face
		Acromegaly	Acromegalic morphology
		Hypoadrenalism	Hyperpigmentation if Addison's disease
		Osteomalacia	Common in older people
		Carcinoma/paraneoplastic neuromyopathy	Weight loss
		Alcohol	History
		Hypophosphataemia	Phosphate level
Genetic myopathies	Muscular dystrophies	Muscular dystrophies with predominant axial or limb girdle weakness	See text
		Non-limb girdle muscular dystrophies with cranial muscles involvement	
		Distal myopathies	
	Congenital myopathies	Many, e.g. centronuclear myopathy	Distal weakness
		Tend to be non-progressive	Long, thin face
			High-arched palate
	Muscle ion channel disorders	Myotonic dystrophy (DM1)	Myotonia (impaired muscle relaxation)
			Distal weakness
		Proximal myotonic myopathy (PROMM or DM2)	Proximal weakness
		Non-dystrophic myotonias and periodic paralyses	Myotonia and/or periodic paralysis
	Genetically determined metabolic myopathies	McArdle's disease and storage diseases	Myalgia on exercise
		Mitochondrial disorders	Isolated or with central nervous system symptoms
		Rarities, e.g. malignant hyperthermia	

Box 3.68 Causes of myositis

Idiopathic myositis

- Primary idiopathic polymyositis
- Primary idiopathic dermatomyositis
- Polymyositis/dermatomyositis associated with neoplasia
- Polymyositis/dermatomyositis associated with autoimmune disease
- Inclusion body myositis

Infection

- Viral, e.g. influenza virus, hepatitis B virus, coxsackievirus, echovirus, human immunodeficiency virus
- Bacterial, e.g. staphylococcus, streptococcus, clostridium, mycobacterium
- Parasitic, e.g. toxoplasmosis

Drugs

- Cholesterol-lowering agents, e.g. statins, fibrates
- Antibiotics, e.g. rifampicin, sulphonamides, zidovudine
- Other, e.g. angiotensin-converting enzyme inhibitors, colchicines, penicillamine

---

What are the similarities and differences between the common types of myositis?

These are outlined in Table 3.53.

How would you screen for malignancy in polymyositis/dermatomyositis?

There is no absolute consensus as to what is appropriate. Chest X-ray, abdominal and pelvic ultrasound, breast examination and mammography, and measurements of ovarian tumour markers or prostate-specific antigen are performed by many physicians, with possibly a computed tomograph of the chest in smokers. A barium swallow and endoscopy are needed for dysphagia.

Does magnetic resonance imaging have a place in investigating myositis?

It can help to localise inflammation and target biopsy.

Does biopsy usually further the diagnosis in myositis?

Biopsy is very helpful but should be from a likely site, such as deltoid or quadriceps, and very weak muscle should be avoided because burnt out fibrosis may be all that is seen. Prior arrangement with a pathologist is essential because specimens should be handled immediately, as fresh specimens for biochemistry and frozen specimens for light and electron microscopy.

Does electromyography (EMG) further the diagnosis in myositis?

Spontaneous muscle fibrillation, complex repetitive discharges, positive sharp waves at rest and short duration, decreased amplitude discharges on contraction are all common, non-specific features.

What do you know about the muscular dystrophies?

This is a group of disorders characterised by fibre necrosis and replacement of muscle by fat and fibrous tissue.

Muscular dystrophies with predominant axial or limb girdle weakness

◾ **Duchenne muscular dystrophy**   This is X-linked; the gene responsible is on the short arm of the X chromosome. A translocation at the locus Xp21 prevents production of a protein called dystrophin. Patients develop severe proximal myopathy and pseudohypertrophy of the calf muscles in early childhood with difficulty in rising to standing position – the hands 'walk up' the front of the legs to assist standing (Gower's sign). In childhood the gait is waddling but patients are invariably wheelchair-bound before their teens. Death is common in the second or third decades from respiratory infection. Tall R waves may be present on the ECG and cardiac failure is not unusual. Becker's muscular dystrophy is a milder form, with dystrophin produced in smaller quantities than normal. In neither is facial weakness predominant.

◾ **Limb girdle muscular dystrophies (LGMDs)**   These are the commonest muscular dystrophies in adults, presenting in the second or third decade, and are a heterogeneous group involving the upper and lower limbs, generally starting proximally. Neck muscles may become weak but facial and bulbar muscles are not affected. The group is inherited in an autosomal recessive fashion. Life expectancy is normal.

Non-limb girdle muscular dystrophies with cranial muscle involvement

◾ **Fascioscapulohumeral muscular dystrophy**   This affects the face and shoulder girdle. There is marked facial weakness with impaired expression and difficulty smiling, whistling and closing the eyes. The lips at rest are slack, the mouth open. There is dysarthria because of weakness of the buccal muscles. The neck muscles are weak, as are the shoulder girdle muscles with winging of the scapula. Onset is often in early adult life with a normal life expectancy. It is autosomal dominant.

◾ **Oculopharyngeal muscular dystrophy**   This presents with ptosis and weakness of extraocular muscles and bulbar muscles.

Why do glycogen storage diseases cause myalgia?

In McArdle's disease, the commonest storage disorder, deficient myophosphorylase results in a failure to break down glycogen to glucose. Severe myalgia develops soon after the start of exercise with cramp (electrically silent muscle contracture) until alternative energy sources are mobilised.

What are mitochondrial cytopathies?

These can affect muscle specifically or may act as part of a multisystem disorder, typically involving the central nervous system. Large deletions or point mutations in mitochondrial DNA cause Kearns–Sayre syndrome, a chronic, progressive external ophthalmoplegia, MELAS

Table 3.53 Common types of myositis

		Polymyositis	Dermatomyositis	Inclusion body myositis
Age of onset		Older age group > 50 years	Younger adults Children	The most common inflammatory myopathy > 50 years
Cause		Unknown		Unknown
Pathology		Autoimmune to muscle antigen Th1 proinflammatory disease IFN-γ, IL-2 and TNF-α provoke interstitial, intracellular muscle damage	Immune mediated by complement Perivascular damage	Minimal inflammation Inclusion bodies within vacuoles or within cells – though vacuoles may be empty, commonly staining for β-amyloid
Muscle symptoms	Onset	Insidious and subacute over weeks to months		Slowly progressive Often present for years before diagnosis
	Weakness (the most common symptom)	Symmetrical Proximal (distal rare)		Asymmetry common Proximal and distal Finger flexion weakness and foot drop are common
	Atrophy	Uncommon		Marked, especially distally, similar to amyotrophic lateral sclerosis
	Myalgia	Painful in about 50%		Painless
	Facial/bulbar involvement	Rare e.g. dysphagia, hoarseness, dysphonia		Does not occur
	Ocular involvement	Never		
Extramuscular involvement	Skin	No	With or without myositis Heliotrope rash – violaceous eyelids, malar area, 'V' area of anterior chest and upper back Gottron's papules – purple-red, scaly plaques on knuckles and fingers often extending to forearms	No
	Calcinosis	Occasional, intracutaneous, subcutaneous, fascial and intramuscular		No
	Joints	Common Symmetrical large joints		No
	Gastrointestinal	Dysphagia		No
	Lung	Diffuse parenchymal lung disease Aspiration		No
	Cardiovascular	Raynaud's phenomenon Myocarditis Pericarditis		No
	Renal	Proteinuria Nephrotic syndrome Mesangial proliferative glomerulonephritis		No
	Constitutional symptoms	Fatigue Fever Anorexia Weight loss		Less likely
Complications	Malignancy	Risk increased, especially dermatomyositis/men over 45 years Estimated 5% prevalence		No increased risk
Investigations	Creatine kinase	5–50× normal Other muscle enzyme, e.g. transaminases, LDH may be raised		Normal since limited inflammation
	ESR/C-reactive protein	Usually moderately elevated		
	ANA	> 80% positive ENAs include Ro (SS-A), U1 (ribonucleoprotein, centromere, mitochondria) and tRNA synthase. Other myositis-specific autoantibodies include anti-signal recognition particle (anti-SRP), anti-M2 and anti-PM-Scl (a subset with systemic sclerosis)		Positive in small minority

Table 3.53 Common types of myositis—cont'd

	Polymyositis	Dermatomyositis	Inclusion body myositis
Treatment	Good response to steroids (high dose initially, e.g. 60 mg prednisolone) Steroid-sparing agents, e.g. azathioprine, methotrexate, ciclosporin	Intravenous immunoglobulin effective in steroid-resistant dermatomyositis	No effective treatment
	At this stage a specialist (rheumatologist, neurologist or immunologist) should be involved		
Monitoring	Muscle power Creatine kinase For treatment complications, e.g. DEXA scan		
Prognosis	80% 5-year survival About one-third die of disease, one-third remain weak and one-third return to normal		Inevitable progression

ANA, antinuclear antibodies; ENA, extractable nuclear antigen; ESR, erythrocyte sedimentation rate; IFN-γ, interferon-γ; IL-2, interleukin-2; LDH, lactate dehydrogenase; TNF-α, tumour necrosis factor-α.

(mitochondrial encephalopathy, lactic acidosis and strokes) and MERRF (myoclonus, epilepsy and ragged red fibres).

How is polymyalgia usually distinguished from myositis or other myopathies?

Polymyalgia typically causes stiffness and weakness, and is less tender than myositis. Muscle enzymes are normal, but the erythrocyte sedimentation rate is generally higher than that of myositis.

CASE 3.50

MYOTONIC DYSTROPHY

Instruction

Please examine this patient's muscle strength and proceed as you think best.

Recognition

The *face is myopathic* (it looks sad, sleepy and lifeless) with *bilateral ptosis*. There is *wasting of temporalis muscles* causing hollowing of the temples, and there may be wasting of other facial muscles, neck muscles and muscles of the shoulder girdle. There is *distal weakness* and *wasting*. There is *frontalis muscle wasting* and the *forehead is smooth*, with *frontal balding* (Fig. 3.95).

When you shake hands you may notice *slow release of grip*. The same occurs if the patient is asked to make a fist, and is worse if the patient is cold or excited. *Percussion myotonia* is present on the thenar eminences – when you percuss, a dimple appears which is slow to resolve. There is also slow eyelid opening after firm closure. Tendon reflexes may be attenuated.

Speech is *dysarthric* and *nasal*.
Myotonic dystrophy is also illustrated in Figs 3.96–3.98.

Interpretation

Confirm the diagnosis

Unlike muscular dystrophies, myotonic dystrophy is a multisystem disorder with an assortment of presentations. Classic myotonic dystrophy patients have myotonia, weakness and a range of other features by early to mid-adult life; mild myotonic dystrophy can present in later adult life with subtle myotonia and weakness, or other features such as cataracts or diabetes.

What to do next – assess other systems

Look for cataracts or evidence of cataract surgery, and blepharitis, and then tell the examiners that you would:

- Check for gynaecomastia and testicular atrophy
- Also expect percussion myotonia of the tongue
- Ask about gastrointestinal symptoms, which include dysphagia, delayed gastric emptying, bowel dysmotility and small bowel bacterial overgrowth

Consider severity/decompensation/complications

Tell the examiners that:

- Disease progresses very slowly; grip myotonia is often the first symptom, muscle weakness and wasting then starting distally and at the sternocleidomastoids with proximal involvement a late sign.
- Diabetes mellitus is increased four-fold.
- Cardiac conduction abnormalities are common; cardiomyopathy can occur but is less common.
- Respiratory complications account for 30–40% of deaths.
- Patients are at increased risk from general anaesthesia.

Case 3.50   Myotonic dystrophy

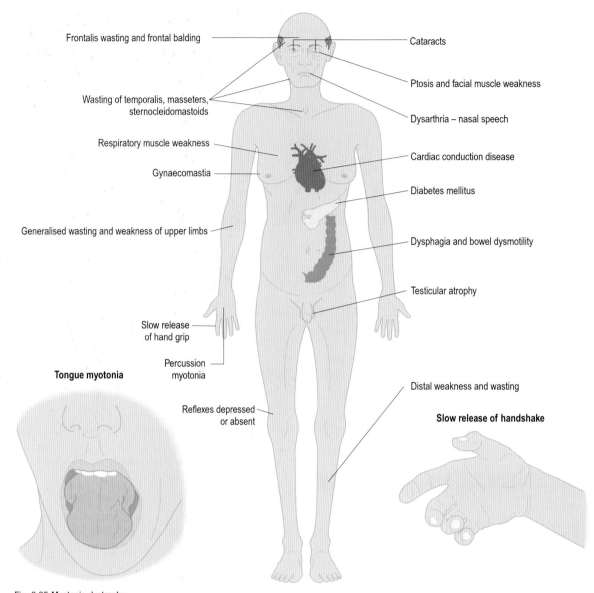

Frontalis wasting and frontal balding

Cataracts

Wasting of temporalis, masseters, sternocleidomastoids

Ptosis and facial muscle weakness

Dysarthria – nasal speech

Respiratory muscle weakness

Cardiac conduction disease

Gynaecomastia

Diabetes mellitus

Generalised wasting and weakness of upper limbs

Dysphagia and bowel dysmotility

Testicular atrophy

Slow release of hand grip

Tongue myotonia

Percussion myotonia

Distal weakness and wasting

Slow release of handshake

Reflexes depressed or absent

Fig. 3.95 Myotonic dystrophy.

Consider function

The non-neuromuscular symptoms described above can be disabling. Hypersomnolence is also common, and does not correlate with the severity of muscle involvement.

Discussion

What do you understand by the term myotonia?

Myotonia implies continued contraction of muscles after voluntary contraction with slow, delayed relaxation.

What is the genetic basis of myotonic dystrophy?

Myotonic dystrophy type 1 (other types are rare) is a progressive, inherited muscular dystrophy with a prevalence of about 1 in 8000. It is an autosomal dominant condition on chromosome 19, with an equal male : female ratio; it is also one of numerous neurogenetic disorders caused by expansion in the size of a three base-pair (triplet or trinucleotide) repeat sequence. In myotonic dystrophy the triplet repeat is CTG, occurring up to 35 times in unaffected individuals but more than 50 times in myotonic dystrophy; generally, 50–100 repeats is mild, 200–500 repeats results in classic myotonic dystrophy and those

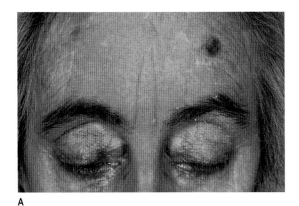

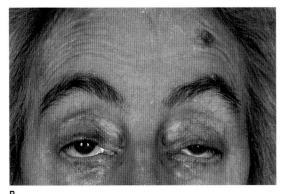

Fig. 3.96 Myotonic dystrophy: (A) eyes closed, (B) eyes open with bilateral ptosis.

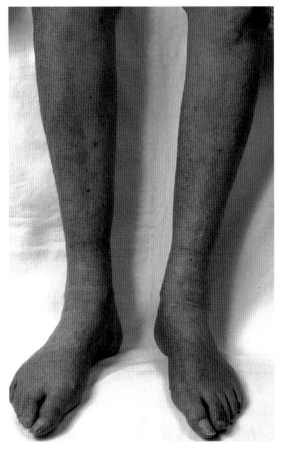

Fig. 3.97 Myotonic dystrophy – distal wasting of lower limbs.

with more than 1000 repeats have congenital or childhood onset disease. Triplet expansion increases with successive generations, a phenomenon known as genetic anticipation.

How does the triplet repeat cause disease?

The CTG repeat mutation on the *DMPK* gene is outwith the sequence of mRNA that is translated into protein, but many effects are the result of the abnormal, expanded mRNA binding to nuclear proteins that in turn affect processing of other genes. Changes affecting insulin receptor mRNA and muscle chloride mRNA cause insulin resistance and myotonia, respectively. Reduced DMPK protein due to the mutation affects ion channels, altering skeletal and cardiac muscle excitability. The mutation affects the amount of protein made by adjacent genes, and reduced levels in of one of these, *SIX5*, is implicated in cataract development.

Are mildly affected adults easy to miss?

Mild weakness of grip or myotonia in late adulthood is often overlooked by the patient.

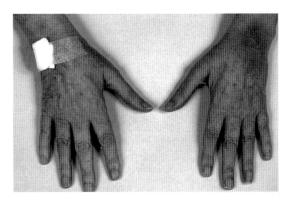

Fig. 3.98 Myotonic dystrophy – diffuse wasting of hand muscles.

Do mildly affected adults have an increased cardiac risk?

Cardiac complications still occur and surveillance is required.

What is myotonia congenita?

This refers to delayed relaxation after muscle contraction, without other features of myotonic dystrophy.

References and further reading

Cardiovascular system

Mitral stenosis

American College of Cardiology/American Heart Association Task Force on Practice Guidelines, Society of Cardiovascular Anesthesiologists, Society for Cardiovascular Angiography and Interventions, Society of Thoracic Surgeons, et al. ACC/AHA 2006 guidelines for the management of patients with valvular heart disease: a report of the American College of Cardiology/American Heart Association Task Force on Practice Guidelines (writing committee to revise the 1998 Guidelines for the Management of Patients With Valvular Heart Disease): developed in collaboration with the Society of Cardiovascular Anesthesiologists: endorsed by the Society for Cardiovascular Angiography and Interventions and the Society of Thoracic Surgeons. Circulation 2006; 114:e84–e231

Iunge B, Gohlke-Barwolf C, Tornos P et al. Recommendations on the management of the asymptomatic patient with valvular heart disease. Eur Heart J 2002; 23:1253–1266

Special Writing Group of the Committee on rheumatic fever, endocarditis and Kawasaki disease of the Council on Cardiovascular Disease in the Young of the American Heart Association. Guidelines for the diagnosis of rheumatic fever. Jones criteria, 1992 update. JAMA 1992; 268:2069

Mitral regurgitation

American College of Cardiology/American Heart Association Task Force on Practice Guidelines, Society of Cardiovascular Anesthesiologists, Society for Cardiovascular Angiography and Interventions, Society of Thoracic Surgeons, et al. ACC/AHA 2006 guidelines for the management of patients with valvular heart disease: a report of the American College of Cardiology/American Heart Association Task Force on Practice Guidelines (writing committee to revise the 1998 Guidelines for the Management of Patients With Valvular Heart Disease): developed in collaboration with the Society of Cardiovascular Anesthesiologists: endorsed by the Society for Cardiovascular Angiography and Interventions and the Society of Thoracic Surgeons. Circulation 2006; 114:e84–e231

Enrique-Sarano M, Avierinos JF, Messika-Zeitoun D et al. Quantitative determinants of the outcome of asymptomatic mitral regurgitation. N Engl J Med 2005; 352:875–883

Iunge B, Gohlke-Barwolf C, Tornos P et al. Recommendations on the management of the asymptomatic patient with valvular heart disease. Eur Heart J 2002; 23:1253–1266

Otto CM. Timing of surgery in mitral regurgitation. Heart 2003; 89:100–105

Aortic stenosis

American College of Cardiology/American Heart Association Task Force on Practice Guidelines, Society of Cardiovascular Anesthesiologists, Society for Cardiovascular Angiography and Interventions, Society of Thoracic Surgeons, et al. ACC/AHA 2006 guidelines for the management of patients with valvular heart disease: a report of the American College of Cardiology/American Heart Association Task Force on Practice Guidelines (writing committee to revise the 1998 Guidelines for the Management of Patients With Valvular Heart Disease): developed in collaboration with the Society of Cardiovascular Anesthesiologists: endorsed by the Society for Cardiovascular Angiography and Interventions and the Society of Thoracic Surgeons. Circulation 2006; 114:e84–e231

Cowell SJ, Newby DE, Boon NA et al. Calcific aortic stenosis: same old story? Age and Ageing 2004; 33:538–544

Cowell SJ, Newby DE, Prescott RJ et al. A randomised trial of intensive lipid-lowering therapy in calcific aortic stenosis. N Eng J Med 2005; 352:2389–2397

Iunge B, Gohlke-Barwolf C, Tornos P et al. Recommendations on the management of the asymptomatic patient with valvular heart disease. Eur Heart J 2002; 23:1253–1266

Ramaraj R, Sorrell VL. Degenerative aortic stenosis. BMJ 2008; 336:550–555

Aortic regurgitation

American College of Cardiology/American Heart Association Task Force on Practice Guidelines, Society of Cardiovascular Anesthesiologists, Society for Cardiovascular Angiography and Interventions, Society of Thoracic Surgeons, et al. ACC/AHA 2006 guidelines for the management of patients with valvular heart disease: a report of the American College of Cardiology/American Heart Association Task Force on Practice Guidelines (writing committee to revise the 1998 Guidelines for the Management of Patients With Valvular Heart Disease): developed in collaboration with the Society of Cardiovascular Anesthesiologists: endorsed by the Society for Cardiovascular Angiography and Interventions and the Society of Thoracic Surgeons. Circulation 2006; 114:e84–e231

Evangelista A, Tornos P, Sambola A et al. Long-term vasodilator therapy in patients with severe aortic regurgitation. N Engl J Med 2005; 353:1342–1349

Iunge B, Gohlke-Barwolf C, Tornos P et al. Recommendations on the management of the asymptomatic patient with valvular heart disease. Eur Heart J 2002; 23:1253–1266

Mitral valve prolapse

Hayek E, Grigg CN, Griffin BP. Mitral valve prolapse. Lancet 2005; 305:507–518

Permanent pacemaker

Bleasdale RA, Frenneaux MP. Cardiac resynchronisation therapy: when the drugs don't work. Heart 2004; 90(Suppl. 6):2–4

Grubb N. Device therapy. J R Coll Physicians Edinb 2006; 36:136–140

Harris S. Implantable cardioverter defibrillators. Clin Med 2007; 7:397

Hohnloser SH, Kucj KH, Dorian P. Prophylactic use of an implantable cardioverter-defibrillator after acute myocardial infarction. N Engl J Med 2004; 351:2481–2488

Josephson M, Wellens HJ. Implantable defibrillators and sudden cardiac death. Circulation 2004; 109:2685–2691

Linde C. Implantable cardioverter-defibrillator treatment and resynchronisation in heart failure. Heart 2004; 90:231–234

National Institute for Health and Clinical Excellence (NICE). Implantable cardioverter defibrillators for arrhythmias. London: National Institute for Health and Clinical Excellence NICE; 2006

National Institute for Health and Clinical Excellence (NICE). Clinical Guideline. Heart failure: Cardiac resynchronisation. London: NICE, 2007. Available: www.nice.org.uk

Priori SG, Aliot E, Blomstrom-Lundqvist C et al. Task force on sudden cardiac death of the European Society of Cardiology. Eur Heart J 2001; 22:1374–1350

Infective endocarditis

Durack DT, Lukes AS, Bright DK. New criteria for diagnosis of infective endocarditis: utilization of specific echocardiographic findings. Duke Endocarditis Service. Am J Med 1994; 96:200–209

Mylonakis E, Calderwood SB. Infective endocarditis in adults. N Engl J Med 2001; 345:1318–1330

National Institute for Health and Clinical Excellence. Prophylaxis against Infective Endocarditis. London: NICE, 2008

Rhys P Beynon, Bahl VK, Prendergast BD. Infective endocarditis. BMJ 2006; 333:334–339

Hypertrophic cardiomyopathy

Elliot P. Investigation and treatment of hypertrophic cardiomyopathy. Clin Med 2007; 7:383–387

Elliot P, McKenna WJ. Hypertrophic cardiomyopathy. Lancet 2004; 363:1881–1891

Maron BJ, McKenna WJ, Danielson GK et al. American College of Cardiology/European society of Cardiology clinical expert consensus document on hypertrophic cardiomyopathy. A report of the American College of Cardiology Foundation Task Force on Clinical Expert Consensus Documents and the European Society of Cardiology Committee for Practice Guidelines. J Am Coll Cardiol 2003; 42:1687–1713

Spirito P, Autore C. Management of hypertrophic cardiomyopathy. BMJ 2006; 332:1251–1255

Nervous system

Examination

Fletcher N. Other movement disorders. Medicine 2004; 32:97–99

Folstein MF, Folstein SE, McHugh PR. 'Mini-mental state' practical method for grading the cognitive state of patients for the clinician. J Psychiatr Res 1975; 12:189–198

Patten JP. Neurological differential diagnosis, 2nd edn. Berlin: Springer; 1996

Weatherall MW. The mysterious Weber's test. BMJ 2002; 325:26 [responses: Mbubaegbu CE. Physics renders Weber's test not so mysterious. BMJ 2002; 325:1117; Kroukamp G. And a collaborative group of otorhinolaryngologists reports its findings. BMJ 2002; 325:1117]

Cerebellopontine angle syndrome

Bennetto L, Patel NK, Fuller G. Trigeminal neuralgia and its management. BMJ 2007; 334:201–205

Facial nerve palsy

Holland NJ, Weiner GM. Recent developments in Bell's palsy. BMJ 2004; 329:553–557

Wareham DW, Breaer J. Herpes zoster. BMJ 2007; 334:1211–1215

Anterior circulation stroke syndromes

Albers GW, Olivet J. Alteplase in ischaemic stroke. Lancet 2007; 369:249–250

Bamford J, Sandercock P, Dennis M et al. Classification and natural history of clinically identifiable subtypes of cerebral infarction. Lancet 1991; 337:1521–1526

Batty GD, Lee I-Min. Physical activity for preventing strokes. BMJ 2002; 325:350–351

Bruins SK, Berge E, Dorman M et al., on behalf of the Oxfordshire Community Stroke Project, the International Stroke Trial (UK), and the Lothian Stroke Register Collaborative Groups. Impact of functional status at six months on long-term survival in patients with ischaemic stroke: prospective cohort studies. BMJ 2008 [editorial: Rodgers H, Thomson R. BMJ 2008; 336:337–338]

Candilese L, Gattinoni M, Bersano A. Stroke-unit care for acute stroke patients: an observational follow-up study. Lancet 2007; 369:299–305

Clinical Effectiveness and Evaluation Unit, Royal College of Physicians, London. National Sentinel Stroke Audit 2006. Available: www.rcplondon.ac.uk/pubs/books/stroke-audit/

Department of Health / Vascular Programme / Stroke. National Stroke Strategy. London: Department of Health, 2007

Diener HC, Bogousslavsky J, Brass LM. Aspirin and clopidogrel compared with clopidogrel alone after recent ischaemic stroke or transient ischaemic attack in high-risk patients (MATCH): randomised, double blind, placebo-controlled trial. Lancet 2004; 364:331–337

Donnan GA, Dewey HM, Davis SM. MRI and stroke: why has it taken so long? Lancet 2007; 369:252–254

Halkes PH, van Gijn J, Kappelle LJ, Koudstaal PJ, Algra A; ESPRIT Study Group. Aspirin plus dipyridamole versus aspirin alone after cerebral ischaemia of arterial origin (ESPRIT): randomised controlled trial. Lancet 2006; 367:1665–1673

Jarret D. Acute ischaemic stroke. J R Coll Physicians Edinb 2007; 37:36–39

Khaja AM, Grotta JC. Established treatments for acute ischaemic stroke. Lancet 2007; 369:319–330

Mayer SA, Brun NC, Begtrup K et al. Recombinant activated factor VII for acute intracerebral hemorrhage. N Engl J Med 2005; 352:777–785

Mendelow AD, Gregson BA, Fernandes HM et al. Early surgery versus initial conservative treatment in patients with spontaneous supratentorial intracerebral haematomas in the international surgical trial in intracerebral haemorrhage (STICH): a randomised trial. Lancet 2005; 365:387–397

PROGRESS Collaborative Group: randomised trial of a perindopril based blood pressure lowering regimen among 6105 individuals with previous stroke or transient ischaemic attack. Lancet 2001; 358:1033–1041

Ramachandran VS. Phantoms in the brain. Reith lectures 2003: the emerging mind. London: Profile Books; 2003

Rothwell PM. Atherothrombosis and ischaemic stroke: unstable plaque is the main mechanism of stroke in patients with carotid stenosis. BMJ 2007; 334:379–380

Royal College of Physicians Intercollegiate Stroke Working Party. National Clinical Guideline on the Management of People with Stroke (incorporating the NICE Acute Stroke and TIA guidelines). In press 2008

The Lancet. Editorial. Stroke – prevention is better than cure. Lancet 2007; 369:247

Agnosias and apraxias

Ramachandran VS. Phantoms in the brain. Reith lectures 2003: the emerging mind. London: Profile Books; 2003

Ramachandran VS. Synapses and the self. Reith lectures 2003: the emerging mind. London: Profile Books; 2003

Ramachandran VS. Purple numbers and sharp cheese. Reith lectures 2003: the emerging mind. London: Profile Books; 2003

Posterior circulation stroke syndromes

Savitz SI, Caplan LR. Vertebrobasilar disease. N Engl J Med 2005; 352:2618–2626

Parkinson's disease

National Collaborating Centre for Chronic Conditions (NCC-CC, of the Royal College of Physicians). Parkinson's Disease. National guideline for diagnosis and management in primary and secondary care (funded by NICE). Royal College of Physicians. London 2006

Motor neurone disease

McDermott CJ, Shaw PJ. Diagnosis and management of motor neurone disease. BMJ 2008; 336:658-662

Carpal tunnel syndrome

Fuller G. Diagnosing and managing mononeuropathies. Clin Med 2004; 4:113–117

Ulnar nerve lesion

Fuller G. Diagnosing and managing mononeuropathies. Clin Med 2004; 4:113–117

Radial nerve lesion

Fuller G. Diagnosing and managing mononeuropathies. Clin Med 2004; 4:113–117

Spastic paraparesis

Fuller G. Diagnosing and managing mononeuropathies. Clin Med 2004; 4:113–117

Peripheral neuropathy

England JD, Asbury AK. Peripheral neuropathy. Lancet 2004; 363:2151–2161

Fuller G. Diagnosing and managing mononeuropathies. Clin Med 2004; 4:113–117

Guillain–Barré syndrome

Hughes RAC, Cornblath DR. Guillain–Barré syndrome. Lancet 2005; 366:1653–1666

Myasthenia gravis

Hilton-Jones D, Palace J. Disorders of the neuromuscular junction. In: Warrell DA, Cox TM, Firth JD et al., eds. Oxford textbook of medicine, 4th edn. Oxford: Oxford University Press; 2003.

Myopathy and myositis

Choy EH, Isenberg DA. Treatment of dermatomyositis and polymyositis. Rheumatology 2002; 41:7–13

Myotonic dystrophy

Longman C. Myotonic dystrophy. J R Coll Physicians Edinb 2006; 36:51–55

Cardiovascular and nervous system

Station 4

Communication skills and ethics

INTRODUCTION TO COMMUNICATION SKILLS AND ETHICS

Communication skills 486

Ethics 487

Cases

DISCUSSING CLINICAL MANAGEMENT

4.1 Explaining a diagnosis 488
4.2 Explaining an investigation 489
4.3 Discussing treatment 492
4.4 Discussing management, prognosis and possible complications in a patient with multiple problems 494
4.5 Discussing diagnostic uncertainty 496
4.6 Discussing risk and treatment effect 497
4.7 Negotiating a management plan for a chronic disease/long-term condition 500
4.8 Encouraging concordance with treatment and prevention 502

COMMUNICATION IN SPECIAL CIRCUMSTANCES

4.9 Cross-cultural communication 505
4.10 Communicating with angry patients or relatives 506
4.11 Communicating with upset or distressed relatives 508
4.12 Discharge against medical advice 509
4.13 Delayed discharge 511

BREAKING BAD NEWS

4.14 Cancer – potentially curable 514
4.15 Cancer – probably incurable 516
4.16 Cancer – patient not fit for active treatment 518
4.17 Chronic disease 520
4.18 Discussing an acutely terminal situation with relatives 522

CONFIDENTIALITY, CONSENT AND CAPACITY

4.19 Legal points in confidentiality 524
4.20 Breaching confidentiality when a third party may be at risk 526
4.21 Breaching confidentiality in the public interest 527
4.22 Confidentiality when talking with relatives and other third parties 529
4.23 Consent for investigation or treatment 530
4.24 Consent and capacity 533
4.25 Refusal of consent 537
4.26 Deliberate self-harm 540

END-OF-LIFE ISSUES

4.27 Resuscitation-status decision-making – discussion with patient 543
4.28 Resuscitation-status decision-making – discussion with relative 547
4.29 Appropriateness of intensive therapy unit transfer 548
4.30 Withholding and withdrawing life-prolonging treatments – antibiotics and drugs 550
4.31 Withholding and withdrawing life-prolonging treatments – artificial hydration and nutrition 553
4.32 Percutaneous endoscopic gastrostomy feeding 556
4.33 Palliative care 558
4.34 Advance directives/decisions 561
4.35 Persistent vegetative state 563
4.36 Brainstem death 565
4.37 Discussing live organ donation 568
4.38 Requesting an autopsy (post mortem) 569

CLINICAL GOVERNANCE

4.39 Critical incident 572
4.40 Managing a complaint and the question of negligence 575
4.41 Fitness to practise – poor performance in a colleague 578
4.42 Fitness to practise – misconduct in a colleague 580
4.43 Fitness to practise – health problems in a colleague 582
4.44 Recruitment to a randomised controlled trial 584

OTHER COMMUNICATION, ETHICAL AND LEGAL SCENARIOS

4.45 Genetic testing 589
4.46 HIV testing 590
4.47 Needlestick injury 591
4.48 Medical opinion on fitness for anaesthesia 593
4.49 Fitness to drive 595
4.50 Industrial injury benefits 596

References and further reading 598

INTRODUCTION TO COMMUNICATION SKILLS AND ETHICS

Communication skills

Effective communication

Effective communication in medicine means simply that doctor and patient (relative, colleague, etc.) understand each other. We could, broadly, consider two stages to an encounter with a patient. The first stage is concerned with information gathering. The aim is to answer the question *What is the problem or what are the problems?* The second stage is concerned with developing a management plan, aiming to answer the question *How do I solve this problem or these problems?* Management plans should be developed not just *for* patients but also *with* patients. A plan is seldom a case of saying:

> *You have an overactive thyroid; you will need to take a tablet called carbimazole,*

but more a case of

> *Let's look at how we could treat your overactive thyroid.*

It is a two-way process of information sharing. The doctor does not so much know the solution to the problem (although may know what is clinically best), but reach a solution through communicating with the patient. This method of problem-solving is more patient centred.

Doctor-centred and patient-centred communication

At first sight, allowing patients to be involved in management decisions might seem to be relinquishing medical expertise and merely facilitating what patients want. This would be unprofessional, and we could deservedly question how patients can know what they want without medical knowledge and training. Were you to say to the thyrotoxic patient,

> *We could treat your overactive thyroid with tablets called carbimazole or we could use radiotherapy or we could arrange for you to have an operation. Now which will it be?*

she would be likely to respond with

> *Well, I don't know what's best. You're the doctor.*

Patient-centred communication does not mean abdicating decision-making to patients. It is the process of providing patients with the appropriate knowledge and understanding to enable them to make informed decisions and take appropriate responsibility for their care. Such an approach combines the professional knowledge and opinions of the doctor with respect for the autonomy of the patient. A better way to approach the thyrotoxic patient would be

> *There are a number of ways to treat an overactive thyroid. One would be to take tablets for a few months to see if they settle it down. They are often very effective, although some patients do eventually need to have an operation. Another choice would be to consider surgery at the outset, but in my experience most surgeons prefer to operate if tablets don't work. A third option would be something called radiotherapy, but this may not be a good idea if you were planning to become pregnant in the near future. I usually prefer patients to take advice from a doctor who specialises in thyroid problems before deciding, but wonder if you have any immediate thoughts about these treatments.*

The degree to which we engage in open discussion depends upon the patient. At one end of the spectrum are patients with seemingly very little interest in decision participation – *I'll go with whatever you think is best, doctor.* At the other extreme are patients who ruminate over everything that happens to them, and want to know everything – *How many stitches would the surgeon need to use, doctor?*

Patients differ. Yet when we look for evidence-based management of disease, we find management plans that focus on disease and not on the permutations of our patients. Traditionally, doctors have been *disease centred*, but diseases are wrapped in packages that are patients and a fundamental clinical skill is applying evidence-based medicine to the spectrum of different patients. Guidelines might advise against radioactive iodine in pregnancy and the patient might say

> *I was thinking about having a family soon.*

But she might also say

> *My mother had a thyroidectomy 30 years ago and had terrible swallowing problems afterwards until the day she died.*

Those swallowing problems may not have been associated with the thyroidectomy. One could also say that surgery has moved forward in 30 years but the patient may nevertheless have decided she does not want to contemplate surgery. The point is that the *apparently optimal management of a disease is not automatically the optimal management for a patient with that disease.*

Taking into account how a patient feels about their disease and its management is what is meant by *patient centredness*. Pure *doctor centredness* is doctor controlled and tends to be inflexible from patient to patient. Management decisions are made by the doctor and the patient is expected to comply. The key to patient centredness is not to abandon the strengths of disease-centred and doctor-centred practice, but to share information so that decisions about management are shared with and acceptable to the patient. Patient centredness and doctor centredness should work together, the latter relating to clinical knowledge of disease and how it should be managed, the former a means of harnessing the patient's perspective to convert that knowledge into an acceptable management plan. Patients have a fundamental ethical right to be involved in decisions about managing their disease so doctors have a duty to be patient centred.

Patient centredness is central to helping patients decide what is best for them. Consider that the surgeon of the thyrotoxic patient felt thyroidectomy to be the best course of action. It would certainly be right to explore her understandable concerns about the operation. Negotiating the best course of action for her should address these concerns. A balanced explanation by the surgeon may emphasise the low incidence of serious complications, despite her fears, and include an expectation of what may happen if she does not proceed to surgery now. Despite this process of shared understanding, if the patient, competent to decide and aware of the risks, declines surgery, she is exercising her autonomy. More likely, she will be reassured and begin to find surgery an acceptable option.

Patients have a right to be involved in decisions that affect them. Practising modern medicine is not just about knowledge, but about the skills to share that knowledge in ways that encourage patients to make sound, informed choices. Patients, in general, value our ability to guide. When they are guided, rather than pushed, they are far more likely to keep going along the treatment path we suggest.

Ethics

The importance of ethical decision-making

Every day in medicine we make ethical decisions. Some of these decisions are based on documented professional or legal frameworks. Most are less clearly defined. How much information about the side effects of a drug should we give a patient, for example?

Ethical decision-making involves the application of ethical principles. Often, the decisions we reach seem intuitively right; however, intuition, while valuable, may alone be inadequate and even detrimental to a patient's care. For one thing, a purely intuitive approach alone may lead to inconsistent behaviour in the way we care for patients, especially with complex issues. If we aspire to provide the best care, we need to be more analytical.

Ethical principles

Four broad ethical principles underlie ethical decision-making (Box 4.1).

Applying ethical principles

Specific cases have a vital role in ethical argument. Ethics is not a science where we agree upon a set of principles and then deduce what is right or wrong from these. Rather, the *implications* of the principles in specific cases must be explored.

Ethical reasoning is an interactive process that involves consideration of individual situations and application of

---

Box 4.1 Ethical principles

1. Respect for persons

We have a duty to respect the rights, autonomy and dignity of the person. This duty incorporates concepts such as honesty, truthfulness, sincerity and trust. In medicine, respecting a patient's autonomy is a fundamental ethical principle.

Autonomy is the capacity to think and decide, and to act on the basis of such thought and decision, freely and independently. This requires health professionals to provide the necessary information to help patients reach decisions for themselves and respect such decisions even if these do not appear to be the best course of action.

2. Justice

Justice refers to our duty of universal fairness or equity. It incorporates our duty to avoid discrimination, abuse or exploitation of people.

3. Beneficence

The duty to do good (in the medical context, to our patients) is a fundamental guiding ethical principle. It entails doing what is best for patients, but raises the question as to who is the judge of what is best.

Beneficence is often seen as being applied in practice when a health professional determines, by objective assessment, what is in a patient's best interests. The patient's views are encapsulated in the principle of autonomy. Usually, that which the health professional determines and the patient's views lead to the same conclusion, because most patients choose what is objectively in their best interests.

In a sense, beneficence is the first duty of a doctor – to alleviate symptoms and suffering, usually, but not always, through diagnosis and treatment.

4. Non-maleficence

The duty to avoid doing harm runs, in most situations, parallel to the duty to do good. Most treatments carry some risk of doing more harm than good but it does not follow that such treatments should be avoided on grounds that avoiding harm takes priority over doing good.

---

ethical principles. One logical requirement to this process is consistency. If what you believe to be right in one situation seems inconsistent with what you believe to be right in another, you must either identify a morally relevant difference between the two situations or change your view. When considering individual patients and applying ethical principles, foremost in our minds in decision-making should be what is deemed in the patient's best interests. It helps, when making a decision, to ask why you have made it and to be able to justify it.

A word on dignity

In recent years the notion of dignity, emerging primarily from palliative care, has been more formally applied across the spectrum of medicine. The core values of kindness, respect and dignity are indispensable and invariably, although not automatically, allow ethical practice to flourish. Awareness of the A,B,C,D of dignity in healthcare is of value to some: attitudes (largely about appreciating the patient's situation and your own impact on it), behaviours (professional and respectful disposition and clinical examination, and facilitation of communication), compassion and dialogue. The Royal College of Physicians rightly emphasises the importance of dignity in both clinical practice and professional examinations.

DISCUSSING CLINICAL MANAGEMENT

CASE 4.1

EXPLAINING A DIAGNOSIS

Candidate information

Role

You are a doctor in the medical outpatient clinic. Please read this summary.

Scenario

> Re: Mrs Elizabeth Wright, aged 45 years
>
> Mrs Wright has systemic lupus erythematosus (SLE). She has had a malar rash and pain in her hands for 12 months. Her clinical presentation, together with results of extensive investigations including autoimmune serology and radiology, supports the diagnosis of SLE confined to skin and joints without other multi-systemic involvement. She is here today for results. She is a hospital secretary and very concerned that she may need to stop working.
>
> Your task is to explain the diagnosis, addressing her concerns.

Your examiners will warn you when 12 minutes have elapsed. You have 14 minutes to communicate with the patient/subject followed by 1 minute of reflection. There will then follow 5 minutes of discussion with the examiners. Do not take the history again except for details that will help in your discussion with the patient/subject. You are not required to examine the patient/subject.

Patient/subject information

Mrs Elizabeth Wright is a 45-year-old hospital secretary with two sons. For the last year she has had intermittent but slowly worsening pain in the joints of her hands and a facial rash that is sensitive to sunlight. She is previously very well, takes no medications and is a non-smoker. She has been investigated recently in the outpatient clinic and informed that systemic lupus erythematosus (SLE) is a possibility. She is here today for the results of tests. She is very concerned that she may need to stop working, which she can ill afford as a single mother. She is also concerned because she is aware of a patient in her workplace needing dialysis, and an internet search advised that SLE was not a curable disease and could cause kidney failure. Otherwise she knows very little about SLE.

How to approach the case

Communication skills (conduct of interview, exploration and problem negotiation) and ethics and law

1 Introduction

Introduce yourself and confirm her identity.

2 Clarify the task

Be clear in your own mind what problem or diagnosis needs to be discussed.

> The tests confirm that SLE has very probably been the cause of your problems.

3 Establish previous experience

Stronger candidates are guided by patients when giving explanations. They operate within a patient-centred framework. Weaker candidates think 'Oh no! What do I know about SLE?' and proceed to tell their patients very little or far too much, often in a disorganised fashion. Try to establish what your patient knows about the diagnosis before launching into your explanation. Rather than saying

> SLE is a condition which . . .

a better approach would be one of

> Have you heard of this condition before?
> I wonder if you know anything about this condition before we start?
> Have you any ideas about this condition?
> What have you been told so far about this condition?

A specific, uncommon condition like SLE may mean very little to a patient. Other diagnoses, such as multiple sclerosis, cancer and rheumatoid arthritis, are well known but often poorly understood. Establishing prior knowledge or preconceptions helps to determine at what level the explanation should start. She might not know that SLE can be a multi-system disease affecting more than skin and joints. Alternatively, she might say

> I was reading that it can affect the kidneys and that some patients end up on dialysis. Is that likely to happen to me?

4 Be alert to ideas, concerns and expectations

Establishing prior experience can help you understand any specific fears that may relate to it. Throughout your explanation, try to take account of any ideas, concerns and expectations you elicit. Examples of concerns that a patient with SLE might have include no longer being able to go out in the sun, an unsightly rash, arthritis, needing to take drugs or serious complications such as renal failure. Effects of a diagnosis on work, finances and home life are often central concerns.

5 Frame the explanation

Try to provide a framework or order to your explanation. You might talk about why SLE occurs ('misdirected' immune system), possible clinical problems and the likely natural history, with and without treatment.

6 Keep it clear

Keep your explanation as clear as possible. Use language she will understand (without being patronising), avoiding complex medical terminology. Sometimes it helps to use similar phrases to the patient

> *How does it look on the whole, doctor?*
> *It looks alright, on the whole. Most patients with your condition live a very normal life.*

7 Repeat important information

This can be an effective way of emphasising 'take home' messages

> *I should emphasise again that most people do not end up with kidney problems or need dialysis. Most patients have skin and joint problems similar to yourself, and these tend to get better with treatment.*

8 Confirm understanding

It can sometimes be useful to ask the patient to recount what they feel to be the important points of the discussion.

9 Encourage feedback and invite questions

> *I appreciate we've covered rather a lot there. Is there anything you would like me to go over again or are there any questions you would like to ask me?*

Be honest in your explanations and be prepared to admit uncertainty (with assurance you will seek the answer) if she asks something you cannot answer.

10 Agree a way forward

Ensure that there are arrangements for treatment and follow-up.

Discussion

Would you tell her that her condition is incurable, if she asked?

The approach to explaining any diagnosis depends upon the diagnosis itself and should be tailored to the patient. Many conditions are potentially serious but treatable, and in this case potentially 'incurable' in that it may return

without treatment but nonetheless likely to be fully treatable. Other conditions are more palpably 'incurable', such as disseminated malignancy. Few if any conditions are untreatable because palliation is always possible. Words like incurable are unhelpful, and it is more helpful to tell her that her condition can usually be fully suppressed with treatment.

CASE 4.2

EXPLAINING AN INVESTIGATION

Candidate information

Role

You are a doctor on the medical ward.
  Please read this summary.

Scenario

> Re: Mr Roger Thornhill, aged 74 years
>
> Mr Thornhill has been losing weight for five months, and feeling slightly breathless on exertion. He has hitherto been a well man, playing golf every day until admission to hospital last week with cough and possible pneumonia. He feels the antibiotics have helped. However, his chest X-ray showed mediastinal widening and a computed tomography (CT) scan confirmed a mass arising from the left hilum, probably primary lung cancer but possibly lymphoma. He was aware that the chest X-ray showed an abnormal shadow but does not know the results of his CT scan. He has not smoked for 20 years.
>
> Your tasks are to explain the results of the CT scan and discuss bronchoscopy as the best next step.

Your examiners will warn you when 12 minutes have elapsed. You have 14 minutes to communicate with the patient/subject followed by 1 minute of reflection. There will then follow 5 minutes of discussion with the examiners. Do not take the history again except for details that will help in your discussion with the patient/subject. You are not required to examine the patient/subject.

Patient/subject information

Mr Roger Thornhill is a 74-year-old man admitted to hospital last week with cough and pneumonia. He has been losing weight for five months. Although he feels a little better after antibiotics, he has been told that his chest X-ray shows an abnormal shadow that may not be purely attributable to infection. A chest CT scan has been performed and he is awaiting the results. He has been worried that the scan might show something sinister, like cancer. He has been an active man, playing golf daily. He was widowed six years ago. He gave up smoking 20 years ago.

How to approach the case

Communication skills (conduct of interview, exploration and problem negotiation) and ethics and law

1 Introduction

Introduce yourself and confirm his identity.

2 Clarify the task

Be clear in your own mind what investigation needs to be discussed, and the purpose for which it is being performed.

3 Establish previous experience

Try to establish what he knows about the problem before explaining the investigation. Rather than saying

> *You need to have a test called a bronchoscopy*

a better approach might be

> *The chest specialist feels that we should look more closely into this problem of coughing up blood. He suggests some further tests. May I ask you what you've been told about the results of your tests so far?*
> *I know the X-ray wasn't completely normal. What tests does he suggest?*
> *He suggests a test called a bronchoscopy. Have you heard of a bronchoscopy before?*

4 Be alert to ideas, concerns and expectations

Establishing prior experience can help you to understand any specific fears relating to the potential diagnosis or to the test itself. These should be addressed before proceeding.

> *What do you think the X-ray means, doctor? The other doctor said it could be a growth in the lung. I've smoked all my life so I wouldn't be surprised, to be honest with you. Is it bad?*
> *The X-ray does suggest the possibility of a growth in the lung. A bronchoscopy is the best way of knowing this for certain. It's very hard to say what it means for you until we know for sure what it is. Once we know, we are in a much better position to know the best way forward.*

5 Frame the explanation

Try to provide a framework for your explanation of the investigation (Box 4.2).

> *The bronchoscopy involves passing a flexible telescope with a light on the end into the airways, usually*

Box 4.2 Explaining an investigation

- The purpose of the investigation (usually to further a diagnosis, assess the severity or extent of a disease, or monitor response to treatment)
- The nature of the proposed investigation
- Any risks that may be involved

> *under sedation. If there is anything seen, such as a growth, then the specialist would take a biopsy, a small piece of tissue, from it for closer examination. It is a very common test these days, and generally very safe.*

6 Keep it clear

Keep your explanation as clear as possible. Use language he will understand.

7 Repeat important information

This can be an effective way of emphasising 'take home' messages.

8 Confirm understanding

It can sometimes be useful to ask the patient to recount what they feel to be the important points of the discussion.

9 Encourage feedback and invite questions

> *I appreciate we've covered rather a lot there. Is there anything you would like me to go over again or are there any questions you would like to ask me?*

10 Seek consent

Remember that you are explaining the reason for an investigation and not telling a patient they must have it. Following explanation, you should seek informed consent to proceed.

Discussion

An 86-year-old lady with moderately severe dementia has a suspicious lesion on chest X-ray. Would you recommend bronchoscopy?

Guidelines for investigating and treating suspected lung cancer suggest bronchoscopy or percutaneous biopsy to guide appropriate treatment – surgery, chemotherapy, radiotherapy or palliation; however, guidelines often fail to address significant comorbidity. Here, assessment of cognition, functional and social support and symptom control probably supersede attempts to confirm a diagnosis, but investigation may be warranted if likely tumour-related symptoms develop to allow more secure planning of palliative measures. Her capacity to understand the issues should be explored, ideally in the presence of next of kin, and empirical treatment considered if she does not accept investigation. If she accepts investigation, the least likely to cause distress should be arranged, for example a CT scan rather than bronchoscopy.

What do you understand by the terms sensitivity, specificity, positive predictive value (PPV) and negative predictive value (NPV) of tests?

Sensitivity and specificity are to do with finding or not finding disease. Sensitivity is concerned with finding disease, and specificity with not detecting disease in those without the disease. Disease positives and negatives are based on 'gold standard tests' (ultimate diagnostic tests as the profession sees them). Predictive values are to do with diagnostic/screening tests. If a test is positive, the question is whether or not it is good at detecting disease; if a test is negative, the question is whether or not it is good at not missing disease. Sensitivity and specificity are not affected by the prevalence of a disease; predictive values are (Table 4.1).

Sensitivity

Sensitivity refers to the ability of a test to detect disease. It considers all those with disease (disease positives) and is the proportion of true disease positives $(a + c)$ that the test detects (a). A highly sensitive test is able to detect disease or target substance in trace amounts and so misses few that have the disease, i.e. a low false-negative rate. For example, bone marrow aspiration and soluble transferrin receptor assay are highly sensitive tests for confirming iron deficiency, whereas ferritin may be misleading.

Specificity

Specificity refers to the ability of a test to exclude disease. It considers all without disease (disease negatives) and is the proportion of true disease negatives $(b + d)$ that the test correctly identifies as negative (d). A highly specific test is able to detect a single disease or target substance and no other and seldom misdiagnoses disease, i.e. a low false-positive rate. For example, mammography screens a defined age population with higher specificity for detecting breast cancer. Lowering the age threshold for screening may lower specificity and increase false-positive results because younger women tend to have lumpier breasts.

PPV

PPV considers all those who test positive and is the proportion of people with a positive test $(a + b)$ who have the disease in question (a). A high PPV is desirable for diagnostic tests, i.e. a low false-positive rate.

NPV

NPV considers all who test negative and is the proportion of people with a negative test $(c + d)$ who do not have the disease in question (d). A high NPV is desirable for diagnostic tests, i.e. a low false-negative rate.

Explain the terms pre-test probability and post-test probability

Pre-test probability refers to the proportion of people with a target disorder in the population at risk and is simply another term for prevalence. Pre-test probability may be calculated using the formula $(a + c)/(a + b + c + d)$. Post-test probability refers to the proportion of patients with a particular test result who have the target disorder.

What criteria are important in determining whether to implement a screening test for a disease?

Ideally, the disease should be common, important and diagnosable by an accepted method. There must be a latent interval between disease onset and important manifestations during which effective intervention is possible. The screening test should be simple, cheap (cost-effective) and performed on a group deemed by policy to be at high risk. It should have a high sensitivity and specificity.

What is meant by a valid and reliable test?

A valid test is one that measures what it sets out to measure. A reliable test is one that produces repeatable results.

Which factors may influence a decision to investigate older people?

Guidelines for investigating conditions can fail to address individual factors that should be considered when assessing the potential benefits and risks of investigation; such factors become more common with advancing age. Co-morbidity and multiple pathologies become more likely in older patients, with an increase in chronic diseases, and it can be more appropriate to identify problems and use problem-solving than seek single unifying diagnoses, and more appropriate to make judgements as to which problems are most likely to be affecting quality of life. Cognitive impairment, either mild or dementia, may preclude informed consent for an investigation. Physical disability such as osteoarthritis can, for example, thwart exercise tolerance testing. Patients' views and wishes are of course most valuable in deciding the best way forward. A common example is the extent of investigation for anaemia in an older person once a basic 'blood screen' has been completed.

Table 4.1 Sensitivity, specificity and predictive values			
	Disease positive	**Disease negative**	
Test positive (abnormal)	a	b	PPV = a/(a + b)
Test negative (normal)	c	d	NPV = d/(c + d)
	Sensitivity = a/(a + c)	Specificity = d/(b + d)	
NPV, negative predictive value; PPV, positive predictive value.			

Communication skills and ethics

A pragmatic way of decision-making for investigating older people is to select investigations that are most likely to change management or yield prognostic information. If a patient is competent to give informed consent to an investigation then it is possible to proceed; if not then it may be discussed with those close to the patient, or a decision can be made in the patient's best interests as judged by the doctor. If either a competent patient or those close to a patient not competent refuse investigation then empirical treatment might be offered.

Automatic investigations that will not benefit patients are inappropriate but discrimination against older patients by restricting access to investigations is equally unacceptable. Decisions should be made by balancing potential benefits and risks, and not determined by age.

CASE 4.3

DISCUSSING TREATMENT

Candidate information

Role

You are a doctor on the cardiology ward.
   Please read this summary.

Scenario

Re: Mr James Bonde, aged 80 years

Mr Bonde is recovering well from a non-ST elevation myocardial infarction. Although well before admission, coronary angiography is not being considered and he is keen to go home. He is currently taking aspirin. Beta blockade is deemed risky on account of sinus bradycardia. Blood pressure is 160/90. You think he might benefit from clopidogrel, a statin and an angiotensin-converting enzyme (ACE) inhibitor to further modify risk.

Your task is to explain these treatments to him, and allow him to make an informed choice about whether or not to take them.

Your examiners will warn you when 12 minutes have elapsed. You have 14 minutes to communicate with the patient/subject followed by 1 minute of reflection. There will then follow 5 minutes of discussion with the examiners. Do not take the history again except for details that will help in your discussion with the patient/subject. You are not required to examine the patient/subject.

Patient/subject information

Mr James Bonde is an 80-year-old man who has never before been in hospital. He was admitted to hospital four

days ago with a heart attack. His wife died of heart disease six years ago, having taken many medications for her heart. He feels he has had a good life. He does not want to be kept in hospital for further tests or treatments if he can be allowed home more quickly without these, and fully accepts he might be declining potentially optimal, 'cutting edge' approaches. He feels simply that he has done all that he wants to in life and 'will accept the end when it comes, with or without treatment'. He will consider treatment that keeps further chest pains at bay, but does not want 'anything too complicated'.

How to approach the case

Communication skills (conduct of interview, exploration and problem negotiation) and ethics and law

1 Introduction

Introduce yourself and confirm his identity.

2 Explain the reasons for considering treatment

I'm glad to see that you are recovering from your recent heart attack. Your test results are largely encouraging but your blood cholesterol level and blood pressure are still a little high. When the cholesterol is high and we don't treat it, this can increase the risk of future heart attack, as can high blood pressure. Fortunately, the risk can be reduced with medication and I think we should discuss starting this medication in your case.

3 Give the patient a chance to react to the need for treatment

Remember that a lot has happened to him recently. His world has been changed by the heart attack. He probably had an enormous fright when admitted, and is still coming to terms with the repercussions of his diagnosis. He will have received a great deal of advice from doctors, nurses and members of the cardiac rehabilitation team. He will be on a range of tablets indefinitely. It is important to recognise that his hopes and yours may not immediately be the same. There may be a mismatch of agendas. You want him to start more tablets and then see your next patient but he desperately wants some good news. Yet more tablets may not be what he had in mind. Going home may be. Give him a chance to react to what you see as the most important next step, and appreciate his.

4 Be alert to ideas, concerns and expectations

Establishing prior experience (e.g. of his wife) can help you understand any specific beliefs. Throughout your explanation, try to take account of any ideas, concerns and expectations you elicit.

5 Explain the likely benefits of treatment

Explain these as accurately as possible, without over-whelming him with outcomes of studies. It often helps to reassure patients that others are taking the same drug and that your advice is commensurate with the larger body of current medical opinion.

6 Explain what the treatment involves

Explain the frequency of dosing of tablets, the duration of therapy and any special instructions (e.g. when tablets should be taken). Any requirements for blood monitoring, if relevant, should be discussed.

7 Explain likely side effects of treatment

Mention side effects that are common or serious. Try to explain the balance of risk (benefits versus side effects). Explain what should be done if a side effect occurs. Many patients know that aspirin can cause ulcers, but carry on taking it if they have bleeding symptoms. Patients have not worked in medical units. Do not assume that what is obvious to you is obvious to your patient.

8 Encourage feedback and invite questions

I appreciate we've covered rather a lot there. Is there anything you would like me to go over again or are there any questions you would like to ask me?

9 Seek consent

Remember that you are explaining the reasons for tablets and not telling him he must have them.

10 Respect autonomy

Ultimately, the decision to accept treatment or stay in hospital is his, and his informed decision should be respected.

Discussion

Are you more reluctant to prescribe medications for older people?

Treating older people must aim for maximum benefit (it is older people who often derive most benefit from a particular drug) and minimal adverse effects by avoiding excessive or inappropriate medications. To achieve this balance, individualised prescribing that considers comorbidity, co-prescription and social aspects of care, and careful judgement of overall frailty and likelihood of benefit, are crucial. Older people are often inappropriately under-represented in therapeutic trials, and so the size of benefit might be under-appreciated in an older person, but so might the absolute risk increase. Six rules in prescribing for older people are shown in Box 4.3.

> **Box 4.3 Prescribing for older people**
>
> **Consider the indication**
>
> This includes stopping drugs when investigations do not support a diagnosis. It is not uncommon for patients whose results do not support ischaemic heart disease to be continued on antiplatelet and antihypertensive treatment and to be readmitted with anaemia and hyponatraemia!
>
> **Be alert to possible side effects and limit prescribing**
>
> Almost any drug can provoke confusion. Extrapyramidal side effects are not uncommon with antipychotics, anti-emetics and anti-histamines; depression can be triggered by beta blockers and calcium channel blockers; constipation can be the result of opiates, diuretics and anticholinergics. Broad-spectrum antibiotics, antipsychotics, benzodiazepines, beta blockers and phenytoin are just some drugs that may be better avoided in older people.
>
> **Do not withhold treatments that work**
>
> Warfarin, for example, is often inappropriately withheld. Bisphosphonates are under-prescribed, and although evidence in the management of osteoporosis over the age of 80 years is limited, ongoing benefits are likely. Calcium and vitamin D are under-prescribed.
>
> **Stop inappropriate medications**
>
> The aim should be symptom relief, for example in patients who are dying, who should not be given a diet of statins and aspirin.
>
> **Be imaginative with routes of administration**
>
> Use intramuscular gentamicin, for example, in an agitated, confused patient with a urinary infection, with haloperidol if there is an absolute need to sedate.
>
> **Consider concordance**
>
> Ideally patients should be discharged with a list of their treatments and the reasons for each.

Is treatment for coronary syndromes the same for older as younger patients?

Thrombolytic agents provide a greater absolute benefit in older people and should only be withheld if there are contraindications, although these are more likely in older people. Meta-analyses of aspirin trials show around 25% reduction over two years in secondary prevention of major vascular occlusive events, relative risk reduction being similar in younger and older people but absolute benefit greatest for high-risk patients over 65 (but the risk : benefit ratio tips aspirin out of favour for low-risk older people in primary prevention). Beta blockers after myocardial infarction reduce mortality from ischaemia and arrhythmias with evidence up to 75 years but beyond this age benefit can only be extrapolated and older people are more likely to have relative or absolute contraindications, such as sinus pauses or postural hypotension. ACE inhibitors reduce mortality and morbidity in cardiovascular disease but again older patients are more likely to have contraindications such as hypotension, moderate aortic stenosis or vulnerable renovascular disease.

Is treatment for hypertension the same for older as younger patients?

Absolute benefit from antihypertensive treatment is much greater in older people.

Is treatment for hyperlipidaemia the same for older as younger patients?

The benefits of statin therapy are deduced from overall risk rather than lipid concentration. The Heart Protection Study showed significant reductions in first event rates (around 25%, $P < 0.0001$) for myocardial infarction and stroke each year after the first year and these rates were similar in those under or over 70 years. Statins should be considered for patients with occlusive arterial disease or diabetes where life expectancy is greater than one year and quality of life is positive.

Is warfarin justified in patients aged over 75 years with atrial fibrillation?

Warfarin in atrial fibrillation reduces stroke risk by 68%, compared with 21% with aspirin. The high rate of intra-cranial haemorrhage with warfarin in patients aged over 75 years does not quite negate its benefit, but co-morbidities limiting life expectancy may limit its potential benefit.

CASE 4.4

DISCUSSING MANAGEMENT, PROGNOSIS AND POSSIBLE COMPLICATIONS IN A PATIENT WITH MULTIPLE PROBLEMS

Candidate information

Role

You are a doctor in the medical outpatient clinic.
Please read this summary.

Scenario

Re: Mr John Rowe, aged 76 years

Mr Rowe had a partial gastrectomy for gastric cancer two years ago. It was diagnosed very early by oesophagogastroduodenoendoscopy (OGD) for dyspepsia. After surgery and a course of *Helicobacter pylori* eradication he had no further symptoms and his surgeon told him all appeared to be clear. He now has recurrence of dyspepsia and is seeing you urgently in clinic and wants to know if the cancer might have returned. He has recently seen the cardiologists because of suspected angina and had a positive exercise tolerance test and awaits

angiography. He has been started on aspirin, a statin and an angiotensin-converting enzyme (ACE) inhibitor but not a beta blocker because of mild chronic obstructive pulmonary disease (COPD), for which he takes inhalers. He also wishes to talk to you about his angina and breathing because he feels the cardiologists did not tell him very much. He has recently had two episodes of fresh rectal bleeding, but he is not too troubled by this. You may assume systematic enquiry otherwise unremarkable.

Your task is to address his concerns and discuss a way forward.

Your examiners will warn you when 12 minutes have elapsed. You have 14 minutes to communicate with the patient/subject followed by 1 minute of reflection. There will then follow 5 minutes of discussion with the examiners. Do not take the history again except for details that will help in your discussion with the patient/subject. You are not required to examine the patient/subject.

Patient/subject information

Mr John Rowe is a 76-year-old gentleman who had an operation for gastric cancer 2 years ago. It was diagnosed very early, by investigation for indigestion. After surgery he had no further symptoms and his surgeon told him 'all was clear'. He now has recurrence of indigestion. He has also recently seen the cardiologists because of suspected angina and had a positive exercise tolerance test and awaits angiography. He has been started on aspirin, simvastatin and ramipril. He has mild emphysema for which he takes inhalers, and gave up smoking 20 years ago. He also wishes to talk about his angina and breathing because he feels the cardiologists did not tell him very much. He is worried about the risks of an angiogram but also worried that without further tests he could have a heart attack. He wonders what his risk of a heart attack might be. He recently had two episodes of fresh rectal bleeding, but is not too troubled by this.

How to approach the case

Communication skills (conduct of interview, exploration and problem negotiation) and ethics and law

1 Introduction

Introduce yourself and confirm his identity.

2 Know how to deal with multiple problems

It is increasingly common in general internal medicine to face numerous problems in a single consultation. Patients with multiple problems are often uncertain about what is really wrong. They might not know why certain tests are being arranged. They might not know exactly why they are taking medications. In the era of increasing specialisation they might also be attending multiple specialist clinics, sometimes punctuated by acute admissions to hospital after which they are discharged on different tablets, and they might have difficulty organising and retaining sometimes seemingly conflicting advice from the different health professionals they have seen.

3 Take one step at a time

Your task is to arrange the puzzle into a series of boxes, and address each of these on the basis of which you see as priorities. In this case an appropriate way forward is to address the dyspepsia first and consider further endoscopy (which he has had before), and reassure him that you will move on to discuss his angina and breathing problems afterwards, and not forget his rectal bleeding.

4 Obtain the facts

Dyspepsia is often hard to differentiate from cardiac chest pain. He has had a positive exercise tolerance test but equally a history of gastric malignancy and recently starting aspirin and so has two compelling reasons to proceed to OGD (balanced against minor procedural risks posed by stable angina).

5 Explore concerns

Make sure you explore any specific concerns he may have, for example about proceeding to the angiogram.

6 Discuss management options with a clear framework

> I think we should strongly consider looking into the stomach again with the endoscopy you had before. This will quickly tell us whether or not there is anything we need to be worried about. I'd hope it would simply show some ulceration that we can treat with tablets, and this would not be uncommon in people taking aspirin. But I think you should continue the aspirin for the time being, because it gives some protection to the heart. In the unlikely event that the endoscopy showed anything more untoward then we would be in a better position to know what to do sooner rather than later.

7 Discuss potential prognoses and possible complications of any diagnoses (with and without treatment) or treatments

It can be easy to be drawn into discussion of possible outcomes but as far as possible try to avoid hypothetical discussion of what has not been diagnosed. With respect to his angina, it would be best to leave management in the hands of the cardiologists, but it would be appropriate to comment on the reasons for angiography (to consider if a procedure such as stenting would help his angina) and the importance of medications in reducing the risk of a heart attack.

8 Prioritise . . . but do not forget unturned stones

It is important at this stage not to ignore his rectal bleeding, which he considers less important. Unturned small stones can sometimes turn out to be very significant.

> I do not think we should ignore the bleeding you have had from the tail end, and it may be preferable for us to consider examining the tail end with a flexible telescope with a light on the end – similar to the endoscopy you have had before – to be certain we are not missing something.

Assuming rectal examination is normal, colonoscopy might be a crucial test, and the decision is where to place it in the overall sequence. One way forward would be to request it provisionally (waiting lists may preclude rapid access!).

9 Encourage feedback and invite questions

> I appreciate we've covered rather a lot there. Is there anything you would like me to go over again or are there any questions you would like to ask me?

10 Agree a way forward and ensure follow-up arrangements are in place

Reassure him of follow-up arrangements, and that you would happily review sooner at any time at his or his general practitioner's request if there are questions or concerns.

Discussion

What issues should you generally be aware of when managing older people?

Many of the scenarios in this book deal with older patients, and appropriately so since general internal medicine is managing an increasingly older population. A mnemonic for issues you should be particularly aware of is given in Box 4.4.

Box 4.4 Issues to be aware of in managing older people

- **R**educed body reserve
- **A**typical presentations
- **M**ultiple problems/pathologies
- **P**olypharmacy
- **S**ocial adversities

CASE 4.5

DISCUSSING DIAGNOSTIC UNCERTAINTY

Candidate information

Role

You are a doctor in the medical outpatient clinic.
Please read this summary.

Scenario

> Re: Miss Melissa Hamilton, aged 24 years
>
> You have been seeing Miss Hamilton in clinic for
> follow up of Crohn's disease. She has been
> asymptomatic for six months. At the end of the
> consultation she mentions that she has had pain in
> her right calf for the past week. She hoped you
> might take a quick look at it. Examination is
> unremarkable.
>
> Your task is to discuss management options with her.

Your examiners will warn you when 12 minutes have
elapsed. You have 14 minutes to communicate with the
patient/subject followed by 1 minute of reflection. There
will then follow 5 minutes of discussion with the examiners. Do not take the history again except for details that
will help in your discussion with the patient/subject. You
are not required to examine the patient/subject.

Patient/subject information

Miss Melissa Hamilton is a 24-year-old lady with Crohn's
disease that has been well controlled on treatment for six
months. At the end of her outpatient consultation she
mentions that she has had pain in her right calf for the past
week. She did not want 'to bother her GP' and hoped you
might take a look at it. She is not particularly concerned
about it but wonders what might be causing it. She is otherwise well. She started the combined oral contraceptive
pill (COCP) two months ago while touring in Australia
with her boyfriend. They returned home 10 days ago. She
has no family history of thromboembolic disease.

How to approach the case

Communication skills (conduct of interview, exploration and problem negotiation) and ethics and law

1 Introduction

Introduce yourself and confirm her identity.

2 Clarify the task

Confirm that the problem is calf pain, and nothing else.

3 Obtain the necessary facts

Gather information that is necessary to discuss management. Crucially, this includes additional symptoms and
risk factors for venous thromboembolism – personal or
family history, long-haul travel, COCP.

4 Be alert to ideas, concerns and expectations

She probably has no concerns about a deep venous thrombosis (DVT).

5 Outline the possibilities

She appears to lead an active lifestyle, has no signs of a
DVT, and the absolute risk of thromboembolic disease
on the COCP is very low. Conversely, she has two
possible risk factors, the COCP and a long-haul flight, and
thromboembolic disease, although unlikely, can be life-
threatening and is treatable.

6 Share the probability and potential seriousness of a diagnosis

Probability is discussed in Box 4.5.

> *This is most likely to be harmless muscle pain. There
> is a small possibility that the pain is the result of
> a clot of blood in one of the deeper veins of the
> leg. It is difficult to exclude this without further
> tests. Although I think a blood clot very unlikely,
> there is a risk that an untreated blood clot could
> travel to the lungs and cause serious harm. We
> could arrange a blood test and then possibly a scan
> of the leg to be more sure, if you wanted us to.*

This sounds straightforward, but in practice there can
be a problem with sharing information in this way. Patients
frequently do not warm to the idea of being asked to make
a decision and *if you wanted us to* may be too open-ended
to actually help her decide. She might respond

> *Well, you're the doctor, I'll take your advice. Do you
> think it's really necessary?*

Sharing information is more than showing patients the
menu!

Box 4.5 Probability and potential seriousness of diagnosis

A symptom may have a low probability of representing serious
pathology but a high probability of serious consequences if ignored.
Such information should always be shared with a patient. The
management of disease in theory is often clear-cut: investigation A for
suspected disease B; treatment Y for disease Z. In practice, whether
or not to embark on an investigation in the face of limited evidence
is a complex decision that should involve sharing your knowledge,
concerns and expectations with the patient.

7 Give an honest professional opinion

If these decisions are difficult for us, with medical training, then they can be enormously difficult for patients, given only small quantities of distilled information. Since there is no clear history of muscle strain, the potential serious- ness of a DVT may persuade you to say

> *I'd advise a blood test called a D-dimer. If this is negative we can be reassured that a blood clot is highly unlikely. If it is positive, we should go on to arrange a scan of the leg to be sure.*

8 Confirm understanding

It can sometimes be useful to ask the patient to recount what they feel to be the important points of the discussion.

9 Encourage feedback and invite questions

> *I appreciate we've covered rather a lot there. Is there anything you would like me to go over again or are there any questions you would like to ask me?*

10 Cast a 'safety net'

If a patient decides not to pursue tests, always have a safety net, such as follow up by the general practitioner or to seek medical advice if symptoms develop further. Any decision that involves waiting for something else to happen before acting should be 'safety netted' and you should be clear about which symptoms should prompt reassessment.

Discussion

An 85-year-old man has had a large cortical stroke causing dysphasia and dense hemiplegia. Routine tests reveal a haemoglobin of 9 g/dl with a low ferritin. Would you investigate this further or accept diagnostic uncertainty?

Oesophagogastroduodenoscopy (OGD) and colonoscopy are the standard investigations used to look for a source of chronic blood loss in iron deficiency anaemia. However, the balance of risk of proceeding with these might not be in the patient's best interests immediately. OGD might increase the risk of hypoxia, colonoscopy might be imprac- tical and, depending upon the type of dysphasia, informed consent could be an issue. Investigations should probably be delayed until the outcome of the stroke is clearer, and as an interim measure exclusion of other haematic defi- ciencies, supplemental iron and possible withholding of antiplatelet treatment are appropriate. If recovery is satis- factory, investigations could be instituted a few weeks later, and even if colorectal cancer is diagnosed and inop- erable or declined because of operative risk, then such information may influence placement or the type of future care provision. If there is severe residual disability from the stroke, then investigations should probably not be pursued and perhaps only considered if severe blood loss

demands repeated transfusion. Myelodysplasia is common in older people and anaemia is not usually a contraindica- tion to antiplatelet therapy if monitored closely, or even anticoagulation if there is an embolic source and high risk of further stroke in a recovering patient.

A 70-year-old woman has new onset exertional chest pain. She has severe osteoarthritis, walking only a limited distance, and Parkinson's disease. Would you attempt to further the diagnosis of angina with a stress test?

A stress test would define risk more precisely and identify whether coronary angiography and potential revasculari- sation are likely to be of benefit. An alternative to treadmill testing, such as pharmacological testing with dipyridamole, dobutamine or adenosine, would be needed. The likely net benefits of investigation and possible treatments should be explained and her views should be sought as to whether to proceed to testing or a more conservative strategy.

A 48-year-old non-smoker is being discharged from your ward today following investigation for chronic diarrhoea. No cause has been found. He tells you that a few weeks ago he had a single episode of 'coughing up a teaspoonful of blood' that he'd forgotten to mention until now. His chest X-ray was normal. What are the important issues?

There is probably no sinister cause. It has not recurred and he is a non-smoker with a normal chest X-ray. Nevertheless, the haemoptysis remains unexplained. There are numerous potential approaches to the problem. At one extreme he might be reassured and told that no further tests are needed; at the other extreme he could be advised to have a bronchoscopy to exclude a tumour. Each doctor has his or her own 'risk threshold' for undertaking inves- tigations, but the problem with each is that they do not involve the patient. It would be important to share with him that a small lesion may not show up on chest X-ray and that the only way to be certain of excluding this would be with further tests. Teamwork is integral to good clinical care and when you feel out of your depth in making a decision then you should seek advice.

CASE 4.6

DISCUSSING RISK AND TREATMENT EFFECT

Candidate information

Role

You are a doctor in the emergency medical admissions unit.

Please read this summary.

Scenario

> Re: Mr Christopher Roberts, aged 47 years
>
> Mr Roberts was admitted with atypical chest pain and is about to be discharged on a statin because of a cholesterol level of 6.5 mmol/l. He is obese with a body mass index (BMI) of 32, and has numerous other risk factors for cardiovascular disease (CVD) including smoking, alcohol consumption on the edge of safety and borderline hypertension. You are aware of evidence that stopping smoking, statin therapy, targeting his hypertension (alcohol reduction playing a part), exercise and a 'Mediterranean' diet will significantly reduce his relative risk of CVD and developing type 2 diabetes.
>
> Your task is to discuss his perceived risks and the benefits of these treatments and lifestyle modifications with him.

Your examiners will warn you when 12 minutes have elapsed. You have 14 minutes to communicate with the patient/subject followed by 1 minute of reflection. There will then follow 5 minutes of discussion with the examiners. Do not take the history again except for details that will help in your discussion with the patient/subject. You are not required to examine the patient/subject.

Patient/subject information

Mr Christopher Roberts is a 47-year-old travel agent admitted with chest pain initially thought to be angina. He is very relieved to be told that investigations have not shown evidence of a heart attack or angina and that his pain is now thought to be muscular resulting from poor posture and a sedentary lifestyle coupled with a lot of driving and a recent minor whiplash accident. He is about to be discharged on a statin because of a cholesterol level of 6.5 mmol/l. He is obese, with a BMI of 32, and has numerous other risk factors for coronary heart disease (CHD) including smoking, 42 units of alcohol per week and high blood pressure. His father died of a heart attack at the age of 55.

How to approach the case

Communication skills (conduct of interview, exploration and problem negotiation) and ethics and law

1 Introduction

Introduce yourself and confirm his identity.

2 Review the history

Recap to him that the tests did not show that he had had a heart attack but that it was very clear on assessing him that he had significant risk factors for heart disease.

3 Clarify the task

Make it clear that reducing his risk of future heart attacks is the aim of the discussion, and that this is a very achievable goal.

4 Be alert to ideas, concerns and expectations

That his father died relatively young from a heart attack may be very much on his mind, but he may not know that it puts him at increased risk or that overall risk relates to the interplay with other, modifiable risk factors. Risk perception is discussed in Box 4.6.

5 Clarify risk

Having established his risk perception, clarify exactly what his risk factors are – smoking, alcohol, deficient exercise, high cholesterol and blood pressure – and potential health consequences of these.

6 Risk communication

Frame advice around the benefits of risk modification (Box 4.7).

7 Optimise the likelihood of concordance

Concordance is more likely when risk perception is realised, and he realises risk can be modified and that he can do it. The message can be reinforced through gentle repetition and a plan of action and support.

8 Confirm understanding

Confirm his understanding not just that he is at risk but that his risk can be substantially reduced.

9 Encourage feedback and invite questions

> *I appreciate we've covered rather a lot there. Is there anything you would like me to go over again or are there any questions you would like to ask me?*

Box 4.6 Risk perception

- Risk perception can determine risk-reducing behaviour. People who *perceive themselves at increased risk of coronary heart disease are more likely to adopt risk-reducing behaviours* such as smoking cessation, taking a Mediterranean diet, increased exercise and taking medication. Risk perception consists of two judgements, the *perceived likelihood* of an event and the *perceived severity* of that event.
- Risks can be discussed in verbal categories such as likely, probable and possible, and in absolute probabilities, such as a 10% chance of having the event. Verbal categories mean different things to different people. *People tend to downplay risk and make overly optimistic judgements of risk in comparison with others of the same age and sex.*
- The *perception of being at increased risk is unlikely to motivate people to adopt risk-reducing behaviours.* It is *also necessary to perceive that one has control over the risk* of an event and this has two components – *response efficacy* is the perception that risk-reducing behaviour will be effective and *self-efficacy* is having confidence in one's ability to adopt it.

Box 4.7 Risk communication

Risk communication involves sharing information about risk, how to reduce it and ensuring patients have the confidence to change their behaviour.

Response efficacy

It is helpful to outline not just the benefits in terms of coronary heart disease, but also the more widespread benefits of disease-modifying behaviours.

- Stopping smoking will of course also reduce respiratory disease and exercise intolerance and be financially advantageous.
- Statin therapy has well-established primary and secondary preventive outcome benefits.
- Targeting hypertension reduces stroke, coronary heart disease, renovascular disease and peripheral vascular disease.
- Exercise not only reduces the risk of vascular disease but also improves physical dexterity and overall well-being.
- A Mediterranean diet produces similar benefits.

Self efficacy

Habits are hard to break. Patients must not only be aware of the benefits of trying to improve their situation, but also should be instilled with the belief that they can. Motivation can be assisted by trying to identify which consequences of failing to modify behaviour resonate most with a patient (e.g. not being able to walk into the garden without feeling breathless by the age of 55, erectile dysfunction) and support networks and agencies to assist, such as specialist cardiac and respiratory nurses, smoking advice services and so forth.

10 Agree a way forward and ensure follow-up arrangements are in place

This might include writing to his general practitioner and suggesting follow-up with the practice nurse, seeing a dietitian and attending a smoking cessation advice service.

Discussion

What is meant by the term prevalence?

This refers to the proportion of individuals in a population with the condition of interest at a point in time.

$$\text{Prevalence} = \text{number with the condition/number in the population}$$

What is meant by the term incidence?

Incidence is concerned with the rate of new occurrences. There are three principle measures of incidence – *risk*, *odds* and *rate*.

What is meant by the term risk?

Risk is simply the *proportion* (a 1 in 2 or 50% chance of a coin landing heads or tails) of disease-free individuals who develop the condition during the study period.

$$\text{Risk} = \text{number of new cases in the period/number of disease-free individuals at the start}$$

It is the probability that a disease-free individual will develop the disease over the period.

What is meant by the term odds?

This is the *ratio* (a 1 to 1 odds of the coin landing heads or tails) of the probability of getting the disease to the probability of not.

$$\text{Odds} = \text{number of new cases in the period/number who remain disease-free during the period}$$

Odds against disease simply inverts the formula.

If 20 people have a stroke out of 100 in a population studied (i.e. 80 do not), the *risk* of stroke is 20/100 = 0.2 or 20% and the *odds* of a stroke is 20/80 = 0.25 or 25%. We could also think of odds as 'this versus this' and risk as 'this versus the whole population'.

What is meant by the term rate?

Risk and odds assume that all individuals are present throughout the period. In practice, some enter after the start and some leave before the end.

$$\text{Incidence rate} = \text{number of cases/total person time at risk}$$

What is meant by the term risk ratio?

Risk ratio is also referred to as *relative risk*.

$$\text{Relative risk} = \text{risk in exposed group/risk in unexposed group}$$

The risk of an event in an exposed or intervention group is sometimes called the experimental event rate (EER). The risk of an event in the unexposed or control group is sometimes called the control event rate (CER). Assume the risk of myocardial infarction in those treated with lipid-lowering therapy is 1 in 100 (EER) and the risk in the control group is 2 in 100 (CER). The relative risk of myocardial infarction with treatment is (1/100)/(2/100) or 0.5. Equally, the risk without treatment is doubled or 2.

What is meant by the term odds ratio?

$$\text{Odds ratio} = \text{odds in exposed group/odds in unexposed group}$$

What is meant by the term rate ratio?

$$\text{Rate ratio} = \text{rate in exposed group/rate in unexposed group}$$

If these ratios are 1 there is no difference between exposed and unexposed groups. If < 1, the exposed group is at lower risk, if > 1 at higher risk.

How does relative risk (RR) differ from absolute risk (AR)?

Absolute risk refers to the risk difference between exposed (e.g. treated) and unexposed.

$$\text{Risk difference} = \text{risk in exposed group} - \text{risk in unexposed group}$$

similarly

$$\text{Rate difference} = \text{rate in exposed group} - \text{rate in unexposed group}$$

These absolute measures are generally referred to as measures of *attributable risk*.

Relative risk should be interpreted in the context of the prevalence of the condition in question. If, for example, a study showed that the risk of a disease x were doubled by a particular drug y (e.g. the risk of venous thromboembolism is increased by hormone replacement therapy), then it is important to place that increased risk in the context of the likelihood of an event (absolute risk). If the natural prevalence or absolute risk of disease x is 1 in 1 million, then the absolute risk in the presence of treatment y is still only 1 in 500 000. A decision to treat will depend upon the risk : benefit ratio of treatment y.

Conversely, relative risk may not, at first sight, seem high, but 10 extra strokes per 1000 people, for example, would be clinically substantial.

What is meant by the term relative risk reduction (RRR)?

RRR is an illustration of how the risk of an event has been reduced by intervention.

$$RRR = 1 - RR$$

If, for example, RR = 0.2, then RRR = 1 − 0.2 = 0.8 or 80%.

What is meant by the term absolute risk reduction (ARR)?

ARR refers to the number of additional people who benefit from an intervention out of 100 and is the absolute arithmetic difference in rates of bad outcomes between control and experimental groups in a trial. ARR is therefore useful in determining if the RRR is important. If CER = 2% and EER = 1%, ARR is therefore 1% and so 1 in 100 people benefit from treatment. If the CER is much smaller, say 0.001%, the ARR achieved by the same RRR of 50% is 0.0005%. This ARR would warrant a much higher 'number needed to treat'.

What is meant by the term number needed to treat (NNT)?

NNT refers to the number of patients who need to be treated to prevent one bad outcome (or achieve one additional favourable outcome and benefit one additional patient). NNT is the reciprocal of ARR, i.e. 1/ARR.

What is meant by the term number needed to harm (NNH)?

NNH refers to the number of patients who need to be treated to cause one bad outcome. The lower the NNH, the more harmful the treatment.

NEGOTIATING A MANAGEMENT PLAN FOR A CHRONIC DISEASE/ LONG-TERM CONDITION

Candidate information

Role

You are a doctor on the medical ward.
Please read this summary.

Scenario

Re: Mr Henry Jackson, aged 45 years

Mr Jackson was admitted with a large anterior myocardial infarction and subsequent heart failure, requiring initial ionotropic support. His echocardiogram showed moderate systolic dysfunction and angiography showed a critical lesion in his left anterior descending artery for which he received percutaneous coronary intervention. He has been established on numerous secondary preventive drugs [aspirin, clopidogrel, a statin, an angiotensin-converting enzyme (ACE) inhibitor, a beta blocker and eplerenone]. He is being discharged and has some concerns about going home.

Your task is to discuss his concerns and negotiate a management plan for him following discharge from hospital.

Your examiners will warn you when 12 minutes have elapsed. You have 14 minutes to communicate with the patient/subject followed by 1 minute of reflection. There will then follow 5 minutes of discussion with the examiners. Do not take the history again except for details that will help in your discussion with the patient/subject. You are not required to examine the patient/subject.

Patient/subject information

Mr Henry Jackson is a 45-year-old man admitted 14 days ago with a large anterior myocardial infarction. He was very unwell for the first few days, and developed subsequent heart failure. He has had a stent inserted in one of his coronary arteries. His echocardiogram shows that he has significant damage to the left ventricle. He is now taking six different medications. He is very concerned that he still cannot walk far around the hospital without feeling a little short of breath. He wonders if he will get back to a normal life. He is very concerned that he was a previously very well man working as a manager for an IT company. He has a wife and two children and could not afford to give up work. He is a little overweight. He used to smoke 30 cigarettes per day.

How to approach the case

Communication skills (conduct of interview, exploration and problem negotiation) and ethics and law

1 Introduction

Introduce yourself and confirm his identity.

2 Clarify the task

Reassure him that your task and expectation are to guide him back to as normal a life as possible.

3 Establish the facts

In practice you would establish as much history as possible but because your communication skills are being assessed you should explore the concerns as soon as possible.

4 Explore concerns

The key word is *concerns*. It is very easy to assume what a patient's concerns are likely to be and then address assumptions. It is not uncommon to overlook a patient's concerns when giving advice after, for example, a coronary syndrome because there are standard areas that are usually discussed relating to medications. Patients do not always voice their concerns, thinking the doctor is 'too busy' or because they are afraid or simply do not know how to. It is important to ask.

> *There are a number of things to explain before you go home, but before we start is there anything worrying you in particular?*

Concerns will include return to a normal life, return to work, impact on family life, likelihood of taking tablets indefinitely, whether it could happen again and the way forward from here.

5 Share management options

Patients vary in the extent to which they wish to be involved in management decisions, but most want to be informed of possible options. It is worth stating your position if there appears to be a strongly 'right' option clinically and a patient is not keen to concord (for example, in taking secondary preventive drugs). Where there is a range of clinically acceptable options you could deploy 'thinking aloud' skills, observing the patient's reactions or asking, encouraging good ideas and gently countering bad ones.

> *I wonder . . .*
> *It might help if . . .*
> *I expect that if we . . .* (never say what will happen, only what seems likely)

Explicit categorisation can help, telling your patient that there are three things, for example, you want him or her to know, and that they are as follows.

6 Frame your suggested management plan

Being patient centred is shepherding rather than abdicating all responsibility for decisions to the patient. As well as exploring concerns, you will have a framework of things you need to discuss that might include reasons for each medication (offering to write these down), need for follow-up (hospital and cardiac rehabilitation nurse) and secondary preventive modifications to lifestyle. Most patients prefer doctors who are open, informative and consider their concerns, but with one proviso – that their doctor appears to be *actively in control of the problem*. A good analogy is with active and passive listening. A doctor who sits forward, makes good eye contact and seems attentive is more likely to inspire confidence than one who sits back and appears uninterested. Equally, a doctor who is actively trying to negotiate the best management strategy through considered, informed discussion is more likely to achieve a better outcome.

7 Respond to patient cues

Throughout, be alert to his reactions or ask what he thinks, encouraging good ideas while gently countering bad ones.

8 Confirm understanding

It can sometimes be useful to ask the patient to recount what they feel to be the important points of the discussion.

9 Encourage feedback and invite questions

> *I appreciate we've covered rather a lot there. Is there anything you would like me to go over again or are there any questions you would like to ask me?*

10 Agree a way forward and ensure follow-up arrangements are in place

Reassure him of follow-up arrangements with your team, including the cardiac rehabilitation team, that you will contact his general practitioner (GP) about his condition and that you would happily review sooner at any time at his or his GP's request if there were questions or concerns.

Discussion

What do you understand by the term chronic disease or long-term condition (LTC)?

A 2005 Department of Health document, Supporting People with Long Term Conditions (a term deemed favourable to chronic disease) highlighted the problems faced by the NHS. LTCs generally last longer than a year, are incurable, require ongoing care and often progress. They include diabetes, arthritis, asthma, coronary heart disease and chronic heart failure.

Should LTCs be managed by primary or secondary care?

Integration is crucial! Multiple areas of care have evolved separately in the NHS (primary care, secondary care, outpatient clinics, social care, mental health, intermediate care), but the assumption in the past was that GPs would coordinate all care. An ageing population and proliferation of LTCs make this an increasingly difficult task. Ideally, secondary-care admissions should fit as acute episodes within a continuum of care for a chronic process that is integrated between multiple services in close liaison. The three broad contexts of managing LTCs are acute care, disease management (monitoring, treatment adjustments, secondary prevention) and frailty management (recognising when patients, often with multiple LTCs, and often in the last year or two of life, can no longer adapt to their environment).

Is there a role for community geriatricians?

The proportions of elderly people with LTCs and of frail elderly are expanding with a predicted doubling of people aged over 80 in the next 20 years. The British Geriatrics Society in 1994 reinforced the need for the role of community geriatricians. These are consultants working mostly in the community in teams with physiotherapists, occupational therapists, specialist nurses and other allied health professionals, with access to acute hospital beds. Their roles include community clinics providing easy access and immediate liaison with primary care, community hospital ward rounds with primary care, intermediate care (hospital at home, rapid response teams, residential rehabilitation, domiciliary rehabilitation), domiciliary visiting, telephone linkage and an advisory service. In common with elderly care physicians working in acute hospital trusts, they also advise on investigations and treatments and on the limits of treatments, can provide specialist clinics and have important roles in clinical governance and education.

A major role of day hospitals, where patients could receive low-intensity investigation, treatment and care was to preserve frail people in the community, but this, sadly, was largely eroded by the advent of private nursing home care.

Are domiciliary visits still important?

Domiciliary visits generally serve one of three purposes – the assessment of patients too unwell or frail to visit outpatient clinics, to assess patients in their own environment and understand the medical and social context and, rarely these days, to provide the human face of the hospital – seen by many as a place of no return to be feared – and reassure that the aim is to enable rather than be the thin end of the wedge that culminates in nursing home placement.

CASE 4.8

ENCOURAGING CONCORDANCE WITH TREATMENT AND PREVENTION

Candidate information

Role

You are a doctor in the medical outpatient clinic.
  Please read this summary.

Scenario

> Re: Mr Mark Davey, aged 46 years
>
> Mr Davey was in hospital two months ago with severe hypertension (240/120 on admission) and renal impairment. Investigations did not reveal a secondary cause for hypertension and urinalysis revealed isolated proteinuria. The renal team decided against renal biopsy and thought it very likely he had nephrosclerosis from hypertension. He was established on an angiotensin-converting enzyme (ACE) inhibitor and calcium channel blocker. His ECG showed left ventricular hypertrophy. His blood pressure on discharge was 140/85 but today in clinic is 180/100. He told the nurse that he has not been taking his medications because he has felt well.
>
> Your task is to discuss ways to improve his blood pressure control.

Your examiners will warn you when 12 minutes have elapsed. You have 14 minutes to communicate with the patient/subject followed by 1 minute of reflection. There will then follow 5 minutes of discussion with the examiners. Do not take the history again except for details that will help in your discussion with the patient/subject. You are not required to examine the patient/subject.

Patient/subject information

Mr Mark Davey is a 46-year-old gentleman being reviewed in clinic. He was in hospital two months ago with headaches, severe hypertension and resulting kidney damage. Investigations did not reveal a secondary cause for hypertension. He was started on perindopril and amlodipine to control his blood pressure but stopped taking these soon after discharge because he developed an irritating cough. He has felt well since and did not see a need to continue medications. The hospital team had told him it was important to continue taking tablets but he does not remember the reason. He has a wife and two children and enjoys life. He is not overweight, but has successfully given up smoking. He manages a vineyard, but does not consume excess alcohol.

How to approach the case

Communication skills (conduct of interview, exploration and problem negotiation) and ethics and law

1 Introduction

Introduce yourself and confirm his identity.

2 Clarify the task

Make it clear that achieving better control of his blood pressure is the aim of the discussion. Do not assume at the start that you are dealing with poor concordance.

3 Explore whether poor concordance could be a problem

The term concordance is often preferred to compliance because the former suggests agreement between patient and doctor. Concordance should always be checked before evaluating the effectiveness of a treatment. Non-concordance with antihypertensives is common, and it is important not to apportion blame. Patients do not take medications for many reasons and the discussion should begin with this premise and not by highlighting this patient's 'failure'. Before you attempt to influence him in taking his medications, consider the three questions in Box 4.8.

4 Be alert to ideas, concerns and expectations

His cough is probably the result of the ACE inhibitor but he may think it a side effect of all antihypertensives. He may, at the time, have appreciated the severity of his illness but may not understand that despite feeling well, hypertension could lead to worsening chronic kidney disease and an ultimate need for renal replacement therapy. He may also not understand the other effects of uncontrolled hypertension, notably stroke.

5 Counter misunderstandings

Explain that ACE inhibitors can cause cough, but not amlodipine, and that there are alternatives (e.g. angiotensin receptor blockers). Explain the risks of uncontrolled hypertension.

6 Discuss management options within a clear framework

Frame the discussion around advantages that are likely to be important to him – retarding progressive chronic kidney disease, reduction in stroke risk, need for future hospital admissions and so on. Such *gift-wrapping* of treatments can be highly effective. Sometimes illustrating the point with reference to a similar case can help. Explain that all blood pressure tablets can have side effects but that these are usually mild and if problematic a different tablet can always be considered.

7 Repeat important information

This is especially important when poor concordance may be the result of misunderstanding or previous poor explanation.

8 Confirm understanding

It can sometimes be useful to ask the patient to recount what he or she feels to be the important points of the discussion.

9 Encourage feedback and invite questions

> *I appreciate we've covered rather a lot there. Is there anything you would like me to go over again or are there any questions you would like to ask me?*

10 Agree a way forward and ensure follow-up arrangements are in place

Reassure him of follow-up arrangements and that you would happily review sooner at any time at his or his general practitioner's request if there are questions or concerns.

Discussion

A 34-year-old man being treated for a high-grade non-Hodgkin's lymphoma on your haematology ward is three days into a chemotherapy regimen involving high-dose steroids. This morning, according to your house officer, he was in a strange mood, tearful but also declaring he believed himself cured. He left the ward in pyjamas and overcoat and has not returned. What should be done?

Patients have the right to decide how they are going to be treated and indeed whether they are going to be treated. Such autonomy should be respected. However, where declining treatment is likely to have serious consequences it is imperative to explore a patient's reasoning. Here, iat-

---

Box 4.8 Questions about concordance

Are you dealing with poor concordance?

Often the importance of taking medications has not been carefully explained or sufficiently emphasised. Even when explained, patients may still not fully understand or may forget the importance of medication.

Is poor concordance the result of iatrogenic symptoms?

Always consider drug side effects or drug–drug interactions as a reason for a patient not taking prescribed medication.

Is there another reason for the poor concordance that needs to be explored?

Very often, poor concordance is the result of a discrepancy between what the doctor sees as important and what the patient sees as important.

Box 4.9 Discussing smoking cessation

Ask about current smoking status

This includes asking about whether other household members smoke.

Advise about the benefits of smoking cessation

These include physical, social, financial and cosmetic. Emphasise the health benefits of stopping rather than the risks of continuing smoking. Reinforce the patient's own motivation for wanting to stop.

Ask about reasons for wanting to stop and assess motivation

Ask if the patient really wants to stop and if they would be prepared to stop now or within the next few weeks. Find out about previous attempts to stop and what measures helped or hindered. Ask if other household members are also willing to stop.

Discuss ways of assisting

These could include setting a date and stopping completely, enlisting the help of family and friends, enlisting the help of health promotion services and general practitioner, nicotine replacement therapy (best avoided in severe cardiovascular disorders) and amfebutamone. It helps many patients to consider themselves 'non-smokers' rather than 'ex-smokers'.

---

rogenic mood disturbance from high-dose steroids must be considered, and his 'autonomy' questioned until further assessment has been made. Informing ward staff, the consultant, the patient's general practitioner, relatives, and, on discussion with the consultant, involving hospital security and the police (restraint under the Mental Health Act is generally a last resort but may need to be instituted), are steps which may be needed to ensure his safety.

How might you help persuade a patient to stop smoking?

As well as its serious cardiac, respiratory and neoplastic risks, smoking carries considerable social harms and promotes premature ageing. Smoking cessation (Box 4.9) carries immediate benefits, including mortality reduction, and reduces the risk of many diseases including cardiovascular disease, chronic obstructive pulmonary disease, cancer of lung, mouth, throat, larynx, oesophagus, pancreas, bladder and cervix, peptic ulcer disease and complications of pregnancy. Nicotine addiction is now acknowledged as a treatable condition and there is substantial evidence of the effectiveness and cost-effectiveness of behavioural and pharmacological interventions.

COMMUNICATION IN SPECIAL CIRCUMSTANCES

CASE 4.9

CROSS-CULTURAL COMMUNICATION

Candidate information

Role

You are a doctor in the medical outpatient clinic.
Please read this summary.

Scenario

> Re: Mr Ash Khan, aged 38 years
>
> Mr Khan is an asylum seeker. He has been in the UK for one year with his family and was referred to your clinic with sweats, fevers and painful joints, although language differences have thwarted some elements of history taking on previous occasions. On one occasion you had an interpreter in clinic but he is not here today. However, Mr Khan's English comprehension has improved steadily over the last year. After extensive investigations he appears to have chronic osteomyelitis of his knee. Tuberculosis has not been suggested by chest X-ray or other results so far.
>
> Your task is to explain the likely diagnosis to him and propose referral to your orthopaedic colleagues for further treatment and possible bone biopsy and surgery.

Your examiners will warn you when 12 minutes have elapsed. You have 14 minutes to communicate with the patient/subject followed by 1 minute of reflection. There will then follow 5 minutes of discussion with the examiners. Do not take the history again except for details that will help in your discussion with the patient/subject. You are not required to examine the patient/subject.

Patient/subject information

Mr Ash Khan is a 38-year-old asylum seeker. He has been in the UK for one year with his wife and two children and has found work in a restaurant. He was referred to clinic with sweats, fevers and painful joints, although language differences have thwarted good history taking on previous occasions. On one occasion there was an interpreter in clinic but he is not here today. However, Mr Khan's English comprehension has improved steadily over the last year. After extensive investigations he appears to have chronic osteomyelitis affecting his knee. Tuberculosis is

possible but not likely on the basis of tests so far. Mr Khan simply wants to be relieved of pain and has been taking a lot of tablets from a local herbalist.

How to approach the case

Communication skills (conduct of interview, exploration and problem negotiation) and ethics and law

1 Introduction

Introduce yourself and confirm his identity. Inevitably if there are language differences a consultation has the potential to take longer and ideally in practice (not in PACES) you would allow more time for this.

2 Remember to treat patients equally and do not do very much differently!

When people communicate, there is a vast array of cultural influences. Cultural background, health beliefs and expectations affect all health-care encounters with patients. These differences may seem stark when there is an additional language difficulty, but perhaps most important is to remember that we are usually more similar to each other than we are different! The range of human beliefs, concerns and expectations that we must be aware of with any patient needs to be considered, and perhaps with heightened awareness when treating people from different cultures. Beware of the tendency to stereotype people – to assume they have characteristics because they appear to belong to a certain group. When stereotyped, people can become victims of prejudice – opinions, often unfavourable, formed without good reason. This can jeopardise good care.

3 Establish as far as possible the patient's concerns and give non-verbal reassurance

This patient might simply want to have his pain relieved, and you should indicate that this too is a concern of yours, but that you wish to treat the underlying cause.

4 Frame your suggested management plan

The medical steps are fairly clear – continuing to relieve pain, and urgent referral to orthopaedic colleagues. Sometimes religious reasons mandate an approach to management. During Ramadan, for example, Muslim patients may not eat anything, including tablets, during daylight hours and often eat a large meal after dark. Type 2 diabetes is common in Asian people and, if Muslim, there may be important repercussions on the style of management chosen.

5 Keep explanations clear and simple, avoiding jargon

The same principles of good communication apply when dealing with patients from different cultures. In other words, you should try to do more of the same, rather than treat such patients differently. In this case, as well as explaining the way forward with respect to input by the knee specialists, you might need to counter the herbal remedy beliefs. You might also need to explore his work further, particularly if tuberculosis is still in question!

6 Repeat important information

This can be particularly important when communicating with people whose first language is not English.

7 Respond to patient cues

Throughout, be alert to his reactions or ask what he thinks, encouraging good ideas while gently countering bad ones.

8 Confirm understanding and acceptance

It would be important to ask him to recount what he understands to be the main points of the discussion.

9 Encourage feedback and invite questions

Is there anything you would like me to go over again or are there any questions you would like to ask me?

10 Agree a way forward and ensure follow-up arrangements are in place

Ensure that there are arrangements for treatment and follow-up.

Discussion

What do you understand by the term culture?

'Culture' refers to the shared beliefs, values and attitudes that guide the behaviour of a social group. It is applied most commonly to describe people of a shared national, ethnic or regional origin, but there is a dynamic social context for every individual's culture that embraces age, gender, education, socio-economic background, language, family, occupation, religion and so forth.

What potential problems may arise when using interpreters?

These are outlined in Box 4.10.

Box 4.10 Potential problems when using interpreters

- Assuming the patient cannot understand any of what is being said – beware of assumptions and seek to find out what a patient can and cannot understand
- Failure to address both the patient and the interpreter
- Failure to communicate simply and in small chunks
- Incorrect understanding or transmission of information
- Avoidance of delicate topics
- Domination of the patient by the interpreter
- Failure to allow enough time (at least a doubling of time is often required)

CASE 4.10

COMMUNICATING WITH ANGRY PATIENTS OR RELATIVES

Candidate information

Role

You are a doctor on the medical ward.
    Please read this summary.

Scenario

Re: Mr Charlie Buchanan, aged 69 years

Mr Buchanan has a left hilar mass on his chest X-ray, discovered during the course of investigations for pneumonia. The computed tomography (CT) scan suggests a potentially operable bronchial carcinoma, with lymphoma the main differential diagnosis. Although recovered from his pneumonia, and now feeling well, he was kept as an inpatient because the respiratory team had a slot for bronchoscopy at the end of the week. However, you have now been informed it has been postponed because of a full list of urgent bronchoscopy appointments. You are also aware that the respiratory team is thin on the ground next week because of a conference in Italy and have been informed by the respiratory specialist registrar that it will be the week after next. He advises you to send Mr Buchanan home in the meantime. Mr Buchanan is angry.

Your tasks are to listen to his concerns and discuss possible solutions.

Your examiners will warn you when 12 minutes have elapsed. You have 14 minutes to communicate with the patient/subject followed by 1 minute of reflection. There will then follow 5 minutes of discussion with the examiners. Do not take the history again except for details that will help in your discussion with the patient/subject. You are not required to examine the patient/subject.

Patient/subject information

Mr Buchanan is a 69-year-old gentleman with possible lung cancer discovered on chest X-ray during the course of investigations for pneumonia. The CT scan suggests a potentially operable tumour. Although recovered from pneumonia, and now feeling well, he was kept in hospital because the respiratory team had arranged his broncho-scopy at the end of the week. However, the respiratory specialist nurse advised him that this has now been postponed and that it might be best if he went home because the respiratory team will not be around next week. Mr Buchanan does not think he should be told 'what is best for him'. Mr Buchanan lives alone and his son and daughter-in-law are going on holiday next week. He has a history of anxiety and depression and feels that going home without all of this being resolved and without support will be hard. His wife died from oesophageal cancer two years ago and he recalls similar delays with her investigations. He is worried that each day missed is a day when the cancer could be spreading. He has always been an avid supporter of the NHS but his support is now beginning to waver and with this news he feels angry. He is particularly upset that the respiratory team are going to be 'sunning themselves' while he waits for vital tests.

How to approach the case

Communication skills (conduct of interview, exploration and problem negotiation) and ethics and law

1   Introduce yourself

Introduce yourself and confirm the name/identity of the patient.

2   Make it clear that you want to help

Show from the outset that you are here to try to help. Remain polite. The nature of medical training equips most doctors well with the skills of negotiation. Some patients simply do not have these skills. People are capable of acting out of character and appearing aggressive when upset. His primary motivation is likely to be fear or distress and he is depending on you to help. Do not take any criticisms of the system personally.

3   Remember to deal with emotions before facts and that anger is not usually anger

Always try to calm emotions before dealing with any facts and remember that anger is usually secondary to another emotion such as fear, guilt or uncertainty. Discovering the underlying emotion is far more likely to achieve resolution than taking anger at face value. Since minor disagreement can explode unpredictably into more serious confrontation, dialogue should, from the start, work towards de-escalation and resolution.

4   Acknowledge the concerns

Legitimising rather than confronting his understandable concerns will help bridge the gap between his initial anger and your remit to help.

Obviously you are very upset by this. I understand. I can understand fully why you are upset. I am very concerned, too, that you are having to wait.

5   Explore the emotions and concerns

In this case, fear of cancer spreading and opening of the old wounds of his wife's experiences will doubtless be at the forefront of his mind.

I agree that we must sort this out as quickly as possible. I will do everything I can to help. It will help me if I understand what you fear most if the investigations are delayed.

6   Work towards resolution, weaving in the facts

Steer away from areas of conflict – comments from other staff that may have upset him, for example. Good communication and finding common ground are the keys to successful resolution. Focus on constructive ways forward.

7   Try to ameliorate concerns that can honestly be ameliorated

Give clear advice and honest professional opinions about the implications of delay. Delays in investigations are unhappily part of everyday experience in the NHS, and not always with as devastating implications as patients imagine.

8   Never criticise colleagues

Avoid comments that might incriminate colleagues. It would not help to focus on the fact that the respiratory team are in Italy next week, as educational events are inevitable and essential components of medicine and you are not responsible for how another team has organised itself or at liberty to comment. Criticism of any colleague or department or service is always counterproductive. Most NHS employees are stretched and working together is paramount.

9   Encourage feedback and invite questions

I appreciate we've covered rather a lot there. Is there anything you would like me to go over again or are there any questions you would like to ask me?

10   Agree a way forward

Assure him that you will find out exactly when his test is going to be.

Discussion

Would you encourage him to make a formal complaint?

He is perfectly at liberty to complain, but more imperative is to find a mutual way forward than potentially drive the divide further by encouraging a complaint. However, if he requests help in making a complaint you should direct him to the local complaints procedure. If you feel that there may be a system failure (unlikely in this case) a Clinical Incident report could be forwarded to Trust Risk Management.

Box 4.11 Handling threatening, abusive and violent behaviour

- Unhappily abuse by patients to staff is increasingly common, often threatening words but sometimes physical or even sexual.
- Doctors must avoid the temptation to take the law into their own hands, and first and foremost must appreciate that there are often medical reasons for this (confusion due to infection or metabolic disturbance, for example) and such patients cannot be left without treatment.
- If threats are towards a particular staff member they should no longer be involved in that patient's care.
- Sedation may be considered if violence is a symptom of illness and it is necessary to prevent injury to patient or staff.
- Restraining measures are occasionally necessary, but may inflame or worsen a situation and cot-sides are frankly dangerous.
- Advice from a psychiatrist may be sought, especially if anti-psychotic medication is needed.
- Security should be called immediately if a patient is physically violent but removal by the police is not acceptable if there are medical reasons underlying the behaviour.
- Empathy and practical support might need to be given to nursing and other staff.

What do you do if a patient is threatening, abusive or violent?

Strategies are outlined in Box 4.11.

CASE 4.11

COMMUNICATING WITH UPSET OR DISTRESSED RELATIVES

Candidate information

Role

You are a doctor in the emergency medical admissions unit.

Please read this summary.

Scenario

Re: Mr George Tilner, aged 63 years

Ms Tilner is the sister of a 63-year-old gentleman, Mr George Tilner, who has just died in the emergency department. He had advanced non-Hodgkin's lymphoma, no longer responsive to chemotherapy and recently received palliative radiotherapy. He was admitted two hours earlier from a peripheral hospital with sepsis and peri-arrest but your rapid perusal of his case notes showed that he had spinal and renal metastases and you decided that a decision to resuscitate would not be appropriate if he had a cardiac or respiratory arrest despite fluids and antibiotics. He was an accountant and his last wish was that he completed his clients' work and that his briefcase be brought with him in the ambulance. You

know that his sister is in the relative's room, and is very upset. Your personal feeling is that an advance decision should have been made to manage any deterioration at the peripheral hospital.

Your tasks are to explain to her that he has died, and manage the emotional situation.

Your examiners will warn you when 12 minutes have elapsed. You have 14 minutes to communicate with the patient/subject followed by 1 minute of reflection. There will then follow 5 minutes of discussion with the examiners. Do not take the history again except for details that will help in your discussion with the patient/subject. You are not required to examine the patient/subject.

Patient/subject information

You are the sister of Mr George Tilner, a 63-year-old man admitted to the emergency department two hours ago from a peripheral hospital. He has advanced non-Hodgkin's lymphoma, no longer responsive to chemotherapy and he recently received radiotherapy. You have just arrived at the hospital, having received a call from nursing staff at the peripheral hospital to say your brother was very unwell with infection and was being transferred to the emergency department. He was an accountant and his last wish was that he completed his clients' work. Although you knew he was very unwell, you are still awaiting news from the doctor about his condition. You hope the doctors will do all that they can to save his life, but your sister-in-law is a district nurse and has gradually persuaded your over recent weeks that in the event of a deterioration from which recovery seems remote it might be best to 'let him go' peacefully. You are about to speak to the doctor.

How to approach the case

Communication skills (conduct of interview, exploration and problem negotiation) and ethics and law

1 Preparation and scene setting

Introduce yourself and confirm the identity of the relative. Ideally, you would ensure that a member of nursing staff is there, and talk in a setting where interruptions are very unlikely to occur. Sit at the same level as the relative, and use a calm tone.

2 Give vital information early

Do not give a detailed account of events up to his death, other than making it clear that he was very unwell.

Ms Tilner, your brother was very unwell – comatose – when he arrived, and I am very sorry to tell you that he has passed away.

While bad news communicated to patients should be delivered gently with attention to cues from the patient, communicating the death of a patient to a relative should be equally gentle but not delayed, with attention to cues guiding subsequent discussion.

3 Deal with emotions before facts

She is unlikely to take in much more, if any, information immediately. Allow her time to exhibit emotions.

4 Acknowledge distress and support ventilation of feelings

Above all, people need to know that you understand, and you can do so non-verbally, practically (e.g. by offering tissues) or by acknowledging that emotions are understandable (legitimising). Remember that at this point patients are too preoccupied to assimilate further information.

5 Respond to patient cues

Throughout, be alert to any cues.

6 Gently explain what happened

Usually, distressed relatives say what they need to say, and you are there to support, acknowledge and provide whatever additional comfort seems intuitive.

> I know that he was very ill. And I know he wouldn't have wanted to suffer. His wife, my sister-in-law, knew that he didn't have very long. It's just such a shock. But he wouldn't have wanted things to drag on and be in pain, I know that.

It might be right to say, at this point

> I know it may not be of any great comfort now, but I think it is important you know that I do not believe that he was in any pain . . . or even aware of things.

Keep all explanation clear and straightforward.

7 Do not raise personal concerns

Your feeling that acute admission might have been avoided with advance planning is not helpful at this time. Focus on supporting her through what has happened.

8 Identify patient support systems

Try to establish who, if anyone, is going to be available to be with her.

9 Check present information needs

While it is generally good practice to encourage feedback and invite questions, this is one situation where asking a relative if she has further questions can sound a little pressurising if handled as a direct question. It might be preferable to give an assurance that you can answer questions now but are available to talk further at any time later.

10 Make clear what support is available

> I'll leave you with sister/staff nurse for now, but I am here, and my team are here, at any time.

Discussion

How might you detach yourself from distressed relatives?

It can sometimes be difficult to detach yourself from relatives who are very distressed or upset, although largely there is a discernible point when all that is to be said has been said and relatives are not ready or able to ask more questions. You should always leave relatives with a point of contact, usually a nurse, and express your willingness to come back at any time if there is anything you might help with or answer.

CASE 4.12

DISCHARGE AGAINST MEDICAL ADVICE

Candidate information

Role

You are a doctor on the medical ward.
    Please read this summary.

Scenario

Re: Miss Sarah Walker, aged 23 years

Miss Walker was admitted 12 days ago with high fevers, subsequently confirmed as acute bacterial endocarditis. She has been on intravenous antibiotics four times daily with advice from microbiology. She was taking intravenous heroin until the date of admission and with assistance from the drug and alcohol advisory service is now on an appropriate methadone replacement regimen. She now wishes to discharge herself from hospital. She says that she feels better. She spends considerable time off the ward smoking, and the nursing staff have expressed concerns about possible ongoing drug misuse, as her partner meets her outside the hospital. Your medical plan is to keep her in hospital until her inflammatory markers are much improved, with repeat echocardiography. There remains the possibility of cardiothoracic surgery being needed if her valve decompensates.

Your tasks are to explore her reasons for wanting to self-discharge, discuss the medical reasons for her staying and find alternative solutions if she cannot be persuaded to stay.

Your examiners will warn you when 12 minutes have elapsed. You have 14 minutes to communicate with the patient/subject followed by 1 minute of reflection. There will then follow 5 minutes of discussion with the examiners. Do not take the history again except for details that will help in your discussion with the patient/subject. You are not required to examine the patient/subject.

Patient/subject information

Miss Sarah Walker is a 23 year old admitted 12 days ago with high fevers, subsequently confirmed as acute bacterial endocarditis. She has been on intravenous antibiotics four times daily. She was taking intravenous heroin until the date of admission and with assistance from the drug and alcohol advisory service is now on a methadone replacement regimen but does not feel the dose adequate because she still feels psychological withdrawal. She is very keen to try to stop heroin altogether. She has two young children at home, both currently being looked after by her partner. She has little confidence in him doing so because he was the person who introduced her to drugs and continues to keep unreliable hours at home. She is meeting him regularly outside the hospital to try to negotiate his agreeing to her sister, whom she trusts, caring for the children. She now wishes to discharge herself from hospital because of her concerns. She spends considerable time off the ward smoking, but feels the attitudes of the nursing staff are prejudiced against this, while she feels it is currently her only enjoyment. Venous access is poor and although she has 'had enough' of treatment she might be persuaded to continue if she knows her children are safe.

How to approach the case

Communication skills (conduct of interview, exploration and problem negotiation) and ethics and law

1 Introduction

Introduce yourself and confirm her identity.

2 Make it clear you want to help

It is crucial to start with the premise that she may have fully understandable reasons for wanting to leave hospital, and show that you are prepared to listen to these.

3 Explore concerns and reasons for wanting to self-discharge

Patients' stated reasons for wanting to self-discharge may mask deeper or more personal reasons. Fears for family members are often high on the list. Frequently a list of factors conspires to make the hospital unpalatable – uncomfortable investigations and treatments, poor communication, noisy wards, other patients, disturbed sleep, unpalatable food . . .

4 Explain the medical reasons for wanting the patient to stay

This is essential for her to reach an informed decision because she might be unaware that the microorganisms must be fully eradicated (and that this usually requires a few weeks of intravenous antibiotics) otherwise the problem will recur, with worsening damage to the valve. Explain also that the diseased valve must be reassessed after treatment. Confirm her knowledge that intravenous drug use is a high-risk practice for developing endocarditis.

5 Aim to address the patient's concerns

It would be wise to ask the social worker to review the welfare of the children. This could be presented in a non-judgemental way to her partner. He would have a right to look after his children if he is the father and he is fit to do so but if he is not the father, or if there are concerns as to his fitness to do so, then social workers could become involved on the presumption of assistance but in parallel explore the children's safety. It might also be possible for the children to visit hospital more or for her to be allowed home for periods of time between antibiotic treatment, although not wise to send her into the community with an intravenous cannula. Addressing her other concerns could also lessen the impact of hospitalisation.

6 Accept that the patient may self-discharge

It is, ultimately, a competent, informed patient's acceptable choice to self-discharge if she or he wishes.

7 If self-discharge seems inevitable, try to reach the best compromise

This might include discussing with the microbiologist the possibility of less frequent intravenous antibiotics delivered by a district nurse and/or oral antibiotics and early follow-up in clinic.

8 Confirm understanding and acceptance

Confirm that she is fully informed to make her decision.

9 Encourage feedback and invite questions

I appreciate we've covered rather a lot there. Is there anything you would like me to go over again or are there any questions you would like to ask me?

10 Agree a way forward and ensure follow-up arrangements are in place

Ensure that she signs a self-discharge form taking legal responsibility for her own care, document all discussions clearly and inform your consultant and her general practitioner of arrangements.

Discussion

Is a discharge against medical advice form a legal necessity?

It is not legally necessary, although it may enhance future evidence, to obtain signed declaration by the patient that discharge is against advice. It is important to document that the patient had capacity and was fully informed and understood the medical reasons for staying.

CASE 4.13

DELAYED DISCHARGE

Candidate information

Role

You are a doctor on an elderly care ward.
    Please read this summary.

Scenario

Re: Mrs Anna Clare, aged 93 years

Mrs Clare was admitted to your ward one month ago with numerous medical problems – inoperable peripheral arterial occlusive disease, anaemia due to aspirin-induced gastritis, dizziness induced by antihypertensives and back pain caused by osteoporosis. She has a past history of recurrent strokes and may have had a further one while in hospital. She is now very unsteady even with a walking frame and assistance and is unsafe to go home. She accepts that she may need nursing home care. Her daughter, Mrs Kenton, is keen on this but wants her to stay in hospital until the 'right one comes up'. An interim place is available in a home that is not the daughter's favoured choice.

Your task is to discuss potential discharge solutions with the daughter.

Your examiners will warn you when 12 minutes have elapsed. You have 14 minutes to communicate with the patient/subject followed by 1 minute of reflection. There will then follow 5 minutes of discussion with the examiners. Do not take the history again except for details that will help in your discussion with the patient/subject. You are not required to examine the patient/subject.

Patient/subject information

You are the daughter of Mrs Anna Clare who is aged 93 years. Mrs Clare was admitted to hospital two weeks ago with numerous medical problems (previous strokes, poor circulation, anaemia after aspirin use, dizziness caused by antihypertensives and osteoporosis). The major issue is that she is no longer safe either from the point of view of her mobility or to be at home and has accepted long-term residential care. You have inspected numerous nursing homes on the advice of the social work department and have a very definite favourite where a bed will not be available for an indeterminate time, possibly many weeks. An interim bed is available and has been suggested by the discharge team in an alternative nursing home, but your father died in that nursing home and you do not want your mother to go there. You feel that your mother would receive better care in hospital until the favoured placement becomes available but would be amenable to considering alternatives that did not carry sad and emotive memories. You hope that the doctor will agree to this and feel that your mother deserves such care.

How to approach the case

Communication skills (conduct of interview, exploration and problem negotiation) and ethics and law

1 Introduction

Introduce yourself and confirm the name/identity of the relative.

2 Make it clear that you want to help

Establish from the outset that you want to work with her to find the best possible solution that provides the optimum care her mother deserves. The fastest way to dissolve rapport and thwart a way forward is to give the impression that you are there to tell her what to do.

3 Start by listening and agreeing

Ask her if she understands exactly what has happened to her mother during her lengthy hospital admission, and offer to summarise it. Then state grounds where you are likely to both agree.

> That's right. We are, of course, very pleased that she has recovered somewhat from the problems that brought her into hospital. But there have been significant problems, as I know you are very much aware, some of which are unlikely to go away and some of which could even get worse over time. So it is the opinion of our nursing staff, our therapists, ourselves, and most importantly of course, herself and yourself, that she would be safer in the longer term in a place where full-time care could be provided.

4 Explore ideas, concerns and expectations

Explore any specific fears she has about particular nursing homes. There is a clear reason she does not want to proceed with one nursing home and that is very reasonable to accept.

> *I understand. I am sorry that that one was suggested to you.*

5 State a suggested management plan

> *I understand that you have a favoured nursing home. We would of course support her getting a place there. What may be less easy is to get it quickly, and if that is the case then we need to think very carefully about finding a way forward that is acceptable to her and which provides for her needs.*

She may say that hospital is surely the best place for her mother until such time.

> *Hospital has certainly been the best place for her while she has been so unwell. But an acute hospital setting is not necessarily the best place at this stage. Because our nursing staff and therapists are so necessarily occupied with their acutely unwell patients, they do not always have that much time with less acutely unwell patients, who by their very nature may be more stimulated to do things in a more streamlined setting. There are also risks to being in hospital that we often take for granted but which should not be ignored – the fact that a hospital bed in a ward of acutely unwell patients carries by its very nature an increased risk of developing hospital-acquired infections.*

6 Be alert to cues

She is likely to show acceptance or disappointment at your suggestions. Look out for cues, and respond if necessary.

7 Do not criticise hospital managers

Managers generally want to help and must give patients choice until the multidisciplinary team (MDT) confirms the need for a specific transfer. Never tell patients or relatives you would like patients to stay in but managers will not allow it. We all have a duty to discharge or transfer care as soon as appropriate. Managers are often prepared to come and talk with patients, explaining the number of acute coronary syndromes waiting in emergency departments (there has been an appreciable increase in medical admissions since the mid-1990s but an unparalleled and relentless sharp upstroke, especially in the elderly, since autumn 2004 – with complex reasons but perhaps in part related to a decrease in out-of-hours primary care) and assuring patients that they will get the bed they want but that they cannot wait for it in an acute hospital bed. What they cannot do is put a patient in an exiting ambulance against their will (assault) or evict (not legally tested and brave the Trust that tries!). There will always be the difficult or resistant 1% of patients or relatives (but with the best of intentions and at an emotional time).

8 Encourage feedback and invite questions

> *I appreciate we've covered rather a lot there. Is there anything you would like me to go over again or are there any questions you would like to ask me?*

9 Confirm understanding and acceptance

Make sure that she is generally accepting of your suggestions so far.

10 Agree a way forward

Agree, for example, to speak to the hospital discharge team and discuss appropriate interim alternatives.

Discussion

What is an integrated care pathway (ICP)?

ICPs aim to map a patient's journey from admission to discharge or beyond and have been used for many conditions including stroke but have not been shown to improve outcome measures where a unit already functions well. ICPs are more useful in setting up a new unit from scratch. Clerking pro formas for particular diseases such as stroke, however, may be useful.

Hospital trust managers are very keen on discharge planning. Do you think you should be as concerned as your hospital managers?

Discharge planning is a crucial part of modern hospital practice, and often badly managed. Depending upon the patient, it might include information to patients and carers, training of carers, pre-discharge home visits by the multidisciplinary team (initially to assess the home and subsequently to assess the patient in their home), pre-discharge case conferences for patients with complex care packages, clear instructions of who to contact should there be problems, further community rehabilitation at home or in a day hospital and follow-up arrangements.

What is early supported discharge?

Early discharge of selected patients is cost effective and safe (shown by Langhorne and colleagues in a meta-analysis published in the *Lancet* in 2005). It might include three to seven daily visits per week for up to a month by the multidisciplinary team (e.g. occupational therapy assistant, physiotherapy assistant, health-care assistant).

Is there a role for discharge assessment teams (DATs)?

Increasing pressure on ward staff with acute admissions within a target-driven health service, and in the context of changing community resources, and a thrust towards patient choice have led to difficulties in finding time for optimum discharge planning. DATs take referrals for patients when a complex discharge is likely. Such patients might be elderly, need rehabilitation, have social problems including homelessness, or have palliative care needs. Concerns might also be raised by the family. DATs help patients through the system by ensuring maximum utilisation of community hospital beds, identifying rehabilitation needs, ensuring timely paperwork, working with, for example, social work and palliative care, and generally acting as a resource for discharge-related dilemmas. Patients will generally be discharged to one of three settings:

Home

A good social history is vital, and DATS may work to integrate this information, for example by using a booklet at the end of the bed for the patient and family to fill out, along with:

- assessing the realism of patient's expectations
- ensuring early referral to occupational therapy, physiotherapy or social work
- prompting multidisciplinary discussion
- prompting specialist assessment of care needs (SACN) and care packages
- identifying community resources such as nurse specialists, the voluntary sector, the housing department and interim placement.

Rehabilitation or other interim settings

DATs co-ordinate rehabilitation or other community beds for patients who might benefit from rehabilitation or for patients with chronic diseases, who have palliative care needs or who are awaiting care packages or assessment for entry into long-term care.

Care home

This may be residential or nursing, but the term care home has been adopted since 2003.

Ideally the patient, the family and the MDT should agree on this. Once medically ready for discharge and the SACN has been given to the social work department, a patient's discharge is officially delayed, and there then arises:

- pressure on the patient and family to find a care home (or accept interim placement) based on advice from social workers as to which may be appropriate based on the SACN (if a nursing home is needed then the nursing home also assesses the patient)

- pressure on the social work department whose reimbursement starts dwindling for each day lost and pressure on the hospital because an acute bed is blocked.

What is meant by delayed transfer of care (DTOC)?

DTOC occurs when a patient is ready for discharge from an acute bed (clinical decision, multidisciplinary team decision, safe to do so) and there is no medical reason for the delay. There are various categories, depending on the reason for DTOC, such as lack of availability of onward placement, delayed funding, delay in arranging domiciliary packages or delay in community equipment. It incurs bills immediately to social services. The conflicting mantras imposed on the NHS of expanding patient choice (which often drives unrealistic expectations) and targets for acute care (with four-hour movement through emergency departments but prompt discharge if there is not an acute problem) mean that doctors and managers must work together towards the same goal.

What is meant by the term intermediate care?

This refers to care outside the acute setting that occupies a transition period to another setting. It includes rehabilitation after an acute event, responses to an overt crisis and care while long-term care is being considered or assessed.

How is a patient assessed for entry into long-term care?

Individual trusts have developed pro formas assessing not just the medical diagnosis and treatment but multidisciplinary team assessment of breathing, feeding and diet, gut function, bladder, toileting, dressing, mobility and transfer, stair assessment, skin, pain, sensation (hearing, vision), communication, comprehension, sleep, memory, depression and anxiety, initiative and involvement, relationships, past roles and physical behaviours. Pro formas also consider requirements for equipment.

What is meant by the term 'continuing care'?

This refers to a situation where, following a thorough assessment of needs, a person's overall health needs are judged so great that the NHS will manage and pay for all the care they need. An NHS professional supervises the agreed care plan, which can be in any setting, for example a person's own home, a hospice, care home or hospital.

BREAKING BAD NEWS

CASE 4.14

CANCER – POTENTIALLY CURABLE

Candidate information

Role

You are a doctor on the medical ward.
Please read this summary.

Scenario

> Re: Mr James Oakley, aged 58 years
>
> Mr Oakley is a previously well gentleman on your ward with recent night sweats, weight loss and abdominal discomfort. He works as an information technology consultant and has been under a lot of work stress recently, travelling a lot and under pressure to meet sales targets. He attributed his symptoms to this but his GP admitted him with high fever and marked splenomegaly. He was initially treated for possible atypical pneumonia but his full blood picture suggests possible chronic myeloid leukaemia. The haematology team plan to perform a bone marrow aspirate and trephine but he wants to know the diagnosis you suspect.
>
> Your task is to discuss the possible diagnosis, addressing his concerns.

Your examiners will warn you when 12 minutes have elapsed. You have 14 minutes to communicate with the patient/subject followed by 1 minute of reflection. There will then follow 5 minutes of discussion with the examiners. Do not take the history again except for details that will help in your discussion with the patient/subject. You are not required to examine the patient/subject.

Patient/subject information

Mr James Oakley is a previously well 58-year-old gentleman with a history of recent night sweats and abdominal discomfort. He works as an information technology consultant and has been under a lot of work stress recently, travelling a lot and under pressure to meet sales targets. He attributed his symptoms to this but his GP admitted him with high fever and marked splenomegaly. He was initially treated for pneumonia but his blood tests are apparently not so straightforward. The haematology doctors plan to perform a bone marrow aspiration but he wants to know why, and what diagnosis his doctors suspect. He is married with two children and is keen to get back to work soon.

How to approach the case

Communication skills (conduct of interview, exploration and problem negotiation) and ethics and law

1 Preparation and scene setting

'Bad news' is any information that drastically changes a patient's view of their future for the worse. The way in which it is communicated affects their perception of the situation and, crucially, their attitude to living with an illness and the ability to adjust. Many candidates are naturally adept at creating rapport and building a feeling of trust with patients. Important components of preparing include:

- Having the time and privacy to talk without interruptions
- Being clear about the diagnosis, problem or test results so far and suitable ways forward
- The presence (not in PACES) of a supportive co-worker such as a named nurse or ward sister
- The presence (not in PACES) of a relative or close person if a patient wishes
- Sitting close enough for good eye contact and detection of non-verbal cues; sitting at the same level as the patient rather than above (or worse, standing), is less threatening to an already apprehensive patient
- Opening with a neutral statement

> *How are you feeling today?*
> *You and I know that you have had these pains in your tummy for some time now.*

- Active listening, being attentive to what you hear and showing concern and empathy through eye contact, head nodding and other natural body language

In short, your patient should feel that this discussion is the most important thing on your agenda, and not that you are distracted.

2 Establish what the patient knows already

Establishing previous experience and knowledge is crucial. The rule is to ask before telling with such questions as:

> *Can you tell me what you understand about your illness?*
> *I believe you put your symptoms down to stresses at work. Did any other possibilities cross your mind?*
> *Have you thought about any other possibilities for the cause of your symptoms?*

Such a question both explores ideas and concerns and prepares for more serious news. He might elaborate his concerns about the possibilities. Non-verbal skills such as silence, active listening and simple words such as *yes, and then* and *hmm*, and repeating and reflecting back information you are told can be very effective.

So you had been worried about something like that?

He might indicate immediately that he has an idea of what might be wrong.

I'm worried it might be cancer.

If he already suspects a diagnosis then it is possible to gently confirm rather than break bad news at this stage.

3 Establish what the patient wants to know

A very useful step if handled well. Possible questions are

You said you wanted me to be honest and open with you. Are you the sort of person who likes to know everything about his condition?
Would you like me to explain the problem as we understand it so far?
We can't be certain of what is wrong from the tests so far. But are you the sort of person who likes to know all the possibilities?

Patients tend to declare outright or indicate that they do not want to talk about their disease (in which case it may be appropriate to ask if they would like you to explain things in more detail to a relative) or they want to know more.

4 Give a warning shot

When a patient is apparently unaware of potential bad news, the skill is in conveying information without provoking overwhelming distress or pushing them into denial

I'm afraid that things look a little more complicated than we had thought/hoped.
I'm afraid it doesn't look like a straightforward infection.

The next thing to do is wait! Allow time for the warning shot to sink in. He can signal that no further information is wanted

Just tell me what we have to do next.

or that more information is wanted

What do you mean not straightforward?

5 Break bad news gently

When the pathologist looked at the blood samples he found some abnormal cells.

Again, he can signal 'enough'

What do you need to do next?

or 'go on'

What do you mean by abnormal? I need to know if you mean what I think you do?

At this point be as honest and informative as possible

There is a possibility that they might be cancerous, a form of blood cancer or leukaemia.

Bad news should always be broken gently but not be unduly delayed. It should be given in clear, simple, small pieces and patients should be given plenty of opportunity to respond or question at any stage. Important information should be repeated and patient understanding might need to be checked, remembering that patients are likely to experience a heavy impact and that repeating the word 'cancer' is not necessary unless it is very clear that it has not been understood. Such fear words are best used only when a diagnosis is established beyond doubt or is a strong possibility.

6 Acknowledge distress and support ventilation of feelings

Above all, people need to know that you understand, not that you feel sorry for them. You can do this non-verbally, practically (e.g. by offering tissues) or by acknowledging that emotions are understandable (legitimising).

It's normal to be upset. I understand that this is very hard.

Never rush in with immediate optimism or reassurance *(I'm sorry to tell you it's cancer but the good news is/let me tell you what we can do . . .)*. Always remember that at this point patients are too preoccupied to assimilate further information. Research shows that subduing or not allowing ventilation of feelings and concerns thwarts recall of what you tell patients next.

7 Identify and prioritise concerns

It may be appropriate, after a while, to ask

What are the particular things you are thinking about?
How does this news make you feel?

It is always important to elicit all concerns before giving advice or information. When concerns are not explored or patient needs not established patients are more likely to remain preoccupied with their concerns, fail to assimilate what is said, perceive information as inadequate and develop anxiety or depression that will hinder the control of future symptoms such as pain.

8 Check present information needs

Is there anything else you want to ask me about?
Do you want to tell me anything more?

Research shows that too much information can cause as big a problem as too little.

9 Identify patient support systems

Who is at home with you?
What about family/friends/others?

Box 4.12 Mistakes when breaking bad news
• Avoiding it in the first place and expecting that someone else will do it
• Not scene setting appropriately, e.g. not enough time or not in privacy
• Not establishing background knowledge
• Not establishing how much the patient wants to know
• Giving the bad news too quickly, rather than gently
• Hesitating too long before getting to the bad news, e.g. a junior emergency department doctor goes to speak to anxious parents about the accident their child has had; the doctor explains what happened in detail, what was done in the resuscitation area and only after considerable time tells them that the outcome of their efforts to resuscitate was unsuccessful
• Not acknowledging the patient's distress
• Not exploring the patient's concerns
• Not exploring the patient's information needs
• Being dishonest, e.g. 'We think you'll be all right.'

10 Make clear what support is available and what is going to happen

Never remove all hope, however bad a diagnosis, giving absolute assurance of what can be done and what should be done next – further investigations or treatments, support of hospital staff, GP, nursing staff, support groups and so forth and follow-up arrangements (making it clear that the patient can be seen at any time before this if there are questions or concerns).

Discussion

Can you think of some common mistakes when breaking bad news?

These are listed in Box 4.12.

CASE 4.15

CANCER – PROBABLY INCURABLE

Candidate information

Role

You are a doctor in the medical outpatient clinic.
Please read this summary.

Scenario

Re: Mrs Jean Paget, aged 86 years

Mrs Paget is a previously well lady with mild hearing difficulty, in clinic for the results of recent investigations for iron deficiency anaemia. She was discharged from hospital three weeks ago following a transfusion to correct her anaemia. Subsequent urgent outpatient investigations comprised an oesophagogastroduodenoscopy (OGD) and an abdominal computed tomography (CT) scan. Colonoscopy was not performed, jointly agreed by patient and doctor on account of her being physically frail and it being against her wishes. The OGD showed an isolated, large gastric ulcer for which she has started a proton pump inhibitor and preliminary histology confirms malignancy but not the type. The CT scan shows two large cystic masses in the pelvis, likely arising from an ovary. The radiology report suggests these may be malignant, but you have not had an opportunity to discuss the scan in any more detail with the radiologist. Mrs Paget's daughter and son-in-law are present, supportive family members with whom Mrs Paget lives.

Your examiners will warn you when 12 minutes have elapsed. You have 14 minutes to communicate with the patient/subject followed by 1 minute of reflection. There will then follow 5 minutes of discussion with the examiners. Do not take the history again except for details that will help in your discussion with the patient/subject. You are not required to examine the patient/subject.

Patient/subject information

Mrs Jean Paget is an 86-year-old lady who lives with her daughter and son-in-law, supportive family members accompanying her in clinic today. She has come for the results of outpatient tests. She was discharged from hospital three weeks ago following a transfusion to correct anaemia. The urgent outpatient tests were performed to look for a reason for anaemia and were upper gastrointestinal endoscopy and an abdominal CT scan. Colonoscopy was not performed, jointly agreed by her and the doctor when in hospital on account of her frailty and it being against her wishes. Mrs Paget has mild hearing difficulty but has previously been well and is not taking any regular medications. Cognition is normal but she is functionally limited by arthritis and dependent on her family to assist her with dressing and meals. She has not really considered possible diagnoses but feels that 'at her time of life' she can accept any bad news.

How to approach the case

Communication skills (conduct of interview, exploration and problem negotiation) and ethics and law

1 Preparation and scene setting

Introduce yourself, ensuring she can hear all that is said. You may need to speak up. Ensure that she and her family do not sense that you are pressured for time. Sit forward, remembering that your first duty is to her, aiming for good eye contact and active listening. Ask if she agrees to your speaking openly with her and her family.

> *May I take it that you are happy for us to speak openly in front of your family?*

2 Establish what the patient knows already

At this point it is appropriate to seek her knowledge of the reasons for investigation so far

> *Could I ask, first of all, what you understand about the reasons for your recent tests?*

It may be helpful to summarise

> *You will recall that we recently found you to be anaemic – your blood count to be low – and that one of our concerns was that there might be a reason for this in the tummy, giving rise to a slow leakage of blood internally. That is why we agreed to have a look into the tummy with the endoscopy, together with a scan.*

3 Establish what the patient wants to know

The rule is to ask before telling, but not to delay breaking bad news. In this situation it may be appropriate to say

> *We have the preliminary results of those tests, and I take it you would want me to be frank with you about everything that we know.*

4 Give a warning shot

> *There was an ulcer in the stomach . . . and, in addition, two lumps in the pelvis were seen on the scan . . . and the early signs are that these findings may not be nice.*

Wait for a few seconds for this to register!

5 Break bad news gently

The key here is to continue explaining results clearly and slowly, taking account of her reaction as each piece of information is related.

> *The biopsy – when they took a small piece of tissue from the stomach – suggests that the problem may be a growth.*

6 Acknowledge distress and support ventilation of feelings

At this point there may be little value and further distress in giving more details unless she asks for more information. Now respond to reactions with appropriate gestures (it may be reasonable to touch on the forearm, for example, during the above explanation).

7 Identify and prioritise concerns

Be open to any questions that she or her family might have.

8 Check present information needs

At the end of this, she might ask what needs to be done. You do not have enough information to suggest a definite course of action, but you can hypothesise

> *We are still waiting for the final pieces of information from the biopsy. And I would also like to see the pictures of the scan myself and discuss these in more detail with the radiologist. But if this is what we suspect, then you and I will need to discuss the way forward. It seems likely that the lumps in the pelvis are connected to what we have found in the stomach, but even if they are not, then I do not think it likely that an operation on the stomach would be the answer. An operation is, I think, unlikely to be possible and even if it were, it would not be without considerable risk. There is a possibility that we might hold things at bay for a period of time with some other form of treatment – drug treatment. But the other consideration that would be for you and your family to think about is that if you are having no symptoms, it may be reasonable to leave things alone.*

She might then ask

> *And what would happen then, doctor?*

You would need to make it very clear that you would have a plan to support her

> *We would talk with your doctor (general practitioner) and let him/her know of the situation in full, so that treatment can be given for any symptoms that arise. But in the first place, I think it would be sensible for us to meet again in a week or so, by which time we should have the final results of the biopsy and I should have had an opportunity to review your scan in more detail with the radiologist.*

In other words, it is often desirable to discuss the diagnosis of cancer at the first appointment, but defer any definite decisions about the way forward (especially if results are still pending) until a second appointment (or subsequent ward round for inpatients), by which time patient and family will have had time to discuss the implications among themselves.

9 Identify patient support systems

Find out a little about how things are at home.

10 Make clear what support is available and what is going to happen

Agree to meet again in the very near future to consider the best way forward.

Discussion

What information would you need before seeing her again?

A review of the CT scan with the radiologist, the final histology report and possibly a CA125 blood test.

The radiologist, at a second view, thinks the pelvic masses could be simple cysts and are likely unrelated to the gastric malignancy. The histopathology of the latter, surprisingly, reports a high-grade non-Hodgkin's B-cell lymphoma, rather than carcinoma. When you see her again, will you attempt to persuade her to have treatment?

You would, of course, discuss the results and reach a shared management plan. You might suggest that the only way to be sure about the pelvic lumps would be to obtain a biopsy, and this would require further hospital intervention. This does not escape the fact that there is, involving the stomach, a form of growth called lymphoma that is not treatable by operation. There may be a possibility of treatment involving chemotherapy or radiotherapy, but to know the absolute answer to this one would need to obtain more information and to seek advice from a specialist who treats lymphoma.

She asks if she will die without treatment. How might you respond?

It is sometimes worth exploring why patients ask this question. It might seem obvious, but it is important to know what patients are thinking. Saying

> *I can answer that. But could I first ask you why you've asked me that?*

might help you to understand her main concerns or fears. She might tell you that her husband had chemotherapy and that she doesn't want any treatment if it is not going to make her better or cure her. She might ask

> *Could we do anything else, doctor?*

to which you could reply

> *We could make sure you were as comfortable as possible and try to let you spend as much time as possible at home.*

She says that she does not wish more hospital tests or treatments. She says 'When my time has come, my time has come; I'd rather take my chances than have any more tests or treatment.' Would you accept this?

If this is her informed choice, yes.

CASE 4.16

CANCER – PATIENT NOT FIT FOR ACTIVE TREATMENT

Candidate information

Role

You are a doctor on the medical ward.
Please read this summary.

Scenario

> **Re: Mrs Rose Broadley, aged 79 years**
>
> Mrs Broadley has been under your team's care for almost a week, and is receiving anticoagulation for two large pulmonary emboli diagnosed on admission. She has been non-specifically unwell for the past two months, feeling tired and losing a little weight and admission to hospital was arranged when she developed worsening breathlessness. Unfortunately, she also has a swollen left thigh and groin with an ulcerated patch from which methicillin-resistant *Staphylococcus aureus* (MRSA) has been cultured and is receiving intravenous antimicrobials. Inflammatory markers have been high, perhaps not surprisingly, but because of the systemic symptoms and the absence of any clear precipitating cause for her pulmonary emboli, a computed tomography (CT) scan of thorax, abdomen and pelvis was arranged that revealed a large caecal mass and para-aortic lymphadenopathy. The diagnosis is almost certainly cancer. Mrs Broadley asked earlier in the week if the reason for the scan was to look for cancer, which you confirmed.
>
> Your task is to explain results, and discuss possible ways forward.

Your examiners will warn you when 12 minutes have elapsed. You have 14 minutes to communicate with the patient/subject followed by 1 minute of reflection. There will then follow 5 minutes of discussion with the examiners. Do not take the history again except for details that will help in your discussion with the patient/subject. You are not required to examine the patient/subject.

Patient/subject information

Mrs Rose Broadley is a 79-year-old lady who has been in hospital for almost a week, and is receiving anticoagulation for two large pulmonary emboli diagnosed on admission. She has been tired and losing weight for two months and was admitted to hospital when she developed worsening breathlessness. Unfortunately, she also has a swollen left thigh and groin with ulceration from which methicillin-resistant *Staphylococcus aureus* (MRSA) has been cultured and is receiving intravenous antibiotics. Her doctors were concerned as to why she developed pulmonary emboli and a CT scan of her thorax, abdomen and pelvis was arranged. Mrs Broadley is a pragmatic lady who likes to know the facts, is aware there is a suspicious lump that can be felt in her abdomen and that the scan was to look for evidence of cancer. She is about to speak to the doctor who has the results.

How to approach the case

Communication skills (conduct of interview, exploration and problem negotiation) and ethics and law

1 Preparation and scene setting

This case combines confirming bad news to a patient who already knows it is a possibility, with making a management plan. The problems are complex, and the discussion should focus on possibilities rather than making absolute decisions now. In real life discussion might be with her alone or with relatives if that is her wish, and ideally in the presence of her nurse. It seems very likely she has colorectal cancer with lymph node spread and that this explains her thromboembolic tendency. The challenge is that you do not have a tissue diagnosis, and the need for anticoagulation and the sepsis make further investigation (colonoscopy, biopsy) and potential treatments (curative surgery or surgery to debulk tumour and reduce the likelihood of obstruction and/or chemotherapy) difficult. These facts need to be included in your discussion.

2 Establish what the patient knows already

You know that she understands what has been happening, but it is still helpful to summarise

> *As you know, it has been a difficult sequence of events. You have been feeling unwell for some time, and when you first came into hospital we suspected, and confirmed, a blood clot on the lung. This was compounded, as I know you are all too well aware, by the infection in the upper part of the leg. And you know, as we have discussed, that we were rather worried that there might be some underlying reason for all of this happening to you . . . hence, the scan.*

She will be likely to show acknowledgement to all of this. While vital not to delay giving the results of the scan, a preamble like this not only leads seamlessly into breaking the bad news but also shows that you are fully aware of her case and this is crucial to maintaining her confidence.

3 Establish what the patient wants to know

Here you may assume that she wants to know everything.

4 Give a warning shot

> *The scan does give us a reason for all of this. It does show an abnormality, and one that may not be nice.*

5 Break bad news gently

> *It shows a lump, within the bowel – within the lower part of the bowel – that is of considerable size.*

She will probably register understanding. It may be appropriate to confirm, because patients cannot start to ventilate feelings until you do

> *It is very likely to be a growth.*

Occasionally, if you choose to use the word growth rather than cancer, patients will rephrase this by asking *Cancer?* to which it is appropriate to confirm that single word.

It may then be appropriate to say that there are also lumps in glands adjacent to the bowel.

6 Acknowledge distress and support ventilation of feelings

Now give her time to come to terms with this news.

7 Identify and prioritise concerns

As a pragmatic lady who has already suspected serious possibilities, she will probably want to know what needs to be done. The following is an outline of areas that your discussion should explore. Speak clearly and not too quickly and be ready to address questions or clarify information throughout.

> *There are a number of things to consider. The first is that although it seems very likely that this is what we suspect it is, the way to be certain would be to look directly into the bowel with a flexible telescope with a light on the end – a test called a colonoscopy – and that would enable us to take a needle sample from it.*
> *The problem is that the blood thinning medication you are taking makes it a little tricky, though by no means impossible.*
> *We strongly suspect that the colonoscopy would show a growth, and a nasty one. The reason that we would do it would be to consider what to do about it, including surgery or other forms of treatment.*
> *I would suggest that we do not make any decisions now but simply say that ultimately we have to decide – and in the last analysis you have to decide – what is the right thing to do.*

8 Check present information needs

She might want to know more about possible treatments

> *We might be in a position to consider an operation. And what we would like to do, if you agree, is ask one of our specialist surgical doctors to see you and talk through what they think possible. An operation would not be without considerable risk,*

because of the blood clots and because of the infection, and because of the infection it is not something we could consider immediately.

An operation, depending upon what was found, might carry a possibility of getting rid of it, but also the possibility of not getting rid of it completely. On the other hand, you might decide that even if surgery were possible, you would not wish it. And simply accept that things are likely to progress.

We would fully understand, if you were to say 'if you're not sure it's going to make it go away, I don't want to go through the pain of an operation'. On the other hand, if you were to say 'I know it's risky but if it's the only way to possibly make things go away . . .' we would do our best to bring everything, and everyone, together to make that happen.

One thing that you should be aware of is that if surgery cannot remove it completely, it might be possible to remove some of it and that without surgery there is a possibility that things could, at some stage, become obstructed.

We will respect whatever you decide/We will do our best whatever you decide. It's not an easy decision to make, I know.

She may want to know what would happen without further treatment.

We would simply keep a very close eye on things, and do whatever we can to ease/alleviate the situation.

9 Identify patient support systems

Find out a little more, if you don't already know, about her home circumstances.

10 Make clear what support is available and what is going to happen

What I would suggest, if I may, is that we think about this a little more and talk again. Meantime, if you agree, we will ask the surgeon to give an opinion on surgery. And we are here at any time, before we next meet, if there is anything you want to discuss, or if you would wish us to sit down with you and your family . . . I am here, other members of my team are here, and ward Sister is here.

Discussion

An elderly lady has liver metastases from an unknown primary site. She is frail, deemed medically unfit to undergo more than palliative treatment, and wishes to know 'just what I need to know, doctor, but no more'. You judge her mental capacity to be borderline. What might you tell her?

She could be told that the news is not good; that there is trouble in the liver that is not nice (to use the word growth

or cancer would very much depend upon feedback from her); that a lot of tests could be done to try to find out where it came from, but that there would not seem to be any ground gained by subjecting her to uncomfortable tests; that the fact is the growth is here, and that it seems best now to try to get her home, perhaps with a period of convalescence, with the support of family, and to keep a close eye on things, treating any symptoms such as pain if and when they arise.

An 88-year-old man has been losing weight. He smokes and has a recent Horner's syndrome and a Pancoast's tumour clinically. He was informed that this is worrying. The chest X-ray now confirms it. What would you tell him?

Using the ten-step framework for breaking bad news, he might be told

Remember how we discussed that we were very worried about things. The X-ray confirms our worries. What we are seeing may not be nice.

If he does not indicate that he has heard enough

We must wait until we know exactly what we are dealing with, but there is a high possibility of a growth.

When he is ready, he will want direction, but may not know what to say. He may say something as open-ended as

Not good, is it?

You must not leave him without support and you must give him a clear sense of your ownership in helping him

No, but it is here. And what we must now do is decide how we are going to deal with what is here.

CASE 4.17

CHRONIC DISEASE

Candidate information

Role

You are a doctor in the neurology clinic.
   Please read this summary.

Scenario

> Re: Mrs Amy March, aged 28 years
> Mrs March was referred to the neurology clinic two months ago with blurred vision in her right eye, subsequently diagnosed as a second episode of optic neuritis; she had had a similar episode six months previously and attended the eye clinic. During her

last visit, it was suggested by the neurologist, when she asked, that her symptoms could be the result of multiple sclerosis. Magnetic resonance (MR) imaging arranged after that appointment and performed last week has been reported as showing multiple demyelinating plaques in the brainstem and periventricular areas consistent with multiple sclerosis.

Your task is to explain the diagnosis.

Your examiners will warn you when 12 minutes have elapsed. You have 14 minutes to communicate with the patient/subject followed by 1 minute of reflection. There will then follow 5 minutes of discussion with the examiners. Do not take the history again except for details that will help in your discussion with the patient/subject. You are not required to examine the patient/subject.

Patient/subject information

Mrs Amy March is a 28-year-old teacher who presented to the eye clinic six months ago with blurred vision in her right eye, diagnosed as optic neuritis. A second episode occurred two months ago and she was referred to the neurology clinic where it was suggested to her, when she asked, that multiple sclerosis was a possibility. She is at the clinic today for results of an MR scan to look for evidence of multiple sclerosis. She is very concerned about what a diagnosis of multiple sclerosis might mean if she wished to become pregnant, and the future implications of this disease.

How to approach the case

Communication skills (conduct of interview, exploration and problem negotiation) and ethics and law

1 Preparation and scene setting

Introduce yourself, and ask how she has been since the last appointment.

2 Establish what the patient knows already

Establishing previous experience and knowledge is crucial, not least exactly what she was told about the possibility of multiple sclerosis and whether she had still been thinking about it.

3 Establish what the patient wants to know

Establish what has gone through her mind about multiple sclerosis, and if it engendered any particular worries. Here you may assume that she wants to know everything.

4 Give a warning shot

Tell her that the scan does confirm the thoughts that the neurologist had last time.

5 Break bad news gently

Explain the results of the MR scan, that it does suggest multiple sclerosis, and allow her time to take this on board.

6 Acknowledge distress and support ventilation of feelings

Watch for her reactions.

7 Identify and prioritise concerns

When she appears ready, explore particular concerns. Tell her that people with multiple sclerosis can have very healthy pregnancies, indeed that sometimes multiple sclerosis tends to improve during pregnancy, although symptoms can flare up after delivery and so close monitoring is needed by the obstetrician and neurologist. Reassure her that not all patients develop disabling disease and that it can vary greatly from one patient to another but that most patients continue to lead normal lives. Explain that it tends to relapse and remit, but that some patients go for many years between relapses. Explain that her specialist will discuss what, if any, treatments might be desirable at this stage.

8 Check present information needs

Do not overwhelm her with information; at this stage largely respond to her concerns.

Is there anything else you want to ask me about?
Do you want to tell me anything more?

9 Identify patient support systems

Establish who is at home with her and if her symptoms have interfered with her work at all.

10 Make clear what support is available and what is going to happen

Explain that you will speak with the neurology consultant about any treatment and ensure that things are kept under review.

Discussion

Would you allow a patient in denial of their illness to continue in such denial, or attempt to change this?

Occasionally, it is necessary to challenge denial because it hinders their ability to deal with important unfinished business or their treatment. It is sometimes possible to confront patients gently by highlighting the inconsistencies, such as a declared belief they are getting better in the face of increasing disability. Where a patient is in persistent denial, it may be because they are unable to tolerate the pain of reality and leaving them in that defence mode until further opportunities during the illness may be best.

DISCUSSING AN ACUTELY TERMINAL SITUATION WITH RELATIVES

Candidate information

Role

You are a doctor in the emergency medical admissions unit.

Please read this summary.

Scenario

> Re: Mr Frank Wentworth, aged 88 years
>
> Mr Wentworth is an 88-year-old man admitted to hospital two hours ago with a thoracic aneurysm rupture ('mediastinal catastrophe') diagnosed clinically and with a radiologically wide mediastinum on chest X-ray. You wondered about a computed tomography scan but your consultant feels that the diagnosis is beyond significant doubt, that there is no alternative, reversible explanation for his presentation and that a scan would not alter management. A team decision has been reached to keep him comfortable. You have just come back to review him, and his daughter is now with him. You have not spoken with her before but it is clear to her that her father is very unwell and it appears to you that he is deteriorating quickly because he is less alert than two hours ago, with gradually falling blood pressure. You offer to go to the ward Sister's office to discuss her father's case.
>
> Your task is to discuss with her what has happened and what the outcome is likely to be, responding to her distress.

Your examiners will warn you when 12 minutes have elapsed. You have 14 minutes to communicate with the patient/subject followed by 1 minute of reflection. There will then follow 5 minutes of discussion with the examiners. Do not take the history again except for details that will help in your discussion with the patient/subject. You are not required to examine the patient/subject.

Patient/subject information

You are the daughter of Mr Frank Wentworth, an 88-year-old man admitted to hospital two hours ago with a ruptured thoracic aneurysm. You are a schoolteacher, phoned at work by a nurse at the hospital to say that your father was very unwell and that you should come in. You have just arrived. You do not know anything else, but have been at the bedside for a few minutes and can see that your father is clearly critically unwell and barely conscious. You are not really sure what an aneurysm is but fear the worst, although you do not think this means imminent decline. Your husband is also on the way to hospital. Your father has previously been very healthy, playing golf until last year. He has been widowed for two years but has remained independent on his own. You have been invited to the ward Sister's office to talk to the doctor. You are extremely worried and will be very distressed to hear the worst but need to know exactly what the doctor thinks.

How to approach the case

Communication skills (conduct of interview, exploration and problem negotiation) and ethics and law

1 Preparation and scene setting

Introduce yourself, and sit close enough to allow good eye contact and at her level.

2 Establish what the relative knows already

Ask what she knows so far but do not labour it; she will want to know what is going on straight away.

3 Establish what the relative wants to know

This step in the breaking bad news ten-step sequence should be bypassed if it is clear that she is waiting in distressed anticipation of what she needs to know.

4 Give a warning shot

Simply saying

> (I'm afraid) the news is not good

may be enough to start.

5 Break bad news gently

Explain what has happened, clearly and calmly. So that there is little doubt of the critical position, one way to conclude the explanation would be to say

> There may not be an easy way out of this . . . there may not <u>be</u> a way out of this.

pausing between both statements, the first telling her gently that he may not recover, the second building on the first to inform her that you may have run out of options to save his life.

6 Acknowledge distress and support ventilation of feelings

She will be very distressed and now is the time to let your comments sink in, and not the time to give more information.

7 Identify and prioritise concerns

Every case must be treated on its own merit. Sometimes it is appropriate to ask how a patient feels about bad news that has been broken. Here, it would be inappropriate to question her thoughts, which are obvious, and you should simply continue to acknowledge her distress, respond to questions and speak honestly, clearly and with understanding.

She may ask

> *What can you do?*

A suitable reply would be

> *We can only watch and wait and see if the bleeding stops. It is all that we can do. There is simply no way of getting to where the bleeding is. He may be dying.*
> *Right now?*
> *Yes.*

It can be difficult for relatives to accept such abrupt news like this. But it is vital to be straightforward and honest.

> *Things are absolutely critical.*

8 Check present information needs

> *How long do you think he has got?*
> *These hours are critical.*

One concern that it is always helpful to anticipate and mention is about pain and distress.

> *What we can do is make certain that, whatever else, he is not in any pain or distress. As he becomes less conscious it is very unlikely he will feel any pain, not at this stage. But if we had any reason to suspect discomfort at any stage we could treat that with medication, with morphia.*

9 Identify support systems

You may wish to check that her husband is on his way, and whether or not she has other relatives who should be aware of the situation.

10 Make clear what support is available and what is going to happen

Assure her that the doctors and nursing staff are available at any time to speak to her again.

Discussion

Patients with incurable but more chronic conditions often ask about how much time is left. How might you respond?

Clearly it depends upon the situation. It is important to acknowledge that you cannot be certain but patients then often ask you to guess. It may be appropriate, if realistic, to say something such as 'Well, the way things have been going it might be just months', but while it is important to be as honest as possible about prognosis it is important not to give specific time frames. Patients sometimes ask about specific dates like whether they will be here for Christmas. You might say 'I would hope so', but ask if there is any reason they mention Christmas in particular. It might be, for example, that a relative died at Christmas and the patient is worried that it will be particularly hard on other family members.

Why is it important to respond to questions about prognosis?

Patients might otherwise be misled about their outlook and might not use their remaining time to deal with important practical and emotional unfinished business with loved ones. This will also make the bereavement process more difficult for loved ones and increase psychiatric morbidity from, for example, major depressive disorder.

CONFIDENTIALITY, CONSENT AND CAPACITY

CASE 4.19

LEGAL POINTS IN CONFIDENTIALITY

Candidate information

Role

You are a doctor on the medical ward.
  Please read this summary.

Scenario

> Re: Mrs Marcia Smith, aged 30
>
> Mrs Smith, a Thai woman who speaks good English, was admitted to the ward with abdominal discomfort and fatigue, now confirmed to be the result of hepatitis B virus infection. She also has inguinal lymphadenopathy and you have sought her consent for a human immunodeficiency virus (HIV) test. She has lived in the UK for six months with her English husband whom she met and married a year ago. She refuses the test. She also tells you not to tell her husband her diagnosis.
>
> Your tasks are to explore her reasoning, and discuss the importance of the test and possible consequences of refusal.

Your examiners will warn you when 12 minutes have elapsed. You have 14 minutes to communicate with the patient/subject followed by 1 minute of reflection. There will then follow 5 minutes of discussion with the examiners. Do not take the history again except for details that will help in your discussion with the patient/subject. You are not required to examine the patient/subject.

Patient/subject information

Mrs Marcia Smith, a 30-year-old Thai woman who speaks good English, was recently admitted to hospital with abdominal discomfort and fatigue, now confirmed to be the result of hepatitis B virus infection. She also has lymph node enlargement in her groin and her doctors have asked if she might consent to a test for HIV. She has lived in the UK for six months with her English husband whom she met and married a year ago. She is very afraid. A friend of hers died two years ago from HIV in Thailand, although sustained treatment had not been available. She is also very afraid for her two-month-old baby, and her husband. She does not want the doctors to perform the test nor tell her husband of her current diagnosis.

How to approach the case

Communication skills (conduct of interview, exploration and problem negotiation) and ethics and law

1 Introduction

Introduce yourself and confirm her identity.

2 Establish rapport

There is potential conflict between her right to confidentiality and the rights of her husband (and baby) to information and possible treatment in the event that he (they) was (were) infected. From the outset, you may be balancing her confidentiality against potential risks to others. However, avoid giving her 'ultimatums' at this stage. It is vital not to 'rush in'. Your first duty is to her, analysing her perspective and how you may best help. Explain this to her, and assure her you are there to help.

3 Explore patient understanding and concerns

Ensure that she is aware of the problem and try to explore her beliefs, concerns and expectations about the problem.

4 Attempt to discover the patient's reasons for not wanting to disclose

Is she scared about being diagnosed with HIV? If so, why? Is she scared for herself, or for the effect it will have on her family or marriage? Perhaps she knows that she has been exposed to HIV in the past and has always feared this sort of predicament. Is it possible that she has been diagnosed with HIV in the past but has been living in denial?

5 Share your concerns and desired management plan

Your first concern is that she may be infected with HIV in addition to the hepatitis B virus. Try to let her see the importance of excluding or confirming the diagnosis. A supportive approach is essential, letting her see the potential advantages – the HIV test may be negative; were the test positive, it would allow earlier institution of treatment and testing of contacts (who could well be negative). Much better treatments are available for HIV than her friend would have received. Denial will not make the problem go away. She will know this, and her decision to avoid testing and telling is almost certainly motivated by fear.

6 Respond to patient cues

Continuously look for non-verbal as well as verbal cues.

7 Discuss possible consequences of refusal

In a non-threatening way, explain that you have a dilemma of interests. While your first concern is for her, you are very concerned that in the event that she does have a positive test there are wider implications.

8 Confirm understanding

Ensure that she fully understands that your first duty is to her and not her husband, that you will not tell her husband, but that for the best steps to be taken for her health and the potential health of her family she needs to tell him.

9 Allow time to think about what has been discussed and invite questions

Allow her time to think about what has been discussed and to ask questions. She may have initially decided that the worst outcome would be for her husband to know that she has hepatitis or HIV. Your task has been to identify other outcomes for her to consider.

10 Agree a way forward

If she does not immediately agree, it is likely that she needs more time to contemplate what you have discussed and you should at least attempt to end the discussion with a plan to talk again.

Discussion

Why is confidentiality important?

Confidentiality is central to the trust that exists in the relationship between doctor and patient. This has been enshrined in doctors' codes of professional conduct including the Hippocratic Oath, the Declaration of Geneva and General Medical Council (GMC) guidelines. Information that a doctor learns from a patient 'belongs' to that patient. From a legal point of view a patient's case records do not belong to that patient, but from an ethical point of view patients should have the right to determine in general who has access to information they provide. Respect for patient autonomy supports confidentiality and opposes paternalistic attitudes, common in the past, in which doctors 'knew what was in a patient's best interests'.

What is your legal commitment to respect confidentiality?

The general obligation is to keep patient information confidential. This obligation is not absolute; the law may allow or obligate breach of confidentiality, but any breach should only be to the relevant person or authority. The question of whether or not breach of confidentiality is legal is often a matter of balancing harm to the patient if confidentiality is breached, against harm to others if it is not. The equation is seldom simple and the law sees a strong public interest in individual doctor–patient confidentiality being maintained.

GMC guidelines do not have the force of law but are taken seriously by the Courts.

Breach of confidentiality does not occur if a patient is not identifiable or if a patient has consented to disclosure of information.

Doctors have a duty to take reasonable precautions to prevent confidential information from falling into the wrong hands.

Under what circumstances might confidential information be disclosed?

These are outlined in Box 4.13.

What are the possible consequences of breach of confidentiality?

These include loss of trust and breakdown in doctor–patient relationship, disciplinary action by the GMC, investigation of serious professional misconduct by the GMC and civil legal action.

Does information remain confidential after death?

Yes, and information cannot be released without the consent of the patient's executor or a close relative fully informed of the consequences of disclosure.

Box 4.13 Circumstances in which confidential information might be disclosed

Circumstances in which confidential information *must* be disclosed

- When legally required by a Court Order
- When a statutory duty to statutory regulatory bodies, as in communicable disease notification and the reporting of births, deaths, abortions and work-related accidents
- In cases of national security such as terrorism or major crime prevention or in assisting in the solving of a major crime (although you may not disclose detailed information to police officers about any matter)

Circumstances in which confidential information *may*, at a doctor's discretion, be disclosed

- When a third party is deemed to be at risk of harm, e.g. at risk of contracting a serious infectious disease
- In the public interest, e.g. informing the Driver and Vehicle Licensing Agency in the case of a patient with seizures known to continue to drive illegally
- Through sharing information with the health-care team

When disclosure of relevant information between health-care team members is clearly required for investigation or treatment to which a patient has agreed, the patient's explicit consent may not be required. Such sharing of information is not generally viewed by the law as breaching confidentiality. Examples include passing information to medical secretaries for typing and writing information on request forms for investigations.

Timing of disclosure

Breaching confidentiality should usually be the 'last resort'. The patient should be given an explanation as to why disclosure is intended, and the doctor must be able to justify the decision. Before disclosing, a doctor might sensibly seek advice from colleagues, professional bodies such as the British Medical Association, and their medical defence organisation.

CASE 4.20

BREACHING CONFIDENTIALITY WHEN A THIRD PARTY MAY BE AT RISK

Candidate information

Role

You are a doctor on the renal ward.

Please read this summary.

Scenario

Re: Mr Joe Green, aged 25 years

Mr Green is a builder about to undergo a renal biopsy for suspected immunoglobulin A (IgA) nephropathy. He tells you that he is hepatitis C-positive but instructs you not to share this information with anyone else.

Your task is to discuss this with him and decide whether or not the biopsy should proceed.

Your examiners will warn you when 12 minutes have elapsed. You have 14 minutes to communicate with the patient/subject followed by 1 minute of reflection. There will then follow 5 minutes of discussion with the examiners. Do not take the history again except for details that will help in your discussion with the patient/subject. You are not required to examine the patient/subject.

Patient/subject information

Mr Joe Green is a 25-year-old builder who has been diagnosed with probable glomerulonephritis following an episode of macroscopic haematuria. He has been admitted to hospital for further tests including a renal biopsy. He has previously been well but has sporadically taken intravenous drugs and has had multiple sexually transmitted diseases. He was tested for hepatitis C at the genitourinary medicine clinic two years ago and the test was positive [human immunodeficiency virus (HIV) being negative] but has not required any specific treatment. He was due for follow-up blood tests last year but did not attend. He was afraid of possible progression. His girlfriend works as a nurse at your hospital. She does not know he is hepatitis C-positive and he is afraid that if this information is recorded she could conceivably have access to it. He will tell her about his hepatitis but now is 'not the right time'. He felt he should tell the doctor in case it affected his biopsy but does not want anyone else to know.

How to approach the case

Communication skills (conduct of interview, exploration and problem negotiation) and ethics and law

1 Introduction

Introduce yourself and confirm his identity.

2 Establish rapport

There is potential conflict between his right to confidentiality and the potential risk to colleagues, especially the doctor performing the biopsy and those performing phlebotomy. Start by reassuring him that you will try to help.

3 Explore patient understanding and concerns

It is always best to gather information before reaching conclusions and deciding on a course of action. Ask more about his hepatitis C. How does he know that he has hepatitis C? How did he contract it? What investigations and treatments has he had so far? Who has been supervising his care? He may feel that these are irrelevant questions and that you do not need this information. Explain that it may be important in building a better understanding of his kidney problem and that a renal biopsy can be dangerous if liver function is impaired.

4 Attempt to discover the patient's reasons for not wanting to disclose

Is he scared about his girlfriend finding out because of the impact on their relationship or are there other reasons? You might explore why he has told you of his diagnosis but instructed that others not be informed. Exploring his fears may give you the answer.

5 Share your concerns and desired management plan

Your first concern is that he has a condition that could put colleagues at risk. Although all patients should be deemed potential sources of risk when performing invasive procedures, knowledge of the condition is important both for taking extra vigilance with procedures and in his overall assessment. Certain forms of glomerulonephritis are more common in hepatitis C infection or with HIV (his last test was two years ago). A further concern is for his girlfriend. Explain that it would be important for the medical team involved in the procedure and in his management to know that he has hepatitis C, but that the information would go no further than those involved in his immediate care. Explain that it would be sensible to obtain up-to-date serology for hepatitis B and C and HIV to build up a better picture of his condition, institute early treatment if there is evidence of active disease, and reassure if results are unchanged. Explain why his girlfriend should know.

6 Respond to patient cues

Continuously look for non-verbal as well as verbal cues.

7 Discuss possible consequences of refusal

If he still refuses disclosure, explain that you may need to talk to colleagues on a 'strictly need to know' basis. Discussion with your medical defence organisation may be appropriate.

8 Confirm understanding

Ensure that he understands the reasons for his hepatitis being known, not least that he may be offered the best treatment.

9 Allow time to think about what has been discussed and invite questions

Allow him time to think about what has been discussed and to ask questions.

10 Agree a way forward

The examiners are aware that such a discussion is difficult. They are not looking for a 'model answer' but are checking your awareness of the range of issues provoked and your ability to handle these sensitively and professionally. They would be more concerned if you found such a case clear-cut and chose one of two extremes – agreeing to the patient's instructions or informing him that you intended to breach confidentiality without having had careful discussion around it. If he remains firm in his decision and refuses to allow disclosure, you may conclude that failure to inform some of your colleagues will place them at serious risk. It is then possible to breach confidentiality on the grounds of risk to others and on a strictly 'need to know' basis. You should inform him of what you propose to do.

Discussion

Does his girlfriend have a right to know?

A patient who has decided not to tell contacts at risk must recognise that this decision may have serious outcomes for these contacts and that breach of confidentiality would be a potential ultimate step. Persuading him to share that knowledge is preferable, and other possible routes could be to involve his general practitioner or the genitourinary medicine specialist, ideally with his consent.

A 32-year-old man has presented to your general medical clinic with weight loss and admits to a history of intravenous drug misuse and having multiple sexual partners. He is now living with his girlfriend, who is pregnant. You mention the possibility of HIV infection and he admits to having suspected this but adds 'If I had AIDS I would want to kill myself, doctor'. He also says that he feels angry. How might you respond?

It takes time to come to terms with the possibility of a serious diagnosis like cancer or HIV infection, and very

often anger is a secondary emotion, the primary one fear. At this stage you are not talking to him about having HIV infection, but about the importance of testing for it. Again, you should attempt to explore his fears, and find out why he would want to kill himself. It may be that to him HIV is a 'death penalty' and that he does not fully understand its natural history and current treatments. It may be appropriate to offer him a referral to trained HIV counsellors for further discussion of the implications of the test and its possible result. His partner and the fetus would be at risk and would warrant screening for HIV and the hepatitis B and C viruses were this patient positive. There are also implications for the obstetric team. The difficulty is that this patient has not yet been tested. Although he has not refused to be tested, he has threatened self-harm should the test be positive. Hopefully, exploring his views and reaching a shared understanding of the problem may persuade him of the value of being tested and sharing the problem with his partner.

CASE 4.21

BREACHING CONFIDENTIALITY IN THE PUBLIC INTEREST

Candidate information

Role

You are a doctor in the neurology clinic.
  Please read this summary.

Scenario

> Re: Ms Holly Long, aged 22 years
> Ms Long is a previously well student brought into hospital six weeks ago after a road traffic accident. She lost consciousness at the wheel and drove into a wall. She has had a normal ambulatory electrocardiogram (ECG) and echocardiogram. She says she lost consciousness only transiently after she took a fizzy drink giving rise to severe heartburn. To build in evidence that this was likely situational syncope rather than seizure activity with an aura you feel she also warrants magnetic resonance (MR) brain imaging and an electroencephalogram. She is here for the results of her heart tests and is keen to drive again.
> Your task is to talk with her.

Your examiners will warn you when 12 minutes have elapsed. You have 14 minutes to communicate with the patient/subject followed by 1 minute of reflection. There will then follow 5 minutes of discussion with the examiners.

Do not take the history again except for details that will help in your discussion with the patient/subject. You are not required to examine the patient/subject.

Patient/subject information

Ms Holly Long is a previously well 22-year-old student brought into hospital six weeks ago after a road traffic accident. She lost consciousness at the wheel after a gulp of fizzy drink with immediate heartburn and drove into a wall and has had subsequent tests to exclude a heart problem. She was told she could not drive until after the results. She is here for the results. She has a partner at a different university 100 miles away and desperately wants to be able to drive to visit him at weekends. She feels well and has decided to drive 'whatever the doctor says' and will tell him so.

How to approach the case

Communication skills (conduct of interview, exploration and problem negotiation) and ethics and law

1 Introduction

Introduce yourself and confirm her identity.

2 Establish rapport

Your first duty is to her, analysing her perspective and how you may best help. Show this from the start.

3 Explain the results

Explain that the test results were reassuring. Explain that while this is so, the tests do not exclude a seizure. While physicians might not treat a first seizure, driving regulations do not permit driving within 12 months of unexplained loss of consciousness.

4 Explore patient understanding and concerns

Ensure that she understands this and explore any difficulties it might pose.

5 Attempt to discover the patient's reasons for not wanting to adhere to advice

Show that you appreciate her concerns about not being able to drive to visit her partner.

6 Explain the risks and consider alternatives

Reiterate the dangerous accident she had, threatening both her own life and that of others. Are there alternatives to her, such as public transport? Ensure that she is aware it is only for a period of time.

7 Respond to patient cues

Continuously look for non-verbal as well as verbal cues.

8 Discuss possible consequences of refusal

In a non-threatening way, explain that you have a dilemma of interests. While your first concern is for her, you are very concerned that were she to continue driving, she might be at risk personally and legally, and be a risk to others.

9 Allow time to think about what has been discussed and invite questions

Allow her time to think about what has been discussed and to ask questions. She may have initially decided that the worst outcome would be for her not to be able to drive for six months. She may now see that taking your advice is, on balance, best.

10 Agree a way forward

Remember that patients have a right to a second opinion, although it may be appropriate to advise patients that some decisions are likely to be uniform among doctors, particularly where bound by a professional or legal framework.

Discussion

When may disclosure of confidential information be made in the public interest?

Personal information may be disclosed in the public interest without a patient's consent where the benefits to an individual or society outweigh the patient's interests in keeping that information confidential. Where there is a serious risk to patients or others, disclosures may be justified even where patients have been asked to agree to disclosure but have withheld consent. You should inform patients that disclosure will be made, where practical to do so. Ultimately, the public interest can only be determined by the Courts, and the General Medical Council may require you to justify your actions.

A patient you are seeing in clinic with epilepsy last had a seizure nine months ago and continues to drive. What are the implications?

An epileptic patient who continues to drive has autonomy and a right to confidentiality. Yet breach of this confidentiality may be more important in the greater interests of benefit to society. The Driver and Vehicle Licensing Agency (DVLA) publishes a booklet on driving rules in medical conditions. Current rules for drivers (of non-heavy goods or public vehicles) are that they must have been seizure-free for more than 12 months or free of daytime seizures for more than three years if seizures are purely nocturnal. These rules apply on or off antiepileptic drugs. Patients should not drive for six months following any dose adjustment.

When should you disclose confidential information to the DVLA?

This is outlined in Box 4.14.

Box 4.14 Disclosure of confidential information to the DVLA

- The DVLA is legally responsible for deciding if a person is medically unfit to drive and should know of a condition likely, now or in the future, to affect safety
- Patients should understand that their condition may affect the safety of themselves and others
- Patients have a legal duty to inform the DVLA about their condition
- If a patient refuses to accept the diagnosis or its safety implications, you should suggest a second opinion, assist the patient in obtaining it and advise them to refrain from driving until it has been sought
- If a patient continues to drive when medically unfit, you should make every reasonable effort to dissuade them, which may include informing a next of kin
- If this fails, you may disclose relevant medical information, in confidence, to the DVLA's medical adviser, informing the patient that you intend to do this

---

CASE 4.22

CONFIDENTIALITY WHEN TALKING WITH RELATIVES AND OTHER THIRD PARTIES

Candidate information

Role

You are a doctor on the medical ward.
Please read this summary.

Scenario

Re: Mr Peter Price, aged 34

Mr Price has muscular dystrophy and has been admitted to your ward with lobar pneumonia. He is stable but has a number of signs associated with a high risk (reduced consciousness, hypotension and leucopenia). His carer, who is not a relative, asks how he is. You also would value some background information about his home circumstances, quality of life and any prior expressed wishes in the event of this sort of situation.
Your task is to speak to the carer.

Your examiners will warn you when 12 minutes have elapsed. You have 14 minutes to communicate with the patient/subject followed by 1 minute of reflection. There will then follow 5 minutes of discussion with the examiners. Do not take the history again except for details that will help in your discussion with the patient/subject. You are not required to examine the patient/subject.

Patient/subject information

You are a carer of Mr Peter Price, a 34-year-old man with muscular dystrophy. He has just been admitted to hospital

with lobar pneumonia. His condition is unstable. You have cared for Mr Price for four years in his own home, but despite physical disabilities, notably his being unable to move his limbs, his general health has been very good. You are very anxious that he is now so unwell.

How to approach the case

Communication skills (conduct of interview, exploration and problem negotiation) and ethics and law

1 Introduction

Introduce yourself and establish the carer's identity.

> *I'm sure you will understand that out of respect for (patient's name), I need to be sure to whom I'm speaking.*

2 Acknowledge a valued contribution

Your primary responsibility is to the patient, whose medical details remain confidential. It is very easy to forget this when a patient is unable to speak. It is equally important, however, to respect the concerns of a third party and the valued information they can often provide. Show respect for the carer's expertise (and experience with this particular patient), and acknowledge the interdependence between patient and carer. The case records may be a valuable source of information and even demonstrate the patient's willingness for information to be shared with the carer.

3 Explain a little

State, in broad terms, that the situation is not good. Listen to responses and look for cues. It is remarkable how worried relatives and carers end up doing much of the talking and by disclosing very little you can often open the door to a lot of information from them. Frequently the relative or carer knows, or has suspected, a lot more than you may think.

4 Ask a little

Additional questions may open the door much wider!

5 Explain in more depth, directed by responses

You may then be in a position to speak more freely about the condition, again respecting your first duty to the patient and making sure anything you say is strictly information that will be of use to the carer in her role, and ultimately beneficial to the patient.

6 Involve the carer in the desired management plan

Involve the carer as far as you can in making decisions, without compromising the autonomy of the patient. Asking 'What do you feel he would want us to do?' is not asking the carer to make a decision but inviting her valued insights to help guide your own decision-making.

7 Respond to cues

Continually look for non-verbal as well as verbal cues.

8 Consider other issues

It may or may not be appropriate, depending upon how well you feel she knows him, to establish if she is aware of any prior wishes regarding resuscitation in the event of a cardiopulmonary arrest.

9 Allow time to think about what has been discussed and invite questions

Allow her time to think about what has been discussed and to ask questions.

10 Agree a way forward

Assure her that you will do all that you can to get him better, and that now you have established her involvement you would be happy to update her at any time on his progress.

Discussion

Under which circumstances may implied consent be sufficient for disclosure of confidential information to third parties?

Implied consent (Case 4.23) is appropriate for sharing information in the health-care team, provided that wishes are respected if a patient objects to a particular person or agency being made aware and this would not put others at risk, or when disclosing information for clinical audit, including identifiable information if patients have been informed that their information may be used for such purposes and have not objected.

Under what circumstances must express consent be sought to disclose information to third parties?

Express consent (Case 4.23), verbal or written, is needed for disclosure of information to a third party under most other circumstances, including to a nearest relative.

What type of consent is needed when disclosing information to third parties such as employers, lawyers and insurance companies?

Verbal consent from patients is usually sufficient when giving information to relatives, but written consent should be obtained when communicating with employers and in any legal matters. Patients must be aware of the purpose of disclosure, the obligation a doctor has to the third party and that this may include disclosure of personal information.

Can information about a patient be disclosed for education and research without consent?

Information about patients can be useful for such purposes as education, research, audit, administration, monitoring, epidemiology and public-health surveillance. Express consent is generally preferable for disclosure, whether or not it is judged that patients can be identified from the disclosure and even although disclosure is unlikely to confer personal consequences. Anonymised data without patient consent may be acceptable for education and audit, and in research where it is not practicable to contact patients, a research ethics committee should decide whether the likely benefits of research outweigh the loss of confidentiality. Express consent should be sought when publishing material such as case histories or photographs of a patient, whether or not that patient is clearly identifiable.

An 80-year-old man has just recovered from a stroke. He lives independently and is to be discharged from your ward later this week. One of the nurses on your ward asks if you'll speak to his daughter. You are asked by a woman over the phone, 'What has happened to my father?' Would you tell her?

You would establish the caller's identity. Clearly, if you have met her on the ward, recognise her voice, and know that her father has always been happy to share his medical problems with her, you would be less guarded. If you had no prior knowledge that he consents to divulging of information, you should explain why you could not without his permission.

The daughter now requests that you not tell him anything more about his condition without her prior permission – 'he is a worrier'. Would you agree to this?

You should not be willing to withhold information from him based solely on his daughter's wishes. You should explain that he has a right to know what has happened (respecting his autonomy) and to make his own decisions based on that information. You could reassure her that you would not force information on him, explaining only as much as he appeared to want to know. You might also suggest that discussion by phone is not ideal and offer to speak to her if she comes in to hospital to visit her father. You should avoid stating legal rights in these sorts of situations. Relatives never warm to being told 'I'm within my rights not to tell you'. Phrases like 'I share your concerns', 'I understand how concerned you must be', or 'I appreciate how you must feel' offer empathy and show that you are listening.

CASE 4.23

CONSENT FOR INVESTIGATION OR TREATMENT

Candidate information

Role

You are a doctor in the emergency medical admissions unit.

Please read this summary.

Scenario

Re: Ms Kate Morland, aged 23 years

Ms Morland was admitted last night with a severe occipital headache of sudden onset. She is a normally fit and well young woman, who works at your hospital as a nurse. She sustained a minor whiplash injury three days previously in a minor road traffic accident. Her headache came on suddenly at a party. It was the worst headache she has ever experienced and reduced her to tears. Her computed tomography (CT) brain scan is normal.

Your tasks are to explain the reasons for performing a lumbar puncture (to exclude subarachnoid haemorrhage) and obtain her consent.

Your examiners will warn you when 12 minutes have elapsed. You have 14 minutes to communicate with the patient/subject followed by 1 minute of reflection. There will then follow 5 minutes of discussion with the examiners. Do not take the history again except for details that will help in your discussion with the patient/subject. You are not required to examine the patient/subject.

Patient/subject information

Ms Kate Morland, a 23-year-old nurse, was admitted to the emergency medical admissions unit last night with the worst headache she has ever experienced. She is a normally fit and well young woman, who works at this hospital. She sustained a minor whiplash injury three days ago in a minor road traffic accident. She is very scared. She has never felt this unwell. She is afraid that colleagues have witnessed her tears and distress. She has been told that a lumbar puncture is necessary but is afraid of further investigations involving needles and does not understand why she needs to stay in hospital because her brain scan was normal.

How to approach the case

Communication skills (conduct of interview, exploration and problem negotiation) and ethics and law

1 Introduction

She is very apprehensive, probably a cumulative effect of recent personal stresses, being admitted to her own workplace and fear of needles. Patients' fears are multiplied significantly if they feel, as they often do, uncertain about what is happening to them, what is planned and why. Establish an aura of calm. Explain that before you do anything else, you would like to recap on the reasons for the scan, the desirability of doing one further test – the lumbar puncture – and to talk this through with her so that she can decide whether or not to go ahead. Make it very clear that in the last analysis it is her decision.

2 Explain the situation so far

Reassure her that the test results so far are good and that nothing bad, such as a brain tumour, has been seen. Explain the main unresolved concern.

The main concern in this situation is the possibility of a small bleed, known as a subarachnoid haemorrhage. This is usually detected by the scan, but a small number of cases, perhaps around 10%, may not be picked up. Although it is generally small bleeds that are not picked up, the concern is that subarachnoid bleeds arise from a weakness in the wall of a blood vessel, and if not detected can recur with much more serious consequences. If detected, there are possible treatments to correct the underlying cause.

3 Explain the best way forward

The only way to detect a smaller bleed is with a test called a lumbar puncture, these days a relatively straightforward test without too much discomfort.

4 Establish previous experience and be alert to ideas and concerns

Before explaining the test in more detail, establish any specific ideas or concerns. Many patients have heard exaggerated stories about lumbar punctures and big needles. Alternatively, she might have personal knowledge of someone close to her who had a difficult lumbar puncture for a serious disease.

5 Explain the nature of the investigation or treatment

Explain that a lumbar puncture involves, with local anaesthetic, a small needle inserted in to the lower part of the back to draw off spinal fluid. In the case of a subarachnoid bleed, this should be bloodstained. She will need to lie curled up on her side during the procedure and remain in bed for around four hours afterwards.

6 Explain the risks and benefits of the investigation or treatment

Complications include headache (common) and much more rarely serious complications such as infection.

7 Explain any possible alternatives

In this case the alternative is to do nothing, because subarachnoid haemorrhage may be unlikely. Less optimal tests in patients at higher suspicion of subarachnoid haemorrhage who abjectly decline lumbar puncture might include magnetic resonance cerebral angiography, although this might only detect larger aneurysms.

8 Show respect for autonomy

In respecting her right to decide, you must be sure that she has been informed and understands that the test is ordinarily safe and straightforward and that the possible diagnosis, albeit unlikely, is potentially life-threatening. Without telling a patient what must be done, it is crucial to explain that in your opinion a particular course of action seems to be in that patient's best interests.

9 Confirm understanding and invite questions

Allow her time to assimilate all of this information, confirm that she understands what you have explained and invite any questions.

10 Seek permission to proceed

Use an open question.

How does this sound?

Discussion

What is consent?

Agreement to an action based on knowledge of what that action involves and its likely consequences.

What are the necessary requirements for valid consent?

Consent rests on the principle of respect for patient autonomy. For it to be legally valid three conditions must be met (Box 4.15).

What is battery?

A procedure performed without consent may be grounds for battery. Generally, if a person touches another without consent, this constitutes battery, for which damages may be awarded. Unlike negligence (Case 4.40), proof of harm is not necessary.

What is meant by implied and express consent?

Types of consent are discussed in Box 4.16.

What exceptions are there to informed consent?

Exceptions are where a patient is judged not to have the capacity to give informed consent.

How might doctors be at risk of committing battery when obtaining consent from a competent patient?

By failing to give sufficient information about the nature of the procedure.

How might doctors be at risk of negligence when obtaining consent from a competent patient?

By failing to give sufficient information about common and rare serious side effects, benefits and possible alternatives.

A 65-year-old man has diabetic nephropathy as evidenced by microalbuminuria. You wish to start an angiotensin-converting enzyme (ACE) inhibitor. What type of consent would you obtain?

Rights are so basic yet so easily ignored. This is especially true of the right to consent to treatment or refuse it. In

---

Box 4.15 Valid consent

Requirements for valid consent

1   The patient should be properly informed.
2   The patient should understand that information and be competent (legally, have capacity) to give consent.
3   Consent must be given voluntarily, without coercion.
    A written record of the conversation is necessary.

'Informed consent'

A patient needs a certain amount of information for consent to be legally valid. He or she must be aware of:

- The *nature of the intervention*; avoidance of *battery* requires that the doctor explains, in broad terms, the nature of the procedure.
- The *risks and benefits, and alternative options or treatments*; this relates to the *avoidance of negligence*. In general, a doctor is not negligent if he or she has acted in accordance with the practice accepted as proper by a responsible body of doctors skilled in that art (i.e. what a responsible body of medical opinion would disclose in the same or similar circumstances). This is termed the Bolam test after the relevant legal case. However, the standard of information provision by doctors is evolving in English law, mainly due to General Medical Council guidelines, and is drawing nearer to the prudent-patient test widely used in North America. According to this test, doctors should provide the amount of information that a 'prudent patient' would want.

What most patients would want to know

For an investigation or treatment most patients would want to know:

- The possible or likely diagnosis, and its prognosis with or without treatment.
- The purpose of the proposed investigation or treatment (furthering diagnosis, excluding serious diagnoses, improving prognosis).
- Any common or serious complications or side effects of the proposed investigation or treatment.

Box 4.16 Types of consent

Implied consent

Because touching a patient without consent can constitute battery, consent is needed even when, for example, taking a pulse or examining the chest. Yet doctors seldom obtain consent, either expressed orally or in writing, for such routine tasks, and in law patients could not successfully sue doctors most of the time because the Courts accept the concept of implied consent. If a patient offers their wrist while the doctor takes the pulse, consent is implied by their behaviour. However, the fact that a patient is in hospital for examination does not constitute consent to examination, investigation or treatment.

Express consent

Express consent, explicitly given (usually verbal but sometimes written), for investigation or treatment is preferable when:

- The investigation or treatment is complex or involves significant risks or side effects
- Clinical care is not the primary purpose of the investigation
- The investigation or treatment forms part of research
- There may be significant personal consequences for the patient

theory, consent should always be obtained for any treatment. In practice, there is often an implicit understanding that consent for examination, investigation or treatment is implied. Although such assumptions seldom result in problems, legal justification for them is not inevitable. You should obtain express consent, explaining why you feel the ACE inhibitor would be beneficial (knowledge of disease and its treatment), important side effects (knowledge of drug), any alternatives, and the risks or benefits and likely outcomes of these.

CASE 4.24

CONSENT AND CAPACITY

Candidate information

Role

You are a doctor on the stroke unit.
    Please read this summary.

Scenario

Re: Mr Ashley Wills, aged 77 years

Mr Wills has been on your ward for four weeks following a left total anterior circulation infarct with dense right-sided hemiparesis, expressive dysphasia and a degree of receptive dysphasia. Over the past four weeks recovery has been minimal and his swallow, as assessed by the speech and language therapists, remains unsafe. At least one confirmed episode of aspiration has occurred. He has pulled out his nasogastric tube on numerous occasions and feeding has been erratic because it is difficult to replace. His serum albumin (although not reliably related to nutritional status) has fallen to 26 g/l. Your team feel that a percutaneous endoscopic gastrostomy (PEG) tube is in his best interests to support adequate nutrition and optimise potential recovery. It is increasingly likely that he will require long-term nursing care. You cannot be certain that Mr Wills understands or retains information.

Your tasks are to discuss with Mrs Wills, your patient's wife, why a PEG tube is being considered and obtain her consent.

Your examiners will warn you when 12 minutes have elapsed. You have 14 minutes to communicate with the patient/subject followed by 1 minute of reflection. There will then follow 5 minutes of discussion with the examiners. Do not take the history again except for details that will help in your discussion with the patient/subject. You are not required to examine the patient/subject.

Patient/subject information

Your husband, Mr Ashley Wills, is a 77-year-old gentleman who has been on the stroke unit for four weeks following a large stroke with dense right-sided weakness and loss of speech. His comprehension of anything he is told is variable, and you cannot always be sure of what he understands. Over the past four weeks recovery has been minimal and his swallow remains unsafe. He is sometimes agitated, pulling out his nasogastric feeding tube on numerous occasions and his feeding has been erratic. You can see that his nutritional state is not optimal and the doctors have told you that this is confirmed on blood tests. The doctors feel that a percutaneous endoscopic gastrostomy (PEG), a feeding tube passed directly into the stomach, would support adequate nutrition and optimise potential recovery, but you have also been told that he is unlikely to get home again. Your husband has always feared 'ending up in a nursing home' and you are not sure that he would want further intervention.

How to approach the case

Communication skills (conduct of interview, exploration and problem negotiation) and ethics and law

1 Introduce yourself and establish the relative's identity

Introduce yourself and confirm that she is Mr Wills' wife.

2 Establish background knowledge

Find out what she understands about her husband's condition and the problems faced (rehabilitation challenges, nutrition compromised) to get an idea of where to start your explanation.

3 Explain the problem

Explain that the stroke has led to swallowing problems, preventing adequate nutrition and putting him at risk of further episodes of aspiration. Explain that he has pulled out the nasogastric tube on numerous occasions and that it has proved challenging to replace and that in any event this is not an ideal long-term solution to meeting his nutritional needs. Explain that with time and without adequate nutrition her husband will inevitably decline.

4 Explain possible solutions

Explain that one option is a PEG tube, and explain that this involves insertion of a small feeding tube directly into the stomach through the abdominal wall. This can be performed in various ways but the most common method is via endoscopic guidance, under local anaesthetic and with a degree of sedation. Explain the potentially serious complications (infection, perforation, death). PEG tubes carry a modest but significant mortality as well as significant morbidity.

5 Be alert to cues

You may perceive how she feels about your proposed strategies from non-verbal cues.

6 Ask how the relative feels, and how she thinks the patient would feel about this

Sometimes patients' relatives are reluctant to give a view because they feel it is too much responsibility for a loved one to take. More often, relatives have concerns. They simply want what is best for their loved one but find it hard to make decisions because there seem to be risks with every choice. Reassure her that you will always try to do what is in the patient's best interests, but that it is important to know if to her knowledge her husband might have had any strong wishes one way or the other.

7 Attempt to address concerns

Relatives struggle, understandably, to come to terms with major changes such as the likelihood of nursing home dependency. However, in coming to terms with this there are many smaller hurdles or decisions to be negotiated along the way. Apart from the general wishes of most people not to be ill or to face nursing care or mental incapacity, most will not have thought in detail and discussed specific wishes like PEGs and even with valid advance directives the devil is often in the detail. When faced with a choice between nutrition to optimise whatever recovery is possible, and certain decline, most relatives will agree to a PEG tube unless decline seems inevitable even with nutrition, in which case doctors would not consider it.

8 Relative agrees or relative disagrees with what you see as in patient's best interests

Most relatives agree to PEG feeding if it is clinically indicated. In those uncommon circumstances where there is a major differing view between relatives and medical staff you should consider two possibilities. If you can be convinced that information provided by his wife confirms his advance refusal of consent to a feeding tube, this should be respected. If you cannot be convinced of this, and feel that these are exclusively his wife's wishes then you should resolve to seek further advice from senior colleagues and ultimately, may need to contemplate a course of action that is at odds with a relative's wishes but that is seen as in that patient's best interests by the medical team; such a course of action should generally be followed gently, allowing relatives time to question the issue themselves and see things from your perspective.

9 Confirm understanding and invite questions

Be clear that she understands the issues raised, and invite questions.

10 Agree a way forward

A likely way forward will be to request PEG insertion, with the understanding that this decision might be revised if he were to deteriorate in the next few days but proceed if he remains stable.

Discussion

What are the key aspects, based on case law, of capacity to give or withhold consent?

For a patient to give valid consent to a procedure or treatment, she or he must be *competent* or, *in legal terms, have the capacity* to do so. The key aspects of capacity are listed in Box 4.17.

Incapacity must be proven. All adults are assumed by law to have capacity unless proven otherwise. Further, a person may not be globally competent or incompetent. It is 'function or decision specific'. For example, a patient may be capable of declining surgery but incapable of judging their safety at home. Capacity may also fluctuate over time. Even where capacity may be limited, a doctor has a duty to give an account in simple terms to a patient of what is being proposed. According to the Mental Capacity Act (below) a person lacks capacity if because of 'an impairment of, or a disturbance in the functioning of, the brain and mind' (which can be permanent or temporary) he or she is unable to fulfil any of the four criteria in Box 4.17.

Can any doctor judge a patient's capacity?

It is the personal responsibility of any doctor proposing an investigation or treatment to establish whether a patient has the capacity to give valid consent. Where incapacity is being judged it is wise to seek agreement from colleagues and other members of the team involved in the patient's care, and where there is any doubt to seek the opinion of a psychiatrist.

What do you know of the legal necessity to treat incapacitated patients?

The concept of necessity is that not only is a doctor able to give treatment to an incapacitated patient when it is clearly in that patient's best interests, but it is also common law to do so. This still only applies to treatment aimed to

Box 4.17 The key aspects of capacity
Each of the following must apply for a person to have capacity: 1. The ability *to understand information* relevant to the decision (proposed interventions such as investigations or treatments, alternative options, the intervention's possible benefits and risks, and the consequences of non-treatment); the person should also of course believe that information to be true   2. The ability to *retain that information* (for how long depends upon what the information is)   3. The ability to *weigh up the information* to reach a decision   4. The ability to *communicate* a decision

---

Box 4.18 Guidance when making decisions for a patient without capacity

- Doctors may act in what they see as a patient's *best interests*. The doctrine of necessity underpinning the treatment of people who lack capacity requires that there must be a necessity to act and that such action must be in the best interests of the person concerned. Under current law, *best interests will be served when a doctor acts in accordance with accepted medical opinion (Bolam test)*. When more than one option seem reasonably in a patient's best interests (including non-treatment) that which *least restricts that patient's future choices* should be chosen.
- Doctors may be guided by any expressed wishes or *advance decisions* made at a time when the patient had capacity. Losing capacity, such as losing consciousness, does not negate previous wishes and a valid advance directive overrides best interests if these are discrepant.
- Doctors may be guided by *third parties who have more knowledge of the patient* (partner, family, carers), who may be sources of information but who cannot, under common law, give or refuse consent to a treatment. However, there is now proxy for this in English law under the *Mental Capacity Act*.
- The rights of an incapacitated patient to such principles as non-discrimination, confidentiality, liberty and dignity are of course identical to those of a patient with capacity.

Box 4.19 The five key principles of the Mental Capacity Act

1. People are assumed to have capacity unless proven otherwise.
2. Before deciding that someone lacks capacity, all steps should be taken to enhance his or her decision-making abilities.
3. Someone cannot be said to lack capacity simply because he or she is making what might be seen as an eccentric or unwise decision.
4. A person's best interests should always be taken into account in making a decision on his or her behalf.
5. The least restrictive option (of basic rights and freedoms) should always be used.

Box 4.20 Determining best interests

The person making a decision must

- Consider when/if the person is likely to regain capacity.
- Encourage patient participation (repeatedly pulling out a nasogastric tube may be indicative of wishes).
- Consider past and present feelings, previous beliefs and values and other relevant factors.
- Consult others (account should be taken, where practicable and appropriate, of the views of at least one of: anyone named by the person to be consulted on matters of the kind; anyone engaged in caring for the person or interested in their welfare; any donee with lasting power of attorney (LPA) granted by the person; any court appointed deputy). For people who lack capacity and who lack a spokesperson (no relative, friend, carer, LPA or deputee) an independent consultee arrangement is possible.

---

improve or prevent deterioration in health. If the patient is known to have prior objections to all or some parts of a treatment, doctors are not justified in proceeding, even in emergency situations. If incapacity is temporary (e.g. anaesthesia, intoxication, unconsciousness), doctors should not proceed beyond what is essential to preserve life or prevent deterioration in health.

How may doctors be guided when making decisions for a patient without capacity?

Doctors, not relatives, are responsible for making medical decisions about incapacitated patients. Any procedures requiring a consent form should be consented to by doctors, not a next of kin. Guidance when making decisions for patients without capacity is given in Box 4.18.

What are the key principles and innovations of the English Mental Capacity Act 2005?

The Mental Capacity Act provides a statutory framework to empower and protect vulnerable people who are not able to make their own decisions. It makes it clear who can take decisions, in which situations, and how they should go about this. It is underpinned by five key principles (Box 4.19).

Key innovations of the Mental Capacity Act are outlined in Table 4.2.

Are there any differences in Scotland?

'Those close' to a patient may include a partner, a family member, a professional or other carer or an informal advocate. In Scotland the phrase also includes a 'proxy decision-maker' appointed under the *Adults with Incapacity (Scotland) Act 2000* (which defines incapacity but not capacity). This may be a 'nearest relative' or a 'person claiming an interest' such as a public guardian or mental welfare commissioner (as referred to in the Act or under Scottish mental health legislation).

Does the Mental Capacity Act aid determination of best interests?

It provides a best interests checklist (Box 4.20).

Can incapacity be inferred from a particular medical illness or diagnosis?

No. Alzheimer's disease, for example, does not necessarily imply incapacity.

What do you know about legal representation for incapacitated adults?

Social services can provide *agency* or *appointeeship* for handling the financial affairs of an incapacitated adult. Doctors may sign letters confirming mental incapacity; psychiatrists may become involved where mental state assessment is challenging.

Power of attorney (PA)

PA gives someone the legal right to act on behalf of another. PA is only applicable for people who can

Table 4.2 Key innovations of the Mental Capacity Act

Key innovation	What it means		Relevance to doctors
Definition of incapacity	A clear test of incapacity (Box 4.17)		Not really differing from previous legal definitions
Designated 'proxy' decision-makers may act on behalf of someone who lacks capacity under two mechanisms	Lasting power of attorney (LPA)	A person who still has capacity may donate an LPA to one or more people. This is similar to enduring power of attorney (EPA) which preceded it, but now allows for the donor's (that person giving power of attorney) care, including medical care, to be decided by the donee (that person given power of attorney) although an LPA cannot refuse life-sustaining treatment unless expressively given this power and is bound by advance directives.	The key change for doctors to be aware of; while these two forms of proxy may become increasingly common, it is likely that most patients will continue to have no such provision and will be treated as previously by doctors making 'best interests' decisions
	Court-appointed deputies	The Court can appoint a deputy or deputies who can make welfare, health and financial decisions on behalf of a person who lacks capacity but are not able to refuse consent to life-sustaining treatment. They can only be appointed if the Court cannot make a one-off decision to resolve issues	
Development of two public bodies to support the statutory framework designed around the needs of those who lack capacity	A new Court of Protection	Has jurisdiction relating to the whole Act and final arbiter for capacity matters	Awareness
	A new Public Guardian	Registering authority for LPAs and deputies	Awareness
Greater emphasis on decisions being made in the patient's best interests	Applies both to doctors and to any proxy decision-makers		No change
Three further provisions to protect vulnerable people	Independent Mental Capacity Advocate (IMCA)	Someone appointed to support a person who lacks capacity but has no-one to speak for them. Makes representations about feelings, beliefs and values and brings relevant facts to attention of decision-maker. Can challenge decision-maker	Awareness
	Advance decisions to refuse treatment	Statutory support of advance directives and decision-making	Does not apply to any treatment a doctor considers necessary to sustain life unless strict formalities have been complied with that include a decision in writing that is signed and witnessed and that includes an express statement that the decision stands 'even if life is at risk'
	Criminal offence	For ill treatment or neglect of a person who lacks capacity	Awareness
Clear parameters for research	Research may be lawful if approved by relevant bodies (e.g. Ethics Committees) and cannot be performed as effectively on those with capacity. Carers or nominated third parties must be consulted and agree that patient would approve		Awareness

understand and not for people with incapacity (compare with proxy decision-making in Scotland). A solicitor, for example, may act as PA to sell your house while you are on holiday. PA formerly lapsed if a person became incapacitated but in 1985 a special type of PA known as *enduring power of attorney (EPA)* changed this. PA can be revoked. Sometimes PA representatives can try to take PA too far. PA does not give the right to make medical decisions, which remain up to the patient, or, if the patient is incapacitated, the doctor acting in the patient's best interests, except in those circumstances where *lasting power of attorney (LPA)*, now replacing EPA, has been invoked allowing for proxy decision-making under the Mental Capacity Act.

Court of Protection/Court Appointed Deputies

Court of Protection (C.o.P.) (now a system of Court Appointed Deputies) applies to circumstances in which EPA (now LPA) has not been given and a patient has become incapacitated. It is concerned mostly with property, and requires medical evidence. C.o.P. applications can be made by a solicitor (usual) or the state (Director of Social Services). Solicitors then request details as to why a doctor feels that a patient is incapacitated. Many doctors (e.g. Care of the Elderly physicians) complete the forms where incapacity is clear (brief, layperson's language is acceptable, e.g. poor memory, deluded); psychiatrists are often involved where incapacity is not so clear. The Court appoints a receiver (e.g. relative, accountant) who acts for the incapacitated person. C.o.P. is not necessarily permanent because it depends more on behaviour than prognosis.

It is common to look after patients in hospital who are vulnerable and lack insight and capacity, for example the elderly lady who lives alone in her own house, has no close relatives and who wanders at night around the house putting on the gas, or outside on to the road. If she lacks insight, she may ask to go home and simply reject all of your concerns. Your responsibility is for her safety. It may be impossible to put in care at home at night and if she has progressive dementia without acute psychosis or depression transferring her to psychiatric care is only shifting the problem. She will probably need gentle ushering to a community hospital bed unless direct care-home placement is available, with her general practitioner on board. Although not urgent, ultimately her house may need to be sold and other affairs attended to. Therefore, concurrently, assuming she has no LPA in a distant relative or in her solicitor, social services should be contacted to start C.o.P. proceedings.

Does the Mental Capacity Act allow restraint of patients?

It is only permitted if it is reasonably believed to prevent harm and must be proportionate to the likelihood of serious harm.

What do you know about safeguarding vulnerable adults in hospital?

Vulnerable adults include those who lack mental capacity, those with cognitive impairment, those disabled mentally or physically, those with sensory impairment, those in institutions, those with no fixed abode and those socially isolated.

Vulnerable adult risk management involves case-specific management, often a multi-agency approach, and involving the patient as far as possible in decision making; where this is not possible and there are no relatives or carers, or if there are concerns about the motives of relatives or carers, an independent mental capacity advocate (IMCA) may aid decision making in best interests, making more robust the traditional doctor 'best interests' decisions. IMCAs may be helpful if there are major medical decisions or if care placement is being planned, and they have the right to use the Court of Protection if they have concerns about decisions being proposed.

Sadly, vulnerable adults are often subject to abuse, most commonly by those 'caring' for them, often in institutions, sometimes in their own home; carers may not be aware of the abuse, and abuse is not always intended; sometimes it has become 'the norm' over many years, and sometimes the patient's needs outgrow well-intentioned carers or institutions.

Signs of abuse may be physical (e.g. bruises, pressure areas), behavioural (e.g. fear, avoidance), loss of financial assets or neglect (e.g. malnutrition, weight loss, dehydration, unkempt appearance).

The clinician's role is an index of suspicion, accurate record keeping, arranging any appropriate medical photography, multidisciplinary team liaison and referral to the Hospital Social Services Team (HSST). The HSST coordinates all subsequent investigation and referral to the Adult Protection (AP) team or the AP police who may determine whether or not an offence has been committed; the AP police take over investigation of any offence, and it is important for clinicians to share information on a need-to-know basis.

CASE 4.25

REFUSAL OF CONSENT

Candidate information

Role

You are a doctor on the medical ward.
Please read this summary.

Communication skills and ethics

Scenario

> Re: Ms Eleanor Dashwood, aged 75 years
>
> Ms Dashwood was admitted to hospital recently with pneumonia. During the course of investigations she was found to have iron deficiency anaemia and subsequently a hard rectal mass was discovered, most probably a carcinoma. She is asymptomatic. She is otherwise well and has no past medical history of note. She has now made a good recovery from her pneumonia and is keen to go home. She refuses any further investigations or treatments for the likely tumour.
>
> Your task is to establish that this is her informed decision.

Your examiners will warn you when 12 minutes have elapsed. You have 14 minutes to communicate with the patient/subject followed by 1 minute of reflection. There will then follow 5 minutes of discussion with the examiners. Do not take the history again except for details that will help in your discussion with the patient/subject. You are not required to examine the patient/subject.

Patient/subject information

Ms Eleanor Dashwood is a previously well 75-year-old, independent lady admitted to hospital with pneumonia. She is recovering from this but during the course of her stay she was found to be anaemic and subsequently a rectal lump was discovered, most probably a cancer. She told the doctors she had no symptoms but has in fact had constipation and episodes of fresh rectal bleeding over the last two months. She has not told anyone because her husband developed similar symptoms a few months before his bowel cancer was diagnosed. His cancer had spread to the liver at diagnosis and was incurable. He died despite a complex array of investigations and treatments. She does not wish to 'go down the same route of hospitals and tests' and would prefer to let nature take its course, even if that means rapidly deteriorating like her husband. She will refuse any further investigations or treatments for the likely tumour.

How to approach the case

Communication skills (conduct of interview, exploration and problem negotiation) and ethics and law

1 Introduction

Introduce yourself and make it clear you are here to help.

2 Explain the situation so far

> As I think you know, you had a rather nasty pneumonia when you came in to hospital that has responded very well to antibiotics. But I think you also know that during the course of our tests we found that you were anaemic – that your blood count was low. We also discovered a lump, in the tail end, and this is very likely the reason for the anaemia, very possibly a lump that may not be nice . . . a form of growth.

She will be likely to acknowledge all of this and may either tell you she has thought about this and decided she does not want anything done or she may be a little more open to your thoughts and ask what you feel ought to be done.

3 Explain the best way forward

The best way forward for her can only be established in conjunction with her.

> That is for us to decide. First of all, we would need to consider some further tests to try to establish accurately what it is.

4 Establish previous experience and be alert to beliefs and concerns

Her husband's experience is clearly pivotal in her decision. Acknowledge this.

> I understand. I do understand.

It may be that she imagines painful tests. It may be that she imagines only chemotherapy, about which she has heard so many dreadful things, but would consider an operation. There are many 'maybes'. The point is that before respecting her wishes (autonomy) for no further tests, you must try to understand precisely what her position is and help to inform her. Her decision may already have been made. But you should try to discover the reasons she made it and whether or not she has sufficient information at her disposal to make an informed decision. She may choose not to receive any more information, but ideally informed consent to no treatment should be obtained and based upon discussion of the acceptability and effectiveness of the various options.

5 Explain the nature of the investigation or treatment

> I understand fully how you must feel. And I'll say immediately that we will respect any decision you make. I should also tell you that at this stage we are by no means certain of the diagnosis and that tests would help us to be more certain – and to more certainly know whether this is a very different situation to that of your husband. It may well be.

Were we to investigate, I would recommend a scan of the tummy, and then very likely a biopsy of the lump – by asking one of our surgical colleagues to take a sample of tissue from the lump via flexible telescope with a light on the end. We would then be in a much better position to know the best way forward.

6 Explain the risks and benefits of the investigation or treatment and the consequences of not pursuing matters

The tests would probably tell us one of two things. Firstly, they might show that this problem is very well localised, and if that is the case then very possibly curable. Secondly, if, and there is always the possibility, things were not as confined as we hoped, then we might well be able to predict future problems and take action to lessen these. One of the more immediate problems that can sometimes arise is a blockage in the bowel, which can be difficult, and far more difficult to treat if it happens without our prior knowledge. There is, of course, a possibility that the lump is not as worrying as we had thought, and the anaemia is caused by something very simple. It would be nice to know this.

7 Explain any possible alternatives

She may ask what would happen next if she chose not to pursue tests.

The alternative is simply to let you go home, perhaps asking your doctor to keep a close eye on things, and arranging for you to see us again at any stage if you were to change your mind. Or we could see you here in clinic in a few weeks to have another talk about things. I would just say, however, that you are a healthy lady in all other respects, and that makes it much more likely that you would find the tests, and perhaps treatment, more straightforward.

Ask if she has any relatives or people close to her with whom she might wish to discuss options, or with whom she might wish you to talk. A common problem, however, is that relatives may take a different view and exert pressure on the physician to act. The primary emotion is almost always desire for the best management of the patient. The physician may explain (if the patient is happy for such a discussion) that the issue has been fully discussed in terms of likely benefits and risks and outcomes, and that as a result of this information an informed decision has been made by the patient. Occasionally, relatives may feel that the patient is unable to make the best decision ('she is old and does not know what is best') to which the physician must explain that there is no evidence she or he does not have the capacity to make informed decisions.

8 Show respect for autonomy

We will do our best, whatever you decide.

9 Confirm understanding and invite questions

Allow her time to assimilate all of this information, confirm that she understands what you have explained and invite any questions.

10 Keep the door open

If she still refuses ongoing investigation, make it very clear that you are happy to see her again. In this situation, where she will have a lot to assimilate, it might be sensible to arrange follow-up in clinic anyway, if she agrees. She might be more likely to miss out on potential treatments unless you set up possible avenues towards these.

Discussion

If a young woman with Grave's thyrotoxicosis wanted to pursue homeopathic treatment, even when the endocrinologist has recommended carbimazole, would you agree?

You may not have the facts in front of you, but feel she 'needs' more than homoeopathic treatment. It is vital to understand why she feels the way she does and explore her reasons for choosing homoeopathy. She may have experience of homeopathy for other conditions, she may have been ready to consider carbimazole before learning of a dangerous side effect (leucopenia), and she may have considered other forms of treatment. You should talk to her about Graves' disease, its complications, the benefits and risks of treatment and the likely natural history without treatment. You might tell her you are unaware of any effective homoeopathic treatments. Is it possible, if she is adamant that homoeopathic treatment will help her, that she would consider conventional treatment as well? Failing this, might she accept switching to conventional treatment within a certain time limit if her approach fails? You would of course inform your consultant of any conversation and document your advice carefully.

You have been seeing a 50-year-old man with tuberculosis in the respiratory clinic. He wishes to pursue homoeopathic treatment rather than continue with antibiotics. Would you agree?

There comes a point where collusion with a patient is wrong, clinically, ethically and legally. Here, you have not just to consider this man's autonomy, but risks to other members of the public from his active tuberculosis. Rather than approaching this dilemma in a dogmatic way, listening to the patient's reasons, beliefs and concerns may avoid confrontation. Perhaps the importance of antibiotic therapy has never been fully explained. Perhaps he has heard that homoeopathy can help a wide range of respiratory conditions. Listening and simple explanation may be

- Any adult with capacity, because of their right of autonomy or self-determination, may refuse investigation or treatment for reasons that are rational, irrational or for no reason.
- Legally, such refusal of treatment supersedes the sanctity of life.
- To treat in these circumstances would constitute trespass or battery.
- Existing consent may be withdrawn at any time and new refusal overrides prior consent.

An example of refusal of treatment with a potentially life-threatening outcome would be that of a patient who is a Jehovah's Witness refusing blood products for whom a blood transfusion might be life-saving. Respect for autonomy (self-determination) means that this refusal must be respected. Notwithstanding this, if an individual chooses an option that not only contradicts what appears to be in his or her best interests and that most people would choose, but also appears to contradict that individual's previously expressed attitudes, then you would be justified in questioning the individual's capacity to make a valid refusal and to wish to exclude a possible depressed or deluded state.

enough to persuade him of his misconception. Perhaps he feels the antibiotics should have worked by now and is concerned that he's still coughing. Perhaps he is frustrated that he cannot return to work and needs to vent his feelings.

Can a patient refuse treatment, even to the point of death?

Refusal of consent is discussed in Box 4.21.

CASE 4.26

DELIBERATE SELF-HARM

Candidate information

Role

You are a doctor on the emergency medical admissions unit.

Please read this summary.

Scenario

Re: Miss Jane Hughes, aged 22 years

Miss Hughes was admitted to the emergency medical admissions unit earlier today after taking an overdose of paracetamol. She reported taking 16 50-mg tablets 12 hours before admission, with the intention of committing suicide. Her paracetamol level was below the treatment line and liver function tests are normal including the international normalised ratio (INR). She is now keen to go home. The ward nurse is concerned that she may be at risk of further suicide attempts, and although a

psychiatry opinion has been requested this might not happen until tomorrow.

Your tasks are to explore the reasons for her suicide attempt, assess her current suicide risk and suggest a way forward.

Your examiners will warn you when 12 minutes have elapsed. You have 14 minutes to communicate with the patient/subject followed by 1 minute of reflection. There will then follow 5 minutes of discussion with the examiners. Do not take the history again except for details that will help in your discussion with the patient/subject. You are not required to examine the patient/subject.

Patient/subject information

Miss Jane Hughes is a 22-year-old primary school teacher with no medical history of note. She was admitted to hospital this morning following an overdose of 16 paracetamol tablets. She has recently moved to the area, having finished her teacher training last year, and although she has no history of psychiatric disease or suicide attempts herself in the past she has suffered recently 'in silence' from the death of her father and taken to getting excessively drunk with new friends in the area on week nights, and, increasingly, drinking alone. Last month one of her class children died in a road traffic accident and she has found herself ruminating over this a lot. She is 'a bright young thing' according to friends, and 'has everything going for her' but suffers from low self-esteem, which she knows is irrational. She has never had any delusions or hallucinations. She does not know why she took the overdose now, only that she told a friend who brought her to hospital. She just wants to go home and forget it happened. She is about to see the doctor.

How to approach the case

Communication skills (conduct of interview, exploration and problem negotiation) and ethics and law

1 Introduction

Introduce yourself and make it clear you are here to help.

2 Show empathy

Deliberate self-harm, unhappily, is an increasing problem for emergency services and it is all too easy to assume that 'just another overdose' has arrived, 'probably with no intention of significant self-harm'. Suicide is an escalating problem and no patient's intentions should be underestimated and every patient's case should be considered on its own unique merit. These cases are complex, and warrant psychiatric appraisal. All doctors should be able to make an initial assessment of the situation and the risk. Firstly,

Questions about the episode

- Events preceding the act
- Reasons for the act
- Suicide intent
- Any psychiatric disorders including previous suicide attempts
- Family history
- Coping resources and support network
- Whether ready to accept help

Factors suggesting suicide intent

- Act undertaken alone
- Act timed that intervention unlikely
- Precautions to avoid discovery
- Active preparation for attempt
- Preparations made anticipating death
- Leaving a note
- Failure to inform potential rescuers afterwards
- Admission of suicidal intent

Factors associated with an increased risk of further suicide attempts

- Male
- Under 19 or over 45 years of age
- Unemployment
- Separated, divorced, widowed or living alone
- Previous suicide attempts with admission to hospital
- Alcohol or drug problems
- Psychiatric disorder
- Chronic disease

tell her that you are sorry she is in hospital and that you understand things must have been very difficult to have reached this stage.

3 Establish ideas and concerns

There are clearly background issues, which she may or may not allude to.

4 Assessment of patient following a suicide attempt

All doctors should be able to perform an initial psychosocial assessment following attempted suicide (Box 4.22).

5 Explain what should be done next

Reassure her that you are satisfied medically but that you are concerned for her overall welfare.

6 Reassure that information given is confidential

Give absolute reassurance of this.

7 Reassure that the psychiatrist will help to identify problems

Explain that the reasons for seeking a psychiatrist's help are that it is not your area of expertise and that you wish to protect her from future self-harm by dealing with issues that hold her back so that she can get on with life.

8 Explain possible alternatives

She may ask what would happen if she chose not to wait to see a psychiatrist. This depends on your assessment of

her risk. Options include trying to arrange for more immediate psychiatric assessment by a liaison psychiatrist or member of the liaison psychiatric team or to seek telephone advice from a psychiatrist as to whether it is felt that she could be allowed home with early review. If risk is sufficiently worrying, you should be honest with her and explain that you have a duty of care to ensure that she does not leave until she has seen a psychiatrist. Application of the Mental Health Act should be a last resort.

9 Invite further questions

Is there anything you would like me to go over again or are there any questions you would like to ask me?

10 Agree a way forward

The examiners are aware that such a discussion is difficult. They are not looking for a 'model answer' but checking your awareness of the range of issues provoked and ability to handle these sensitively and professionally.

Discussion

What would you do if a patient wants to leave hospital before being assessed by a mental health professional?

Doctors have a duty of care that includes protecting patients as best as possible from ongoing risk. If a patient refuses to stay for mental health assessment following an episode of deliberate self-harm, you should if possible make your own assessment of risk (see Box 4.22). If you are still concerned, you should try to persuade the patient to stay and if they still refuse you may detain them under common law pending formal psychiatric assessment. If you are satisfied that risk is low, you may allow the patient to be discharged with appropriate information to the general practitioner (ideally after telephone approval from and perhaps follow-up with a psychiatrist).

What does common law allow in the matter of detention or treatment of patients?

It allows doctors to act in a patient's best interests in emergency situations where consent cannot be given (patient unconscious or lacks capacity). It allows detention pending assessment or treatment against a patient's will if in that patient's best interests (by saving life or to ensure improvement or prevent deterioration of physical or mental health). It should be documented that you are treating in best interests under common law.

Can you detain or treat against a patient's will if they have capacity?

Detention or treatment against a patient's will under common law or under the Mental Health Act is not possible if a patient has capacity. To do so may constitute a criminal offence. Where there are doubts about capacity (which may be function-specific rather than global and may change over time) it is usually better to treat than not treat. In the case of deliberate self-harm, patients frequently do have capacity but you may equally be concerned that capacity is temporarily lost by a psychiatric illness such as depression and if your assessment deems a patient to be at serious risk then you are unlikely to be criticised. Detention and treatment may be given under common law.

Table 4.3 Sections of the Mental Health Act	
Section	Provision
2	Allows assessment and/or treatment for up to 28 days Requires two appropriately qualified doctors and a social worker
3	Allows extension for up to six months (may follow Section 2)
4	Allows patient to be brought to hospital in an emergency Requires a doctor and social worker
5 (2)	Allows any hospital doctor to detain an inpatient under the nominated hospital consultant if psychiatric assessment likely to be delayed Patient may be detained for 72 hours pending full Mental Health Act assessment Initiated by a form available on the wards that is submitted to the local Mental Health Act administration team Does not allow treatment of any kind, which must be under common law if a patient does not consent (herewith a 'best interests' decision based on presumed current incapacity allows attempted treatment)
5 (4)	Allows a nurse to detain for six hours pending the arrival of a doctor to detain under Section 5 (2)
136	Allows police to bring a patient to the emergency department where doctors may decide to informally assess or arrange for a Section 2 or 3

Which aspects of the Mental Health Act are relevant to general medicine?

The Mental Health Act 1983 permits compulsory detention and/or treatment of patients with a mental illness and/or mental impairment of a nature and/or degree that requires inpatient treatment against their wishes. If a patient needs to be in hospital because of a risk to self or others he or she may be detained or brought into hospital if appropriate people agree. But the Act does not allow treatment of mentally impaired patients for physical problems against their will, even if the physical problem is a result of deliberate self-harm such as self-poisoning. Therefore psychiatrists, often asked to 'section' such a patient for compulsory treatment, cannot do so, although treatment may be given under common law. The Act does, however, allow treatment where a physical condition causes the mental condition, as in an organic psychosis. Relevant sections of the Mental Health Act are listed in Table 4.3. Although there is a different legal system in Scotland, the principles are the same.

An elderly lady takes a lethal ingestion with the intention of suicide. She declines intervention. She is assessed by the psychiatric team who feel that she has capacity to make this decision. Would you accept this?

At first sight it may seem that any patient attempting suicide must lack capacity because of depressed mood but this is by no means necessarily so. Some patients do feel that life is so miserable for intractable reasons and see no hope, such that, notwithstanding possible depression, they have the capacity to decide they no longer wish to live. While every opportunity must be given to allow the patient to change their mind, and it must be clear that the patient fully understands the implications of the decision, if a psychiatrist has confirmed capacity and declared that the decision should be respected, the patient's autonomy should be respected.

END-OF-LIFE ISSUES

CASE 4.27

RESUSCITATION-STATUS DECISION-MAKING – DISCUSSION WITH PATIENT

Candidate information

Role

You are a doctor on the respiratory ward.
Please read this summary.

Scenario

> Re: Mr Robert Churchill, aged 75 years
>
> Mr Churchill has severe chronic obstructive pulmonary disease. He has a home oxygen cylinder. For the last three years he has been confined to his house, with twice-daily carers to assist with bathing, meals and housework. Breathlessness is his main limitation. Over the last year he has been admitted to hospital five times with increasing frequency with exacerbations of breathlessness, sometimes precipitated by infection. Investigations for pulmonary emboli have been negative. He was readmitted yesterday with breathlessness and responded to initial non-invasive ventilation from which he has been successfully weaned. However, his resuscitation status has not been documented.
>
> Your task is to discuss his resuscitation status with him. You may assume that you were involved in his care yesterday and on previous admissions and that he knows who you are.

Your examiners will warn you when 12 minutes have elapsed. You have 14 minutes to communicate with the patient/subject followed by 1 minute of reflection. There will then follow 5 minutes of discussion with the examiners. Do not take the history again except for details that will help in your discussion with the patient/subject. You are not required to examine the patient/subject.

Patient/subject information

Mr Robert Churchill is a 75-year-old gentleman who has severe chronic obstructive pulmonary disease. He has a home oxygen cylinder. For the last three years he has been confined to his house, where he lives alone, having been widowed for five years. He has twice-daily

carers to assist with bathing, meals and housework. Breathlessness is his main limitation. Over the last year he has been admitted to hospital five times with increasing frequency and with exacerbations of his breathlessness. He was readmitted yesterday with breathlessness and required a tight breathing mask to improve respiratory distress. He is better today but knows things are not going to get any better in the long run. He has two children, but they live a long distance away. He has considered the future and 'doesn't want to go on indefinitely like this' but the issue of whether or not he should be resuscitated in the event of a cardiac or respiratory arrest has never been discussed.

How to approach the case

Communication skills (conduct of interview, exploration and problem negotiation) and ethics and law

1 Introduction, setting and rapport

A discussion about resuscitation should be between a patient and ideally a doctor who has already created a rapport with that patient, even if brief. The setting should ideally be quiet, and without distractions.

2 Ensure the patient has enough information about their condition

A resuscitation discussion should only come once he has a full grasp of his condition and its likely prognosis even with treatment.

3 Then come directly to the reason for the discussion

> *Mr Churchill, there is one thing I should discuss with you, that relates to what we might do in the event – not that I'm expecting it – but in the event of things going very wrong (with your health) on this admission to hospital.*

4 Pace the explanation slowly and carefully, and in words the patient will understand, allowing him to assimilate what you are saying

> *You have been in hospital rather a lot over the last year, and now you're back in hospital sooner than you and your doctors had hoped. Someone with a lung condition as bad as yours may suddenly take a turn for the worse. I know you know this, having used the breathing apparatus last night and on other occasions in the past. We will of course do all that we can to improve the situation for you this time. But there is always the possibility, as with any unwell patient, that things could go very wrong. That the heart could stop, or the breathing stop, altogether. Have you ever thought about what your wishes might be in that situation?*

5 Many patients immediately understand all of this, and pre-empt further discussion by declaring clearly pre-considered wishes. Some patients wish to go further and may ask about resuscitation

> *If things were to go horribly wrong, and your heart or breathing were to stop, would you wish us to try to restart things with heart-starting machines or breathing tubes and so forth?*

6 Be prepared to deal with emotions before facts if you sense the discussion is causing distress

> *I can see that you find this difficult. We could talk about it later, if you prefer, or, if you wish, with members of your family here (if you know there are family members) or some patients simply prefer that we do what we think is the very best for them.*

7 Many patients prefer to leave the decision to their doctors

> *I would leave it in your hands, doctor. Do as you think best.*

8 Some patients might ask what you think

> *Well, we would have great concerns that in the event of things getting to that stage, trying to rescue the situation would be in vain. It simply would not work.*

It is not inappropriate to tell patients or relatives that you think resuscitation extremely unlikely to be successful or to be futile or that invasive ventilation would be very unlikely to bring recovery. Many patients do not appreciate, until it is explained, that resuscitation and the potential consequences of temporary revival without meaningful recovery or longer-term survival might simply be increasing the distress of an inevitable natural death, prolonging death rather than sustaining life, or increasing the likelihood of 'two deaths'.

9 Confirm patient understanding and explore any other concerns

Ensure that he is clear about the course of action, be prepared to explore any other concerns and ask if he would like anything clarified.

10 Conclude with assurances

Always conclude with an assurance that if a decision is made not to resuscitate, you and your team will continue to do all that you can to actively treat his condition and to relieve symptoms. Make it clear, where appropriate, that a decision can be reviewed and altered at any time.

> *Meantime, we will do all that we can to get you better (up to the brink).*

Discussion

Do you know of any guidelines relating to 'do not attempt resuscitation' (DNAR) decision-making?

All establishments (e.g. hospitals, care homes) that face decisions about attempting cardiopulmonary resuscitation (CPR) should have local policies for decision-making. A joint statement by the British Medical Association, Resuscitation Council (UK) and the Royal College of Nursing has provided guidelines outlining ethical and legal considerations for such decision-making. The guidelines embrace decisions made in advance that form part of a patient's care plan, and the emergency where no advance plan has been made. The guidelines can assist local policies for DNR decision-making, for example those produced by NHS Trusts, and should be understood by and accessible to all relevant staff and available to patients.

Why do we need policies for DNAR decision-making?

At the time of a cardiac or respiratory arrest, there is neither time to deliberate about its appropriateness nor opportunity to ascertain a patient's wishes, because he or she would now lack the capacity to consent to or refuse it. CPR can be attempted on anyone whose cardiac or respiratory functions cease. Since there comes a time for every person when death is inevitable, it is essential to deliberate in advance and seek a patient's wishes in advance – either to identify patients for whom cardiopulmonary arrest would represent a terminal event in their illness and for whom CPR is inappropriate, or patients who would not wish CPR and competently refuse it. The decision-making principles are the same for all patients in all settings, but no guideline can embrace the complex clinical considerations that health teams face, and the way decisions are made may vary with the setting; a hospital emergency department may adapt guidelines in a different way to a care home, for example. The wide range of scenarios may mean that the decision reached for one case may be inappropriate in another superficially similar case.

Do you know of any legal statements that underpin DNAR decision-making?

The Human Rights Act 1998, implemented in 2000, incorporates the bulk of rights set out in the European Convention on Human Rights into UK law. Health professionals must be able to demonstrate that decisions are compatible with human rights set out in the Articles of the Convention. Particularly relevant provisions include the rights to life (Article 2), freedom from inhuman or degrading treatment (Article 3), respect for privacy and family life (Article 8), freedom of expression, which includes the right to hold opinions and receive information (Article 10) and freedom from discriminatory practices in respect of these rights (Article 14).

What challenges are there to implementing DNAR decision-making guidelines in practice?

There is often failure to appreciate that the justification for attempting resuscitation rests on a reasonable balance to harms and risks, which is difficult to judge in advance. There is obvious difficulty in making advance decisions if the circumstances of a future cardiopulmonary arrest cannot be envisaged, in which case the balance of benefits and risks cannot be judged. There is often uncertainty about the role of the patient or relatives in decision-making. There is often lack of appreciation that an advance decision about CPR should be implemented under the same principles and ethical and legal guidance as any other advance statement.

Is prolonging a patient's life the most important goal?

The goal of treatment is to benefit patients, by restoring or maintaining health as far as possible, thereby maximising benefit and minimising harm. If treatment fails, or if it ceases to provide a net benefit, or if a competent patient refuses treatment, this goal cannot be realised and treatment is no longer justified. Prolonging a patient's life is usually to their benefit, but is not an appropriate goal at all cost with disregard to quality of life and burdens of treatment.

Some *competent* patients (in legal terms, those with *capacity*) decide that a stage has been reached when prolonging life, although possible, is not appropriate. Some competent patients identify a future point when this may be so through an advance directive.

Where a patient is *not competent* (in legal terms, *incapacitated*) and there is no advance directive, a decision must be made that is in the *best interests* of that patient.

What factors should be considered in resuscitation decision-making?

A DNAR order is a specific example of a limitation of treatment. The joint statement by the British Medical Association, Resuscitation Council (UK) and Royal College of Nursing has the following underlying principles:

- Timely support for patients and relatives with effective communication
- Decisions must be based on individual circumstances and reviewed regularly – any decision can be changed at any time
- Sensitive discussion in advance should be encouraged but not enforced
- There needs to be a realistic chance of success in using CPR

Decisions should ideally be made in advance as part of an overall care plan, after consultation and after consideration of all relevant aspects of the patient's condition (Box 4.23).

Box 4.23 Factors to be considered in resuscitation decision-making
The likely clinical outcome
This includes the likelihood of successful CPR and the overall benefit achieved from successful CPR.
The patient's known or ascertainable wishes
A valid and applicable advance refusal is legally binding but a patient cannot legally demand resuscitation.
Capacity
Even in patients with cognitive impairment, capacity to make decisions can vary greatly.
Rights of partners or relatives
Partners and relatives do not have a legal right to demand, consent to or refuse treatment on a patient's behalf.
The patient's views expressed contemporaneously or in an advance statement override those of partner or relatives.
The patient's human rights
Under the European Human Rights Act.
Second opinion
Any request for a second opinion should be respected.
Communication
The views of the patient, all members of the health-care team and people close to the patient are valuable in making the decision. Once made, the decision should be communicated to all relevant parties and documented, signed and dated.

What do you understand by the presumption in favour of attempting resuscitation?

For the vast majority of patients in hospital the likelihood of cardiopulmonary arrest is small and no advance decision has been made. CPR should be attempted where no explicit advance decision has been made about the appropriateness of attempting CPR, and where a patient's express wishes are unknown and cannot be ascertained. Although this is a general presumption, it is unlikely to be considered reasonable to attempt CPR in the terminal phase of illness in patients for whom the burdens of treatment clearly outweigh potential benefits.

Under which circumstances is it appropriate to consider a DNAR order?

Circumstances are described in Box 4.24.

Is it always necessary to discuss resuscitation status with a patient?

Patients have ethical and legal rights to be involved in decisions relating to them. Their views about the level of burden or risk they consider acceptable carry considerable weight in deciding whether or not to give a particular treatment. Therefore, decisions about whether the likely benefits from successful CPR outweigh the burdens should also involve patients. There are generally three circumstances

---

Box 4.24 Circumstances in which it is appropriate to consider a do not attempt resuscitation (DNAR) order

1. The health-care team is as certain as it can be that CPR will not restart heart and breathing

The term *futility* has been used, but here refers very specifically to the immediate intervention, CPR. The concept of futility is gradually being abandoned because it makes a complex value judgement sound like one that a doctor can make alone on objective criteria when in fact it necessarily involves a value judgement about what chance of success is worth taking, and doctors, patients and families may disagree about this.

2. There is no benefit in restarting the patient's heart and breathing

No benefit is gained if only brief extension of life can be obtained and if comorbidity is such that imminent death cannot be averted.

Similarly, no benefit is gained if a patient will never have awareness or the ability to interact and therefore cannot experience benefit.

3. The expected benefit is outweighed by the burden

Attempting to prolong life is often justified despite a treatment carrying side effects, burdens and risks. CPR itself carries side effects, burdens and risks (e.g. rib fracture, intubation, admission to intensive care, brain damage if delay in CPR, traumatic death). Where a reasonable quality of life seems likely, most patients would risk some disadvantages. It is lawful, however, to withhold CPR where it is deemed (upon consideration of medical factors and whether or not treatment may provide reasonable quality of life) that CPR would not confer benefit. Where patients suffer profound disability, or have minimal or no awareness and no hope of recovering it, or suffer severe unmanageable pain or other distress, the question arises as to whether prolonging life would provide benefit. It is also appropriate to consider whether CPR is likely to fail repeatedly. Doctors must also weigh up human rights issues and refrain from artificially preserving life where a patient would consider the resulting situation an 'inhumane' or 'degrading' state.

4. CPR is not in accord with a competent patient's recorded and sustained wishes

The situation here is clear.

5. CPR is not in accord with a valid advance decision

The situation here should be clear, but the validity of advance directives or decisions is not always unequivocal.

---

that form a framework for making CPR decisions (Table 4.4).

Although discussions can be difficult and distressing for all concerned, more distress can be created later on than by a sensitive pre-emptive discussion handled at the outset.

What would you do if a patient requests CPR when you feel that it would be inappropriate?

Some patients request that CPR be attempted even when the clinical evidence suggests it is likely to be ineffective. Sensitive efforts should be made to provide a realistic view of the procedure without causing undue alarm. A patient does not have a legal right to demand any treatment, including resuscitation, and the general requirement is for discussion rather than agreement, and although it might seem medico-legally more attractive to concord with such a patient's wishes, the ethical dilemma is that it may not seem in their best interests and resources could be put to the test in the unfortunate scenario of a concurrent cardiac arrest elsewhere in the unit. In practice, fortunately, patients and doctors reach the same view the vast majority of the time, but if a patient explicitly requests resuscitation and the medical view is that it would not be of benefit then most doctors would choose to accord with that patient's wishes and make a sensible judgement about how far to take that resuscitation attempt at the time it happens.

What if a patient does not wish to discuss the issue?

This should be respected, and you may consider discussion with family to help reach a judgement. If length and quality of life after resuscitation are likely to be worse than death, then a DNAR order is appropriate, but if length and quality of life after resuscitation are likely to be worthwhile then no DNAR should be made.

Table 4.4 Framework of circumstances for making a CPR decision

Circumstance	Appropriate action	
Impossible to anticipate particular circumstances in which CPR is proposed	Since for the vast majority of patients in hospital the likelihood of cardiopulmonary arrest is small, advance decisions need only be made where cardiopulmonary arrest is a foreseeable likelihood	
Medical team as certain as can be that CPR could help the patient	Patient with capacity	Discussion with patient and any advance refusal accepted
	Patient without capacity	Medical team should act in best interests of patient unless there is clear ascertainment of other wishes from patient based on valid advance refusal or information from partner or relatives
Medical team as certain as can be that CPR would not help the patient	The general requirement is to discuss a do not resuscitate (DNAR) decision with patients but where death is expected as an inevitable consequence of disease and the team are as certain as can be that resuscitation would not restart heart or breathing or extend life significantly (points 1 and 2 in Box 4.24), discussion may unnecessarily burden the patient, partner or family. A DNAR decision can be made and a natural death should be allowed with an appropriate palliative pathway when that time approaches	

CPR, cardiopulmonary resuscitation.

CASE 4.28

RESUSCITATION-STATUS DECISION-MAKING – DISCUSSION WITH RELATIVE

Candidate information

Role

You are a doctor in the emergency medical admissions unit.

Please read this summary.

Scenario

> **Mr Chris Ryder, aged 55 years**
>
> Mr Ryder has advanced Huntington's disease. For the last year he has required full-time care in a nursing unit with specialised psychiatric skills because of behavioural disturbance. He is not competent to make decisions for himself. He has been admitted with aspiration pneumonia and has worsening acute renal failure due to sepsis. Haemodialysis may be the only way to manage his renal failure in the short term, but in the context of his comorbidity you have to decide if this is appropriate. His sister is here to talk with you. She is not genetically affected.
>
> Your task is to discuss the appropriateness of haemodialysis and intensive care, along with resuscitation status, with his sister.

Your examiners will warn you when 12 minutes have elapsed. You have 14 minutes to communicate with the patient/subject followed by 1 minute of reflection. There will then follow 5 minutes of discussion with the examiners. Do not take the history again except for details that will help in your discussion with the patient/subject. You are not required to examine the patient/subject.

Patient/subject information

You are the sister of Mr Chris Ryder, a 55-year-old man with advanced Huntington's disease. For the last year he has required full-time care in a nursing unit with specialised psychiatric skills on account of behavioural disturbance. He is not competent to make decisions for himself. You have lived with the knowledge of his inevitable decline for many years and anticipated situations from which he may not recover. You do not carry any risk of developing the disease yourself. He has now been admitted with aspiration pneumonia and has severe renal failure caused by his infection. Your brother did not make a written advance directive about his future wishes,

but your feeling is that he would not wish to be kept alive if there were no possibility of long-term cure of the underlying cause. You are a trained nurse and feel that intensive-care transfer, if it came to that, would not be in his best interests.

How to approach the case

Communication skills (conduct of interview, exploration and problem negotiation) and ethics and law

1 Introduction

Introduce yourself and establish that she is Mr Ryder's sister.

2 Establish what the relative knows

Firstly, establish a rapport with a relative you have not met before, establishing what she knows, and what she thinks, before moving to a gentle explanation of where you are in terms of her brother's medical condition and possible ways forward.

> *What have you been told so far about his condition since admission to hospital?*

3 Seek further information about the patient

Relatives are highly valuable sources of information. She may know intimately the duration and nature of his decline, his care needs and, in a chronic condition such as this, may well have anticipated what his wishes might be in the event of a precipitous acute episode of illness, and established her own views.

4 Don't forget empathy

No matter how pragmatic she may seem about his illness, remember that even expected declines often still strike harshly. Remain empathetic and pace your explanations slowly and carefully, and in words relatives will understand.

5 Explain the situation

Explain that his pneumonia is in itself treatable, but that it has provoked kidney failure that may or may not be recoverable. Explain that pneumonia is a more likely event in patients with advancing chronic conditions like Huntington's disease but that the kidney problem is now the most threatening. Explain that it is being managed with careful fluid replacement and monitoring of blood chemistry.

6 Approach the issue of more invasive interventions

> *The next, very difficult question that I know you know I'm coming to, is if things were to deteriorate*

sharply, what we might do. We are treating as energetically, as vigorously, as we can, with fluids and antibiotics and by correcting the abnormalities in the blood which arise from the kidney failure. And we hope that things may improve. But he is at serious risk, and there is no getting away from that.

7 Ensure that your explanation does not conflict with any ideas, concerns and expectations

Most importantly, ensure that she understands that his life is threatened and if she makes it clear that she does and that she does not think that he would wish for more complex interventions it is appropriate to reinforce her views.

I would have to agree. And my strong feeling and advice to you is that if there were further deterioration/a disaster, I would not be inclined to go down the route of dialysis or ventilators and intensive care . . . because I just do not think he would come through it. And the trouble is that even if he were to come through it all, without a clear way forward beyond all of this, without seeing him getting better, I think it would be putting him through unnecessary distress.

8 Many relatives worry that the decision is theirs and theirs alone

It may be important to highlight that the decision is ultimately yours, but that her views of what his wishes might be are highly valuable.

9 Confirm understanding and invite questions

Make it clear that you are happy to answer questions now or later.

10 Conclude with assurances

Always conclude with an assurance that if a decision is made not to resuscitate, you and your team will continue to do all that you can to actively treat his condition and to relieve symptoms. Make it clear, where appropriate, that a decision can be reviewed and altered at any time.

But we will do all that we can, keeping a very close eye and treating all that is treatable here on the ward. And we are here, if there are any questions at any time.

Discussion

What is the approach to do not resuscitate (DNAR) decision-making with incapacitated adults?

This is described in Box 4.25.

Box 4.25 Do not resuscitate (DNAR) decision-making with incapacitated adults

People close to patients often perceive that they have the 'final say' or that the 'burden of responsibility' rests with them. Yet in England, Wales and Northern Ireland no person has been* legally entitled to give consent to medical treatment on behalf of a patient who lacks decision-making capacity.

Doctors have authority to act in their patients' best interests where consent is not available. *Best interests* (Box 4.20, Case 4.24) embraces clinical interests and any previously expressed wishes and preferences. Where no information is available, decisions must be consistent with a patient's interests and rights.

People close to the patient often understandably feel they are the natural decision-makers, and it is good practice to involve them as fully as possible. They should be kept informed and should be involved in decision-making to reflect a patient's views, wishes and preferences. It is important to be as clear as possible that information provided is that which the patient would have wanted as opposed to that which those consulted would like for the patient or would want for themselves.

In Scotland, the Adults with Incapacity (Scotland) Act allows people over 16 to appoint a proxy decision-maker who has the legal power to consent to medical treatment when the patient loses capacity and in England the Mental Capacity Act* has opened the gateway to this. Proxy decision-makers cannot, however, demand treatment that is judged to be against a patient's best interests.

CASE 4.29

APPROPRIATENESS OF INTENSIVE THERAPY UNIT TRANSFER

Candidate information

Role

You are a doctor on the medical ward.
Please read this summary.

Scenario

Re: Mrs Angela Elliot, aged 62 years

Mrs Elliot has advanced multiple sclerosis. She is immobile, dependent upon carers for transfer from her wheelchair to bed, and unable to feed herself. Bulbar function is significantly impaired whenever she has inter-current infection, its recovery following episodes is incomplete and she can only just tolerate a strict diet. Percutaneous gastrostomy feeding was being considered. Unfortunately, she has been readmitted to hospital with her fourth episode of pneumonia in 12 months. On this occasion admission to the intensive therapy unit (ITU) was considered for the first time, but because of a lack of ITU beds she was observed carefully by the ITU outreach team and 'made it through the night' with high-flow oxygen, suction and antibiotics. She is slowly improving, and no longer breathless. The nursing team have questioned whether she should be considered for ITU next time she has pneumonia, as Mrs Elliot has apparently expressed concerns about 'going on a ventilator' and would like to speak to a doctor.

Your task is to address her concerns.

Your examiners will warn you when 12 minutes have elapsed. You have 14 minutes to communicate with the patient/subject followed by 1 minute of reflection. There will then follow 5 minutes of discussion with the examiners. Do not take the history again except for details that will help in your discussion with the patient/subject. You are not required to examine the patient/subject.

Patient/subject information

Mrs Angela Elliot is a 62-year-old lady who has advanced multiple sclerosis. She is fully dependent upon carers for transfer from her wheelchair to her bed, and unable to feed herself. She can swallow food, albeit very carefully prepared and of the right consistency, but swallowing is further impaired each time she is unwell. Percutaneous gastrostomy feeding has been considered and is acceptable to her. Unfortunately, she has been readmitted to hospital with her fourth episode of pneumonia in 12 months. On this occasion admission to the ITU was considered, but she 'made it through the night' with oxygen, chest physiotherapy and antibiotics. She is slowly improving, and no longer breathless. She has great concerns about a ventilator because she does not want to be 'kept alive indefinitely on an artificial machine'. Her daughter died after spending four months in an ITU following a road traffic accident. She has no other children, and is widowed. She would like to discuss whether ITU would really benefit her in future if this happens again. She has a fear of being ventilated only to die at the end of months of distress.

How to approach the case

Communication skills (conduct of interview, exploration and problem negotiation) and ethics and law

1 Introduction, setting and rapport

Introduce yourself and state that you are glad to see her feeling a little better. Make it clear that you will do everything you can to continue to make her feel comfortable, and treat the chest infection.

2 Acknowledge how unwell the patient has been

Mention that you know how unwell she has been, and that while you feel she should continue to improve on this occasion, she came very close to needing ventilatory support.

3 Explore the patient's concerns

Mention that the nursing staff have told you she had some concerns at being treated in intensive care. Explain that while you are always happy to consider what seems the best treatment at the time, it would be important to know if she has any strong feelings one way or the other about any specific measures, including intensive care.

4 Address the patient's concerns

Patients with long-term conditions have often given thought to what their wishes might be in the event of hypothetical clinical circumstances. While some patients would 'want everything done', many are very clear about circumstances they would not wish to occur, and this will very likely include being artificially ventilated when there is no prospect of recovery (doctors would be unlikely to offer such a treatment in any event). The difficulty is that medicine is seldom clear-cut, and the prospect of recovery is often a case of best judgement rather than absolute certainty one way or the other. It is reasonable, provided the patient wishes it, to consider ventilation when there is a reversible acute cause for respiratory failure such as infection, but the balance of favouring to ventilate is progressively tempered as worsening of the underlying condition thwarts the likelihood of successful weaning from ventilation, and ultimately ventilation is tilted out of favour. Patients may choose not to be ventilated even when the balance seems to be in their favour, provided this is an informed choice. Occasionally, patients will feel guilty about refusing an option that may prolong their life, especially if they have close relatives. Ventilation may carry the prospect of recovery from future infective exacerbations, but the patient will judge if the extent of that recovery is something she wishes to be brought back to. ITU would, of course, decline admission when recovery does not seem likely. Increasingly, non-invasive ventilation has been an alternative to invasive ventilation and can be applied outside ITU, but its best evidence is in the setting of chronic obstructive pulmonary disease (COPD) exacerbations.

5 Discuss resuscitation status

It is often, but not inevitably, appropriate to discuss resuscitation status. Such discussion is usually a logical and natural extension if you have reached a decision about ITU being inappropriate, but should be discussed sensitively.

6 Ensure that the patient is fully informed

If a decision is to be made not to admit to ITU in future, especially if there is still a prospect of ITU benefit outweighing risk, ensure that this is made with adequate understanding of the alternatives and the consequences, and formed without coercion or undue influence.

7 Agree a plan

Agree to respect her informed choice.

8 Confirm understanding

Ensure that she is clear about the course of action and be prepared to explore any other concerns.

9 Invite questions

Ask if there is anything she would like clarified.

10 Conclude with assurances

Always conclude with an assurance that if a decision is made not to admit to ITU in future, you and your team will continue to do all that you can to actively treat her condition and to relieve symptoms.

Discussion

Is invasive ventilation contraindicated in COPD?

Invasive ventilation is more likely to be appropriate where there is a reversible cause and an acceptable quality of life or habitual level of activity. Each case must be assessed individually. COPD is not a blanket reason not to ventilate because of fears about weaning. You should get an idea, for example, of how much oxygen is required at home or what is meant exactly by 'housebound'. Invasive ventilation may be appropriate for a remediable acute cause, if there is no significant other organ failure, for a first episode of respiratory failure or if the patient has made an informed wish for it to be attempted, whereas it would be inappropriate for a patient with end-stage COPD and a high premorbid arterial pCO_2.

How does age affect ITU outcome?

Around 25% of ITU admissions are of patients over 75 years of age, and this is likely to increase. Surgical patients are more likely to need admission than medical, usually related to sepsis and other postoperative complications. Around 80% of patients over 80 years of age who are ventilated with sepsis do not survive. Other adverse factors include poor cognition, decreased consciousness, recent stroke, limited activities of daily living, poor nutrition and unplanned admission. Despite this, age is a risk factor for poor outcome (7%) by only around one-tenth that of the underlying physiology (73%) in the APACHE III scoring system. Physiological problems should be much bigger determinants of admission to ITU than age; single-organ reversible disease even in very old people who were previously healthy (another important determinant of outcome) certainly deserves consideration of ITU involvement.

CASE 4.30

WITHHOLDING AND WITHDRAWING LIFE-PROLONGING TREATMENTS – ANTIBIOTICS AND DRUGS

Candidate information

Role

You are a doctor on an elderly care ward.
Please read this summary.

Scenario

Re: Mrs Eliza Bennett, aged 83 years

Mrs Eliza Bennett has been on your ward for three weeks with unresolving pneumonia. She has significant comorbidity. She has had type 2 diabetes for many years, latterly requiring insulin, with associated chronic kidney disease and advanced diabetic maculopathy. She was admitted with right lower lobe pneumonia, which has failed to respond to two courses of intravenous antibiotics. The microbiologist has suggested a third regimen, but the possibility of non-infective underlying causes, including cancer, is there, although not established, and she has been too unwell for complex investigations. She has steadily declined, with a falling serum albumin and increasing peripheral oedema. She is now too drowsy to engage in discussion. Intravenous access is now not possible peripherally, and your house officer called you to consider a central venous catheter. Mr Bennett is visiting his wife.

Your task is to discuss her treatment options with Mr Bennett, her husband.

Your examiners will warn you when 12 minutes have elapsed. You have 14 minutes to communicate with the patient/subject followed by 1 minute of reflection. There will then follow 5 minutes of discussion with the examiners. Do not take the history again except for details that will help in your discussion with the patient/subject. You are not required to examine the patient/subject.

Patient/subject information

Your wife, Mrs Eliza Bennett, is an 83-year-old lady who has been on the ward for three weeks with pneumonia that is steadily getting worse. She has been unwell, in your view, for the last year. She has longstanding diabetes, requiring insulin as well as tablets, with associated kidney problems and visual impairment. She used to be very active and has been very depressed for the last year, virtually housebound by weakness in her legs and poor vision. To you, and you think to her, this is the last straw. She is not getting better, her legs are swelling up and you have seen her becoming more confused and drowsy since admission. She has always said that she would not want to go on if her diabetes had got the better of her and would not want to be dependent upon carers or nurses. The doctors are concerned that she has not responded to antibiotics and they appear to be running out of options.

How to approach the case

Communication skills (conduct of interview, exploration and problem negotiation) and ethics and law

1 Introduction

Introduce yourself, establish his identity and acknowledge that it is a difficult time.

2 Acknowledge the value of the relative

As his wife is not able to speak for herself, his presence is highly valuable in determining what her wishes might have been. Acknowledging him as closest relative, it may be helpful to ask if there are other family members nearby who might also wish to be involved in discussion.

3 Reassure the relative that any decisions will be carefully considered and that the 'burden of responsibility' for difficult decisions will not rest with him

Reassure him that decisions will consider what is best for his wife, and that his views will be very helpful. Explain that you are very concerned that treatments do not seem to be working as you had hoped, and that you now must contemplate what are reasonable interventions and what may not be reasonable interventions and not in his wife's best interests. Explain that decisions will very much take account of any views he has but that decisions will be made together. Remember that your consultant is there to help with difficult decisions such as this, and you should make difficult decisions with more senior team members.

4 Explain the problem

This should start with a summary of the background, explaining that his wife's pneumonia has not responded. Acknowledge that there is uncertainty as to why this is so. It is likely that her diabetes (hyperglycaemia, small vessel disease, renal failure) is impairing the fight against infection. It may be that there is an underlying reason (including a growth) predisposing to infection, but his wife has been too unwell for more complicated investigations. Explain that as time goes on, the prospects

of recovery from the pneumonia diminish, particularly as other things start to go wrong (drowsiness, hypoalbuminaemia, oedema). Explain that all you have been able to do recently is continue with antibiotics, attempt to correct any abnormalities in the blood chemistry and watch and wait, trying to ensure that she is comfortable. Explain that the new problem is that it is no longer possible to secure peripheral intravenous access for delivery of antibiotics.

5 Explain your view

Explain that the next step could be to consider intravenous access via a catheter inserted into a larger vein in the neck, but that this is more invasive. Acknowledge that this is not without complications, and not always comfortable to insert, but is an effective way of ensuring that treatment continues, although you cannot say if treatment will work. It is unlikely that she is able to take tablets at the moment, but if she were to improve and show the ability to take things orally, then oral antibiotics could be considered.

6 Explore what the relative feels the patient would have wanted

He may request, based on his knowledge of his wife's values and views, that this would be a step too far.

7 Explore any concerns the relative may have

A common concern is that the patient may suffer or be in pain. When a patient is not responding to treatment, it is crucial to reassure relatives that one thing you can do is ensure their comfort.

8 Consider and justify, or plan to change, any apparent discrepancies such as delivering some medications but not others

If a decision is made to withdraw antibiotics, the issue of continuing insulin may need to be discussed. If she cannot take tablets, and is already insulin-dependent, then withdrawal of insulin would be likely to lead to rapid spiralling of hyperglycaemia and possible death from hyperglycaemic coma. This could be avoided with subcutaneous insulin and this may still be a reasonable intervention while nature confirms its likely course without antibiotics. If and when it becomes certain that she is dying then it may be appropriate to withdraw insulin in favour of purely symptomatic palliative measures.

9 Confirm understanding and invite questions

Make it clear that you are happy to answer further questions now or at any time.

10 Give strong reassurance about continuing with care

Make it clear that the team will continue to care for his wife with very close attention to what is reasonably treatable and to alleviation of symptoms. Tell him that you are happy to answer questions at any time.

Discussion

Do you know of any guidelines on withholding and withdrawing life-prolonging treatments?

A General Medical Council (GMC) guideline covers the principles of withdrawing and withholding life-prolonging treatment that are summarised in Box 4.26. Thorough assessment of the diagnosis and likely prognosis must precede any treatment decision. Treatment options should be based on clinical evidence of efficacy, side effects and risks, and a considered judgement should be reached on the likely clinical and personal benefits, burdens and risks of each treatment (or non-treatment). A clinician with relevant experience should be consulted if the responsible doctor has limited experience of the condition.

Must you provide treatment to a patient who demands it but which you do not think is in that patient's best interests?

Whilst English law allows a competent patient to refuse life-sustaining or other treatment, it does not require a doctor to provide treatment that a patient demands but which the doctor does not feel is in the patient's best interests.

How might you be guided in making decisions about limitation of treatment for patients without capacity?

A doctor should act in what is considered to be the best interests of a patient. There is a reason not to treat if there will be no significant benefit (e.g. insignificant likelihood of successful resuscitation or insignificant prolongation of life) or if the patient will be harmed (burdens outweigh benefits). Doctors might also question if treatment requires an unfair allocation of scarce resources.

There is no legal duty to preserve life at all cost and the law recognises that best interests may be best served by withholding or withdrawing life-prolonging treatments that would be overall burdensome, or by providing palliative treatment that could shorten life. However, it would be illegal to act with the intention of shortening life (see doctrine of double effect – Case 4.33).

In the USA, respect for self-determination is embodied in the notion of 'substituted judgement', which attempts to forge a hypothetical preference if the patient were competent now, based largely on previously expressed views and values. English law gives some weight to this notion, but only when applied directly to the clinical situation. Clearly the views of family and friends, the general practi-

Box 4.26 Principles on withholding and withdrawing life-prolonging treatments

Respect for human life and best interests

Prolonging life will usually be in a patient's best interests if treatment is not excessively burdensome or disproportionate to expected benefits. Not continuing or starting treatment is in a patient's best interests when there is no net benefit. Life has a natural end and doctors should not strive to prolong the dying process with no regard to patient wishes.

Patients with capacity

Patients with capacity have the right of autonomy to decide how much weight to attach to the benefits, burdens and risks and overall acceptability of treatment. They have the right to refuse treatment. Desires regarding treatment must of course be made with an adequate understanding of the alternatives and the consequences, and formed without coercion or undue influence.

Incapacitated patients

Any valid advance refusal of treatment must be respected. Without this, assessment of the benefits, burdens and risks and overall acceptability of treatment must be made on a patient's behalf by the doctor, taking into account what is known of the patient and information from those closest to the patient.

Differing views about best interests

Applying principles may result in different decisions in each case because patient's assessments of benefits, burdens and risks, and the weights and priorities attached to these, will differ according to values and beliefs. Some patients will want everything possible done; others will want to avoid too much medical intervention. Where doctors and members of a health-care team take different views about an incompetent patient, independent legal advice may be necessary.

Starting then stopping treatment

Where it is decided that treatment is not in a patient's best interests, there is no ethical or legal reason to provide it and thus no need to distinguish withdrawal of treatment from not starting treatment. Where a patient lacks capacity and there is uncertainty about appropriateness of treatment, treatment that may be of some benefit should be started until clearer assessment is made. This is particularly important in emergencies where there may be doubt about the severity of a condition or the benefit of a treatment.

Artificial hydration and nutrition (AHN)

This can be difficult, because benefits and burdens may not easily be known. AHN is discussed in Case 4.31.

Other principles

Other principles include non-discrimination, equal respect and care for the dying, respect for conscientious objection but with the onus on the conscientious objector to ensure care from a suitably qualified colleague without delay, and accountability by doctors to patients, society, the GMC and the Courts. Clinical responsibility for decisions rests with a consultant or the general practitioner.

tioner, and any advanced statement can be valuable and if the patient would have freely refused treatment in the circumstances, based on his or her (most recent) values and knowing all the relevant facts, then there is a reason to limit life-prolonging treatment.

CASE 4.31

WITHHOLDING AND WITHDRAWING LIFE-PROLONGING TREATMENTS – ARTIFICIAL HYDRATION AND NUTRITION

Candidate information

Role

You are a doctor on the stroke unit.

Please read this summary.

Scenario

Re: Mr Harold Hunt, aged 86 years

Mr Hunt was admitted to your ward three days ago following a left total anterior circulation stroke. He remains unconscious and the consensus opinion of all members of the health-care team is that his prognosis is very poor. His daughter feels that he should be 'left in peace'. He is on 'a drip' but one of the nurses mentioned the possibility of a 'feeding tube' to her. She is now not sure if he is being starved.

Your task is to discuss the issue of artificial hydration and nutrition with his daughter.

Your examiners will warn you when 12 minutes have elapsed. You have 14 minutes to communicate with the patient/subject followed by 1 minute of reflection. There will then follow 5 minutes of discussion with the examiners. Do not take the history again except for details that will help in your discussion with the patient/subject. You are not required to examine the patient/subject.

Patient/subject information

Mr Harold Hunt, your father, is an 86-year-old gentleman who was admitted to the ward three days ago following a very large stroke. He remains unconscious and the consensus opinion of all members of the health-care team is that his prognosis is very poor. You feel that he should be 'left in peace'. He had a very active life in the army, but since being widowed three years ago became rather withdrawn and always said he would want 'to have all of his faculties'. He has been on 'a drip' since admission but one of the nurses mentioned the possibility of a 'feeding tube'. You do not see the value of feeding your father if he is going to die, but are worried that if he is being starved it may be uncomfortable for him. You wonder if the drip should continue, and if so whether it might be delaying an inevitable death.

How to approach this case

Communication skills (conduct of interview, exploration and problem negotiation) and ethics and law

1 Introduction

Introduce yourself, establish his identity and acknowledge that it is a difficult time.

2 Acknowledge the value of the relative

As her father is not able to speak for himself, her presence is highly valuable in determining what his wishes might have been. It is always useful to establish if there are other people who might wish to be involved in discussions.

3 Reassure the relative that any decisions will be carefully considered and that the 'burden of responsibility' for difficult decisions will not rest with her

Reassure her that decisions will always consider her father's best interests first, aided by her better knowledge of her father. Although relatives often wish strong account be taken of their views, they may also need to be reassured that ultimately the 'burden of responsibility' for decisions rests with the medical team. She will wish to express the perceived values and preferences of her father but may well feel uncomfortable if she feels that a life and death decision about a family member is hers.

4 Explain the reasons for and against artificial hydration and nutrition

Explain that where a patient cannot take fluids or food orally, an assessment is always made of the requirements for hydration and nutrition, and the appropriateness of instituting these. Explain that in this situation intravenous fluids were started initially because it could not be determined whether her father would recover and if so, how long this would take, but that supportive fluids are necessary early on if there is to be some recovery. Explain that artificial nutrition is less immediate, but should be started via a tube passed through the nose directly into the stomach (nasogastric tube) within the first few days in patients showing signs of recovery. Acknowledge that it is a very sensitive issue and not one with absolutely right or wrong answers, but that the generally accepted view is not to institute artificial nutrition unless a patient is showing signs of recovery. Specifically, a patient should be conscious and able to sit up and ideally aware of the reasons for the tube.

5 Explain your view

It is often best, particularly where you feel relatives are showing agreement, to suggest what you think might be appropriate, provided this is not dogmatic and you demonstrate willingness to be fluid in your decisions depending upon feedback. You might consider artificial nutrition if there were a spontaneous change for the better, but now it is entirely reasonable to watch and wait.

6 Explore what the relative feels the patient would have wanted

She will probably agree with withholding nutrition.

7 Explore any concerns the relative may have

She may need to be reassured that there is no evidence that withholding nutrition causes distress by 'starvation'. She may not see the logic of maintaining intravenous fluids when nutrition is being withheld.

8 Consider and justify or plan to change any apparent discrepancies such as delivering hydration but withholding nutrition

The British Medical Association (BMA) and General Medical Council (GMC) have stated that withdrawing a life-prolonging treatment may not be ethically distinguishable from withholding it, although the former can seem more difficult. Whilst intravenous or subcutaneous fluids could be withdrawn, there are reasons for continuing their provision, although these cannot be evidence-based. In this case three days may seem too soon to withdraw a relatively non-invasive treatment, especially if access for fluids is not causing distress. Unlike nutrition, fluids pose little risk. Nasogastric feeding may provoke aspiration and may be uncomfortable and is not suitable for unconscious or agitated patients or for patients who cannot sit up. Percutaneous endoscopic gastrostomy (PEG) feeding is not suitable unless patients demonstrate potential for longer-term survival. Hydration may avert distress, although there is no convincing evidence for this and indeed the Liverpool Care Pathway for palliation specifically excludes hydration and nutrition.

9 Confirm understanding and invite questions

Make it clear that you are happy to answer further questions now or at any time.

10 Give strong reassurance about continuing with care

Explain that needs and symptoms may change, and that he will be carefully assessed regularly.

Discussion

What is meant by artificial hydration and nutrition (AHN)?

Artificial hydration and artificial nutrition may involve intravenous or subcutaneous fluids, nasogastric feeding or gastrostomy feeding. It does not include oral hydration and nutrition, generally considered part of nursing care.

When are AHN appropriate?

In deciding which of the options are appropriate, full account should be taken of the opinions of the patient (where competent), members of the health-care team (not least speech and language therapists), and, where a patient's wishes cannot be determined, those close to the patient.

Generally, the benefits and burdens of artificial hydration and artificial nutrition are different and should be assessed separately. Where there is uncertainty about benefits or burdens a trial of artificial hydration or nutrition may be appropriate.

Where death seems imminent, it would not usually be appropriate to start artificial hydration or nutrition, although artificial hydration may be appropriate where it is considered to provide symptom relief.

Where death is imminent and artificial nutrition or hydration is already in use, it may be appropriate to withdraw it if it is considered that burdens outweigh possible benefits.

Should a competent patient not have the right to determine whether or not to receive, or refuse withdrawal of, a life-prolonging treatment?

In 2004 Mr L. Burke, a patient with a progressive, degenerative brain disease, wanted assurance that GMC guidance in *Withholding and Withdrawing Life-prolonging Treatment* did not allow or authorise doctors to withdraw life-prolonging AHN from him, as a competent patient in contradiction to his expressed views, when he reached a stage in his illness that left him unable to communicate his views and decisions.

In the original judgement, Justice Munby found limited aspects of the GMC's guidance unlawful. However, this area of the law is complex and continues to evolve, especially in light of the European Convention on Human Rights.

The GMC appealed against the judgement (Justice Munby granting that there was compelling public interest in so doing), primarily because it seemed to make important changes to the law that needed further testing. Firstly, it made competent patients' wishes in principle 'determinative' of the treatment they should receive and whether or not treatment was in their best interests; secondly, it re-defined the best interests test – used where a patient is incapacitated – so that the 'touchstone' for deciding best interests would be the 'intolerability' of providing or not providing a treatment; thirdly, it made it a legal requirement, in a range of situations, to seek the Court's view before withdrawing a life-prolonging treatment.

The Court of Appeal concluded that Mr Burke's fears were already addressed under common law, that GMC guidance was not unlawful and that it was unnecessary and inappropriate to have applied for declarations by the Court. Each of the declarations made by the High Court Judge was thus overturned. The key conclusions of the Court of Appeal are outlined in Box 4.27.

How are the best interests of a patient without capacity determined when considering life-prolonging treatments?

The position was also affirmed by the Court of Appeal, its conclusions summarised in Box 4.28.

Box 4.27 Update to guidance on withholding and withdrawing life-prolonging treatments – withholding and withdrawing life-prolonging treatment against a patient's express wishes

- Decisions about end-of-life care should be approached with a strong presumption in favour of prolonging life.
- Current GMC guidance on *Withholding and Withdrawing Life-Prolonging Treatment* is lawful, at least as it concerns withdrawal of life-prolonging artificial nutrition and hydration (AHN) from competent patients who express a wish to continue to receive it.
- A doctor who withdraws AHN from such a patient with the intention of hastening death would find no defence in the common law charge of murder.
- The crucial consideration is not the patient's wish to receive treatment but that the doctor has a duty of care that involves the duty to provide treatment in a patient's best interests, and generally to take steps that are reasonable to keep the patient alive.
- While a patient's right to autonomy gives an absolute right to refuse treatment, there is no comparable right to treatment on demand, whether AHN or other treatment. What is in a patient's best interests does not automatically equate with that patient's wishes.
- The decision as to what treatment is clinically indicated remains with the doctor; the decision as to whether to accept it is with the patient.
- If AHN is needed to sustain life, it is impossible to suggest that AHN is not a clinically indicated treatment. Where AHN cannot prolong life, but may cause suffering or hasten death, the patient cannot, by requesting such treatment, oblige the doctor to treatment that is not clinically indicated.
- There is no legal obligation to refer any decision to withdraw AHN to the Court. Where a decision is controversial, it may be good practice to seek legal advice and for an application for a declaration to be made.

Box 4.28 Determining the best interests for a patient without capacity

- For a patient without capacity, a doctor's decision as to what is in that patient's best interests (Box 4.20, Case 4.24) is determinative of the treatment that patient receives.
- A decision as to whether it is in the patient's best interests to withdraw artificial nutrition and hydration (AHN) is not limited to circumstances where continued life with treatment can be considered 'intolerable'. It is not possible to define what is in the best interest of any patient by reference to a single test applicable in all circumstances. 'Intolerability' does not replace 'best interests' as the appropriate test, nor should it be considered the 'touchstone' of best interests in every case.
- A distinction should be drawn between cases where life can be prolonged indefinitely by treatment but only at the cost of great suffering, and cases where a patient is in the final stages of life and although treatment could prolong the dying process, this would be at the cost of comfort and dignity. In both cases the doctor should consider all the circumstances of the case and take an objective decision. In the former, doctors should follow guidance, and in the latter they should consider that the goal of treatment 'may properly be to ease the suffering and, where appropriate, to ease the passing, rather than to achieve a short prolongation of life'.

A 68-year-old man with advanced Lewy Body dementia is admitted with an unsafe swallow and multiple failed nasogastric feeding attempts because he pulls out the tubes. He is receiving intravenous fluid. His essential medical therapy is warfarin for a metallic heart valve. What are the options?

Broadly, there are three options:

- To allow comfort feeding; in other words, to allow him to take what he wishes orally and accept the risks of aspiration
- To simply withhold nutrition; in other words, to allow him to starve to death
- To withhold nutrition and, additionally, withhold intravenous hydration

Percutaneous gastrostomy feeding would probably not be appropriate in this situation. Blood tests are appropriate to guide a life-saving treatment (warfarin) until a definitive decision for no further active management has been made.

How would you decide which option to choose?

The option to comfort feed may seem the most appropriate to medical staff, but his family's views on his perceived wishes may help. Withdrawal of hydration before discussion would seem least correct immediately, particularly while his family are coming to terms with a difficult situation. His family are likely to be strongly in agreement that no further attempts should be made to feed via nasogastric tube. It may be decided that if no future can be envisaged beyond this admission to hospital, no further intravenous or subcutaneous access for hydration would be appropriate once the current cannula 'tissues'. A decision should then also be made not to give antibiotics in the event of aspiration. Assurance of preservation of his dignity should be given, with a shift in care exclusively to comfort and suppression of distress. Warfarin should be withdrawn and the possibility of sudden valve obstruction accepted as a potential mode of death.

He shows signs of improvement with comfort feeding but has choking episodes with comfort feeding. What would you do now?

There are two, at first glance conflicting, options but each one depends upon the type of improvement. If he is showing signs of returning to his pre-admission self, then it may well be appropriate to revise decisions, and this could include stopping comfort feeding, administering artificial hydration and considering percutaneous gastrostomy feeding, although there are enormous concerns about the risk : benefit ratio of the latter in dementia. If, however, he shows the day-to-day minor undulation that is true of many hospital patients, then it is vital for his family not to be given false hope or to burden the patient or family with swinging decisions in the context of an inevitable end.

CASE 4.32

PERCUTANEOUS ENDOSCOPIC GASTROSTOMY FEEDING

Candidate information

Role

You are a doctor on the medical ward.
  Please read this summary.

Scenario

> Re: Mr James Hawkins, aged 82 years
>
> Mr Hawkins was admitted to your ward a week ago with aspiration pneumonia. On admission the prognosis seemed poor and resuscitation in the event of cardiac or respiratory arrest was not considered appropriate. He has idiopathic epilepsy (since childhood, and currently treated with phenytoin, carbamazepine and sodium valproate) and Parkinson's disease, on treatment for eight years. A year ago he had a stroke after which he spent six weeks in a rehabilitation hospital before returning to his wife at home. She is his main carer, and he requires help with washing, dressing, meals and mobility around the house. Following antibiotic treatment he has recovered to the point of cardiorespiratory stability, but cannot swallow. The speech and language therapist assessing him believes he might never safely swallow because this was significantly impaired before admission and the balance has now been tipped. Unfortunately, Mr Hawkins has not tolerated numerous attempts to pass a nasogastric feeding tube and the speech and language therapist has suggested that a percutaneous endoscopic gastrostomy (PEG) would enable him to receive nutrition. Unfortunately, Mr Hawkins is unable to participate in such a discussion because he has been too cognitively impaired for the last year. His wife fears that he will starve without a PEG and wishes to discuss the issues with you.
>
> Your task is to discuss the options with her and help her reach a decision.

Your examiners will warn you when 12 minutes have elapsed. You have 14 minutes to communicate with the patient/subject followed by 1 minute of reflection. There will then follow 5 minutes of discussion with the examiners. Do not take the history again except for details that will help in your discussion with the patient/subject. You are not required to examine the patient/subject.

Patient/subject information

Mr James Hawkins, your husband, is an 82-year-old man admitted to hospital a week ago with aspiration pneumonia. On admission the prognosis seemed poor and resuscitation in the event of cardiac or respiratory arrest was not considered appropriate. He has epilepsy (on treatment since childhood) and Parkinson's disease (on treatment for eight years). A year ago he had a stroke after which he spent six weeks in a rehabilitation hospital before returning home. You are his main carer, and he requires help with washing, dressing, meals and moving around the house. He is confined to a wheelchair much of the time, but sometimes can walk with a stick. Following antibiotic treatment he has recovered somewhat, but cannot swallow. The speech and language therapist believes he might never safely swallow again. Unfortunately, he has not tolerated numerous attempts to pass a nasogastric feeding tube and the speech and language therapist has suggested that a PEG feeding tube would enable him to receive nutrition. Unfortunately, he is unable to participate in such a discussion because he has been too cognitively impaired for the last year. You fear that he will ultimately starve without a tube and will not receive his usual medications, and wish to discuss the issues with the doctor.

How to approach the case

Communication skills (conduct of interview, exploration and problem negotiation) and ethics and law

1 Introduction

Introduce yourself, confirm her identity and say that you would like to respond to her concerns about feeding and discuss possible ways to tackle this.

2 Explain the current situation as you see it

Explain that despite some improvement, the position remains very serious. Explain the reasons for considering a PEG tube, in this case delivery of medications and administration of feeding.

3 Explain the main issues relating to PEG tubes

Discuss the issues relevant to PEG tube insertion in more detail. Explain that it might not be a means of improving or prolonging life. Explain there is no good evidence that it would do so where there are problems with memory and understanding. There would be a small but significant risk of complications including peritonitis (around 2%) and an increased risk of aspiration, which in this case is particularly relevant.

4 Try to establish the patient's wishes

Ask if she and her husband have ever discussed what his wishes might be if such a scenario ever arose.

5 Explain alternatives

Explain that the alternative is to administer medications via alternative routes (phenytoin intravenously, diazepam rectally), but that not all drugs can be delivered, and for practical purposes there would be no feeding and so inevitably there would be a starvation factor. Point out that fluids can be given intravenously or subcutaneously (a small needle under the skin of the abdomen).

6 Be alert to cues

Do not simply deliver your spiel without being aware of any reactions she may have.

7 Explore her concerns

Understand that it is a heart-rending decision. Ask if she has any particular feelings about things at this stage. Explain that a decision does not have to be made now. Patients' and relatives' expectations from PEG tube feeding are often improved nutrition, prevention of aspiration, extension of life, improvement of pressure sores, comfort, strength and help in overcoming an acute illness. The evidence is that rarely do patients achieve these expectations; in 70% there may be no improvement and there is no prevention of aspiration; in the frail elderly there is a 30-day mortality of 22% and 1-year mortality of 50%.

8 Respond to questions

She might ask for your advice. You might say that putting everything together, without seeing a clear way forward to long-term improvement, it may not be in his best interests to 'go there'. If that is what she decides then assure her that there is no evidence that he would suffer from things like hunger pains, not at this stage.

9 Confirm understanding and agree a way forward

Make sure that she has enough information and either agree a way forward or allow her more time to think things over.

10 Reassure that decisions are not irreversible

Make it clear that no decision that she or the medical team makes is irreversible and of course if the situation were to change then any decision could be reviewed.

Discussion

A 68-year-old man has a left total anterior circulation stroke with right hemiparesis and dysphagia. His swallow is deemed unsafe by the speech and language therapist (SLT). His family want to know if you will be feeding him to keep his strength up. When is enteral feeding recommended and what methods are there?

Enteral feeding in adult hospital patients is indicated if feeding is likely to be delayed more than five to seven days.

Earlier instigation is favoured in malnourished patients. Methods for enteral feeding are nasogastric tube (NGT) feeding or percutaneous endoscopic gastrostomy (PEG) or less commonly jejunostomy (PEJ) feeding. Of 30 patients with a stroke randomised to PEG or NGT feeding, two out of 16 with a PEG died within six weeks, compared with eight of 14 with a NGT. Six with a PEG were discharged at three months compared with none with a NGT. However, there are more complications with a PEG and the higher mortality in patients with a NGT may simply represent a more unwell population who were not well enough to be considered for PEG feeding.

At day two the SLT team feel his swallow is still unsafe and NGT feeding is suggested. What are the complications of NGT insertion?

These include discomfort, epistaxis, oesophageal stenosis, aspiration and complications from enteral feeds.

At day 10 the SLT team feel his swallow has shown little sign of improvement. A gastrostomy tube is recommended. What are the indications for gastrostomy feeding?

A gastrostomy tube is considered when nutritional intake is likely to be impaired for more than two to four weeks or when an NGT is not tolerated or is contraindicated. A functioning gut distal to the stomach is a prerequisite. Common conditions for consideration of gastrostomy feeding include stroke, degenerating neurological conditions (e.g. multiple sclerosis, motor neurone disease, Parkinson's disease, cerebral palsy), head injury, and head and neck cancers.

What are the contraindications to gastrostomy feeding?

These include confusion, dementia, active peptic ulcer disease, infection and bleeding diatheses. In the United States 30% of PEG tubes are in patients with dementia. There is, however, no evidence to support their use and there is evidence of possible harm; we should continue to counsel strongly against PEG tubes at least in advanced dementia. There is no evidence that PEG tubes reduce the risk of aspiration and pneumonia (they may even increase them) or pressure ulcer rates or enhance healing or make patients live longer; quality of life markers are harder to prove but a substantial proportion of patients report that it improves quality.

What are the complications of gastrostomy feeding?

Immediate complications include failure to place the tube (2–5%), and other procedural complications such as bleeding and perforation (1%). Early complications include wound infection (10–20%), bleeding, perforation (especially colonic), displacement, leakage, reflux/aspiration, lower respiratory tract infection (20%), nausea and vomiting, bloating, pain, diarrhoea (very common, related to feeding), metabolic complications (refeeding syndrome, hyperglycaemia, fluid overload, electrolyte disturbance) and death (21% hospital mortality and 34% 12-month mortality). Late complications also include, in addition, 'buried bumper syndrome' (avoided by daily twirling) and hypergranulation. The 30-day mortality is high at around one-quarter of all patients for all causes of PEG insertion and half of all patients with dementia and at one-year mortality is 90% in dementia.

How should PEG tubes be managed immediately after insertion?

Vigilance for signs of bleeding, perforation or peritonitis with monitoring of vital signs and any abdominal pain should be routine immediate management. At 6–12 hours the patient should be assessed for absence of abdominal pain or distension and signs of bowel function; 50-ml sterile water flushes through the PEG should not cause distress. Feed can then be commenced at the dietitian's recommended rate. To prevent gastric leakage and peritonitis, the external disc should not be released until around day three. The tube should be flushed before and after feeds. The tube should be rotated (by unclamping the triangular disc, gently pushing the tube 3–5 cm inwards, rotating through 360 degrees, pulling back the tube, leaving a 1-cm gap between skin and flange and reclamping) from day 3 and on a daily basis until the site has healed and then at least once weekly but not more than once daily. It should not be rotated if infection is suspected.

How should PEG tube blockages be managed?

Ensure that all clamps are open and the tube is not kinked, connect a 50-ml syringe to the funnel adaptor and try to aspirate. Flush with 50 ml warm water and leave for 30 minutes to dissolve any fat globules, reflush, flush with carbonated water and leave for 30 minutes. If these measures fail, seek advice.

How might you manage wound infection?

Some major studies show the benefit of broad-spectrum antibiotics immediately or one hour before insertion. For the first 48 hours the stoma should be managed aseptically by cleansing at least twice daily with normal saline and sterile gauze. The triangular retention disc should not be displaced for this. After two days, soap and water may be used and the stoma can be dried gently but thoroughly. Showering is then permissible and bathing is allowed once the stoma has healed, normally at 7–14 days. Methicillin-resistant *Staphylococcus aureus* (MRSA) is common, and if any signs of infection emerge then the wound should be swabbed and a dressing applied over the triangular disc.

How might you manage leakage?

Options include proton pump inhibitors, barrier creams, a PEG on tension (short term) and button gastrostomy.

How might you reduce the risk of aspiration?

Options include feeding at 30 degrees, prokinetic agents or a PEG or PEJ.

How long may a PEG tube remain in situ for?

It should be replaced after several months.

A gastrostomy tube is inserted but the patient becomes confused and it is displaced within a week after insertion. What problems could arise and what action should be taken?

Problems include risk of a stomal tract not forming (it generally forms within 1–2 weeks but tubes should not be routinely removed for 2–4 weeks), gastric contents entering the peritoneum causing peritonitis and healing of the stoma (this occurs within hours). A replacement gastrostomy tube or sterile tube through the stoma should be instituted as soon as possible with inflation of the balloon. It should not be used to feed if the tract is less than four weeks old and contrast examination via the tube (or oesophagogastroduodenoscopy) should ascertain that the tube is in the stomach. If more than four weeks have elapsed feeds can commence immediately.

What are the risks of PEG feeding for major head and neck surgery?

There is a higher complication rate. Seeding of cancer to the stoma site has been reported.

What is refeeding syndrome?

Patients who have not received nutrition for a significant period of time are at risk of life-threatening electrolyte disturbances, not least phosphate, potassium and magnesium, and should receive close electrolyte monitoring with an individualised re-feeding regimen aided by a dietitian.

CASE 4.33

PALLIATIVE CARE

Candidate information

Role

You are a doctor on the medical ward.
  Please read this summary.

Scenario

Re: Mrs Sylvia Earnshaw, aged 85 years
Mrs Earnshaw was admitted to the ward three days ago following an attempt to pass an oesophageal stent. A decision that curative surgery would not be possible for her oesophageal cancer was reached on a previous admission. She was admitted because of drowsiness following the procedure (an intended day

case) and the procedure was not wholly successful, unable to negotiate the distal end of the tumour, and a repeat attempt was not ruled out. However, since admission she has deteriorated with aspiration pneumonia, thus far not responding to antibiotics and is progressively drowsy.

Your task is to discuss the care now appropriate for Mrs Earnshaw with her son.

Your examiners will warn you when 12 minutes have elapsed. You have 14 minutes to communicate with the patient/subject followed by 1 minute of reflection. There will then follow 5 minutes of discussion with the examiners. Do not take the history again except for details that will help in your discussion with the patient/subject. You are not required to examine the patient/subject.

Patient/subject information

You are the son of Mrs Earnshaw, an 85-year-old lady admitted three days ago following an attempt to pass a stent into her oesophagus. You are aware that the procedure was to relieve symptoms, but not really sure if that means an operation to cure things will be possible at a later date. She was admitted because of drowsiness following the stent procedure (an intended day case) and since then she has become more breathless. You are very concerned that she is much worse than before she was admitted, and wonder what is happening to her.

How to approach this case

Communication skills (conduct of interview, exploration and problem negotiation) and ethics and law

1 Introduction

Introduce yourself and establish that he is Mrs Earnshaw's son.

2 Establish what the relative knows

Firstly, establish a rapport with a relative you have not met before, establishing what he knows, appreciating that relatives may either have been told little or have been afraid to ask for more information and may still have false expectations about the future.

What have you been told so far about her condition?

3 Give a warning shot

This is largely a breaking bad news scenario, and before explaining her condition you should say that she is very unwell. A simple statement, followed by a pause, is enough.

Your mother's condition is not good.

4 Explain the situation

Relatives sometimes then volunteer that they are aware of the overall prognosis, but that things have deteriorated more quickly than anticipated, but are sometimes very surprised. Be prepared for any scenario.

Your mother has developed a rather nasty chest infection, almost certainly because of the growth in the oesophagus – the gullet – that means that she has been at very high risk of aspirating or regurgitating food and fluids and saliva down into her lungs. The procedure, as I know you know, was tricky and the gastroenterologist found it impossible to pass the tube beyond the growth.

5 Acknowledge distress and allow ventilation of feelings

Wait for his response before explaining more.

6 Identify and prioritise concerns

He will probably want to know what that means in terms of overall prognosis now.

The fact that the growth was difficult to bypass is of course a real concern. I know the gastroenterologists had hoped that if they could alleviate the obstruction it might enable her to eat and drink for a time. And I know that they have not discounted the prospect of having a further attempt. But clearly, as more complications arise, it becomes harder to see a good way forward. The growth, as you can appreciate, has not been one amenable to removal, or cure, and any treatments have therefore been directed to keeping symptoms at bay for as long as possible.

7 Explain what is likely to happen

Explain that you will continue to treat the infection actively, but there are inevitably limits. Explain that if it becomes inevitable that she is not going to get better, it might be appropriate to switch treatment entirely to controlling pain and breathlessness. You might feel that that stage has already been reached, but at least allow him some time to come to terms with the sudden change in his mother's condition. It may be appropriate to discuss continuation of intravenous fluids for the time being.

8 Identify support networks

It is human to want to discover a little more about the practical implications to him such as what other family members may be nearby, how far it is for him and other family to visit and so forth.

9 Invite questions

Always do this.

10 Conclude with assurances

Always conclude with an assurance that you will do all that you can to keep her comfortable and always be happy to discuss the situation with him or any member of the family.

Discussion

What is the Liverpool Care Pathway?

This care pathway (one of numerous) for the terminal/ dying phase is intended as a guide to treatment and an aid to documenting progress. The multiprofessional team must agree that the patient is dying and that two of the following apply: bed-bound; semi-comatose; only able to take sips of fluids; no longer able to take tablets.

Palliative care teams in many Trusts have produced handbooks and guidelines on managing patients in the palliative phase.

What is the doctrine of double effect?

The doctrine of double effect attempts to distinguish between harms intended and harms foreseen but not intended. In medicine it is often used in palliative care, such as when administering high doses of morphine to relieve pain, foreseeing that it may shorten life by depressing respiration. Whereas it would be morally wrong to administer with the intention of hastening death, it would not be so if the intention were to relieve pain. Four (all controversial) conditions must apply for the act not to be wrong:

1.   The act must be good or morally neutral independent of its consequences.
2.   The agent must intend the good effect, but not the bad effect.
3.   The bad effect must not be the means to or the direct casual result of the good effect.
4.   The good effect must outweigh the bad effect.

Consider a patient dying from a malignant brain tumour who develops pneumonia and respiratory failure. A ventilator may prolong life but may also delay an inevitable death. What courses of action are there?

Broadly, there are five options at the end of life (Box 4.29).

> **Box 4.29 End-of-life options**
>
> - The sanctity of life view – to ventilate and therefore prolong life whatever else may apply. He would likely die from progression of his tumour.
> - To withhold life-prolonging treatment – to withhold ventilation, for example. He would likely die from respiratory failure. This is sometimes considered passive euthanasia (very contentiously).
> - To withdraw life-prolonging treatment – to ventilate then withdraw from ventilation. He would likely die rapidly on withdrawal of ventilation. This is sometimes considered passive euthanasia (very contentiously).
> - Assisted suicide. This is illegal.
> - Active euthanasia (performing an action that results in a patient's death). Killing a patient for any reason is normally murder.

Is allowing a person to die different to killing that person?

Many people believe there is a moral difference between killing someone and allowing that person to die but Rachels showed that the distinction is not necessarily clear, describing two cases. In the first, person A stands to gain a large inheritance if his six-year-old cousin dies and sneaks into the child's bathroom and drowns the child in a way that will look like an accident. In the second, person B also stands to gain and plans to drown the child but on approaching the child slips and hit his head, falling face down in the bath; person B watches the child die. A kills; B allows to die; but there seems no moral difference here.

The question of a moral difference becomes more relevant when applied to withholding or withdrawing life-prolonging treatments. The central idea is that if a doctor kills a patient the doctor causes the patient's death, but if a doctor allows a patient to die the patient's death is the result of disease or 'nature taking its course'. Thus, options 4 and 5 in Box 4.29 seem worse than 2 and 3, which are accepted medical practices. Option 1 is now uncommon. Options 4 and 5 are illegal, and arguments against euthanasia include palliative care obviating its need, concerns about manipulation or exploitation, and 'slippery slope' effects. Although emotionally it may be easier to withhold than to withdraw life-prolonging treatment, the British Medical Association and General Medical Council have indicated that there are no legal, or necessarily moral, differences between the two.

Have you heard of the Assisted Dying for the Terminally Ill Bill and if so, what ethical issues does it raise?

This concerns deliberate acts to end life, not assisting in the natural dying process. The Bill was the subject of a House of Lords Select Committee Report. The idea of deliberately ending life brings intense ethical questions, notably concerning morality, the integrity of the medical profession and social implications of the effects of society permitting direct killing, and so weakening the prohibition against killing, which currently protects us all. Palliative care is concerned with enabling patients with advanced life-threatening conditions to live with the best possible quality of life until death. Clinical experience and research suggest that most requests for euthanasia or physician-assisted suicide arise because of poor symptom control, depression, poor social and family support and loss of autonomy. Palliative care focuses on improving these aspects of a patient's life and many of us believe that The Assisted Dying Bill and attempts to legalise physician-assisted suicide are ethically unsound, fail to appreciate the nature and scope of palliative care and undermine the progress made in the care of the dying in recent years.

One of your patients, a dying man with end-stage renal failure, diabetes and peripheral gangrene has a hypoglycaemic attack. Would you treat him?

This would depend upon any prior wishes he may have made. He may have told his doctors to 'let him go' if he takes any turn for the worse. He may, alternatively, have declined treatment for his renal failure and requested a comfortable death. A scenario such as hypoglycaemia may not have been anticipated or explicitly discussed. A common response to a potentially fatal change in condition that has not been previously discussed is to treat the current episode and later discuss with the patient what they would wish were it to recur. This said, because hypoglycaemia, unlike other potentially fatal changes in his condition, is caused by the medication and easily reversed, there may be legal risks in not treating, whatever the patient says.

A lady has breast cancer with cerebral metastases. She asks you how many of her anticonvulsant pills she would need to take to end her life. How might you respond?

We sometimes hasten death in clinical practice. The crucial distinction is intention, which may be to hasten death or relieve suffering. Frequently, doctors set out to relieve pain and suffering but see that life may be shortened. Foreseeing is not necessarily the same as intending. This has been tested in law and held to be permissible and in keeping with the duties of a doctor. It is one aspect of the doctrine of double effect, which makes a distinction between harms that are intended and harms that are foreseen but not intended. Telling the patient how many pills would be required to kill herself could be seen as assisting suicide and a criminal act. Your communication skills should endeavour to elicit key aspects of her suffering as she sees them and explore alternative ways of relieving them.

CASE 4.34

ADVANCE DIRECTIVES/DECISIONS

Candidate information

Role

You are a doctor on the medical ward.
    Please read this summary.

Scenario

Re: Dr Max Winter, aged 79 years

Dr Winter is a retired microbiologist with chronic obstructive pulmonary disease (COPD). Four months ago he prepared an advance directive in conjunction with his family. This stated that in the event of worsening respiratory problems requiring admission to hospital he would not wish cardiopulmonary resuscitation or any form of ventilation including non-invasive ventilation. He was admitted to hospital a few minutes ago with an acute exacerbation of COPD and marked hypoxia. He is confused, probably a result of his hypoxia, and now says that he will accept any treatment to make him better, although this is at odds with his advance directive. The emergency team have ignored his advance directive and just instituted non-invasive ventilation, with apparently good effect. His wife wishes to discuss the advance directive with you.

Your task is to discuss his management with his wife, taking into account the issue of the advance directive.

Your examiners will warn you when 12 minutes have elapsed. You have 14 minutes to communicate with the patient/subject followed by 1 minute of reflection. There will then follow 5 minutes of discussion with the examiners. Do not take the history again except for details that will help in your discussion with the patient/subject. You are not required to examine the patient/subject.

Patient/subject information

You are a retired general practitioner. Your husband, Dr Max Winter, is a 79-year-old retired microbiologist with COPD. Four months ago he prepared an advance directive in conjunction with his family. This stated that in the event of worsening respiratory problems requiring admission to hospital he would not wish cardiopulmonary resuscitation or any form of ventilation including non-invasive ventilation. He was admitted to hospital a few minutes ago with an acute exacerbation of COPD and marked hypoxia. He is confused, probably a result of his hypoxia, and now says that he will accept any treatment to make him better, although this is at odds with his advance directive. The emergency team have ignored his advance directive and just instituted non-invasive ventilation, with apparently good effect. You have mixed feelings. On the one hand you are pleased to see your husband less distressed but on the other are concerned about his prior wishes being ignored. You wonder if the advance directive has any validity.

How to approach the case

Communication skills (conduct of interview/problem exploration and negotiation), ethics and law

1 Introduction

Introduce yourself and establish that she is Dr Winter's wife.

2 Establish rapport and be alert to cues

Firstly, establish a rapport with a relative you have not met before, establishing what she knows, and if she does not volunteer the fact it may become clear that she is a professional colleague.

3 Seek further information about the patient

Relatives are highly valuable resources of information. She will know intimately the nature of his condition and his wishes in the event of a precipitous acute episode of illness.

4 Be sure that you understand the principles of advance directives

Advance directives are summarised in Box 4.30.

Box 4.30 Advance directives ('advance statements', written advance decisions or 'living wills')

- These are statements made by adults when they have capacity to decide for themselves about treatments they wish to accept or refuse, in circumstances in the future, when they are no longer able to make decisions or communicate their preferences. To make an advance directive, a patient should have sufficient information to understand the consequences of any decision as well as being legally competent (having capacity).
- The premise of an advance directive is that patients have the right to consent to or refuse specific treatments or procedures although basic care and hygiene cannot be refused and specific interventions cannot be demanded.
- There are different types of advance directive. *Instruction directives* set down a patient's wishes in highly specific circumstances. Defining circumstances is clearly difficult. It may be difficult to draw conclusions, for example, from an advance directive made in the event of a stroke, where the particular type of disability has not been stated. *Value directives* provide more general guidelines. Directives may be oral as well as written.
- Advance directives may not always be legally binding or unambiguous, although an informed advance directive can potentially be regarded in the same way as contemporaneous consent or refusal and ignoring it could constitute negligence or battery. Advance refusal of treatment made when a patient had capacity, on the basis of adequate information about the implications of his/her choice, is legally binding and must be respected where clearly applicable to the patient's present circumstances and where there is no reason to believe that the patient has changed his/her mind. Doctors, however, should not delay emergency care or withdraw basic care and cannot be forced to act against conscience.
- Advance directives are most useful with reference to specific treatments. Broad statements about life-saving treatments may be open to interpretation. What, for example, constitutes treatment? Does treatment include feeding a patient in a persistent vegetative state? Even with an advance directive, obtaining legal advice before withdrawing treatment may be advisable.
- To make an advance directive, a competent patient must have sufficient information to understand the consequences of any decision. Advance directives must be free from coercion and not the result of illness, fatigue or drugs.
- Patients are free to amend their advance directive at any time.

---

5 Explain the situation

Be honest about what has happened. In this case there is a possibility that he is temporarily incapacitated by hypoxia and the previous advance directive, made when he had capacity, means there is a risk that the doctors applying non-invasive ventilation are committing battery. However, it seems very reasonable to have erred on the side of the possibility of his having changed his mind. Where there is uncertainty it is always preferable to make the choice that preserves future choice as much as possible. His wife will probably fully accept this, provided you are open with her and any court (it would be very unlikely to go that far) would almost certainly see it that way, too!

6 Have a plan

The best way forward is likely to be to continue to treat non-invasively, stopping short of invasive ventilation, until her husband is able to competently confirm his wishes about any subsequent institution of non-invasive ventilation.

7 Ensure that your suggestions do not conflict with any ideas, concerns and expectations

Most importantly, ensure that she understands that where there was doubt the emergency team had little choice but to act in what they saw as being his current wishes or in his best interests but that you will be very sure to ascertain his wishes as soon as he is able to communicate these.

8 Seek acceptance of this plan

Highlight that the decision was ultimately that of the medical team, but that in future you will ensure that any unequivocal wishes will be confirmed and respected.

9 Invite questions

Make it clear that you are happy to answer questions now or later.

10 Conclude with assurances

Always conclude with an assurance that you will do your best to keep her husband comfortable and accord with his wishes as soon as these can be confirmed.

Discussion

An elderly lady with dementia, living alone but with carers, fractures her neck of femur. She is admitted to hospital with an abbreviated mental test score (AMTS) of 4/10. Her son says she would not wish any treatment. Would you agree to his request?

Regarding her autonomy, the patient is probably not competent and her AMTS is likely to represent a pot pourri of background cognitive impairment, pain and possible analgesia. On the principle of justice, most patients are more likely to do well with repair of their fractured neck of femurs and the benefits of surgery may outweigh the risks. It may be desirable to go ahead with treatment, with efforts to explain the rationale and get her family 'on board'.

A young woman with a history of asthma, necessitating multiple admissions to ITU, and depression is admitted with a further exacerbation of asthma requiring immediate ITU support. A handwritten letter in her notes addressed to her chest physician states that she wishes no treatment in the event of future collapse. Should she be admitted to ITU?

The answer is almost certainly yes. The validity of the advance directive may be in question for numerous reasons. It might have been written while she was depressed and her capacity may have been in question. The details may be sparse rather than specific. There may not be evidence that it was written by her. In case law there is a potential risk of battery if she receives treatment against the instructions of a valid advance directive but not treating puts her doctors at risk of manslaughter and because of the uncertainty the correct course of action is almost certainly to treat because of the uncertainty.

CASE 4.35

PERSISTENT VEGETATIVE STATE

Candidate information

Role

You are a doctor on the medical ward.
   Please read this summary.

Scenario

Re: Mr Roger Hunt, aged 19 years

Mr Hunt is a 19-year-old patient with type 1 diabetes who sustained severe cortical brain damage from an episode of prolonged hypoglycaemia while out drinking with friends at New Year. He breathes spontaneously but has been on your ward for four months and not shown any signs of interacting with his environment. He receives percutaneous gastrostomy feeding. He has had two episodes of aspiration pneumonia. His father is convinced he will get better one day, but is concerned that the doctors will label his son as being in a persistent vegetative state and seeks your reassurance that you will not stop actively treating future infections or providing artificial hydration and nutrition.

Your task is to address his father's concerns.

Your examiners will warn you when 12 minutes have elapsed. You have 14 minutes to communicate with the patient/subject followed by 1 minute of reflection. There will then follow 5 minutes of discussion with the examiners. Do not take the history again except for details that will help in your discussion with the patient/subject. You are not required to examine the patient/subject.

Patient/subject information

Your son, Roger Hunt, is 19 years old and has type 1 diabetes. Four months ago he sustained severe brain damage from an episode of prolonged hypoglycaemia while out drinking with friends. He breathes spontaneously but, according to the doctors, has not shown any signs of interacting with his environment. However, you are certain that he occasionally smiles and even seems to shed tears in your and your wife's company. He receives percutaneous gastrostomy feeding. He has had two episodes of pneumonia. You are convinced he will get better one day, but are very concerned that the doctors will label him as being in a persistent vegetative state. You want reassurance that the doctors will not stop actively treating future infections or providing artificial hydration and nutrition.

How to approach the case

Communication skills (conduct of interview, exploration and problem negotiation), ethics and law

1 Introduction

Introduce yourself and establish that he is Mr Hunt's father.

2 Establish what the relative knows

Firstly, establish what he knows about his son's condition, so that you have a basis for addressing his concerns.

3 Elicit ideas, concerns and expectations

Explore his ideas, concerns and expectations, actively listening.

4 Address ideas, concerns and expectations

Start with an immediate reassurance that there are no plans to withdraw care for his son. Note his remark about a persistent vegetative state. Explain that at this stage in his son's illness there would be every attempt to vigorously treat any infection, manage his diabetes carefully and of course provide full hydration and nutrition in conjunction with appropriate colleagues. Explain that certain movements and facial gestures are not uncommon in this situation, and that while you do not have the expertise to be sure that they are not signs of awareness, your understanding is that they could very well be involuntary reflex movements. The point is that you do not want to unequivocally remove hope and yet you want to truthfully reinforce what seems likely.

5 Be alert to cues

Throughout your explanation, be alert and ready to address any cues suggesting concern or disagreement. Above all, be empathetic and at no point challenge his desire to see his son get better, even though you may be less certain of its likelihood.

6 Elaborate on the meaning of the term persistent vegetative state

Offer to explain more about a persistent vegetative state. In particular explain that a diagnosis cannot be made this early on in the illness and can only be made later by certain specialists.

7 Be honest about the prognosis as it appears now

At the same time, do not reinforce what you feel to be excessive hope. Explain that you and the medical and nursing team would have hoped that more definite signs of improvement would have started to develop by now, and that as time goes on the prospects of the recovery that you would all wish for become less easy to envisage.

8 Concede uncertainty

Despite this, concede that at this stage there are no certainties; that in itself is often a heart-rending thing to wrestle with.

9 Invite questions

Make sure there are no areas that have not been discussed and express that you are willing to address any issues at any time with him.

10 Conclude with assurances

Reiterate that at this stage a diagnosis of persistent vegetative state has not and cannot be made, and that you will continue to actively treat his son's condition and any complications.

Discussion

What is meant by the term persistent vegetative state (PVS)?

A patient in a PVS shows no behavioural evidence of awareness of self or the environment, although there is a spectrum from unawareness to awareness. Features of PVS are outlined in Box 4.31.

Since the brain damage is cortical and the brainstem is preserved, awareness and consciousness are lost but breathing and circulation are spontaneous and support in an intensive care unit is not usually required.

> **Box 4.31 Features of a persistent vegetative state**
>
> - The absence of voluntary action or cognitive behaviour of any kind
> - An inability to communicate or interact purposefully with the environment
> - Brain damage consistent with the diagnosis of persistent vegetative state, and no reversible causes identified
> - At least six months and usually 12 months in this state from the initial insult to diagnosis

Why do we provide life-sustaining treatments to patients in a PVS?

The Terri Schiavo case in the United States is the most famous in recent history of a PVS and illustrates the dilemma of continuing to provide life-sustaining measures to a patient in a PVS. In 1990 Mrs Schiavo suffered severe brain damage from cerebral hypoxia following a cardiac arrest. She went into a coma and subsequently spent 15 years in an irreversible PVS. The cause of her cardiac arrest was never irrefutably established but electrolyte disturbance was implicated, her serum potassium being low on admission to hospital. She had suffered from an eating disorder that she had attempted to hide, causing presentation to obstetric services for fertility problems.

Despite rehabilitation attempts, Mrs Schiavo showed no signs of regaining awareness and required 24-hour care. She received hydration and nutrition via a gastrostomy tube. Her parents disputed the diagnosis of PVS and ultimately seven neurologists agreed that Mrs Schiavo was in a PVS, but a further neurologist disagreed.

There are well-documented cases of recovery from an apparent PVS, which is why it tends to be referred to as a persistent rather than permanent vegetative state. This said, it usually is permanent because of the nature of the underlying damage.

In 1994, after established and experimental therapies, Mr Schiavo accepted his wife's diagnosis, and when she developed a urinary tract infection, in conjunction with her physician, much therapy was halted and a do not resuscitate (DNAR) order was made. This was later rescinded when Mrs Schiavo's parents and her nursing home protested.

The case went on. Terri Schiavo had not made an advance directive, and, like most young people, had no reason to. While her husband eventually accepted the idea of her dying 'naturally' rather than remain in the non-cognitive, vegetative state, her parents disagreed. They video-recorded Mrs Schiavo with facial gestures which they felt exhibited signs of awareness, although it was generally held by clinicians that these were reflex movements. Patients in PVS may exhibit behaviours that can be construed as arising from partial consciousness including reflexive or random behaviours such as grinding teeth, swallowing, grunting, smiling or shedding tears.

Mrs Schiavo's parents stated up to and even after her death in early 2005 (when the Courts decided that hydration and nutrition should be withdrawn) there was 'no evidence she wanted to die of dehydration, or that she believed that the level of one's disability gives anyone the moral and legal right to end another's life'.

Important considerations in the future care of a patient in a PVS are therefore summarised in Box 4.32.

Why is PVS not the same as coma?

Coma patients do not respond to stimuli or show signs of awareness and thus appear to be asleep. Frequently, severe brain damage does result in coma but the sub-group who enter a PVS show wakefulness without signs of consciousness or awareness. They may experience sleep–wake cycles or be in a state of chronic wakefulness. Wakefulness is determined by nuclei in the hypothalamus that coordinate the circadian rhythm and is a prerequisite for consciousness and awareness, but in the event that higher centres (the cerebral cortex) are severely damaged or destroyed the wakefulness is without consciousness or awareness. Apparent awareness in this state of wakefulness, including opening of eyes, movements, swallowing and even emotional outbursts, are automatic reflexes.

How is coma measured?

The depth of unconsciousness is measured by the Glasgow Coma Score (Table 4.5).

Box 4.32 Considerations in the future care of a patient in a persistent vegetative state

- Establishing the diagnosis
- Deciding on its permanence
- The presence of any valid advance directive
- Deciding whether or not to withdraw life-prolonging treatments, which even in the presence of an advance directive often has to be decided in the Courts

---

Table 4.5 Glasgow Coma Score

	Score
Eye opening	
Spontaneously	4
To speech	3
To pain	2
No response	1
Best verbal response	
Orientated	5
Disorientated	4
Inappropriate words	3
Incomprehensible sounds	2
No response	1
Best motor response	
Obeys verbal commands	6
Localises painful stimuli	5
Withdrawal to pain	4
Flexion to pain (decorticate posturing)	3
Extension to pain (decerebrate posturing)	2
No response	1

Does spontaneous eye opening always indicate awareness?

Spontaneous eye opening indicates intact brainstem arousal mechanisms but not necessarily awareness.

What is 'locked-in' syndrome?

Locked-in syndrome refers to a state of awareness or consciousness with spontaneous breathing and circulation in the setting of severe brain damage rendering most other activity impossible. Numerous anatomical and aetiological types are possible, but a classic locked-in syndrome occurs with basilar territory infarction sparing respiratory drive centres but damaging long tracts and cranial nerve nuclei in the brainstem bilaterally. The cortex is unimpaired but cannot deliver any of its actions. Patients can breathe and think normally but can perform few if any actions.

Why is PVS not the same as brain death?

In brain death there is loss of brainstem activity. Brainstem reflexes are absent and spontaneous breathing and circulation cannot occur and can only be maintained artificially.

CASE 4.36

BRAINSTEM DEATH

Candidate information

Role

You are a doctor on the medical ward.
Please read this summary.

Scenario

Re: Mrs Anne Daly, aged 58 years

Mrs Daly is a previously well 58-year-old lady admitted to hospital two days ago with collapse. She was intubated on arrival to hospital but subsequent brain imaging confirms that she has had a spontaneous subarachnoid haemorrhage. She has not received sedation since initial ventilation and shows no signs of recovery. Two consultants have confirmed brainstem death. She was previously well and normotensive. Her daughter, Mrs Watts, is in the waiting room, aware that brainstem testing is being carried out although not completely aware of the implications of this.

Your task is to discuss the results with her daughter.

Your examiners will warn you when 12 minutes have elapsed. You have 14 minutes to communicate with the patient/subject followed by 1 minute of reflection. There will then follow 5 minutes of discussion with the examiners. Do not take the history again except for details that will help in your discussion with the patient/subject. You are not required to examine the patient/subject.

Patient/subject information

You are the daughter of Mrs Daly, a previously active 58-year-old lady. She was admitted to hospital two days ago following a fall while walking her dogs on the moor. She sustained a significant head injury. She was artificially ventilated on arrival to hospital and subsequent brain scans showed that she had sustained a large subarachnoid haemorrhage. She has subsequently shown no signs of recovery. She was previously well and normotensive. You are aware that brainstem testing is being carried out and, although not completely aware of the implications of this, sense that the news will be bad and that your mother is not going to recover. You are surprised that she is so desperately unwell, however, because her heart appears so good on the monitor and she looks well but asleep. She carried a donor card, and you will tell the doctor this.

How to approach the case

Communication skills (conduct of interview/ problem exploration and negotiation), ethics and law

1 Introduction

Introduce yourself and establish that she is Mrs Daly's daughter.

2 Establish what the relative knows

Ask her what she knows about her mother's condition.

3 Explain the situation

Explain that there have been no signs of recovery of consciousness and that this has been the major concern.

4 Explain brainstem death

Explain sensitively and empathetically that because of the injury, she has sustained irreversible brain damage, and this has just been confirmed by the specialists. Explain that she will not wake up and that this means that she has died from her injuries. Point out that the ventilator is sustaining her breathing and that when turned off her heart would stop soon afterwards.

5 Acknowledge distress and allow ventilation of feelings

Wait for her response before giving any more details.

6 Explain what will happen now

Explain that the medical team have to make the decision to turn off the ventilator, that it will not cause her mother

any distress, and that she need not feel any responsibility for this decision.

7 Discuss organ donation

Thank her for being able to mention this at this time. Assure her that as it is her mother's wish you will arrange for the transplant team to assess her mother for suitability, and until such time as any organ retrieval were to take place ventilation would be continued.

8 Identify support networks

It is human to want to discover a little more about the practical implications to her such as what other family members may be nearby.

9 Invite questions

Ask if she has any immediate questions.

10 Ensure that the relative has a point of contact

Ideally there would also be a nurse present to attend to her now but be prepared to meet her again later in the day or week if she has further questions.

Discussion

How might brainstem function be assessed?

Assessing brainstem function is vital to managing coma, raised intracranial pressure, brainstem strokes and confirming brain death.

Pupils assess midbrain integrity. Pupil size and reactivity assess third nerve function through the superior colliculus and connections to the Edinger Westphal nucleus (midbrain) and efferent parasympathetic outflow.

The corneal reflex assesses the fifth and seventh nerves, connected in the pons.

Resting eye position might suggest asymmetric brainstem dysfunction, dysconjugate position a disorder of the third, fourth or sixth nerves or their nuclei (third and fourth in midbrain and sixth in pons). Spontaneous saccadic (fast) horizontal and vertical eye movements suggest that the brainstem mechanism for generating this is intact and there is no need to test for oculocephalic or oculovestibular responses. Horizontal saccades rely on an intact paramedian pontine reticular formation (pons), third nerve nucleus, sixth nerve nucleus and median longitudinal fasciculus connecting these. Vertical saccades rely on the dorsal mid-brain.

Swallowing requires intact glossopharyngeal and vagus nerves and connections including the swallowing centre in the reticular formation of the medulla.

Respiratory pattern is sometimes useful in localisation. Apneustic breathing (prolonged inspiration followed by a period of apnoea) and cluster breathing (closely grouped respirations followed by a period of apnoea) imply pontine damage. Ataxic breathing (chaotic) and gasping breathing (gasps followed by variable apnoea) occur when the medullary respiratory centre is damaged and are precursors to respiratory arrest. Cheyne–Stokes breathing (often used to describe a range of brainstem damage patterns of breathing) can be the result of cortical damage but is mostly caused by cardiovascular or respiratory disease. Slow, shallow breathing may occur when drugs depress medullary function. Central neurogenic hyperventilation (rapid, deep continuous breathing at a rate of around 25 cycles/minute) is not localising but suggests deepening coma and worsening prognosis.

Long tract signs can occur and may be crossed with cranial signs because of decussation.

What are oculocephalic and oculovestibular responses?

Passive head rotation stimulates vestibular and neck receptors which in comatose patients with intact brainstems leads to reflexive slow conjugate eye movements mediated by the vestibulo-ocular reflex (VOR) pathway in the brainstem in the direction opposite to head rotation. Ice water irrigation of the ear switches off this pathway, leading to the unopposed contribution of the contralateral vestibular system, and the eyes deviate towards the ice. Both the oculocephalic (doll's head manoeuvre) response and the oculovestibular (caloric) response test the VOR, but the latter is more sensitive.

Major brainstem pathology is unlikely with normal VORs. An absent horizontal VOR with an intact vertical VOR may indicate pontine damage. If both are absent there may be wider brainstem pathology or a metabolic disturbance, the latter more likely if pupils react. A very small number of drugs depress brainstem function. VOR testing may be difficult if there are dysconjugate eye movements (when brainstem dysfunction is likely) or if there are fast saccades (when brainstem dysfunction is unlikely).

Which brainstem syndromes arise from brain shift?

There are four important syndromes (Box 4.33).

How is brain death determined?

There is irreversible loss of capacity for consciousness and capacity to breathe. Both of these are lost without the stem. Because it is possible to maintain circulation and ventilation with ventilators in patients with irreversible brain damage without brainstem function, criteria for brain death were developed (Box 4.34). Testing should be by two experienced clinicians, at least one a consultant.

Is there a legal definition of death?

There is no legal definition of death. Death is usually defined by irreversible loss of capacity for consciousness together with irreversible loss of capacity to breathe due to cessation of brainstem function. Brainstem death therefore equates to death of an individual.

Box 4.33 Brainstem syndromes arising from brain shift

Central herniation

A supratentorial mass displaces the diencephalons (cerebral peduncles, thalamic areas and related structures between cerebral hemispheres and upper brainstem) through the tentorium to compress the upper midbrain, then the pons, then the medulla. Signs such as unilateral hemiplegia, together with paratonia (gegenhalten) and extensor plantars (diencephalic stage), precede diminished alertness and Cheyne–Stokes breathing. The pupils are small, perhaps because of hypothalamic sympathetic dysfunction, but reactive. There is decorticate (flexor) posturing to pain. Progression from midbrain to upper pontine dysfunction causes temperature fluctuation, unreactive pupils in mid-position, loss of vertical eye movements (doll's head manoeuvre), diminishing vestibulo-ocular reflex (VORs) and apneustic or cluster breathing or central hyperventilation. Decerebrate posturing to pain develops. Progression to lower pontine and upper medullary damage causes chaotic breathing and absent VORs. Tone is flaccid. Progression to medullary damage is terminal. Heart rate may fall and blood pressure rise (Cushing response), breathing is chaotic or gasping, and pupils become dilated and fixed.

Lateral (uncal) herniation

Lesions in the lateral middle fossa or temporal lobe push the medial edge of the uncus and hippocampal gyrus over the free lateral edge of the tentorium. The first sign is a unilateral dilating pupil as the third nerve is compressed, followed by a third nerve palsy. Midbrain compression with diminished alertness and coma and the sequence as for central herniation can follow, without an initial diencephalic stage and decorticate responses.

False localisation

Expanding supratentorial lesions may distort structures and produce signs because of traction from afar, often affecting cranial nerves V to VIII.

Tonsillar herniation

Subtentorial lesions may cause herniation of the cerebellar tonsils through the foramen magnum to compress the pons and midbrain directly. There may also be upward compression, giving rise to supratentorial effects, but the rostrocaudal sequence of damage typical of central herniation is lacking.

Box 4.34 Brain death criteria

Preconditions

- Irreversible brain damage, e.g. head injury, brain haemorrhage, anoxia
- Apnoeic coma
- Absence of reversible factors such as drugs or metabolic or temperature disturbance

All brainstem reflexes absent

- Pupils fixed and unresponsive to bright light (not necessarily dilated)
- Absent corneal reflexes
- Absent vestibulo-ocular reflexes
- No motor responses within the cranial nerve distribution to stimulation of any somatic area
- No reflex response to touching the pharynx (gag reflex) or a suction catheter in the trachea (cough reflex)

Apnoea

- No respiratory movements without the ventilator

CASE 4.37

DISCUSSING LIVE ORGAN DONATION

Candidate information

Role

You are a doctor in the renal clinic.
    Please read this summary.

Scenario

> **Re: Mr Stephen Wells, aged 45 years**
>
> Mr Wells, a solicitor, has chronic kidney disease due to diabetes mellitus on a background of poor renal reserve caused by damage from sepsis as a child. He currently receives haemodialysis. He is on the transplant list. His sister is with him today because they have both discussed the idea of live organ transplantation, having read of its success. Her concerns are the risks to her and her brother.
>
> Your task is to discuss live organ transplantation.

Your examiners will warn you when 12 minutes have elapsed. You have 14 minutes to communicate with the patient/subject followed by 1 minute of reflection. There will then follow 5 minutes of discussion with the examiners. Do not take the history again except for details that will help in your discussion with the patient/subject. You are not required to examine the patient/subject.

Patient/subject information

You are the sister of Stephen Wells, a 45-year-old solicitor who has chronic kidney disease from diabetes mellitus and kidney damage as a child. He currently receives haemodialysis. He is on the transplant list. You are with him today because you have both discussed the idea of live organ transplantation, having read of its success. Your concerns are the risks to yourself and your brother, but you would prefer your brother to have your kidney than one from an unknown source, and feel his body would not reject an organ from a relative.

How to approach this case

Communication skills (conduct of interview, exploration and problem negotiation) and ethics and law

1 Introduction

Introduce yourself. Both potential recipient and donor should be present (in PACES only one subject but the principles are the same).

2 Establish background knowledge

Find out what they know about organ donation.

3 Explore ideas, concerns and expectations

Explore their understanding of the advantages of live organ donation. Explain that there are very clear advantages but that the complications of transplantation, including rejection, remain a risk.

4 Explain the principles of live organ donation

Explain briefly there would be a dual hospital stay for the operation but that the surgical procedure is not your area of expertise and you would arrange a meeting with the transplant surgeon were they to decide to go down this route.

5 Respond to ideas, concerns and expectations

Explain that matching is a potential problem but that it needs not be perfect nor, indeed, need it be a relative. Her being a sibling does not remove the possibility of rejection and he will still need to take immunosuppression with its attendant risks.

6 Explain potential benefits to recipient and donor

Explain that outcome is better with donation from a live than a deceased person. While on the waiting list there is no guarantee of when a suitable organ will be available and his health might deteriorate in the meantime; live organ donation would remove this problem. There may be significant psychological satisfaction in donating to a relative.

7 Explain potential risks to recipient and donor

Risks to the donor include operative and perioperative risks (major surgery requiring around a week in hospital and some weeks off work), and having a single kidney (although compatible with a normal life). Risks to the recipient are immediate surgical complications and rejection.

8 Other matters

There may be insurance issues for the donor.

9 Invite questions

> *I appreciate we've covered rather a lot there. Is there anything you would like me to go over again or are there any questions you would like to ask me?*

Be honest in your explanations and prepared to admit uncertainty (with assurance you will seek the answer) if there are questions you cannot answer.

10 Explain what would happen next

Explain that if they decide to take things further, formal assessment by the transplant team would be needed.

Discussion

How is organ transplantation governed in the UK?

Organ transplantation in the UK is governed by the Human Tissue Act (1969) and the Human Organ Transplant Act (1989). Following the retained organs controversy (Case 4.38), a Human Tissue Act in 2004 introduced new legislation and regulation for all human material, whether from living or deceased people. It applies to England, Wales and Northern Ireland and the Scottish Assembly passed similar legislation in 2006.

Is there a shortage of organ donors?

There is a worldwide shortage of cadaveric donor organs, and a living related donor is more likely to provide the best histocompatibility but more likely to feel pressure to donate. Shortage of organs is doubtless in part the result of the understandable reluctance of staff to approach relatives for consent after a patient dies.

How might the supply of organ donors be increased?

The situation could be improved by educating the public to leave evidence of their wishes, reducing the need to broach the subject with grieving relatives. The default position of a population opting in to donate is mooted by governments.

Does the Human Tissue Act aim to improve the number of organ donors?

Currently, even if the deceased carries a donor card, a relative's objections can prevent transplantation. The new Act will ensure that the patient's recorded wishes, or the decision of a representative nominated by the patient, must be followed. Failing this, consent from a person in a 'qualifying relationship' is necessary (there is a hierarchical list). The Act unambiguously outlaws all commerce in human bodies and body parts.

Can dying patients who are potential donors be 'kept alive' in intensive care while consent is being sought for organ donation?

Donor ventilatory and circulatory support is essential before heart transplantation and desirable for other organs. Transplantation procedures can only occur when brainstem death has been determined, and this should be by a team separate to that caring for the patient. 'Elective ventilation', the concept of sustaining the life of a dying patient for the sole purpose of transplantation, appears to be illegal, but the Act authorises methods to preserve organs of deceased individuals while consent is being sought.

Are there advantages of live organ donation?

Carefully selected living related donors are more immunologically compatible and the chances of graft rejection are reduced.

Box 4.35 Criteria for live organ donors

- The risk to the donor must be low.
- The donor must give full informed consent.
- The consent must be given freely and without coercion or pressure.
- The donor must understand that he or she may withdraw consent at any time before the procedure.
- The offer of the organ must be without any inducements, including financial.
- There must be a good chance of a successful outcome for the recipient.

What ethical criteria should be met by live organ donors?

These are listed in Box 4.35.

Is there a place for unrelated live transplants?

A donation may be obtained from a non-genetically related person provided no payment is involved. Historically, live unrelated donors of kidneys were seldom considered because there was no greater chance of graft survival but modern immunosuppression means that less well-matched grafts can now survive. The Human Organ Transplants Act restricts transplants between unrelated people and approval must be given through an independent authority, the Unrelated Live Transplant Regulatory Authority (ULTRA), set up under the Act.

CASE 4.38

REQUESTING AN AUTOPSY (POST MORTEM)

Candidate information

Role

You are a doctor on the medical ward.
   Please read this summary.

Scenario

Re: Mrs Jane Ayre, aged 76 years

Mrs Ayre was a 76-year-old lady who died yesterday on your ward. She had been admitted with weight loss, vomiting and hypotension. She was awaiting further investigation after an abdominal computed tomography (CT) scan showed bilateral adrenal masses. The concern had been whether she might have adrenal metastases and secondary hypoadrenalism. Her daughter is here, and your consultant has asked you to seek permission for an autopsy to clarify cause of death, but is happy for a death certificate to be issued if she does not consent.

Your task is to request permission for an autopsy.

Your examiners will warn you when 12 minutes have elapsed. You have 14 minutes to communicate with the patient/subject followed by 1 minute of reflection. There will then follow 5 minutes of discussion with the examiners. Do not take the history again except for details that will help in your discussion with the patient/subject. You are not required to examine the patient/subject.

Patient/subject information

Your mother, Mrs Ayre, died yesterday on the hospital ward, aged 76. The cause of death was unclear but very possibly cancer. She had been admitted from home following one week of vomiting and dizziness. She had been losing weight for a few months before this. She and you had been told that cancer was a possibility although you had not expected her to die so suddenly. The doctor is about to ask your permission for an autopsy. You are not happy for an autopsy, feeling that if cancer was likely there is no reason to explore further. You are also worried that an autopsy could delay funeral arrangements and cause disfigurement. After consideration, you will agree to an autopsy.

How to approach this case

Communication skills (conduct of interview, exploration and problem negotiation) and ethics and law

1 Introduction

Introduce yourself and confirm her identity.

2 Acknowledge that it is a difficult time

Tell her how sorry you are that her mother has died and that staff were saddened by the news. Pause to allow her to express her emotions. Asking permission to carry out an autopsy at a time when relatives may be distressed is not always easy and not a task that should be delegated to the most junior member of the team. Before approaching relatives, it is important to establish if the patient had made any prior wishes.

3 Retrace the relevant background

Explain the medical team's thoughts about what might have been wrong with the patient and why.

4 Explain the reasons for requesting an autopsy

Common reasons for requesting an autopsy are listed in Box 4.36. Additional benefits include education and training, research and audit.

5 Explain the autopsy consent form

Explain that she will need to sign a consent form. This includes an option for relatives to request a limited autopsy, with separate sections for permission for organ retention,

---

> **Box 4.36 Common reasons for requesting an autopsy**
>
> - The cause of death was not clear.
> - While the cause of death may have seemed clear, some features of the disease remain unusual.
> - The disease was rare and an autopsy could shed new light on it.
> - The information from the autopsy might help the management of other patients (in some cases family members) who suffer from the same condition.

permission for education and training and permission for the use of retained tissue in research.

6 Explore concerns

She may have concerns about further examination when all she wants, and she feels her mother wants, is to be left in peace.

7 Be prepared to discuss arrangements about the body

Explain that an autopsy will not (usually) delay funeral arrangements. Relatives sometimes ask if the body can be viewed after autopsy and might need to be reassured that in hospital autopsies standard incisions are used that are not visible when the body is gowned and that the body can be viewed after autopsy.

8 Invite questions

> *I appreciate we've covered rather a lot there. Is there anything you would like me to go over again or are there any questions you would like to ask me?*

9 Explain what would happen next

Explain that nothing needs to be done by the daughter, and that the hospital would arrange everything and that the funeral director would liaise with the hospital directly.

10 Seek consent or accept refusal

And thank her for discussing this.

Discussion

What changes have occurred in recent years in the law regarding retention of human tissue and organs?

The public inquiries at Bristol Royal Infirmary and Alder Hey Children's Hospital found organ retention without the knowledge or consent of relatives to be common practice. The Chief Medical Officer subsequently arranged a consensus that revealed 105 000 retained organs, body parts, stillbirths and fetuses within English Hospital Trusts and The Retained Organs Commission was set up to oversee the return, donation for research or disposal of retained material according to the wishes of relatives who enquired, and to advise on future legislation.

The Human Tissue Act makes it a criminal offence to remove, retain or use tissue or organs without consent and covers all material containing human cells removed from the living or dead (gametes or embryos are covered by separate legislation). Thus no research or teaching is now possible without consent. Use for clinical or public health audit, education or research using anonymised material does not require consent if the material comes from the living, but will always be needed if the material is from deceased persons. The Act is not retrospective, but the Human Tissue Authority, the regulatory body for the Act, issues codes of practice for dealing with material already retained.

What is the role of the Human Tissue Authority?

It is to regulate the removal, storage, use and disposal of human bodies, organs and tissue from the living and deceased.

What are the implications for hospital autopsies?

Most Hospital Trusts have guidelines for autopsy requests. Most autopsies in hospital are hospital requested and performed by a hospital pathologist, and for these relatives must grant permission.

Consent forms usually cover the option for relatives to request a limited autopsy, and separate sections for permission for organ retention (usually brain or lungs), permission for education and training (often a clause stating that information may be used for such purposes unless relatives disagree) and permission for the use of retained tissue in research.

Organs retained can either be disposed of by the pathology department or returned to the funeral director at the family's request.

There is concern that hospital autopsies will decline in number, and training will suffer, although the legislation

---

Box 4.37 Deaths that should be reported to the coroner

- Deaths that are sudden or unexplained
- Deaths where the deceased had not been attended by a medical practitioner for their last illness and within 14 days before death
- Deaths not due, or not entirely due, to natural causes, e.g. accidents, deaths occurring after an operation, occupational disease, lack of care, self-neglect, suicide and self-harm, violence
- Deaths involving septicaemia if originating from injury or medical intervention
- Dead on arrival at hospital
- Death in police custody or prison or following admission from these
- Deaths where the cause is natural but unknown and the doctor cannot issue a death certificate

---

acknowledges that people expect clear information and partnership with the medical profession. Hospital Trusts must therefore produce clear procedures and consent forms and provide adequate training in gaining consent from relatives.

In which circumstances might the Coroner (in Scotland Procurator Fiscal) wish to perform an autopsy?

While the statutory duty to report a death to the Coroner resides with the Registrar of Births and Deaths, doctors should be aware of the circumstances in which a registrar is required to report a death and should report a death themselves in those circumstances listed in Box 4.37.

Does a Coroner's autopsy need consent?

No. Relatives do not have the right to either grant or refuse permission for an autopsy requested by the Coroner, nor any organ retention, although the Act will make it necessary for consent to be obtained for retention or use of material after investigations are concluded.

CLINICAL GOVERNANCE

CASE 4.39

CRITICAL INCIDENT

Candidate information

Role

You are a doctor in the emergency medical admissions unit.

Please read this summary.

Scenario

> Re: Mrs Jane Parker, aged 84 years
>
> Mrs Parker was admitted three days ago with life-threatening haematemesis. She had a history of a stroke from which she had made a partial recovery. You resuscitated her with blood. The gastroenterologist requested central access for monitoring purposes while preparations were made for endoscopy. This was a difficult procedure because her systolic blood pressure was < 80 mmHg. Eventually you obtained flashback of dark red blood in the left internal jugular region and gained access. At endoscopy a bleeding gastric ulcer was injected and she was admitted to the high-dependency unit (HDU).
>
> The gastroenterologist met you yesterday to let you know of a critical incident. The day after admission to the HDU Mrs Parker suffered a further stroke with dense left-sided weakness and a computed tomography (CT) scan showed a very large right parietal infarction, probably from watershed ischaemia. It was also noticed in the HDU that your central line was positioned in the left carotid artery. It had not been used, although for reasons not yet established had not been removed despite a chest X-ray showing malposition. Unhappily, the HDU doctor told Mrs Parker's daughter that arterial catheterisation should never occur because it can cause a stroke. You honestly cannot recall reviewing the chest X-ray.
>
> The gastroenterologist is convinced that the stroke was caused by hypotension on a background of a cerebrovascular disease, not least because the stroke occurred on the wrong side to implicate the catheter. He is also very irritated by the careless remarks of the HDU doctor. However, he feels that the incident should be reported because although unlikely to be causative, and a well-recognised complication of the procedure, a system failure led to the potentially dangerous situation of

non-removal of the malpositioned line. He has spoken to the daughter and given these views. However, the patient's daughter, with whom you spoke on admission, would also like to talk to you. Your task is to talk to the daughter and respond to her concerns.

Your examiners will warn you when 12 minutes have elapsed. You have 14 minutes to communicate with the patient/subject followed by 1 minute of reflection. There will then follow 5 minutes of discussion with the examiners. Do not take the history again except for details that will help in your discussion with the patient/subject. You are not required to examine the patient/subject.

Patient/subject information

Your mother, Mrs Jane Parker, is an 84-year-old lady who was admitted to hospital three days ago with a bleeding stomach ulcer. She had a stroke two years ago, leaving her relatively immobile and she lives with you. She has continued to have 'mini-strokes' with effects on mobility and memory and you have been concerned about her quality of life. At endoscopy the bleeding ulcer, which you accepted as life-threatening, was treated and she was admitted to the HDU because of very low blood pressure. You were very happy with the admitting doctor's (the candidate's) communication to you of events. Subsequently, your mother has had a stroke and is now very unwell. You were not surprised by this although you were upset when another doctor, in the HDU, told you that the admitting doctor had placed a catheter incorrectly into the artery of her neck and that this probably caused the stroke. The consultant has subsequently made you feel easier, explaining that the line was placed incorrectly, but that it does not seem to have been the cause of the stroke but that the matter will be looked into thoroughly. You believe the consultant, have no wish to make a complaint because you have been very happy with the care given to your mother over the years and accept that she has been unwell for some time. However, you would like to speak to the admitting doctor, both to hear his view of events and to be further reassured that the HDU doctor was 'out of line'.

How to approach the case

Communication skills (conduct of interview/ exploration and problem negotiation), ethics and law

1 Introduction and setting

Show that you are willing to listen, explain and help in whatever way you can. Angry or upset patients and relatives should never feel threatened.

2 Listen to concerns

Allow her to say what she wants to, without interruption. Find out the exact nature of her concerns. More often than not, venting of emotions is what people want, in this case concern and likely confusion created by the careless words of a colleague.

3 Acknowledge concerns

First and foremost, make her see that you understand her concerns. Make it very clear that you and the consultant are concerned about the incident. Tell her that she has a right to know exactly what happened.

4 Apologise, if appropriate

Where it is clear that a mistake has been made, say how sorry you are that the incident occurred. In this case, however, you should not admit to the allegation of the HDU doctor but you do want to concede that a recognised complication of the procedure occurred. You may also need to say how sorry you are that she has been upset and confused by apparently conflicting comments.

5 Do not criticise colleagues but give your view

Colleagues have the same rights to be consulted and given the opportunity to seek advice, and ill-considered remarks could lead patients or relatives to misleading conclusions and prejudice a colleague's interests. Colleagues should never be criticised openly, but this does not necessarily mean dismissing or excusing a patient's or relative's expressed concern or complaint. While you should not criticise the HDU doctor (no matter how you may feel about his careless remarks) it is appropriate to say you agree with the comments made by the consultant, reinforcing what you see as correct information. Overall, you need to let her see how sorry you are that her mother's condition has deteriorated, without focusing so much on the HDU doctor's view.

6 Explain how the incident occurred

Explain, as clearly as possible, how the incident occurred. Explain that your action was in good faith in the best interests of her mother, who was very unwell, and that you were deeply concerned to learn that you had placed the catheter in the artery as soon as it became known to you.

7 Work with facts – do not speculate!

Since you should work with facts, do not speculate as to why the catheter was left incorrectly in situ until the facts have been established.

8 Give an assurance of further action

Explain that normally mechanisms should be in place to recognise such a complication (chest X-ray ± blood gases). Tell her that the incident will be reported as a 'critical incident' to the risk management team, who will investigate it further and decide what action might be taken to avert such an incident in future (the use of Doppler-guided central line placement is now considered best practice).

9 Invite questions and provide further information if needed

Ask if there are any other specific concerns she has not mentioned. Hopefully she accepts your candid response to the incident but if she wishes to make a formal written complaint she should be informed of to whom to write. In any event, you should offer to be of further assistance should she have further questions or concerns.

10 Document everything fully and carefully

The vast majority of critical incidents are errors not of one person but of a system within which fallible people operate. Discuss the incident with your consultant, document everything clearly and depending upon the significance of the incident discuss it confidentially with your medical defence organisation.

Discussion

What do you understand by the term clinical governance (CG)?

The full definition, from the government paper *A First Class Service 2000*, is 'a framework through which NHS organisations are accountable for continuously improving the quality of their services and safeguarding high standards of care by creating an environment in which excellence in clinical care will flourish'. In short, it means striving for the best quality, minimising harm and maximising benefit within budget and resources.

CG was given impetus by health-care disasters like Shipman and the Bristol Enquiry. Key areas of CG are outlined in Box 4.38. Ideally, CG should be proactive, but it often needs to react to complaints, claims and incidents.

What is a critical incident?

A critical incident is an event that gives rise to, or has the potential to produce, unexpected or unwanted effects

---

Box 4.38 Key areas of clinical governance

- Clinical risk management, e.g. incident reporting
- Education and training, e.g. standardised outcomes and assessments
- Patient and public involvement, e.g. expert patients, copying letters to patients
- Staffing, e.g. appropriate selection
- Effective communication and use of information, e.g. use of computerised imaging and electronic patient records
- Audit, e.g. local, national
- Research, evidence-based practice and clinical effectiveness, e.g. use of NICE guidelines

involving the safety of patients. It is a serious event that harmed or could have harmed and as such would be likely to give rise to public concern or criticism of the service involved. Annually in the NHS there are known to be around 850 000 adverse events and 28 000 complaints. This may be the tip of the iceberg. Trusts have Clinical Risk Management teams to aid investigation of clinical incidents and many have their own legal department and solicitors.

Should you report all incidents?

All incidents should be reported, but because of the enormous number of them, grading systems or risk matrices have been introduced that incorporate both their likelihood and their consequence, to give priority to the more serious.

What do you understand by the term system error?

Seldom is one individual wholly responsible for a critical incident. The role of risk management teams is to investigate the system within which individuals operate to identify gaps that expose it to errors. The above case illustrates such gaps (e.g. the use of Doppler-imaging for inserting central venous catheters, chest X-ray confirmation post-procedure and the question of who is responsible for checking it if a patient moves to a different team's care). Incidents happen because of failures in the organisation's management, local conditions (e.g. under-staffing, tiredness, under-resourced), individual unsafe acts (e.g. missing out a step in a procedure because short of time or multitasking) and what has been called 'the final defence barrier breach' (e.g. in an adequately staffed procedural room, a doctor may have omitted to check the date and label on the local anaesthetic but a nurse might have noted it). For these reasons alone, it is never acceptable to rush to blame.

What is the National Patient Safety Agency (NPSA)?

Everyone makes mistakes. The questions are why are they made repeatedly, how can we learn from them and can we eliminate some of them. The NSPA takes a seven-themed approach to this (Box 4.39).

How is a hospital managed?

A Trust Board has overall responsibility for scrutinising trust policy, implementing national/government policies and advising the Trust Executive. The Trust Board comprises a chief executive together with executive and non-executive directors. Board executives are usually ex-bankers or lawyers or business people, and sometimes nurses.

The Trust Executive is the hospital's functioning body. It comprises Clinical Directorates and Corporate Directorates.

Clinical Directorates typically include Medicine (usually enormous), General Surgery, Specialist Surgery, Trauma

---

Box 4.39 National Patient Safety Agency approach

Promoting a safety culture

This includes enhancing awareness and building safety into daily work with such activities as induction, handovers and audit.

Leading and supporting staff

This includes clinical leadership and supporting staff ideas.

Integration of risk management activity

This includes working across teams, departments, trusts and the NHS, e.g. the tracking of blood for transfusion from source to patient. It embraces all information such as incidents, complaints, litigation and audit, and balances costs with levels of risk. It is not feasible, for example, for all surgical instruments to be single-use. Risk management at the directorate level includes risk and medical management, critical incidents and audit, and at the governance committee level are a Health and Safety Committee, evidence-based practice, infection control and so forth.

Promotion of reporting

This includes reporting of incidents, near misses and methods for investigation and review (information, mapping of event, barriers to safety). Barriers to safety include discontinuity of care, communication failure and the different layouts of each ward, and barriers to reporting include fear of blame, no clear benefit, 'not my job', no feedback or 'a waste of time'. A non-punitive atmosphere is essential to promote reporting.

Communication with patients and public

Key principles are honesty, apology, explanation and thorough investigation.

Learning and sharing lessons

Information needs to be disseminated, by, for example, email, written memos, policy documents and discussion.

Implementation of solutions

A National Confidential Enquiry into Patient Outcomes and Deaths (NCEPOD), for example, under the National Patient Safety Agency (NPSA), recommends more consultant involvement in clinical care to recognise and manage critical illness.

---

and Orthopaedics, Child and Women's Health, Critical Care/Emergency Medical Services, Diagnostic Services and Professional Services. Each Clinical Directorate provides services, e.g. the disciplines of general medicine and specialist medicine within the Medicine Directorate, and physiotherapy, occupational therapy, speech and language therapy and dietetics within the Professional Services Directorate. Each clinical directorate comprises a Clinical Director (CD), directorate manager, a lead nurse and a directorate accountant. These are all responsible to the Medical Director (MD), who in turn is answerable to the Chief Executive. These people tend to meet monthly. The CD is usually a doctor, who relies very much on the directorate manager as he or she usually struggles to combine CD work with clinical work. Two or three sessions per week are usually recommended for CD work, but it invariably demands much more. Roles include ensuring clinical and operational performance, changing strategies within the trust in line with national policies and working with Primary Care Trusts. Much work is 'fire fighting' – handling complaints, approving study leave and so forth.

Each Corporate Directorate comprises a director and provides certain services. Corporate Directorates might typically include the Chief Executive, the Medical Director, Finance and IM&T, Human Resources (staffing, occupational health), Operations (e.g. clinical directorate management, operational performance, business planning, emergency preparedness), Facilities (e.g. estates, catering, laundry, parking, security, fire, bookshop), Nursing and Service Improvement (e.g. complaints handling) and Planning.

The flow of NHS money is from the Department of Health, which feeds it to primary care trusts, which feed via the Planning Directorate to NHS trusts (linked to Strategic Health Authorities) who set their own budgets.

What do you know about the Access to Health Records Act?

This gives patients the general right to see their medical records, obtain copies thereof and have the records explained to them. It only applies to records after 1 November 1991. A doctor may deny access (it is not that the whole record should be withheld but only specific information within it) on the grounds that it is 'likely to cause serious harm to the physical or mental health of the patient or any other person, or could lead to the identification of another individual (other than the health professional) who has been involved in the care of the subject'. An application must be in writing and made by a patient, person authorised by the patient, person appointed by the Court or an executor. When application for access is made by an individual on behalf of a patient who is incompetent or deceased, no information can be given that the patient had considered confidential and the holder is not required to explain why any part of the record has been withheld. Viewing of the records should be provided within 21 days (40 days for records at least 40 days old). A reasonable fee may be charged.

CASE 4.40

MANAGING A COMPLAINT AND THE QUESTION OF NEGLIGENCE

Candidate information

Role

You are a doctor on the medical ward.
  Please read this summary.

Scenario

> Re: Mr Jeremy Finch, aged 64 years
> Mr Finch is a 64-year-old man on your ward who last week had an endobronchial biopsy for a suspicious lung lesion. Yesterday evening he was told by a member of staff (you are not yet sure who), in the presence of his daughter, that the lesion might well be benign, and yet this morning you received the formal report suggesting it is an adenocarcinoma. You discussed this sensitively and Mr Finch seemed to accept the diagnosis but his daughter now wants to talk to you.
> You task is to address his daughter's concerns.

Your examiners will warn you when 12 minutes have elapsed. You have 14 minutes to communicate with the patient/subject followed by 1 minute of reflection. There will then follow 5 minutes of discussion with the examiners. Do not take the history again except for details that will help in your discussion with the patient/subject. You are not required to examine the patient/subject.

Patient/subject information

You are the daughter of Mr Jeremy Finch, a 64-year-old man who has been told by his doctor this morning that the result of his lung biopsy is that he has lung cancer. You are understandably upset although you had been concerned for some time that he had been coughing up blood and it took you some months to persuade your father to come to hospital. You are, however, very upset that yesterday evening a junior doctor on night shift came to take blood from your father with you present and commented that very often these turn out to be benign. You are concerned because this is not the first 'disaster'. When your father was first admitted he was told he had pneumonia and given a dose of penicillin when it was documented very clearly in his general practitioner's referral that he was allergic to penicillin. You feel that the hospital makes one mistake after another and want to complain and may consider suing the hospital for negligence.

How to approach the case

Communication skills (conduct of interview/ exploration and problem negotiation), ethics and law

1 Introduction and setting

Introduce yourself and confirm her identity. Show that you are willing to listen, explain and help in whatever way you can. Angry or upset patients and relatives should never feel threatened.

2 Listen to concerns/complaint

Allow her to say what she wants to, without interruption. Do not take any criticism personally. Find out the exact nature of her complaint. More often than not, venting of feelings to a sincere and responsible listener is enough for patients or relatives. Progression to a complaint is less likely if you can facilitate this.

3 Acknowledge concerns

Let her see that you understand her grievances, and are dedicated to responding to these appropriately.

4 Apologise, if appropriate

Where it is clear that a mistake has been made, say how sorry you are that this incident occurred. Unless it is very clear that a complaint is unreasonable, it is always best to offer a sincere apology, and if unreasonable, to say you are sorry the person feels that way.

5 Do not criticise colleagues but give your view

Focus on any problem in the system, not on any individual.

6 Explain how the incident occurred

Explain, as clearly as possible (if you know), how the incident occurred.

7 Work with facts – do not speculate!

It is inappropriate to speculate (or worse, ascribe blame) when you do not have all the facts; these should be established, if need be, by proper inquiry. Emphasise the clinical imperatives – to now seek advice from the respiratory and cancer specialist about the best way to treat her father's condition.

8 Give an assurance of further action about the complaint

Tell her that you will share the information with your consultant and report the incident as a 'critical incident' to the risk management team, who will investigate things further and decide what action might be taken to avert such an incident in future.

9 Invite questions and provide further information if needed

Hopefully she accepts your candid response to the incident but if she wishes to make a formal written complaint she should be told to whom to write. In any event, you should offer to be of further assistance should she have any further questions or concerns.

10 Document everything fully and carefully

The vast majority of critical incidents are errors not of one person but of a system within which fallible people operate. Discuss the incident with your consultant, document everything clearly and depending upon the significance of the incident discuss it confidentially with your medical defence organisation.

Discussion

Why do people make a complaint?

People complain to vent anger, seek changes, receive an apology, feel better, blame someone else and stop the same thing happening again. Sometimes they complain seeking compensation. People complain about clinical care, staff attitudes, outpatient delays, poor communication, discharge and aspects of non-clinical care.

How might complaints be avoided or minimised?

Knowing why people complain can help minimise complaints. Every effort should be made to avoid dispute or altercation. The General Medical Council recommends that patients and relatives have a right to expect prompt, open, constructive and honest responses to their concerns. This will include an explanation of what has happened and, where appropriate, an apology. Communication is the key to 'damage limitation', while withholding facts or retreating behind a wall of silence can inflame concerns. Clear documentation is the key to defending actions now that may be questioned at any time in the future. Happily, gratitude is overwhelmingly more common than complaints.

Must you cooperate with a complaint, even if you disagree with the person making the complaint?

You must cooperate fully with a complaint or formal enquiry, although any complaint made that demands more than an initial verbal response should be handled by the complaints procedure. You must provide information as to whom to write – the complaints manager/complaints department, through whom all complaints are managed.

What are the purposes of NHS complaints procedures?

These are to resolve a patient's complaints (e.g. by explanation or apology) and to improve NHS services. Where compensation is sought, this is no longer a complaint to be managed by the complaints department, but a claim, and the patient must seek legal representation.

What are the general levels of complaints procedures?

There are three levels to which a complaint might go (Box 4.40). Most are locally resolved, with a response within 20 days.

Can an NHS complaints procedure be used to discipline a doctor or award compensation?

No.

Box 4.40 Levels of complaint

Local procedures

- Attempt to resolve complaints by local staff and managers

Independent review panel

- Comprises professional and lay members
- Investigates complaints not resolved locally if convenor (a non-executive director of the health authority) decides the panel should be set up
- Panel sends reports to complainants and the investigated NHS body

NHS ombudsman

- Can investigate, if certain criteria are fulfilled, usually in matters of maladministration
- Ombudsman decides whether to investigate, conducts investigation and reports to the NHS body involved, disseminating findings widely and implementing action needed

---

Box 4.41 Conditions for negligence

1 The professional had a duty of care to the patient

The law imposes an onus on a doctor only if a professional relationship exists between the doctor and the patient. The doctor has particular knowledge and skills and the patient consults them, as when a patient consults their GP or is cared for by a doctor in hospital. A duty of care does not exist for strangers ('Good Samaritan' acts) although a doctor may become liable if he or she proceeds to treat improperly or causes harm. It is usually easy to establish if a duty of care exists.

2 The professional was in breach of the appropriate standard of care

A patient must show that the doctor did not fulfil his or her duty. Doctors have a broad range of duties including making appropriate diagnoses, giving appropriate treatments and ensuring that patients are fully informed so that consent is valid. However, it is well known that equally knowledgeable, skilled and experienced doctors may tackle a case differently. Therefore the courts have used the 'Bolam test' to decide whether a duty of care has been breached – that duty not breached if a 'responsible body of medical opinion would have acted in the same way in the same situation'. It is also accepted that experts differ in opinion (e.g. treating cough, sputum and fever with antibiotics or considering it viral) and either may be acceptable. The test, however, must be that other experts would have done the same, and not 'that could have happened to me, I could easily have found myself in that situation', the latter analogous to driving at 40 mph in a 30 mph zone.

3 Harm resulted

Negligence cannot be considered if no damage was incurred, even if there was a breach of duty.

4 The breach of duty caused the patient's harm

The patient must show that the doctor's mistake or failure or action caused the injury or other losses. This is the most difficult condition to prove, as breach of duty and harm may both have occurred, but that the former caused the latter does not necessarily follow.

What are the conditions for negligence?

People often use the term professional negligence loosely to mean bad clinical practice. The legal definition is much more precise. Legal action for negligence is the patient's claim for compensation for losses caused by the professional. For a successful claim, all of the conditions in Box 4.41 must be proved.

These four conditions may be summarised as 'Duty, Deviance, Damage and Due to'.

Is there a time limit for suing for an act of alleged negligence?

A patient must sue within three years of the act of alleged negligence. For a complaint the time limit is six months, often extended to a year.

Are individual doctors or Trusts sued?

Before 1990 a patient or relative who wished to make a civil claim as a result of NHS care sued an individual, named doctor or health-care professional and the defence of the claim was handled by the relevant defence organisation. Since then 'Crown Indemnity' has been introduced, and it is the Trust which is sued and the case is investigated and defended by the hospital's legal team, solicitors and the NHS Litigation Authority. The NHS Litigation Authority has developed as a powerful centralised legal body for the NHS. It decides on the basis of the four 'D's if it thinks the case if defendable, which in most cases it will be. Where clearly indefensible (e.g. wrong finger amputated), it will attempt to settle out of court rather than proceed to civil court proceedings. Doctors are therefore witnesses in proceedings and not personally liable for payment of legal costs or damages but their involvement in a claim may be considered as a separate issue by the Trust's consultants or directorates.

Are damages awarded in cases of negligence punitive?

Any damages awarded aim to meet losses incurred, but not to exceed them. In other words, punitive damages are not awarded.

What are vicarious liabilities?

NHS employers may be covered for cases of negligence by the Crown Indemnity Scheme. Patients may sue health professionals personally, but provided certain conditions are fulfilled, they may choose to seek compensation from the employer. The advantages of vicarious liability to patients is that more substantial claims for damages may be affordable to employers and, if action is brought many years after an event, the health professional may be harder to trace.

What is an inquest?

This is a fact-finding enquiry about a reported death, conducted by the coroner, who requests written and sometimes verbal evidence from a variety of sources. It is not a trial. There are no parties, and there is no indictment, prosecution or defence. Possible verdicts include natural causes, unlawful killing, accidental death or industrial disease. The verdict for a patient who has died from complications following an operation may be accidental death because the operation was planned but the outcome was not. An open verdict is returned if the coroner believes there is insufficient evidence to reach a decision. The coroner's court is a public court and the press may attend, as do a hospital's legal team.

CASE 4.41

FITNESS TO PRACTISE – POOR PERFORMANCE IN A COLLEAGUE

Candidate information

Role

You are a doctor on the medical ward.
   Please read this summary.

Scenario

Re: Dr Stephen Cotton, aged 25 years

Dr Cotton has been your F1 doctor (house officer) for one month, having worked on a different ward for three months beforehand. He has a further two months with you. You think his medical knowledge is sound and do not doubt his genuine intention to be a good doctor because he clearly works very hard and stays late after work to complete tasks he has been unable to complete during the day. However, his work is ineffective. You believe his main problem is inability to prioritise tasks. He tends to respond to every request made of him by nursing and other staff immediately, although dropping what he is doing in the process. If he is on your ward round, for example, and a nurse tells him a drug chart needs to be written in the next bay, he will leave to rewrite the drug chart. He seems to see every task as equally weighted. Furthermore, when he is on your ward rounds he does not appear to listen to instructions or advice because he seems too nervous about all of the jobs he has to do. You can cope with a weaker member of the team, but are aware that colleagues are increasingly frustrated by his performance. Some laugh about it behind his back. You feel he could benefit from confidential support and advice.

Your tasks are to explore his poor performance and offer constructive advice.

Your examiners will warn you when 12 minutes have elapsed. You have 14 minutes to communicate with the patient/subject followed by 1 minute of reflection. There will then follow 5 minutes of discussion with the examiners. Do not take the history again except for details that will help in your discussion with the patient/subject. You are not required to examine the patient/subject.

Patient/subject information

Dr Stephen Cotton has been an F1 doctor (house officer) for four months. He found his first three-month post enormously difficult because there was simply too much work, and he was constantly being bleeped with more of it. Other staff seemed not to be pulling their weight. He felt out of his depth, and he found the F2 doctor (senior house officer) was never there to help or advise him. He felt he did not know what he was doing much of the time, and so simply did what everyone – usually nursing staff – told him to do. This frustrated him, as he was a very good student and had great hopes of being a good doctor. For the past month he has been in a different post where the senior doctor is very helpful, but he is still not sure that he is performing well. He has heard colleagues in the hospital mess laughing about him because of his inefficiency but he does not know how he could work any harder. His senior colleague is about to talk to him about his performance.

How to approach the case

Communication skills (conduct of interview/ exploration and problem negotiation), ethics and law

1 Introduction and setting

Ensure you have time to talk with him, in a non-pressured environment, and make it clear the discussion is confidential.

2 Open diplomatically

Telling someone they are no good does not open dialogue. Tell him that you wanted to discuss his experiences of the post so far. Explain that it is often difficult to judge how a relatively new doctor is feeling about the job, although it has become apparent to you that he works exceptionally hard and feels a sense of duty to respond immediately to every request.

3 Make it clear you are there to offer constructive help

Explain that this is an impossible task for any doctor and if there are strategies to make the burdens of the job seem easier, and the remaining two months as educationally valuable as possible, you would like to try to identify these.

4 Listen to the experiences of the poorly performing doctor

Listen supportively, as the last thing he needs is for everybody to takes sides against him. Allow him to tell you how he sees the job, which might be very different to how you or your colleagues see it.

5 Share the good points

Show understanding of how a house officer's job is difficult – doctors must adjust from the learning environment of medical school to the intensely practical and often mundane tasks of clinical work; when emergencies happen you can feel out of your depth; support can sometimes seem lacking; there always seems to be too much work and not enough time; and beyond all of this all doctors, as all people, need personal time and a life outside work. Tell him that you are in no doubt that he is a very hardworking doctor.

6 Be honest about where you think performance falters

Explain that where you think this falters is in his desire to do everything, and now. Medicine, more than many jobs, requires many generic skills, and one of these is prioritisation. Explain that this is not a comment on his medical knowledge, which is perfectly satisfactory.

7 Identify problems and possible solutions

Explain that the transition from medical school to house officer means seeking and using the support of more senior staff. Perhaps explain that on your next ward round he should not leave unless a job is urgent, and that you and he can decide this together. Offer to supervise his work more closely, constructively correcting any problems and regularly teaching on ward rounds. Offer to meet at the end of shifts to see what work is remaining and of this, what needs to be done now, what can wait and what should be handed over. Ensure that he is taking all leave to which he is entitled.

8 Invite further questions

Invite him to discuss anything not covered.

9 Agree a plan

Make and agree a definite plan, using the list of identified problems and possible solutions.

10 Offer ongoing help

Ensure he knows you will be an ongoing source of confidential help.

Discussion

Do you have a duty to identify poorly performing doctors?

Poorly performing doctors should be identified and supported in a proper manner. There should be a sense of responsibility for these doctors, even where performance is not considered abjectly dangerous because doctors are just as susceptible to personal problems and work difficulties as anyone else and need support rather than being left to languish in this and subsequent posts. Where patient care is considered to be at risk, these doctors should be identified with a view to further training or re-education. A plan for this should be constructed in a tailored way in conjunction with the consultant in charge and sometimes the postgraduate deanery. Reappraisal will be necessary.

What types of problem-doctor can you identify?

The General Medical Council (GMC) identifies the broad categories of poor performance (incompetence), misconduct (bad behaviour) and problems of physical or mental health (sickness), although each of these is of variable significance and often these overlap.

What are the causes of poor performance?

These are wide-ranging, e.g. poor knowledge or skills, difficulty putting theory into practice, arrogance or failure to know limitations (usually poor insight or overcompensated insecurity), poor communication, poor teamwork, offhand attitudes, laziness and dishonesty (almost undoubtedly the worst). Often one problem suggests that a cluster may be present. Interestingly, those who think they are good tend to overestimate themselves, and those who think they are not so good, underestimate! Good doctors can be bad doctors, e.g. the perfectionist who cannot delegate, and in general there are five working styles and we tend to each have a couple – 'hurry up', 'be strong', 'be perfect', 'try hard' or 'please people'.

What should be done when a poorly performing doctor is identified?

The principles with any poorly performing doctor are:

* Ensure patient safety (training is always a balance between patient safety and learning opportunity).
* Let the doctor know; too commonly he or she is the last to know.
* Be objective.
* Discover the cause (trainee, team or external factors?).
* Decide what action needs taking.

Action at your stage is to speak to your consultant. Further action depends on the problem, ranging from informal action to, at the other extreme, a formal hearing. The people who might become involved to help with educational issues are the clinical and educational supervisor, the clinical director, and if ongoing the postgraduate dean; sometimes the National Clinical Assessment Service, an organisation which supervises doctors with performance or educational problems (often communication problems), acts on a strictly need-to-know basis with that doctor, retaining considerable confidentiality for the doctor.

Box 4.42 Duties of a doctor

- Make the care of your patient your first concern
- Protect and promote the health of patients and the public
- Provide a good standard of practice and care
- Keep your professional knowledge and skills up to date
- Recognise and work within the limits of your competence
- Work with colleagues in the ways that best serve patient's interests
- Treat patients as individuals and respect their dignity
- Treat patients politely and considerately
- Respect patients' right to confidentiality
- Work in partnership with patients
- Listen to patients and respond to their concerns and preferences
- Give patients the information they want or need in a way they can understand
- Respect patients' right to reach decisions with you about their treatment and care
- Support patients in caring for themselves to improve and maintain their health
- Be honest and open and act with integrity
- Act without delay if you have good reason to believe that you or a colleague may be putting patients at risk
- Never discriminate unfairly against patients or colleagues
- Never abuse your patients' trust in you or the public's trust in the profession

---

Box 4.43 Good medical practice

- Good clinical care (this includes providing a good standard of practice)
- Maintaining good medical practice (this includes keeping up to date and maintaining performance)
- Teaching and training, appraising and assessing
- Relationships with patients (this includes obtaining consent, maintaining confidentiality and trust, good communication, dealing with problems in professional practice, the conduct and performance of colleagues and handling complaints)
- Working with colleagues (this includes treating colleagues fairly, working in teams, leading teams, arranging cover, taking up appointments, sharing information with colleagues, delegation and referral)
- Probity (this includes providing information about services, writing reports, giving evidence and signing reports, research, financial interests and conflicts of interest)
- Health

List some duties of a doctor

The GMC advises that to maintain a good standard of practice and show respect for human life doctors should respect those duties listed in Box 4.42.

List some key components of good medical practice

The GMC advises that good medical practice involves the seven key components listed in Box 4.43.

A colleague is making small clinical errors. Who should be made aware?

This starts internally by involving your consultant. The colleague should be asked for his or her side of the story from the outset. Depending upon the level of concern, the

matter might be referred to the lead clinician of your department, the clinical director, the medical director or the chief executive. It is also possible to report concerns anonymously to the National Patient Safety Agency, which can conduct a non-judgemental investigation.

CASE 4.42

FITNESS TO PRACTISE – MISCONDUCT IN A COLLEAGUE

Candidate information

Role

You are a doctor on an elderly care ward.
 Please read this summary.

Scenario

> Re: Dr Harry Winter, aged 28 years
>
> Dr Winter, your new junior colleague, is developing a reputation as a rather arrogant doctor who wants to be an emergency physician. He has just come from the intensive therapy unit (ITU), where his advice to colleagues was either that their referred patients were too sick to come to ITU ('wouldn't survive anyway') or too well to warrant ITU and he seldom if ever took a patient. He has just rotated to working on your elderly care ward. One of your patients, an 84-year-old lady with a total anterior circulation stroke developed aspiration pneumonia and was very distressed. While you were assessing her you asked that Dr Winter ensure that 5 mg of morphine be prepared and then administered to relieve her distress. He administered the injection and wrote up 5 mg on the drug chart. Later, the nurse told you that Dr Winter had asked her for 15 mg. She is sure that she made up 15 mg with him and it is documented accordingly on the controlled drugs record. You are aware that not infrequently larger doses of opiates are prepared than are used and the remnant amounts discarded. But this is not the first time the same issue has been noted with Dr Winter.
>
> Your task is to discuss the incident with Dr Winter.

Your examiners will warn you when 12 minutes have elapsed. You have 14 minutes to communicate with the patient/subject followed by 1 minute of reflection. There will then follow 5 minutes of discussion with the examiners. Do not take the history again except for details that will help in your discussion with the patient/subject. You are not required to examine the patient/subject.

Patient/subject information

Dr Harry Winter is a competent, and very confident doctor, so much so that he often feels his senior colleagues need to re-train. He has read a lot, knows a lot and gets very frustrated when senior colleagues waste time with what he sees as meaningless interventions and drug doses that do not seem to make a difference. He wants to be an Emergency Physician. He hates his current post on the elderly care ward, where things are too slow. In fact, he has contempt for most elderly care physicians, perceiving that a lot of resources are 'wasted' on older people who do not seem to get better. Yesterday, an 84-year-old lady with a total anterior circulation stroke developed aspiration pneumonia and was very distressed. While his senior colleague was assessing her he asked Dr Winter to ensure that 5 mg of morphine was prepared and administered. Dr Winter felt this dose stupidly low and had given much higher doses to young trauma patients in the Emergency Department. Dr Winter decided to give 15 mg and although the lady became extremely drowsy she is still alive today and this, he feels, vindicates his decision. He only prescribed 5 mg, however, knowing his senior colleague would not have approved. The nurse with whom he prepared the morphine challenged him about the discrepancy between what he had asked for and what he had prescribed. Dr Winter does not feel it is a nurse's place to question a doctor but to appease her said that he discarded 10 mg as it was subsequently not needed. This is not the first time he has given bigger doses than recommended or requested, but he feels he is right. The senior doctor now wishes to talk to Dr Winter about these episodes, and he will have to admit the truth, albeit exposing his contemptuous convictions, because the alternative is that he is perceived as taking the morphine himself, which he is not. In fact, he thinks drug addicts should be shot.

How to approach this case

Communication skills (conduct of interview/ exploration and problem negotiation), ethics and law

1 Introduction and setting

Ensure you have time to talk with him, in a non-pressured environment, as much for your sake as his.

2 Open diplomatically

Tell him that you wish to discuss the discrepancy between the dose of morphine apparently administered and the dose given. Make it clear that you are not being judgemental, and that there are of course numerous potential reasons this could occur. You should be aware, however, that if he is lying about drug doses that will be a very serious issue of honesty and probity.

3 Make it clear you are there to offer constructive help

Explain that whatever the motives, you would hope to be able to offer constructive help (it is of course more difficult to do this when a doctor with poor conduct does not seem to appreciate this).

4 Listen to the experiences of the doctor with poor conduct

Allow him to tell his story. Try to identify, if he admits to the act, his reasoning behind it and ask him if he saw any alternatives, such as discussing his thoughts with his senior colleagues first.

5 Share any good points

Acknowledge that he is generally a knowledgeable and competent doctor.

6 Be honest about where you think performance falters

Explain that you feel his ethical decision-making is leading him into territory that is dangerous to patients and risking his professional integrity; explain that these actions could have very serious repercussions, not least threatening his future career.

7 Identify problems and possible solutions

With a lesser issue you might advise him that you would wish him to discuss all treatment decisions while attached to the elderly care ward with you. Tell him that medical decisions are always within a framework that puts patient safety first. Here, you must inform your consultant.

8 Invite further questions

Invite him to question your suggestions. ·

9 Agree a plan

Make and agree to a definite plan, using the list of identified problems and possible solutions. Tell him that the matter is not one that you can keep to yourself, and you will need to also discuss it with your consultant.

10 Offer ongoing help

Offer to be a source of advice and help during his attachment to the elderly care ward.

Discussion

What types of professional misconduct do we sometimes hear about in doctors?

These include (not in any order of importance):

- Lack of probity or honesty
- Lack of reliability and poor time keeping
- Acting under the influence of alcohol or drugs

- Inappropriate or criminal behaviour
- Inappropriate use of NHS facilities
- Failure to follow organisational policies
- Bullying
- Sexual or racial harassment
- Neglect of or disregard for responsibility to patients
- Breach of confidence
- Unprofessional attitudes to work

What are the possible outcomes of challenges to a doctor's actions?

Possible outcomes are listed in Table 4.6. Your first duty is to speak to your consultant if you have concerns about a doctor. Depending upon the seriousness of the problem, others involved include the medical director, the chief executive, the deanery and the General Medical Council. The police may be involved if there is criminal action. In the event of improper use of internet sites, Trust IT departments may not inform the individual but have direct links to the police who will take it extremely seriously. Other people who may be involved in misconduct investigations are outlined in Table 4.6. Depending upon the action, restriction of practice or exclusion may ensue before investigations start. It is not acceptable to apply different outcomes to doctors as to other members of staff. If dismissal is appropriate for a porter, then it is for a doctor.

Should you accept a gift from patient?

The general answer is no. Gifts that should not politely be returned, such as chocolates, might be shared with other members of the team; money should never be accepted and the patient might be advised to contact the Trust Patient Advice Service if they wish to make a charitable donation.

Should you always see a patient if a junior asks you to?

Patient safety comes first and if there are concerns about a junior's level of competence this should be handled second and your conduct in protecting patients will be paramount. You should see that patient.

CASE 4.43

FITNESS TO PRACTISE – HEALTH PROBLEMS IN A COLLEAGUE

Candidate information

Role

You are a doctor in the emergency medical admissions unit.

Please read this summary.

Table 4.6 Possible outcomes of challenges to a doctor's actions

Procedure	Who or what instigates	Who conducts	Purpose	Criteria	Possible outcomes
NHS complaints	Patients or relatives	Hospital managers or independent panel	To resolve complaints and improve service		Explanation or apology from managers
Negligence claim	Patients	Civil court with a judge	Compensation	'Bolam test'	Financial compensation to patients
Employer's disciplinary proceedings	Reports from staff	Trust managers	Protection of patients	Breach of employment contract or law	Warning, suspension or dismissal
Professional bodies such as GMC	Health professionals	Professional committees	Assessing fitness to practise	Guidance such as GMC guidance	Admonition, registration with conditions, suspension from medical register or erasure from medical register
Criminal negligence	Crown Prosecution Service	Criminal court	Punishment	Gross negligence	Absolute or conditional discharge, suspended imprisonment or imprisonment
Coroner's inquest	A reported death	Coroner	To determine cause of death		Verdict on cause of death

GMC, General Medical Council.

Scenario

> Re: Dr Emma Wood, aged 26 years
>
> Dr Wood, your new F1 doctor, has worked with you for three months and is persistently late for work. When at work, her performance is highly substandard. Notably, she is extremely slow, being able to clerk in one or two patients on days she is 'on take'. Initially, you gave her the benefit of the doubt as she told you she found work very stressful. She feels that doctors do not give enough time to patients, declaring that patients have 'emotional needs as well as physical'. But you now think this a thin excuse. She arrives at work smelling of alcohol, and colleagues have told you how she is often at parties all night or in her room with dubious friends drinking until an hour before work. On two occasions you have sent her home because she was intoxicated.
>
> Your tasks are to confirm that she has an alcohol problem and find ways to manage the problem.

Your examiners will warn you when 12 minutes have elapsed. You have 14 minutes to communicate with the patient/subject followed by 1 minute of reflection. There will then follow 5 minutes of discussion with the examiners. Do not take the history again except for details that will help in your discussion with the patient/subject. You are not required to examine the patient/subject.

Patient/subject information

Dr Emma Wood has been an F1 doctor in medicine for three months. She was an average student, performing well in psychiatry, but finds being a doctor exceptionally difficult. Initially she found it a culture shock to have to see so many patients, and felt that most doctors did not spend enough time talking to their patients. She was told by one consultant that this is the modern NHS, there is a service commitment to see patients and it is better to 'get around all patients missing irrelevances' than to see one or two in depth. She found this infuriating and against what she found as a student in psychiatry, when she would frequently put in a whole afternoon talking with one patient. She now feels contempt for physicians. She cannot be bothered working with the team, which she thinks just runs around in circles, and feels she is 'destined for better things'. She has been drinking more and more alcohol in recent months – she always drank a lot as a student – and is aware that she comes to work after one or two morning drinks 'to steady her frustration' but does not think her colleagues have noticed. In any event, she enjoys it, and has increasingly been feeling that alcohol is a good thing for young people earning money and hates being criticised by people who tell her differently. Her senior is about to speak to her

Box 4.44 CAGE questions

- Have you ever felt you ought to **C**ut down your drinking?
- Have people **A**nnoyed you by criticising your drinking?
- Have you ever felt bad or **G**uilty about drinking?
- Have you ever had a drink first thing in the morning, an **E**ye opener?

about his concerns, and she may eventually see that there could be a problem and agree to seek advice.

How to approach the case

Communication skills (conduct of interview/ exploration and problem negotiation), ethics and law

1 Introduction and setting

Ensure you have time to talk with her, in a non-pressured environment, and make it clear that the discussion is confidential.

2 Ask if the sick doctor recognises the problem

Tell her that you are concerned she may be drinking heavily. Ask if she feels there may be a problem.

3 Make it clear you are there to offer constructive help

Explain that you are concerned and that you would like, and may need, to help or intervene if there is a problem.

4 Listen to the experiences of the doctor

Listen supportively, but be aware that she may not admit to having a problem. She may not see that she does.

5 Ask specific questions

Ask the CAGE questions (Box 4.44). Ask if anyone else has hinted that there may be a problem. Crucially, you are exploring whether or not she has insight into the problem. Explore the possibility of depression.

6 Be specific about your concerns

If she denies a problem, suggest the evidence. Explain you are concerned that continuing in this way may put patients at risk. Explain you are also very concerned about the possible implications for her, including not adequately making it through house year and, ultimately, a risk of not obtaining General Medical Council (GMC) registration. Explain that if patients are at risk she has a duty to seek help and if she does not then it is necessary for colleagues to intervene. Explain that you are obliged to speak to her consultant.

7 Explore any other concerns

Invite her to discuss anything not covered.

8 Discuss possible solutions

These include support from you, and help from her registered GP and/or the occupational health service, and confidential services for sick doctors including the British

Medical Association, The Sick Doctors' Trust and the Doctors' Support Network.

9 Agree a plan

Make and agree a definite plan.

10 Offer ongoing confidential help

Ensure she knows that you will be an ongoing source of confidential help.

Discussion

If you suspect a colleague's sickness is putting patients at risk, how do you decide when 'whistle-blowing' overrides the confidentiality of the colleague?

You must protect patients from harm posed by another health-care professional's health, conduct or performance and this includes problems of alcohol or drug misuse. Patient safety comes first. Serious concerns should provoke immediate action to establish if they are well founded. You must give an honest explanation to an appropriate person in your health-care organisation, such as your consultant or the medical director. If local systems do not or cannot resolve the issue, then a professional organisation such as the GMC may need to be informed of your concerns.

If a colleague smells of alcohol and it is difficult to judge if he or she is drunk, and this is a first time, then it is more likely a case of local help and discipline with close observation. But any professional who smells of alcohol cannot see patients.

In recent years, gambling has also become a health-related concern.

In all cases, important considerations are:

- To alert the individual of your concerns
- To ensure patient safety, e.g. is immediate exclusion from work needed?
- To involve your consultant, who should act upwards depending upon the level of concern – medical director, chief executive, GMC
- The health of the individual, e.g. occupational health department

CASE 4.44

RECRUITMENT TO A RANDOMISED CONTROLLED TRIAL

Candidate information

Role

You are a doctor in the emergency medical admissions unit.

Please read this summary.

Scenario

> Re: Mr John Walker, aged 54 years
>
> You are conducting a randomised controlled trial (RCT) with your consultant on inpatient insomnia. You have designed the RCT to involve four groups – no treatment, an eye-shield alone, earplugs alone, and an eye-shield plus earplugs. Patients will be randomised to one group for one night only and report their sleep satisfaction on the basis of a rating scale.
>
> Your task is to ask Mr Walker, a patient admitted with dehydration and acute renal impairment, if he might agree to participate in the trial and counsel him about it.

Your examiners will warn you when 12 minutes have elapsed. You have 14 minutes to communicate with the patient/subject followed by 1 minute of reflection. There will then follow 5 minutes of discussion with the examiners. Do not take the history again except for details that will help in your discussion with the patient/subject. You are not required to examine the patient/subject.

Patient/subject information

Mr Walker is a 54-year-old mathematician who has been admitted with acute renal impairment caused by gastroenteritis and dehydration. He is about to be asked if he might consider participating in a treatment trial, and will be very interested to know all about it, not least about the safety aspects and the ethics of it being conducted.

How to approach the case

Communication skills (conduct of interview/ exploration and problem negotiation), ethics and law

1 Introduce yourself and the topic for discussion

Explain that research is vital in improving the care of patients and that you would like to invite your patient to participate in research and the reason why. Ask if he is happy to discuss your project.

2 Explain the nature of the study

Explain the nature of the research, its aims and an outline of the method. For such an RCT, the nature of the randomisation and any reasons for it should be explained, although by its very nature this RCT cannot be a double-blind RCT in which neither patient nor researcher know whether patient is receiving treatment or placebo.

3 Discuss ethical approval

Explain that ethical approval has been obtained and that the research does not come before the best interests of a patient and that there are legal rights and safeguards. Any foreseeable risks must never outweigh potential benefits and developing new knowledge or treatment should never take precedence over a patient's interests. An RCT is not ethical if there is evidence that an intervention is dangerous and an RCT must be stopped if evidence emerges for a benefit or risk before completion. Doctors involved in research have an ethical duty to respect human life and people's autonomy (if that research is an experimental study into the causes, treatment or prevention of disease, involving people or their tissues, organs or data; audit is not experimental study).

4 Explain potential benefits and risks

There may be potential benefits and risks. Explain these, and any arrangement for dealing with adverse events. Explain that the results are not predictable.

5 Explain data handling

Explain that you will record and report all results accurately. Explain that you will aim to complete the research unless evidence emerged of a risk or no potential benefit to participants. Information about outcomes will be available.

6 Discuss confidentiality

Explain that all information will fully respect your patient's right to confidentiality. Where data or patient information is needed for research, doctors must seek consent for its disclosure whenever practicable, anonymise data where this will suffice and keep all disclosures to the minimum necessary. If consent is not practicable, then the ethics committee may need to decide if the likely benefits of the research outweigh the loss of confidentiality.

7 Discuss consent

If he would like to proceed then you would wish to obtain consent. Sometimes it is preferable to give patients time to think about things. On no account must a patient feel coercion. They also have the right to withdraw from research at any time without reason. Any additional information given, other than that required to fulfil a doctor's obligation to provide informed consent, will depend very much upon the individual. It should be determined by effective communication, by not making assumptions and by asking about specific concerns. An information leaflet is often very helpful before discussing research with patients.

8 Consider conflict of interest

Any conflict of interest should be declared from the outset and research should not be motivated by financial, per-sonal, political or other interest. Ethical approval is mandatory.

9 Confirm understanding and invite questions

I appreciate we've covered rather a lot there. Is there anything you would like me to go over again or are there any questions you would like to ask me?

10 Seek consent or refusal

And do not question his decision if he refuses.

Discussion

What do you understand by the term evidence-based medicine (EBM)?

EBM refers to the conscientious, explicit and judicious application of current best evidence in making decisions about the care of individual patients. Practising EBM must integrate external evidence with clinician's expertise and patient's beliefs, concerns, expectations, values and informed choice. Evidence-based health-care extends the application of principles of EBM to all professions involved in health-care.

What do you understand by the term critical reading or critical appraisal?

The ability to evaluate scientific literature, analyse data, and base management decisions on the basis of evidence.

What broad types of research are there?

Quantitative research

This is concerned with inferences about populations and testing theories. A collection of numerical data is subject to statistical analysis to test hypotheses. Things that are measurable by quantitative studies include *disease frequency* (incidence and prevalence), *factors that modify risk of disease*, methods for *detection and diagnosis* of disease, *costs and consequences* of health states and *effects of treatments and interventions* (clinical trials).

Qualitative research

This is concerned with understanding the experiences of individuals and using this to build theories. It is guided not by hypotheses, but by questions and issues and seeks to describe culture, beliefs and attitudes and to understand behaviour. It may generate hypotheses for testing using survey or intervention designs. It may utilise, for example, case reports, interviews (structured and non-structured), health diaries, audio recordings, focus groups or group interviews.

What types of study design are there?

Study designs may be non-interventional (case reports, cross-sectional studies, case–control studies, cohort studies) or interventional, which measure 'before' and 'after' (RCTs, systematic reviews, meta-analyses). Study designs are listed below in the order of their ascending hierarchy of evidence:

Case report

This reports a single patient's story. A report on a series of patients with an outcome of interest is a case series.

Cross-sectional (descriptive) study

A representative sample of people ('subjects') is studied at a single point in time. It may be used to determine the prevalence of a particular disease. Subjects are selected without regard to the outcome of interest.

Case–control (retrospective) study

This involves identifying subjects with a particular condition of interest (*cases*) and comparing or 'matching' these with subjects without the condition of interest (*controls*). Retrospective data are collected from patient records to try to identify a past exposure or potential causal agent of interest that discriminates between the two groups. It is not possible to demonstrate causality from a case–control study; the association of A with B does not prove that A causes B. Subjects are selected based on the outcome of interest.

Cohort (prospective) study

This is an observational study of subjects without the condition of interest; they are selected and then followed up to monitor the occurrence of the outcome. Two or more groups (*cohorts*) are selected on the basis of a *difference in exposure to a particular agent of interest* (e.g. drug, potential toxin, smoking) and followed up to see how many in each group develop a *disease or other outcome*. Cohort studies may take years. A famous cohort study was that by Sir Richard Doll to investigate smoking as a risk factor for lung cancer. Subjects are selected before the outcome of interest is observed. It is not strictly possible to determine causality from a cohort study (something which tobacco companies have used in their defence in the face of overwhelming evidence) but strength of association may be used as a marker of risk. An RCT is needed to prove causality, but may not be ethical in the face of a strong association. Cohort studies may be used to determine prognosis.

Clinical trial

This is a planned experiment designed to assess the efficacy of a treatment in humans. The RCT is the most powerful experimental design to obtain evidence of causation or the impact of an intervention. Patients are randomly allocated or randomised into an experimental group to receive an intervention and a control group to receive standard treatment or placebo. These groups are followed up and compared for differences in outcomes of interest and any differences are tested for significance. The process of inference from an RCT will typically result in signifi-

cance tests (*P* values), estimates of risk or treatment effect and confidence intervals (below). Advantages of an RCT include the rigorous evaluation of a single variable in a defined patient group, the prospective nature eliminating bias, the search to falsify rather than confirm its hypothesis and the facility for meta-analysis at a later date. Disadvantages include time and cost, hidden biases such as imperfect randomisation, funding sometimes by pharmaceutical companies, and the use sometimes of surrogate endpoints.

Systematic review and meta-analysis

A systematic review is a summary of the medical literature that uses explicit methods to perform a thorough literature search and critical appraisal of individual valid studies and that uses appropriate statistical techniques to combine these studies. Meta-analyses pool data from numerous trials, and the Cochrane Collaboration is one body that has standardised this approach.

What is a clinical practice guideline?

A systematically developed statement designed to assist clinicians and patients in appropriate decision-making.

Are there guidelines for critically appraising papers?

Checklists to assist critical appraisal have been developed for many different types of study and may include a clearly specified *objective*, a *design* appropriate for the objective, a definition of the *target population* and whether *generalisation* from the study to the target population is possible, *subject selection* (how the subjects were selected for inclusion), clearly defined *treatments/interventions*, whether *randomisation* was used for allocation (including treatment masking/blinding and if not whether this could affect outcomes), justification of the *sample size*, the *outcome measures* (primary and secondary, with statement of reliability and validity) and *completeness* (compliance, drop-outs or missing data). Checklists to assist critical appraisal have been developed specifically for RCTs. One such is the Consolidated Standards of Reporting Trials (CONSORT) checklist.

What is bias?

Bias refers to deviation of results from the truth, or processes leading to such deviation. *Selection bias* in a sample is an error caused by systematic differences between groups of subjects or between those selected and those who are not. For example, volunteers may differ from non-volunteers in health terms (motivated, free time, well). Selection should really be random. *Information bias* refers to a flaw in measurement that results in a difference in the quality of information between groups. There are many types of information bias:

- *Inter-observer bias* resulting from different observers classifying outcomes

- *Recall bias* resulting from incomplete recall, worse in a case–control study
- *Lead time bias*, important in measuring survival if a new procedure has been introduced (i.e. is an apparent increase in survival because of early intervention or a parallel diagnosis?)
- *Performance bias*, resulting from differences in care provided apart from the intervention (e.g. a doctor may or may not counsel as well as prescribing antidepressants)
- *Exclusion bias*, which implies systematic differences in trial withdrawals
- *Detection bias*, which implies a systematic difference in outcome assessment

What information might you need to determine the sample size necessary for a study?

Sample size should be calculated by a statistician before embarking on a study. A larger sample may yield a more significant result. Sample sizes are determined from:

- An *estimation of prevalence* of the outcome of interest in the population being studied or the control group.
- *'Clinical intuition'* to decide the minimal clinical difference or smallest change in outcome between treatment and control groups that would be deemed clinically relevant.
- The *significance level*, which refers to the probability of a significant result, when in fact there is no difference. The smaller the better, but it could never be 0% unless we were to study the entire population. By convention the significance level is 5% or 0.05, represented as the '*P*' value (below).
- *Power*, which refers to the probability that a study of a given size statistically detects a real difference. The bigger the better, and the more likely to detect smaller differences, but power could never be 100% unless we were to study the entire population; 80% or 90% are by convention the standards.

What is the null hypothesis?

That there is no real difference between intervention and control (relative risk = 1 or absolute risk = 0). Trials start with this presumption, and then set out to disprove it. In other words, evidence is based on an innocent until proven guilty basis, a rather tortuous approach that requires a '*P*' value to be < 0.05 to be beyond reasonable doubt. We can never prove the null hypothesis, but only try very hard to reject it.

What is a '*P*' value?

The *P* value relates to the confidence that a difference between intervention and control groups is not the result of chance alone. Its value is arbitrary, and by convention < 0.05 (i.e. a < 0.05 or < 1 in 20 chance of the difference being due to chance alone) is deemed statistically significant. Sometimes tiers are considered, < 0.01 being yet stronger evidence and < 0.001 being very strong evidence. The smaller the *P* value, the less likely the difference is the result of chance alone and the more likely it is to be significant (but only if the sample size is large enough). A significant result suggests that the author reject the null hypothesis, and a non-significant result implies either no difference or too small a sample. The *P* value must always be read in the context of the sample size and confidence intervals. Formerly, *P* values were often given alone when reporting studies but now, confidence intervals tend to be given also. Importantly, statistical significance need not necessarily imply practical, real or clinical significance. Furthermore, absence of evidence is not the same as evidence of absence!

What do you understand by the term confidence interval (CI)?

If we were to repeat a trial hundreds of times, we would not get the same results each time but on average we would establish a level of difference between the two arms of the trial. In 90% of the trials the difference between the two arms would lie within certain broad limits; 95% of the trials would lie within certain, even broader limits and 99% within broader limits still. *The CI is the range within which we would expect the true value of a statistical measure to lie. It is basically the degree of wobble in a result that is based on a small sample population (those in the study) rather than the entire population.* The CI is usually accompanied by the percentage value for the *level of confidence* that the true value lies within this range. For example, a number needed to treat (NNT; see Case 4.6) of 20 with a 95% CI of 15 to 25 implies that we are 95% confident that the true NNT is between 15 and 25. It is standard to have 95% CIs. CIs can be applied to any statistical test, e.g. NNT, relative risk (RR), absolute risk (AR), odds ratio (OR), sensitivity. A *P* value might be 0.05, but if, for the sake of example, the CI for that *P* value were 1.1 to 25 then the result could be of almost no significance because this CI is wide and 1.1 is close to the line of no significance. A wide difference in results (a wide CI), especially if close to or crossing the line of no significance, is less significant. A narrow difference in results (a narrow CI) distant from the line of no significance, is more significant. The line of no significance is 1 for ratios (negatives are not possible), such as relative risk or odds ratio, and 0 for absolutes, such as absolute risk.

What is a type 1 error?

The intervention is shown to work but it does not! This is equivalent to the *P* value.

What is a type 2 error?

The intervention is shown not to work but it does! This is more common than a type 1 error.

What do you understand by the term generalisation?

Making inferences from a clinical trial involves a process of generalisation from the sample to the target population. The extent to which this is appropriate is known as generalisability.

What do you understand by the term confounding factors?

Mixing of two or more factors so that their individual effect upon an outcome cannot be separated.

What do you know about intention to treat (ITT) analysis?

Drop-outs or non-respondents can alter a sample size and conclusions significantly. ITT is an analysis in which the results in the control and treatment groups are analysed with respect to the numbers of patients entering the study (regardless of whether or not they received treatment or completed participation in the RCT). By including for analysis all entrants to the study, ITT analysis avoids biases because of a failure of concordance and admits side effects of a treatment causing subjects to drop out. ITT analysis provides a pragmatic estimate of the overall benefit of intervention in the population studied.

OTHER COMMUNICATION, ETHICAL AND LEGAL SCENARIOS

CASE 4.45

GENETIC TESTING

Candidate information

Role

You are a doctor on the neurology ward.
Please read this summary.

Scenario

> **Mr Roger Molton, aged 58 years**
>
> Mr Molton was recently admitted to the neurology ward for assessment of a movement disorder. Genetic testing has recently confirmed Huntington's disease and you are about to speak to his son, who wants to know more about the condition, particularly whether or not it is inherited and whether or not he and his siblings should be tested.
>
> Your task is to explain the diagnosis and counsel him about testing for this condition.

Your examiners will warn you when 12 minutes have elapsed. You have 14 minutes to communicate with the patient/subject followed by 1 minute of reflection. There will then follow 5 minutes of discussion with the examiners. Do not take the history again except for details that will help in your discussion with the patient/subject. You are not required to examine the patient/subject.

Patient/subject information

You are the son of Mr Roger Molton, a 58-year-old man who has recently been diagnosed with Huntington's disease. You know a little about the effects of the disease and have heard that it might be inherited. You wish to discuss the likelihood of being affected and if there is a test that you could have. You currently have no children but are concerned about the possible risk of passing the condition on to any children in future.

How to approach the case

Communication skills (conduct of interview/ exploration and problem negotiation), ethics and law

1 Introduction

Introduce yourself and establish his identity.

2 Establish area for discussion and background knowledge

Discover his pre-existing knowledge of Huntington's disease.

3 Establish any family history

Try to obtain a family tree and ask if he knows of anybody in the family who has had similar symptoms.

4 Explore ideas, concerns and expectations

Ask if he wishes to know anything else about the disease or its implications.

5 Respond to ideas, concerns and expectations

Explain that Huntington's disease is caused by an abnormal gene that is passed on to 50% of children. Explain that the disease may not become apparent until later life in affected offspring, but that there is a tendency for successive generations to be affected at an earlier age. Explain that offspring who do not carry the gene cannot ever be affected or pass on the condition.

6 Advise about genetic testing

Explain that genetic testing can determine whether he carries the abnormal gene. Explain that false-positive and false-negative tests do occur, but are very unusual. Point out that there are potential medical, family, occupational, insurance and financial implications of a positive result. Point out that there is no current prevention or cure for those carrying the gene. Point out that for those carrying the gene there is no means of predicting age of onset of symptoms, severity of symptoms or rate of progression.

7 Advise about counselling for genetic testing

All doctors should have a grasp of the principles and be able to respond to immediate questions and concerns. However, counselling for genetic testing is a specialised skill and counsellors should be specifically trained and part of a multidisciplinary team with psychosocial support. Having confirmed his understanding of Huntington's disease, explored and responded to his concerns, and explained the nature of testing, advise that a decision about the test is something he should not make now, but consider discussing with those close to him. Advise that he might discuss the implications of the test and the condition further at a regional genetic centre if he wished, and in the company of someone close to him, but at the very least your neurology consultant should be involved in the process. A minimum of one month is desirable between initial pre-test information and testing and results should always be given in person by the counsellor. Post-test counselling is mandatory whatever the result.

8 Consider legal aspects

As with human immunodeficiency virus (HIV) testing, testing for Huntington's disease should never be performed without counselling and explicit informed consent. Counselling must include up-to-date information about the condition and the implications of testing that allow a patient to make an informed choice. The test is available only to those who have reached the age of maturity. Ownership of the test result is with the subject who requested it but ownership of the stored DNA is with the patient. DNA from another affected family member may be needed, who of course must give consent, but asking an affected family member who is unaware of or unwilling to acknowledge their symptoms may be considered an invasion of privacy. Care should be taken when a test result may provide information about a third party who has not requested a test. Oral and written information should be provided by the team providing the testing service.

9 Invite questions

Ask if he has any other questions or concerns that have not been addressed.

10 Agree a way forward

This may well be for him to think about the above before contemplating next steps.

Discussion

What is the genetic basis of Huntington's disease?

It is an autosomal dominant condition with a mutation on the distal short arm of chromosome 4. Huntington's disease exhibits genetic anticipation with an increasing number of trinucleotide repeat sequences in affected offspring. It is a genetic disease but of course spawned by a sporadic index case.

CASE 4.46

HIV TESTING

Candidate information

Role

You are a doctor on the medical ward.
   Please read this summary.

Scenario

Re: Mr Julian Lyons, aged 36 years
Mr Lyons is a 36-year-old ex-intravenous drug user, who has abstained from drugs for three years. He has been admitted to your ward with a respiratory illness, mild hypoxia and X-ray findings that would be consistent with *Pneumocystis* pneumonia. He has also been losing weight. Your consultant has asked

that you discuss a human immunodeficiency virus (HIV) test with him.
Your tasks are to explain the possible diagnosis, approach the possibility of HIV infection and counsel him for an HIV test.

Your examiners will warn you when 12 minutes have elapsed. You have 14 minutes to communicate with the patient/subject followed by 1 minute of reflection. There will then follow 5 minutes of discussion with the examiners. Do not take the history again except for details that will help in your discussion with the patient/subject. You are not required to examine the patient/subject.

Patient/subject information

Mr Julian Lyons is a 36-year-old who used intravenous heroin until three years ago. He admits to having shared needles. He has been admitted to hospital with a short respiratory illness and his doctors suspect HIV infection as a possible underlying cause. He has been slowly losing weight over the last few months. He is heterosexual, currently unemployed, and lives with a dog. He smokes 20 cigarettes a day and drinks a moderate amount of alcohol. He has never had an HIV test. The possibility of HIV has crossed his mind and he is willing to undergo an HIV test but first would like to know more about the implications of the test.

How to approach the case

Communication skills (conduct of interview/ exploration and problem negotiation), ethics and law

1 Introduction

Introduce yourself, confirm his identity and ask how he is.

2 Explain the results of tests

Explain that the chest X-ray suggests pneumonia, and that there are a number of possibilities underlying it.

3 Explore risk factors, suggesting possible implications of the results

Ask about his heroin use. Did he share needles? Were any of his associates known to be HIV positive? When did he stop using intravenous drugs? Ask about other risk factors for HIV acquisition, especially the sexual history. These questions suggest that HIV is on your mind and if he does not respond suggest that HIV is something that must always be considered.

4 Explore ideas, concerns and expectations

Ask him if this is something that has crossed his mind, or if he has ever considered the possibility of HIV infection.

5 Respond to ideas, concerns and expectations

Explain what HIV and acquired immunodeficiency syndrome (AIDS) are, and how HIV is transmitted (and how transmission can be reduced).

6 Counsel with respect to HIV testing

Pre-test counselling should prepare an individual for receiving, understanding and managing a result. Discussion should embrace the consequences of a positive result, including impact on partners, pregnancy, employment and insurance (Box 4.45).

7 Give an assurance of confidentiality

This is essential.

8 Invite questions

Ask if he has any other questions or concerns that have not been addressed.

9 Seek consent to proceed with the HIV test

Agree that he should decide whether or not to go ahead with the test, and if he goes ahead who will inform him of and explain the result, and that you will continue to investigate and treat his pneumonia.

10 Discuss what would happen after the test

Post-test counselling is mandatory, whether a positive or negative result, and the pre- and post-test counsellor should really be the same person.

Discussion

Does a negative test exclude HIV infection?

No. The window period means that testing must be repeated if there is a possibility that infection has been acquired in the last few months. The management of HIV infection is further discussed in Case 2.39.

CASE 4.47

NEEDLESTICK INJURY

Candidate information

Role

You are a doctor in the emergency medical admissions unit.

Please read this summary.

Scenario

Re: Dr Tess Martin, aged 25 years

Dr Martin is an F1 doctor (house officer) working with you. She comes to you extremely upset because she has sustained a needlestick injury while taking blood from a patient she has just clerked, who is an intravenous drug user.

Your tasks are to calm the situation and advise about managing the needlestick injury.

Your examiners will warn you when 12 minutes have elapsed. You have 14 minutes to communicate with the patient/subject followed by 1 minute of reflection. There will then follow 5 minutes of discussion with the examiners. Do not take the history again except for details that will help in your discussion with the patient/subject. You are not required to examine the patient/subject.

Patient/subject information

Dr Tess Martin is an F1 doctor (house officer) working on the emergency medical admissions unit with her senior (the candidate). She has just sustained a needlestick injury from a patient who is a known intravenous drug user, admitted with a soft tissue infection. The patient told her that tests for human immunodeficiency virus (HIV) and hepatitis two years previously were negative, but that his status had not been checked since and he has continued to use intravenous drugs. Dr Martin wore two pairs of gloves for the procedure. After withdrawing the green needle it punctured her gloves and 'pricked the end' of her left index finger, drawing blood. She immediately, quite correctly, washed the area with soap and water without scrubbing, and allowed the injury site to bleed freely. She is not sure about the risks of HIV and hepatitis C in this situation, nor what she should do next. She is fully immunised against hepatitis B with an excellent antibody response.

How to approach the case

Communication skills (conduct of interview/ exploration and problem negotiation), ethics and law

1 Introduction

Ask Dr Martin exactly what happened and reassure her that you will help and follow the hospital guidelines for dealing with a needlestick injury.

2 Advise on immediate management

Advise her to wash the contaminated area thoroughly and allow the wound to bleed freely (if she has not already done so).

3 Establish details of the incident

Establish the nature of the injury, the type of needle used and the time of the incident.

4 Establish details about the patient and the staff member

Establish if HIV and hepatitis B and C status are known. Ask if Dr Martin has been immunised against hepatitis B.

5 Remain calm

Explain immediately that the risk of infectious disease transmission is not all that high from a positive patient, and that she has acted quite correctly so far to reduce any risk even further.

6 Explain what you will do next

Explain that you will counsel and take a blood sample from the patient for HIV and hepatitis B and C (this should not be done by the individual who was exposed). Explain to Dr Martin that she should be encouraged to have a blood test also for HIV and hepatitis B and C and offer to counsel her to do this.

7 Respect confidentiality and consent

Assure her of confidentiality. Advise that without a test now, if she were later found to be positive it might be difficult to claim compensation (industrial disablement benefit). Confidentiality for both parties is essential and of course counselling and consent for HIV testing are mandatory.

8 Explore outstanding concerns

Explore any other concerns she may have or if there is anything she is not sure about.

9 Invite questions

Ask if she has any other questions.

10 Consider the remainder of the shift

Suggest that she might wish to go off duty and that you will arrange the necessary cover.

Discussion

What is the risk of HIV transmission from a positive patient following needlestick injury?

Around 0.3%, but individual risk depends upon the nature of the inoculation and viral load transmitted, together with the HIV subtype and immunological factors in the person sustaining the injury.

What action is indicated in the setting of needlestick injury if a patient is known to be positive for HIV?

Action points are listed in Box 4.46.

What factors increase the risk of occupationally acquired HIV transmission?

These include deep injury, visible blood on the device causing the injury, injury with a needle that has been inserted in the source patient's vein or artery and terminal HIV-related illness in the source patient.

Box 4.46 Action for needlestick injury from an HIV-infected individual

- An anti-HIV triple therapy starter pack should be given within the first hour. The occupational health department can advise on up-to-date local guidelines (national guidelines have been developed on postexposure prophylaxis for health-care workers by the Chief Medical Officer's Expert Advisory Group on AIDS), and if outside normal working hours the hospital senior nurse should know where the latest guidelines are and where treatments are kept.
- Health-care workers exposed to infectious patients should be given the opportunity to discuss the balance of risks with appropriate psychological support, particularly allowing informed decisions about postexposure prophylaxis.
- Treatment for HIV is with two nucleoside reverse transcriptase inhibitors (e.g. zidovudine, lamivudine, zalcitabine) and *either* a non-nucleoside reverse transcriptase inhibitor (e.g. nevirapine) or one or two protease inhibitors (e.g. indinavir, nelfinavir). Postexposure prophylaxis similarly employs combination therapy and is for four weeks. Common side effects are rash and nausea. Be aware of drug interactions listed in the British National Formulary. Any symptoms that might suggest seroconversion (fever, malaise, myalgia, lymphadenopathy, rash) should be explained.
- Pending follow-up and absence of seroconversion, health-care workers need not modify their work.
- All exposed individuals should be given advice on safe sex and avoiding blood donation.
- Follow-up is through the occupational health department and HIV retesting is performed at six months.

Would your management be any different if your house officer were pregnant?

She should tell her obstetric consultant of the incident, and this is essential if the incident involves an infected patient. Zidovudine and lamivudine are considered safe in the second and third trimesters of pregnancy but experience with other treatments is limited. However, the advantages are generally deemed to outweigh the risks and reduce the risk of vertical transmission.

CASE 4.48

MEDICAL OPINION ON FITNESS FOR ANAESTHESIA

Candidate information

Role

You are a doctor on the medical ward.
    Please read this summary.

Scenario

> Re: Mrs Beth Evans, aged 80 years
>
> Mrs Evans was admitted to hospital 10 days ago under the care of the orthopaedic surgeons following a fractured neck of femur. On admission her course was complicated by right lower lobe pneumonia from which she is recovering well on your ward. Her past medical history includes osteoporosis, ischaemic heart disease and heart failure and current medications are antibiotics, aspirin, frusemide, a nitrate spray and topical hormone replacement therapy. Blood pressure is currently 160/90 mmHg, heart sounds are normal with no added sounds or murmurs and there are bibasal crackles. Renal function and blood haematobiochemistry are normal, and her total cholesterol is 5.6 mmol/l.
>
> Your task is to assess the lady's medical condition with a view to whether she might undergo hip surgery.

Your examiners will warn you when 12 minutes have elapsed. You have 14 minutes to communicate with the patient/subject followed by 1 minute of reflection. There will then follow 5 minutes of discussion with the examiners. Do not take the history again except for details that will help in your discussion with the patient/subject. You are not required to examine the patient/subject.

Patient/subject information

Mrs Beth Evans is an 80-year-old widowed lady, hitherto living alone in a bungalow. She was admitted to hospital

10 days ago following a fall on her steps (there are three steps up to the front door of her bungalow). She has fractured her left neck of femur and this requires surgery. Surgery has, however, been postponed so far because of pneumonia, confirmed when she came into hospital. This has been treated successfully, and now the orthopaedic team would like a medical assessment, mostly to see if Mrs Evans is fit to undergo surgery. Her past medical history comprises osteoporosis, confirmed by a bone densitometry scan, angina (only on exertion) and heart failure, and her medications are aspirin, frusemide and a nitrate spray. She also takes a hormone replacement patch, and has done so for 20 years because it relieves hot flushes and she was once told it helped osteoporosis. Her general practitioner once suggested stopping it but she does not think 'she could live without it'. Mrs Evans will accept the opinion of the medical team as to whether she is yet fit for surgery but is worried about her heart and will ask the doctor for an honest view.

How to approach the case

Communication skills (conduct of interview/ exploration and problem negotiation), ethics and law

1 Introduction

Introduce yourself, confirm her identity and ask how she is.

2 Clarify the task

Explain that you are a physician and are here to advise on her medical problems and help optimise her treatment before any operation. Explain that you are not the anaesthetist, who would be responsible for deciding whether she is fit for an anaesthetic.

3 Explore symptoms

Explore the symptoms of ischaemic heart disease and heart failure and how these may limit her and what medications she has taken in the past.

4 Explore the past medical history

Explore the history of her osteoporosis, how it was first diagnosed (e.g. previous fractures, strong family history of osteoporosis or fractures) and enquire about the hormone replacement therapy – how long she has been on it, and for what reason (osteoporosis, symptoms of oestrogen deficiency such as flushes). Ask about other medical problems or medications. Ask about previous operations and anaesthesia. Ask about any allergies.

5 Explore ideas, concerns and expectations

Explore any concerns she may have about her medical problems or the operation.

6 Explain and advise as clearly as possible

Suggest that you would like to examine her, especially her heart and lungs, and review the electrocardiogram (ECG) and chest X-ray. Suggest that you may recommend optimising treatment of her problems, notably with a view to reducing the future risk of heart attacks and fluid on the lungs. Ask if she is willing for you to adjust her medication regimen, and explain that the adjustments will probably include adding in a drug known as an angiotensin-converting enzyme (ACE) inhibitor (beware preoperatively) and a statin (to reduce cholesterol and stabilise endothelium) and possibly another diuretic (spironolactone). A beta blocker may be considered later. An echocardiogram would be useful. Explore the past diagnosis of osteoporosis (presumptive or confirmed by bone densitometry) and the reason for her taking hormone replacement therapy (osteoporosis or symptoms of oestrogen deficiency such as flushes and atrophic vaginitis). Suggest that you would strongly advise the withdrawal of the hormone replacement therapy because the risks (venous thromboembolism, arterial disease, breast cancer) now very much outweigh any potential benefits (osteoporosis prophylaxis) and there are now better treatments for osteoporosis than hormone replacement therapy (a bisphosphonate with calcium and vitamin D supplementation).

7 Repeat important information

This can be an effective way of emphasising 'take home' messages.

8 Confirm understanding

Ensure that she understands your advice.

9 Encourage feedback and invite questions

I appreciate we've covered rather a lot there. Is there anything you would like me to go over again or are there any questions you would like to ask me?

10 Agree a way forward

Physicians are frequently asked to give an opinion on whether or not a patient is 'fit for surgery' or 'fit for anaesthesia', although the crucial decisions as to whether the patient would tolerate anaesthesia and the appropriate mode of anaesthesia must be made by an anaesthetist. Explain to patients (and the team making such a request) that you are not an expert in anaesthesia nor are you the right person to judge anaesthetic fitness, but that you are delighted to advise on optimising medical care. Your role is to give a medical opinion that can be used to optimise a patient's health before surgery.

Discussion

List some risk factors for anaesthesia

Age is an independent risk factor (a strong predictor for adverse cardiorespiratory outcomes such as arrhythmias,

Table 4.7 Exercise tolerance measured in metabolic equivalents (METs)	
MET	**Activity**
1	Self care Using toilet Walking 2–3 mph Light housework
4	Climbing a flight of stairs or a hill Walking at 4 mph Running a short distance Dancing, golf
> 10	Highly strenuous sports – swimming, football

hypotension and death) but anaesthetists look more closely at factors such as comorbidity, obesity, reflux and a difficult airway. Exercise tolerance in daily life reflects biological age and functional status can be measured in metabolic equivalents or METs (Table 4.7): 1 MET corresponds to oxygen consumption of 3.5 ml/kg/min (in a 70-kg, 40-year-old man at rest). Excellent functional reserve is > 7, moderate 4–7 and poor < 4.

Why are surgery and anaesthesia such a threat?

Surgery causes blood loss and fluid shifts. Postoperatively, surgery causes pain (with reduced coughing and increased risk of respiratory infection), limits movement and triggers the stress response of sympathetic activity, glucocorticoid activity and fluid and salt retention. There is also reduced enteral absorption, altered immune function and altered coagulation. These changes peak in the first two days but linger for weeks.

Most intravenous anaesthetic drugs have adverse cardiovascular effects, reducing afterload and having negative ionotropic effects. They cause apnoea, necessitating positive pressure ventilation and inhibit mucociliary function for 24 hours. They adversely affect renal function. Propofol, a modern induction agent, reduces systolic pressure by 40% on average in elderly patients. Regional anaesthesia vasodilates the affected area and interrupts sympathetic innervation of the heart and can result in marked bradycardia and hypotension if near the higher thoracic outflow.

Anaesthesia affects thermoregulation. A drop of 2°C centrally in the first 20 minutes is normal but can take an hour or two to recover with active warming. This hypothermia has a profound effect on cardiorespiratory, cerebral clotting and immune function.

What cardiovascular problems are provoked by anaesthesia?

Increased arterial stiffness with age increases afterload such that there is little change in cardiac output with an increase in stroke work and a longer systolic and shorter diastolic time. Late diastolic filling is increasingly important as the left ventricular end diastolic volume increases. Consequently:

- Atrial systole is even more important in situations where it is less likely (!) and anaesthetists do not like to anaesthetise patients with fast or variably controlled atrial fibrillation except in emergencies.
- Reduced diastolic time reduces coronary flow and ST changes on the ECG are common, especially at induction. These changes, often associated with hypotension and tachycardia, may respond to fluid challenges but the sting in the tail is that elderly patients are less tolerant of this.

Postoperative myocardial ischaemia remains the biggest cause of death and morbidity in elderly patients. Myocardial infarction tends (anecdotally) to occur on the second postoperative night. Systolic murmurs are extremely common. A good exercise tolerance and ECG are usually reassuring preoperatively, but significant aortic stenosis combined with anaesthesia can lead to a disastrous drop in afterload. Heart failure does not blend well with anaesthesia for all of the reasons outlined.

Is hypertension a risk factor for anaesthesia?

For every 10 mmHg in systolic pressure above 140, there is an odds ratio of 1.2, such that a systolic pressure of 180 mmHg doubles the risk of infarction.

What medical problems are relevant to anaesthesia?

Other important problems include respiratory problems with reduced functional residual capacity or low oxygen saturation (higher inspired oxygen is needed and positive pressure ventilation increases ventilation/perfusion mismatch), respiratory tract infection, reflux, confusion, alcohol misuse, electrolyte disturbance, obesity, hypothyroidism and drugs.

CASE 4.49

FITNESS TO DRIVE

Candidate information

Role

You are a doctor in the diabetes clinic.
Please read this summary.

Scenario

> Re: Mrs Julie Blyth, aged 36 years
>
> Mrs Blyth has type 1 diabetes and takes insulin. She has problems with hypoglycaemic unawareness. She is still driving and you are immediately concerned by this.
>
> Your task is to explore the issue of driving with her and make some recommendations.

Your examiners will warn you when 12 minutes have elapsed. You have 14 minutes to communicate with the patient/subject followed by 1 minute of reflection. There will then follow 5 minutes of discussion with the examiners. Do not take the history again except for details that will help in your discussion with the patient/subject. You are not required to examine the patient/subject.

Patient/subject information

Mrs Julie Blyth is a 36-year-old single mother of three children. She has type 1 diabetes and takes the combination of long- and short-acting analogues glargine and novorapid. She is very afraid of long-term diabetes complications and runs her blood glucoses very tightly between 3 and 4 mmol/l, which she believes to be the normal range. She has frequent hypoglycaemic symptoms (sweats, light-headedness), but does not recognise these as such. She feels she must drive. She drives a car to pick her children up from school and a small delivery van for an income. She is very concerned that the doctor in the diabetes clinic could 'take her licence away'.

How to approach the case

Communication skills (conduct of interview/exploration and problem negotiation), ethics and law

1 Introduction

Introduce yourself and confirm her identity.

2 Provide initial reassurance

Reassure her that you wish to try to establish why she is having symptoms and aim to correct these, rather than recommend that she does not drive.

3 Review her diabetes treatment and any complications to date

Be aware that insulin is a contraindication only to driving a heavy goods vehicle and not to other driving provided that she is not having hypoglycaemic episodes.

4 Be alert to ideas, concerns and expectations

Establish the discrepancy between her idea of normal blood glucose readings and what are in fact normal.

5 Reframe her ideas

Explain that she should be aiming for blood glucose readings of 4–7 mmol/l, and that she is currently aiming too low and this is probably giving rise to symptoms. Reassure her that resetting her target should not increase her risk of long-term complications.

6 Keep it clear

Keep your explanation as clear as possible.

7 Repeat important information

If she is anxious this may be especially important.

8 Confirm understanding

Ensure that she understands that her blood glucose target was too low.

9 Encourage feedback and invite questions

I appreciate we've covered rather a lot there. Is there anything you would like me to go over again or are there any questions you would like to ask me?

10 Agree a way forward

Assure her that she will be able to drive, but only when her blood glucose levels are normal. Ensure that there are arrangements for treatment and follow-up.

Discussion

Who is legally responsible for deciding whether a patient is unfit to drive?

The Driving and Vehicle Licensing Authority (DVLA) is responsible. The DVLA should be informed if a patient who holds a driving licence has a medical condition that now or at some future date may affect driving safety. The legal basis of fitness to drive lies in the Road Traffic Act of 1988 and subsequent regulations.

When might it be a doctor's responsibility to inform the DVLA?

These are outlined in Box 4.47.

Do you know the differences between a prescribed disability, a relevant disability and a prospective disability?

- A prescribed disability is a condition that legally bars the holding of a driving licence unless certain conditions are met, e.g. epilepsy.
- A relevant disability is a condition that probably renders a person unsafe to drive, e.g. visual field defect.

Box 4.47 Situations when a doctor might need to inform the DVLA

- If a patient lacks capacity to understand advice not to drive, e.g. dementia.
- If a doctor is aware that a patient continues to drive against medical advice, every reasonable step may be made to persuade the patient to stop, and this may include breaching confidentially and speaking with a relative. If a doctor is unable to persuade, or becomes aware that such a patient is continuing to drive, then the relevant medical information should be disclosed immediately to a medical adviser at the DVLA. Before disclosure, a patient should be informed of the decision to do so, and afterwards informed by letter. The patient's general practitioner should also be informed.

- A prospective disability is a progressive or intermittent condition that may in future lead to a relevant or prescribed disability, e.g. type 1 diabetes.

May a patient with a prospective disability drive?

Yes, subject to medical review at defined intervals.

What are the visual requirements for driving?

The visual acuity requirement for driving a private car is based on the number plate test. A person should be able to read in good light a number plate of letters or numbers 79.4 mm high (binocular vision with correction for any refractive error) at 20.5 m. This equates to a visual acuity of between 6/9 to 6/12 on a Snellen chart. Failing to meet the requirement constitutes a prescribed disability and a licence must be refused or revoked. The minimum field of vision for safe driving is at least 120° on the horizontal measured by the Goldmann perimeter using III4e settings.

What are the rules on driving after a seizure?

Current legal rules for drivers (of non-heavy goods or public transport vehicles) are that they must be seizure-free for more than 12 months or free of daytime seizures for more than three years if seizures are purely nocturnal. These rules apply on or off anti-epileptic drugs. Patients must not drive for six months following any dose adjustment. Patients have a legal duty to inform the DVLA of their condition. Driving regulations are further discussed in Cases 2.41 and 2.44.

CASE 4.50

INDUSTRIAL INJURY BENEFITS

Candidate information

Role

You are a doctor in the respiratory clinic.
Please read this summary.

Scenario

Re: Mr Andrew Hopkins, aged 77 years

Mr Hopkins is a retired shipyard worker, and has been progressively breathless. His chest X-ray suggests pulmonary fibrosis and there is pleural thickening with calcified pleural plaques. Pulmonary function tests reveal moderate restrictive lung disease and a thoracic computed tomography (CT) scan confirms interstitial lung disease. All of this suggests asbestos-related lung disease. Mr Hopkins is here for results and says that a friend told him he might claim industrial disablement benefit were asbestos the cause.

Your task is to explain the results and discuss the way forward for industrial disablement benefit.

Your examiners will warn you when 12 minutes have elapsed. You have 14 minutes to communicate with the patient/subject followed by 1 minute of reflection. There will then follow 5 minutes of discussion with the examiners. Do not take the history again except for details that will help in your discussion with the patient/subject. You are not required to examine the patient/subject.

Patient/subject information

Mr Andrew Hopkins is a 77-year-old retired shipyard worker, exposed to asbestos for at least 25 years of his working life during handling of construction materials. He has been progressively breathless over the last 18 months and a chest X-ray, pulmonary function tests and thoracic CT scan have confirmed asbestos-related lung disease. He is aware that industrial disablement benefit is available from the Department of Social Security (DSS) and wishes to discuss this.

How to approach the case

Communication skills (conduct of interview/ exploration and problem negotiation), ethics and law

1 Introduction

Introduce yourself and ask how he is.

2 Explain the results of tests

Explain that there is thickening of the lining of the lungs with plaques (hard patches) due to asbestos exposure, and scarring of the lungs almost certainly caused by asbestos (asbestosis).

3 Explore occupational history

Obtain details of different occupations and length of exposure with each.

4 Explain the implications of the results

Explain that treatment options are limited and that asbestosis tends to progress, albeit slowly. However, reassure him that there is no evidence of lung cancer or of cancer to the lining of the lung (mesothelioma), which can occur in asbestos lung disease.

5 Establish knowledge of eligibility for compensation

Ask if he is aware of his eligibility to claim for industrial disablement benefit.

Box 4.48 Asbestos lung disease eligible for compensation

- Mesothelioma
- Asbestosis
- Bilateral diffuse pleural thickening to a thickness of 5 mm or more at any point on chest X-ray
- Primary lung cancer with evidence of asbestosis or diffuse pleural thickening

---

6 Explain the legal position

Explain that people with asbestos lung disease are entitled to compensation. Explain that a DSS medical officer would visit to assess the degree of disability and that this information would help determine the level of benefit. Explain that benefit may be backdated up to three months. Explain that he could appeal within three months, if he disagreed with the verdict.

7 Explain what to do in practice

Explain that he should go to his local social security office and collect form B1 (100Pn). This covers occupational lung diseases. Say that you will write this down for him later.

8 Explore any outstanding concerns

Ensure that you have addressed all of his concerns.

9 Invite questions

Ask if he has any other questions.

10 Agree a way forward

Agree a clear course of action, ensuring that medical follow-up at clinic or with his general practitioner is in place.

Discussion

What types of asbestos lung disease make a patient eligible for compensation?

These are listed in Box 4.48.

Can compensation be considered for any other lung diseases?

Patients with a wide range of pneumoconioses, including coal worker's pneumoconiosis and silicosis, are eligible.

Can patients sue previous employers?

Yes, but many patients will have been exposed to asbestos from various workplaces and it may be difficult to prove that exposure in one workplace caused disease. Furthermore, many employers no longer exist and legal expenses make legal action untenable.

References and further reading

Communication skills and ethics
British Medical Association, www.bma.org.uk
Chochinov HM. Dignity and the essence of medicine: the A, B, C and D of dignity conserving care. BMJ 2007; 335:184–187
General Medical Council, www.gmc.org
Hope T. Medical ethics; a very short introduction. Oxford: Oxford University Press; 2004
Hope T, Savulescu J, Hendrick J. Medical ethics and law: the core curriculum. Edinburgh: Churchill Livingstone, Elsevier Science; 2003
Neighbour R. The inner consultation. Lancaster: MTP Press; 1987
The Oxford Centre for Ethics and Communication in Health Care Practice, www.ethox.org.uk
Tate P. The doctor's communication handbook. Oxford: Radcliffe Press; 1984
The UK Clinical Ethics Network, www.ethics-network.org.uk

Discussing clinical management
Explaining an investigation
Adler BJ, Stott DJ. How far to investigate older people? Clin Med 2003; 3:418–422

Discussing treatment
Stroke Prevention in Atrial Fibrillation II Study. Warfarin versus aspirin for prevention of thromboembolism in atrial fibrillation. Lancet 1994; 343:687–691
Wynne HA. Sensible prescribing for older people. Clin Med 2003; 3:409–412

Communication in special circumstances
Delayed discharge
Langhorne P, Taylor G, Murray G, et al. Early supported discharge services for stroke patients: a meta-analysis of individual patients' data. Lancet 2005; 365(9458):501–506

Breaking bad news
Buckman R. How to break bad news. A guide for healthcare professionals. London: Pan Books; 1992
Kaye P. Breaking bad news. A ten step approach. Northampton: EPL Publications; 1996
Maguire P. Breaking bad news: talking about death and dying. Medicine 2005; 33:29–31
Maguire P, Faulkner A. How to do it – communicate with cancer patients: handling bad news and difficult questions. BMJ 1998; 297:907–909
Maguire P, Faulkner A, Booth K, et al. Helping cancer patients disclose their concerns. Eur J Cancer 1996; 32A:78–81

Confidentiality, consent and capacity
General Medical Council. Consent and Confidentiality. Manchester: GMC; 2001
General Medical Council. Research: The Role and Responsibilities of Doctors. Manchester: GMC; 2001
General Medical Council. Confidentiality: Protecting and Providing Information. Manchester: GMC; 2004
General Medical Council. Confidentiality: Protecting and Providing Information: Frequently asked questions. Manchester: GMC; 2004
Hotopf M. The assessment of mental capacity. Clin Med 2005; 5:580–584
Lockwood G. Confidentiality. Medicine 2005; 33:8–11
Mental Capacity Act 2005. London: Department of Health. Available: www.dh.gov.uk/

End of life issues
Resuscitation status decision-making
A joint statement by the British Medical Association, the Resuscitation Council (UK) and the Royal College of Nursing. Decisions relating to cardiopulmonary resuscitation. London: British Medical Association; January 2002
British Medical Association, www.bma.org.uk

Regnard C, Randall F. A framework for making advance decisions on resuscitation. Clin Med 2005; 5:354–360
Resuscitation Council (UK), www.resus.org.uk
Royal College of Nursing, www.rcn.org.uk

Withholding and withdrawing life-prolonging treatments
General Medical Council (GMC). Withholding and withdrawing life-prolonging treatments. Good practice in decision-making. Manchester: GMC; August 2002. Available online at www.gmc.org

Percutaneous endoscopic gastrostomy feeding
Callahan CM, Haag, KM, Weinberger M, et al. Outcomes of percutaneous endoscopic gastrostomy among older adults in a community setting. J Am Geriatr Soc 2000; 48:1048–1054
Hoffer LJ. Tube feeding in advanced dementia: the metabolic perspective. BMJ 2006; 333:1214–1215
Monteleoni C, Clark E. Using rapid cycle quality improvement methodology to reduce feeding tubes in patients with advanced dementia: before and after study. BMJ 2004; 329: 491–494
Norton B, Homer-Ward M, Donnelly MT, Long RG, Holmes GK. A randomised prospective comparison of percutaneous endoscopic gastrostomy and nasogastric tube feeding after acute dysphagic stroke. BMJ 1996; 312:13–16
Sanders DS, Carter MJ, D'Silva J, James G, Bolton RP, Bardhan KD. Survival analysis in percutaneous endoscopic gastrostomy feeding: a worse outcome in patients with dementia. Am J Gastroenterol 2000; 95:1472–1475

Palliative care
Beauchamp TL, Childress JF. Principles of biomedical ethics, 5th edn. New York: Oxford University Press; 2001
Jeffrey D. The Assisted Dying for the Terminally Ill Bill: an inappropriate response to the challenge of caring for the dying. J R Coll Physicians Edinb 2005; 35:195–198
Rachels J. Active and passive euthanasia. In: Singer P, ed. Applied ethics. Oxford: Oxford University Press; 1986:29–37
Savulescu J. End-of-life decisions. Medicine 2005; 33:2: 11–15

Requesting an autopsy
Bristol Royal Infirmary. Interim report: removal and retention of human material. London: Central Office of Information; 2000
Royal Liverpool Children's Inquiry. London: HMSO; 2001

Clinical governance
Fitness to practise
General Medical Council. Good Medical Practice; 2006

Recruitment to a randomised controlled trial
Fowkes FGR, Fulton PM. Critical appraisal of published research: introductory guidelines. BMJ 1991; 302:1136–1140
General Medical Council. Research: the role and responsibilities of doctors; 2002
Greenhaugh T. How to read a paper: the basics of evidence based medicine. London: BMJ Books; 1997
Moher D, Dchulz KF, Altman DG. The CONSORT Statement: revised recommendations for improving the quality of reports of parallel-group randomisation trials. Ann Intern Med 2001; 134:657–662
Sackett DL, Strauss SE, Richardson WS, et al. Evidence-based medicine: how to practice and teach EBM, 2nd edn. Edinburgh: Churchill Livingstone; 2000 (associated website http://www.library.utoronto.ca/medicine/ebm/
The Centre for Evidence-based Medicine, http://cebm.jr2.ox.ac.uk

Other communication, ethical and legal scenarios
Fitness to drive
DVLA. At a glance guide to the current medical standards of fitness to drive. Available: www.dvla.gov.uk/ at_a_glance/aag_contents.htm

Station 5

Skin, locomotor system, eyes, endocrine system

SKIN

Examination of the skin   600

Cases

5.1   Psoriasis   600
5.2   Dermatitis   605
5.3   Lichen planus   607
5.4   Blistering skin disorders   608
5.5   Facial rash   612
5.6   Scleroderma, vitiligo and autoimmune skin
        disease   617
5.7   Oral lesions   619
5.8   Nail lesions   620
5.9   Shin lesions   621
5.10 Neurofibromatosis   625
5.11 Tuberose sclerosis   627
5.12 Neoplastic skin lesions   628
5.13 Skin vasculitis   630
5.14 Xanthomata and xanthelasmata   631
5.15 Skin and soft tissue infection   632

LOCOMOTOR SYSTEM

Examination of the joints – overview   635

Examination of the hands and arms   635

Examination of the legs   640

Examination of the spine   642

Cases

5.16 Rheumatoid hands and rheumatoid
        arthritis   643
5.17 Ankylosing spondylitis and
        spondyloarthropathies   652
5.18 Systemic lupus erythematosus   655
5.19 Scleroderma   659
5.20 Crystal arthropathy   662
5.21 Osteoarthritis   664
5.22 Paget's disease   666
5.23 Marfan's syndrome   668
5.24 Ehlers–Danlos syndrome   670
5.25 Osteogenesis imperfecta   671

EYES

Examination of the eyes   673

Cases

5.26 Diabetic retinopathy   675
5.27 Hypertensive retinopathy   678
5.28 Swollen optic disc and papilloedema   679
5.29 Optic atrophy   680
5.30 Chorioretinitis   682
5.31 Retinitis pigmentosa   682
5.32 Central retinal vein occlusion   683
5.33 Central retinal artery occlusion   684
5.34 Retinal detachment and vitreous
        haemorrhage   685
5.35 Drusen and age-related macular degeneration
        (asteroids)   686
5.36 Angioid streaks   688
5.37 Myelinated nerve fibres   688
5.38 Glaucoma   689
5.39 Cataracts   690
5.40 Uveitis and red eye   691

ENDOCRINE SYSTEM

Examination of the thyroid   693

Cases

5.41 Hyperthyroidism and Graves' disease   693
5.42 Hypothyroidism   697
5.43 Goitre and neck lumps   699
5.44 Hypopituitarism   700
5.45 Acromegaly   703
5.46 Cushing's syndrome   705
5.47 Hypoadrenalism and Addison's disease   707
5.48 Hirsutism and polycystic ovarian
        syndrome   711
5.49 Hypogonadism and gynaecomastia   712
5.50 Pseudohypoparathyroidism   713

References and further reading   714

SKIN

Examination of the skin

Introduction

Skin comprises an inner dermis of collagen and elastic tissue lying on subcutaneous fat, and an outer, continuously replenishing epidermis extending from a basal layer of cells with scattered melanocytes to a top layer of protective keratinocytes. These continuously degenerate and slough off to be replaced by cells from beneath. The epidermal–dermal junction is demarcated by a basement membrane. Skin disease can originate in any of these structures and skin, the only visible organ, can be a window to the world of systemic disease. In skin cases, be prepared to do two things:

- Look at the distribution of a rash (pattern recognition is important, e.g. photosensitivity).
- Describe lesions (the morphology may be diagnostic, e.g. psoriasis; if it not diagnostic, comment on differential diagnoses).

Distribution of skin lesions

You are likely to be asked to examine a particular region, e.g. the scalp, face, mouth, hands, nails or shins. If not, work from scalp to sole. Always attempt to describe the distribution of skin lesions, noting particularly if they are bilateral or symmetrical. As a rule, endogenous causes are more likely to produce bilateral lesions (e.g. psoriasis, see Fig. 5.1; Case 5.1) and exogenous causes produce a more random distribution.

Description of skin lesions

Central to dermatology is your ability to describe skin lesions (Table 5.1).

Summary

A summary of the skin examination sequence is given in the Summary Box.

SUMMARY BOX – SKIN EXAMINATION SEQUENCE

- Look at the distribution of the rash, e.g. bilateral, symmetrical, photosensitive areas
- Be able to describe lesions (Table 5.1); the morphology may be diagnostic, e.g. psoriasis; if not diagnostic, comment on differential diagnoses
- Look for relevant non-cutaneous signs, e.g. psoriatic arthropathy

---

CASE 5.1

PSORIASIS

Instruction

Please examine this patient's knees and any other areas of skin you think appropriate. Discuss your findings and propose some management options.

Table 5.1 Terminology for skin lesions

Term	Description
Macule	Flat area of discoloration ranging from pale (loss of melanin) to brown or black (increased melanin); many macules are red, indicating vascular dilatation or an inflammatory process
Patch	Large macule
Papule	Raised lesion < 1 cm in diameter
Nodule	Raised lesion > 1 cm in diameter
Plaque	Raised lesion with a flattened top, or plateau
Vesicle	Fluid-filled lesion or 'blister' < 0.5 cm in diameter
Bulla	Larger blister
Pustule	Vesicle filled with neutrophils (not necessarily infection)
Telangiectasia	Dilated, superficial blood vessels (capillaries, postcapillary venules) – idiopathic or associated with cold outdoor exposure, pulmonary hypertension, scleroderma, systemic lupus erythematosus, rosacea, lupus pernio or necrobiosis lipoidica diabeticorum
Discoid	Flat and disc-like lesion (term sometimes overlapping with nummular or coin-like lesions)
Annular	Ring-shaped
Reticular	'Net-like' lesions, e.g. erythema ab igne (Granny's tartan) and livedo reticularis (physiological or associated with sepsis, connective tissue disease or malignancy)
Atrophy	Loss of tissue – loss of dermis or subcutaneous fat usually leaves a depression in the skin; loss of epidermis causes wrinkling and a translucent, hypopigmented appearance
Lichenification	Characteristic skin thickening (resembling lichen on rocks or trees) often produced by chronic inflammation or rubbing
Erosion	Area of lost epidermis that generally heals without scarring
Excoriation	Linear erosions often produced by scratching
Ulcer	Area of skin loss involving the dermis
Fissures	Slit through whole thickness of skin

Recognition

Chronic plaque psoriasis

Skin

There are numerous symmetrically distributed plaques (Fig. 5.1) most prominent on *extensor surfaces (elbows, knees)*, the *scalp* and *hairline* and *behind the ears*, the *lower back (sacrum)* and the *shins*. Plaques may range in size from a few millimetres to a large area of the limbs or trunk. These are *sharply marginated* and *pink/red* with *silvery white scaling surfaces* (sometimes said to resemble limpets).

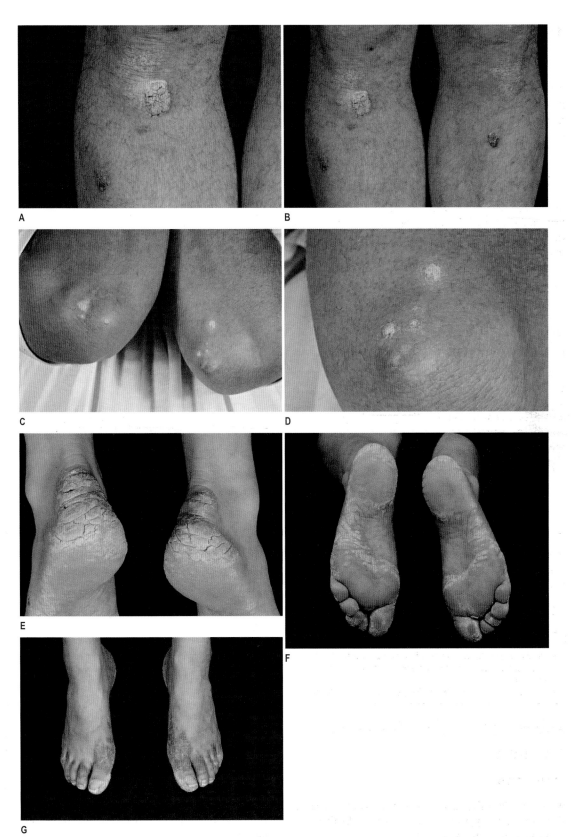

Fig. 5.1 Psoriasis: (A,B) knees, (C,D) elbows, (E–G) symmetrical distribution on heels, soles and dorsum of feet respectively.

Hands and nails

There may be *nail pitting* and *onycholysis* and *arthropathy* of the hands.

Auspitz sign and Köbner's phenomenon

The predominance of erythema or scaling can vary from patient to patient. Scratching of scales may result in a *waxy* appearance, although lesions are not usually itchy. Lifting larger scales (do not do this) may result in capillary bleeding (*Auspitz sign*). Occasionally, instead of scaling, the surfaces of plaques are covered by hard, thickened firmly adherent keratin. *Köbner's phenomenon*, in which lesions often appear at sites of minor trauma (e.g. surgical wound, trivial scratch, abrasion, burn), is a helpful diagnostic feature, and sometimes the first sign of psoriasis. Other causes of Köbner's phenomenon include lichen planus, pemphigoid and certain viruses, but it does not occur in dermatitis.

Psoriasis variants

Eighty per cent of psoriasis is the chronic plaque variety. Rarer variants are described in Table 5.2.

Interpretation

Confirm the diagnosis

Chronic plaque psoriasis is characteristic.

What to do next – assess other systems

Psoriatic arthropathy affects up to 10% of patients with psoriasis and may precede or follow skin disease by months or even years. There are, in theory, five types, although overlap is common (Table 5.3). If there is arthropathy, consider the tendency for HLA B27 spondyloarthropathies to overlap, common features being sacroiliac discomfort and enthesopathies such as plantar fasciitis.

Consider severity/decompensation/complications

Note the extent of skin involvement and any variants.

Consider function

Severe hand or foot psoriasis or psoriatic arthropathy affects function. Psychological morbidity and quality of life effects are very important in such a chronic, currently incurable disease. Share these points with the examiners.

Table 5.2 Psoriasis variants

Variant	Features	Differential diagnosis
Guttate psoriasis	Acute eruption of small plaques typically < 1 cm in diameter over trunk and limbs; these look like drops of rain or paint Common in adolescence Usually triggered by upper respiratory infection, e.g. streptococcal pharyngitis	Pityriasis versicolor Pityriasis rosea
Palmoplantar pustular psoriasis	Often chronic relapsing and remitting More common in females Scattered crops of pustules resembling 'raindrops' turn from white to 'autumn-brown' colour then fade Severe erythema, scaling and soreness Not generally associated with other forms of psoriasis	Pompholyx Dermatophyte infection
Generalised pustular psoriasis	Life-threatening acute eruption with systemic illness Sheets of pustules may merge to form lakes of pus over an erythematous and oedematous base Commonly affects flexures but spreads widely Usually no psoriasis history Sometimes associated with corticosteroid withdrawal	Acute exanthematous toxic pustuloderma
Flexural psoriasis	More erythematous than scaly May be exudative Axillae, groins, umbilicus and genitalia	Candida Seborrhoeic dermatitis Allergic contact dermatitis
Erythrodermic psoriasis	Exfoliative dermatitis with severe erythema and scaling over entire body Usually pre-existing psoriasis that is difficult to control	Drug eruption Eczema Icthyoses Cutaneous lymphoma
Nail involvement psoriasis	Pitting Oncycholysis Dystrophy Subungual hyperkeratosis Features reflect psoriasis in the nail matrix and bed Often pink or yellowish area beneath nail, adjacent to free margin or an area of onycholysis (oil-drop sign)	Dermatitis (pitting) Alopecia areata (pitting) Drug or phototoxic reaction during psoralen UVA therapy (onycholysis) Dermatophyte infection (subungual hyperkeratosis)
Facial psoriasis	Uncommon but frontal hairline may be affected Sebopsoriasis, a variety of the Köbner's phenomenon, may occur in seborrhoeic dermatitis	Seborrhoeic dermatitis Contact dermatitis Atopic dermatitis

Table 5.3 Psoriatic arthropathy	
Type	**Features**
Rheumatoid-like hands	The commonest type; seronegative
Asymmetrical distal interphalangeal joint arthropathy	Relatively uncommon but the form most strongly associated with psoriasis; affected digits often show nail changes such as pitting
Asymmetrical large joint mono- or oligoarthropathy	Large joint pain or swelling
Spondyloarthropathy and sacroiliitis	Low back pain
Arthritis mutilans	Very uncommon, severely destructive type

Discussion

What causes psoriasis?

This is unknown. There are two peaks of incidence of onset – before 40 years and 55–60 years, the former more likely to have a family history (association with HLA Cw6). Psoriasis may be precipitated by physical (e.g. trauma, pregnancy, infection, drugs, steroid withdrawal) or psychological stress and is attenuated by sunlight.

What standard treatments are used in psoriasis?

These are outlined in Table 5.4. Cognitive behavioural therapy is effective in psoriasis triggered by psychological stress.

What is the immunopathology of psoriasis?

Psoriasis is now viewed as a predominantly T helper type 1 (Th1) cytokine-mediated pro-inflammatory disease. $CD45RO^+$ memory effector T cells, interleukin-12 (IL-12), which promotes deviation to Th1 lymphocyte production, and the Th1 lymphocyte-derived cytokines IL-2 and interferon-γ (IFN-γ) are abundant in plaques.

Tumour necrosis factor-α (TNF-α) is a key proinflammatory cytokine, and, along with IL-1 and IL-6, a final common mediator in the Th1-driven proinflammatory pathway.

Leucocyte function-associated antigen 1 (LFA-1), a member of the integrin family of chemokines, is expressed on the surface of leucocytes; it comprises CD11a (α) and CD18 (β) integrin subunits and aids leucocyte (including T-cell) activation and extravasation from blood to tissues. In pustular psoriasis, migration of neutrophils into the epidermis is especially pronounced, causing multiple, small, sterile pus deposits. CD11a binds intercellular adhesion molecule 1 (ICAM-1), ICAM-2, and ICAM-3 on endothelial cells, other leucocytes, fibroblasts and keratinocytes. Expression of ICAM-1 is induced by numerous cytokines, including TNF-α, IL-1 and IL-6.

The proinflammatory response in psoriasis leads to epidermal keratinocyte proliferation and thickening of the epidermis with thick keratin. However, rapid turnover prevents adequate differentiation into normal keratin and the

Table 5.4 Standard treatments in psoriasis	
Treatment	**Comment**
Topical therapy (first line for limited chronic plaque psoriasis) Emollients	
Coal tar ointments and pastes	Easier to apply in hospital; safe and effective for stable plaques but salicylic acid may also be needed to dissolve thick keratin
Short contact dithranol	Useful in incremental concentrations as first-line treatment for stable plaques; stains plaques and hair and must not be applied for longer than directed, usually 30 minutes
Vitamin D3 analogues, e.g. calipotriol, tacalitol	Useful for mild to moderate stable plaques; remission duration short so treatment is constant; high doses (extensive psoriasis) may cause hypercalcaemia
Corticosteroids	Tachyphylaxis (rebound on withdrawal) is a major drawback
Retinoids, e.g. tazarotene	Clean and convenient; experience limited; teratogenic
Calcineurin inhibitors, e.g. tacrolimus (unlicensed in UK)	Effective only on thin plaques (face and flexures); should not be combined with phototherapy
Phototherapy Ultraviolet B (UVB)	Useful in widespread plaque or guttate psoriasis
Oral (or topical psoralens), followed by irradiation with long-wave ultraviolet A (PUVA)	Useful in widespread plaque psoriasis
Systemic therapy Ciclosporin	Rapid acting and highly effective; inhibits calcineurin; side effects are immunosuppression, hypertension and nephrotoxicity
Methotrexate	Widely used in extensive plaque psoriasis, generalised pustular psoriasis, erythrodermic psoriasis and psoriatic arthropathy; side effects bone marrow suppression and hepatotoxicity
Acitretin	A treatment of choice for psoriasis as monotherapy or in combination with PUVA; teratogenic
Hydroxycarbamide	Less commonly used

keratin produced is scaly and readily removed. An equivalent process in the nail leads to thickening, pitting and onycholysis. Angiogenesis is also prominent, and when scales are removed a red vascular layer with capillaries reaching upwards is characteristic (*Auspitz sign*).

What immunomodulatory therapies are there in psoriasis?

These are outlined in Fig. 5.2 and Table 5.5. They are currently very expensive, and time to, extent of and duration of response varies. Ways of assessing response include the Psoriasis Area Severity Index (PASI).

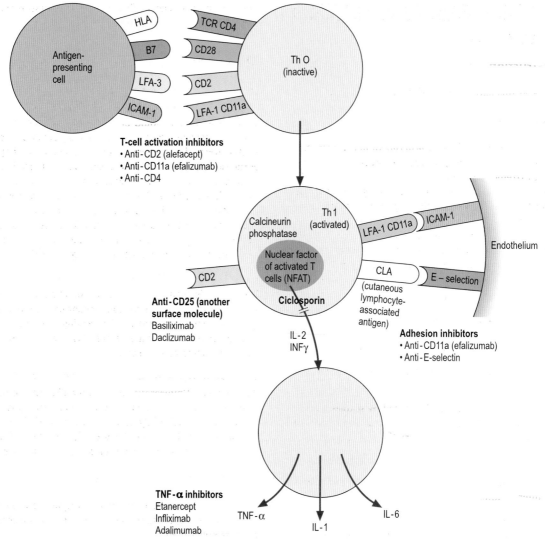

Fig. 5.2 Current and proposed immunomodulatory therapies or 'biologics' in psoriasis.

Table 5.5 Current immunomodulatory therapies or 'biologics' in psoriasis

Biologic		Why it works/should work	Comment
TNF-α inhibitors	Etanercept	Human recombinant fusion protein comprising TNF-α p75 receptor fused to Fc portion of immunoglobulin G1 Binds to and inactivates TNF-α	Twice weekly subcutaneous injection Immunosuppression monitoring needed
	Infliximab	Chimeric monoclonal antibody Binds to and inactivates TNF-α	Intravenous injection schedule Immunosuppression monitoring needed
	Adalimumab		
T-cell activation inhibitors	Alefacept	Binds T-cell receptor CD2 and inhibits T-cell activation that follows binding to LFA-3 on antigen-presenting cells	Intravenous or intramuscular injection schedule
	Efalizumab	Humanised IgG1 monoclonal antibody against CD11a subunit of LFA-1, blocking LFA-1 binding to ICAM-1 and inhibiting both T-cell activation and adhesion of circulating T cells to ICAM-1-expressing endothelial cells and keratinocytes, thus preventing cutaneous T-cell trafficking	Weekly subcutaneous injection

ICAM-1, intercellular adhesion molecule 1; IgG1, immunoglobulin 1; LFA-1, leucocyte function-associated antigen 1; TNF-α, tumour necrosis factor-α.

CASE 5.2

DERMATITIS

Instruction

Look at this patient's skin. Discuss your findings.

Recognition

The skin is *red, swollen and blistering* or *dry, thickened and leathery, with erythema, scaling and evidence of scratching*. Both extremes are *itchy*.

Dermatitis and eczema are interchangeable terms. The term 'eczema' means skin 'boiling over'. There are many types of dermatitis and the clinical appearance can fall anywhere between the two extremes. Pathologically, there is breakdown in the skin's horny barrier and there may be oedema high in the dermis. Any blisters tend to have a honeycomb, multiloculated core, not typical of other blistering diseases such as pemphigus.

Interpretation

Confirm the diagnosis

Although you are unlikely to meet infectious diseases in PACES:

- Acute 'dermatitis' may be caused by scabies and is often intensely itchy and worse after hot showers or baths and at night. Burrows of the scabies mite *Sarcoptes scabei* may be seen.
- *Tinea pedis* should be considered before diagnosing foot dermatitis. It is often unilateral, dry, scaly and interdigitate.

What to do next – consider causes

Dermatitis may have endogenous or exogenous causes, the latter generally contact dermatitis and photosensitivity (Table 5.6). Bilateral dermatitis is more likely to have an endogenous cause and unilateral dermatitis an exogenous cause (but contact dermatitis commonly affects both hands if dipped in chemical irritants). Tell the examiners the features of the history that you would explore, especially atopy (hay fever, asthma), occupation and exposure to irritants (Fig. 5.3).

Consider severity/decompensation/complications

Dermatitis can be severe and even life-threatening, especially with secondary infection. Apparent dermatitis occasionally represents a more sinister aetiology. In adults, an eruption resembling flexoral atopic dermatitis is occasionally the result of agammaglobulinaemia, coeliac disease or mycosis fungoides.

Consider function

Consider occupational causes of contact dermatitis and whether or not dermatitis could have an impact on occupa-

tion. The psychological effects of severe dermatitis can be incalculable.

Discussion

How is atopic eczema treated?

Patients should avoid identified allergens (e.g. vacuuming, damp dusting) but should be informed that improvement may take many months (e.g. after changing bedding). Emollients and emollient bathing promote skin hydration. Topical corticosteroids (Box 5.1) are the main treatment for inflammation and pruritus. Less potent drugs should be used on the eyelids, face and flexural surfaces because of the risk of cataracts, skin atopy and telangiectasia. More potent treatment is allowable for these areas for a few days before stepping down to less potent maintenance treatment. Topical/systemic antibiotics and antihistamines may be needed.

How do ointments and creams differ?

These vary in their grease:water ratio. The epidermis can absorb both greasy and aqueous preparations. Generally, greasy ointments are best for dry, scaling skin and watery creams for crusted weeping lesions. Pastes may be used for sustained action or occlusion.

Do topical immunomodulators have a place?

Tacrolimus and pimecrolimus are very effective for intermittent use in mild to moderate atopic dermatitis, but should be applied thinly and only when needed to limit neoplastic risk. They do not cause skin atrophy and there is minimal absorption. They may be used on the face.

How is severe, refractory atopic dermatitis treated?

Systemic corticosteroids and immunosuppressant therapy with ciclosporin, azathioprine or mycophenolate mofetil are sometimes used.

Mention some other itchy skin conditions

Primary skin diseases causing itch include all types of dermatitis, lichen planus, blistering disorders, especially dermatitis herpetiformis (pemphigoid does not itch), fungal infection or mite infestation, flea/tick bites and ichthyosis (dry skin with fish-like scales, with a genetic basis or associated with malignancy). Systemic causes include cholestasis, uraemia, diabetes, hyper/hypothyroidism, polycythaemia vera, lymphoma, parasitophobia and certain drugs.

What types of drug-induced rash are there?

These include exanthematous, urticarial, blistering (e.g. Stevens–Johnson syndrome), fixed drug eruptions (macules, papules or blisters tending to occur at the same site with each exposure), vasculitic or photosensitivity (e.g. amiodarone).

What is meant by the term urticaria?

This refers to wheals (oedema) surrounded by flares of erythema. It may be caused by drugs, heat, cold, pressure,

Table 5.6 Types of dermatitis

Type	Cause	Features
Atopic eczema	Th2-weighted allergic process House dust mite important (its faeces contributes hugely to weight of old pillows!); it likes moist, sweaty atmospheres, preferring beds to curtains and carpets, but cannot survive in high, dry atmospheres above 3000 metres Other allergens include pollen, animal dander and pollution, and interact with a genetic tendency Diagnosis aided by radioallergosorbent tests (RASTs) to identify allergen specific IgE in serum Alternatively, skin prick testing introduces allergen into the skin, where it interacts with IgE bound to mast cells and causes histamine release and a consequent 'wheal and flare' (oedema and erythema) response	At least 50% of all dermatitis, prevalence increasing *Validated UK-refined Hanifen and Rajka diagnostic criteria* *Itchy skin in last 12 months* *plus three or more of:* *Onset before two years of age; typically develops in infancy, when a trial of milk and egg exclusion may be warranted; may wax and wane through adult life* *History of flexural involvement* *History of generally dry skin* *History of other atopic disease* *Visible flexural dermatitis; tends to affect flexors, with itch, erythematous macules, papules or papulovesicles which may become lichenified and excoriated* Superimposed staphylococcal or streptococcal infection, impeding response to steroids, common Herpes simplex type 1 may cause rapid worsening of dermatitis, especially atopic (eczema herpeticum/'Kaposi's varicelliform eruption')
Irritant contact dermatitis (ICD)	Usually due to daily, regular exposure to trigger factor (thus more readily identifiable), e.g. hand dermatitis due to soaps, solvents or chronic skin wear and tear Thus early intervention crucial to successful treatment; the more chronic the process, the less likely to remit and if it does can rapidly reappear with re-exposure Atopic dermatitis predisposes to ICD	Often sub-clinical skin damage before skin begins to dry, crack and develop a smooth, shiny atrophic appearance Oedema and blistering may develop
Allergic contact dermatitis (ACD)	Type IV hypersensitivity reaction to previously tolerated substance, e.g. nickel (clothing, including underwear, keys and money), cosmetics (including 'hypoallergenic' cosmetics!), occupational chemicals (e.g. epoxy resins, chromate, rubber), nail varnish, glues, pine trees Patch testing screens for common triggers ICD may predispose to ACD, because disturbance of skin barrier function allows allergen penetration. ICD and ACD exhibit identical inflammatory cell and cytokine profiles but memory T cells have no role in ICD	Unlike irritant contact dermatitis, often sudden reaction to trace quantity of allergen May become widespread, spreading to areas of body not recently exposed
Photosensitive dermatitis	True sun-induced dermatitis rare. Much more common are other forms of dermatitis aggravated by sunlight and other photodermatoses such as polymorphic light eruption	Dermatitis in photosensitive distribution
Discoid/nummular dermatitis	Likely infection (staphylococcal superantigens)	Intensely itchy coin-shaped lesions on limbs, often distributed symmetrically Affects middle-aged to older adults
Venous dermatitis	Venous stasis	Swelling, sclerosis or atrophy on lower leg (often starting at medial malleolus) Haemosiderin deposition from extravasated blood causes brownish discoloration May be ulceration
Seborrhoeic dermatitis (see Fig. 5.3)	Likely genetic predisposition, mediated by several factors, e.g. hormonal, dietary May be inflammatory response to *Pitysporum ovale*, a yeast in human scalp	Erythematous plaques or patches on scalp, preauricular area, nasolabial folds, glabella or eyelids; may be otitis externa Despite the name, lesions dry, often with scaling surface, and not associated with excess sebum May be part of spectrum that includes dandruff Blepharitis (itchy lids and crusting lid margins with a dandruffy appearance and broken lashes) strongly associated with seborrhoeic dermatitis or staphylococcal infection; conjunctivae are glistening and swollen with excess lipid secretion and foaming of the lid margins

Table 5.6 Types of dermatitis—cont'd

Type	Cause	Features
Pompholyx	Seasonal or without obvious trigger Contact dermatitis affecting palms sometimes also referred to as pompholyx	Intensely itchy blisters on palms
Juvenile plantar dermatosis	Not known but prevalence seems to be increasing *Tinea pedis* should be excluded by microscopy of skin scrapings	Shiny, glazed appearance to aspects of the soles of the feet in contact with footwear
Neurodermatitis	Trigger usually historical, the signs due to habitual rubbing and scratching	Chronic lichenified skin (lichen simplex chronicus)
Asteatotic dermatitis (eczema craquelé)	Not known	Dry, crazy paving pattern of fissuring, especially on the limbs

IgE, immunoglobulin E; Th2, T helper type 2.

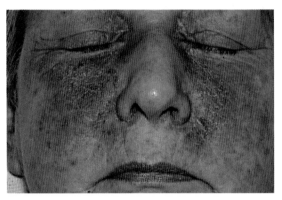

Fig. 5.3 Seborrhoeic dermatitis.

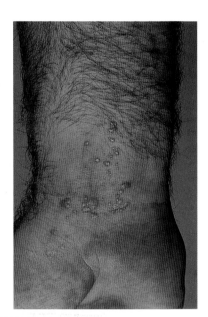

Fig. 5.4 Lichen planus.

Box 5.1 Potency of some typical corticosteroids

Mild
- Hydrocortisone
- Fucidic acid and hydrocortisone (*Fucidin H*)

Moderate
- Clobetasone butyrate (*Eumovate*)

Potent
- Hydrocortisone butyrate (*Locoid*)
- Betamethasone valerate (*Betnovate*)
- Fucidic acid and betamethasone (*Fucibet*)
- Mometosone furoate (*Elocon*)

Very potent
- Clobetasol proprionate (*Dermovate*)
- Clobetasol proprionate, neomycin and nystatin (*Dermovate NN*)

water, food substances, infections, insect bites or dermatographism. More severe reactions may lead to angiooedema. Urticaria pigmentosa refers to itchy red-brown macules/papules, which are the dermal manifestation of systemic mastocytosis.

CASE 5.3

LICHEN PLANUS

Instruction

Look at this patient's wrists/ankles and discuss what you see.

Recognition

There are *well demarcated, polygonal, raised plaques on the flexor surfaces*, especially the *wrists* and *ankles* (Fig. 5.4). Their *flat tops* are *shiny* with a *violaceous colour*, interrupted by *milky white streaks – Wickhams's striae*. They are very likely to be *intensely itchy*. There may be Köbner's phenomenon. Lesions usually resolve over a period of months to leave brownish macules.

Interpretation

Confirm the diagnosis

Lichenification is a feature of many skin diseases such as eczema and itchy drug eruptions. The shiny, purplish flat tops of lichen planus, and their distribution, usually aid diagnosis.

What to do next – assess other systems

There may be white, 'net-like' lesions on the buccal mucosa (Fig. 5.5) or tongue (Fig. 5.6), often with ulceration.

Atrophy and longitudinal grooves may affect the nail plates; sometimes nails disappear altogether.

Consider severity/decompensation/complications

Lichen planus is not life-threatening, but white oral lesions may not be lichen planus; differential diagnoses include candidiasis and leucoplakia (hyperkeratotic lesions associated with Epstein–Barr virus), both more common in human immunodeficiency virus (HIV) infection.

Consider function

Function is likely to be normal.

Discussion

What causes lichen planus?

The cause is uncertain. There is no family history and no definite association with stress.

How does lichen planus arise?

The epidermis is thickened, with increased keratin. The white streaks imply a thickened granular layer and underlying cellular infiltrate. The basal layer is infiltrated with T lymphocytes in a band pattern.

How may lichen planus be treated?

Moderately potent topical (occasionally systemic) steroids are effective. Lichen planus is self-limiting but tends to relapse and remit over months or even years.

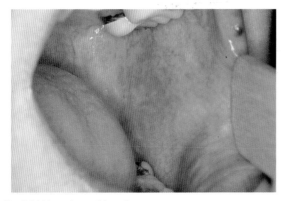

Fig. 5.5 Lichen planus of buccal mucosa.

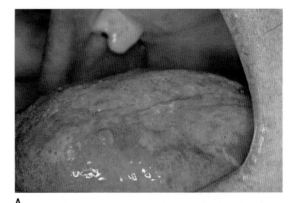

A

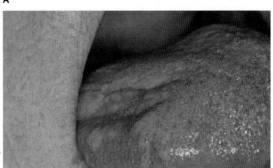

B

Fig. 5.6 Lichen planus of tongue.

What is pityriasis rosea?

Pityriasis is Greek for 'bran' and refers to a fine scaly appearance. In pityriasis rosea the scales are on top of pale pink oval patches. There is often a 'herald patch'. It affects young adults, is of unknown cause, and self-limiting.

What is pityriasis versicolor?

This refers to white macules on tanned skin or pale brown patches on non-tanned skin, in the absence of inflammation or vesicles, suggesting yeast infection.

CASE 5.4

BLISTERING SKIN DISORDERS

Instruction

Please inspect this patient's skin and discuss the possible causes.

Recognition

Bullous pemphigoid

There are *tense blisters* of *variable size* (much more variable than pemphigus, from a few millimetres to a few centimetres, but large, tense blisters up to 3 cm in diameter are typical) on the *flexor surfaces* spreading to the *trunk* (Fig. 5.7) on an erythematous base. Blisters may be broken because of excoriation. Early disease may appear as a pruritic, urticarial rash. Oral lesions are less frequent than in pemphigus, occurring in around one-third of patients and seldom a presenting feature. The anus, vagina and oesophagus are occasionally involved.

Pemphigus

There is a *bullous eruption* (in a middle-aged/older patient) comprising *flaccid, fragile, thin-walled blisters* on the *trunk* 1–2 cm in diameter (Fig. 5.8). Many have *burst*, leaving *red, exuding, tender patches* (even rubbing of normal skin

can cause sloughing of the epidermis – Nikolsky sign). *Oral erosions* are common and painful and may precede the rash. *Pemphigus foliaceous* is characterised by superficial blisters that affect only the skin. *Pemphigus vulgaris* is characterised by mucosal involvement and subsequent skin involvement with blisters and erosions.

Interpretation

Confirm the diagnosis

Pemphigoid blisters are tense and pemphigus blisters are flaccid. Inspect the mouth for erosions (Fig. 5.9).

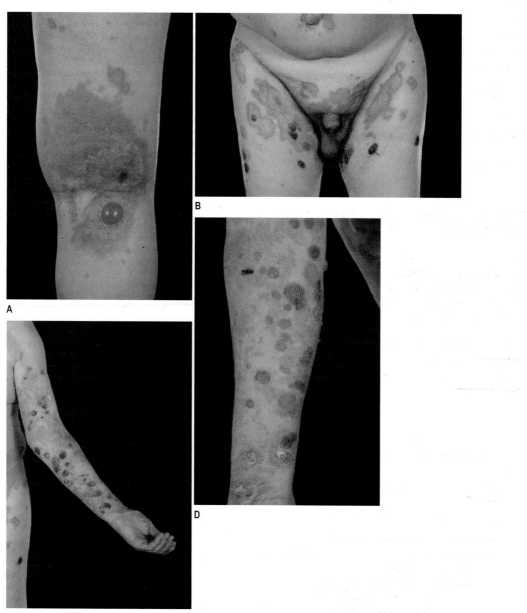

Fig. 5.7 Pemphigoid (A–D).

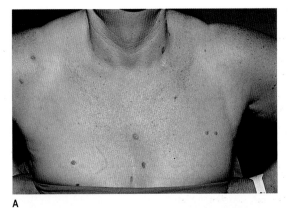

A

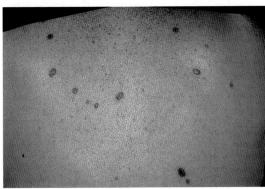

B

Fig. 5.8 (A,B) Pemphigus – trunk.

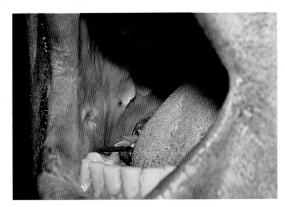

Fig. 5.9 Pemphigus – intraoral.

What to do next – consider causes

Important differential diagnoses are listed in Table 5.7.

Consider severity/decompensation/complications

Note if lesions are widespread or confluent. Note Cushingoid features (prolonged corticosteroids). Pemphigus is gen-

erally more serious than pemphigoid, although mucous membrane pemphigoid is a variant with predominant mucous membrane involvement, severe scarring and risk of blindness and laryngeal stenosis. Blistering diseases may be complicated by secondary bacterial infection.

Consider function

Blistering diseases can be very disabling.

Discussion

What are the differences between pemphigoid and pemphigus?

These are described in Table 5.8.

How do porphyrias arise and what are the possible skin manifestations?

Haem comprises a tetramer porphyrin ring with an iron molecule in its ferrous form. Porphyrias are enzyme disorders in the stepwise chain to haem synthesis (Table 5.9). These lead to loss of the production line ahead and accumulation of pre-haem metabolites (porphyrin precursors or porphyrins) behind the metabolic 'dam'. Accumulated metabolites early in the stepwise chain to haem synthesis tend to be water soluble, appearing in urine, and those later in the chain tend to appear in the stool. Important molecules early in the chain include aminolaevulinic acid (ALA) and porphobilinogen (PBG).

What are the neuropsychiatric or acute porphyrias?

Porphyrias causing neuropsychiatric manifestations include acute intermittent porphyria, hereditary coprophorphyria and variegate porphyria. These are also known as the acute porphyrias or the hepatic porphyrias because they arise from enzyme abnormalities in the liver.

What are the cutaneous porphyrias?

Skin disease is a feature of most porphyrias (acute intermittent porphyria is a notable exception) because porphyrins become toxic when exposed to light. Photons of violet light electronically excite porphyrin molecules, which produce reactive oxygen species causing tissue damage directly and via other molecules such as metalloproteinases. Cutaneous porphyrias thus share common skin manifestations, including marked photosensitivity, blistering, erosions, pigmentation and scarring. Sunscreens are essential.

What are the acquired porphyrias?

Most porphyrias are genetic, but porphyria cutanea tarda is often acquired; it is essentially a liver disorder presenting in the skin.

Table 5.7 Important differential diagnoses of blistering diseases

	Conditions	Clinical clues
Immunological	Pemphigoid	Described above
	Pemphigus	Described above
	Dermatitis herpetiformis	Symmetrical, intensely itchy vesicles or urticarial plaques on trunk and extensor surfaces, buttocks and occasionally the face and scalp
		Associated with gluten-sensitive enteropathy (coeliac disease) and granular deposition of IgA
		Responds to dapsone
	Lichen planus	White lacy pattern characteristic
Genetic	Epidermolysis bullosa (EB)	A group of hereditary disorders with blistering and erosions on minimal trauma
		EB simplex a range of diseases with suprabasal splitting and blistering of limbs, healing without scarring
		Junctional EB rare and often lethal
		Dystrophic EB a range of diseases with subepidermal blisters below the dermo-epidermal junction; scarring common; squamous cell carcinoma a late complication
Inflammatory	Infection (staphylococcal, streptococcal, herpes simplex virus, herpes zoster virus, coxsackievirus, fungal)	e.g. impetigo with staphylococcus, dermatomal distribution with herpes zoster
	Dermatitis	Case 5.2
	Insect bites	History
	Erythema multiforme and Stevens–Johnson syndrome (severe bullous form)	Crops of maculopapular erythema on limbs and trunk
		Lesions may expand, leaving a pale centre, the classic target lesion
		Bullae/vesicles and/or necrosis may develop within targets and in mucous membranes
		Causes include herpes simplex virus, *Mycoplasma*, infectious mononucleosis, HIV, sulphonamides, penicillin, SLE, Wegener's granulomatosis, sarcoidosis
Physical	Heat and cold	History
	Irradiation	History
	Contact with irritants	History
	Friction/rubbing	History
	Oedema	History
Drug reactions	Fixed drug eruption	Drug history, e.g. aspirin
	Erythema multiforme	Drug history, e.g. sulphonamides, NSAIDs
	Photosensitive eruption	Drug history, e.g. phenothiazines
	Toxic epidermal necrolysis	Drug history, e.g. sulphonamides, NSAIDs
Systemic	Porphyria cutanea tarda	Described below
	Carcinoma	

HIV, human immunodeficiency virus; IgA, immunoglobulin A; NSAIDs, non-steroidal anti-inflammatory drugs; SLE, systemic lupus erythematosus.

Which factors predispose to development of porphyria cutanea tarda?

Porphyria cutanea tarda is a result of acquired inhibition of hepatic uroporphyrinogen decarboxylase. Inhibitors form in the presence of iron and oxidative environments, and so a significant proportion of people with porphyria cutanea tarda have associated haemochromatosis. Other associations include the hepatitis C virus, oestrogen in the contraceptive pill or hormone replacement therapy, and excessive alcohol.

How are porphyrias diagnosed?

Porphyrin precursors can now be accurately analysed using high-performance liquid chromatography; assays of the enzymes are straightforward and molecular genetic studies are in widespread use.

Table 5.8 Pemphigoid and pemphigus

	Pemphigoid	Pemphigus
Age of onset	Over 50 years	Wide range; peak 60–70 years
Cause	Autoimmune Target antigens at dermo-epidermal junction in hemidesmosome (or a protein traversing the plasma membrane, linking to anchoring filaments and inserting to lamina densa)	Autoimmune Target antigens desmosomal – desmoglein 3 (pemphigus vulgaris) and desmoglein 1 (pemphigus foliaceous)
Clinical features	Described above	Described above
Histology	Level of splitting basement membrane	Level of splitting, and thus site of blister formation, within epidermis Intra-epidermal separation of keratinocytes, forming split between lower and upper portion of epidermis, and acantholysis (separation of individual epidermal cells from surrounding cells) Level of split subdivides two types of pemphigus – just above basal layer in pemphigus vulgaris and superficial epidermal split in pemphigus foliaceous
Direct immunofluorescence	Linear band with IgG or C3	Intra-epidermal IgG between cells throughout epidermis
Serology	IgG or C3 antibody to basement membrane in 75%	Positive in most patients, titre reflecting disease activity and can monitor disease
Complications	Most morbidity and mortality due to treatment – tendency now to treat less aggressively	Mucous membrane involvement may never fully resolve
Management	Oral then topical corticosteroids Occasionally azathioprine as steroid-sparing agent	Oral corticosteroids (higher dose than pemphigoid) Azathioprine More potent immunomodulatory drugs may be needed
Prognosis	Often remits after 2–5 years	Mortality 15–25% (100% without treatment)

IgG, immunoglobulin G.

Do porphyrias carry malignant potential?

Both acute intermittent porphyria and porphyria cutanea tarda are associated with an increased risk of hepatocellular carcinoma because of their links with liver disease, but the cutaneous porphyrias are not associated with increased skin malignancy.

Do any other conditions lead to porphyrin accumulation?

Lead poisoning causes accumulation of porphyrins by inhibiting several steps in haem synthesis, which may lead to abdominal pain, motor neuropathy, a blue line on the gum and sideroblastic anaemia with basophilic stippling.

How may acute porphyria be treated?

Avoiding precipitating factors is essential. Carbohydrate and intravenous haem therapy are synergistic in reversing the biochemical changes in acute attacks. Intravenous haem arginate inhibits ALA synthase, the initial and rate-limiting enzyme in the haem synthetic pathway. Liver transplantation is a potential treatment for those with recurrent, disabling attacks.

CASE 5.5

FACIAL RASH – SYSTEMIC LUPUS ERYTHEMATOSUS, DISCOID LUPUS ERYTHEMATOSUS, ROSACEA, SEBORRHOEIC DERMATITIS, DERMATOMYOSITIS, LUPUS PERNIO, LUPUS VULGARIS

Instruction

Please look at this patient's facial rash. Describe what you see and comment on your differential diagnosis and the likely cause.

Recognition

Systemic lupus erythematosus (SLE)

There is a *'butterfly distribution' malar rash* (Fig. 5.10). There are *raised or flat patches of malar erythema, sparing the nasolabial folds*. Other areas such as the forehead and

Table 5.9 Porphyrias

Type	Enzyme block	Mode of inheritance	Clinical features	Diagnosis
Doss porphyria	ALA dehydratase (PBG synthase)	Autosomal recessive (AR)	Abdominal pain	↑ urinary ALA and copro III Normal faecal porphyrins
Acute intermittent porphyria (AIP)	PBG deaminase (HMB synthase)	Autosomal dominant (AD)	Abdominal pain Tachycardia Hypertension or postural hypotension Constipation Motor peripheral neuropathy Muscle pain and weakness Chronic kidney disease Rhabdomyolysis Hyponatraemia Neuropsychiatric Most never develop symptoms	May be precipitated by drugs or infection Porphyrins that cannot be metabolised by the liver accumulate in the urine (even between attacks) turning it dark red on light exposure – ↑ urinary ALA and PBG
Congenital erythropoietic porphyria (CEP)	Uroporphyrin III synthase	AR	Severe skin lesions with scarring Haemolysis	Normal ALA and PBG ↑ urinary and faecal porphyrins
Porphyria cutanea tarda (PCT)	Uroporphyrinogen decarboxylase	AD	Non-acute Marked skin lesions – blisters, erosions, pigmentation, scars and milia, especially of face, and secondary scarring Often secondary to chronic liver disease, especially alcohol or haemochromatosis	Normal ALA and PBG ↑ urinary and faecal porphyrins
Hereditary coproporphyria (HC)	Coproporphyrinogen oxidase	AD	Acute Skin vesicles Neuropsychiatric	↑ ALA and PBG ↑ urinary and faecal copro III
Variegate porphyria (VP)	Protoporphyrinogen oxidase	AD	Acute Skin vesicles Neuropsychiatric	↑ faecal protoporphyrins
Erythropoietic protoporphyria (EPP)	Ferrochelatase	AD	Photosensitivity	↑ red cell and faecal protoporphyrin IX

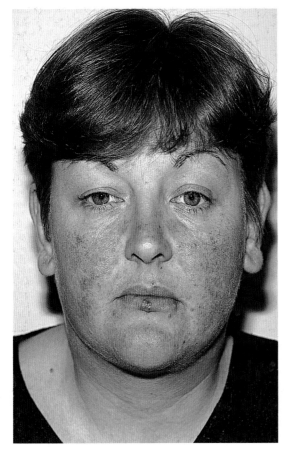

Fig. 5.10 Malar rash.

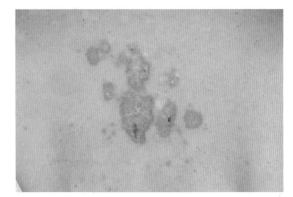

Fig. 5.11 Discoid lupus erythematosus.

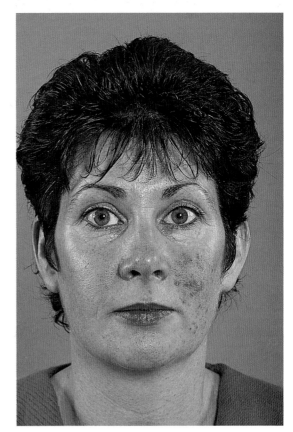

Fig. 5.12 Rosacea.

neck are often affected. There may be marked *photosensitivity*. There may be *mouth ulcers*.

Discoid lupus erythematosus (DLE)

DLE is a skin-limited disease, with well-defined erythematous papules or plaques on light exposed areas including the head, neck, hands and arms. Mostly affected are the cheeks, nose and forehead (Fig. 5.11). Like SLE, the rash is photosensitive, and more common in females. Lesions are scaling and hyperkeratosis of hair follicles gives these scales a dotted, 'nutmeg' appearance. If you were to remove the scales and inspect their under-surface, you would see spicules projecting from them. This is known as follicular keratosis or plugging (also known as the 'carpet track' sign) and no other scaling condition does this; it is specific to lupus. There may be patches of depigmentation. Once affected areas heal and the scab falls off, the skin beneath is often scarred, hypopigmented and atrophic.

Rosacea

There is an *erythematous, 'acneiform' papular eruption* on the *flush areas* or convexities of the face – *forehead, nose, cheeks, chin* (Fig. 5.12). The distribution is usually symmetrical; occasionally one side of the face is affected, and rarely, other sites – the 'V' of the chest, upper arms and back.

There are two main clinical components to rosacea, vascular (episodic flushing, erythema and telangiectasia) and inflammatory (erythematous papules and pustules). *Pustules* within the eruption are almost pathognomonic. Later

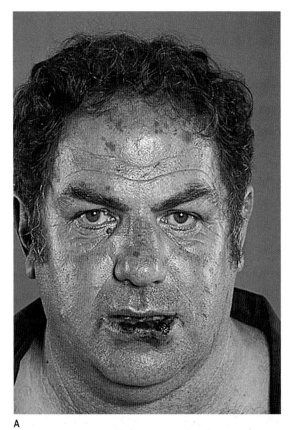

A

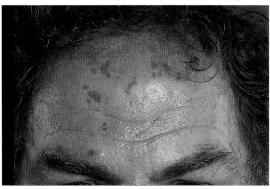

B

Fig. 5.13 (A,B) Lupus pernio

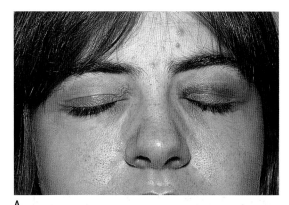

A

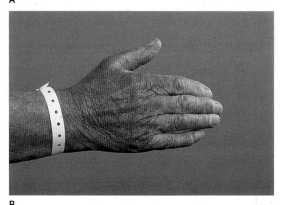

B

Fig. 5.14 (A,B) Dermatomyositis.

in disease, there is sebaceous hyperplasia, but seborrhoea and comedones (features of acne) are not features.

Seborrhoeic dermatitis

Seborrhoeic dermatitis is discussed in Case 5.2.

Dermatomyositis

There is a *heliotrope* (referring to the distinctive lilac colour of the flower so named) *rash* around the *eyelids* (Fig. 5.13). It may also affect the malar region, limb extensors, knuckles and trunk.

Gottron's papules may be present on the dorsum of the hands (notably metacarpophalangeal joints and interphalangeal joints) and occasionally elsewhere. *Nail-fold erythema* due to *dilated capillaries (telangiectasia)* is often present, and the cuticles may be ragged.

Lupus pernio

There are *purple/red/violaceous plaques on the nose, cheeks and earlobes* with *telangiectasia over and around the plaques* (Fig. 5.14). The plaques may have a yellowish translucency. They tend to flatten with time.

Lupus vulgaris

This is the skin manifestation of tuberculosis and is rare in the UK. The lesion has an 'apple jelly' consistency when a translucent slide is rested upon it.

Pulmonary hypertension/mitral stenosis

This is another cause of a malar rash.

Interpretation

Confirm the diagnosis

Some distinguishing features are shown in Box 5.2.

Box 5.2 Distinguishing features of facial rashes

Systemic lupus erythematosus (SLE)

- Spares the nasolabial folds
- Pustules not a feature

Discoid lupus erythematosus (DLE)

- Spares the nasolabial folds
- Pustules not a feature
- Scaling, follicular plugging and scarring are features of lupus but not rosacea

Rosacea

- May not spare the nasolabial folds
- Pustules characteristic
- Scaling unusual

Seborrhoeic dermatitis

- Involves the scalp, nasolabial folds or eyelids
- Scaling characteristic
- However, seborrhoeic dermatitis and rosacea may coexist

Dermatomyositis

- Characteristic colour
- Not pustular

Lupus pernio

- Not pustular
- Surface of nose thickened in lupus pernio, although telangiectactic, smooth and lacks the rugose peau d'orange surface of rhinophyma

Lupus vulgaris

- Not pustular

Pulmonary hypertension

- Other signs, e.g. signs of mitral stenosis

Box 5.3 Worrying associations of facial rashes

Systemic lupus erythematosus (SLE)

- Multi-organ involvement, e.g. kidneys, lung, nervous system

Discoid lupus erythematosus (DLE)

- Not associated with multi-organ involvement

Rosacea

- Complications (more common in males)
- Rhinophyma (overgrowth of fibrous tissue and glands on nose, often seen in elderly men as thickened erythematous skin with enlarged follicles)
- Lymphoedema (particularly under the eyes)
- Ocular involvement (blepharitis, conjunctivitis, episcleritis and keratitis)

Seborrhoeic dermatitis

- Marginal keratitis

Dermatomyositis

- Occasionally associated with neoplasms, e.g. colorectal, ovarian, breast, lung

Lupus pernio

- Multi-organ involvement, e.g. lungs, central nervous system

Lupus vulgaris

- Unrecognised or untreated tuberculosis

Pulmonary hypertension

- Cardiac decompensation

What to do next – assess other systems

SLE is a multisystem disease; DLE is limited. Rosacea is not a multi-system disease. Seborrhoeic dermatitis is discussed in Case 5.2. In dermatomyositis, look for symmetrical weakness in a proximal muscle distribution (polymyositis). Lupus pernio is a manifestation of sarcoidosis.

Consider severity/decompensation/complications

Some worrying associations of facial rashes are listed in Box 5.3.

Consider function

Burning symptoms, itching and dryness can be distracting. Facial rashes can, of course, be psychologically damaging.

Discussion

Which treatments may be used for the rash of lupus erythematosus?

Treatments include moderately potent topical steroids and hydroxychloroquine. Sunscreens are essential.

What causes rosacea?

Rosacea is a common, chronic inflammatory skin disease tending to affect middle-aged patients (mostly 30–50 years), especially females. Precipitating factors include heat, sun, alcohol, spicy foods, emotion/embarrassment and corticosteroids. A *Demodex folliculorum* theory implicates pilosebaceous follicular mites as an underlying cause, but this is not certain.

How is rosacea treated?

Corticosteroids should not be used. They are not effective in the long term and tend to cause skin addiction and 'flares' of severe rebound erythema, which do not easily settle. Avoidance of precipitating factors is seldom helpful except for the use of sunscreens. Topical treatments include metronidazole or erythromycin gel, with an emollient.

Systemic treatments include tetracycline (often prolonged as low-dose maintenance treatment), minocycline and doxycycline. Although remissions with treatment occur, long-term treatment is usually needed. Topical tretinoin helps vascular features and, in severe cases, pulsed dye laser therapy is used.

What is acne vulgaris?

The aetiology and pathology of acne and rosacea are not related. Acne vulgaris is a chronic inflammatory disorder of the sebaceous glands associated with hair follicles, characterised by comedones (non-inflamed lesions), erythematous papules, pustules and nodules (inflamed lesions) and scarring. Scarring tends to be hypertrophic and keloid (trunk) or 'ice pick' (cheeks). Acneiform lesions are mostly distributed on the face, back, chest and anogenital region, the distribution of pilosebaceous structures, although sebaceous glands are also distributed in areas not associated with hair follicles, including the eyelids (whose follicles are separate structures) and these do not give rise to acne. Sebaceous glands contain holocrine cells which secrete triglycerides, fatty acids, wax and sterols as sebum. Four main factors conspire to cause acne:

- There is primarily an increase in androgen-induced seborrhoea or sebum production by the sebaceous glands, although testosterone levels are not increased, and there is a correlation between sebum excretion rate and acne severity.
- Abnormal proliferation and differentiation of pilosebaceous ductal keratinocytes is central to increased sebum production and leads to formation of the primary acne lesion, the microcomedone (commonly present in normal looking skin). Thickening (cornification) of the keratin lining of the duct is associated with an increase in sebum lipid content and keratinocyte comedogenesis. Larger lesions are visible as closed or open comedones, comedones representing retention of hyperproliferating ductal corneocytes. Comedones may be open forming 'blackheads' (the colour mainly caused by melanin, not dirt) or closed forming 'whiteheads'.
- Duct occlusion leads to enlargement of the sebaceous gland, leakage of sebum into the dermis and colonisation of the sebaceous gland and duct with *Proprionibacterium acnes* and other bacteria.
- A significant inflammatory infiltrate is seen around follicles before evidence of comedone formation, but inflammation remains prominent as acne progresses as red papules, pustules and nodules.

How is acne vulgaris treated?

Treatment involves tackling the above four factors.

- Seborrhoea may be treated by reducing either sebaceous gland size with isotretinoin or androgen drive with anti-androgens and oral contraceptives.
- Sebaceous gland blockage may be treated with retinoids or benzoyl peroxide.
- Bacterial colonisation is treated with antibiotics, benzoyl peroxide or azelaic acid.
- Inflammation is treated with retinoids, antibiotics and, in severe cases, oral or topical corticosteroids.

For mild acne, topical retinoid targets comedogenesis and in combination with a topical antimicrobial such as benzoyl peroxide or erythromycin may help. Moderate acne may require oral antibiotics (or hormonal therapy) in addition to topical therapy. For severe acne oral isotretinoin may be indicated after a few unsuccessful courses of antibiotic, although persistence for some months with the latter is needed; high-dose antibiotics may also be needed.

What is isotretinoin?

It is a dietary metabolite of vitamin A with anti-inflammatory, regulatory and inhibitory effects on sebaceous glands, and the gold standard for severe recalcitrant cystic acne. It is teratogenic.

CASE 5.6

SCLERODERMA, VITILIGO AND AUTOIMMUNE SKIN DISEASE

Instruction

Please examine this patient's hands and face and report your findings.

Recognition

Scleroderma – face

There is facial *telangiectasia*. The skin is *smooth*, *shiny* and *tight*. There is *perioral skin puckering* (Fig. 5.15).

Scleroderma – hands

There is *sclerodactyly, nail-fold erythema due to dilated nail-fold capillaries* (telangiectasia), *nail-fold infarction, ragged cuticles, digital ischaemia, pulp atrophy, calcinosis* and *Raynaud's phenomenon*.

Interpretation

Confirm the diagnosis

Skin signs are characteristic, but serology is needed for confirmation.

What to do next – assess other systems

Skin signs are common in autoimmune connective tissue diseases (Box 5.4, Fig 5.16).

Consider severity/decompensation/complications

Lung disease (pulmonary hypertension and interstitial lung disease) is an important cause of morbidity and mortality (Case 1.18).

Consider function

Sclerodactyly can restrict hand function and Raynaud's phenomenon causes pain. Restrictive lung function may cause breathlessness.

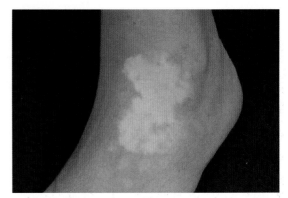

Fig. 5.16 Vitiligo.

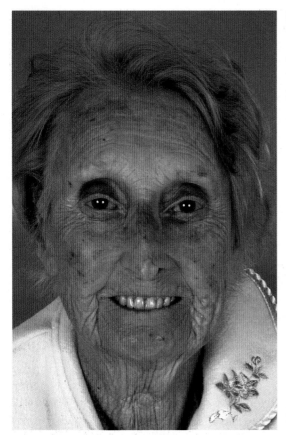

Fig. 5.15 Scleroderma.

Box 5.5 Causes of alopecia

Non-scarring alopecia

- Male pattern (androgenic) baldness
- Stress
- Hypopituitarism
- Thyroid disease
- Hypoparathyroidism
- Diabetes mellitus
- Pregnancy
- Drugs, e.g. cytotoxics, antithyroid drugs, anticoagulants, cyclosporin

Scarring alopecia

- Psoriasis
- Dermatitis
- Lichen planus
- Fungal and other infections
- Trauma and burns
- Lupus erythematosus
- Morphea
- Sarcoidosis

Box 5.4 Skin signs in autoimmune connective tissue diseases

Raynaud's phenomenon

- Part of scleroderma spectrum
- Cold white hands (ischaemia), turn blue (stasis) then red (reactive hyperaemia) with pain

Rheumatoid arthritis

- Cutaneous/nail-fold vasculitis
- Nodules
- Pyoderma gangrenosum

Systemic lupus erythematosus (SLE)

- Malar erythema, sparing nasolabial folds

Dermatomyositis

- Heliotrope rash (especially of eyelids)
- Gottron's papules
- Nail-fold erythema

Vitiligo

- Often idiopathic
- Often associated with autoimmune disease (see Fig. 5.16)

Discussion

What is alopecia areata?

This causes diffuse, patchy hair loss and does not scar (the hair follicles are not destroyed) and 'exclamation mark' hairs may be seen 'sprouting in the desert'. It is associated with nail pitting, vitiligo and autoimmune disease.

List some other causes of non-scarring alopecia

These are listed in Box 5.5.

List some causes of scarring alopecia

These are listed in Box 5.5.

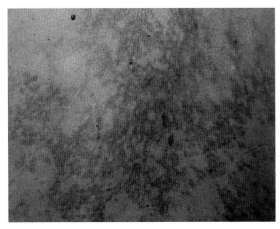

Fig. 5.17 Telangiectasia.

> **Box 5.6 Causes of mouth ulceration**
>
> - Aphthous ulcers
> - Traumatic ulcers
> - Lichen planus
> - Infection, e.g. candidiasis, herpes simplex virus
> - Stevens–Johnson syndrome
> - Pemphigus
> - Carcinoma
> - Behçet's disease
> - Crohn's disease

CASE 5.7

ORAL LESIONS – HEREDITARY HAEMORRHAGIC TELANGIECTASIA, PEUTZ–JEGHERS SYNDROME

Instruction

Please examine this patient's mouth and comment on your findings.

Recognition

Hereditary haemorrhagic telangiectasia (HHT)

There are *dilated capillaries/venules of the lips and tongue* and *around the mouth* (Fig. 5.17), *nail beds, hands* and frequently elsewhere. There may be evidence of recent epistaxis.

Peutz–Jeghers syndrome

The *lips* are *pigmented*.

Other

Other oral lesions you could encounter include perioral dermatitis, lichen planus, leucoplakia, candida, pemphigus and Addison's disease pigmentation.

Interpretation

Confirm the diagnosis

HHT is usually unmistakable (when overt, but mild forms with expression in later life occur, for example with iron deficiency anaemia). The circumoral and mucosal pigmentation of Peutz–Jeghers syndrome is usually less diffuse than that of Addison's disease.

What to do next – assess other systems

In HHT there may be arteriovenous malformations – direct connections between arteries and veins – throughout the gastrointestinal tract, liver, lungs and nervous system. Tell the examiners you would check for:

- Pallor (iron deficiency anaemia due to gastrointestinal haemorrhage)
- Hepatic bruits
- Dyspnoea/tachypnoea/cyanosis (polycythaemia)
- Chest bruits

Consider severity/decompensation/complications

Tell the examiners that you would ask about neurological problems in HHT. These may result from an intracranial arteriovenous malformation (subarachnoid haemorrhage is one the most serious complications of HHT) or from an embolic stroke arising from a pulmonary arteriovenous malformation. Gastrointestinal bleeding and malignancy may complicate Peutz–Jeghers syndrome.

Consider function

Any disability depends upon the disorder. For example, HHT may cause fatigue due to anaemia.

Discussion

What causes hereditary haemorrhagic telangiectasia?

HHT refers to a group of autosomal dominant diseases genetically linked to chromosomes 9 and 12. In some families the implicated gene encodes endoglin, a protein on endothelial cells that binds transforming growth factor-β (TGF-β).

What is Peutz–Jeghers syndrome?

This is an autosomal dominant disorder characterised by mucocutaneous melanosis (lentigo) and gastrointestinal hamartomas.

List some causes of mouth ulcers

These are listed in Box 5.6.

CASE 5.8

NAIL LESIONS

Instruction

Please look at this patient's nails and comment on the possible cause.

Recognition

Psoriasis

There is *pitting*, *onycholysis* and *subungual hyperkeratosis*.

Lichen planus

Occasionally lichen planus may cause *atrophy of the nail plate* (which may disappear altogether or exhibit longitudinal furrows) and the cuticle may advance forwards.

Nail lines

Beau's lines are *transverse* depressions representing altered growth rate and are a non-specific sign of previous illness or physiological change. *Onychomedesis* refers to shedding of the nail, which may occur in severe illness. *Longitudinal* depressions or ridges may occur in lichen planus, alopecia areata and Darier's disease (dystrophy with a series of longitudinal streaks which end in triangular nicks at the free margin).

Clubbing

Clubbing progresses through four phases (Box 5.7).

Leuconychia

The nails appear *white*.

Koilonychia

The nails (especially the fingernails) are *brittle* and *concave* or 'spoon-shaped'.

Interpretation

Confirm the diagnosis

Some distinguishing features of nail lesions are shown in Box 5.8.

What to do next – assess other systems

What to do next is outlined in Box 5.9.

Consider severity/decompensation/complications

This depends upon the underlying disease.

Consider function

This depends upon the underlying disease.

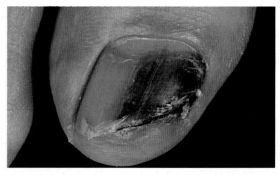

Fig. 5.18 Onychomycosis.

Box 5.7 Phases of clubbing

1. Swelling of the soft tissues of the terminal phalanx with fluctuant nail beds.
2. A permanently decreased angle between the nail plate and the posterior nail fold (this defines clubbing)
3. Increased curvature of the nails due to soft tissue hypertrophy Shamroth's sign may be used to confirm 2 and 3 – when the distal phalanges of corresponding digits of opposite hands are directly apposed, fingernail to fingernail, a small diamond-shaped window is apparent between the nailbeds; if obliterated, the test is positive and clubbing is present
4. Hypertrophic pulmonary osteoarthropathy (HPOA), a rare and most extreme form

---

Box 5.8 Distinguishing features of nail lesions

Psoriasis
- Pitting characteristic but not pathognomonic
- Onycholysis (often with discoloured, thickened, hyperkeratotic but brittle, dystrophic nails) may also be caused by fungal infection (onychomycosis, see Fig. 5.18), trauma, dermatitis, peripheral vascular disease, thyrotoxicosis (Plummer's nails) or may be idiopathic, sometimes associated with excessive wetting of nails and chronic bacterial paronychia

Lichen planus
- No pathognomonic features

Beau's lines
- History of systemic illness

Clubbing
- Defined by the angle between the nail plate and the posterior nail fold

Leuconychia
- A little subjective

Koilonychia
- Characteristic shape

Box 5.9 Assessing other systems in nail lesions

Psoriasis
- Look at the joints for evidence of psoriatic arthropathy

Lichen planus
- Look in the mouth for intraoral lichen planus

Beau's lines
- Tell the examiners you would explore systemic illness

Clubbing
- Tell the examiners that clubbing may be caused by chronic suppurative lung disease, lung cancer, idiopathic fibrosing alveolitis, infective endocarditis, congenital cyanotic heart disease, chronic liver disease and inflammatory bowel disease; it may be congenital or idiopathic

Leuconychia
- Look for signs of chronic liver disease

Koilonychia
- Consider iron deficiency anaemia

Table 5.10 Nail discoloration

Discoloration	Cause
Yellow/brownish tinge	Dystrophic nails of any cause Chronic kidney disease
Leuconychia	Chronic liver disease
'Half and half' nails in which proximal halves are pale and the distal halves pink	Chronic kidney disease
Isolated pigment discoloration beneath a nail	Subungual melanoma (melanin may also cause brown longitudinal streaks)
Blue-tinged lunula	Wilson's disease
Yellow, curved nails	Yellow nail syndrome (associated with pleural effusion, bronchiectasis, nephrotic syndrome, malignancy, lymphoedema, thyroid disease and rheumatoid disease)
Drug staining	Tetracyclines (yellow) Antimalarials (blue)

Discussion

How do the nail changes in psoriasis arise?

Nails comprise a nail bed, on top of which grows the highly keratinised nail plate (between the posterior and lateral nail folds and anterior free margin) from the nail matrix beneath the lunula and cuticle. Psoriasis causes keratin thickening of the nail. Loss of minute plugs of normal keratin results in characteristic *pitting* and sometimes the thickened, dystrophic nail separates from its nail bed (*onycholysis*).

What is onychogryphosis?

This is hypertrophy of the nail plate, often resulting from chronic trauma.

What other causes of nail discoloration do you know?

Causes of nail discoloration are listed in Table 5.10.

CASE 5.9

SHIN LESIONS – ERYTHEMA NODOSUM, PYODERMA GANGRENOSUM, NECROBIOSIS LIPODICA DIABETICORUM, PRETIBIAL MYXOEDEMA

Instruction

Please examine the rash on this patient's legs and discuss your findings.

Recognition

Erythema nodosum

There are *erythematous* (progressing through the colour changes of a bruise), *warm, nodular* (flatten with healing) *lesions over the anterior aspect of both shins* (Fig. 5.19). They may be single or multiple, of various sizes, and may occur elsewhere. Ask if they are *tender* (before you examine them!). Lesions evolve slowly, changing from acute red nodules to residual bruises over a period of weeks.

Pyoderma gangrenosum

Several variants of pyoderma gangrenosum exist. *Classic pyoderma gangrenosum* is a *deep ulcer* with a *well-defined border* that is usually violet or blue (Fig. 5.20). The ulcer edge may be undermined (worn and damaged) and the surrounding skin may be erythematous and indurated. The ulcer often starts as a red papule or nodule or collection of papules, which break down to form small ulcers with a 'cat's paw' appearance; these coalesce and the central area becomes necrotic and forms the ulcer. Lesions are painful. Pyoderma gangrenosum can occur at any site, but the face and legs are common sites. Healing often leaves a papery scar.

Variants include *peristomal* pyoderma gangrenosum (around 15% of all cases), *pustular pyoderma gangrenosum* (a rare, superficial variant), *bullous pyoderma gangrenosum* (a superficial variant that tends to affect the upper limbs or face and often associated with haematological malignancy) and *vegetative pyoderma gangrenosum* (a less aggressive superficial form).

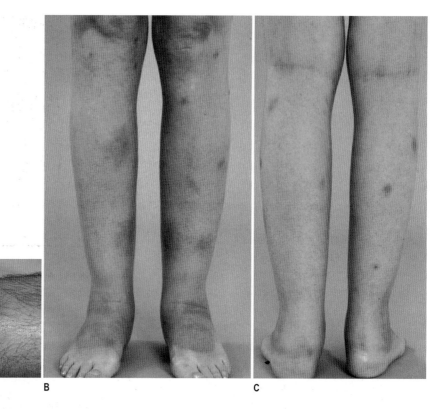

A   B   C

Fig. 5.19 (A–C) Erythema nodosum.

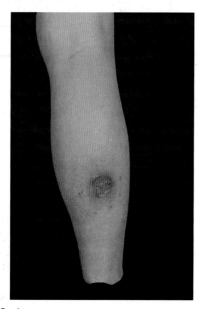

Fig. 5.20 Pyoderma gangrenosum.

Box 5.10 Features to help confirm diagnosis	
Erythema nodosum	characteristically tender
Pyoderma gangrenosum	characteristically ulcerated
Necrobiosis lipoidica	characteristically exhibits telangiectasia
Pretibial myxoedema	characteristic 'orange-peel' surface

Necrobiosis lipoidica (diabeticorum)

There are *well-demarcated (often oval) non-scaling plaques* on the shins (Fig. 5.21). Characteristically they occur on the legs but they may occur anywhere else. They have a *shiny, atrophic surface, red/brown margins* and *yellow waxy*

centres. Surface telangiectasia is characteristic. Trauma often results in persistent ulceration (Fig. 5.22).

Pretibial myxoedema

There are *elevated symmetrical shin lesions* (Fig. 5.23). Such lesions may occur at other sites. They are *coarse, purplish red or brown,* with *well-defined edges.* The *skin is shiny,* with an *orange peel appearance.* The lesions may be asymptomatic or painful. Coarse hairs tend to occur in the vicinity of the lesions.

Interpretation

Confirm the diagnosis

Some confirmatory features are listed in Box 5.10.

What to do next – consider causes

Causes of erythema nodosum and pyoderma gangrenosum are listed in Table 5.11.

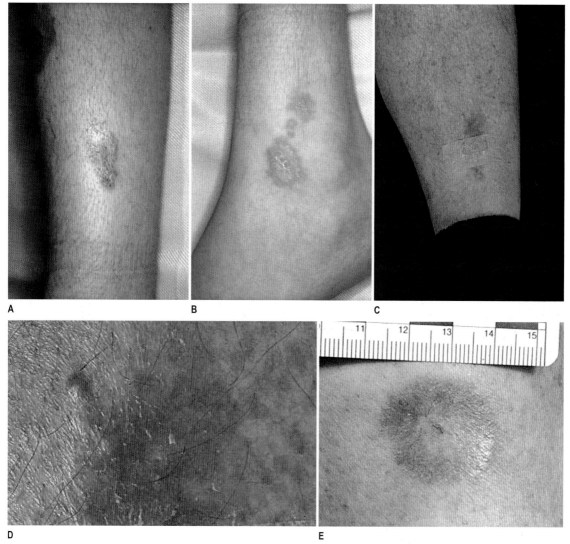

A   B   C

D   E

Fig. 5.21 (A–E) Necrobiosis lipoidica diabeticorum.

Pretibial myxoedema is specific to Graves' disease. Necrobiosis lipoidica may occur in diabetes.

Consider severity/decompensation/complications

This depends upon the underlying disease.

Consider function

This depends upon the underlying disease.

Discussion

What is the histology of pretibial myxoedema?

The superficial layer of the skin is infiltrated with muco-polysaccharides and hyaluronic acid. Keloid scarring occurs post biopsy.

How does necrobiosis lipoidica diabeticorum arise?

Necrobiosis lipoidica diabeticorum affects < 0.5% of diabetes patients and there is, in essence, degeneration and thickening of collagen bundles within the dermis with a palisading granuloma (similar to another condition, granuloma annulare, which may also occur in diabetes). Lesions progress slowly and seldom resolve. There is no effective treatment but topical or intralesional steroids occasionally help. Lesions often recur at the sites of skin grafts.

List some other skin manifestations of diabetes

- Infection
- Arterial foot ulcers
- Vitiligo
- Lipoatrophy

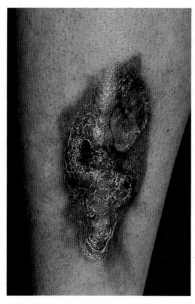

Fig. 5.22 Necrobiosis lipoidica diabeticorum – ulcerated.

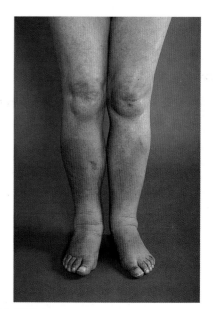

Fig. 5.23 Petibial myxoedema.

Table 5.11 Causes of erythema nodosum and pyoderma gangrenosum		
	Erythema nodosum	Pyoderma gangrenosum
Infection	Viral Streptococcus (sore throat) Salmonella or Campylobacter (enteritis) Primary tuberculosis Leprosy Fungi	Uncommon, but pyoderma gangrenosum should be in the differential diagnosis of any non-healing ulcer
Drugs	Oral contraceptive pill Sulphonamides Tetracyclines Penicillin	Uncommon
Inflammation	Ulcerative colitis Crohn's disease	Ulcerative colitis Crohn's disease
Other systemic disease	Sarcoidosis, commonly with arthralgia and bilateral hilar lymphadenopathy	Rheumatoid arthritis Ankylosing spondylitis Chronic active hepatitis Primary biliary cirrhosis Sclerosing cholangitis Sarcoidosis Diabetes mellitus Thyroid disease
Malignancy	Lymphoma	Lymphoproliferative and myeloproliferative disorders
Other	Pregnancy	

Mention some causes of leg ulceration

These include infection, chronic venous insufficiency, peripheral vascular disease, vasculitis, neuropathy (often with Charcot's joints), pyoderma gangrenosum, sickle cell disease and malignancy.

How is pyoderma gangrenosum treated?

Strategies include topical or systemic corticosteroids, immunosuppressants such as ciclosporin, azathioprine and tacrolimus, and potentially anti-tumour necrosis factor-α agents.

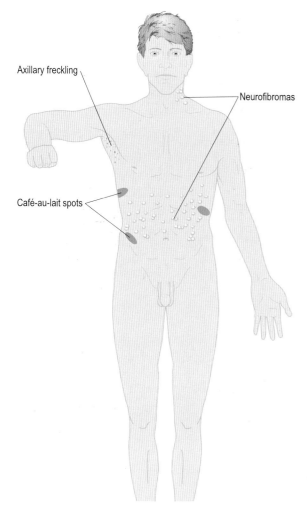

Axillary freckling

Neurofibromas

Café-au-lait spots

Fig. 5.24 Café-au-lait spots, neurofibromas and axillary freckling.

CASE 5.10

NEUROFIBROMATOSIS

Instruction

Please look at this patient's skin and axillae and discuss your findings.

Recognition

There are multiple *café au lait spots*, each more than 15 mm in greatest diameter. There is *axillary and skin-fold freckling*. There are multiple *neurofibromas*. These may be soft mobile subcutaneous lumps or nodules along peripheral nerves (Fig. 5.24).

> **Box 5.11 Diagnostic criteria for neurofibromatosis 1 (NF1)**
>
> Two or more of the following are diagnostic:
>
> - Six or more café-au-lait spots (> 5 mm in diameter prepubertal or > 15 mm in diameter postpubertal)
> - Two or more neurofibromas of any type or one plexiform neurofibroma
> - Axillary or inguinal freckling
> - Optic glioma
> - Two or more Lisch nodules
> - Osseous lesion, e.g. sphenoid dysplasia, thinning of long bone cortex
> - First-degree relative with NF1 by above criteria

Interpretation

Confirm the diagnosis

There are two types of neurofibromatosis – NF1 and NF2; NF1 is much more common. The diagnostic criteria for NF1, based on the 1987 NIH consensus, are shown in Box 5.11.

Other causes of abnormal pigmentation include Addison's disease, Peutz–Jeghers syndrome, haemosiderin deposition, haemochromatosis, uraemia and amiodarone, but neurofibromatosis should be obvious.

What to do next – assess other systems

Look for those features in Table 5.12. Lisch nodules are melanocytic hamartomas of the iris, appearing as well-defined, yellow-brown, dome-shaped elevations on the surface of the iris. They might only be visible on slit lamp examination.

Consider severity/decompensation/complications

Around 50% of people with NF1 develop complications (Box 5.12). By far the commonest are learning problems, often with coordination and behavioural disturbance. Plexiform neurofibromas are also common. All other complications are unusual, with a frequency under 5%. Complications cannot be predicted, even within families.

Consider function

Tell the examiners that function may be affected by learning difficulties, peripheral nerve involvement or orthopaedic complications. Epilepsy affects driving.

Discussion

What is neurofibromatosis?

Neurofibromatoses are a group of disorders characterised by tumours of the nervous system and characteristic skin pigmentation. The type of peripheral nerve tumour (neurofibroma versus schwannoma), the presence or absence of café-au-lait spots and skin-fold freckling and the presence of certain ophthalmic features characterise each type. Two main types – NF1 and NF2 – are different at molecular and clinical levels.

Table 5.12 Clinical features of neurofibromatosis 1 (NF1)

Major defining features	Frequency	Significance
Café-au-lait spots	> 99%	Cosmetic
Freckling (skin fold)	> 99%	Cosmetic
Peripheral neurofibromas	67%	Two types, each comprising all elements of a peripheral nerve
		Dermal neurofibroma — **Nodular neurofibroma**
		Most patients — 5–10% of patients
		Arise from dermis and epidermis — Arise from major peripheral nerve
		Move with skin
		Discrete
		Soft
		Violatious colour — Firm
		Usually asymptomatic — Neurological symptoms common
		No malignant potential — Higher risk of malignant peripheral nerve sheath tumours (MPNSTs)
Lisch nodules (iris hamartomas)	90–95%	Cosmetic

Box 5.12 Complications of neurofibromatosis 1 (NF1)

Learning problems
- Usually minor

Plexiform neurofibroma (fusiform enlargement rather than subcutaneous nodules)
- Large lesion of head and neck
- Limb or trunk lesions associated with skin and bone hypertrophy

Epilepsy
- Central nervous system tumours
- Optic gliomas
- Spinal neurofibromas
- Other

Aqueduct stenosis

Orthopaedic
- Scoliosis
- Pseudoarthrosis of tibia and fibula
- Vertical scalloping
- Sphenoid wing dysplasia

Malignancy
- Malignant peripheral nerve sheath tumours (MPNSTs)
- Pelvic rhabdomyosarcomas

Other tumours
- Gastrointestinal neurofibromas
- Phaeochromocytomas
- Duodenal carcinoid
- Glomus tumours of nail beds

Vascular
- Renal artery stenosis
- Cerebrovascular disease

How common are the neurofibromatoses?

NF1 is one of the most common autosomal dominant conditions, with an incidence of around 1 in 3000 births. Its major features – café-au-lait spots, neurofibromas and Lisch nodules – are not associated with other problems. NF2 is much less common with an incidence of around 1 in 30 000 to 1 in 40 000.

What is the genetic basis of the neurofibromatoses?

Inheritance of both NF1 and NF2 is autosomal dominant, but about 50% of cases of NF1 and NF2 are first cases within a family; penetrance is 100% by age five such that if no café-au-lait spots are present by then it can be inferred that NF1 has not been inherited. The genes in both types normally act as tumour suppressors. The NF1 gene is on chromosome 17 and encodes the protein neurofibromin, a GTPase-activating protein for the p21 ras protein family that normally inhibits ras by converting active ras-GTP to inactive ras-GDP. Neurofibromin absence thus leads to cell growth activation. The NF1 gene is large, with many mutations with slightly varying clinical manifestations, whereas NF2 tends to cause predictable features within a family. The NF2 gene is on chromosome 22 and encodes the protein merlin (schwannomin), part of the Ezrin–Radixin–Moexin (ERM) sub-group of the protein 4.1 super family. Merlin is a negative growth regulator and affects cell signalling.

Do café-au-lait spots occur in unaffected people?

Around 10% of people have one or two café-au-lait spots. A small number of patients with NF1 have fewer than six spots, and disease can be identified by a positive family history and observation to teenage years for neurofibromas, or by genetic testing.

Is genetic testing used routinely in diagnosing neurofibromatoses?

Genetic testing is not routine because clinical diagnosis is usually straightforward and there is a large array of possible genetic mutations. It may be used in prenatal counselling or to establish diagnosis in rare situations where NF1 diagnostic criteria are fulfilled but with very limited evidence of disease – NF1 limited to a segment with just six café-au-lait spots and axillary freckles, known as mosaic NF1 and which may not be inheritable as gonadal tissue may be unaffected, or a rare homozygous recessive disorder of mismatch repair genes in which there are six or more café-au-lait spots and an affected sibling, but no other features.

What are the features of NF2?

The hallmark of NF2 is bilateral vestibular schwannomas, this term now preferred to acoustic neuromas because they are schwannomas histologically and arise from the vestibular branch of the VIIIth nerve. They are usually diagnosed with magnetic resonance imaging. Meningiomas and other cranial nerve and spinal root schwannomas are also common. The most sensitive and specific criteria are the Manchester criteria (Box 5.13).

Box 5.13 Diagnostic criteria for neurofibromatosis 2 (NF2)

Any one of the following is diagnostic:

- Bilateral vestibular schwannomas
- First-degree relative with NF2 and unilateral vestibular schwannoma or any two of: mengingioma, schwannoma, glioma, neurofibroma, posterior subcapsular lenticular opacities
- Unilateral vestibular schwannoma and any two of: mengingioma, schwannoma, glioma, neurofibroma, posterior subcapsular lenticular opacities
- Multiple meningiomas (two or more) and unilateral vestibular schwannoma and any two of: schwannoma, glioma, neurofibroma, cataract

---

Unlike NF1, NF2 is associated with significant morbidity and mortality in all patients (Table 5.13).

How may NF2 be distinguished from NF1?

NF2 is usually easy to distinguish from NF1, except in a small number of cases of NF2 with a few café-au-lait spots and peripheral nerve tumours indistinguishable from those in NF1. However, histologically these are schwannomas in NF2. NF2 does not cause skin-fold freckling but does cause a unique skin lesion, the NF2 plaque. NF2 also causes ophthalmic complications (see Table 5.13).

How are neurofibromatoses managed?

NF1 management in adults is largely education-based, teaching patients about possible complications. NF2 is managed in multidisciplinary specialist centres.

CASE 5.11

TUBEROSE SCLEROSIS

Instruction

Please look at this patient's face and discuss your findings.

Recognition

There are multiple small skin lesions on the face. There are several flesh coloured or pink papules on the nose and cheeks. These are *angiofibromata* (Fig. 5.25) (once incorrectly called adenoma sebaceum). Leathery, lumpy, flesh-coloured *shagreen patches* may be present, often on the trunk. There may also be *hypopigmented macules* in an *oval or mountain ash leaf configuration. Periungual fibromata* arise from the proximal nail folds of the fingers or toes.

Table 5.13 Clinical features of neurofibromatosis 2 (NF2)

Major defining features	Frequency	
Nervous system tumours	Bilateral vestibular schwannomas	85%
	Meningiomas	45%
	Peripheral nervous system involvement	70%
	Other, e.g. ependymomas, astrocytomas	
NF2 plaques	Discrete, well circumscribed, slightly raised lesions, usually < 2 cm in diameter	Around 50%
Café-au-lait spots	Four or more	Nearly 50% (six very rare)
Ophthalmic features	Cataracts (posterior capsular or cortical or both)	80%
	Retinal hamartomas	

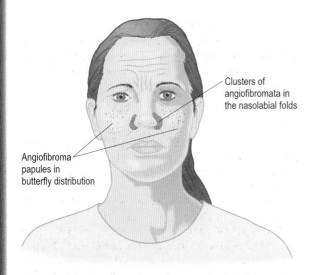

Clusters of
angiofibromata in
the nasolabial folds

Angiofibroma
papules in
butterfly distribution

Fig. 5.25 Angiofibromata.

Table 5.14 Organ involvement in tuberose sclerosis	
Organ	**Problems**
Skin hamartomata	Angiofibromata
Cerebral cortex hamartomata	Epilepsy Learning difficulties
Retinal hamartomata	Visual disturbance
Renal hamartomata	Cysts including polycystic kidney disease
Cardiac hamartomata	Arrhythmias Heart failure
Lung hamartomata	Cystic lung disease Pneumothorax
Bone hamartomata	

Interpretation

Confirm the diagnosis

Angiofibromata are very similar to adenoma sebaceum. They tend to be symmetrical, e.g. nasolabial folds, butterfly rash.

What to do next – assess other systems

Tell the examiners that you would ask about other organ involvement (Table 5.14).

Consider severity/decompensation/complications

This depends on the distribution of hamartomata.

Consider function

Tell the examiners that epilepsy occurs in most cases of tuberose sclerosis.

Discussion

What is the genetic basis of tuberose sclerosis?

It is an autosomal dominant condition (TSC1 gene at 9q34 and TSC2 gene at 16p13.3) in which hamartomatas occur in multiple organs.

CASE 5.12

NEOPLASTIC SKIN LESIONS

Instruction

Please examine this skin lesion and suggest some differential diagnoses.

Recognition

This lesion has a *rolled, pearly edge* and is characteristic of a basal cell carcinoma (Fig. 5.26).

Interpretation

Confirm the diagnosis

Tell the examiners that you would take a history for sun exposure.

What to do next – consider causes

Important neoplastic skin lesions arising in the epidermis are malignant melanoma, squamous cell carcinoma (often with a keratotic surface) and basal cell carcinoma (pearly tendency, but may be raised red patches or ulcerated). Less common skin tumours arise from blood vessels (e.g. angiosarcoma) or connective tissue (e.g. dermatofibromasarcoma); lymphoma can also arise in the skin.

Consider severity/decompensation/complications

Basal cell carcinoma may become deeply invasive if untreated. Metastases are more likely with malignant melanoma and squamous cell carcinoma.

Consider function

This depends upon site and spread of tumour.

Discussion

What is meant by the term pigmented lesion?

Pigmented lesion usually implies melanocytic naevi (moles). Non-melanocytic lesions can appear pigmented such as seborrhoeic keratoses or vascular lesions. Blue

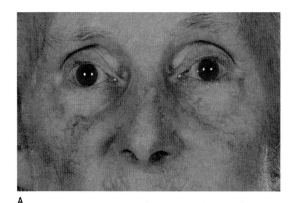

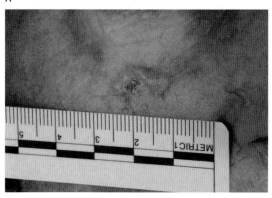

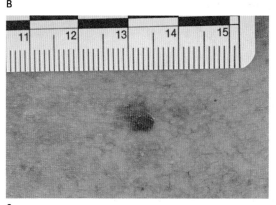

C

Fig. (A–C) 5.26 Basal cell carcinoma.

naevi (well-circumscribed blue nodules) or halo naevi (pigmented lesions with a white 'atoll') are benign. The crucial decision is whether a pigmented lesion could be malignant melanoma (Table 5.15).

Do you know of any premalignant sun-related lesions?

These include solar keratoses, cutaneous horns, actinic chelitis, disseminated superficial actinic parakeratosis and Bowen's disease.

What is malignant melanoma?

This is a malignant tumour arising from melanocytes, the pigment-producing cells of the epidermis. It has high metastatic potential. The incidence continues to rise sharply.

Do you know of any factors that increase the risk of melanoma?

Sun (UV) exposure is the major risk factor, and while incidence is highest in parts of the world with the longest hours of sunlight, the pattern of exposure is important.

Skin type is important, white people with red hair, freckled and pale skin phenotype at greater risk.

Dysplastic naevus syndrome increases the risk. More than 50 atypical naevi increases the risk almost 200-fold, and a family history increases it 500-fold. Even one to four atypical moles has a fivefold increased risk. The atypical mole syndrome affects around 2% of the population with a lifetime risk of melanoma of around 1 in 20. More then 50 benign naevi > 2 mm in diameter also carry a moderately increased risk of melanoma. Congenital naevi, especially giant naevi > 20 cm, carry considerable risk.

Family history confers a modestly increased risk, and there is increasing genetic understanding of this.

Where does malignant melanoma tend to arise?

Melanoma arises on any part of the body, commonly the legs in women and back and trunk in men.

What types of malignant melanoma are there?

Types of melanoma are listed in Table 5.16.

How is malignant melanoma managed?

Prognosis directly relates to depth of invasion, measured histologically from the cornified layer to the deepest invading malignant cell – the Breslow thickness. Sentinel lymph node biopsy also adds prognostic information. Surgical excision is the only curative treatment but if caught early has an excellent prognosis, a Breslow thickness, under 1-mm, a five-year survival of 95–100%. Suspicious lesions are excised under a maximum two-week wait system and if histologically confirmed as melanoma a wider excision then performed. Avoidance of sunburn, and the sun between the most risky hours of 11 a.m. and 3 p.m., is crucial, as are public health measures such as the Slip-Slop-Slap campaign in Australia in the 1990s – slip on a shirt, slop on some sunscreen and slap on a hat. For a condition that is common (about 1 in 100 people have melanoma), curative if detected early, and relatively easy to detect (skin examination), screening might seem logical, although it would need to be undertaken regularly; currently only high-risk people are screened, and privately funded clinics offering skin photography with computerised annual comparisons of lesions are sparsely available.

Table 5.15 Assessing possible melanoma

Assessment	Features of concern		
Lesions that could be melanoma	New lesion (almost two-thirds of melanomas arise de novo), especially over the age of 30 Change in existing mole in size, shape, colour or symptoms		
Risk factors for melanoma	Familial dysplastic naevus syndrome (atypical naevi are 3–15 mm in diameter with variable colour, and an irregular edge) Multiple melanocytic naevi (more than 50 > 2 mm in diameter) Congenital naevus Personal or family history of melanoma Immunosuppression Type 1 skin (red hair, burns easily, never tans) Significant sun exposure (UV exposure in the UK is underestimated) Previous sunburns		
Examination findings	Modified American Cancer Society ABCD system		
	A	Asymmetry	Divide lesion into four quadrants; asymmetry if lack of mirror image in any of the quadrants
	B	Border	Irregularities of border
	C	Colour variation	Two or more colours within lesion Lack of even pigmentation throughout Blue or black pigment highly suspicious
	D	Diameter	> 6 mm in diameter
	E	Evolution of lesion/elevation/erythema	Definite change in size, shape or colour

Table 5.16 Types of melanoma

Type	Features
Superficial spreading and nodular melanoma	Commonly history of change in size, shape or colour of pre-existing mole or freckle May arise de novo Usually asymmetrical, irregular border, contains more than one colour and over 0.6 mm diameter May be inflamed, crusty, ulcerated or bleeding
Lentigo maligna and lentigo maligna melanoma	Typically sun-exposed areas of face in older people Resembles large, irregular freckle Tends to grow slowly May be regarded as malignant melanoma in situ Malignant transformation to invasive lentigo melanoma uncommon, but can occur at any time with prognosis then as for any other melanoma
Acral lentiginous melanoma	Non-hair bearing skin of soles and palms and under nails (subungual melanoma) Often late diagnosis
Amelanocytic melanoma	Melanoma without pigment Often mistaken for squamous cell carcinoma or pyogenic granuloma

CASE 5.13

SKIN VASCULITIS

Instruction

Please examine this patient's feet and hands and report your findings.

Recognition

There is a *non-blanching, purpuric rash*. This is skin vasculitis, and the purpura *may be palpable* (Fig. 5.27).

Interpretation

Confirm the diagnosis

The clinical appearance is usually obvious, but the type may be confirmed by biopsy.

What to do next – consider causes

Causes of skin vasculitis are listed in Box 5.14.

Consider severity/decompensation/complications

Tell the examiners you would check urinalysis, renal function and obtain a chest X-ray.

Consider function

Any functional problem depends upon the cause.

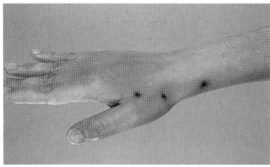

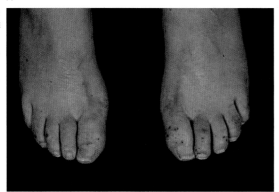

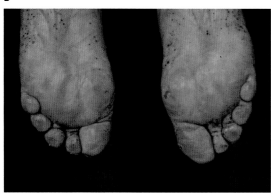

C

Fig. 5.27 Vasculitis: (A) hand, (B) dorsum, (C) soles of the feet.

Box 5.14 Causes of skin vasculitis

- Primary systemic vasculitis (Case 2.28)
- Autoimmune connective tissue disease, e.g. rheumatoid arthritis, systemic lupus erythematosus, scleroderma
- Drug reactions
- Infective endocarditis
- Henoch–Schönlein syndrome
- Prothrombotic disease, e.g. antiphospholipid syndrome
- Cryoglobulinaemia
- Lymphoproliferative disease

Discussion

What is leucocytoclastic vasculitis?

This is cutaneous vasculitis that may occur in isolation or in association with systemic disease including antineutrophil cytoplasmic antibody-associated vasculitis, connective tissue disease, infection (e.g. infective endocarditis, hepatitis B virus, hepatits C virus), inflammatory bowel disease or paraproteinaemia.

What is immunoglobulin A (IgA) vasculitis?

This is an IgA-mediated vasculitis causing a linear immunofluorescent pattern histologically. It is seen in IgA disease such as Henoch–Schönlein purpura.

CASE 5.14

XANTHOMATA AND XANTHELASMATA

Instruction

Please examine this gentleman's eyes and report your findings.

Recognition

There are multiple *tendon xanthomata* on the *extensor surfaces* (dorsum of hand, elbow, Achilles tendons, patella tendons). There may be xanthelasmata (Fig. 5.28).

Interpretation

Confirm the diagnosis

Tendon xanthomata should be distinguished from rheumatoid nodules or lipomas. Tendon xanthomata indicate familial hypercholesterolaemia, and sometimes raised and nodular tuberous xanthomata may also occur over the extensor surfaces and buttocks. Eruptive xanthomata are yellow papules on the extensor surfaces associated with hypertriglyceridaemia.

What to do next – consider causes

Types of dyslipidaemia are discussed in Case 2.13. Xanthelasmata and corneal arcus do not necessarily imply hyperlipidaemia.

Consider severity/decompensation/complications

Tell the examiners you would assess cardiovascular disease risk (Case 2.7).

Consider function

This relates to cardiac status.

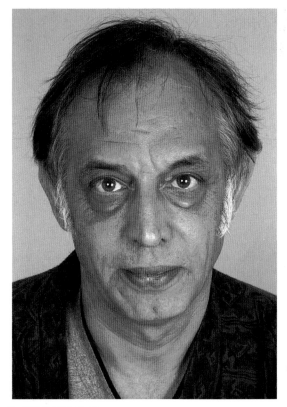

Fig. 5.28 Xanthelasmata.

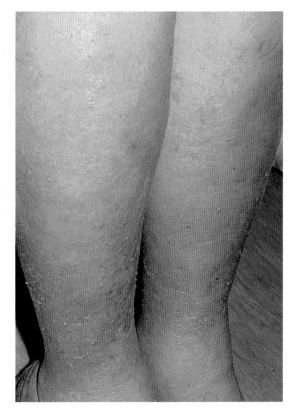

Fig. 5.29 Cellulitis.

Discussion

What are the common types of dyslipidaemia?

These are discussed in Case 2.13.

CASE 5.15

SKIN AND SOFT TISSUE INFECTION

Instruction

Please examine this lady's legs and discuss your findings.

Recognition

There is *erythema* over the anterior aspect of the lower leg, which is *warm*, and slightly swollen (Figs 5.29 and 5.30).

Interpretation

Confirm the diagnosis

The two main differential diagnoses are:

- Deep venous thrombosis (DVT), which causes circumferential swelling of the leg, often with erythema or discoloration with calf predominance and calf tenderness; Wells' criteria for diagnosing DVT are discussed in Case 2.36.
- Bilateral erythema in the setting of lower limb oedema; although commonly treated as soft tissue infection, bilateral swollen legs are seldom infected.

What to do next – consider causes

Tell the examiners that cellulitis is usually caused by staphylococcal or streptococcal infection. The term erysipelas is often used to describe deeper, often streptococcal, infection with greater demarcation of erythema. In practice it may be hard to distinguish the type of soft tissue infection.

Consider severity/decompensation/complications

Tell the examiners that you would always consider necrotising fasciitis (Fig. 5.31). Pain and tenderness is disproportionately predominant and visible signs may be minimal, especially early on. Necrotising fasciitis refers to infection that spreads rapidly through fascial layers, often extending through a limb within hours. Erythema is minimal and not always present. Bullae or vesicles are

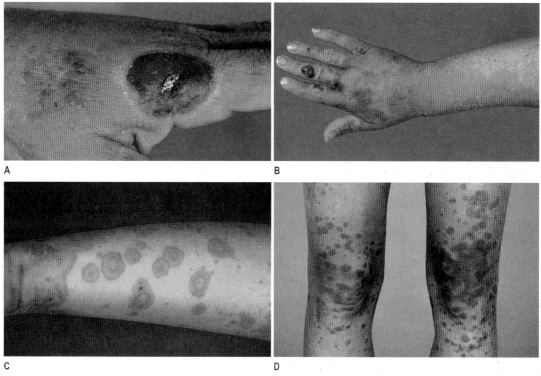

Fig. 5.30 (A–D) Erythema multiforme due to orf with secondary soft tissue infection.

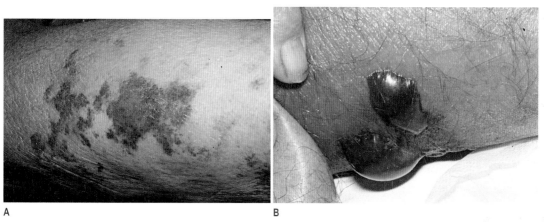

Fig. 5.31 (A,B) Necrotising fasciitis.

common, but late, signs. Black, necrotic skin is also a later sign, and often more obvious than erythema. Although traditionally streptococcal organisms are responsible, many cases of necrotising fasciitis are of mixed growth, and some cases may be caused by less rapidly progressive organisms (relatively) such as streptococcal group G

organisms. Both creatine kinase and C-reactive protein serum levels may be raised but are unreliable in excluding necrotising fasciitis if normal.

Consider function

Tell the examiners you would assess pain and mobility.

Table 5.17 Pressure ulcers

Grade 1	Grade 2	Grade 3	Grade 4
Non-blanchable erythema of intact skin Discoloration, warmth, oedema, induration or hardness	Partial thickness skin loss involving epidermis or dermis or both Superficial, appearing as abrasion or blister	Full thickness skin loss involving damage or necrosis of subcutaneous tissue that may extend down to, but not through, fascia	Extensive destruction, tissue necrosis, or damage to muscle, bone or supporting structures with or without full thickness skin loss

Discussion

How is necrotising fasciitis treated?

Urgent fasciotomy is needed to establish diagnosis and extensive surgery is the only potential cure, aided by appropriate antimicrobials.

What is a pressure ulcer?

This is a breach in the skin and underlying tissue secondary to unrelieved pressure, shear or friction. Pressure may be high for a short time or low for a longer time, as in sacral pressure ulcers caused by immobility in a chair or bed. Friction pressure ulcers commonly occur at the heels, elbows and knees, and may be associated with poor manual handling or positioning, and are common in agitated patients. Shearing, when gravity overcomes friction as when a patient slides down the bed, commonly causes pressure ulcers on the buttocks, sacrum or back. Other factors conspire to increase pressure ulcer risk or worsen pressure ulcers such as poor nutrition, body weight, incontinence and comorbidity such as cardiovascular disease.

How are pressure ulcers graded?

The European Pressure Ulcer Advisory Panel classification system describes four grades of pressure ulcer (Table 5.17).

What are the surgical treatments for ulcers?

Treatments depend upon the cause. Some examples are shown in Table 5.18.

Table 5.18 Treatments for ulcers

Type of ulcer	Treatments
Pressure	Pressure-relieving devices Modern dressings, e.g. hydrocolloids, hydrogels, foams, films, alginates, soft silicones Antimicrobials as necessary
Venous	Appropriate compression bandages, especially in prevention (light, moderate, high or extra-high compression)
Arterial	Surgery Vasodilators, e.g. pentoxylline, iloprost
Vasculitic	Treatment of underlying cause Immune suppression
Ulcer with lymphoedema	Compression bandages Intermittent pneumatic compression device
Exuding cavity	Vacuum-assisted closure
Ulcer with slough and non-viable tissue	Debridement, e.g. sharp, mechanical, enzymatic, biosurgery (maggots)
Necrobiosis lipoidica	Psoralen and ultraviolet light therapy

LOCOMOTOR SYSTEM

Examination of the joints – overview

The GALS screen

The locomotor system comprises bones, joints and muscles with associated ligaments, tendons and bursae. A gait, arms, legs, spine (GALS) screen (Fig. 5.32) is useful for rapidly detecting most musculoskeletal problems and some neurological problems, and assesses function. Abnormalities should prompt a full regional examination. Most physicians have developed their own GALS screen.

The GALS screen is recorded as in Table 5.19.

Regional examination

In PACES you are most likely to be asked to perform a regional examination. This is most commonly of the hands and wrists, but you should be prepared to examine the shoulders, ankles and feet, knees, hips or spine. Regional examination should follow the Look-Feel-Move format (Table 5.20).

Joints may be flexed, extended, abducted, adducted, externally rotated, internally rotated, supinated, pronated, inverted, everted and circumducted; only ball and socket joints (hip and shoulder) can do the latter. In general, pain and stiffness caused by synovitis occurs with both active and passive movements; pain from tendonitis is worse with active movements, and pain due to movements of a tendon

over an inflamed bursa (e.g. impingement in subacromial bursitis) occurs with passive and active movements.

Further assessment

Symptoms

Common rheumatological symptoms are pain, stiffness and joint swelling (Table 5.21).

Autoimmune tests

Diagnosis in rheumatology may take time, the clinical picture often emerging over months or even years. When the history and examination meet a number of diagnostic criteria, serological tests can seek to confirm the diagnosis. This is the purest view, but in practice serology is often requested in the absence of clinical assessment meeting defined criteria. For example, an 18-year-old lady might develop pericarditis as the first manifestation of systemic lupus erythematosus (SLE), and positive auto-antibodies are then highly suspicious.

■ **Antinuclear antibodies (ANAs)** ANAs are autoantibodies (usually immunoglobulin G) directed against cellular proteins or nucleic acids; despite their name, several of these antigens are confined to the cytoplasm. The most common ANAs react with DNA–protein or RNA–protein complexes. ANAs are detected by immunofluorescence (increasingly by enzyme-linked immunosorbent assay testing); staining may show a predominantly homogeneous (e.g. SLE – dsDNA), speckled (e.g. Sjögren's syndrome – Ro, La; mixed connective tissue disease – U1RNP), nucleolar (scleroderma – Scl-70) or centromere (scleroderma) pattern. A titre $\geq 1:160$ is regarded as high. Subsequent detection of antibodies to extractable nuclear antigens (ENAs) is useful in diagnosing specific autoimmune diseases (Table 5.22).

Examination of the hands and arms

The hands and wrists

- Be careful before shaking a patient's hand. Ask if there is pain before examining, and preferably examine the hands rested on a pillow on your seated patient's lap.
- Proceed to look, feel and move (Table 5.23; Figs 5.33 and 5.34).

Swelling, tenderness and crepitus are found over the tendon sheaths in stenosing tenosynovitis (trigger finger), usually a consequence of persistent inflammation. De Quervain's tenosynovitis is a form that affects abductor pollicis longus and extensor pollicis brevis, with symptoms around the base of the thumb and pain aggravated by movements at the wrist or thumb, often with marked crepitus. Osteoarthritis of the carpometacarpal joint may cause similar pain. Finkelstein's test is positive in De Quervain's tenosynovitis – the wrist is deviated in an ulnar direction while the thumb is held flexed in the palm by the fingers

Table 5.19 Record of GALS screen		
	Appearance	Movement
G	√	√
A	√	√
L	√	√
S	√	√

Table 5.20 Look – Feel – Move	
Look	At the skin, e.g. erythema, scars For swellings For deformities, e.g. joints, shape and position of the limbs and digits For muscle wasting
Feel	The skin (warmth) and surrounding tissues (fluid, soft tissue or bone) The joints (at rest)
Move	The joints Movements may be *active* (involving active muscle contraction) or *passive* (especially if active movement limited)

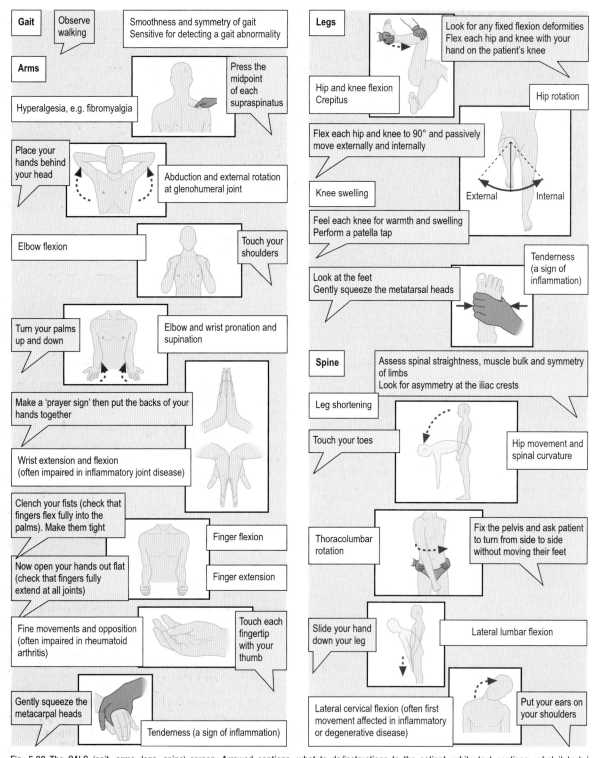

Gait — Observe walking — Smoothness and symmetry of gait / Sensitive for detecting a gait abnormality

Arms — Press the midpoint of each supraspinatus — Hyperalgesia, e.g. fibromyalgia

Place your hands behind your head — Abduction and external rotation at glenohumeral joint

Elbow flexion — Touch your shoulders

Turn your palms up and down — Elbow and wrist pronation and supination

Make a 'prayer sign' then put the backs of your hands together

Wrist extension and flexion (often impaired in inflammatory joint disease)

Clench your fists (check that fingers flex fully into the palms). Make them tight — Finger flexion

Now open your hands out flat (check that fingers fully extend at all joints) — Finger extension

Fine movements and opposition (often impaired in rheumatoid arthritis) — Touch each fingertip with your thumb

Gently squeeze the metacarpal heads — Tenderness (a sign of inflammation)

Legs — Look for any fixed flexion deformities / Flex each hip and knee with your hand on the patient's knee

Hip and knee flexion / Crepitus — Hip rotation

Flex each hip and knee to 90° and passively move externally and internally — Knee swelling — External / Internal

Feel each knee for warmth and swelling / Perform a patella tap

Look at the feet / Gently squeeze the metatarsal heads — Tenderness (a sign of inflammation)

Spine — Assess spinal straightness, muscle bulk and symmetry of limbs / Look for asymmetry at the iliac crests

Leg shortening

Touch your toes — Hip movement and spinal curvature

Thoracolumbar rotation — Fix the pelvis and ask patient to turn from side to side without moving their feet

Slide your hand down your leg — Lateral lumbar flexion

Lateral cervical flexion (often first movement affected in inflammatory or degenerative disease) — Put your ears on your shoulders

Fig. 5.32 The GALS (gait, arms, legs, spine) screen. Arrowed captions, what to do/instructions to the patient; white text captions, what it tests/detects.

Table 5.21 Differentiating rheumatological disorders by symptoms

Symptoms	Causes	
Diffuse pain not localised to joints and without stiffness	Chronic pain syndrome (Polymyalgia rheumatica causes diffuse symptoms but is characterised by stiffness)	
Pain and stiffness localised to joints without joint swelling (Arthralgia without arthritis)	Osteoarthritis Systemic lupus erythematosus Viral infections (Tendonitis may give rise to pain in the region of a joint, and bursitis to swelling in the region of a joint)	
Pain and stiffness with joint swelling (Arthralgia with arthritis/synovitis)	Monoarticular swelling	Palindromic rheumatoid, usually short lived (days) and occasionally the first manifestation Crystal arthropathy Spondyloarthropathy Septic arthritis Osteoarthritis
	Polyarticular symptoms	Rheumatoid arthritis Crystal arthropathy Spondyloarthropathy Systemic lupus erythematosus Viral infections

Table 5.22 Autoantibody tests

Disease	Autoantibodies to ENAs	Prevalence in this disease	Specificity	Clinical associations
Systemic lupus erythematosus (SLE)	Double-stranded DNA (dsDNA)	70%	High (unlike antibodies to single-stranded DNA)	Lupus nephritis
	Sm	5% (white) 30–50% (African Caribbean)	High	Central nervous system (CNS) lupus
	Ro (SS-A)	40%	High	Sjögren's syndrome, congenital heart block
	La (SS-B)	15%	High	
	U1 ribonucleoprotein (RNP)	30%	Low	Overlap/mixed connective tissue disease – arthritis, Raynaud's phenomenon, myositis
	rRNP	15%	High	CNS lupus
	PCNA (cyclin)	5%	High	
	Phospholipid	30–40%	Low	Antiphospholipid syndrome
	C1q	40%	Moderate	Lupus nephritis
Systemic sclerosis (SSc)	Topoisomerase 1 (Scl-70)	30%	High	Diffuse cutaneous SSc
	Centromere	60%	Moderate	Limited cutaneous SSc
	RNA polymerases	20%	High	Diffuse cutaneous SSc
	PM-Scl	5%	High	
Sjögren's syndrome	Ro (SS-A)	75%	High	Not predictive of particular features but tendency for extraglandular disease
	La (SS-B)	50%	SSA positive before SSB because SSA peripheral to SSB and exposed to autoantibodies first	
Polymyositis	Jo-1 (a tRNA synthetase)	30%	High	Myositis, interstitial lung disease, Raynaud's phenomenon
	Signal recognition peptide (SRP)	5%	High	Severe myositis
	Mi-2	10%	High	Dermatomyositis
Vasculitis	PR3 (associated with cANCA)	90%	High	Wegener's granulomatosis
	MPO (associated with pANCA)	50%	Moderate	Microscopic polyarteritis Churg–Strauss syndrome

Table 5.23 Examining the hands and wrists

Look	At the skin	Erythema suggests acute inflammation, e.g. crystal arthropathy, septic arthritis, tendon sheath infection, soft tissue infection. Look for palmar erythema, vasculitis, digital ischaemia, telangiectasia, purpura (corticosteroids) or scars (arthrodeses or previous carpal tunnel release) Look at the nails for pitting or evidence of vasculitis – nail fold erythema or infarction		
	For swellings	Swelling of the interphalangeal (IP) joints or metacarpophalangeal (MCP) joints suggests synovitis; there is loss of interdigital indentation of the MCP and IP joints when the fingers are flexed ('loss of mountains' sign).		
	For deformities	Swan neck and boutonnière deformities, Z-shaped thumbs and ulnar deviation of the MCP joints are typical of rheumatoid arthritis Anterior (volar) displacement of the wrist from partial dislocation (subluxation) is also common in rheumatoid arthritis A mallet finger or thumb, in which the terminal phalanx cannot be actively extended, is caused by rupture of the extensor tendon, usually from trauma or rheumatoid arthritis Arachnodactyly suggests Marfan's syndrome		
	For muscle wasting	Look for wasting of the thenar or hypothenar muscle groups or both		
Feel	The skin and surrounding tissues	Feel for warmth		
	The joints (at rest)	Bony swellings of the distal or proximal IP joints are likely Heberden's or Bouchard's nodes of osteoarthritis 'Squaring' of the wrist is due to osteophytes at the first carpometacarpal (CMC) joint Soft tissue swelling suggests synovitis, a fusiform swelling Feel the flexor tendon sheaths for localised swelling or tenderness; if present look for triggering or locking during extension Feel for crepitus of the opening and closing fingers with your index finger		
Move	The joints	Make a 'prayer sign'		Test wrist extension to 90°
		Now do the opposite		Test wrist flexion to 90°
		Make a fist Now tighten it	Note that flexion of the MCP rather than the IP joints is better tested as shown below	Test finger flexion Incomplete fist formation may be due to a problem with the IP or MCP joints or thickening of the flexor tendons – asking the patient to grip your fingers may detect thickening that is not visible
		Spread your fingers apart		Test the extensor tendons

(Fig. 5.35). This causes pain. In osteoarthritis, grinding the extended thumb causes pain at the thumb base.

The elbow

- Ask about any pain.
- Proceed to look, feel and move (Table 5.24).

The shoulder

To know what you are examining for, you should be aware of shoulder joint anatomy (Fig. 5.36). It comprises the glenohumeral joint and the acromioclavicular joint, but movement of the shoulder is also facilitated if the scapula rotates outwards against the chest wall, notably in shoulder abduction. The subacromial joint beneath the acromial head of the scapula is sometimes called the subacromial bursa. Shoulder movements can also move the sternoclavicular joint (Table 5.25).

Shoulder problems arise from any of these joints. Common glenohumeral joint problems are adhesive capsulitis and osteoarthritis. A common subacromial joint problem is rotator cuff disease.

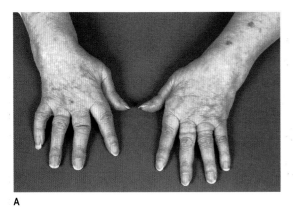

A

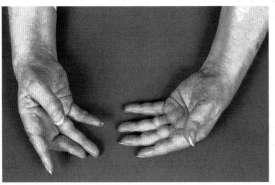

B

Fig. 5.33 Rheumatoid hands – synovitis.

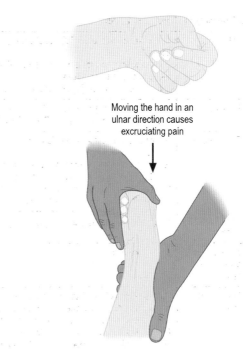

Moving the hand in an ulnar direction causes excruciating pain

Fig. 5.35 Finkelstein's test.

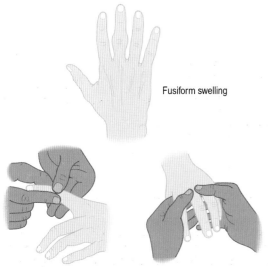

Fusiform swelling

Palpation of interphalangeal joint for synovitis

Palpation of metacarpophalangeal joint for synovitis

Fig. 5.34 Examining for synovitis. Press both sides of the joint with the index finger and thumb of one hand and any swelling will 'bulge up'. Now press on the swelling (it has a spongy feel) with the fingers of your other hand. You should normally be able to feel the bony margins of each metacarpophalangeal (MCP) joint and the gaps between them, especially when the patient makes a fist, like mountain peaks and valleys. In inflammatory joint disease the valleys are filled with synovial fluid.

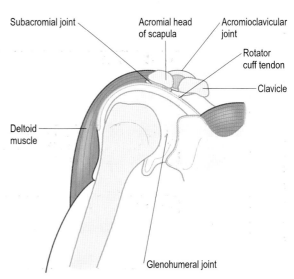

Subacromial joint · Acromial head of scapula · Acromioclavicular joint

Rotator cuff tendon

Clavicle

Deltoid muscle

Glenohumeral joint

Fig. 5.36 The shoulder.

- Ask the patient to point to any site of pain, although this is not a reliable guide for localising the structure from which it arises. Shoulder pain may be referred from cervical roots, thoracic viscera and from structures adjacent to the diaphragm. Patterns of stiffness or loss of movement are more helpful diagnostically; removal of a garment requires external rotation at the glenohumeral joint, for example.
- Proceed to look, feel and move (Table 5.25).

639

Table 5.24 Examining the elbow

Look	At the skin	Look for rheumatoid nodules or psoriatic plaques
	For swellings	Synovitis or an effusion appears as a bulge between the olecranon and the lateral epicondyle.
	For deformities	Look for olecranon bursitis
	For muscle wasting	Look for any valgus or varus deformity
Feel	The skin and surrounding tissues	Feel for bursitis
		Feel for rheumatoid nodules
		Feel for focal tenderness, laterally for a lateral (tennis elbow) epicondylitis causing pain over the lateral elbow and forearm and medially for a medial (golfer's elbow) epicondylitis causing pain over the medial elbow and forearm
	The joint (at rest)	Feel the bony contours of the elbow
		Feel for synovitis
Move	The joint	Flex and extend the joint, and feel for crepitus
		Test supination and pronation

Subacromial disease – rotator cuff disease

This is common under 50 years of age, often de novo or due to repetitive strain. The rotator cuff tendons may tear, often partially, or become inflamed, and often a combination of tearing and inflammation give rise to symptoms. Chronic inflammation in rheumatoid arthritis can also lead to atrophy of the rotator cuff muscles, with symptoms. The rotator cuff muscles and tendons are:

- Supraspinatus – allows abduction and elevation of the shoulder via the deltoid
- Infraspinatus – allows external rotation of the shoulder
- Subscapularis – allows internal rotation of the shoulder

Supraspinatus tendonitis is the most common problem. Rotator cuff tears tend to cause pain at the deltoid insertion, often worse at night, with weakness of overhead activity and outreach fatigue. There may be wasting of rotator cuff muscles over the scapula (supraspinatus and infraspinatus) and restricted movement, particularly active movement. The rotator cuff, notably supraspinatus, initiates abduction. Its presence between the glenohumeral and subacromial joints means that during abduction of the humeral head the tendon has to slide under the acromion where it rubs against the acromion's bony undersurface. Any tear or damage or focus of inflammation in the tendon will be exacerbated by the constant rubbing against bone, and a vicious cycle is set up. Because of the restricted space, the tendon may reach a point of being stuck ('impingement'), particularly as the humeral head and acromion come together. Once the tendon has passed through the space, the remainder of abduction is painless and easier (Table 5.25). This contrasts with acromioclavicular joint disease, usually more symptomatic with high arc abduction. Plain X-rays may show tendon calcification, and atrophy demonstrated by subacromial space narrowing (decreased vertical height between the humeral head and the acromion). Ultrasound or magnetic resonance imaging is helpful. Treatments include steroid injections, physiotherapy and surgery, although a degree of rotator cuff pathology is almost inevitable in most people at some stage, not necessarily symptomatic.

Glenohumeral disease – adhesive capsulitis ('frozen shoulder') and osteoarthritis

Distinguishing these two common differential diagnoses is outlined in Table 5.26.

Summary

A summary of the hands and arms examination sequence is given in the Summary Box.

SUMMARY BOX – HANDS AND ARMS EXAMINATION SEQUENCE

For each region:

- Look at the skin
- Look for swellings
- Look for deformities
- Look for muscle wasting
- Feel the skin and surrounding tissues
- Feel the joints at rest
- Move the joints

Examination of the legs

The hip

The hips are less likely to be involved in inflammatory arthritis and are usually a source of pain rather than swelling; such pain is often referred to the groin or downward to the knee.

- Ask if there is pain.
- Proceed to look, feel and move (Table 5.27).

Table 5.25 Examining the shoulder

Look	At the skin	Erythema and signs of inflammation are rare
	For swellings	Although swelling is unusual, rotator cuff tears with bleeds, rheumatoid arthritis effusions, pseudogout and sepsis can all affect the shoulder. A chronic effusion occurs in a peculiar destructive apatite arthritis of the shoulder (Milwaukee shoulder)
	For deformities	Anterior glenohumeral dislocation (depressed shoulder) and complete acromioclavicular joint dislocation (elevated acromion) are usually obvious, but posterior dislocation can be subtle Elevated or depressed scapulae occur in rare syndromes. Winging of the scapula suggests paralysis of the nerve to serratus anterior
	For muscle wasting	Look at the shoulder contours, especially at the supraspinatus and infraspinatus muscles overlying the upper and lower segments of the scapula; flattening suggests rotator cuff muscle atrophy due to a chronic tear in their tendons
Feel	The skin and surrounding tissues	Feel the supraspinatus tendon by extending the shoulder to bring supraspinatus anterior to the acromion process
	The joint (at rest)	Feel from the sternoclavicular joint and along the clavicle to the acromioclavicular joint. Clavicular or acromioclavicular fractures produce deformity and tenderness Feel the acromion and scapula spine Feel the glenohumeral joint by feeling for the humeral head and sliding your finger into the anterior groove, which is tender in a capsulitis but not in osteoarthritis

Move	The joint Neutral Extension Flexion Flexion and extension 180° 90° Abduction Internal External Rotation External Internal Rotation in abduction	As a screening test stand behind the patient and ask them to put their hands behind their head and then their hands behind their back reaching upwards to touch their shoulder blades Pain or limited movement warrant full examination

	Ask the patient to flex and extend the shoulder as far as possible		
	Test the abduction arcs by asking the patient to abduct the shoulder in the neutral (palm to leg) position B A	Rotator cuff lesions	Pain and restricted movement, especially active movement May be exacerbated by gentle resistance Pain starting in early abduction very suggestive, around 40° to 120°
		Glenohumeral joint disease, usually a capsulitis	Scapular movement starts early, confirmed by palpating the inferior border of the scapula whilst patient abducts
	Normally the scapula swings out and rotates on the chest wall after about 70° of abduction, but the first 70° requires the glenohumeral joint alone	Acromioclavicular arthritis	Pain during a high arc of movement (even passive) – 90° to 180°
	Test active external rotation, a function of the rotator cuff and painful and restricted in rotator cuff disease – returning to the neutral position with elbows flexed at 90° and held at the side, place your hands outside the patient's and ask them to push their hands outwards whilst keeping their elbows tucked in		

Thomas's test

A flexion deformity of the hip can be masked if the patient tilts the pelvis forward and increases the lumbar lordosis. Thomas's test can be used to obliterate the lumbar lordosis and unmask hip flexion (Fig. 5.37). The unaffected hip is flexed to its limit (do not do this if there is a hip replacement, as it may dislocate) to straighten the lumbar spine. An affected hip rises from the couch to reveal the degree of abnormal flexion.

Trendelenberg's test

Standing on one leg on the side of a diseased hip may cause the contralateral hemipelvis to fall below the horizontal.

The knee

- Ask if there is pain.
- Proceed to look, feel and move (Table 5.28).

Table 5.26 Glenohumeral disease – adhesive capsulitis versus osteoarthritis

	Adhesive capsulitis	Osteoarthritis
Age	Uncommon under 40 Peak 56	Older people Less common than adhesive capsulitis
Pathology	Fibrosis	Degeneration and osteophytes
Symptoms	Severe pain, often worse at night Insidious stiffness, often over several months	Pain Stiffness
Signs	Near complete loss of passive and active external rotation (hands behind head) of the shoulder The arm is held in adduction and internal rotation	Stiff, often creaky joint
Progress	Three clinical phases Painful freezing (lasts 3–9 months) Adhesive phase (lasts 4–12 months) Resolution phase (lasts 12–24 months)	Can wax and wane
Investigations	Diagnosis is clinical	Plain radiograph
Treatment	Non-steroidal anti-inflammatory drugs (NSAIDs) are often ineffective. Steroid injections and physiotherapy are used in the painful freezing phase Manipulation under anaesthesia and surgical release occasionally warranted in the adhesive phase	NSAIDs Steroid injections Physiotherapy Surgery
Prognosis	Mean duration 30 months	Slowly progresses

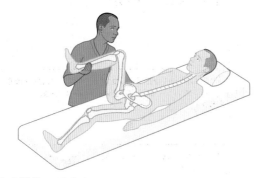

Fig. 5.37 Thomas's test.

The ankles and feet

- Ask if there is pain.
- Proceed to look, feel and move (Table 5.29).

Summary

A summary of the legs examination sequence is given in the Summary Box.

SUMMARY BOX – LEGS EXAMINATION SEQUENCE

For each region:

- Look at the skin
- Look for swellings
- Look for deformities
- Look for muscle wasting
- Feel the skin and surrounding tissues
- Feel the joints at rest
- Move the joints

Examination of the spine

Neurological examination of the limbs for signs referable to the spinal cord is described in Station 3. The look, feel and move approach (Table 5.30) is also appropriate for examining the spine.

Further assessment

Nerve stretch tests for sciatic and femoral nerve impingement are an important part of spinal examination. In the *sciatic nerve stretch test* the supine patient's straight-leg raising is limited by pain produced by tension of nerve roots supplying the sciatic nerve (L4–S2), commonly tensed over a prolapsed disc (commonly at vertebral level L4/5 or L5/S1). Pain may be in the back of the leg, sometimes radiating to the lumbar region. Tension is increased by dorsiflexion of the foot (which tugs the distal component of the sciatic nerve, the posterior tibial nerve) and relieved by flexion of the knee. In the *femoral nerve stretch* test the prone patient's femoral nerve roots (L2–4) are tightened by flexion of the knee, causing pain radiating into the back. The femoral roots may be further tensed by extending the hip joint, producing increasing pain.

Summary

A summary of the spine examination sequence is given in the Summary Box.

Table 5.27 Examining the hip

Look	At the skin	Look for scars, sinuses, dressings or skin changes around the hip
	For swellings	Swelling is seldom present
	For deformities	With the patient standing, note any pelvic tilt (which may mask leg shortening), and whether the spine is straight Apparent shortening of the leg can arise because of a flexion or adduction deformity True shortening is common in neck of femur fractures
	For muscle wasting	Look for quadriceps or gluteal wasting
Feel	The skin and surrounding tissues	Trochanteric bursitis, associated with numerous inflammatory arthritides, produces tenderness over the lateral thigh and pelvis
	The joint (at rest)	Usually unhelpful
Move	The joint The hip is a ball and socket joint that flexes, extends, abducts, adducts, externally and internally rotates and circumducts	Test flexion – normal to 120°
		Test abduction – normal to 45°
		Test adduction – normal to 25°
		Roll the fully extended leg and observe rotation of the foot, flex the knee and hip to 90°, then test external and internal rotation
		Roll the patient onto their back to test extension – normal to 20°

SUMMARY BOX – SPINE EXAMINATION SEQUENCE

For each region:

- Look at the skin
- Look for swellings
- Look for deformities
- Look for muscle wasting
- Feel the skin and surrounding tissues
- Feel the joints at rest
- Move the joints
- Consider performing nerve stretch tests

CASE 5.16

RHEUMATOID HANDS AND RHEUMATOID ARTHRITIS

Instruction

This patient has painful hands. Please examine them and discuss your findings.

Table 5.28 Examining the knee

Look	At the skin	Look for scars, sinuses or erythema
	For swellings	Look for any obvious swellings or effusion including prepatellar and infrapatellar bursitis and popliteal (Baker's) cysts; if the latter ruptures, swelling may track into the calf Knee bursae: a) sites of bursae; b) popliteal cyst Look for distension of the suprapatellar pouch, reflecting a large effusion
	For deformities	Look for a valgus, varus or flexion deformity
	For muscle wasting	Look for quadriceps wasting, common with knee pathology
Feel	The skin and surrounding tissues	Feel for warmth
	The joint (at rest)	 Examining for a large knee effusion	The patellar tap tests for the presence of fluid squeezed back into the joint space from the suprapatellar bursa; squeeze any excess fluid out of the suprapatellar pouch with your thumb and index finger, sliding them distally from a point some 15 cm above the knee to the upper border of the patella; with your other hand feel for the presence of a click by jerking the patella quickly downwards; the click may not be present with either a small or a tense effusion The bulge test, an addition to the patellar tap, is performed by a sudden pincing movement of the upper hand, which displaces fluid inferiorly and this fluid is palpated by a bulging apart of the fingers of the lower hand
		 Examining for a small knee effusion	A smaller effusion may be detected by fluid displacement or the ripple effect; evacuate the suprapatellar pouch as for the patellar tap; the medial side of the joint is then stroked to displace any excess fluid in the main joint cavity to the lateral side of the joint; then stroking the lateral side moves the excess fluid back across the joint resulting in a visible bulge or ripple
Move	The joint	Flex and extend the knees, and palpate for crepitus. Test the stability of the cruciate and collateral ligaments (although more likely to be unstable in orthopaedic settings, e.g. sports injuries) Examining the ligaments of the knee

Table 5.29 Examining the ankles and feet

Look	At the skin	Look for erythema, scars, sinuses, nail changes or vasculitis	
	For swellings	Look for synovitis or gout	
	For deformities	Note pes planus (flat foot) or pes cavus (high arch) and any abnormal forefoot appearances such as hallux valgus, hallux rigidus or dactylitis	
	For muscle wasting	Usually reflects peripheral nerve disease	
Feel	The skin and surrounding tissues	Feel for tenderness; flexor and extensor tendonitis is common in inflammatory arthritis and overuse, plantar fasciitis is common in the spondyloarthropathies	
	The joints (at rest)	Feel for synovitis	
Move	The joints	Active	Test the active range of plantar and dorsiflexion at the ankle and inversion and eversion
		Passive There are three main sets of joints in the ankle and foot • The hindfoot – the true ankle or tibiotalar joint (dorsiflexes by anterior tibialis and plantar flexes by gastrocnemius/soleus) and the talocalcaneal joint • The midfoot • The metatarsophalangeal and interphalangeal joints	Test dorsiflexion and plantar flexion Failure of plantar flexion when patient kneels on a chair and calf is squeezed is pathognomonic of Achilles rupture Stabilise the hindfoot (cupping the patient's ankle in dorsiflexion) and then invert and evert
			Cup the calcaneum in your hand and test flexion/extension and inversion/eversion
			Flex and extend the toes

Recognition

There is *deforming polyarthritis* of both hands.

Skin

There may be *palmar erythema. Cutaneous vasculitis* appears as crops of small brown spots at the nail folds, and as digital pulp infarcts.

Swellings

There is marked *soft tissue swelling* of the *metacarpophalangeal (MCP) joints* and *wrists.* The *proximal interphalangeal (PIP) joints* may be *swollen* (the IP joint of the thumb behaves as a PIP joint). The *distal interphalangeal (DIP) joints* are *spared.* There may be *active synovitis* with *fusiform spongy swelling* of joints.

Soft tissue swelling around a joint is the hallmark of inflammatory joint disease and associated stiffness is worse after inactivity and relieved by movement. Pain, stiffness (early morning lasting > 30 minutes) and warmth are the other features of synovial inflammation, but erythema is rare. Pain originates predominantly from the joint capsule, abundantly supplied with pain fibres.

Deformities

There may be:

- *Ulnar deviation* of the fingers due to subluxation or dislocation at the MCP joints (ulnar deviation also results from displaced extensor tendons)
- *Swan neck deformities* of the fingers (flexion deformity of the DIP joint, with a hyperextended PIP joint)

Table 5.30 Examining the spine

Look	At the skin	Usually no signs
	For swellings	Usually no signs
	For deformities	Look for kyphosis, marked lordosis or scoliosis Note the 'question mark' posture of ankylosing spondylitis
	For muscle wasting	
Feel	The skin and surrounding tissues	Feel the midline spinous processes and confirm alignment. Prominence, especially in the thoracic spine, may indicate anterior wedge compression of a vertebra Feel the paraspinal soft tissues for tenderness
	The joints (at rest)	Lightly percuss the spine for tenderness
Move	The joints	Neutral Flexion and extension Lateral flexion Rotation — Test flexion, extension, lateral flexion and rotation at the cervical spine Flexion Extension Lateral bending Rotation (Left / Right) — Test flexion, extension, lateral flexion and rotation at the thoracic and lumbar spine

- *Boutonnière deformities* of the fingers (extended DIP joint caused by rupture of the extensor tendon slip, with a flexed PIP joint)
- *Z-shaped thumbs* (flexed MCP joint, with extended IP joint)

These deformities are shown in Figs 5.38 and 5.39.

Muscle wasting

This is usually generalised, predominantly from disuse. There is thenar and hypothenar wasting (compare with isolated median or ulnar neuropathies); interosseous wasting is very common.

Interpretation

Confirm the diagnosis

Do not confuse with osteoarthritis, which affects small and large joints and may be symmetrical. Heberden's (DIP joint) and Bouchard's (PIP joint) nodes are bony swellings, not soft synovial swellings. Osteoarthritis commonly affects the knees and hips.

Psoriatic arthritis may mimic rheumatoid arthritis in the hand. Look at the elbows for rheumatoid nodules (Fig. 5.40) or psoriatic plaques to help differentiate.

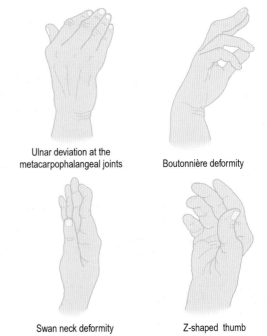

Ulnar deviation at the metacarpophalangeal joints

Boutonnière deformity

Swan neck deformity

Z-shaped thumb

Fig. 5.38 Finger deformities in rheumatoid arthritis.

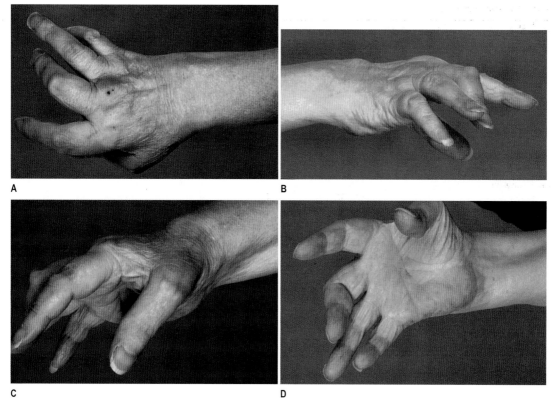

Fig. 5.39 (A–D) Finger deformities in rheumatoid arthritis.

Psoriatic arthritis commonly involves the DIP joints and causes nail pitting.

What to do next – assess other systems

Tell the examiners of extra-articular features of rheumatoid arthritis (Table 5.31). These affect about one-third of patients and are generally associated with rheumatoid factor positivity.

Consider severity/decompensation/complications

Numerous factors are associated with a less favourable prognosis (Box 5.15).

Box 5.15 Factors associated with a less favourable prognosis in rheumatoid arthritis

- High titre rheumatoid factor positivity (70% of patients)
- Many active joints at presentation
- Extra-articular disease (e.g. nodules, vasculitis)
- Severe disability at presentation
- Joint erosions/deformity early in disease
- High erythrocyte sedimentation rate or C reactive protein at presentation
- HLA DR4 presence, especially homozygosity
- Family history
- Psychosocial problems

Subluxation of the atlantoaxial joint because of laxity of the transverse ligament of the atlas is a serious skeletal complication. Synovitis of the facet joints may also contribute to instability. Subluxation is shown by flexion and extension radiographs demonstrating an increased distance between the posterior aspect of the C1 vertebral body and the anterior aspect of the odontoid process of C2.

Consider function

Function can be assessed by a simple screen of pincer, grip and arm movements and by asking about routine activities such as fastening buttons, using keys, writing, taking coins out of pockets, holding cups, opening jars, cleaning teeth, combing hair, getting dressed and reaching into kitchen cupboards.

Tell the examiners you would explore symptoms of disease activity, including joint pain and swelling, weight loss, overall activity during the day (occupation, and if patient can can still work – 50% of patients are unable to work after 10 years) and afternoon tiredness. Rheumatologists have specific ways of assessing disease activity (Box 5.16).

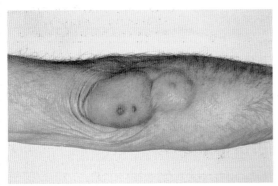

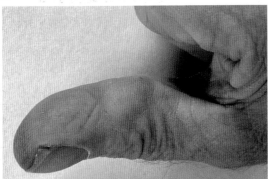

A

B

Fig. 5.40 Rheumatoid nodules: (A) elbow, (B) thumb.

Discussion

What causes rheumatoid arthritis?

It is a chronic inflammatory, autoimmune disease, mediated by proinflammatory cytokines. There is a strong HLA DR4 association. It affects around 1% of people and its onset is commonly in the fifth decade.

What patterns of onset are recognised?

The usual pattern is insidious, over weeks to months, starting with fatigue, anorexia and vague musculoskeletal symptoms. Less frequently it appears over a week or two, and rarely over a few days. A palindromic refers to episodic features with complete resolution in between, such as acute, self-limiting swelling of a knee. Extra-articular onset is recognised.

Which joints may be affected other than those in the hands?

These include the shoulder, the elbow (flexion contractures), the wrist, the knee (synovial hypertrophy, ligament laxity, chronic effusion, and sometimes popliteal cysts), the ankle, the foot (e.g. eversion at the subtalar joint, plantar subluxation of the metatarsal heads, widening of the forefoot, hallux valgus and lateral deviation/dorsal subluxation of the toes), the cervical spine and the temporomandibular joint. Tenosynovitis and bursitis commonly accompany joint disease, e.g. rotator cuff tendonitis, subacromial bursitis, De Quervain's tenosynovitis, hand extensor and flexor tendonitis, trochantric bursitis.

Do you know of any diagnostic criteria for rheumatoid arthritis?

The revised American College of Rheumatology (ACR) criteria are listed in Box 5.17.

List some radiological features of rheumatoid arthritis

- Soft tissue swelling together with juxta-articular osteoporosis in early disease
- Joint space narrowing
- Joint erosions
- Cyst formation
- Joint destruction
- Subluxation/dislocation

What is in synovial fluid in rheumatoid arthritis?

Fluid is often turbid, with low viscosity, high protein concentration, low or normal glucose concentration, low complement levels and an elevated white cell count (5–50 000 cells/ml). There is seldom a place for synovial fluid examination other than to exclude infection.

What is rheumatoid factor (RF)?

RFs are antibodies against the Fc portion of immunoglobulin G. They may be of any isotype but only immunoglobulin M was traditionally detected by the now superseded latex agglutination test. An easy way to consider RF is to first consider that antibodies directed against other antibodies is a normal phenomenon. New antibodies are created continuously in response to an infinite variety

Table 5.31 Extra-articular features of rheumatoid disease

System or feature involved	Possible manifestations	Comment
Neurological	Entrapment neuropathies (carpal tunnel syndrome, foot and wrist drops)	Entrapment by synovial swelling
	Cervical myeloradiculopathy	Cricoarytenoid arthritis
	Dysphonia (rare)	Synovial involvement of ossicles
	Hearing loss (rare)	Due to vasculitis
	Sensory polyneuropathy	Due to mononeuritis multiplex
Lung (findings more common at autopsy than clinically apparent; tend to affect males more than females)	Pleuritic pain	
	Pleural effusions	
	Interstitial lung disease	Methotrexate also causes fibrosis and nodules
	Pulmonary nodules	In Caplan's syndrome, massive fibrotic nodules coexist with coal dust exposure
Cardiac	Constrictive pericarditis	
	Pericardial effusion	Up to 50% at autopsy have a pericardial effusion; usually asymptomatic
	Mitral regurgitation	
Vascular and vasculitis (small vessel)	Usually restricted to skin, e.g. nail folds	Rheumatoid factor highly positive
	Digital gangrene	
	Cutaneous ulceration including pyoderma gangrenosum	
	Peripheral neuropathy	
	Mononeuritis multiplex	
	Coronary, renal, cerebral or mesenteric vasculitis (all very rare)	
	Raynaud's phenomenon	
Rheumatoid nodules (soft tissue nodules, not to be confused with tendon xanthomata)	Sites:	Rheumatoid factor invariably positive
	Extensor tendons of hand	
	Trigger finger (thickening, usually without nodules, of flexor aspect)	
	Pressure points, e.g. elbows, Achilles tendons, bridge of nose if spectacles	
	Lungs	
	Pericardium	
	Sclera (rare)	
Eye	Episcleritis	
	Scleritis	Recurrent scleritis may progress to scleromalacia perforans
	Keratoconjunctivitis sicca (40%)	
Skin	Palmar erythema	
	Livedo reticularis	
	Pyoderma gangrenosum	
Felty's syndrome	Rheumatoid arthritis	
	+ Splenomegaly	Hypersplenism not invariable
	+ Leucopenia	Severe neutropenia (even thrombocytopenia and anaemia) may occur without hypersplenism
Kidney	Nephrotic syndrome	Due to amyloid deposition
Systemic features	Malaise	Not specific to rheumatoid arthritis; due to proinflammatory immune response
	Weight loss	
	Anaemia	
	Lymphadenopathy	
	Amyloid accumulation	

of antigens in the environment; some antibodies, when newly formed, may also be seen by the immune system as foreign and 'anti-antibodies' are produced against them. Sometimes a cascade of antibody against antibody may be triggered.

Some of the anti-antibodies produced in this way are RFs and, hence, RFs are not specific to rheumatoid arthritis. They may be detected transiently after many acute infections, may be present in low titres in chronic infections, and are sometimes found in chronic inflammatory disorders like systemic lupus erythematosus (SLE) and scleroderma. RFs are detectable in 5% of the normal population and in up to 25% of elderly people – simply because elderly people have been exposed for a longer time to the environmental stimuli which engender such antibodies. Up to 70% of patients with rheumatoid arthritis are RF positive.

What is anti-cyclic citrullinated peptide (anti-CPP)?

It has recently been discovered that anti-CPP antibodies are detected in many RF-negative patients, offering a more sensitive test than RF itself. Anti-CPP antibodies occur in 80% of patients with established RA and have a specificity of 95% and a sensitivity of around 65%. Like RF, they also seem to predict development of erosive RA.

List some causes of anaemia in rheumatoid arthritis

- Anaemia of chronic disease
- Non-steroidal anti-inflammatory drug (NSAID)-related gastritis/peptic ulceration
- Bone marrow suppression from disease-modifying anti-rheumatic drugs
- Splenomegaly in Felty's syndrome

- Megaloblastic anaemia (associated pernicious anaemia or methotrexate-related folate deficiency)

What is Sjögren's syndrome?

Sjögren's syndrome is a chronic inflammatory, lympho-proliferative disease with autoimmune exocrinopathy. Primary Sjögren's syndrome is defined by xerostomia (dry mouth caused by decreased salivary gland secretion) and xerophthalmitis (dry eye, also known as keratoconjunctivitis sicca, caused by decreased lacrimal secretion) without other autoimmune disease. Secondary Sjögren's syndrome occurs with rheumatoid arthritis, SLE or other autoimmune connective tissue disease. Sjögren's syndrome is the second commonest autoimmune rheumatic disease after rheumatoid arthritis and may affect up to 3–4% of the adult population with a female:male ratio of 9:1.

Sjögren's syndrome is multifactorial. Genetic predisposition includes *HLA DR3* and *DR52* and *DQ*. Environmental agents including herpes viruses, cytomegalovirus and Epstein–Barr virus, and retroviruses may play a role. Hepatitis C is more common in people with sicca syndrome without Sjögren's syndrome autoantibodies.

Clinical manifestations of Sjögren's syndrome are shown in Table 5.32.

Table 5.32 Clinical manifestations of and diagnostic criteria for Sjögren's syndrome			
	Manifestation	**Symptoms and signs**	**Diagnosis**
Glandular	Ocular	Dry mouth – xerostomia Lack of saliva pool on floor of mouth Swelling of salivary glands Dysphagia	European diagnostic criteria require at least four of six items:
	Oral	Dry, gritty eyes – xerophthalmitis Scleritis Inflammatory nodules Sterile corneal ulcers	• Ocular symptoms • Oral symptoms • Evidence of xerophthalmitis
Systemic Many manifestations caused by vasculitis or tissue lymphoid infiltration	Joint involvement	Symmetrical, small joint arthralgia with mild synovitis	(Schimer's test or Rose–Bengal staining); Schimer's test uses standardised test strips placed
	Vasculitis of small or medium-sized vessels	Purpuric rash Skin ulceration Urticaria Neuropathy	between eyeball and lateral part of inferior lid, positive if < 5 mm of wetness at 5 minutes
	Gastrointestinal Primary biliary cirrhosis or autoimmune hepatitis may be associated	Dysphagia (dry pharynx or oesophageal dysmotility) Chronic atrophic gastritis	• Focal sialedenitis from minor salivary gland involvement (lip biopsy)
	Pulmonary	Chronic bronchitis Mucus plugging Lymphocytic interstitial pneumonitis Pleural effusions Pulmonary hypertension	• Instrumental evidence of salivary gland involvement (salivary flow rate – clinical setting, parotid sialography) • Autoantibodies present (anti-Ro or anti-La)
	Renal Tubular dysfunction and renal tubular acidosis	Renal calculi Nephrocalcinosis Hypokalaemic muscle weakness	
	Neurological	Peripheral neuropathy Mononeuropathy	Positive antibodies or a positive lip biopsy should be mandatory for diagnosis

Between 5% and 10% of patients with Sjögren's syndrome develop non-Hodgkin's B-cell lymphoma. Pseudo-lymphoma, with nodular infiltrates in lungs, also occurs. The erythrocyte sedimentation rate is commonly elevated, diffuse hypergammaglobulinaemia is usually present and antinuclear antibody testing and/or rheumatoid factor is usually positive. Specific autoantibodies – anti-Ro (SSA) and anti-La (SSB) – are often positive, especially anti-Ro.

What do you know about treatment in rheumatoid arthritis?

Treatment goals

Treatment goals are pain relief, reduction of inflammation, limitation of joint damage, control of systemic disease and maintenance of function. No treatment is curative.

When to start treatment

Within three months of onset 10–26% of patients have joint erosions. Treatment is best instituted early in disease, and the early use of disease-modifying anti-rheumatic drugs has been shown to significantly improve efficacy parameters such as Health Assessment Questionnaire scores and swollen joint counts, and reduce radiographic progression.

NSAIDS

Simple analgesics and NSAIDs help pain but do not control inflammation. Potential side effects are peptic ulceration, interstitial nephritis, fluid retention and worsening of asthma.

Disease-modifying antirheumatic drugs (DMARDs)

DMARDS (methotrexate, sulfasalazine, hydroxychloro-quine, gold, ciclosporin, leflunamide) delay disease progression and reduce subsequent disability, and are introduced early in disease. All agents are of similar efficacy at optimum dosage except for hydroychloroquine and auranofin, which are slightly less effective. Methotrexate and sulfasalazine are most widely used but monotherapy with any agent wanes in effect with time. Combinations have therefore been used to sustain benefit and approaches include:

- Sustained combination therapy, which appears to have sustained effect at three years
- Step-down combination therapy, in which several DMARDs are started and then withdrawn, which appears to not maintain long-term benefit
- Step-up combination therapy, a more intuitive approach
- Tight control of rheumatoid arthritis, a predefined treatment strategy

Combinations involving methotrexate may have superior efficacy to monotherapy.

Many DMARDs can cause bone marrow suppression and skin rashes. Gold and penicillamine may cause nephrotic syndrome. Penicillamine is associated with drug-induced lupus and autoimmune disease.

Biological agents

These are novel DMARDs, discussed in Box 5.18.

Corticosteroids

Low-dose oral corticosteroids attenuate the acute-phase response but do not appear to modify disease and their use is carefully balanced against side effects.

Box 5.18 Biological agents in rheumatoid arthritis

Rationale

Rheumatoid synovitis contains predominantly T lymphocytes (CD4+ T helper type 1), macrophages and fibroblasts with secretion of pro-inflammatory cytokines [interleukin 1 (IL-1), IL-6 and tumour necrosis factor-α (TNF-α)] and metalloproteinases, which mediate tissue damage. TNF-α mediates proliferative and inflammatory aspects, while IL-1 mediates cartilage destruction and bone erosion. The IL-6 mediates many actions of TNF-α and IL-1 but also recruits B cells. Most T helper type 1 cells are memory cells but some mediate B-cell help, enhancing local auto-antibody formation. Plasma cells secreting rheumatoid factor are also present.

Agents

- Three monoclonal antibody antagonists to TNF-α are available – infliximab (a chimeric immunoglobulin G antibody), etanercept (a recombinant TNF receptor immunoglobulin G fusion protein) and adalimumab (a fully humanised monoclonal antibody)
- Interleukin receptor antagonists are being developed for clinical use
- Rituximab, a B cell-targeted treatment acting on CD20, is now available for patients with severe active rheumatoid arthritis failing to respond to DMARDs including TNF-α modification therapy

Risks

These include:

- Immediate – infusion reactions
- Intermediate – infection, e.g. tuberculosis reactivation, human immunodeficiency virus, hepatitis B or C; systemic lupus erythematosus syndromes or autoimmunity; heart failure; demyelination
- Late – malignancy, e.g. lymphoma

Indications

The National Institute for Health and Clinical Excellence (NICE) guidelines for biological agents suggest that eligible patients must:

- Satisfy the American Rheumatism Council diagnostic criteria
- Have active disease
- Have failed standard therapy with at least two standard disease-modifying anti-rheumatic drugs

An adequate therapeutic trial would be treatment for at least six months, at least two months at target dose.

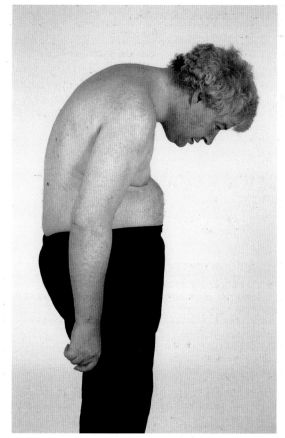

Fig. 5.41 Ankylosing spondylitis.

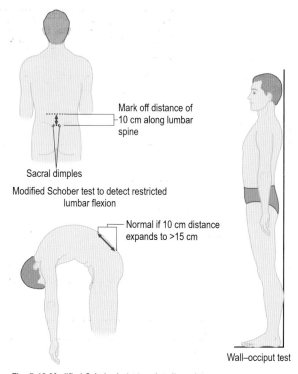

Mark off distance of 10 cm along lumbar spine

Sacral dimples

Modified Schober test to detect restricted lumbar flexion

Normal if 10 cm distance expands to >15 cm

Wall–occiput test

Fig. 5.42 Modified Schober's test and wall–occiput test.

Box 5.19 Typical features of spondyloarthropathy back pain

- Worse sitting, lying and resting
- Worse with prolonged immobility
- Improved by exercise
- Associated with prolonged (> 1 hour) morning stiffness.

    These symptoms also tend to be true for joint symptoms in any inflammatory arthritis.

CASE 5.17

ANKYLOSING SPONDYLITIS AND SPONDYLOARTHROPATHIES

Instruction

Please examine this patient's spine and any other systems you feel relevant, and then discuss your findings.

Recognition

There is *kyphosis* with a characteristic *question mark* posture (Fig. 5.41). There is *restriction of spinal movement in all directions* (extension, lateral flexion, rotation) and a *positive modified Schober's test* (mark the level of the posterior iliac spines and sacral dimples, and a point 10 cm above this in the midline; when the patient flexes forward, the distance between the two points normally increases to at least 15 cm but not if the test is positive). Upper spine involvement is demonstrated by the *wall–occiput* test (Fig. 5.42).

Interpretation

Confirm the diagnosis

Confirm this is a spondyloarthropathy. Some differentiating articular signs are shown in Table 5.33. Tell the examiners that you would ask about those features of back pain listed in Box 5.19. The back pain of spondyloarthropathies, unlike mechanical back pain, has typical features. Remember that ankylosing spondylitis is the primary spondyloarthropathy, but there are others.

What to do next – assess other systems

Some 'A's are associated with ankylosing spondylitis (Box 5.20). Look for these or mention these to the examiners, but apart from tendonitis/fasciitis and anterior uveitis, they are rare – look at the eyes and listen to the aortic area in expiration and to the lung apices and tell the examiners you would ask about heel pain.

Table 5.33 Articular signs differentiating a spondyloarthropathy from rheumatoid arthritis and osteoarthritis

	Spondyloarthropathy	Rheumatoid arthritis	Osteoarthritis
Symmetry	Asymmetrical	Symmetrical	Asymmetrical/symmetrical
Joints affected	Peripheral arthritis affecting mostly large joints, e.g. knees, hips, ankles	Peripheral arthritis affecting mostly small joints, e.g. metacarpophalangeal joints, wrists	Small and large joints affected, e.g. hips, first carpometacarpal joint, knees, hips
Spinal involvement	Spondylitis Sacroiliitis	Atlanto-axial subluxation	Lumbar and cervical degeneration

---

Box 5.20 'A's associated with ankylosing spondylitis

- **A**chilles tendonitis and plantar fasciitis
- **A**nterior uveitis
- **A**ortic regurgitation and aortitis
- **A**pical lung fibrosis
- **A**trioventricular heart block
- **A**myloidosis

Box 5.21 The major spondyloarthropathies

- Ankylosing spondylitis
- Psoriatic arthritis
- Reactive arthritis (including Reiter's syndrome)
- Enteropathic arthritis

Box 5.22 New York criteria for diagnosing ankylosing spondylitis

The presence of at least one clinical criterion plus one radiological criterion is required.

Clinical

The main clinical criteria are:

- Low back pain of at least three month's duration, with inflammatory characteristics (improved by exercise, not relieved by rest)
- Limitation of lumbar spine mobility in both sagittal and frontal planes
- Limitation of chest expansion relative to normal age- and sex-matched values

Radiological

- Unilateral sacroiliitis (grades 3–4) or bilateral sacroiliitis (grade 2)
  - Grade 0 – normal
  - Grade 1 – suspicious changes
  - Grade 2 – minimal sacroiliitis
  - Grade 3 – moderate sacroiliitis
  - Grade 4 – ankylosis

Consider severity/decompensation/complications

Look for signs of severe aortic regurgitation if you detect aortic regurgitation. Tell the examiners that you would arrange pulmonary function tests if you detect pulmonary fibrosis.

Consider function

Note the extent of postural deformity and stiffness. Enquire about activities such as driving; even being a passenger in a car can be difficult.

Discussion

What are the major seronegative spondyloarthropathies?

The seronegative spondyloarthropathies (Box 5.21) lack rheumatoid factor positivity and are associated with human leucocyte antigen (HLA) B27. A family history is common. Environmental triggers and genetic susceptibility probably provoke disease. HLA B27 is positive in 5–10% of the white population and in 90% of patients with ankylosing spondylitis, 70% with Reiter's syndrome and up to 50% with other spondyloarthropathies. Serology is not used widely in diagnosis, which should rely on clinical and radiological assessment.

Overlap of clinical features may occur between spondyloarthropathies, e.g. a patient with psoriatic arthritis may develop anterior uveitis. Symptoms that should raise clinical suspicion of a seronegative arthropathy include:

- Morning stiffness of the lumbar or dorsal spine
- Alternating buttock pain
- Sausage digits
- Asymmetrical inflammatory arthritis
- Plantar fasciitis
- Iritis
- History of psoriasis or inflammatory bowel disease and/or family history

Ankylosing spondylitis

Ankylosing spondylitis is the primary spondyloarthropathy (absence of features to suggest one of the other conditions and symmetrical pain). Age of onset is 15–40 years and the male:female ratio is around 4:1. The New York criteria for diagnosing ankylosing spondylitis are outlined in Box 5.22.

Psoriatic arthritis

Psoriatic arthropathy (Fig. 5.43) affects up to 10% of patients with psoriasis (Fig. 5.44) and may precede or

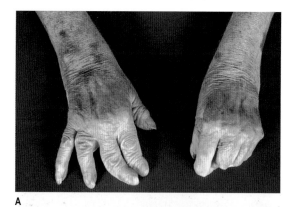

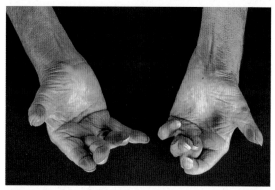

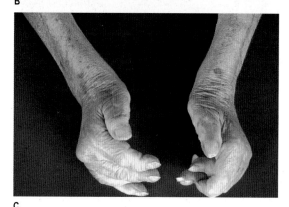

Fig. 5.43 (A–C) Psoriatic arthropathy.

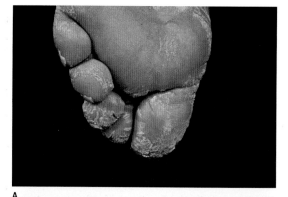

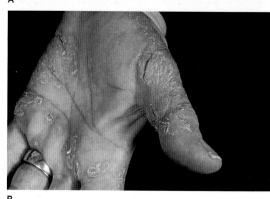

Fig. 5.44 (A,B) Psoriasis.

Reiter's syndrome

Reiter's syndrome, a form of reactive arthritis, often follows urethritis/cervicitis (e.g. *Chlamydia*) or dysenteric infections (e.g. *Shigella*, *Salmonella*, *Campylobacter*, *Yersinia* species). The classic triad is arthritis, urethritis and conjunctivitis/anterior uveitis. The classic triad is not always complete, and common additional findings include mouth ulceration, circinate balanitis, persistent plantar fasciitis and keratoderma blennorrhagica (hyperkeratotic vesicles, often on soles or palms).

Which musculoskeletal features are shared by the spondyloarthropathies?

These are described in Box 5.23.

Which investigations may be useful in a spondyloarthropathy?

Diagnosis is based on clinical and radiological evidence. The radiological features of established spondylitis and sacroiliitis are useful but in acute disease X-rays are normal; symptomatic sacroiliitis can precede radiological changes by years and magnetic resonance imaging of the sacroiliac joints is increasingly used to detect early disease. Inflammatory markers are often elevated in active disease.

follow skin disease by months or even years. There are, in theory, five types of arthropathy (Case 5.1); radiologically, there may be erosions and severe joint destruction.

Reactive arthritis

Reactive arthritis refers to arthritis after any infection. It may affect small or large peripheral joints, with features of a spondyloarthropathy.

Box 5.23 Musculoskeletal features of ankylosing spondylitis and the spondyloarthropathies

Spondylitis (inflammatory spine disease)

This is characterised by an insidious onset, persistence for > 3 months, morning stiffness and improvement with exercise. Enthesitis contributes to spondylitis because destruction of the insertion sites of vertebral discs to vertebrae leads to squaring of the vertebrae. Syndesmophytes (reactive bone formation) sometimes link vertebrae. Calcification within the anterior and posterior spinal ligaments gives rise to the characteristic but rare bamboo spine.

Sacroiliitis

This often causes alternating buttock pain, especially at night. Sacroiliitis tends to be symmetrical in ankylosing spondylitis but asymmetrical or unilateral in the other spondyloarthropathies. Severity is graded radiographically by the extent of joint distortion (Box 5.22).

Peripheral large joint monoarthritis or oligoarthritis

This tends to be asymmetrical and to affect the lower limbs (hip, knee or ankle). It may predate or follow spine disease by several years.

Enthesitis

Many symptoms in spondyloarthropathies are the result of enthesitis, which refers to inflammation (± fibrosis, calcification and ossification) at the insertion site (enthesis) of a tendon, ligament or joint capsule to bone. Heel pain, worse when starting to walk in the morning and associated with a 'burning sole', is the result of plantar fasciitis and is the commonest enthesopathy. Other sites include the insertion of the Achilles tendon to the calcaneus (Achilles tendonitis), the capsular insertions of the costovertebral, sternoclavicular, manubriosternal and costochondral junctions, the capsules and ligaments around finger joints, and finger tendon sheaths.

Dactylitis

This refers to the sausage swelling of a digit resulting from joint and tendon/tendon sheath swelling.

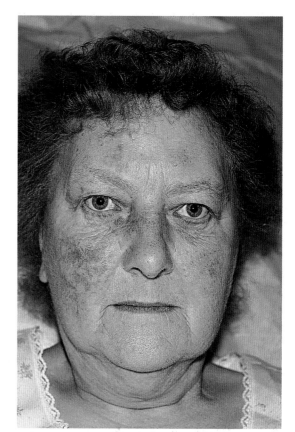

Fig. 5.45 Malar rash typical of systemic lupus erythematosus.

Which treatments are beneficial in spondylarthropathy?

A dramatic improvement with non-steroidal anti-inflammatory drugs (NSAIDs) is typical in early disease. Good posture, physiotherapy and home exercises including extension exercises are important. Disease-modifying anti-rheumatic drugs (DMARDs) similar to those used in rheumatoid arthritis may help large joint arthritis, but seem to have less effect on spine (axial) disease.

What is the place of anti-tumour necrosis factor (TNF) therapy in treatment?

Ankylosing spondylitis does not 'burn out'. It persists through life and fatigue may be a major symptom that is difficult to treat. Furthermore, there is no evidence that NSAIDs or physiotherapy alter progression.

Evidence for the benefit of 'biologics' has emerged, mostly with ankylosing spondylitis but also for psoriatic arthritis, prompting guidelines by the Assessment in Ankylosing Spondylitis (ASAS) Working Group and the British Society of Rheumatology (BSR).

TNF-α mRNA has been identified in inflamed sacroiliac joints in patients with ankylosing spondylitis and joints of patients with psoriatic arthropathy. As with rheumatoid arthritis, infliximab, etanercept and adalimumab may have increasing roles in seronegative arthropathy, especially for axial disease, although indications for use are still emerging; adalimumab is now recommended for active, progressive psoriatic arthropathy with at least three tender, swollen joints where multiple DMARDs have been ineffective.

CASE 5.18

SYSTEMIC LUPUS ERYTHEMATOSUS

Instruction

Please examine this patient's face and hands. Discuss your findings and how you might further assess this patient.

Recognition

There are raised or *flat patches of malar erythema ('butterfly rash'), sparing the nasolabial folds* (Fig. 5.45).

1. Malar rash (raised or flat red patches, nasolabial fold sparing)
2. Discoid rash (red papules on head and neck with scaling, follicular keratosis, atrophic scarring and depigmentation)
3. Photosensitivity
4. Oral/nasopharyngeal ulcers (painless)
5. Arthritis (non-erosive, more than two joints)
6. Pleuritis or pericarditis
7. Renal disorder (proteinuria or casts)
8. Neurological disorder (seizures or psychosis)
9. Haematological disorder (haemolytic anaemia, leucopenia, lymphopenia or thrombocytopenia)
10. Immunological serology (anti-dsDNA, anti-Sm antibody, antiphospholipid antibody)
11. Positive antinuclear antibody

Four criteria are required (only one skin manifestation may be used).

Interpretation

Confirm the diagnosis

Tell the examiners you would ask about photosensitivity. The differential diagnosis of a facial rash is described in Case 5.5. The widely recognised presentation of a young woman with both a butterfly rash and inflammatory arthritis is only part of the spectrum of disease. Tell the examiners that non-specific symptoms such as fatigue, photosensitive skin rashes, mild hair loss, Raynaud's phenomenon, oral ulcers, dry eyes and mouth, arthralgia or pleuritic chest pain are equally likely presentations. The American Rheumatism Council criteria for diagnosis are outlined in Box 5.24.

Presentation may be with major organ dysfunction that can affect virtually any organ.

What to do next – assess other systems

Given the above, the key to early diagnosis is a complete systems review (Table 5.34) with appropriate investigations. Be aware of these possible manifestations of systemic lupus erythematosus (SLE) and share some with the examiners.

Consider severity/decompensation/complications

Disease damage and activity indices are now assessed by various validated disease activity scores, e.g. the SLE Disease Activity Index. Lupus nephritis presents insidiously, and if not detected early has a high risk of progression to renal failure. Myocardial infarction and cerebrovascular disease are common, important causes of morbidity and mortality.

Consider function

Tell the examiners that you would explore fatigue. Fatigue is an often under-appreciated, debilitating symptom, contributed to by depression, pain, arthralgia, poor sleep quality, poor physical fitness and disease activity.

Discussion

What is SLE?

SLE is a multi-system autoimmune connective tissue disease with numerous clinical presentations. It is characterised by flares and remissions. The female:male ratio is at least 9:1 and onset tends to be between 15 and 45 years of age. It is more common in people with African or Asian ancestry.

What causes SLE?

There is no single cause for SLE, although factors such as sunlight and drugs may exacerbate it and there is a complex genetic basis. There is an increased prevalence of human leucocyte antigen (HLA) A1 B8 DR2 and DR3 in whites with SLE. Deficiencies in the classical complement pathway components C1q, C2 and C4 are strongly associated with lupus-like disease. Immunoglobulin G (IgG) receptors on phagocytes cells clear IgG and IgG-containing immune complexes from the circulation, but low-affinity receptors have been found in African American patients.

What is the pathogenesis of SLE?

Anti-dsDNA antibodies may be directly pathogenic. Auto-antibodies may be present for many years before symptoms but often rise in titre just before symptoms develop. Circulating immune complexes are characteristic and are formed or deposited in the skin, kidney and brain; these activate complement and certain complement fragments (e.g. C3a) and induce release of pro-inflammatory cytokines. An increase in B-cell activity is also seen, with production of autoantibodies. Defective clearance of apoptotic cells may contribute to the pathogenesis.

Do any drugs cause SLE?

Drug-induced lupus – e.g. minocycline, hydralazine, procainamide, penicillamine – is more common in males, tends to spare the nervous system and kidneys, resolves on stopping the drug and is anti-dsDNA negative, but histone positive. Exogenous oestrogens may have a lower risk of lupus flares than previously thought but are still associated with thrombotic risk.

Which serological tests may be positive in SLE?

Autoantibodies are directed against several intracellular and cell surface antigens, but not all are clinically relevant. An antinuclear antibody titre > 1:80 is present in around 95% of patients. Anti-dsDNA is the most common antibody to an extractable nuclear antigen, positive in most patients. Anti-Sm antibody is highly specific for SLE but only positive in around 10% of patients. Other important antibodies variably present include anti-Ro, anti-La, anti-RNP and anti-phospholipid antibodies (anti-cardiolipin and lupus anticoagulant). There is increasing awareness of the probable role of

Table 5.34 System review in systemic lupus erythematosus (SLE)

System	Possible features
Non-specific	Fever, fatigue, anorexia, weight loss, lymphadenopathy C-reactive protein usually normal in SLE
Skin (skin involvement affects most patients)	Butterfly rash Alopecia Raynaud's phenomenon Vasculitis, and sometimes widespread erythroderma and skin breakdown Discoid lupus
Musculoskeletal (arthralgia affects most patients)	Symmetrical, flitting and polyarticular arthralgia without synovitis Non-erosive, deforming Jacoud's arthritis more common than erosive arthritis Avascular necrosis of the hip Osteoporosis (vitamin D deficiency, menstrual dysfunction, corticosteroids)
Renal (affects 30%)	Six types of lupus nephritis (LN) (I minimal mesangial LN, II mesangial proliferative LN, III focal LN, IV diffuse LN, V membranous LN, VI advanced sclerosis LN)
Central nervous system lupus/neuropsychiatric SLE (NPSLE)	Traditionally classified as seizures or psychosis Now the American Rheumatism Council classifies central nervous system lupus into 19 syndromes, with clear distinction between manifestations of lupus and those caused by antiphospholipid syndrome Manifestations include strokes, transient ischaemic attacks, seizures, movement disorders (e.g. chorea), headaches including migraine, cognitive disorders, visual loss, transverse myelopathy and demyelination syndromes, (acute demyelinating polyradiculopathy), plexopathy, mononeuropathy, cranial neuropathy Seizures due to lupus cerebral vasculitis rare
Haematological	Around two-thirds have anaemia, usually normochromic normocytic Around one-third have antiphospholipid antibodies Antiphospholipid syndrome
Cardiovascular	Pericarditis commonly subclinical; symptoms in 25% at some stage Myocarditis rare Accelerated atherosclerosis (e.g. coronary, carotid), independent of traditional cardiovascular disease risk factors, now recognised as major cause of morbidity and mortality; relative risk increase appears to be around 50
Respiratory	Pleuritic chest pain common, with or without effusions Acute pneumonitis rare but dangerous Chronic pneumonitis common and seldom severe Pulmonary hypertension due to thrombosis or vasculitis 'Shrinking lung syndrome' characterised by dyspnoea and small lungs
Gastrointestinal disease	Oral lesions discoid, erythematous or ulcerative Small vessel vasculitis can affect gut causing ischaemia, infarction, perforation and peritonitis

anti-C1q antibodies in lupus nephritis; it may be useful in detecting flares.

Are any autoantibodies associated with specific complications or disease activity?

Anti-dsDNA is closely associated with renal disease and increased titres may herald a disease flare. Anti-Ro correlates with photosensitive skin rashes and anti-Ro and La with Sjögren's syndrome.

Is the C-reactive protein usually raised in active SLE?

A normal C-reactive protein with a raised erythrocyte sedimentation rate is characteristic.

What treatments are used in SLE?

These are outlined in Table 5.35. In general, mild disease with skin or joint involvement is treated with topical treatments or hydroxychloroquine, moderate disease with non-life-threatening organ involvement (e.g. pericarditis) is treated with corticosteroids and/or steroid-sparing agents and severe disease with life-threatening organ involvement, such as lupus nephritis or central nervous system lupus, is treated with high-dose immunosuppression.

Do you know of any future potential therapies for severe lupus?

Biologic therapies, as in rheumatoid arthritis, are evolving in SLE. Rituximab is a chimeric human–murine monoclo-

Table 5.35 Treatments in systemic lupus erythematosus (SLE)

Problem	Treatments	Comments
Fatigue	Exercise programmes Anti-malarials (anecdotal evidence)	
Skin rashes and arthralgia	Sunscreens Topical steroid preparations combined with hydroxychloroquine Topical tacrolimus and pimecrolimus (limited evidence yet) Non-steroidal anti-inflammatory drugs and cyclo-oxygenase-2 selective agents avoided because of gastrointestinal, renal and cardiovascular risks	Patients with isolated cutaneous, including discoid, lupus are unlikely to progress to systemic disease Hydroxychloroquine is the mainstay for mild SLE with arthralgia, skin rashes, alopecia and oral or genital ulceration; it is well tolerated, disease modifying, has weak antithrombotic action, benefits lipid and glucose profiles and has a low risk of cataracts Oral dapsone is used in resistant skin disease
Lupus nephritis	Long-term, high-dose monthly or quarterly intravenous 'pulse' cyclophosphamide traditionally used Short courses of low-dose pulse cyclophosphamide followed by azathioprine produce similar results with less toxicity Mycophenolate mofetil as induction and maintenance therapy in severe proliferative lupus nephritis may supersede cyclophosphamide	Lupus nephritis is a powerful prognostic indicator
Central nervous system lupus/ neuropsychiatric SLE (NPSLE)	Corticosteroids Immunosuppression (cyclophosphamide, methotrexate, azathioprine) Antipsychotics Anticoagulation for thrombotic manifestations, e.g. stroke, transient ischaemic attacks, seizures or cognitive dysfunction associated with antiphospholipid antibodies	Treatment depends on syndrome
Cardiovascular disease	Role of corticosteroid and immunosuppression unclear	Chronic inflammatory disease activity likely causes endothelial and vascular damage leading to atherosclerosis

nal antibody against CD20 on B cells and their precursors, but not plasma cells. It is widely used in lymphoma treatment and is relatively well tolerated and safe. It may have a place in treating SLE, in combination with methylprednisolone and cyclophosphamide, that has not responded to alternative immunosuppression. Anti-dsDNA antagonists have been mooted.

What is the relationship between SLE and antiphospholipid syndrome (APS)?

APS or Hughes' syndrome was initially described in SLE but is a syndrome that may complicate other autoimmune disorders or present in its own right (see Case 2.37). The key features are arterial and venous thromboses and recurrent morbidity in pregnancy, often with livedo reticularis and thrombocytopenia. Features are often the result of thrombosis in any organ system. More recently described potential manifestations of APS include renal artery stenosis, metatarsal fractures, avascular necrosis and vascular dysfunction. Heart valve disease, sometimes progressing rapidly to need for replacement, distinguishes APS from other thrombotic disorders. Catastrophic APS, with severe, widespread thrombosis, occurs in around 1% of patients. Pulmonary hypertension is rare in lupus but may be the result of APS. Primary APS seldom progresses to SLE,

while APS presenting in patients with SLE significantly increases morbidity and mortality.

What are the treatments for APS?

Treatments for APS include plasma exchange, corticosteroids and intravenous immunoglobulin. Immunosuppression increases mortality. Anticoagulation aims for an international normalised ratio (INR) of 2.0–3.0 for recurrent venous thrombosis but higher targets, such as 3.0–4.5, may be warranted in recurrent arterial thrombosis.

What is the relationship between SLE and pregnancy, the contraceptive pill and hormone replacement therapy?

In general, pregnancy outcomes are good if SLE is in remission at conception, but there may still be a higher risk of complications. Risk is higher if antiphospholipid antibodies are present. Risk is much higher if active disease, hypertension or lupus nephritis are present at conception, and pregnancy should be deferred until remission. Complications include recurrent early pregnancy loss, fetal death, pre-eclampsia, intrauterine growth restriction and preterm delivery. Maternal thrombosis is increased postpartum, especially in the puerperium. Pulmonary

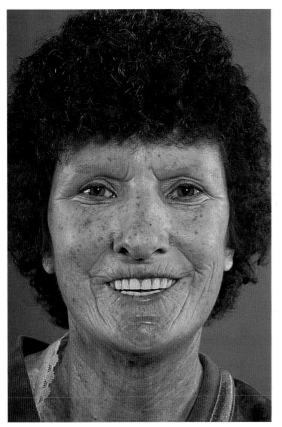

Fig. 5.46 Scleroderma.

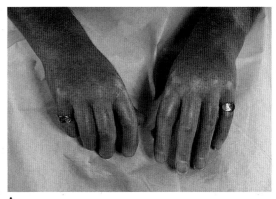

A

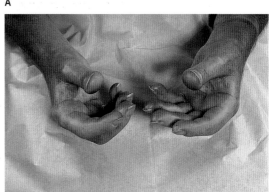

B

Fig. 5.47 (A,B) Scleroderma.

hypertension, although uncommon in lupus, increases maternal mortality.

The role of exogenous oestrogen in SLE is uncertain. Oestrogen might increase the risk of disease flares, but this does not appear to be overt, and the bigger risk is that of thrombotic disease in those with antiphospholipid antibodies.

CASE 5.19

SCLERODERMA

Instruction

Please examine this patient's face and hands and discuss your findings.

Recognition

Face (Fig. 5.46)

There are *dilated capillaries (telangiectasia)*, and the *skin appears smooth, shiny and tight*. The nose may appear beaked. There may be *perioral skin puckering* with microstomia and restricted mouth opening.

Hands (Fig. 5.47)

The *skin over the fingers is also smooth, shiny and tight (sclerodactyly)*. There may be *dilated nail-fold capillaries (telangiectasia)*, *nail-fold infarcts, ragged cuticles, evidence of digital ischaemia with ulceration, infarcts and pulp atrophy* (± amputations), and calcinosis (with subcutaneous calcium deposits in the digits and fingertips).

Interpretation

Confirm the diagnosis

Distinguish limited from diffuse cutaneous systemic sclerosis. The latter extends above the elbows or knees or involves the trunk. Tell the examiners that you would confirm the diagnosis and stratify risk using hallmark antibodies (see Table 5.38).

What to do next – assess other systems

Tell the examiners you would like to:

- Ask about Raynaud's phenomenon
- Examine the lungs for evidence of interstitial lung disease
- Examine for signs of pulmonary hypertension

Table 5.36 Pathogenesis in scleroderma

Pathogenesis	Possible therapies
1. Vascular Microcirculatory endothelial cell activation	Vascular therapies Vasodilators Vascular remodelling, e.g. angiotensin-converting enzyme inhibitors Prostacyclin analogues Antioxidants
2. Immunological Perivascular inflammation with monocyte and subsequent lymphocyte infiltration	Immunomodulatory therapies Methotrexate Cyclophosphamide Azathioprine Mycophenolate mofetil Low-dose corticosteroid Antithymocyte globulin Stem cell transplantation Anti-tumour necrosis factor agents
3. Fibrosis Subsequent fibroblast activation Fibroblasts deposit extracellular matrix in affected tissues and organs	Antifibrotic therapies Anti-transforming growth factor antibody Endothelin receptor antagonists

Table 5.37 Scleroderma classification and spectrum of disease

Type	Subtype
Raynaud's phenomenon	Primary Autoimmune
Systemic scleroderma now more appropriately termed systemic sclerosis (SSc)	Limited Limited cutaneous (Lc) SSc Diffuse cutaneous (Dc) SSc SSc *sine* scleroderma Scleroderma overlap syndromes, e.g. arthritis, polymyositis, systemic lupus erythematosus
Localised scleroderma	Plaque morphea Generalised morphea Linear scleroderma (*en coup de sabre*)

- Ask about gastrointestinal symptoms
- Assess renal function

Consider severity/decompensation/complications

Tell the examiners you would investigate for important complications:

- Interstitial lung disease
- Pulmonary hypertension
- Gastro-oesophageal reflux and Barrett's oesophagus
- Scleroderma renal crisis

Consider function

Tell the examiners that severe sclerodactyly, painful digital ischaemia and breathlessness commonly compromise function.

Discussion

How common is scleroderma?

The prevalence may be around 1–2/10 000. The female : male ratio is 5 : 1.

What is the pathogenesis of scleroderma, and does it have therapeutic implications?

The pathogenesis is incompletely understood, but three mechanisms are involved, with therapeutic implications (Table 5.36).

Is there a genetic basis to scleroderma?

Genetic abnormalities in anti-fibrillin-1 are implicated.

How is scleroderma classified?

Although the terms scleroderma and systemic scleroderma (SSc) are often used synonymously, SSc is a heterogeneous disease within the spectrum of scleroderma disorders, SSc being used to describe conditions involving fibrosis of the skin and internal organs with microvasculopathy. SSc is relatively rare. Scleroderma disorders share several clinical features, notably skin thickening from dermal fibrosis and a high incidence of episodic peripheral vasospasm. The classification of scleroderma is shown in Table 5.37.

Why is Raynaud's phenomenon classified under scleroderma?

In Raynaud's phenomenon there is evidence of microvasculopathy on nail-fold capillaroscopy and/or serum antibodies against nuclear antigens (autoimmune Raynaud's phenomenon), and there is a 10–15% chance of developing a connective tissue disease, including SSc, in the long term. Raynaud's phenomenon affects virtually all patients with SSc, with variable severity. In limited cutaneous (Lc) SSc, it typically precedes other features, but in diffuse cutaneous (Dc) SSc is more likely to be contemporaneous.

What are the differences between LcSSc and DcSSc?

Most SSc may be classified as either LcSSc or DcSSc depending upon the extent of skin involvement. Both forms involve other organs.

LcSSc

This is typically preceded by a long history, often many years, of Raynaud's phenomenon, leading to what used to be referred to as the acronym CREST syndrome (calcinosis, Raynaud's phenomenon, oesophageal dysmotility, sclerodactyly and telangiectasia); the acronym is misleading because it ignores important manifestations of LcSSc such as pulmonary hypertension and gastrointestinal disease.

Table 5.38 Scleroderma hallmark antibodies

Antigen	Immunofluorescence	Clinical association
Centromere	Centromere	LcSSc almost exclusively (and occur in 60% of LcSSc) Pulmonary hypertension and gut disease; less likely to have interstitial lung fibrosis
Topoisomerase 1 (Scl-70)	Nucleolar (diffuse fine speckles)	35% of DcSSc, 10–15% of LcSSc Renal disease in DcScc Lung fibrosis in LCSSc or DcSSc
RNA polymerases I and III	Nucleolar (punctuate)	20% of DcSSc Renal disease in LcSSc or DcSSc
PM-Scl	Nucleolar (homogenous)	5% of patients – myositis
U1 RNP	Nuclear (speckled)	10% of patients, often black
Fibrillarin (U3 RNP)	Nucleolar (clumpy)	5% of LcScc or DcSSc Poor outcome in DcScc (cardiac disease, pulmonary hypertension, renal disease)

SSc, systemic sclerosis; LcSSc, limited cutaneous SSc; DcSSc, diffuse cutaneous SSc.
Autoantibody profiles for scleroderma are evolving as the pathogenicity and prognostic implications of some of these are better understood; topoisomerase 1, for example, carries a poorer prognosis.

DcSSc

This is defined by sclerosis proximal to the elbows or knees or involving the trunk.

Is SSc always symptomatic?

The term SSc has recently been applied to patients without skin involvement but who have SSc-specific antibodies or scleroderma-associated capillaroscopic changes.

What is SSc *sine* scleroderma?

This refers to a small group of patients with vascular symptoms and SSc-specific antibodies and major organ complications in the absence of significant skin sclerosis.

What is morphea?

Morphea refers to plaques of sclerosis, often with a purplish edge, that are usually localised but occasionally generalised.

Can scleroderma complications be predicted?

Scleroderma hallmark antibodies are associated with certain types of scleroderma (Table 5.38) and can identify patients at increased risk of major complications.

How are the organ complications of scleroderma managed?

Management of common features is outlined in Table 5.39.

Would you always treat skin complications?

Only methotrexate currently has evidence of benefit. Alternative new strategies may include anti-thymocyte globulin followed by mycophenolate mofetil and high-dose cyclophosphamide and then autologous peripheral stem cell transplantation. However, treatment is considered in context, because diffuse SSc can sometimes strikingly improve by three years without treatment. Ultimately, diffuse SSc may benefit from more targeted cytokine or chemokine treatments.

What do you know about lung involvement in scleroderma?

Interstitial lung disease (SSc-ILD) and pulmonary hypertension (PAH) are major causes of mortality and morbidity in SSc.

SSc-ILD

Symptoms of fibrosis are usually late. Other contributors to breathlessness may include anaemia, chest wall restriction and drugs, e.g. methotrexate. Cyclophosphamide is the current drug of choice.

PAH

The prevalence of PAH in SSc is probably 7–15% with a five-year survival of 10% compared with 80% in those without PAH. The PAH may occur with both classic limited SSc with anti-centromere antibody positivity and diffuse SSc with antifibrillarin antibodies (U3RNP). Exertional dyspnoea is the major symptom, but diagnosis is often delayed, with subsequent right heart failure. General measures include oral anticoagulation, diuretics and oxygen. Intravenous prostacyclin (epoprostenol) improves exercise capacity, cardiac output and survival but is limited by catheterisation/pump problems and side effects. Other prostacyclin modes of administration (e.g. inhaled, subcutaneous) appear less effective. PDE5 inhibitors (e.g. sildenafil) may be used. The oral endothelin receptor antagonist (bosentan) may be used, sometimes combined with intravenous prostacyclin and sildenafil in severe disease.

Can PAH be predicted?

Patients with SSc should have annual echocardiography and pulmonary function tests, because a reduced TLCO (< 60% predicted) with a normal forced vital capacity may indicate subsequent development of PAH.

Table 5.39 Management of scleroderma

Organ involved or complication	Clinical manifestations	Investigation	Current treatments
Raynaud's phenomenon (Vasospasm + structural changes)	Painful ischaemia Digital ulceration Digital infarction	Capillaroscopy	Vasodilators, e.g. calcium channel blockers Antibiotics Prostacyclin analogues Digital sympathectomy Bosentan Phosphodiesterase inhibitors
Skin	Calcinosis, Raynaud's phenomenon, sclerodactyly, telangiectasia	Biopsy seldom needed	Topical emollients ?Anti-tumour necrosis factor-α agents for calcinosis Methotrexate for diffuse SSc
Lung	Interstitial lung disease (SSc-ILD)	Pulmonary function tests (DLCO the best predictor of survival) High-resolution CT scan (correlates well with DLCO) Bronchoalveolar lavage (heavy neutrophil counts associated with severe disease)	Cyclophosphamide
	Pulmonary hypertension (PAH)	Echocardiography Cardiac angiography (mean PAP > 25 mmHg at rest and > 30 mmHg on exercise)	Long-term oxygen therapy Diuretics Anticoagulation Epoprostenol Bosentan Atrial septostomy Lung transplantation (late stage)
Gastrointestinal tract	Gastro-oesophageal reflux Oesophageal dysmotility Bacterial overgrowth Vascular mucosal lesions Constipation/diarrhoea	Endoscopy	Proton pump inhibitors Prokinetic agents Antibiotics
Kidney	Scleroderma renal crisis (SRC)	Urinalysis Renal biopsy (fibrinoid necrosis; true vasculitis rare)	Angiotensin-converting enzyme inhibitors
Cardiac	Conduction disturbance		Permanent pacemaker

CT, computed tomography; DLCO, diffusing capacity of the lung for carbon monoxide; PAP, pulmonary artery pressure; SSc, systemic sclerosis.

What is a scleroderma renal crisis (SRC)?

This is the most important renal complication, and was the major cause of mortality before angiotensin-converting enzyme (ACE) inhibitors (survival 10% at one year without treatment to 65% at five years with treatment). It is most common in early diffuse SSc with rapid skin progression. Other associations include anaemia, anti-RNA polymerase I and III antibody positivity and antecedent use of high-dose steroids, NSAIDs and ciclosporin. It presents with abrupt severe hypertension with headache and visual disturbances and accelerated oliguric renal failure with a nephritic picture. Flash pulmonary oedema, heart failure and pericardial effusions may occur. Microangiopathic haemolytic anaemia or thrombocytopenia are possible.

CASE 5.20

CRYSTAL ARTHROPATHY

Instruction

Please examine this patient's feet/other joints/ears; discuss your findings and any tests you would like to arrange.

Recognition

Acute gout

There is *swelling of the first metatarsophalangeal (MTP) joint* (or knee, ankle or other joints). The patient reports that the joint has been *exquisitely painful and tender* (ask before examining!). Weight bearing is very painful.

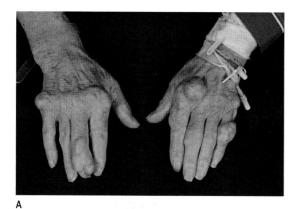

A

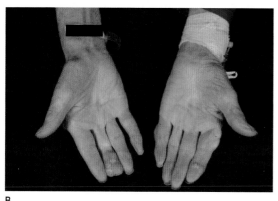

B

Fig. 5.48 (A,B) Tophaceous gout.

Table 5.40 Gout – causes and risk factors

Cause or risk factor	Examples
Sex	Male > female
Family history	Genetics and ethnicity, more common in Maori population (gout was also common in Tyrannosaurus rex)
Metabolic syndrome	Obesity, increased cholesterol and hypertension within metabolic syndrome
Drugs	Alcohol Diuretics Low-dose aspirin/salicylates Cyclosporin/cytotoxics Levodopa Ethambutol, pyrizinamide
Diet (usually in setting of underexcretion)	Excess purines, e.g. beer, shellfish, liver
Underexcretion of urate (the major group of causes)	Chronic kidney disease (creatinine clearance < 30% of normal) Hypothyroidism Drugs Lead
Overproduction of urate	Myeloproliferative or lymphoproliferative disease Tumour lysis/chemotherapy Chronic haemolysis Inborn errors increasing purine levels

Chronic tophaceous gout (Fig. 5.48)

There are *painless tophi* – cheesy, chalky lesions that may ulcerate – at extra-articular sites (helix, olecranon/patellar bursa, ulnar surface of forearm, Achilles tendon, etc.). Polyarticular involvement is also common, e.g. knees, first MTP joint, ankles, hands.

Interpretation

Confirm the diagnosis

An acute monoarthritis that is exquisitely tender and with associated erythema is invariably the result of gout or septic arthritis. Acute gout is the result of an intense inflammatory response in joints (tophaceous gout is non-inflammatory) and there may be fever and systemic upset. Diagnostic aspiration might be needed.

What to do next – consider causes

Many cases of gout are apparently idiopathic. Common causes and risk factors are listed in Table 5.40.

Acute gout is most readily induced when serum urate levels are in a state of rapid flux, rather than by absolute levels. It can occur when the urate level is falling. Factors precipitating attacks include dehydration, alcohol, trauma, sepsis (lactic acid competes with urate excretion), diuretics and allopurinol.

Chronic tophaceous gout tends to affect an older age group and is more readily associated with longstanding high serum urate levels. There tend to be exacerbations and remissions. Uric acid is less soluble at lower temperatures, which may explain the tendency for tophi to occur at sites exposed to cold.

Consider severity/decompensation/complications

Consider the possibility of nephrolithiasis and renal failure caused by urate crystals formed by prolonged hyperuricaemia and hyperuricuria.

Consider function

Acute limitation of movement by the pain in acute gout is characteristic. Chronic loss of function due to erosive joint disease occurs in tophaceous gout.

Discussion

What are the crystal arthropathies?

These are listed in Table 5.41.

How is gout diagnosed?

Synovial fluid should be aspirated whenever possible (large joint) and demonstrates inflammation (often with a very high white cell count); polarised microscopy reveals needle-shaped, negatively birefringent intracellular (especially acute) and extracellular (especially ulcerated tophi) crystals. Serum urate levels can be misleading. Inflammatory markers are raised; a C-reactive protein in the range 50–150 is typical; higher levels suggest possible sepsis. X-rays may show periarticular punched out erosions and eventually joint destruction. Tophi are usually radiolucent but sometimes calcified.

How would you treat acute gout?

Rehydration is important. Any implicated drug should be stopped. Non-steroidal anti-inflammatory drugs (NSAIDs) alleviate symptoms; indomethacin 50 mg four times daily for three days, decreasing by 50 mg every two days thereafter, is very effective (perhaps because most toxic). Cyclo-oxygenase 2 (COX-2) agents (etoricoxib) are of proven efficacy but contentious. Colchicine is useful if NSAIDs are contraindicated, e.g. 0.5 mg twice or thrice daily (not more frequently as was once recommended). Prednisolone 15 mg, reducing over 10 days, is also effective, and corticosteroid joint injections can be used. Painful acute attacks would last several weeks without treatment.

How would you treat recurrent gout?

As well as tackling reversible causes or risk factors, allopurinol is effective. Treatment should be covered for six weeks or so with colchicine or NSAIDs because allopurinol can precipitate acute gout; colchicine has gained favour in recent years. Allopurinol titration to serum urate levels is currently favoured, a typical dose is 300 mg but up to 600 or 900 mg may be needed and a reduction to 100 mg can be required in patients with chronic kidney disease.

When would you consider prophylaxis?

It should be decided with the patient, but two to three attacks is generally a convincing reason. Joints become irreversibly damaged by repeated attacks of inflammation.

Other indications include a single polyarticular attack, tophaceous gout, urate calculi and renal disease.

Does allopurinol cause tophi to recede?

It can sometimes do this, over a few years.

What is 'pseudogout'?

Calcium pyrophosphate arthropathy can mimic gout and often affects the wrist, knee or shoulder but may be polyarticular. Chondrocalcinosis (calcium deposition in cartilage) is an essential precursor, but also occurs in gout, primary hyperparathyroidism, hypothyroidism and haemochromatosis – states promoting cartilage calcification. Synovial fluid is similar to that of gout but crystals are polymorphic, often rhomboid or rectangular, sometimes needle-shaped, and positively birefringent. It is very rare under the age of 50 years. Treatment is as for acute gout, but prophylaxis is unavailable.

What is Milwaukee shoulder?

This is a very severe and rapidly destructive calcium hydroxapatite shoulder arthritis in older people. The other major calcium hydroxapatite arthritis is calcific periarthritis, a rotator cuff problem that tends to occur in midlife.

CASE 5.21

OSTEOARTHRITIS

Instruction

Please examine this patient's hands and discuss your findings.

Recognition

There is *bony swelling* of the *distal interphalangeal (DIP) joints (Heberden's nodes)* (Fig. 5.49) and *proximal*

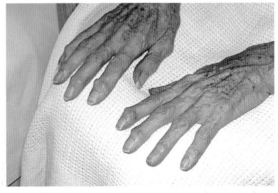

Fig. 5.49 Heberden's nodes.

Table 5.41 The crystal arthropathies	
Arthropathy	**Crystal**
Gout	Urate in joint or soft tissues
Pseudogout	Calcium pyrophosphate (shed from joints)
Basic calcium phosphate arthropathies – calcific periarthritis, Milwaukee shoulder	Calcium hydroxyapatite

interphalangeal (PIP) joints (Bouchard's nodes). There is not usually evidence of synovitis. There may be crepitus and restricted range of movement. There is no apparent systemic upset.

Interpretation

Confirm the diagnosis

Osteoarthritis pain is worse with activity. Any morning stiffness is transient. Pointers to other diagnoses are listed in Table 5.42.

Morning stiffness is usually brief, unlike inflammatory arthritis.

What to do next – consider causes/assess other systems

Osteoarthritis is restricted to synovial joints, typically in the hands and spine (especially C5, L3, L4), and the hips and the knees. Risk factors as well as age and 'wear and tear' are listed in Box 5.25.

Consider severity/decompensation/complications

Tell the examiners that complications of osteoarthritis include pain, deformity, ankylosis, peripheral nerve entrapment and cervical spondylosis with cervical myeloradiculopathy.

Consider function

Tell the examiners that pain, deformity and nerve compression can thwart normal function.

Table 5.42 Pointers to other diagnoses

Clinical features	Associations
Age < 45 years	Inflammatory arthritis
Marked early morning stiffness	Inflammatory arthritis
Joint locking/giving way	Meniscal tear
Regional pain	Fibromyalgia
Swelling adjacent to joint	Bursitis

Box 5.25 Risk factor for osteoarthritis

Generalised predisposition
- Age
- Gender (females > males for hand and knee, females = males for hip)
- Hereditary (genes not yet identified)
- Obesity

Localised/biomechanical
- Joint injury/'wear and tear'
- Surgery
- Muscle weakness

Discussion

What is the prevalence of osteoarthritis?

This is high, but depends upon how osteoarthritis is defined. Almost all people over 50 years of age will have some osteophytes; progression to loss of joint space and subchondral bone sclerosis and ultimately a 'smashed up joint' are characteristic of osteoarthritis.

What is the natural history of osteoarthritis?

Osteoarthritis is a disease of joint damage and joint repair via osteophyte formation, bone remodelling, synovial responses and capsular change – only synovial joints are affected, with loss of cartilage and damage beneath.

What provokes this process is unclear. One theory is that osteoarthritis is equivalent to diverticulitis, with flares and remissions; another is that we are looking at the wrong pathology radiologically – appearances of which do not correlate with symptoms – some researchers think there is a microvascular basis to osteoarthritis. The natural history varies between individuals and joint sites, e.g. symptoms and disability are usually minimal when interphalangeal nodes have evolved, whereas knee osteoarthritis can worsen rapidly.

Osteoarthritis is now viewed as a disease where risk factors (see Box 5.25) induce subtle changes in joint shape and stability leading to attempted repair. This may have one of two possible outcomes – a successful, compensated joint without pain or disability, or a failed, decompensated joint with symptoms and disability. There seem to be three categories of patient – those with developing disease (painful), those with stable disease (painless) and those with progressive disease (painful) – all of which have the same radiological appearances.

What is the cause of symptoms in osteoarthritis?

The cause of pain is less certain, e.g. the ankle is never really affected but often painful; the elbow is often affected but seldom painful; the knee can be highly symptomatic with minimal damage. Pain tends to occur only when joint anatomy is changing, for example by osteophyte formation, perhaps from subchondral pressure or capsular stretching; synovitis is not relevant. Osteoarthritis may be a disorder of accelerated evolution – affected joints tend to be those that have changed as we have evolved from tree-dwelling monkeys and apes to upright humans, and there is no evolutionary pressure to protect joints after reproductive age. Animals tend not to develop osteoarthritis, or if they do it involves specific types, e.g. hip dysplasia in dogs and horses of certain breeds.

List some treatments for osteoarthritis

These are listed in Box 5.26. Prevention is important. Some types of physical activity are associated with an increased risk of arthritis in certain joints. Previous knee injury, surgery and even occupational or habitual

Box 5.26 Treatments for osteoarthritis

Non-pharmacological

- Education
- Weight reduction
- Physiotherapy

Oral and topical drugs

- Paracetamol
- Non-steroidal anti-inflammatory drugs (NSAIDs) or cyclo-oxygenase-2 inhibitors, co-prescribed with a proton pump inhibitor
- Topical NSAIDs for hand or knee arthritis
- Intra-articular steroids

Corticosteroids

Hyaluranons

- Intra-articular viscosupplemtenation not deemed beneficial

Dietary

- Glucosamine sulphate (synthetic cartilage matrix molecule) and chondroitin – modest benefit, discontinue if no improvement after some months

Surgery

- Total joint replacement
- Arthroscopic lavage and debridement not deemed useful unless mechanical locking

kneeling and squatting can, for example, predispose to osteoarthritis.

Is industrial compensation possible for osteoarthritis?

Occupations that at least double the risk of osteoarthritis may confer eligibility, e.g. coal miners (knee), farmers (hip).

CASE 5.22

PAGET'S DISEASE

Instruction

Please examine this patient's face/legs and discuss any further assessment you would make.

Recognition

There is *enlargement of the skull* (Fig. 5.50) or there is *bowing of the tibia* (Fig. 5.51), and the skin over the leg is warm. There may be kyphosis.

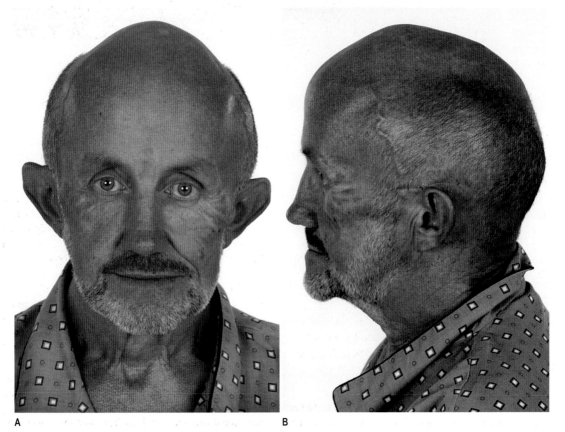

A   B

Fig. 5.50 (A,B) Paget's disease of the skull.

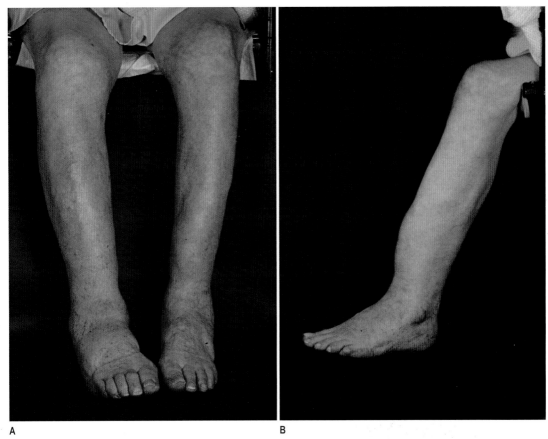

A   B

Fig. 5.51 (A,B) Paget's disease of the tibia.

Interpretation

Confirm the diagnosis

Tell the examiners that you would like to check an alkaline phosphatase level, which would be raised, and obtain X-rays.

What to do next – assess other systems

Neurological compression syndromes may be caused by bone enlargement, e.g. closure of skull foramina causing deafness. Look for a hearing aid.

Consider severity/decompensation/complications

Important serious consequences of Paget's disease include high output cardiac failure. Check for the bounding pulse of hyperdynamic circulation. Osteosarcoma is rare.

Consider function

Tell the examiners you would ask about bone pain. Other common problems are skeletal deformity, secondary osteoarthritis and an increased risk of fractures.

Discussion

How common is Paget's disease?

Radiographic evidence is seen in around 2.5% of men over 55 years of age, and a little less in women. Less than 10% of those have symptoms. It occurs predominantly in people of English origin, including those in North America and Australasia. It may be declining in prevalence.

What happens to bone in Paget's disease?

Paget's disease is caused by focal or multifocal areas of bone resorption by large osteoclasts, followed by increased bone formation, but the new bone is abnormal, with a mosaic appearance on microscopy. It is expanded in size, deforms and fractures more easily and is highly vascularised. Fractures may be complete or 'incremental' along the convex surface of deformed bones. Pathological changes tend to progress through bone at a rate of around 1 cm per year, and do not advance from bone to bone; thus the bony distribution tends to be fixed.

Case 5.23 Marfan's syndrome

List some serum or urine biochemical changes in Paget's disease

- Raised alkaline phosphatase
- Raised serum osteocalcin (but often normal, and not used in practice)
- Raised urinary hydroxyproline and pyridinolone (markers of bone resorption, and not used in practice)

List some other causes of raised alkaline phosphatase

- Hyperparathyroidism
- Bone metastases
- Growth
- Osteomalacia
- Liver disease

Are any other investigations useful?

Radiology confirms Paget's disease by bone expansion. This is rare in metastases, which tend to be sclerotic but not expanded. Uncertainty is occasionally resolved by bone biopsy, for example in a case of isolated rib expansion.

What are the common indications for treatment of Paget's disease?

Bone pain or hypercalcaemia (tends to occur only in immobilised patients) are the usual indications.

Should asymptomatic Paget's disease be treated?

There is no absolute consensus, but indications include skull disease (risk of deafness), long bone disease (risk of deformity, fracture and arthritis) or spinal disease (risk of cord compression or vascular steal syndrome).

What is the current treatment of choice for Paget's disease?

Bisphosphonate therapy (intravenous pamidronate, oral risedronate or intravenous zolendroic acid) is the treatment of choice, with a view to normalisation of alkaline phosphatase levels (achieved in around 75% of patients); this is associated with marked pain reduction.

CASE 5.23

MARFAN'S SYNDROME

Instruction

Please examine this young man's stature and arms and briefly any other systems you feel relevant and report your diagnosis.

Recognition

This gentleman is *tall*, with a *thin body habitus*, *long limbs*, *arachnodactyly* and a *pectus deformity*. There is a *high arched palate* with dental crowding (Fig. 5.52).

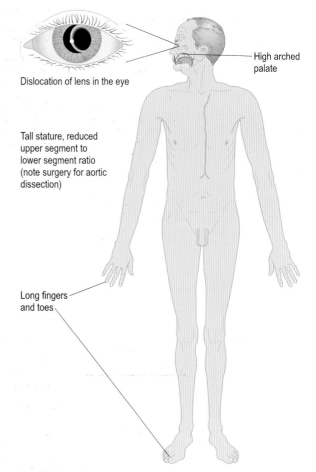

Dislocation of lens in the eye

High arched palate

Tall stature, reduced upper segment to lower segment ratio (note surgery for aortic dissection)

Long fingers and toes

Fig. 5.52 Marfan's syndrome.

Interpretation

Confirm the diagnosis

Recognising the possible Marfan's phenotype is all that is needed. To formally confirm the diagnosis, reference should normally then be made to the Ghent diagnostic nosology devised in 1996 (not to be memorised!), in which clinical features are assessed as part of seven body 'systems' (Table 5.43) to determine whether that system provides a major criterion or simply system involvement. The cardiovascular assessment requires measurement of the aortic diameter at the sinuses of Valsalva, usually by echocardiography.

What to do next – assess other systems

Tell the examiners of other possible features of Marfan's syndrome (Table 5.43). Differential diagnoses on the basis of skeletal, cardiac and ocular manifestations include a range of genetic disorders such as homocystinuria, Ehlers–Danlos syndrome, ectopia lentis, Beal's syndrome, Marshall–Stickler syndrome and the MASS phenotype (see below).

Table 5.43 Diagnostic criteria for Marfan's syndrome

	Major criteria	Minor criteria	For involvement	Diagnosis
Skeletal system	Four or more of: Pectus carinatum Pectus excavatum needing surgery Reduced upper-segment to lower-segment ratio or arm span to height ratio Wrist and thumb signs Scoliosis > 20° or spondylolisthesis Reduced extension of elbows (<170°) Medial displacement of medial malleolus causing pes planus Protrusio acetabulae of any degree on X-ray	Pectus excavatum Joint hypermobility High arched palate with crowded teeth Facial appearance (dolichocephaly, malar hypoplasia, enophthalmos, retrognathia, down-slanting palpebral fissures)	Two or more features contributing to major criteria or one feature contributing to major criteria and two minor criteria	
Ocular system	Ectopia lentis	Flat cornea Increased axial length of globe Hypoplastic iris or ciliary muscle causing decreased miosis	Two or more minor criteria	**Index case** If family/genetic history not contributory, major criteria in two or more different organ systems and involvement of a third are needed; if a mutation is identified, one major criterion in an organ system and involvement of a second are needed for diagnosis **Relative of an index case** meeting diagnostic criteria The presence of a major criterion in the family history, one major criterion in an organ system and involvement of a third are needed for diagnosis
Cardiovascular system	*Either* dilatation of ascending aorta with or without regurgitation, and involving at least sinuses of Valsalva *or* dissection of ascending aorta	Mitral valve prolapse with or without regurgitation Dilatation of main pulmonary artery without alternative cause if younger than 40 years Calcified mitral annulus if younger than 40 years Dilatation or dissection of descending thoracic or abdominal aorta if younger than 50 years	One minor criterion	
Pulmonary system	None	Spontaneous pneumothorax Apical blebs	One minor criterion	
Skin and integument	None	Striae atrophica (stretch marks) without marked weight gain, pregnancy or repetitive stress Recurrent or incisional herniae	One minor criterion	
Dura	Lumbosacral dural ectasia (very common and identified by magnetic resonance imaging if presence would make diagnosis)	None		
Family/genetic history	Parent, child or sibling meeting criteria independently Mutation in *FBN1* Haplotype around *FBN1* associated with Marfan's syndrome in family	None		

Consider severity/decompensation/complications

Tell the examiners that progressive aortic dilatation and associated aortic valve incompetence are the key life-threatening features. Aortic dissection is associated with an aortic diameter exceeding 5.5 cm, a rate of dilatation exceeding 5% or 2 mm per year or a history of aortic dissection. Mitral valve prolapse is a very common feature, often with regurgitation. Recurrent pneumothoraces can be life threatening.

Consider function

Common functional problems in Marfan's syndrome are skeletal, including arthritic sequelae of chronic joint laxity, and ocular, especially lens dislocation and myopia.

Discussion

What causes Marfan's syndrome?

Marfan's syndrome is a variable, autosomal dominant connective tissue disorder with an incidence of around 1–2 in 10 000. It affects both sexes equally. A fundamental problem is a decreased elastin content in tissues, and fragmentation of elastic fibres, due to mutations in the extracellular matrix protein fibrillin 1 (FBM1) located on chromosome 15. Mutations are not always detectable in people with Marfan's syndrome and furthermore may be found in people without Marfan's syndrome. Family history is negative in around 25% of cases, probably explained by sporadic mutations. Modern understanding is that many aspects of the disorder are caused by altered regulation of transforming growth factor-β, highlighting a therapeutic potential for transforming growth factor-β antagonists.

What is the MASS phenotype?

There is a range of Marfan-like disorders with the presence of fibrillin mutations without Marfan's syndrome. These have a good prognosis, and include MASS (**m**itral valve prolapse, mild non-progressive **a**ortic dilatation, **s**kin and **s**keletal features).

What is the treatment for aortic root dilatation in Marfan's syndrome?

Beta blockers reduce the elastic fibre degeneration in the aorta that is the cause of progressive dilatation and important complications of aortic valve incompetence, and aneurysms and aortic dissection. The type of fibrillin mutation determines the severity and rate of progression and if medical treatment fails and the aortic root dilates to 5.5 cm or more, prophylactic surgery should be considered. As patients are surviving longer, second aneurysms and second operations are not uncommon. Life expectancy remains 45 ± 17 years, with scope for improvement.

How are ocular manifestations of Marfan's syndrome managed?

Bilateral ectopia lentis occurs in around 25% of patients. Lens dislocation may occur. Myopia is associated with an increased risk of retinal detachment. Regular ophthalmic assessment is needed.

How are skeletal manifestations of Marfan's syndrome managed?

Common problems are joint laxity with arthralgia and myalgia (> 50% of cases), scoliosis and reduced bone mineral density. Avoidance of contact sports protects joints and the lens of the eye from dislocation.

How are respiratory manifestations of Marfan's syndrome managed?

Pectus excavatum occurs in two-thirds of patients, and can sometimes cause restrictive ventilation requiring surgery. Spontaneous pneumothorax occurs in up to 10% of patients, and patient awareness is essential. Scuba diving should be avoided because of the risk of pneumothorax.

Is pregnancy risky in Marfan's syndrome?

The major risk is aortic dissection, greatly increased, especially if the aortic root diameter exceeds 4 cm, probably because of collagen and elastin deposition inhibition by oestrogens and hyperdynamic circulation.

CASE 5.24

EHLERS–DANLOS SYNDROME

Instruction

Please examine the joints and skin of this patient.

Recognition

There may be a combination of three broad clinical features:

- *Purpura* and skin fragility with poor 'tissue-papery' wound healing (Fig. 5.53)
- *Skin 'stretchiness'* which later becomes lax with extensive folds and wrinkles
- *Joint hypermobility*, and kyphoscoliosis

Interpretation

Confirm the diagnosis

The differential diagnosis of hypermobile joints includes osteogenesis imperfecta, Marfan's syndrome, joint hypermobility syndrome and pseudoxanthoma elasticum.

What to do next – assess other systems

Tell the examiners that you would listen to the heart and assess vision.

Consider severity/decompensation/complications

Tell the examiner that potentially serious complications include mitral valve prolapse and aortic dissection.

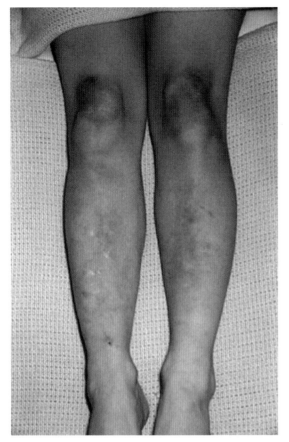

Fig. 5.53 Ehlers–Danlos syndrome – skin changes and bruising.

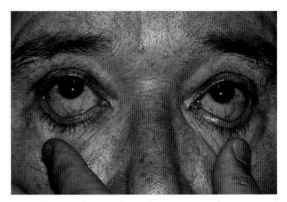

Fig. 5.54 Osteogenesis imperfecta – blue sclera.

Consider function

Tell the examiners that troublesome functional difficulties can arise from myopia, recurrent dislocations and falls.

Discussion

What is the genetic basis of Ehlers–Danlos syndrome?

Ehlers–Danlos syndrome refers to a heterogeneous range of disorders with autosomal dominant, autosomal recessive or X-linked inheritance. In classic Ehlers–Danlos syndrome with gross joint laxity and skin hyperextensibility, disease is principally the result of mutations in genes encoding collagen type V (*COL5A1* and *COL5A2*). In a vascular type of Ehlers–Danlos syndrome, collagen type III (*COL3A1*) results in arterial rupture, e.g. gastrointestinal bleeding.

CASE 5.25

OSTEOGENESIS IMPERFECTA

Instruction

Please look at this patient's eyes and hands and report your findings.

Recognition

The *sclera* have a *blue tinge* (Fig. 5.54). There are multiple finger *deformities* consistent with previous fractures.

Interpretation

Confirm the diagnosis

This should be clear, but tell the examiners that genetic testing may be used.

What to do next – assess other systems

Look at the long bones for deformities and the teeth for dentinogenesis imperfecta with variably coloured, somewhat translucent teeth.

Consider severity/decompensation/complications

Patients with dentinogenesis imperfecta may have accelerated dental caries and are at increased risk of basilar invagination, where the odontoid peg indents the brainstem.

Consider function

Tell the examiners that the severity of bone disease, fracture rate and spinal deformity determine functional abilities and quality of life. Ligament laxity also affects many patients.

Table 5.44 Types of osteogenesis imperfecta		
Type	Severity	Features
I	Mild	Blue sclera, lightening with age Minimal bowing of long bones Dentiginogenesis imperfecta may be present
II	Lethal	Severe fractures
III	Very severe	Triangular face, ocular prominence Fractures in utero, limbs bowed at birth Dentiginogenesis imperfecta
IV	Moderate	Frequent fractures, including vertebral, some deformation
V	Moderate/severe	Progressive deformation, hypertrophic callus formation
VI	Severe	Progressive deformation; growth retardation

Discussion

Are there different types of osteogenesis imperfecta?

The most commonly used classification is that of Sillence, modified by Glorieux (Table 5.44).

What causes osteogenesis imperfecta?

In most case, the underlying genetic abnormality is in genes encoding type 1 collagen (*COL1A1* and *COL1A2*). Several hundred mutations have been described and none are common.

What is the value of radiographs in osteogenesis imperfecta?

These document the degree of limb deformity, the presence of vertebral crush fractures and skull appearances that precede basilar invagination.

What management approaches are used in osteogenesis imperfecta?

Management is multidisciplinary – medical therapy centres on bisphosphonates, surgery helps limb deformity, physiotherapy increases muscle strength and stability, occupational therapy selects aids and optimises fine motor skills, orthotics may be needed and pain may be chronic and unremitting and require specialist pain management.

EYES

Examination of the eyes

Introduction

The eye has two separate visual faculties, served by different parts of the retina:

- Central vision is served by the central retina, dominated by the macula and a super-specialised area of the macula called the fovea.
- Peripheral vision is served by the peripheral retina.

Unlike a camera photographing images in which everything is reproduced with the same detail, the eye fixes on objects using the central retina and everything in the periphery is appreciated in less detail. While central and peripheral vision appear to merge imperceptibly, the retina's functions are discrete. This is why it is possible to lose central vision and preserve peripheral vision and vice versa.

Central image perception is dominated by the cone photoreceptors in the fovea, particularly sensitive to colour. Peripheral images are perceived by rods, particularly sensitive in the dark.

The retina comprises an inner layer of photoreceptors, the neuroretina adjacent to the vitreous, and an outer layer of pigment, the pigment retina, which receives its blood supply from the vascular choroid beneath (Fig. 5.55).

A normal eye brings parallel rays of light to a focus on the retina. Conventionally, beyond 6 m is infinity. Normal distance vision or visual acuity (VA) is said to be 6/6 – meaning that the eye sees at 6 m what it should see at 6 m; 6/24 means it sees only at 6 m what it should be able to see at 24 m. Near vision (< 6 m) is made possible by contraction of the ciliary muscle and alteration in the shape of the lens to shorten the focal length. This is necessary because rays of light entering the eye have diverged slightly from the parallel and, without refractive adjustment by the lens, they would converge to a focal point beyond the retina (too long a focal length). Long sight occurs when the focal length is too long for the eye. In other words, the eye is too short. Short sight occurs when the focal length is too short for the eye. In other words, the eye is too long. Long and short sightedness are merely refractive errors.

Fundoscopy

Neuro-ophthalmological disorders are discussed elsewhere; here the focus is on fundal abnormalities. The retina is the only part of the body where blood vessels and nervous tissue are visualised directly. Fundoscopy is ideally performed in a darkened room with dilating drops. Examiners appreciate the limits of fundoscopy and PACES abnormalities are likely to be overt.

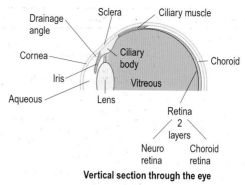

Vertical section through the eye

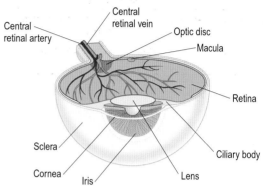

Horizontal section of the left eye, showing relative positions of the pupil, macula and optic disc

Fig. 5.55 Anatomy of the eye.

Approach

- Approach your patient's right eye from the right side, holding the ophthalmoscope in your right hand, and vice versa for the left eye (Fig. 5.56).
- Ask the patient to gaze on a distant object straight ahead at eye level.

Red reflex

- Check the red reflex. This is attenuated or lost in any condition affecting the transparency of structures in front of the retina (such as a cataract or vitreous haemorrhage), and in any condition affecting apposition of the normally transparent retina with the underlying red vascular choroid (such as retinal detachment).

Anterior structures

- Hold the patient's upper eyelid against the orbit (not against the eyeball!) and approach from 30° to the temporal side. This should ultimately bring the optic disc straight into view. Tilting your head sideways gives both the patient and yourself 'breathing space' and enables you to get close to the patient's eye. The closer you are, the easier it is to angle your

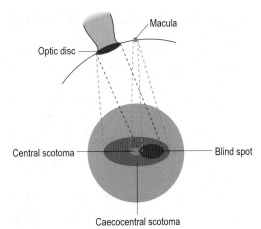

Fig. 5.57 The optic disc, the macula, the blind spot and central scotomas.

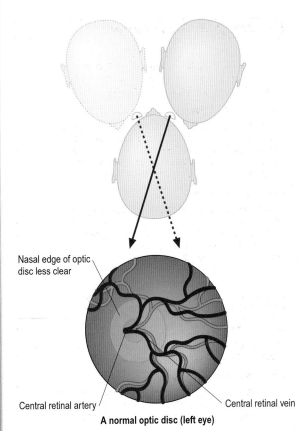

A normal optic disc (left eye)

Fig. 5.56 Fundoscopy.

Box 5.27 Some normal appearances of the optic disc

The nasal margin of the disc is normally less sharply demarcated than the temporal margin, and a rim of pigment seen on the temporal margin is very common. 'Early papilloedema' and 'retinitis pigmentosa' are often suggested apprehensively by candidates hoping to have seen more overt signs!

The centre of the optic disc is normally paler than the rim, and the vessels are seen to plunge into it. The colour of the optic disc varies in adults. Where only the four main vessels are seen on the disc it is normally quite pale. Where the vessels have early branches on the disc itself it appears much pinker. Sometimes elderly patients have very pale discs because of thin vessels.

---

ophthalmoscope into each quadrant and the bigger your field of view of the fundus.

• Before looking at the optic disc, focus through the anterior chamber, lens and vitreous as you proceed. Find '0' on the ophthalmoscope. West of '0' are negative numbers and east of '0' are positive numbers. Dial clockwise so that you start with a short focal length focusing on the cornea. Dialling progressively anticlockwise, through progressively longer focal lengths, will focus through the anterior chamber, lens (detecting any cataract), vitreous and finally on to the fundus.

This takes practice. Remember that short-sighted people have long eyes and '0' will focus on the vitreous; long-sighted people have short eyes and '0' will come to a focus behind the eye; if a patient is wearing their glasses then '0' will come to a focus on the retina.

Optic disc

• Now examine the optic disc. This full-moon-like circle is the optic nerve's head. Note its *margin*, *cup* and *colour*. If only blood vessels come into immediate view, follow them backwards against the angles of their branches. This should bring the optic disc into view.

• Be aware of some normal appearances of the optic disc, which confuse many candidates (Box 5.27).

Blood vessels

• Next pursue the four major vessels into each quadrant.

Macula

• Remember to look temporally at the macula. This can be done by asking your patient to look directly at the light. The *macula* is found two disc diameters from the temporal margin of the disc and appears as a pale yellow spot on a slightly darkened area of retina. It can be difficult to see (Box 5.28; Fig. 5.57).

Summary

The fundoscopy examination sequence is given in the Summary Box.

SUMMARY BOX – FUNDOSCOPY EXAMINATION SEQUENCE

• Check for the red reflex and look for cataracts
• Look at the optic disc and be aware of normal variants
• Follow the blood vessels into each quadrant, noting any abnormalities
• Look at the macula

Box 5.28 Macula, optic disc, central scotoma and blind spot

Candidates are very confused about the *macula*, the *optic disc* (the optic nerve's head), *central scotomas* and *blind spots*. What especially confuses (and is seldom explained in books) is how disease either at the macula or at the optic disc can produce a central scotoma.

The retina comprises a nerve cell (photoreceptor) layer and a deeper pigment layer, its pigment layer lying over the highly vascular choroid. The nerve fibres from the photoreceptors run in an orderly fashion to the optic disc (where they become tightly packed, their millions of converging axons giving rise to the disc's pale appearance) and become the optic nerve. The most important area of the retina is the macula, an area crowded with photoreceptors, whose axons form the most important bundle of fibres entering the optic nerve, the *papillomacular bundle*.

The optic disc, although an area of densely packed nerve fibres, is an area of retina without photoreceptors to receive visual images. The optic disc 'cannot see' and its corresponding visual axis is termed the blind spot (Fig. 5.59). The macula, on the other hand, is an area of densely packed photoreceptors (the fovea being its centre of excellence) and its corresponding visual axis is the area of central vision. Lesions of the macula therefore classically result in a central scotoma (Fig. 5.59).

Sometimes it is not just the macula that is damaged but a wider area of receptors and axons situated between the macula and the optic disc. In such cases the scotoma is large, extending between the visual axes of the macula and the optic disc, and this is called a caecocentral scotoma.

Optic atrophy implies damage to and degeneration of axons entering the optic disc. Because the papillomacular fibres are densely packed and thus vulnerable to a heavy casualty rate, central vision disturbance is marked, and can even result in a central scotoma or caecocentral scotoma.

In the early stages of optic disc swelling (Case 5.28) there is no visual disturbance. Later, retinal oedema may cause blind spot enlargement. Haemorrhages or oedema extending to the macula may cause abrupt central vision disturbance. Chronic scarring resulting from optic disc swelling may cause secondary optic atrophy with a central scotoma and/or progressive visual field restriction as fibres from the periphery entering the optic disc also degenerate.

Arcuate scotomas result from a wide variety of lesions. Arcuate scotomas are scotomas corresponding to damage to a bundle of nerve fibres entering the optic nerve. Primary open angle glaucoma causes a special type of arcuate scotoma that radiates from the blind spot. This is because raised intraocular pressure damages nerve fibres at the disc margins.

CASE 5.26

DIABETIC RETINOPATHY

Instruction

Please examine this patient's fundi and discuss your findings.

Recognition

Diabetic retinopathy (DR) is a microvascular process in which high retinal blood flow induces microangiopathy in capillaries, arterioles and venules, causing vessel occlusion and leakage of plasma contents into the retina itself. DR may be staged separately from diabetic maculopathy.

Box 5.29 Background diabetic retinopathy

Microaneurysms

These are bulges in weakened vessel walls and appear as red dots scattered throughout the fundus, but most commonly temporal to the macula. They arise as a direct result of capillary occlusion.

Hard (leakage) exudates

These are discrete yellow protein–lipid-rich deposits. They represent lipid which has leaked from vessels and been engulfed by macrophages. They commonly occur at the edges of microvascular leakage and may form a circinate pattern around a leaking microaneurysm. They may coalesce to form sheets.

Haemorrhages (dot blot)

Haemorrhages from microaneurysms and weakened vessels appear red but their shape depends upon their site. Deep haemorrhages are round (blots) because they are confined by the tightly packed layers of the deep retina. Superficial haemorrhages are larger and blotchy because they follow the pattern of nerve fibres.

Box 5.30 Preproliferative retinopathy

Cotton wool spots

These indicate ischaemic axons within the retina. They arise because of arteriolar occlusion.

Venous dilatation and changes

Venous dilatation is a sign that retinal blood supply is trying to keep up with demand and venous beading results from sites of complete vessel closure. Venous loops and sausage segmentation also occur.

Intraretinal microvascular abnormalities

The term intraretinal microvascular abnormalities (IRMA) refers to dilated capillaries. Microaneurysms and IRMAs are best seen as black dots and lines against a green background when the ophthalmoscope's green filter is used to eliminate the redness of the choroid.

Non-proliferative diabetic retinopathy (NPDR)

NPDR has traditionally been subdivided into background and preproliferative retinopathy.

Background diabetic retinopathy (BDR)

There are *microaneurysms (dots), hard exudates* and '*dot and blot' haemorrhages* (Box 5.29, Fig. 5.58).

Preproliferative diabetic retinopathy (PPDR)

There are, in addition to background changes, *cotton wool spots* (Box 5.30, Fig. 5.59) and larger blot or 'blotch' haemorrhages. There is *dilatation and beading of retinal veins* (sausage appearance).

BDR and PPDR are now often replaced by the term NPDR, classified in Box 5.31.

Proliferative diabetic retinopathy (PDR)

There is, in addition to NPDR changes, *neovascularisation* (Box 5.32, Fig. 5.60). There may be extensive *laser photocoagulation therapy scarring* (Fig. 5.61).

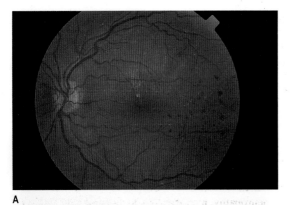

A

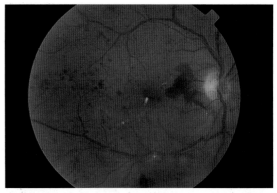

Fig. 5.60 Diabetic retinopathy changes throughout the fundus with neovascularisation at the optic disc. Neovascularisation is also seen notably at 7 o'clock and 11 o'clock (where new vessels have tended to form loops). Note also the large haemorrhage between the optic disc and the macula.

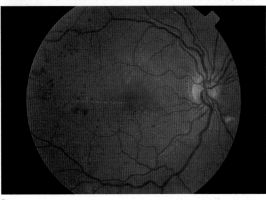

B

Fig. 5.58 (A,B) Microaneurysms, hard exudates and blot haemorrhages. Note that the hard exudates are close to the macula and that the haemorrhages are of different sizes. Sometimes it is difficult to differentiate between smaller 'blot' and larger 'blotch' haemorrhages.

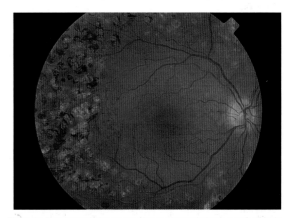

Fig. 5.61 Photocoagulation scars. Note neovascularisation at 8 o'clock.

Box 5.32 Neovascularisation

Neovascularisation occurs in response to occlusive ischaemia (which stimulates angiogenic factors) and affects veins, not arteries. New vessels are usually 'wild' in appearance. They tend to loop off veins and can look like fronds of seaweed.

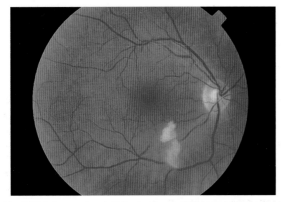

Fig. 5.59 Cotton wool spot. Note also the small blot haemorrhage at 11 o'clock

---

Box 5.31 Non-proliferative diabetic retinopathy (NPDR)

- Mild – microaneurysms
- Moderate – four blots in one quadrant and/or cotton wool spots or venous beading or intraretinal microvascular abnormalities (IRMAs)
- Severe – severe haemorrhage in four quadrants or venous beading in two quadrants or severe IRMA in one quadrant
- Very severe – any two of severe

Advanced eye disease – retinal haemorrhage and retinal detachment

There is, in combination with any of the above features, *preretinal* or *vitreous haemorrhage* and/or (tractional) *retinal detachment* and/or *rubeosis iridis* (Box 5.33, Fig. 5.62).

Diabetic maculopathy

There is evidence of diabetic eye disease near the macula (Box 5.34). This usually takes the form of *hard exudates* (tending to form *circinate rings*) and *oedema* (Fig. 5.63). There may be *neovascularisation*.

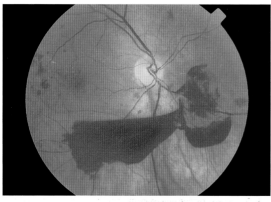

Fig. 5.62 Subhyaloid (preretinal) haemorrhage in diabetic retinopathy. Blood is in the posterior vitreous space and tends to settle inferiorly and outline the attachment of the vitreous to the retina. The appearance has been likened to a bird's nest. A subhyaloid haemorrhage may also be seen with a subarachnoid haemorrhage. Note how a subhyaloid haemorrhage obscures retinal vessels (compare with a choroidal haemorrhage in Fig. 5.78).

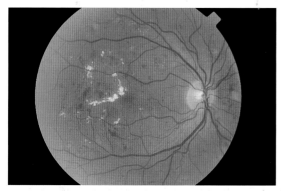

Fig. 5.63 Hard exudates forming a circinate ring at the macula. Note how bright and crisp leaking exudates are compared with cotton wool spots. Note also haemorrhages of varying size.

Box 5.33 Advanced eye disease

Subhyaloid haemorrhages are retained by the hyaloid membrane but may blow into the vitreous, threatening vision completely in the affected eye because they are then restrained only by the limits of the vitreous cavity. Retinal detachment can occur when new vessels exert traction on the retina. Rubeosis iridis (new vessels on the iris) may lead to rubeotic glaucoma.

Box 5.34 Maculopathy

There are three types:

- Focal exudative – hard exudates within 500 μm of the fovea if associated with retinal thickening
- Retinal oedema – within 500 μm (one-third of a disc diameter) of the fovea or one disc diameter or larger, any part of which is within one disc diameter of the fovea
- Ischaemic maculopathy

Interpretation

Confirm the diagnosis

Diabetic eye disease is usually easy to recognise, the main dilemma being to differentiate it from hypertensive retinopathy. Microaneurysms are almost pathognomonic of diabetes, but may occur in venous occlusion. They must be present to diagnose diabetic retinopathy.

What to do next – assess other systems

Tell the examiners you would like to:

- Check for evidence of neuropathy (peripheral neuropathy, mononeuropathy/femoral neuropathy) and nephropathy (proteinuria, serum creatinine).
- Take a history for macrovascular complications, e.g. ischaemic heart disease, stroke.

Consider severity/decompensation/complications

Tell the examiners that:

- You would like to know the level of diabetic control (HbA_{1c}).
- Worsening retinopathy may occur with rapid tightening of glycaemic control.
- Rapid decompensation of eye disease may occur in pregnancy.

Consider function

Tell the examiners that you would assess visual acuity and discuss the impact of any visual loss. This is particularly important in diabetic maculopathy with central vision disturbance.

Discussion

Is retinopathy more likely in type 1 or 2 diabetes mellitus?

Diabetic eye disease is the commonest cause of blindness in the UK for patients of working age, and is related to the duration of and level of control of disease. Two per cent of the UK population have diabetes, 10–13% of which have sight-threatening retinopathy. Type 1 diabetes patients generally have 5–10 years of disease before developing eye signs but eventually nearly all succumb. Type 2 diabetes patients may have eye signs at diagnosis and are more prone to maculopathy.

What are the risk factors for diabetic retinopathy?

These are disease duration, poor glycaemic control, pregnancy, hypertension and nephropathy.

What do you know about screening for diabetic retinopathy?

Screening has been shown to prevent blindness in 80% of patients with PDR and 50–60% of patients with maculopathy. Routine screening of all diabetic patients is

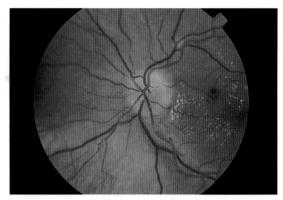

Fig. 5.64 Hypertensive retinopathy. Note arteriovenous nipping, the 'wire' appearance of some vessels, leakage (hard) exudates, haemorrhages and blurring of the optic disc margin.

mandatory at least annually. Screening is performed by digital retinal photography.

What are the management principles in diabetic retinopathy?

These are outlined in Box 5.35.

List some other eye complications that may occur in diabetes mellitus

- Cataracts (early onset age-related variety or snowflake cataracts in poorly controlled type 1 diabetes), or visual changes caused by osmotic alteration in lens shape
- Ocular nerve palsies, especially a sixth nerve palsy
- Increased risk of infection (conjunctivitis, styes, herpes zoster)
- Central retinal artery and vein occlusion

CASE 5.27

HYPERTENSIVE RETINOPATHY

Instruction

Please examine this patient's fundi and discuss your findings.

Recognition

Hypertensive retinopathy may progress through a number of stages:

- *Focal arteriolar attenuation and arteriovenous (AV) nipping* represent the presence of arteriosclerosis of any cause. Thickened arteriolar walls appear like '*silver*' or '*copper*' wires (Fig. 5.64).
- Narrowing of arterioles leads to localised areas of infarction of the superficial retina (*cotton wool spots*)

and *flame-shaped haemorrhages*. Leakages from these vessels result in *hard exudates* (Fig. 5.64).
- *Optic disc swelling*, along with cotton wool spots, flame-shaped haemorrhages and hard exudates, indicates what has been termed '*malignant hypertension*'. Although defined by disc swelling rather than an absolute blood pressure measurement, blood pressure is often above 200/140 mmHg. *Accelerated hypertension* refers to a recent increase over previous hypertensive levels associated with vascular damage on fundoscopy but without disc swelling.

Beware of diagnosing hypertensive retinopathy if disc swelling is unilateral or if it occurs in the absence of other signs of hypertensive retinopathy.

Interpretation

Confirm the diagnosis

The presence of microaneurysms suggests diabetic retinopathy. Tell the examiners you would check the blood pressure.

What to do next – assess other systems

Be aware of the widespread manifestations of hypertension – cardiovascular disease, cerebrovascular disease, renovascular disease and peripheral vascular disease.

Consider severity/decompensation/complications

As well as threatening vision, hypertension may cause target organ failure elsewhere consequent upon poorly controlled chronic hypertension. Additionally, both central retinal artery and central retinal vein occlusion may occur secondary to hypertension with or without hypertensive retinopathy.

Consider function

Tell the examiners you would ask about and discuss the impact of any visual loss.

Box 5.36 Understanding the signs of hypertensive retinopathy

- In childhood, retinal arterioles and venules are of equal width, highly elastic and glisten in the light of an ophthalmoscope. Even normotensive adults lose the sparkling retinal appearances of youth. But hypertension slowly replaces the elastic tissue with fibrous tissue and the glistening disappears. The muscular layer of arterioles is often also replaced and these become rigid. Any remaining arteriolar muscle, still capable of contraction, can give rise to the appearance of *focal arteriolar attenuation*, as the fibrosed segments maintain a static calibre or even dilate.
- *Silver wiring* is an unreliable sign, but *arteriovenous nipping* is the natural progression of arteriolar calibre change and the best sign of arteriosclerosis of any cause. It occurs at sites where dilated arterioles cross over or under venules. The 'compression' or 'nipping' is an illusion.
- *Flame-shaped haemorrhages* occur in the surface layers of the retina (similar to large diabetic haemorrhages) and *hard exudates* are common at the macula, threatening central vision. They often appear as a *star*, following the line of retinal fibres around the macula.
- *Cotton wool spots*, as for diabetes, indicate ischaemia. They may also be a feature of vasculitis, cholesterol emboli, bacterial endocarditis and myeloproliferative disease.
- *Swelling of the optic disc* implies accelerated hypertension.

Discussion

Explain the signs of hypertensive retinopathy
These are explained in Box 5.36.

SWOLLEN OPTIC DISC AND PAPILLOEDEMA

Instruction

Please examine this patient's fundi and discuss your findings.

Recognition

There are many causes of optic disc swelling. Papilloedema, by definition, is swelling of the optic disc due to raised intracranial/cerebrospinal fluid pressure. This should be distinguished from other causes of disc swelling.

A sequence of optic disc signs results from evolving swelling:

- The veins become dilated and tortuous and capillary dilatation leads to hyperaemia of the disc.
- The centre of the disc (the *cup*), becomes *pinker than normal* and *less distinct* as it swells. The *vessels seem to disappear* suddenly in the oedema before reaching the cup. The *disc margins blur* (Fig. 5.65) as the nerve fibre layers swell.

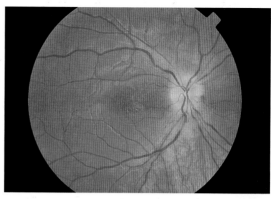

Fig. 5.65 Swollen optic disc (blurring of disc margins).

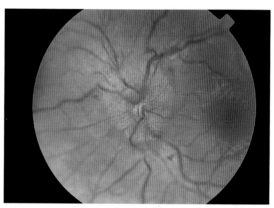

Fig. 5.66 Swollen optic disc (more advanced case).

- The entire disc eventually becomes swollen and raised and the origins of vessels completely disappear. At this stage (Fig. 5.66), retinal *haemorrhages*, *exudates* and *cotton wool spots* may also appear, although any haemorrhages are never as dramatic as in central retinal vein occlusion. *Loss of venous pulsation* implies raised intracranial pressure and is a feature of *papilloedema*. It is difficult to detect and is a normal finding in many individuals. However, *spontaneous venous pulsation excludes papilloedema*.

Interpretation

Confirm the diagnosis
Papilloedema causes loss of venous pulsation.

What to do next – consider causes
Papilloedema is excluded as a cause if spontaneous venous pulsation is seen, but this can be difficult to detect. Other causes of optic disc swelling are given in Box 5.37; see also Fig. 5.67.

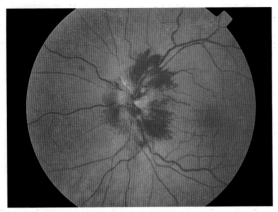

Fig. 5.67 Swollen optic disc. Note the fiery red burst emanating from the optic disc, often seen in retinal vein thrombosis.

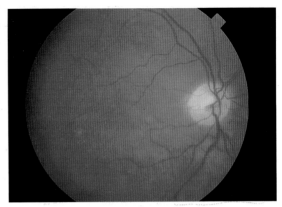

Fig. 5.68 Optic atrophy. Note how the optic disc is instantly eye catching.

Box 5.37 Causes of optic disc swelling

- Papilloedema
- Accelerated hypertension
- Optic papillitis
- Ischaemic optic neuropathy
- Hypercapnia
- Central retinal vein occlusion (Fig. 5.69)
- Hyperproteinaemic disorders, e.g. Waldenström's macroglobulinaemia
- Pseudopapilloedema

Consider severity/decompensation/complications

Check for enlargement of the blind spot by visual field testing. Unless there is also pathology in the optic nerve itself, the visual fields are usually otherwise normal. Chronic untreated hypertension may result in macula oedema (with macula stars), which can rapidly disturb central vision.

Consider function

Tell the examiners you would ask about and discuss the impact of any visual loss.

Discussion

What is the pathophysiology of papilloedema?

The pathophysiology of papilloedema remains obscure but involves transmission of elevated cerebrospinal fluid pressure along the optic nerve sheath, followed by impaired venous drainage from the eye. Papilloedema may take weeks or months to develop, and is therefore a late sign of raised intracranial pressure. Papilloedema may be detected in its early stages by fluorescein angiography.

What is Foster–Kennedy syndrome?

Foster–Kennedy syndrome refers to optic atrophy caused by compression of one optic nerve by an intracranial mass, together with contralateral papilloedema due to raised intracranial pressure.

What is idiopathic intracranial hypertension?

This is possibly caused by microthrombi compromising dural venous drainage. It usually affects young to middle-aged females and has been associated with the oral contraceptive pill and corticosteroids. Raised cerebrospinal fluid pressure is a central feature, causing papilloedema and headaches.

What is pseudopapilloedema?

This is not papilloedema. It occurs in a small, long-sighted and often astigmatic eye where the optic disc appears to be crowded by other structures. Apart from the refractive error, there should be no abnormalities, but doubt can be resolved by fluorescein angiography. Pseudopapilloedema can also result if a disc is raised by drusen.

CASE 5.29

OPTIC ATROPHY

Instruction

Please examine this patient's fundi and any other aspects of eye examination you think appropriate before discussing your findings.

Recognition

The *optic disc* flashes in to view, *bright, white* and *crisp*, like a bright full moon in a dark sky (Fig. 5.68).

Interpretation

Confirm the diagnosis

Look for the five features of optic nerve damage (Box 5.38).

Optic atrophy is not an all or nothing phenomenon. There are 'shades of white' depending upon the degree of

Box 5.38 Five signs of optic nerve damage

1. Relative afferent papillary defect, the most sensitive and specific sign
2. Decreased visual acuity
3. Attenuated colour vision
4. Central or paracentral scotoma
5. Optic atrophy

Box 5.39 Optic neuritis – papillitis and retrobulbar neuritis

In papillitis, inflammation is just behind the optic disc, which may be swollen with blurred margins and floridly coloured because of hyperaemia and haemorrhage. In acute retrobulbar neuritis the optic disc appears normal because the inflammation is further back along the optic nerve. Papillitis is usually distinguishable from papilloedema because papilloedema is usually bilateral and does not give rise to the five signs of optic nerve damage.

Table 5.45 Causes of optic atrophy

Cause	Description
Demyelinating optic neuritis	See text
Ischaemic optic neuritis	See text
Compression	From tumours, aneurysms, glaucoma or Paget's disease
Toxic optic neuritis	From chemicals and drugs such as methanol, tobacco, lead, ethambutol, isoniazid, chloramphenicol and digoxin
Infiltrative lesions	Granulomatous infiltration of the optic nerve in TB, sarcoidosis or syphilis, or from carcinoma
Neurodegeneration	May occur in vitamin deficiencies (especially B_1 and B_{12}), tabes, or hereditary conditions such as Friedreich's ataxia. Leber's hereditary optic neuropathy, a mitochondrial cytopathy, is a rare cause affecting mostly young adult males
Retinitis pigmentosa	This is associated with severe vessel narrowing, which is thought to be the reason for the frequently associated optic atrophy (ischaemic)
Secondary (consecutive) optic atrophy	The term consecutive optic atrophy refers to atrophy due to degeneration of parent ganglion cells and may contribute to the disc pallor in retinitis pigmentosa, chorioretinitis and central retinal artery occlusion. It also occurs as a legacy of papilloedema due to scarring (gliosis) in the optic disc. The disc margin is not usually crisp as it is in primary atrophy

axonal degeneration, and hence degrees of visual disturbance. Patients with multiple sclerosis who have recurrent episodes of optic neuritis develop progressive worsening of the five signs.

What to do next – consider causes

Tell the examiners you would check for signs of demyelination (cerebellar signs, spastic paraparesis, sensory symptoms, ask about bladder disturbance). Multiple sclerosis is the commonest cause of optic atrophy in the UK.

Consider severity/decompensation/complications

Stepwise visual loss accompanies episodes of optic neuritis.

Consider function

Tell the examiners you would ask about and discuss the impact of any visual loss.

Discussion

What are the causes of optic atrophy?

These are listed in Table 5.45.

Episodes of demyelinating optic neuritis (retrobulbar neuritis or papillitis) (Box 5.39)

These are by far the commonest cause of optic atrophy in the UK. While a single episode of optic neuritis does not necessarily imply multiple sclerosis, a high proportion (up to 75%) of patients will develop other signs of multiple sclerosis over time. Visual loss during each episode may be subtle, often described as a 'steamed up' sensation and often only noticeable when the good eye is closed. A key associated symptom is pain, especially on eye movement, often preceding visual disturbance. Recovery from an episode of optic neuritis is usual within a few weeks, although even when the field defect resolves, a defect in sharp colour vision persists. Visual evoked potential (VEP) testing usually detects delayed conduction consistent with demyelination and neuronal loss. Optic neuritis is sometimes treated with corticosteroids, usually intravenously.

Ischaemic optic neuritis

This may be atherosclerotic or vasculitic, notably a complication of untreated giant cell arteritis. It is also common.

What are colobomata?

Colobomata result from persistence of the inferior embryonic cleft of the eyeball which is present during development. A coloboma appears as a white hole in the retina; or if in the disc itself, as a big white patch. Colobomata occasionally extend into the iris. Colobomata may cause central scotomas or arcuate scotomas.

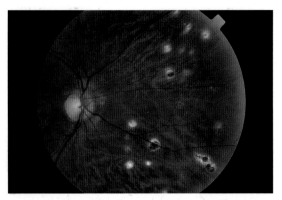

Fig. 5.69 Chorioretinitis.

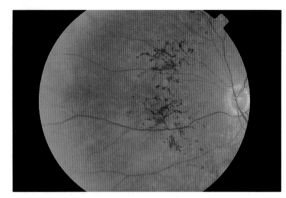

Fig. 5.70 Retinitis pigmentosa.

CASE 5.30

CHORIORETINITIS

Instruction

Please examine this patient's fundi and report your findings.

Recognition

There is evidence of previous inflammation of the chorioretinal layers. Patches of the normal pink chorioretina have been stripped away to reveal the underlying white sclera. Typically, there are *multiple small white and black patches*, the black reflecting proliferation of retinal pigment (Fig. 5.69).

Interpretation

Confirm the diagnosis

Appearances are rather characteristic.

What to do next – consider causes

This is often idiopathic, but may be associated with antecedent infection, e.g. *Toxoplasma*.

Consider severity/decompensation/complications

Check for scotomas/visual field loss.

Consider function

Tell the examiners you would ask about and discuss the impact of any visual loss.

Discussion

List some causes of chorioretinitis

- Usually idiopathic
- *Toxoplasma* infection (often secondary to human immunodeficiency virus)
- Granulomatous diseases

CASE 5.31

RETINITIS PIGMENTOSA

Instruction

Please examine this patient's fundi and visual fields and report your findings.

Recognition

There are webs of *pigment* in the *peripheral retina* (Fig. 5.70).

Interpretation

Confirm the diagnosis

Appearances are absolutely characteristic.

What to do next – consider causes

Look for optic atrophy, which is the result of marked narrowing of arterioles and retinal cell ischaemia/loss.

Consider severity/decompensation/complications

Check the visual fields for *funnel vision*.

Consider function

Tell the examiners you would ask about and discuss the impact of any visual loss.

Discussion

What is retinitis pigmentosa?

Retinitis pigmentosa refers to a group of hereditary, progressive conditions that may be autosomal dominant, autosomal recessive or X-linked and usually begin in childhood.

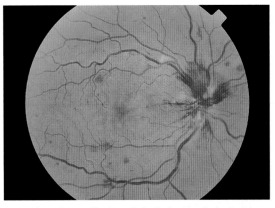

Fig. 5.72 Optic disc swelling in central retinal vein occlusion (in this case caused by hypertension).

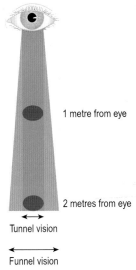

1 metre from eye

2 metres from eye

Tunnel vision

Funnel vision

Fig. 5.71 Funnel and tunnel vision.

List some conditions associated with retinitis pigmentosa

- Laurence–Moon–Biedl syndrome (mental retardation, hypogonadism, obesity, polydactyly, deafness and renal cysts)
- Kearns–Sayre syndrome (mitochondrial cytopathy with ophthalmoplegia, ptosis and heart block)
- Refsum's disease (cerebellar ataxia, peripheral neuropathy and deafness)
- Abetalipoproteinaemia (widespread neurological manifestations)
- Usher syndrome (sensorineural deafness)

What is the difference between 'funnel' and 'tunnel' vision?

Both funnel and tunnel vision refer to the phenomenon of peripheral visual field constriction, with preserved central vision (Fig. 5.71). *Funnel vision* results from disease of the peripheral retina. *Tunnel, or tubular, vision* is always non-organic or psychogenic. In tunnel vision, the visual field defect remains the same size (like looking through a tube) regardless of the distance of a target object. This is physically impossible, because a visual field subtends an arc, such that at double the distance an intact field should be doubled in size.

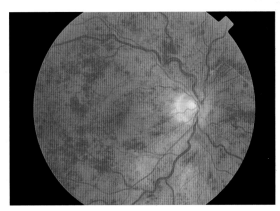

Fig. 5.73 Central retinal vein occlusion.

CASE 5.32

CENTRAL RETINAL VEIN OCCLUSION

Instruction

Please examine this patient's fundi and report your findings.

Recognition

There is *retinal vein dilatation*, together with a flock of *haemorrhages throughout the retina* (an inevitable consequence of the pressure effects of occlusion) and *optic disc swelling* (Fig. 5.72). The overall appearance is like a fiery sunset (Fig. 5.73). The picture may be restricted to one quadrant in branch retinal vein occlusion (BRVO).

Interpretation

Confirm the diagnosis

The blood-orange appearance is rather obvious.

What to do next – consider causes

Tell the examiners that you would like to check for glycosuria and measure the blood pressure.

Consider severity/decompensation/complications

Visual loss is variable, depending upon macula involvement and the extent of retinal ischaemia.

Consider function

Tell the examiners you would ask about and discuss the impact of any visual loss.

Discussion

List some causes of central retinal vein occlusion (CRVO)

- Arteriosclerosis (ageing, hypertension, diabetes mellitus)
- Vasculitis
- Hyperviscosity disorders (hyperproteinaemias, polycythaemia vera)
- Glaucoma (CRVO only)

CRVO is more common in eyes that are prone to primary open-angle glaucoma, but glaucoma may also be a complication of CRVO because neovascularisation may extend to the iris in response to retinal hypoxia.

CASE 5.33

CENTRAL RETINAL ARTERY OCCLUSION

Instruction

Please examine this patient's fundi and report your findings.

Recognition

The *retina is pale*. In the first few days a *cherry red spot is* present at the fovea because the red choroid is visible at the fovea where the retina is rendered especially thin (Figs 5.74 and 5.75). The entire fundus is otherwise *oedematous* with a *milky appearance*. The *arterioles* are *thin*.

Neovascularisation occurs but is never overt, probably because retinal destruction limits the amount of angiogenic factor the retina can produce.

Interpretation

Confirm the diagnosis

There is usually a history of sudden painless visual loss.

What to do next – consider causes

Tell the examiners that you would like to ask about:

- Symptoms of previous temporal arteritis – visual loss in giant cell arteritis is more commonly the result of anterior ischaemic optic neuropathy damaging the optic nerve head
- A history of previous myocardial infarction (mural thrombus) or stroke
- Risks factors for atrial fibrillation, which may be the source of emboli

Occasionally a cholesterol embolus may be visible in a vessel. Cholesterol emboli may occur as a complication of procedures disrupting the endothelium (such as percutaneous coronary intervention). The dislodged emboli may cause visual disturbances, strokes, renal failure or peripheral vascular occlusion.

Consider severity/decompensation/complications

Giant cell arteritis is a medical emergency.

Consider function

Tell the examiners you would ask about and discuss the impact of any visual loss.

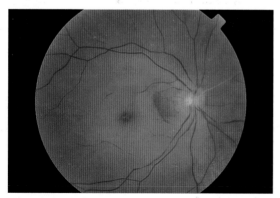

Fig. 5.74 Central retinal artery occlusion. Note the cherry red spot at the macula, the creamy pallor of the fundus and the wispy appearance of the vessels.

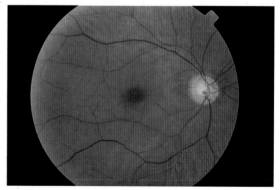

Fig. 5.75 Central retinal artery occlusion. Note how a deeply pigmented retina (which is normal) can alter the colour and appearance of retinal signs.

Discussion

How does a central retinal artery occlusion differ from a branch occlusion?

The central retinal artery divides into upper and lower branches on the disc to supply a 'half moon' of retina above and below the horizontal meridian respectively. Branch occlusion (BRAO) therefore only causes visual field defects in areas corresponding to the retinal supply of the branch and these are limited by the horizontal meridian.

How is central retinal artery occlusion managed?

Retinal artery occlusion is the stroke to the transient ischaemic attack (TIA) that is amaurosis fugax, and should be managed in the same way. Investigations are directed at determining an embolic source (carotid imaging, ECG, echocardiography); neuroimaging is not necessary. Treatment is with dual antiplatelet therapy, consideration of carotid endarterectomy and management of any cardioembolic source with anticoagulation. Secondary prophylaxis of hypertension and hypercholesterolaemia are important, the latter sometimes responsible for cholesterol emboli. Admission to an acute stroke unit, however, is not necessary as aspects of stroke care such as prevention of aspiration and early rehabilitation are not relevant and urgent outpatient investigations are often appropriate.

RETINAL DETACHMENT AND VITREOUS HAEMORRHAGE

Instruction

Please examine this patient's fundi and report your findings.

Recognition

The *retina appears opaque* and its reflex is *grey* rather than pink (the normally transparent retina becomes opaque in any profile other than its normal attached position and obscures the underlying red choroid) (Fig. 5.76). *Rippling* may be visible if the detached retina folds into hills and valleys because of any subretinal fluid.

Interpretation

Confirm the diagnosis

Ask about previous floaters or flashing lights.

What to do next – consider causes

Tell the examiners that you would wish to check for diabetes and hypertension and ask about myopia or previous eye surgery.

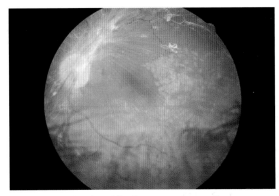

Fig. 5.76 Retinal detachment/traction.

Consider severity/decompensation/complications

Checking the visual acuity and visual fields should reveal an area of visual field loss or scotoma on an axis corresponding to the area of detachment at the retina.

Consider function

Tell the examiners you would ask about and discuss the impact of any visual loss.

Discussion

What are the causes of floaters and flashes?

Floaters

These are usually the result of opacities in the vitreous. They may be caused by:

- Vitreous syneresis (degeneration)
- Posterior vitreous detachment
- Vitreous haemorrhage
- Inflammatory infiltrates, e.g. in posterior uveitis

Flashing lights

The origin of light flashes is less well understood, but they probably result from retinal stimulation by vitreoretinal traction. Flashes are a classic feature of posterior vitreous detachment and incipient retinal detachment but may also occur in migraine with aura.

What is the pathophysiology of retinal detachment?

Retinal detachment refers to separation of the neuroretinal cell layer and its underlying pigment layer. It does not refer to separation of the retina from the underlying choroid. *Posterior vitreous detachment*, in which the posterior vitreous separates from the retina, is the main event predisposing to retinal detachment. As the vitreous collapses, it exerts traction on the neuroretina (with which it is normally in tight adherence) and this may cause a retinal tear, which in turn can lead to separation of the neuroretinal and pigment retinal layers and detachment of the

Table 5.46 Risk factors for retinal detachment

Risk factor	Comment
Age	An intact vitreous of normal viscosity is important in keeping the retina in place; with advancing age viscosity decreases, and the 'fluid vitreous' is capable of creeping behind any small neuroretinal tear that might result from vitreous collapse and posterior vitreous detachment
Myopia	The eye is 'too big' for its retina, which is 'stretched and thinned' and susceptible to tearing
Trauma	May cause direct retinal detachment or produce scarring which can exert abnormal tractional forces on the retina
Cataract surgery	Can alter vitreous volume or shape
Neovascularisation	New blood vessel formation in diabetes may change adhesive forces between the vitreous and retina; vasculitis can cause similar problems
Congenital retinal abnormalities	May sometimes not become manifest until later life
Ocular tumours	Rarely, pressure from behind the retina such as that caused by a choroidal tumour causes retinal detachment

Box 5.40 High-risk features in patients experiencing floaters or light flashes

- Acute onset
- Reduced visual acuity or visual field defect
- Previous history or family history of retinal tear or detachment
- Myopia
- Previous ocular trauma or surgery
- Diabetes

Box 5.41 Causes of vitreous haemorrhage

- Posterior vitreous detachment
- Proliferative diabetic retinopathy
- Retinal vein occlusion
- Subarachnoid haemorrhage (often limited to subhyaloid rather than vitreous haemorrhage)
- Trauma
- Vasculitis

neuroretina. Risk factors for retinal detachment are listed in Table 5.46.

What are the symptoms of posterior vitreous detachment and retinal detachment?

Posterior vitreous detachment may occur acutely, causing *flashes* (vitreoretinal traction) and *floaters* (glial tissue which normally attaches the vitreous to the retina is exposed, and an associated tear in the retina may produce a shower of floaters if specks of blood spurt into the vitreous from torn vessels) or may be of gradual onset with intermittent floaters. If posterior vitreous detachment results in retinal detachment or haemorrhage, visual impairment is very likely, and if the macula is torn or obscured, central vision is abruptly lost. The classic sign of retinal detachment is that of a curtain being drawn across the visual field.

Which patients with floaters or light flashes warrant assessment by an ophthalmologist?

Patients with high-risk features are shown in (Box 5.40). Longstanding intermittent floaters are usually benign and caused by vitreous degeneration, and patients with these warrant review if their floaters change or their vision becomes affected.

How is a retinal tear treated?

Laser photocoagulation; treatment of a detached retina is seldom possible if the neuroretinal layer has become ischaemic and fibrosed.

What are the causes of vitreous haemorrhage?

These are listed in Box 5.41. Vitreous haemorrhages cause floaters and reduced vision. Large bleeds cause loss of the red reflex (other causes of this include cataracts and, rarely, asteroid hyaline bodies and retinoblastomas).

CASE 5.35

DRUSEN AND AGE-RELATED MACULAR DEGENERATION (ASTEROIDS)

Instruction

Please examine this patient's fundi and vision and report your findings.

Recognition

There are *drusen* in the area of the macula, individually or in clusters (Fig. 5.77). These mask the normally transparent retina and its underlying red choroid. There may also be frank *macular atrophy* exposing the white sclera beneath. There may even be areas of *haemorrhage* which mask all underlying structures. The disrupted pigment retinal layer may exhibit areas of *hypopigmentation* or *hyperpigmenta-*

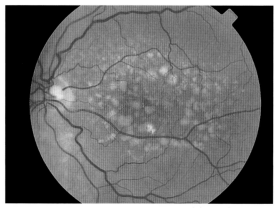

Fig. 5.77 Typical drusen (heralding age-related macular degeneration).

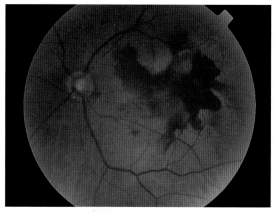

Fig. 5.79 Extensive choroidal haemorrhage.

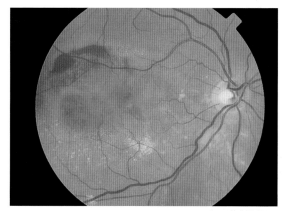

Fig. 5.78 More advanced age-related macular degeneration with choroidal neovascularisation and haemorrhage. This patient would have marked impairment of central vision. Note that with choroidal haemorrhage, the overlying retinal vessels can be clearly seen (compare with pre-retinal haemorrhage in diabetic retinopathy).

tion. The overall appearance of these various changes can be like a *splodge of mixed paints* spilt over the macula (Fig. 5.78). The overall consequence is loss of *central vision*.

Interpretation

Confirm the diagnosis

Visual distortion is a specific and sensitive symptom of choroidal neovascularisation seen in 'wet' age-related macular degeneration (AMD).

What to do next – consider causes

Tell the examiners that causes include genetic predisposition, age and smoking. Drusen are associated with early AMD.

Consider severity/decompensation/complications

AMD is the commonest cause of central vision disturbance and registered blindness in the UK. Visual loss may occur from neovascular abnormalities and haemorrhage ('wet'

AMD) (Fig. 5.79) or non-neovascular abnormalities ('dry' AMD).

Consider function

Tell the examiners you would ask about and discuss the impact of any visual loss.

Discussion

What is the pathophysiology of AMD?

Drusen

Drusen are early features of AMD and appear as small, pale yellow deposits on the retina. They lie between the basement membrane of retinal pigmented epithelium and Bruch's membrane. Their pathogenesis remains uncertain, but they are probably derived from the debris of 'retired' retinal cells. They are commonly detected in people over the age of 65 without other signs of disease.

Wet AMD

In wet AMD (neovascular, exudative or disciform), vessels from the choroid layer (which normally nourish the pigment retina) proliferate across Bruch's membrane and into the subretinal space. Visual distortion (e.g. of printed words or grids) is a specific and sensitive symptom of choroidal neovacularisation. Visual loss occurs as these vessels haemorrhage or leak transudate into the subretinal space, the retina slowly becoming atrophic and fibrosed. Large haemorrhages may even cause retinal detachment. Choroidal neovascularisation itself may not be seen on direct ophthalmoscopy, requiring fluorescein angiography for detection.

Dry AMD (geographic atrophy or non-exudative AMD)

In dry AMD, the retina in the areas of drusen slowly atrophies, and visual deterioration is more gradual, often over many years. Visual distortion is not a feature. Drusen represent dry AMD, which may become confluent or geographic. Wet AMD is a more advanced form of AMD, increasing in prevalence with an ageing population.

How might you determine if a patient with a cataract has AMD?

Even early cataracts may obscure adequate fundoscopy. Typically patients with cataracts find that reading is easier when a light is shone directly onto the page. Visual enhancement with such a simple measure suggests that AMD is not present (of course it cannot exclude AMD).

What treatments are available for AMD?

Laser photocoagulation therapy delivers thermal energy under topical anaesthesia to areas of neovascularisation, but because this treatment also destroys the retina it often cannot be delivered to the areas of greatest need (most patients needing treatment have choroidal neovascularisation extending under the central retina). The closer the treatment to eloquent areas of retina, the higher its risk–benefit ratio. In an attempt to solve this dilemma, photodynamic therapy emerged as a favoured alternative. The principle of this therapy is that a drug which can be photoactivated to destroy tissue locally is given intravenously. When it circulates into the new choroidal vessels, photoactivation is applied. Recently, therapies inhibiting vascular endothelial growth factor (VEGF) (e.g. pegatanib, ranibizumab, bevacizumab) are proving optimal, perhaps combined with photodynamic therapy; pegaptinib specifically blocks VEGF 165, the major angiogenic form of VEGF; some therapies are administered intravitreally, and potential side effects include angina and stroke. In addition to regular outpatient follow-up, patients with drusen may be taught to screen themselves frequently using such techniques as looking at the fine lines on a piece of graph paper for any black spots or areas of distortion which may indicate underlying neovascularisation.

CASE 5.36

ANGIOID STREAKS

Instruction

Please examine this patient's fundi and report your findings.

Recognition

There are *dark red trails or streaks with irregular edges* (Fig. 5.80). They represent cracks in the retina and Bruch's membrane through which the choroid is exposed.

Interpretation

Confirm the diagnosis

Appearances are rather characteristic.

What to do next – consider causes

Angioid streaks are uncommon. Many patients with angioid streaks have *pseudoxanthoma elasticum*. Angioid

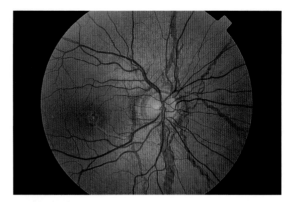

Fig. 5.80 Angioid streaks.

streaks can also be a feature of Ehlers–Danlos syndrome, Paget's disease or sickle cell disease.

Consider severity/decompensation/complications

Visual loss should not occur.

Consider function

Patients are usually asymptomatic.

Discussion

What are angioid streaks?

These are cracks in Bruch's membrane through which choroid is exposed. (The examiners are unlikely to know more about angioid streaks and may ask you about something else!)

CASE 5.37

MYELINATED NERVE FIBRES

Instruction

Please examine this patient's fundi and vision and report your findings.

Recognition

There are *bright white patches with frayed edges* (Fig. 5.81). They can look like an exploding white firework emanating from the optic disc or a bright comet trailing across the retinal sky!

Interpretation

Confirm the diagnosis

Appearances are absolutely characteristic.

What to do next – assess other systems

There is really nothing more to do.

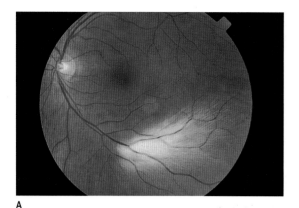

A

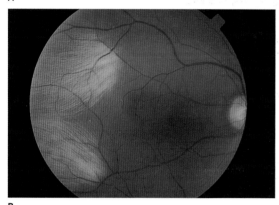

B

Fig. 5.81 (A,B) Myelinated nerve fibres.

Consider severity/decompensation/complications

There may be visual field defects but frequently myelinated nerve fibres are asymptomatic.

Consider function

Tell the examiners you would ask about and discuss the impact of any visual loss.

Discussion

How do myelinated nerve fibres arise?

Myelination of optic nerve fibres is normally arrested before such fibres enter the eye. Failure of arrest during development results in myelinated (or medullated) nerve fibres.

CASE 5.38

GLAUCOMA

Instruction

Please examine this patient's fundi and vision and report your findings.

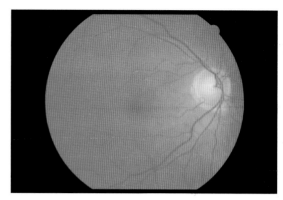

Fig. 5.82 Glaucoma with cupping.

Recognition

There is *cupping* of the *optic disc* (Fig. 5.82).

Interpretation

Confirm the diagnosis

Tell the examiners you would arrange assessment of intra-ocular pressure.

What to do next – consider causes

Tell the examiners you would ask about family history and myopia. The glaucomas are a range of disorders with a characteristic type of optic nerve damage caused by obstruction to flow or drainage of aqueous. The commonest type is primary open-angle glaucoma (POAG), and risk factors include the level of intraocular pressure, age, genetics and family history, Afro-Caribbean origin, a thin cornea, a large cup to disc ratio and myopia.

Consider severity/decompensation/complications

Normal intraocular pressure (IOP) is 10–21 mmHg. Raised IOP with normal visual fields and discs is called ocular hypertension. Glaucoma, untreated, leads to blindness and is the second commonest cause of irreversible blindness.

Consider function

POAG is insidious, often being without symptoms until considerable ocular damage has been sustained. Haloes are a feature of acute closed-angle glaucoma. Patients may present because of visual field loss but are frequently referred from optometrists following the detection of raised intraocular pressure (IOP).

Discussion

How may aqueous flow become obstructed?

Normally the ciliary body secretes aqueous, which flows into the posterior chamber between the lens behind and the iris in front, and then through the pupil into the

Box 5.42 Three cardinal features of primary open-angle glaucoma

- Raised intraocular pressure > 21–22 mmHg (> 30 mmHg warrants urgent referral to an ophthalmologist)
- A cupped optic disc with an increased cup : disc (C : D) ratio
- Visual field loss

anterior chamber. It leaves the eye through the trabecular meshwork, flowing into Schlemm's canal and into epi-scleral veins. In POAG there is resistance to outflow through the meshwork due to partial obstruction and additional, less defined mechanisms. In acute glaucoma, there is complete obstruction to outflow; apposition of the lens to the back of the iris prevents flow of aqueous from the posterior chamber to the anterior chamber. This is more likely when the pupil is semi-dilated at night (iris shortened and fattened). Aqueous then collects behind the iris and pushes it forwards onto the trabecular meshwork and acute block to drainage occurs, leading to rapidly rising intraocular pressure. Acute glaucoma usually arises in long-sighted (hypermetropic) people, who tend to have shallow anterior chambers. It may also occur in rubiosis of the iris and in anterior uveitis (inflammation of the eye) when adhesions may develop between the lens and iris (posterior synechiae).

What are the main features of POAG?

There are three cardinal features of POAG (Box 5.42).

How does POAG arise?

The mechanisms behind the triad of features in POAG can be explained as follows.

- The pathophysiological changes in POAG have traditionally been attributed to raised IOP causing damage to the optic nerve head (optic disc). Increasingly, vascular and toxic damage to optic nerve fibres are thought to contribute, and 'POAG' with normal IOP is recognised. Ageing has a role, and the optic nerve, which at birth contains approximately 10^6 neurons, loses about 10^4 of these per year.
- A normal optic disc contains a central cup, an indentation or cavity from which the blood vessels emanate. It is normally shallow and the ratio of the cup diameter to the disc diameter is normally around 1 : 3. Discs are like shoe sizes, however, varying between individuals and when examining C : D ratios, asymmetry between the eyes and progression over time are more important than a 'snap shot' appearance. As POAG progresses, neurons are lost and the cup becomes a deepening and expanding cave into which the blood vessels appear to dive.
- The classic field defect in POAG is an arcuate scotoma of peripheral visual loss, with relative preservation of macula or central vision (Fig. 5.83); visual acuity may be 6/6. There are two

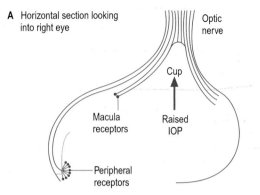

A Horizontal section looking into right eye

Optic nerve

Cup

Macula receptors

Raised IOP

Peripheral receptors

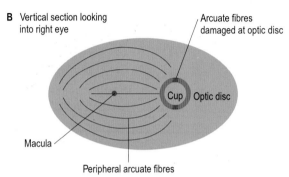

B Vertical section looking into right eye

Arcuate fibres damaged at optic disc

Cup   Optic disc

Macula

Peripheral arcuate fibres

Fig. 5.83 Cupping of the optic disc and arcuate scotoma in primary open-angle glaucoma. IOP, intraocular pressure.

considerations when explaining the field defect. The first is that the ratio of visual receptors (R) to their attached neurons (N) running to the disc is much greater at the periphery (R : N around 8 : 1) than at the macula (R : N 1 : 1). For every neuron lost from peripheral vision, multiple receptors are lost. Secondly, the organisation of nerve fibres is such that those from the macula run directly to the disc while those from the periphery must 'arc' around the macula, tending to reach the disc at its vertical north and south poles. These poles tend to be damaged first in POAG, resulting in an arcuate scotoma. Patients may start bumping into things.

CASE 5.39

CATARACTS

Instruction

Please examine this patient's fundi and vision and report your findings.

Recognition

There is *loss of the red reflex* and the lens appears cloudy (Fig. 5.84).

Box 5.43 Causes of cataract

- Smoking
- Diabetes (most commonly early onset age-related type but occasionally 'snowflake' cortical opacities)
- Corticosteroids
- Wilson's disease (stellate cataracts)
- Hypoparathyroidism
- Congenital (familial, myotonic dystrophy, infection)
- Trauma (including radiation)
- Malnutrition
- Acute dehydration
- Cumulative sunlight exposure

Box 5.44 Symptoms of different types of cataract

Nuclear cataracts

These produce gradually reduced contrast and colour intensity and ultimately difficulty seeing faces, number plates and so forth. It is like looking through a rippled window. Reading is often surprisingly good.

Cortical cataracts

These scatter light from localised opacities and disrupt its smooth transmission. This produces a whitewash behind the window or dirty window sensation, glare when driving, especially from car headlights at night, and difficulty reading. Sunlight is uncomfortable on a winter's day when low in the sky.

Subcapsular cataracts

Opacification of the posterior cortical zone occurs in a posterior subcapsular cataract. These are visually disabling in good lighting but less troublesome in low light when the pupils are dilated. There is difficulty with daytime driving and reading.

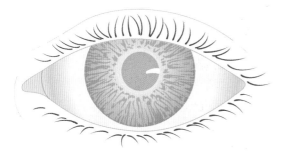

Fig. 5.84 Cataract.

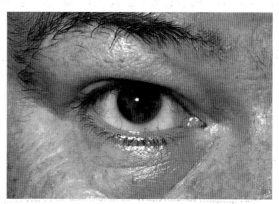

Fig. 5.85 Old iritis.

Interpretation

Confirm the diagnosis

Tell the examiners that you would ask about symptoms (see Box 5.44).

What to do next – consider causes

Tell the examiners that most cataracts arise because of ageing of the crystalline lens. The lens continues to grow through life and new fibres are laid down and old ones not replaced. Yellowing of the nucleus is common with ageing (nuclear sclerosis). The transparency of the lens is a result of many factors, including its chemical consistency. Extrinsic causes of cataract are listed in Box 5.43.

Consider severity/decompensation/complications

The underlying cause is important.

Consider function

Cataracts are classified according to site, with differing effects (Box 5.44).

Discussion

How might a cataract be treated?

Routinely, phacoemulsification with a lens implant can be performed as day surgery and is increasingly 'sutureless'. Yttrium–aluminium–garnet (YAG) laser capsulotomy is also used to eradicate a posterior capsule opacity. In many cases, patients want more than anything to be able to read

and the risks of surgery must be taken into account. A bright light close to a book should improve the vision of an eye with a cataract, but will not improve vision in retinal disease such as age-related macular degeneration. This is often a useful test for dual pathology, because fundoscopy may be precluded by the presence of a cataract.

CASE 5.40

UVEITIS AND RED EYE

Instruction

Please examine this patient's fundi and vision and report your findings.

Recognition

Either there is evidence of previous eye disease with scarring (Fig. 5.85) or the eye is red, predominantly close to the corneoscleral limbus.

Interpretation

Confirm the diagnosis

A distinguishing feature between most of the serious, sight-threatening causes of red eye from non-threatening conjunctivitis is that in the former the redness dominates at the corneoscleral limbus (where blood vessels emerge from the depths of the eye). This is sometimes called ciliary injection. Furthermore, serious causes are usually painful.

What to do next – consider causes

Tell the examiners that the causes of a painful, red eye that are medical emergencies are uveitis (iritis), acute closed-angle glaucoma and keratitis.

Consider severity/decompensation/complications

The major concern is threat to sight.

Consider function

Tell the examiners you would ask about and discuss the impact of any visual loss.

Discussion

What is the uveal tract?

The uveal tract comprises the anterior uvea (iris and ciliary body) and the posterior uveal tract (choroids – the vascular layer which supplies the outer pigment retina).

What do you know about uveitis/iritis?

Uveitis may affect the anterior or posterior uvea or both (panuveitis). Uveitis typically produces a painful, watery, photophobic red eye with blurred vision due to the presence of inflammatory cells. The pupil is small and in spasm in iritis and adhesions between the iris and anterior lens capsule (posterior synechiae) may render it irregularly shaped. There may be keratitic precipitates (clumps of white cells on the inner lining of the cornea and floating in the anterior chamber appear like dust in a beam of light) and precipitation of neutrophils in the anterior chamber may result in a hypopyon. Anterior uveitis is classically associated with human leucocyte antigen (HLA) B27 conditions like ankylosing spondylitis (up to 20% of patients), Reiter's syndrome and psoriatic disease. It occurs in most patients with Behçet's disease (a multisystem vasculitis also causing oral and genital ulceration). Inflammatory bowel disease, sarcoidosis and tuberculosis can cause anterior or posterior uveitis (chorioretinitis), as can a wide range of other infections including toxoplasmosis, toxoca-riasis, human immunodeficiency virus and the herpes simplex and zoster viruses.

What do you know about acute (closed-angle) glaucoma?

This is caused by sudden closure of the drainage angle and is more common in long-sighted people with short eyeballs. It may be precipitated by dilating drops and mydriatics such as tricyclics. It is very painful. The cornea is steamy/cloudy/stormy with a mid-dilated unreactive pupil, and the anterior chamber is narrow. It is an emergency.

What do you know about keratitis?

The cornea may be damaged by trauma (corneal abrasions or penetrating eye injury), foreign bodies and infection. Keratitis and ulceration caused by herpes simplex or zoster infections may assume a punctate or dendritic pattern. Keratitis usually presents with pain, redness and lacrimation. Bacterial ulceration may result in a hypopyon.

What is marginal keratitis?

Keratitis may also arise as a sterile immunological response to antigens. An example is marginal keratitis where staphylococcal exotoxin triggers marginal inflammation of the cornea with ciliary injection. It is often the result of staphylococcal overgrowth in patients with blepharitis. When assessing a corneal problem, the eye should be examined completely with appropriate stains, and a safe rule is that topical steroids should never be commenced without ophthalmological recommendation.

What is corneal melt?

This immunological keratitis tends to be associated with autoimmune conditions such as Wegener's granulomatosis.

What do you know about scleritis?

Scleritis may be a feature of vasculitis, sarcoid, rheumatoid disease, systemic lupus eryhematosus, inflammatory bowel disease and ankylosing spondylitis. Patients with rheumatoid disease may also develop scleromalacia perforans, a necrotising scleritis, which gives the eye a grey-blue tinge. The grey-blue tinge results from thinning of the sclera, faintly exposing the choroid pigment beneath. Osteogenesis imperfecta, Ehlers–Danlos syndrome and Marfan's syndrome may also cause blue sclera.

What is episcleritis?

Episcleritis produces superficial redness, usually without significant pain. It may be associated with rheumatoid disease but is usually an idiopathic self-limiting condition.

ENDOCRINE SYSTEM

Examination of the thyroid

- Ask the patient to sit comfortably at the edge of the bed or on a chair. Stand back and observe, paying particular attention to the face.
- Look at the thyroid gland from the front. Note any scars indicating previous surgery.
- Ask if there is any pain or tenderness, and then feel the thyroid gland from behind (Fig. 5.86). Be gentle, because thyroid examination can be uncomfortable for patients. Feel the isthmus, which overlies the thyroid cartilage, with your right middle and index fingers, and then feel the lobes. Note any diffuse goitre or area of focal nodularity. Note the gland's size and texture.
- Consider asking the patient to swallow a glass of water if you find a goitre, to see and feel if it is readily mobile.
- Feel for lymph nodes – supraclavicular, submandibular, postauricular, suboccipital. If there are palpable nodes, note if they are separate and tender (reactive hyperplasia), hard and clustered together (carcinoma), soft and rubbery (lymphoma), mobile or fixed.
- Auscultate the thyroid gland bilaterally for bruits.
- Examine the eyes for those features in Box 5.45.
- Observe the face, skin and hair for signs of hyperthyroidism or hypothyroidism.
- Feel the pulse.
- Inspect the palms for erythema and feel for sweat. Note any clubbing. Note any tremor with the arms outstretched.
- Ask your patient to abduct their shoulders to assess for proximal muscle weakness.
- Look at the legs for pretibial myxoedema.
- Test the ankle reflexes.

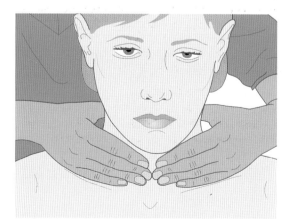

Fig. 5.86 Examining the thyroid and thyroid status.

- You will probably discover early in the course of the examination if you are dealing with a thyroid lump, hyperthyroidism or hypothyroidism, directing your assessment accordingly.

Summary

A summary of the thyroid/endocrine examination sequence is given in the Summary Box.

> **SUMMARY BOX – THYROID/ENDOCRINE SYSTEM EXAMINATION**
>
> Examining the endocrine system in PACES will usually entail examining the thyroid (above), or the face and hands for diagnoses such as Cushing's syndrome or acromegaly

CASE 5.41

HYPERTHYROIDISM AND GRAVES' DISEASE – HYPERTHYROIDISM, EXOPHTHALMOS, PRETIBIAL MYXOEDEMA

Instruction

Please determine this patient's thyroid status and discuss the underlying cause.

Recognition

There may be a triad of groups of signs.

Hyperthyroidism

The hands are *warm and sweaty* with *palmar erythema*. *Tremor* is often obvious (with the arms extended a piece of paper on the hands detects subtle fine tremors). There is *tachycardia* at rest (usually sinus tachycardia, may be atrial fibrillation). There may be *proximal muscle weakness*. These signs may occur in thyrotoxicosis of any cause. A *bruit* bilaterally over the thyroid is specific to *Graves' disease.*

> **Box 5.45 Features to examine for in thyroid disease**
>
> - Proptosis (protrusion of the eyeball, best seen from above, standing behind the patient)
> - Lid retraction (the upper sclera is visible between the cornea and the upper lid)
> - Exophthalmos (the lower sclera is visible between the cornea and the lower lid)
> - Lid lag (move your finger downwards and ask the patient to follow it, while fixing their forehead with your other hand; the movement must be quite fast to elicit lid lag)
> - Ophthalmoplegia
> - Chemosis (if present, mention that you would consider using fluorescein to look for corneal ulceration)

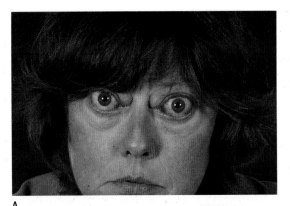

A

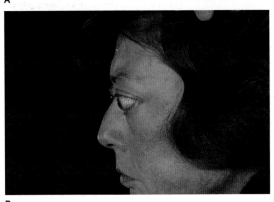

B

Fig. 5.87 (A,B) Thyroid eye disease.

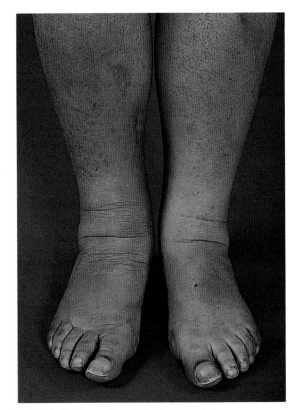

Fig. 5.88 Pretibial myxoedema (note also acropachy).

Box 5.46 Eye signs that occur in Graves' disease but not other causes of thyrotoxicosis

- Grittiness and redness
- Conjunctival oedema (chemosis)
- Periorbital oedema
- Proptosis (occasionally unilateral) and exophthalmos
- Ophthalmoplegia (due to orbital lymphocytic infiltration of the orbit) causing diplopia; often a complex ophthalmoplegia involving numerous ocular muscles

---

Box 5.47 Symptoms of thyrotoxicosis (of any cause)

- Weight loss
- Increased appetite
- Heat intolerance
- Preference for cold and sweating
- Diarrhoea
- Tremor
- Hyperactivity, irritability, insomnia or anxiety
- Depression (especially elderly)
- Oligomenorrhoea and loss of libido
- Polyuria
- Weakness and fatigue

Exophthalmos

This affects around 30–50% of patients. *Lid lag* and *lid retraction* are the result of excess sympathetic activity and not specific to Graves' disease. Eye signs that occur in Graves' ophthalmopathy (Fig. 5.87) but not other causes of thyrotoxicosis are listed in Box 5.46.

Pretibial myxoedema

This is rare (1–2% of Graves' disease) but specific to Graves' disease. There are *elevated shin lesions* with *well-defined edges* (Fig. 5.88). Lesions may be *nodular or plaque-like, purplish red or brown* and the *skin is shiny*, with a *thickened, orange peel appearance*. Lesions can occur at

other sites. They are usually painless. Coarse hairs tend to occur in the vicinity. Look also for thyroid acropachy (clubbing) and onycholysis (Plummer's nails), which affect a small minority of patients.

Interpretation

Confirm the diagnosis

Tell the examiners you would like to ask about symptoms of thyrotoxicosis (Box 5.47).

Table 5.47 Causes of thyrotoxicosis

	Disease	Causes	Distinguishing features
Primary hyperthyroidism	Graves' disease	Thyroid-stimulating immunoglobulin G antibodies (TSI) are TSH receptor antibodies that bind to and stimulate the TSH receptor	Painless diffuse goitre in > 90% Ophthalmopathy Pretibial myxoedema
	Toxic multinodular goitre	Unknown	Painful goitre Most common cause in older people
	Toxic adenoma	Solitary secreting adenoma	Thyrotoxicosis without goitre
	Other	Metastatic thyroid cancer Genetic Ectopic thyroid tissue	{ Rare { Consider if above three causes not confirmed
Secondary hyperthyroidism	TSH-secreting pituitary adenoma Gestational thyrotoxicosis		Possibly part of wider pituitary disease TSH detectable despite high FT4 and FT3 Hyperemesis gravidarum due to high levels of human chorionic gonadotrophin in first trimester, which stimulates the TSH receptor
	Thyroid hormone resistance syndrome		Thyrotoxicosis uncommon Elevated FT4 and FT3 due to peripheral resistance to action
Thyrotoxicosis without hyperthyroidism	Destructive thyroiditis	Subacute (de Quervain's)	Viral Small, tender goitre High erythrocyte sedimentation rate Initial thyrotoxicosis without hyperthyroidism due to release of stored hormone Hypothyroidism within weeks Recovery over three to six months May respond to steroids
		Postpartum thyroiditis Amiodarone	Similar to viral thyroiditis but goitre painless A late complication due to a destructive thyroiditis or effects of excess iodide
		Lithium Other drugs (induce autoimmunity or inflammatory thyroiditis)	Onset abrupt
	Excess thyroid hormone taking		History

FT3, free triiodothyronine; FT4, free thyroxine; TSH, thyroid-stimulating hormone.

What to do next – consider causes

Graves' disease accounts for around 70–80% of all thyrotoxicosis (Table 5.47). Toxic multinodular goitre and thyroid adenoma account for most of the remainder.

Consider severity/decompensation/complications

Tell the examiners that you would be concerned about:

- High output cardiac failure
- Thyroid storm or thyrotoxic crisis (metabolic and haemodynamic instability)
- Fixed gaze (usually painful), a surgical emergency because there is risk of optic nerve compression

Consider function

This relates to symptoms (see Box 5.47).

Discussion

Is there a difference between thyrotoxicosis and hyperthyroidism?

Thyrotoxicosis is the syndrome resulting from excessive circulating free thyroxine (FT4) and/or free triiodothyronine (FT3). Hyperthyroidism refers to thyroid gland overactivity resulting in thyrotoxicosis, but thyrotoxicosis can occur without hyperthyroidism when stored hormone is released from a damaged gland (e.g. subacute thyroiditis) or when excess thyroxine hormone is taken.

How common is ophthalmopathy in Graves' disease?

It affects up to 60% clinically, but 90% of patients on computed tomography or magnetic resonance imaging have fusiform ocular muscle oedema and fibrosis. A small group of patients with ophthalmopathy but without Graves' disease have autoimmune hyperthyroidism or thyroid autoantibodies. Euthyroid and hypothyroid Graves' disease are recognised, both with ophthalmopathy.

Which factors increase the risk of ophthalmopathy in Graves' disease?

Smoking is the most important. Age, male gender and radioactive iodine also increase the risk.

What are the biochemical abnormalities of hyperthyroidism?

The thyroid gland secretes both thyroxine (T4) and the active hormone triiodothyronine (T3), while T4 is also converted to T3 peripherally. In thyrotoxicosis, thyroid-stimulating hormone (TSH) is suppressed unless the cause is a pituitary adenoma or thyroid hormone resistance. Suppressed TSH should prompt assessment of T4 levels. Both T3 and T4 are highly protein bound to T4-binding globulin (TBG) so alteration in TBG levels alters the total (but not free) levels of T4 and T3; oestrogens (pregnancy, combined oral contraceptive pill) and liver disease raise levels and protein-losing conditions lower TBG levels. Thus, measurement of FT4 is more reliable than T4. FT3 should be measured if TSH is suppressed and T4 levels are normal. FT3 toxicosis with normal FT4 occurs in early hyperthyroidism of any cause, followed by combined T3 and T4 toxicosis. Isolated T4 toxicosis is uncommon, but may occur with iodine excess.

In what other situations can TSH be suppressed?

It may be suppressed in euthyroid patients with Grave's ophthalmopathy, large goitres or severe non-thyroid illness, or in patients recently treated for thyrotoxicosis.

What is sick euthyroid syndrome?

This refers to changes in thyroid function in severe non-thyroidal illness. These can include decreased conversion of T4 to T3 with normal T4, decreased T3 and usually normal TSH, and a more extreme fall in T3 levels probably secondary to decreased T4 production in more severely ill patients. In very severe illness changes may be secondary to decreased TSH secretion. Patients are euthyroid.

How can drugs affect thyroid function tests?

Many drugs affect T3 and T4 levels by altering TBG levels or by interfering with conversion of T4 to T3.

What is the pattern of thyroid function abnormality seen with amiodarone?

Patients taking amiodarone have elevated/high-normal FT4, low-normal FT3 and initially high TSH that returns to normal within a few months.

What is the place of autoimmune tests in assessing thyrotoxicosis?

Serum autoantibodies against thyroglobulin and thyroid peroxidase are present not only in 80% of patients with Graves' disease, but also in many healthy people, especially women. Peroxidase is an enzyme needed for thyroid hormone synthesis. TSH receptor-stimulating antibodies are not widely available, but the diagnosis of Graves' disease is usually clinical.

What is the place of nuclear medicine scans in assessing thyrotoxicosis?

Thyroid scintiscanning with technetium-99m or iodine-131 is useful when thyrotoxicosis without hyperthyroidism is suspected, because isotope uptake is low or absent compared to all types of hyperthyroidism in which it is high. It can identify a toxic adenoma by demonstrating uptake in the adenoma with complete suppression of uptake in the rest of the gland. Such hot spots are important to identify as they are less responsive to carbimazole.

What do you know about the current drug treatment of hyperthyroidism?

Antithyroid drugs

Antithyroid drugs, such as carbimazole and propylthiouracil, inhibit iodide organification by thyroid peroxidase, reducing T3 and T4 production. They also reduce TSH receptor-stimulating antibody levels. Carbimazole is most widely used and patients should be warned about symptoms of infection and rashes; the earliest symptom of incipient agranulocytosis is usually a sore throat but fever or mouth ulcers are also common and patients should stop treatment and seek an urgent full blood count. Neutropenia occurs in around 0.1% of patients. More common side effects include rash, fever and cholestasis. Carbimazole may be started in one of two main regimens (Box 5.48).

Treatment is usually continued for 18–24 months, but around half of patients will eventually relapse when it is discontinued.

Beta blockers

Carbimazole takes about a month to improve thyroid status. Symptom control is achieved in the interim with

---

Box 5.48 Antithyroid drug regimens

Titration or reducing regimen

30–60 mg of carbimazole is taken daily in three or four divided doses, reduced over four to eight weeks as the patient becomes euthyroid and guided by free thyroxine (FT4) levels, usually to 5–15 mg daily.

Block replace regimen

40 mg carbimazole is taken daily and maintained, adding T4 when the patient becomes euthyroid, usually at around one month. Fewer clinic visits are required and biochemical control is often smoother.

non-cardioselective beta blockers (e.g. propranolol 80 mg thrice daily, weaning to 40 mg twice daily over 4–6 weeks and ceased once carbimazole has taken effect).

What is the place of radioactive iodine in treating thyrotoxicosis?

Radioactive iodine (^{131}I) acts slowly, and is very effective but can cause early transient hypothyroidism, and later permanent hypothyroidism at a rate of around 10% in the first year and a small percentage increase per year thereafter. It can also cause transient thyroiditis, and although antithyroid drugs can be used to reduce this they increase the need for higher doses of ^{131}I. Lifelong thyroxine replacement is often needed after treatment. Contraindications to ^{131}I include pregnancy, lactation and active ophthalmopathy. Patients with ophthalmopathy should be offered corticosteroids following ^{131}I to reduce the risk of exacerbation of eye disease. ^{131}I is the treatment of choice for toxic multinodular goitre, except for large goitres and those with retrosternal extension requiring surgery.

What is the place of surgery in treating thyrotoxicosis?

Indications for subtotal thyroidectomy in Graves' disease include a large goitre, disease relapse, and situations in which ^{131}I is contraindicated, unavailable or unacceptable to the patient. Hypothyroidism is a common side effect.

What is the treatment for Graves' ophthalmopathy?

Treatment is urgent if full lid closure is not possible, to protect from exposure keratitis. Fixed gaze or visual loss warrants immediate assessment and treatment options include steroids and immunosuppression, surgery and orbital radiotherapy. Surgery may be considered electively for less severe disease, but ophthalmopathy often improves over the years with medical treatment. Artificial tears and ointment can help.

Why is Graves' disease significant in pregnancy?

Graves' disease is significant in pregnancy because TSH receptor-stimulating antibodies can cross the placenta and cause fetal hyperthyroidism and tachycardia. Antithyroid drugs can also cross the placenta and cause fetal hypothyroidism. Where necessary, the lowest possible dose is used. Breastfeeding is possible with a low-dose titration regimen.

How would you manage a thyrotoxic storm?

This is uncommon, but has a mortality of around 50% and should be recognised and treated urgently. Treatments include propylthiouracil 600 mg then 200 mg six-hourly, stable iodine (Lugol's iodine) at least one hour later, propranolol 60 mg four-hourly, dexamethasone and intravenous fluids. Precipitating causes include thyroid surgery, radioiodine, withdrawal of drugs and acute illness.

How would you monitor treated hyperthyroidism?

Thyroid function tests should be checked annually if stable, and after two months following any dose adjustment. It takes several weeks for results to reflect changes in treatment.

What do you know about subclinical hyperthyroidism?

This is suggested by a depressed TSH and high–normal or slightly elevated FT3 or FT4, in the absence of overt symptoms; anxiety or sleep disturbance may be present. Over time, many such patients do develop more pronounced hyperthyroidism. The decision to treat is often determined by a wish to improve subtle symptoms unmasked by closer enquiry, especially if biochemical progression is occuring. Atrial fibrillation is a compelling reason to treat, since it is about three times more common in people with 'subclinical' hyperthyroidism. A small dose of carbimazole, such as 5–10 mg daily, may suffice, indicated if TSH consistently < 0.1 mU/l.

CASE 5.42

HYPOTHYROIDISM

Instruction

Please determine this patient's thyroid status and discuss possible causes.

Recognition

You may miss hypothyroidism and think, 'just another little old lady'. Many of the clinical features are non-specific and insidious. They include *excess weight, myxoedematous facial features* (*thick and coarse, with periorbital oedema* and sometimes *hoarseness*), *dry skin, and fine, brittle hair with loss of the outer eyebrows* (Fig. 5.89). There may be *delayed relaxation of ankle and other deep tendon reflexes.*

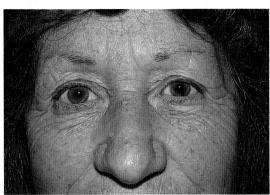

Fig. 5.89 Hypothyroidism.

Box 5.49 Symptoms of hypothyroidism

- Tiredness
- Weight gain
- Preference for warmth
- Mood change including depression
- Constipation
- Menorrhagia
- Myalgia
- Carpal tunnel syndrome

Box 5.50 Causes of hypothyroidism

- Autoimmune Hashimoto's thyroiditis
- Idiopathic atrophic hypothyroidism
- Treatments for thyrotoxicosis – antithyroid drugs, ^{131}I, thyroidectomy
- Destructive thyroiditis
- Secondary to hypothalamic or pituitary failure
- Iodine deficiency

Interpretation

Confirm the diagnosis

Tell the examiners that you would like to ask about symptoms (Box 5.49).

What to do next – consider causes

Tell the examiners the possible causes of hypothyroidism (Box 5.50).

Consider severity/decompensation/complications

Tell the examiners that you would be concerned about:

- Serous effusions (pleural, pericardial, peritoneal, joint)
- Cerebellar signs
- Bradycardia
- Heart failure
- Dyslipidaemia (raised total cholesterol and low-density lipoprotein with increased cardiovascular disease risk)
- Depression or psychosis
- Anaemia (iron deficiency, macrocytic, pernicious, normochromic, normocytic)

Consider function

This relates to symptoms (Box 5.49).

Discussion

What causes myxoedema?

This is the result of local infiltration with hyaluronic acid and mucopolysaccharides.

What is Hashimoto's thyroiditis?

This is the commonest cause of hypothyroidism, in which dense lymphocytic infiltration of the thyroid gland pro-duces a diffuse or finely micronodular goitre. It typically affects middle-aged and older women, presenting with hypothyroidism, a goitre, or both and is autoimmune. Associated conditions include vitiligo, pernicious anaemia, type 1 diabetes, Addison's disease and premature ovarian failure.

How is hypothyroidism confirmed?

Elevated thyroid-stimulating hormone (TSH) with reduced free thyroxine (FT4) or total T4 indicates primary hypo-thyroidism. Measuring free tri-iodothyronine (FT3) or total T3 is usually unhelpful because of increased conversion of T4 to T3. Hypothyroidism secondary to hypothalamic or pituitary disease is associated with low TSH.

Are thyroid autoantibodies helpful in diagnosis?

These can help diagnose the cause, antibodies to thyro-globulin or thyroid peroxidase (microsomal anti-bodies) being usually strongly positive in Hashimoto's thyroiditis.

What do you know about treatment of hypothyroidism?

Young patients, pregnant patients or those patients with evidence of pituitary disease are usually referred to secondary care. Levothyroxine replacement for patients less than 60 years of age without ischaemic heart disease usually starts at 50–100 µg daily. A starting dose of 25 µg daily is often used in patients with high cardiovascular disease risk and titrated upwards to clinical response. Thyroid function should be checked two-monthly, aiming for a normal TSH. Clinical improvement may lag behind TSH normalisation. Levothyroxine is increased in 25-µg increments up to 150 µg daily according to TSH. Larger doses of levothyroxine are seldom necess-ary and if needed should provoke questions about concordance.

What is subclinical hypothyroidism?

Elevated TSH with a normal T4 indicates subclinical hypothyroidism. It is important because treatment, espe-cially with levels of TSH above 10 mU/l, may enhance well-being by erasing hitherto insidious, vague symptoms, improve dyslipidaemic profiles and reduce cardiovascular disease risk.

What is myxoedema coma?

This is an uncommon complication seen in older people, often precipitated by illness such as infection. Reduced consciousness and hypothermia are common, not necessarily with coma. Heart failure, hypotension, hypoventilation and hyponatraemia also occur. Treatment is supportive, with intravenous fluids, slow re-warming, ventilation, antibiotics and intravenous T3 followed by oral or nasogastric T4 once improving. Hydrocortisone is given if hypoadrenalism is also possible.

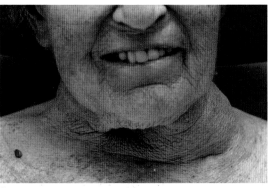

A

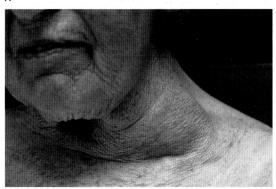

B

Fig. 5.90 (A,B) Neck lump.

Box 5.51 Causes of a thyroid lump

Diffuse goitre

- Simple, non-toxic goitre
- Graves' disease
- Hashimoto's thyroiditis
- Subacute thyroiditis
- Lymphoma

Single nodule

- Adenoma
- Cyst
- Carcinoma

Multinodular goitre

- Toxic multinodular goitre
- Hashimoto's thyroiditis

Worldwide, iodine deficiency is a common cause of goitre.

Table 5.48 Thyroid malignancy

Malignancy	Characteristics
Papillary thyroid carcinoma	Most common Peak incidence young women Locally invasive Prognosis good if detected early
Follicular thyroid carcinoma	Peak incidence in older people Metastases more likely Prognosis still good if detected early
Hurthle cell carcinoma	Uncommon Poor prognosis
Anaplastic carcinoma	Peak incidence in older people Aggressive with high mortality
Lymphoma	Uncommon Good prognosis

CASE 5.43

GOITRE AND NECK LUMPS

Instruction

Please examine this patient's neck/thyroid gland and determine their thyroid status.

Recognition

There is a diffuse goitre/multinodular goitre/single thyroid nodule (Fig. 5.90).

Interpretation

Confirm the diagnosis

Tell the examiners you would ask about symptoms. Most commonly thyroid lumps are asymptomatic and most are euthyroid (endocrine glands generally comprise much redundant tissue). Pressure symptoms (dysphagia, dysphonia, stridor) or pain, especially with bleeding into an adenoma, are possible.

What to do next – consider causes/assess other systems

Tell the examiners you would consider causes (Box 5.51) and assess thyroid status.

Consider severity/decompensation/complications

The key issue is to exclude malignancy (Table 5.48) with further investigations.

Consider function

Swallowing is sometimes affected (see Box 5.52).

Discussion

How would you investigate a thyroid lump?

Thyroid lumps are common, often silent, and increasingly prevalent with age. Nodules may be solid, cystic, mixed (e.g. cystic degeneration within an adenoma) or calcified. The key issue is to exclude malignancy, although this is rare. It is not possible without scanning to determine if a single palpable nodule is part of a multinodular thyroid. Measurement of size and exclusion of tracheal compression are best assessed by computed tomography or magnetic resonance imaging of the neck and thoracic inlet. Radionuclide imaging is less often these days. It does not absolutely exclude malignancy, because most cold nodules are benign and malignant nodules hot, the latter may sometimes be cold. Fine-needle aspiration is the gold standard for diagnosis short of open excision. It is not possible to distinguish between a follicular adenoma and a follicular carcinoma on cytology and all follicular lesions should be excised.

What are the indications for surgery?

Most thyroid lumps are benign. Indications for surgery are listed in Box 5.52.

CASE 5.44

HYPOPITUITARISM

Instruction

Please look at and examine this patient. Discuss your approach to further assessment.

Box 5.52 Indications for surgery for a thyroid lump

- Concerns about malignancy
- Malignancy
- Large cysts (more likely to be malignant)
- Enlarging
- Pressure symptoms (dysphagia, dysphonia, stridor or pain)
- Cosmetic

Recognition

Classic signs of hypopituitarism include *pallor, fine facial skin, decreased axillary and pubic hair, breast atrophy* in females and other signs of *hypogonadism*, reflecting the fact that gonadotrophins tend to be the early hormones lost. Hypopituitarism is shown in Fig. 5.91.

Interpretation

Confirm the diagnosis

The anterior pituitary produces prolactin, growth hormone, adrenocorticotrophic hormone (ACTH), thyroid-stimulating hormone (TSH) and gonadotrophic hormones. Tell the examiners that you would ask about symptoms of hormone deficiency, which are usually those listed in Table 5.49. Posterior pituitary failure is much less common, and disorders of antidiuretic hormone (ADH) are discussed in Case 2.23. Tell the examiners that diagnosis is by combined pituitary function testing and magnetic resonance imaging of the pituitary and sella region.

What to do next – consider causes

Causes of hypopituitarism are listed in Box 5.53. Anterior pituitary dysfunction is much more common than posterior pituitary dysfunction.

Consider severity/decompensation/complications

Tell the examiners that complications are secondary to either pituitary enlargement or dysfunction. Pituitary apoplexy refers to bleeding into pituitary tissue.

Consider function

This relates to symptoms (Box 5.55).

Table 5.49 Symptoms and signs of hypopituitarism

Deficient hormone	Symptoms and signs	Tests of deficiency
Luteinising hormone (LH) and follicle-stimulating hormone (FSH)	Women – oligo/amenorrhoea, infertility, breast atrophy	Low oestradiol with normal or reduced basal LH or FSH
	Men – loss of libido, erectile dysfunction, infertility, loss of body hair	Low testosterone with normal or reduced basal LH or FSH
Growth hormone	Loss of well-being Altered body composition with increased fat mass and central fat Reduced muscle strength	Low insulin-like growth factor (IGF) 1
Thyroid-stimulating hormone (TSH)	Fatigue Cold intolerance Weight gain Dry skin	Low TSH or T4
Adrenocorticotrophic hormone (ACTH)	Fatigue Nausea and vomiting Weight loss Hypoglycaemia	Low morning cortisol (< 100 nmol/l) with normal or low ACTH Hypoglycaemia Insulin-induced hypoglycaemia (failure to stimulate)
Antidiuretic hormone (ADH)	Diabetes insipidus	Water deprivation test (Case 2.30)

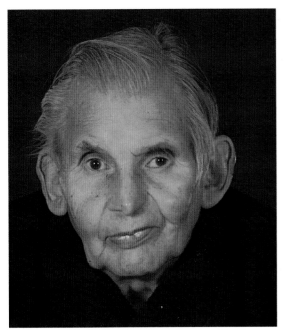

Fig. 5.91 Hypopituitarism.

Discussion

What types of pituitary adenoma are there?

The three common secreting adenomas are outlined in Table 5.50, prolactinomas the most common. Non-functioning adenomas are also common. Rarer functioning adenomas are those secreting TSH or gonadotrophins. Adenomas are usually solitary and monoclonal, and in some, activating mutations in G proteins have been identified, as in many cases of acromegaly in which there is mutation of the G protein linking the growth hormone-releasing hormone receptor to adenylate cyclase in the growth hormone-secreting cells. Pituitary adenomas are sometimes part of multiple endocrine neoplasia (Case 1.43).

How may pituitary tumours present?

The four possible groups of ways in which a pituitary tumour might present are outlined in Table 5.50.

What is Sheehan's syndrome?

Sheehan's syndrome is acute pituitary infarction due to hypovolaemia or septic shock, as in meningococcaemia.

Box 5.53 Causes of hypopituitarism

Pituitary adenoma

- Causes destruction or pressure on pituitary cells, especially macroadenomas

Other masses of the pituitary, sella or suprasellar cistern

- Craniopharyngioma
- Meningioma
- Metastases
- Cysts

- Aneurysm
- Optic glioma
- Granulomatous disease, e.g. sarcoidosis
- Infection

Previous pituitary radiotherapy or surgery

Pituitary haemorrhage or infarction

Table 5.50 Presentations of pituitary adenomas

	Problem	Clinical presentation
Hormone overproduction	Prolactinoma (usually microadenoma in females, macroadenoma in males)	Hyperprolactinaemia
	Growth hormone-secreting (macroadenoma)	Acromegaly
	Adrenocorticotrophic hormone-secreting (microadenoma)	Cushing's disease
Consequence of size	Pituitary compression	Hypopituitarism
	Pituitary mass effect	Headache
	Suprasellar extension	Bitemporal hemianopia
		Stalk displacement – hyperprolactinaemia
		Hypothalamic damage
		Diabetes insipidus
		Hydrocephalus
Incidentaloma	No problem	Discovered during investigation for something else
Pituitary apoplexy	Acute haemorrhage from large adenoma	Acute severe headache and meningism – can present similarly to subarachnoid haemorrhage or meningitis
		Hypotension

What is empty sella syndrome?

This is when an enlarged sella is filled with cerebrospinal fluid, and can be the result of damage from many causes, including infarction, surgery and radiotherapy.

What pituitary replacement treatments are there?

These are outlined in Table 5.51.

What are the causes of hyperprolactinaemia?

Prolactin release from the anterior pituitary is normally inhibited by dopamine derived from the hypothalamus. Causes of hyperprolactinaemia are listed in Box 5.54.

What are the effects of hyperprolactinaemia?

These are galactorrhoea and amenorrhoea in women, who usually present earlier than men. Men may present with loss of libido, erectile dysfunction or reduced facial hair. Galactorrhoea is always the result of hyperprolactinaemia and occurs in 90% of female patients.

What is the treatment for hyperprolactinaemia?

Dopamine agonists such as cabergoline suppress prolactin secretion and cause rapid tumour shrinkage, even of large macroadenomas. Surgery is seldom needed because of the good response to medical therapy.

Table 5.51 Pituitary hormone replacement

Deficient hormone	Treatment	Comments	
Gonadotrophins	Women – oestradiol or conjugated oestrogens plus progesterone	Oral or transdermal	Sex steroids maintain normal body composition, bone mineral density and sexual function
	Men – testosterone	Intramuscular Transdermal Implant Buccal	If fertility is desired in hypogonadotrophic hypogonadism, gonadotrophin-releasing hormone (GnRH) may be used
Growth hormone	Growth hormone	Subcutaneously in evening Improves body composition and quality of life (currently licensed only for severe deficiency)	
Thyroid-stimulating hormone (TSH)	Thyroxine	Treated as for hypothyroidism	
Adrenocorticotrophic hormone	Hydrocortisone	Replaces missing glucocorticoid (much better than prednisolone or dexamethasone) Cortisol has short half life so frequent dosing and small doses desirable Starting dose often 10 mg/5 mg/5 mg Increased dose needed during illness	
Prolactin	Not needed		
Antidiuretic hormone (ADH)	Desmopressin	Intranasal Oral	

Box 5.54 Causes of hyperprolactinaemia

Physiological

- Sleep
- Stress
- Pregnancy/lactation
- Nipple stimulation
- Sexual intercourse

Pituitary tumour

- Prolactinoma (often producing very high prolactin levels)
- Mixed growth hormone/prolactin-secreting tumour

Hypothalamic or pituitary stalk disease

- Mass compressing stalk causing 'disconnection hyperprolactinaemia', e.g. craniopharyngioma
- Infiltration, e.g. sarcoidosis
- Trauma

Drugs

- Dopamine receptor antagonists, e.g. metoclopramide
- Neuroleptics, e.g. haloperidol
- Antidepressants
- Opiates

Hypothyroidism

- Thyroid-releasing hormone stimulates prolactin as well as thyroid-stimulating hormone

Polycystic ovarian syndrome

Post seizure

Idiopathic

- Likely covert microadenoma

CASE 5.45

ACROMEGALY

Instruction

Please examine this patient's face/hands. Assess any other systems you feel relevant and then discuss your findings.

Recognition (Fig. 5.92)

Face

There are *prominent supraorbital ridges*. There is *prognathism* (protrusion of lower jaw), *soft tissue enlargement of the nose, tongue and ears*. The *interdental distances are increased*. There is *general coarsening of features*. The voice may be husky.

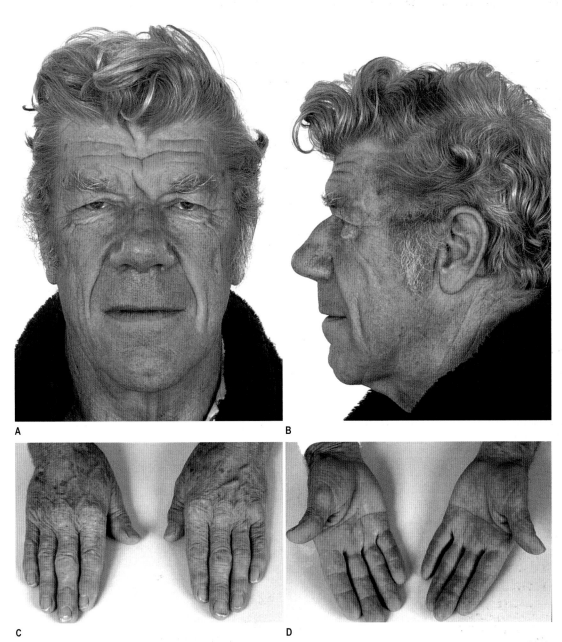

A   B

C   D

Fig. 5.92 (A–D) Acromegaly.

Hands

These are '*spade-like*', squared and large. The skin is *thick*, often with a rubbery texture and moist.

Interpretation

Confirm the diagnosis

Some of the aforementioned terms, beloved of many textbooks, are rather old fashioned, even insulting ('spade-like hands'), and of little practical value. Recognising acromegaly is not likely to be very difficult in PACES, although signs can be subtle as disease slowly and insidiously evolves. Newly diagnosed patients have often had symptoms for years, including increased sweating, increased size of shoes, gloves, rings or dentures, fatigue, joint pains and headaches. It typically becomes apparent between the ages of 40 and 60 years.

What to do next – assess other systems

Mortality is increased two- to three-fold in acromegaly because of cardiorespiratory disease and malignancy (see Table 5.52). Tell the examiners you would check the blood pressure, plasma glucose, and examine for bitemporal hemianopia.

Other symptoms may arise from hypofunction of the compressed anterior pituitary, such as hypogonadism and reduced libido, and local tumour pressure effects. Associated hyperprolactinaemia may contribute to testosterone deficiency.

Consider severity/decompensation/complications

Tell the examiners you would assess for the complications outlined in Table 5.52.

Consider function

This relates to symptoms.

Table 5.52 Complications of acromegaly

Complication	Problems
Hypertension	Cardiomyopathy and heart failure Increased cardiovascular disease mortality
Impaired glucose tolerance and diabetes	Increased cardiovascular disease mortality
Bitemporal hemianopia	Visual loss
Carpal tunnel syndrome	Nocturnal paraesthesia
Obstructive sleep apnoea	Snoring Excessive daytime somnolence Systemic and pulmonary hypertension
Recurrent colorectal polyps	Colorectal cancer Screening advised

Discussion

What causes acromegaly?

Acromegaly is the result of hypersecretion of growth hormone from a macroadenoma.

Which investigations would you consider in the diagnosis and assessment of acromegaly?

Investigations are outlined in Table 5.53.

What treatments are used for acromegaly?

Successful treatment restores life expectancy to normal. Most patients proceed to transphenoidal surgery (transcranial if significant suprasellar extension), by an experienced pituitary surgeon to remove the adenoma. Surgery is invariably complicated by early but transient diabetes insipidus. Larger adenomas may be difficult to completely excise, leaving patients with residual growth hormone excess. Most symptoms and signs of acromegaly do not regress after surgery, except those of disease activity such as sweating and oedema.

External pituitary radiotherapy alone takes several years to achieve growth hormone reduction and often ultimately induces hypopituitarism. It is indicated after incomplete surgery to prevent recurrence and reduce secretion.

Dopamine agonists such as cabergoline are generally less effective at reducing growth hormone secretion and do

Table 5.53 Investigating acromegaly

Diagnosis	Serial growth hormone levels unhelpful since secretion pulsatile Failure of serum growth hormone to suppress to below 1 mU/L in a prolonged 75 g oral glucose tolerance test Elevated serum insulin-like growth factor-1 (IGF-1) level (mediates actions of growth hormone but influenced by many factors such as nutrition and disease)
Anterior pituitary function tests	Serum thyroid-stimulating hormone and thyroxine Serum cortisol Serum gonadotrophins and sex hormones (luteinising hormone-releasing hormone, luteinising hormone, testosterone) Serum prolactin
Pituitary anatomy	Magnetic resonance imaging
Complications	Electrocardiogram Chest X-ray Sleep studies Colonoscopy

not reduce tumour size. Somatostatin analogues such as octreotide, administered by monthly injection, can be effective in inhibiting secretion, but do not cause significant tumour shrinkage. Pegvisomant, a growth hormone receptor agonist, is very effective but there is a small risk of hepatitis.

When might growth hormone be administered therapeutically in adults?

Growth hormone deficiency in adults is increasingly recognised, and can give rise to those features outlined in Box 5.55.

It may improve well-being, bone mineral density and lipid profiles, enhance muscle power and reduce cardiovascular mortality. Unfortunately, it is expensive.

What is ghrelin?

Ghrelin is a gut hormone that is a potent stimulator of growth hormone secretion.

CASE 5.46

CUSHING'S SYNDROME

Instruction

Please look at this patient's face and then assess her condition further. Discuss your findings and the differential diagnosis.

Recognition

As for acromegaly, there are lengthy lists of signs to be found in textbooks, some insulting ('buffalo hump' and 'moon face'), which may best be summarised as signs of corticosteroid excess. Again, recognising these is often not hard (Box 5.56 and Fig. 5.93).

Interpretation

Confirm the diagnosis

Cushing's syndrome results from prolonged exposure to excessive circulating glucocorticoid, and except where the diagnosis is probably iatrogenic, should be confirmed biochemically (see Table 5.53).

What to do next – consider causes

Most patients with Cushing's syndrome are taking long-term corticosteroids for a chronic inflammatory disease such as chronic obstructive pulmonary disease, asthma or inflammatory bowel disease, or a renal transplant. Consider these. Otherwise the three causes of Cushing's syndrome to consider are shown in Table 5.54. Rarely,

---

Box 5.55 Adult growth hormone deficiency

- Impaired well-being
- Altered body composition (increased fat mass and central fat deposition, decreased total body water)
- Decreased bone mineral density
- Altered lipid profile (raised total cholesterol, low-density lipoprotein and triglycerides)
- Cardiovascular effects (hypertension, reduced heart size, raised C-reactive protein and interleukin-6 and reduced fibrinolysis)
- Insulin resistance
- Thin skin
- Decreased sweating
- Reduced glomerular filtration rate
- Reduced red cell mass

Box 5.56 Initial clues to Cushing's syndrome (in order of frequency)

- Obesity/weight gain (centripetal distribution)
- Facial plethora
- Round face
- Decreased libido
- Thin skin
- Menstrual disturbance
- Hypertension
- Hirsutism
- Depression/emotional change
- Easy bruising
- Glucose intolerance
- Weakness (proximal myopathy)
- Osteopenia on X-ray
- Nephrolithiasis

Most discriminating are thin skin, easy bruising and myopathy

---

pseudo-Cushing's syndrome may result from obesity, depression or sometimes alcohol excess.

Consider severity/decompensation/complications

Tell the examiners that hypertension and impaired glucose tolerance or diabetes are associated with Cushing's syndrome. Complications include osteoporosis/wedge fractures (kyphosis) and recurrent infections.

Consider function

Examine briefly for proximal myopathy. Tell the examiners that you would also consider the possibility of depression, psychosis, amenorrhoea and infertility.

Discussion

How could you determine the cause of non-iatrogenic Cushing's syndrome?

There are two steps to investigating clinically suspected non-iatrogenic Cushing's syndrome (Table 5.55).

What treatments are used for Cushing's disease?

Trans-sphenoidal hypophysectomy by an experienced surgeon is the treatment of choice, but potential complica-

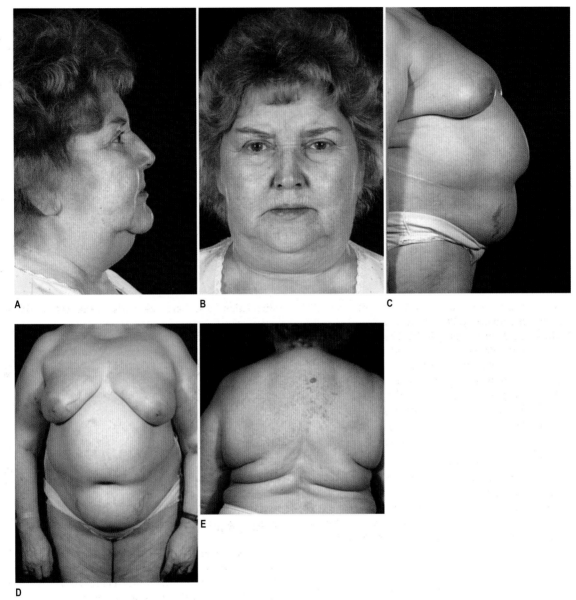

Fig. 5.93 (A–E) Cushing's syndrome.

tions are cerebrospinal fluid rhinorrhoea, diabetes insipidus, hypopituitarism, visual field disturbance, persistent or recurrent disease and death. Lasting remission without other pituitary hormone deficiency is achievable in over 50% of patients.

Pituitary radiotherapy is the next best choice, and used if there is persistent hypercortisolism after surgery. The main complication is progressive anterior pituitary failure, which may be subtle and protracted, sometimes not detect-able for as much as 10 to 20 years. Cortisol levels have usually normalised within a few years, and later growth hormone deficiency, gonadotrophin deficiency and hypoadrenalism are not uncommon.

Drugs are sometimes used before surgery or after failed surgery, and include metyrapone and ketaconazole, which inhibit cortisol synthesis. Metyrapone causes an increase in androgen precursors and hirsutism. Mitotane is sometimes used in adrenocortical carcinoma.

Table 5.54 The three non-iatrogenic causes of Cushing's syndrome

		Cause	Features
Adrenocorticotrophin hormone (ACTH) dependent	**Cushing's disease** (most) **Ectopic ACTH**	Pituitary microadenoma secreting ACTH Often caused by a bronchial carcinoid or small cell lung cancer	The most common non-iatrogenic cause, with typical features of Cushing's syndrome Ectopic ACTH secretion due to carcinoma usually of rapid onset with less florid signs of corticosteroid excess but significant weight loss, hypokalaemia (mineralocorticoid effect due to inhibition of renal tubular 11b hydroxysteroid dehydrogenase) and pigmentation (co-secretion of other peptides) Ectopic ACTH secretion due to an indolent carcinoid tumour can be indistinguishable from Cushing's disease
Adrenal dependent	**Adrenal adenoma** Less commonly carcinoma and rarely hyperplasia	Some adrenal adenomas secrete cortisol	Tend to also secrete androgens, presenting with hirsutism and/or virilisation, e.g. clitoromegaly

There is interest in agents that might inhibit adrenocorticotrophic hormone (ACTH) release.

Unilateral adrenalectomy is the treatment of choice for an isolated adrenal adenoma and bilateral adrenalectomy is reserved for hypercortisolism in Cushing's disease where primary evacuation or treatment is not possible; it may be complicated by Nelson syndrome, in which ACTH levels rise causing melanin-induced hyperpigmentation.

Are all hormones steroids?

Thyroxine, tri-iodothyronine, dopamine and catecholamines are amine hormones. Most other hormones are steroids (cortisol, aldosterone, sex hormones, vitamin D) or peptides (thyroid-stimulating hormone, follicle-stimulating hormone, luteinising hormone, ACTH, vasopressin, insulin, growth hormone).

What hormone changes occur in systemic disease and pregnancy?

As a general rule, 'stress' hormone levels (ACTH, cortisol, growth hormone, catecholamines, glucagon) rise in systemic illness, while the others tend to fall. In pregnancy, most hormone levels rise.

What is the value of a suppression or stimulation test in endocrinology?

Many hormones have a circadian rhythm and isolated levels can be difficult to interpret. Most hormone levels are regulated by other hormones or metabolic substrates via a negative feedback loop, and isolated levels should always be interpreted in their context. Where there is difficulty in interpreting isolated levels, dynamic tests can be useful. Suppression tests are used for suspected hormone excess.

Stimulation tests are used for suspected hormone deficiency.

CASE 5.47

HYPOADRENALISM AND ADDISON'S DISEASE

Instruction

This patient presented with weight loss and weakness. Please examine his hands and face and then discuss your findings.

Recognition

There is *hyperpigmentation*, especially of *skin creases* (*palms*, *elbows*), the *lips* and *mouth*, and *surgical scars* (Fig 5.94). There may be *vitiligo*, and sparse *axillary* (and pubic) *hair*. *Postural hypotension* is possible.

Interpretation

Confirm the diagnosis

Hyperpigmentation is the result of elevated melanocyte-stimulating hormone and adrenocorticotrophic hormone (ACTH) and suggests primary adrenal failure, usually Addison's disease. Tell the examiners that you would ask about symptoms of hypoadrenalism (Box 5.57), which can be insidious.

Tell the examiners that you would arrange a short Synacthen test to determine whether or not administered synthetic ACTH stimulates an appropriate rise in cortisol levels. Measurement of plasma ACTH should be greatly raised in hypopituitarism.

Table 5.55 Investigating Cushing's syndrome

Step	Tests	Interpretation	Diagnosis
1. Diagnosing Cushing's syndrome Three types of test; sometimes repeated tests needed since cyclical secretion of cortisol recognised in some patients	**Low-dose dexamethasone suppression test (LDDST)** Most commonly used test All causes of Cushing's syndrome fail to suppress Normal subjects and those with pseudoCushing's suppress Two types of test		
	Overnight dexamethasone suppression test 1 mg dexamethasone (a synthetic glucocorticoid) administered at 23.00 h	Cushing's syndrome excluded if plasma cortisol < 50 nmol/l at 08.00 to 09.00 h	Cushing's syndrome
	48-hour dexamethasone suppression test More sensitive test 0.5 mg dexamethasone administered six hourly at 09.00, 15.00, 21.00 and 03.00 h for two days	Cushing's syndrome excluded if plasma cortisol < 50 nmol/l	Cushing's syndrome
	Assessment of circadian rhythmicity Normal cortisol levels at 08.00–09.00 h tend to be in the range 150–650 nmol/l, may be in a range around half that at 16.00 h, and can drop to a nadir of < 50 nmol/l at midnight Normal circadian rhythmicity lost in Cushing's syndrome	At 48 hours, single unstressed sleeping midnight plasma cortisol > 50 nmol/l is most sensitive test for Cushing's syndrome but it is generally not practical to admit patients for 48 hours, necessary to allow circadian rhythmicity, before the test (late night salivary cortisol an alternative with slightly lower sensitivity) Test requires admission to hospital – Cushing's syndrome excluded if single sleeping plasma cortisol < 50 nmol/l	Cushing's syndrome
	24-hour urinary free cortisol	Positive if ≥ 275 nmol/24 hours, but low sensitivity (usually tested on up to three occasions)	Cushing's syndrome
2. Establishing the cause	**Plasma ACTH (corticotrophin)** – derived from pro-opiomelanocortin, its gene expressed by ACTH tumours		
	ACTH easily detectable (ACTH-dependent cause)		
	High-dose dexamethasone suppression test (HDDST) or alternatively corticotrophin-releasing hormone (CRH) test	Pituitary adenomas to an extent obey normal physiological rules with HDDST, albeit with higher threshold for suppression than the normal situation – around 80% of Cushing's disease suppress to < 50% of basal levels, i.e. a low sensitivity test. Magnetic resonance imaging now standard but sometimes unsatisfactory since pituitary adenomas can be small and undetectable yet detectable 'incidentalomas' are common Bilateral inferior petrosal sinus sampling (BIPSS) with measurement of ACTH following CRH stimulation can diagnose and permit hemispheric localisation of adenoma, and theoretically permit hemispheric resection with preservation of pituitary function	
	ACTH partially suppressible → Pituitary imaging		**Cushing's disease**
	ACTH not suppressible → Imaging for cause	Ectopic ACTH not suppressible, but exceptions recognised	**Ectopic ACTH**
	ACTH not easily detectable (ACTH independent/ adrenal dependent cause) **Imaging for adrenal tumour**	Adrenal cortisol production suppresses ACTH	**Adrenal tumour**

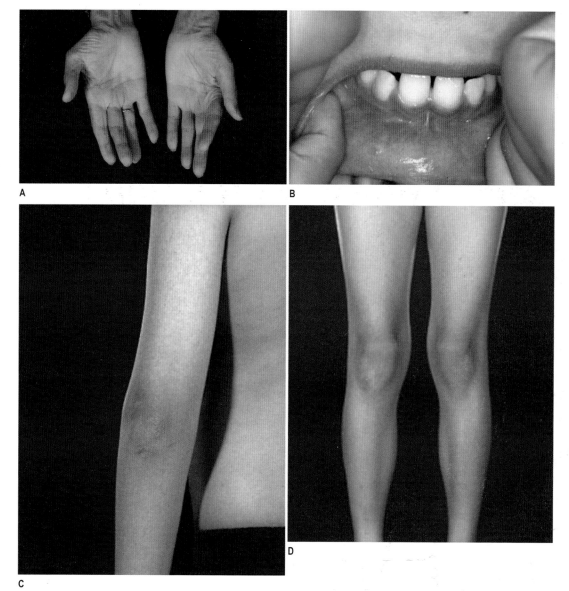

Fig. 5.94 Addison's disease: hyperpigmentation of (A) palms, (B) mouth, (C,D) elbows and knees.

Box 5.57 Symptoms of hypoadrenalism
• Anorexia and weight loss (> 90%)
• Fatigue
• Weakness
• Postural dizziness
• Nausea, vomiting, diarrhoea
• Reduced libido and axillary hair
• Sweating
• Salt craving

What to do next – consider causes/assess other systems

Mention to the examiners some causes of hypoadrenalism/adrenal insufficiency (Table 5.56); these are distinct from secondary pituitary causes.

Consider severity/decompensation/complications

Adrenal crises are associated with haemodynamic instability and life-threatening metabolic disturbances. Tell the examiners you would determine the serum potassium and

Table 5.56 Causes of hypoadrenalism

Cause	Features
Autoimmune destruction (Addison's disease)	Most common cause Hyperpigmentation Increased risk of other organ-specific autoimmune diseases associated with HLA DR3 or DR4, e.g. diabetes
Metastatic disease	Relatively common, e.g. lung, breast, kidney, melanoma, lymphoma Hypoadrenalism less common
Infection	HIV-associated, e.g. cytomegalovirus Tuberculosis Fungal infection, e.g. histoplasmosis, coccidioidomycosis More common in immunocompromised
Infiltration	Granulomatous disease Haemochromatosis Amyloid
Iatrogenic	Ketoconazole, rifampicin, phenytoin
Critical illness	Hypotension can be both the cause (hypoperfusion/infarction) and effect of hypoadrenalism
Haemorrhage	Waterhouse–Friederichsen syndrome (infarction in meningococcal septicaemia)
Congenital/genetic	Adrenoleukodystrophy/other

sodium. Hyponatraemia and hyperkalaemia with type IV renal tubular acidosis are common, due to mineralo-corticoid deficiency. Hypoglycaemia is less common but possible.

Consider function

Fatigue can be disabling.

Discussion

What hormones does the adrenal gland secrete?

The adrenal cortex secretes the glucocorticoid cortisol, the mineralocorticoid aldosterone, and androgens. Aldosterone secretion is predominantly under the control of renin–angiotensin, but around 10% is controlled by ACTH. Glucocorticoid, mineralocorticoid and androgens are reduced in adrenal failure, albeit not until around 90% of functioning tissue is lost, whereas only glucocorticoid activity is affected by ACTH deficiency.

What are the autoimmune polyglandular syndromes?

These are genetically determined syndromes, with various modes of inheritance. Type 1 may involve chronic muco-cutaneous candidiasis, hypoparathyroidism and Addison's disease. Type 2 always includes Addison's disease, and may include thyroid disease (Schmidt syndrome) or diabetes.

How would you confirm hypoadrenalism?

A serum cortisol level of 100 nmol/l at 09.00 h is diagnostic, and elevated ACTH is suggestive. The tetracosactrin or short Synacthen test (SST) is used to confirm a suboptimal response to synthetic ACTH: 250 µg is administered intramuscularly and serum cortisol is measured at 0, 30 and 60 minutes. A normal response is a peak of more than 550 nmol/l, although definitions vary. The result may be less easy to interpret, with a suboptimal response, for people who have just stopped or are on low-dose, long-term prednisolone. Switching to dexamethasone is a potential way of assessing in these circumstances.

How might you determine possible causes?

Adrenal antibodies to adrenal enzymes are present in over 90% of patients with recent adrenal autoimmunity, although most people with adrenal antibodies without symptoms do not develop adrenal insufficiency. Elevated recumbent renin with low or normal aldosterone may be a sign of impending hypoadrenalism where a cause is not confirmed. Other tests include chest and abdominal imaging.

How might you differentiate between hypoadrenalism and hypopituitarism clinically?

Hypoadrenalism and hypopituitarism sometimes seem clinically similar. Addison's disease tends to appear over two to three years with hyperpigmentation, whereas hypopituitarism can take a more protracted course over many more years, especially if radiotherapy is a cause; pallor predominates. An ACTH level resolves the issue, and further tests might include levels of thyroid-stimulating hormone, growth hormone, follicle-stimulating hormone, testosterone and prolactin, computed tomography imaging of the adrenals and magnetic resonance imaging of the pituitary.

What is the treatment for hypoadrenalism?

Treatment involves identification and management of any underlying remediable cause and adrenal replacement therapy with both glucocorticoid and mineralocorticoid. Hydrocortisone is administered at a starting dose of 10 mg on waking (to mimic the physiological peak), 5 mg at lunchtime and 5 mg at 18.00 h. An increased dose may be needed in pregnancy. Fludrocortisone is used to achieve normal sodium homeostasis, as evidenced by normal plasma renin levels. Androgen replacement remains contentious. Increased doses of hydrocortisone are needed in intercurrent illness, generally doubled orally but with high doses intravenously in unstable patients.

How should therapeutic corticosteroids be withdrawn to prevent iatrogenic hypoadrenalism?

If prednisolone has been used for under three weeks at doses of ≤ 40 mg, it can usually be withdrawn abruptly. If this is not the case, gradual withdrawal is needed. After a few weeks of treatment it could be decreased in 2.5 mg decrements for a few days to 7.5 mg and then more slowly, e.g. 2.5 mg every week or every few weeks. After an unknown period it could be decreased in 2.5-mg decrements once or twice monthly to 7.5 mg and then more slowly, e.g. 1–2.5 mg monthly. If disease is likely to recur then reduction is often by 1 mg monthly.

CASE 5.48

HIRSUTISM AND POLYCYSTIC OVARIAN SYNDROME

Instruction

Look at this patient. You may ask her a few questions. Tell the examiners how you would proceed with your assessment.

Recognition

There is *hirsutism*, or excessive hair growth, particularly over the face and limbs (Fig. 5.95). There may be *acne*. There may be other *signs of virilisation*.

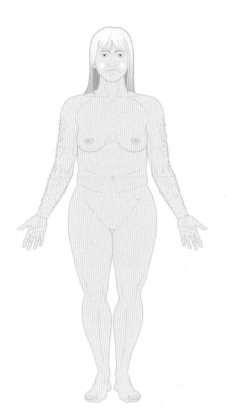

Fig. 5.95 Hirsutism.

Interpretation

Confirm the diagnosis

The diagnosis of polycystic ovarian syndrome (PCOS) rests on a combination of symptoms, clinical findings and biochemical abnormalities. In addition to hirsutism, common associations are acne, obesity, male pattern hair thinning, subfertility and oligomenorrhoea or secondary amenorrhoea (hyperplasia of ovarian thecal cells and multiple cysts). Always consider the possibility of a virilising adrenal tumour causing Cushing's syndrome in your differential diagnosis.

What to do next – assess other systems

Tell the examiners that you would check for glycosuria.

Consider severity/decompensation/complications

Mention that PCOS is often part of the metabolic disorder comprising hyperinsulinaemia, insulin resistance and dyslipidaemia.

Consider function

Hyperandrogenism and regular menses are now recognised as part of the spectrum of PCOS.

Discussion

What is meant by the terms hypertrichosis, hirsutism and virilisation?

Hypertrichosis refers to excess body hair. Hirsutism refers to excess hair in androgen-dependent areas (male pattern). Virilisation refers to male pattern hair loss and other physical changes including voice change, breast atrophy and clitoromegaly. Hirsutism may be constitutional, or it may be the result of adrenal or ovarian disorders, such as androgen-secreting tumours in either of these organs. It may be caused by congenital adrenal hyperplasia (CAH). It may also be caused by drugs. One of the most common causes of hirsutism is PCOS.

What is PCOS?

The pathophysiology of PCOS is incompletely understood. It is a condition of androgen excess, characterised biochemically by:

- Raised testosterone and androstenedione levels
- A raised luteinising hormone : follicle-stimulating hormone ratio with an abnormality in the usual pulsatile secretion of gonadotrophin-releasing hormones
- Normal or elevated oestradiol levels
- Mild hyperprolactinaemia
- Low sex hormone-binding globulin levels
- Low high-density lipoprotein cholesterol
- Insulin resistance with hyperinsulinaemia

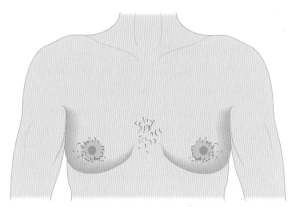

Fig. 5.96 Gynaecomastia.

What treatments are there for PCOS?

These might include induction of ovulation and menstrual regulation in specialist clinics, treatment of hirsutism and treatment of features of the metabolic syndrome. Metformin is widely used.

CASE 5.49

HYPOGONADISM AND GYNAECOMASTIA

Instruction

Look at this patient. You may ask him a few questions. Tell the examiners how you would proceed with your assessment.

Recognition

There is *gynaecomastia* in this *tall* man with *sparse hair* (Fig. 5.96).

interpretation

Confirm the diagnosis

Tell the examiners that Klinefelter's syndrome could be confirmed by chromosome analysis (XXY) and by the finding of small testes, azoospermia and raised gonadotrophins in response to testicular failure.

What to do next – consider causes

Gynaecomastia has many causes (Box 5.58).

Consider severity/decompensation/complications

Tell the examiners that a full hormone, including gonadotrophin, profile would be important, together with assessing for features of testosterone deficiency.

Consider function

Tell the examiners that testosterone deficiency symptoms should be assessed.

Discussion

What is congenital adrenal hyperplasia (CAH)?

These are a group of disorders, all autosomal recessively inherited, the commonest defect being 21-hydroxylase deficiency. There can be a spectrum of clinical manifestations from mild, late-onset signs resembling polycystic ovarian syndrome in females, to ambiguous sexual differentiation at birth. The enzyme defect results in a deficiency of glucocorticoids or mineralocorticoids leading to hyperstimulation of the adrenal gland, which can only respond by producing excess hormones from unaffected pathways – testosterone precursors and testosterone. CAH may cause precocious puberty in males and female virilisation.

What are the causes of testosterone deficiency?

Testosterone deficiency is becoming increasingly recognised, and is not uncommon. It may be a result of a specific hypogonadal disorder or age-related decline. It may be hypergonadotrophic or hypogonadotrophic.

- *Hypergonadotrophic hypogonadism* – refers to primary testicular failure, often with elevated follicle-stimulating hormone (FSH) and luteinising hormone (LH) levels. Acquired causes include mumps, trauma, torsion, surgery, radiotherapy, drugs (spironolactone, chemotherapy, marijuana) and myotonic dystrophy. Congenital disorders include Klinefelter's syndrome and 5α-reductase deficiency (androgen resistance).
- *Hypogonadotrophic hypogonadism* – is gonadal failure secondary to hypothalamic/pituitary disease, usually with low or normal FSH and LH levels.

Systemic disorders including chronic kidney or liver disease, and sickle cell disease can also cause testosterone deficiency. Chronic alcohol excess is a common cause.

How does testosterone deficiency present?

It can present in many ways, most commonly as:

- Reduced libido
- Reduced muscle mass
- Reduced bone mass with an increased risk of osteoporosis
- Reduced facial, body or pubic hair
- Small testes
- Tiredness, depression or non-specific cognitive changes such as poor concentration

What are the features of Turner's syndrome?

Turner's syndrome (45X0) causes primary amenorrhoea, short stature and delayed puberty. There may be a webbed neck and widely spaced nipples. Sometimes there is a horseshoe kidney or aortic coarctation. Oestrogen levels are low with raised FSH and LH levels.

Would you expect galactorrhoea in patients with gynaecomastia?

Gynaecomastia is unrelated to hyperprolactinaemia (the usual cause of galactorrhoea) and is caused instead by a decreased androgen : oestrogen ratio.

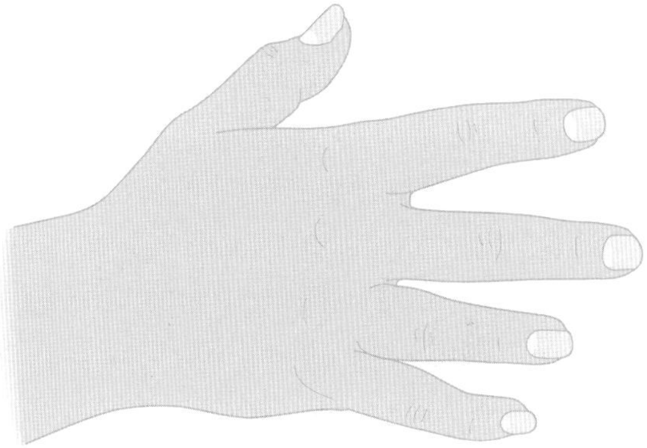

Fig. 5.97 Pseudohypoparathyroidism.

Box 5.59 Causes of short stature

- Familial
- Achondroplasia
- Turner's syndrome
- Noonan's syndrome

CASE 5.50

PSEUDOHYPOPARATHYROIDISM

Instruction

Look at this patient's hands and face and report your findings.

Recognition

There are *short fourth and fifth metacarpals* on both hands. There is short stature, obesity, a round face with frontal bossing of the skull and a short neck (Fig. 5.97).

Interpretation

Confirm the diagnosis

The syndrome with short fourth and fifth metacarpals is likely to be the result of type 1a pseudohypoparathyroidism or pseudopseudohypoparathyroidism.

What to do next – consider causes

Short stature has many causes (Box 5.59).

Consider severity/decompensation/complications

Calcification is a complication of pseudohypoparathyroidism, as might be learning difficulties, hypothyroidism and hypogonadism.

Consider function

Tell the examiners that gonadal function should be assessed.

Discussion

What are the differences between hypoparathyroidism, pseudohypoparathyroidism and pseudopseudohypoparathyroidism?

Hypoparathyroidism is a biochemical condition comprising low levels of parathyroid hormone and calcium and raised phosphate. Pseudohypoparathyroidism is the result of target organ resistance to parathyroid hormone, with high levels of parathyroid hormone, low calcium and raised phosphate. Type 1a or Albright's hereditary osteodystrophy produces the phenotype described above. There is also a morphologically normal phenotype. Pseudohypoparathyroidism has the morphological appearance of type 1a pseudohypoparathyroidism but with normal biochemistry.

References and further reading

Skin

Psoriasis
Ghaffar SA, Clements SE, Griffiths CEM. Modern management of psoriasis. Clin Med 2005; 5:564–568

Dermatitis
British Association of Dermatologists, www.bad.org.uk
Brown S, Reynolds NJ. Atopic and non-atopic eczema. BMJ 2006; 332:584–588

Bistering skin conditions
Peters TJ, Sarkany R. Porphyria for the general physician. Clin Med 2005; 5:275–281

Facial rash
Yates V. Acne: current treatment. Clin Med 2005; 5:569–572

Shin lesions
Brooklyn T, Dunnill G, Probert C. Diagnosis and treatment of pyoderma gangrenosum. BMJ 2006; 333:181–184

Neurofibromatosis
Huson SM. The neurofibromatoses: more than just a medical curiosity. J R Coll Physicians Edinb 2006; 36:44–50

Skin and soft tissue infection
National Institute of Health and Clinical Excellence. Clinical Guideline. The prevention and treatment of pressure ulcers. London: NICE; 2005

Locomotor system

Examining the hands and arms
Dias R, Cutts S, Massoud S. Frozen shoulder. BMJ 2005; 331:1453–1456

Rheumatoid arthritis
Amarasena R, Bowman S. Sjogren's syndrome. Clin Med 2007; 7:53–56
American College of Rheumatology (formerly American Rheumatism Association). Available online: www.rheumatology.org (1987 revised criteria for the classification of rheumatoid arthritis published by Arnett FC et al. Arthritis Rheum 1988; 31:315)
Chee NM, Capell HA, Madhok R. Recent advances in the management of rheumatoid arthritis. J R Coll Physicians Edinb 2005; 35:239–245
Dubey S, Gaffney K. Management of early rheumatoid arthritis. Clin Med 2005; 5:211–214
Östör AJ. Beyond methotrexate: biologic therapy in rheumatoid arthritis. Clin Med 2005; 5:222–226

Ankylosing spondylitis
Khan MA. Spondyloarthropathies. Curr Opin Rheumatol 2001; 13:245–290
Khan MA. Update on spondyloarthropathies. Ann Intern Med 2002; 136:896–907
McVeigh CM, Carins AP. Diagnosis and management of ankylosing spondylitis. BMJ 2006; 333:581–585
Swales C, Bowness P. Anti-tumour necrosis factor therapy in seronegative spondyloarthritis. Clin Med 2005; 5:219–222
Van der Linden S, Valkenburg HA, Cats A. Evaluation of diagnostic criteria for ankylosing spondylitis. A proposal for modification of the New York criteria. Arthritis Rheum 1984; 27:361–368

Systemic lupus erythematosus
D'Cruz DP. Systemic lupus erythematosus. BMJ 2006; 332:890–894
St Thomas Lupus Trust, www.lupus.org.uk

Scleroderma
Ong VH, Brough G, Denton CP. Management of systemic sclerosis. Clin Med 2005; 5:214–219

Crystal arthropathy
Underwood M. Diagnosis and management of gout. BMJ 2006; 332:1315–1319

Osteoarthritis
National Institute of Health and Clinical Excellence. Osteoarthritis: The care and management of osteoarthritis in adults. NICE clinical guidline 59, 2008
Neaem R, Doherty M. Osteoarthritis update. Clin Med 2005; 5:207–210
Osteoarthritis: National Clinical Guideline for Care and Management in Adults. London: Royal College of Physicians, 2008
Zhang W, Moskowitz Rw, Nuki G et al. Osteoarthritis Research Society International (OARSI) recommendations for the management of hip and knee osteoarethritis. Part II: OARSI evidence-based, expert consensus guidelines. Osteoarthritis Cartilage 2008; 16:137–162

Paget's disease
Judge DP, Dietz HC. Marfan's syndrome. Lancet 2005; 366:1965–1976
Selby PL, Davie MWJ, Ralston SH et al. Guidelines on the management of Paget's disease of bone. Bone 2002; 31:366–373

Marfan's syndrome
Dean JCS. Marfan syndrome. J R Coll Physicians Edinb 2006. Available: www.rcpe.ac.uk

Osteogenesis imperfecta
Sillence DO, Senn A, Danks DM. Genetic heterogeneity in osteogenesis imperfecta. J Med Genet 1979; 16:101–116
Glorieux FH, Rauch F, Plotkin H et al. Type V osteogenesis imperfecta: a new form of brittle bone disease. J Bone Miner Res 2000; 15:1650–1658
Glorieux FH, Ward LM, Rauch F et al. Osteogenesis imperfecta type VI: a form of brittle bone disease with a mineralization defect. J Bone Miner Res 2002; 17:30–38

Eyes
Cataracts
Allen D, Vasavada A. Cataract and surgery for cataract. BMJ 2006; 333:128–133

Endocrine system
Hyperthyroidism
Pearce EN. Diagnosis and management of thyrotoxicosis. BMJ 2006; 332:1369–1373
Weetman AP. Abnormal thyroid stimulating hormone levels: when and who to treat. Clin Med 2008; 8:208–211

Cushing's syndrome
Newell-Price J. Cushing's syndrome. Clin Med 2008; 8:204–208
Newell-Price J, Bertagna X, Grossman AB. Cushing's syndrome. Lancet 2006; 367:1605–1617

Hypoadrenalism
Alexandraki KI, Grisman AB. Adrenal incidentaolmas: 'the rule of fours'. Clin Med 2008; 8:201–204
Arit W. Adrenal insufficiency. Clin Med 2008; 8:211–215

Appendix – 100 tips for passing PACES

BEFORE PACES

Timing

1. Many candidates feel that MRCP exams should be sat (and failed) as often as possible in the belief that passing will be the reward of negative but repetitive experience! With the right preparation you can easily pass PACES. Take it when you feel ready and do not listen to pessimistic colleagues.

What the examiners are looking for

2. The examiners want to be satisfied that you are a safe, competent doctor, suitable to enter specialist training.
3. They are not looking for specialist knowledge.
4. They are not looking for the next Professor of Medicine.
5. They want to know that, as your general medical consultant, they could have a sensible discussion with you about the care of a patient.
6. They want to know that, as your consultant, they could entrust the care of their patients to you when away from the wards.
7. They respect a friendly and confident manner, but not arrogance.
8. Many candidates adopt 'victim mode' with head down and victim posture throughout PACES. This concerns examiners, who wonder how a nervous candidate might cope in an emergency. Examiners are likely to be more impressed by the candidate who stands with an upright, confident posture, hands by sides or behind back, and makes good eye contact.

It's in your hands!

9. Passing PACES is well within your grasp.
10. The idea that passing is in your examiners' hands is a negative one.
11. It is in your hands!
12. You can pass with the right preparation.
13. Success is about discipline and desire. You must work to pass, and want to pass.
14. Passing is easier than you think and you probably need to know less than you think. Reading larger textbooks is not a good use of time. Seeing patients is.

Practice

15. Most candidates are competent enough to pass PACES by the exam date. Invariably lack of confidence is the problem. The aim of practice is to build a natural confidence into your already adequate competence.

16. Practise your examination technique for each system at every opportunity (whenever possible in front of senior colleagues).
17. Practise the history-taking skills taught in this book with patients at every opportunity.
18. Practice your communication skills at every opportunity. As well as discussing management and ethical dilemmas with patients and colleagues, some candidates find it helpful to form discussion groups.
19. Be alert to any topical issues in the news and in general medical journals that could be examined and discussed.
20. Read widely. Reading strengthens your communication prowess.
21. Practice does not automatically make perfect. Perfect practice does!
22. When you go into the exam you should appear as though you have performed your examination of each system hundreds of times before, ideally because you have!

ON THE DAY OF PACES

Some formalities

23. PACES requires sustained energy and you must not be so tired through stress and studying as to lose momentum on the day. Meerkats get plenty of sleep each night to be alert and vigilant each day! Try not to work continuously in the run-up to PACES. Have some early nights and avoid caffeine and alcohol.
24. Dress professionally.
25. Arrive at the exam venue in good time.
26. Take your stethoscope. Other equipment should be provided but you may prefer to carry your own ophthalmoscope, tendon hammer and red pin. A case of 'James Bond' gadgets will not impress examiners.
27. Thank your patients and examiners after each case.

At the start

28. Keep in mind that there should be nothing particularly rare and therefore nothing to be particularly scared of throughout the five stations. However, even good candidates find some cases much more difficult than others. A few poor performances can still mean an overall pass and you should be determined from the start to put any difficult cases behind you and give the next one, with different examiners, your best shot.

The patients are more important than the examiners!

29. The patients are your prime concern. Thinking that the outcome of the exam is in the hands of the

examiners is not helpful. The examiners will pass or fail you on the strengths and weaknesses of your performances with patients. Focus on your patients and the exam will take care of itself.

30. Do not hurt patients on any account! This is one of the easiest ways to fail PACES.

31. Be considerate to patients. This is one of the easiest ways to pass PACES. It may seem obvious, but the notion of treating other people as we would like to be treated ourselves is a remarkably effective guiding principle in PACES, as it is in medical practice.

Examiners

32. Examiners come with the full range of personalities. The best advice is not to worry about what sort of examiners you get. Focus instead on doing what you do as well as you can do it.

33. The examiners are not trying to catch you out but want to find out what you know.

Examining patients

34. Be nice to patients! This is worth reiterating. Treat them with respect at all times. A considerate (but not obsequious) approach to patients is the single biggest determinant of success.

35. Ask each patient for permission to examine and if they are in any pain.

36. Ensure that each patient is positioned correctly before you begin.

37. Observation is a vital part of examination!

38. Don't wait for the examiners to keep telling you what to do. Do it spontaneously, using the *Recognition–Interpretation–Discussion (RID)* sequence.

39. Don't look for feedback from the examiners. You will not get it, and looking for it will unnecessarily unnerve you. A good candidate, without appearing to rush, will elicit signs and gather information considerately, swiftly and spontaneously.

40. Remember that you are 'on stage'. Let the examiners see your performance. As in a driving test, your actions should be natural but clearly visible.

41. Remember that from the examiner's perspective you do two things in each case. Firstly, you *examine* your patient. Secondly, you *present* your findings. From your perspective, you are doing much more. While examining, you are looking for signs, deciding how best to interpret these and thinking about how you are going to present your findings. A structured approach is essential. The examination schemes in this book can be performed automatically with practice, allowing you to

concentrate on recognising and interpreting signs and to use this same framework for presenting.

42. At the end of each case ensure that your patient is as comfortable as you found them.

43. Don't forget to thank them.

Examining and presenting

44. Avoid the 'running commentary' approach. Many candidates wonder if they should 'talk as they go' or 'present their findings at the end'. Some candidates believe the running commentary a way of scoring points – such that even if their final diagnosis is incorrect, they may at least have reported some correct findings. This is risky.

45. A running commentary slows you down and fragments the smooth flow of your examination. Examiners do not want to be told that you are examining the pulse to check whether it is collapsing. They want to see you doing it. Examiners are human and easily bored. They will forgive you for omitting things here and there but may be irritated if you do not 'just get on with it'. Constant stops and starts are more likely to draw the attention of examiners to mistakes. Conversely, candidates with competent examination skills who 'get on with it' tend to impress examiners, often lulling them into a sense of security – switching them from hawk to dove mode and blinding them to mistakes.

46. Talking while examining interferes with your *rapport* with a patient. You may think rapport is something you cannot develop within a few minutes but patients in PACES generally have a very good idea of how well a candidate performs, simply because what impresses patients is what impresses examiners – a natural, considerate and considered approach. Be attentive to your patient, not the examiners, while examining. Be completely absorbed by your patient. Tell them what you are doing as you are doing it, smile, look and listen for the subtle cues of cooperation, and above all show that you care. Rapport will come naturally and your examiners, at this stage, should fade into the background.

47. The 'absence' of the examiners allows you to pool all of your mental energy into the case, and should reduce anxiety.

48. The opposite applies when presenting your case. Be decisive in finishing your examination and politely turn away from your patient to give your undivided attention to the examiners. At this point, some candidates are so relieved if they have a diagnosis that they blurt it out and wait for feedback – 'Graves' disease!' Talk through the *Recognition–Interpretation* sequence instead.

49. When presenting, avoid lots of 'ums' and avoid reporting lists of negative findings.

50. Conversely, if you have elicited a sign, mention it. Candidates surprisingly often fail to mention signs they have clearly elicited. Do not assume the examiners know that you have elicited a sign.

51. Never make up signs to conform to an anticipated diagnosis. It is a sure way to fail.

52. If you know the diagnosis, state it and then give the relevant supporting findings.

53. If you do not know the diagnosis, describe what you found.

54. The key to impressing examiners is in ever striving 'to go further'. Examiners prefer candidates who spontaneously present their findings and thoughts.

55. Candidates who lack confidence often look back at their patient when presenting or asked questions as if the findings or answers will magically appear. Try to avoid this.

56. Avoid uncomfortable silences (where no marks can be awarded) by saying something intelligent. For example, if you find a mass in the left upper quadrant and are not sure if it is a spleen, you could describe findings you might expect in support of it being a spleen and findings you might expect in support of it being a kidney. You could also suggest an ultrasound scan to resolve the uncertainty.

57. The key is to try to keep talking, and saying sensible things.

When the diagnosis is not clear

58. Don't always expect a full house of signs. Patients are not from textbooks and examiners frequently disagree about signs before the exam starts. Try to keep calm. Simply blurting out a diagnosis about which you are unsure is hazardous. Remember that describing your findings, even if your diagnosis is incorrect, will allow points to be awarded.

59. There will always be cases where the diagnosis is not clear. Report your findings, telling the examiners which other signs you might have expected to find in support of the important differential diagnoses and what else you could do to resolve the uncertainty. Examiners seldom fail candidates who can demonstrate logical approaches to dilemmas. What often happens is that candidates fail themselves by 'going blank' when they are uncertain.

60. *PACES for the MRCP* has tried to strike a balance between structure and flexibility. It provides a framework for diseases likely to be encountered in PACES, but every patient is different. The same disease is exhibited in different ways in different patients and its impact is individually determined.

You should tailor your knowledge to specific patients. *PACES for the MRCP* is not a substitute for seeing as many patients as possible on the wards, and *Recognition–Interpretation–Discussion* is not something to which you need always adhere. It is simply a map to guide you through cases and bring you back on course if things go wrong.

61. Remember that 'common things are common'. You will have seen most things before.

62. Remember that double pathology can occur.

63. Diagnoses can be difficult. Many candidates struggle especially with neurology and heart valve cases. In cases where you are unsure:
    (i) Describe what you found. Be honest. Never make up signs.
    (ii) Tell the examiner two or three differential diagnoses.
    (iii) Describe what else you might have expected to find in support of these.
    (iv) State some things you could do to help resolve the issue, e.g. dynamic auscultation, arrange echocardiogram.

64. Before this point, many candidates have failed themselves, believing the signs too confusing and their diagnosis to be wrong. Practice often falls far short of theory.

History-taking skills

65. Use the history-taking skills described on pages 116–19.

Communication skills

66. Awareness of the history-taking and communication skills described in this book allows you to further improve your history-taking and communication skills.

67. Watch good communicators at work. See how they handle situations.

68. Try to bring discussion with examiners to life. Add sparkle by appearing enthusiastic and interested in the topic for discussion.

69. Watching politicians and debate programmes on television is a way of seeing negotiation at work. You do not have to like the politicians or agree with their arguments but take an interest in how they communicate. They are usually effective speakers.

70. Remember that we are all more similar to each other than we are different. We share the same molecular ingredients, separated only by a twist of the genetic kaleidoscope! It is never hard to imagine ourselves in other people's shoes. If all the lessons you have learnt seem hard to remember, then one guiding principle should ensure that you never stray

from the right ballpark – that of asking yourself what you would want if you were in your patient's situation.

Answering examiners' questions

71. Listen to the question!
72. Answer the question asked!
73. Try not to repeat the question asked!
74. Take a moment or two before answering it.
75. Look at the examiner and not at the floor. Eye contact is very important.
76. Try to appear confident, yet reflective, giving a well-structured answer. Your examiners will be as impressed by your communication skills as your knowledge.
77. Speak clearly and succinctly. Try to avoid speaking too quickly, and rambling.
78. Some candidates speak very quietly. It is unusual for candidates to speak very loudly. Unless you are one of the latter, it may help to speak up slightly, more *authoritatively*.
79. Do not think of the examiners as examiners. This is easier said than done. Try to think of the examiners as colleagues with whom you are discussing interesting ward cases. Some candidates find it helpful to imagine themselves on a ward round.
80. Curiosity keeps us alert. Let your enthusiasm, curiosity and interest shine through.
81. Difficult questions often reflect a good performance. Examiners will challenge and probe and sometimes make you feel uncomfortable or inadequate.
82. Be confident, if you think you are right, but never argue!
83. Be confident, not arrogant.
84. Avoid casual phrases and abbreviations.
85. Avoid emotive words like 'tumour' in front of patients.
86. Do not be afraid to retract statements you feel are wrong.
87. If you do not know the answer to a question, be honest in your ignorance.
88. Above all, avoid saying anything that would pose a danger to patients.
89. Remember that examiners' questions are often not predetermined but built around what you tell them – 'Would you like to explain that?' You have some opportunity to take control of the areas to be discussed.

Answering examiners' questions at the communication skills and ethics station

90. Don't be too dogmatic. It can be dangerous to go down one route when discussing ethical dilemmas.

It is wiser to state the broad range of issues an ethical dilemma creates, and that there are often numerous viewpoints to consider.

91. Remember that you are not expected to have all the answers. Examiners may be impressed by a mature attitude of self-awareness and a need to discuss an issue further with colleagues, a medical defence organisation and so on. Willingness to communicate with colleagues is considered a strength.
92. While there is often no right or wrong answer, you can state what you think is the best course of action. Examiners may challenge you but it does not mean that your argument is flawed. Provided you feel that your argument is 'safe', run with your convictions. The examiners are usually checking for consistency of your argument, ensuring that it is genuinely your belief, and that you can justify it.
93. Sometimes examiners' questions will be hard! They may be searching, probing and uncomfortable. Again, this does not necessarily mean that you are doing anything wrong. It may mean that you are performing well.
94. Try to be 'patient centred' in your responses.

When you think things are going badly

95. Do not expect feedback from your examiners. They do not give it. This said, a confident, respectful and competent candidate with a friendly but not overly familiar manner is someone examiners warm to immediately.
96. Difficult cases may be genuinely difficult to all candidates (and to examiners!).
97. Difficult questions often reflect a good performance!
98. Examiners may play on your nerves and ask 'Are you sure?' in response to your answers. Often, they are simply testing your confidence and your answer is correct.
99. Each station and case is marked separately. Try not to lose hope if you feel you have performed badly in a particular case. Examiners allow numerous mistakes (provided these would not have overtly dangerous clinical consequences) and a poor performance does not necessarily result in overall failure.

AFTER PACES

100. Most candidates who pass do so despite a few weak performances. Many candidates are convinced that they have failed until they receive the 'Pass' envelope from the College. That is the time to put PACES behind you, watch a movie and relax.

Index

Page numbers in *italics* refer to figures and those in **bold** refer to tables and boxes

AAI pacing, 368
abbreviated mental test score (AMTS),
    305, **305**
    advance directives, 562–563
ABCD scores, 196, **196**
abdominal mass(es), 87, **88**
    palpation, 64–65
abdominal pain
    causes, **138**
    history taking, 136–139
        approach, 137–138
'abdominal' phenotype, 144
abdominal system, 62–111
    ascites, 65, 73–74
    auscultation, 65
    inspection, 62
    palpation, 62–65, **65**
    percussion, 65
    regions, *63*
    scars, *63*
    veins, *63*
    see also specific conditions; specific
        organs
abducens nerve (VI)
    eye movement, 383–384
    lesions, 408, *408*
abductor pollicis brevis (APB) wasting,
    459
abscess(es)
    amoebic, 85
    lung, 23–24
    pyogenic, 85
absolute risk (AR), 499–500
absolute risk reduction (ARR), 500
accessory nerve (XI) examination, 386, *387*
Access to Health Records Act, 575
accommodation reflex, **383**
ACE inhibitors *see* angiotensin-converting
    enzyme (ACE) inhibitors
acetylcholine receptors (AChR),
    myasthenia gravis, 473
acetylcholinesterase inhibitors, 313
achalasia, 130
acid–base balance
    disturbances, 257, **257**
    regulation, 257
acne vulgaris, 616–617
    treatment, 617

acromegaly, *703*, 703–705
    complications, **704**
    face, 703
    hands, 704
    investigations, **704**
    treatment, 704–705
activated partial thromboplastin time
    (APTT), 272
activated protein C, 276
    deficiency, **277**
acute coronary syndrome (ACS), 153
    diabetes, 159
    differential diagnosis, 156
    history taking, 155–161
        approach, 156
    management, *157*, 157–158
    percutaneous coronary intervention, 158
    risk stratification systems, 158
    secondary prevention, 161, **161**
    temporary pacing, 161
acute flaccid paralysis, **470**
acute inflammatory demyelinating
        polyradiculoneuropathy (AIDP),
        470, **471**
acute intermittent porphyria (AIP), **613**
acute motor and sensory axonal
        neuropathy (AMSAN), 470, **471**
acute motor axonal neuropathy (AMAN),
        470, **471**
acute myeloid leukaemia (AML)
    FAB classification, **97**
    treatment, 98
acute promyelocytic leukaemia (APML),
        97
acute renal failure (ARF), **230**
    blood tests, **229**
    chronic kidney disease *vs.*, 236
    fluid status, 228–229, **229**
    history taking, 228–233
        approach, 228–229
    investigations, 229–230
    metabolic status, 229
    pre-renal *vs.* oliguric, 230, **231**
    renovascular disease, **230**
    uraemic symptoms, 228, **228**
acute sensory neuropathy, **471**
acute transverse myelopathy, **445**
acute tubular injury (ATI), 230

acute tubular necrosis (ATN), 230
Addison's disease, 707, 709–711
    hyperpigmentation, *709*
adenosine, SVT treatment, 168
adenosine agonists, 173
adhesion molecules, atherosclerosis, 153
adhesive capsulitis, **642**
adrenal gland hormones, 710
adrenocorticotrophic hormone (ACTH),
        707
    deficiency, **700**
    tumour-produced, **250**
adult respiratory distress syndrome
        (ARDS), 39
advanced glycation end products (AGEP),
        313
advance directives/decisions, 561–563,
        562
aegophony, 12
afferent pupillary defect (APD), **384**
ageing/age-related changes
    disequilibrium, **292**
    miosis, 414
age-related macular degeneration (AMD),
        686–688, *687*
    cataracts and, 688
    pathophysiology, 687–688
    treatment, 688
agglutinins, cold, 324
agnosia(s), **389**, 432–435, **433**
    definition, 432
AIDS-related cancer, 289
AIDS-related dementia, 288
akinetic-rigid syndromes, **393**
alcoholic liver disease, 74–75
alcohol misuse, 75
aldosterone
    Conn's syndrome, 184
    deficiency, renal tubular acidosis, 259
    potassium regulation, **232**
    terminal distal tubule, 259
aldosterone antagonists
    acute coronary syndrome, **161**
    heart failure, **164**
alendronate, 210
alkaline phosphatase, Paget's disease, 668
allergic bronchopulmonary aspergillosis
        (ABPA), **41**

allergic contact dermatitis (ACD), **606**
allergy, 324
allografts, 367
allostasis, 151
alopecia, **618**
alopecia areata, 618
α1-antitrypsin deficiency, 17
α-glucosidase inhibitors, **224**
alpha blockers, hypertension, **186**
Alport's syndrome, 244
Alzheimer's dementia (AD), 309, 311
  vascular dementia *vs.*, 311
American College of Cardiology/American
    Heart Association/European
    Society of Cardiology (ACC/AHA/
    ESC) stroke guidelines, 174
amiodarone, 696
amlodipine, 186
amoebic abscess, 85
amyloidosis, 283, **283**
anaemia, 260–264, **262**
  chronic kidney disease, 237
  definition, 261
  history taking, 260–264
    approach, 260–261
  inherited, 265–266
  rheumatoid arthritis, 650
  signs, 261
  symptoms, 260
  see also specific types
anaemia of chronic disease, 261, **262**
anaesthesia
  patient fitness, 593–595
  risk factors, 594
analgesia, diabetic neuropathy, 467
anaphylaxis, **324**
anergy, 325
angina, 153
  aortic stenosis, 360
  chronic stable, treatment, **155**
  classification, **152**
  history taking, 151–155
    approach, 151–152
  risk factors, 152
  'self-management' strategies, 155
  stable, 154
  treatment
    non-direct coronary intervention, 155
    non-pharmacological, 155
  unstable, 154
  see also chest pain
angiofibromata, *628*
angiography *see specific types*
angioid streaks, 688, *688*
angioplasty, thrombolysis *vs.*, 159
angiotensin-converting enzyme (ACE)
    inhibitors
  acute coronary syndrome, **161**
  angiotensin II receptor blockers and,
    165
  cardiovascular disease, 150, **150**
  chronic kidney disease, 237
  heart failure, **164**, 378
  hypertension, 185–186, **186**

non-diabetic nephropathy, 236–237
older people, 493
renal artery stenosis, 237, *237*
stroke, 429–430
angiotensin II receptor blockers (ARBs),
    165
  angiotensin-converting enzyme
    inhibitors and, 165
  chronic kidney disease, 237
  heart failure, **164**
  hypertension, **186**
  non-diabetic nephropathy, 236–237
  renal artery stenosis, 237
anion exchange resins, **181**
ankle jerks, absent, 447–449
  causes, **461**
  extensor plantar *vs.*, **448**
ankle movement examination, 402, **645**
ankylosing spondylitis, *652*, 652–655,
    653
  diagnostic criteria, **653**
  musculoskeletal features, **655**
annular skin lesions, **600**
anosagnosia, 434
anterior cerebral artery, *423*
anterior circulation stroke syndromes,
    421–431
anterior communicating artery, *423*
anterior fossae, *423*
anterior interosseous nerve lesion, 455
anterior mediastinal mass, 30
antiarrhythmic drugs
  atrial fibrillation, 172
  ventricular arrhythmia, 369
  ventricular tachycardia, 170
antibiotics, withholding treatment,
    550–552
anticholinesterase, myasthenia gravis, 474,
    474
anticoagulation
  acute coronary syndrome, **161**
  atrial fibrillation, 172, 175
  heart failure, **164**
  natural mechanisms, 271
  paroxysmal atrial fibrillation, 175
  reversal, 275
  transient ischaemic attack, recurrent,
    195
anti-cyclic citrullinated peptide (anti-CPP),
    650
anticytoplasmic antineutrophil
    cytoplasmic antibodies (cANCA),
    246
antidiuretic hormone (ADH), 259
  deficiency, **700**
  hyponatraemia, **255**
  tumours, **250**
anti-epileptic drugs, 303–304
  pregnancy, **304**
  side effects, **304**
antigens, 318, *318*
anti-glomerular basement membrane (anti-
    GBM) disease, 247
anti-hyperglycaemic agents, 223

antihypertensive therapy, 185–187
  'beyond blood pressure' benefits,
    185–186
  stroke, 429
antimicrobial therapy
  chronic obstructive pulmonary disease,
    22
  diarrhoea, 141
  pneumonia, 22–23
antineutrophil cytoplasmic antibodies
    (ANCA), 246
antineutrophil cytoplasmic antibody
    (ANCA)-associated systemic
    vasculitis (AASV), 244–247, **245**
  diagnosis, 246–247
  differential diagnosis, 248
  symptoms, 244–245
  treatment, 247, *247*
antinuclear antibodies (ANAs), 635
anti-obesity drugs, 147–148
antiperinuclear antineutrophil cytoplasmic
    antibodies (pANCA), 246
antiphospholipid syndrome (APS), 278
  systemic lupus erythematosus and, 658
  treatment, 658
antiplatelet therapy, 158
  acute coronary syndrome, **161**
  stroke, 428–429
antiresorptive agents, osteoporosis, 208
antiretroviral treatment, 289
anti-T-cell antibodies, renal transplants,
    109
antithrombin, 271, 275
antithrombotic therapy, **149**, 275–276
  atrial fibrillation, stroke prevention,
    173–174, **174**
antithyroid drugs, 696, **696**
anti-tumour necrosis factor, ankylosing
    spondylitis, 655
antiviral drugs, hepatitis B virus, 78
aortic coarctation, 373–375
aortic regurgitation, 361–363
  causes, 362
  investigations, 363
  pathophysiology, **363**
  signs, 362, *362*
  surgical indications, 363
aortic root dilation, 669
aortic sclerosis, 360
aortic stenosis, 359–361
  ACE inhibitor contraindications,
    164–165
  angina, 360
  aortic sclerosis *vs.*, 360
  calcific, 360, 361
  causes, 360
  differential diagnosis, 359–360
  hypertrophic cardiomyopathy *vs.*, **376**
  investigations, 361
  left ventricular outflow obstruction, 360
  pathophysiology, **360**
  progression rate, 361
  severity, **360**
  signs, *359*

surgery, 361
treatment, 361
aortic valve
abnormalities, **365**
replacement, 368
apex beat
abnormalities, **347**
palpation, 347, *350*
aphthous ulceration, Crohn's disease, **88**
aplastic anaemia, 101, 264
apolipoprotein(s), 176
apolipoprotein AI (Apo AI), 176
apolipoprotein B48 (Apo B48), 176
apolipoprotein B100 (Apo B100), 176
apolipoprotein CII (Apo CII), 176
apolipoprotein CIII (Apo CIII), 176
apolipoprotein E (Apo E), 176, 313
Alzheimer's dementia, 311
apparent mineralocorticoid excess (AME), **184**
apraxia(s), **389**, 434, **435**
apraxic gait, **405**, **435**
Argyll Robertson pupils (ARPs), 414, *414*
arm examination, 638–640
cardiovascular system inspection, 346
arrhythmias
syncope and, *297*
ventricular, 369
arterial blood gases (ABG), COPD, **19**
arterial pulse
abnormalities, **349**
hypertrophic cardiomyopathy, 375–376
palpation, 347
arteriovenous fistula (AVF), 239
artificial hydration and nutrition (AHN), 554
withholding/withdrawing treatment, 550–555
asbestos, lung effects, **44**, **45**
asbestosis, 43, **45**
compensation, **597**
ascites, 65, 73–74, **74**
chronic liver disease, 69
decompensation, 73
management, 74
serum:ascites albumin gradient, 74
aspiration pneumonia, myasthenia gravis, 472
aspiration risks
dysphagia, 136
gastronomy feeding, 558
aspirin, 158
atrial fibrillation, 174
heart failure, **164**
hypertension, 187
older people, 493
platelet effects, 270
STEMI management, 159
stroke
acute, 428–429
secondary prevention, 430
transient ischaemic attack, 195
Assisted Dying for the Terminally Ill Bill, 560

asteatotic dermatitis (eczema craquelé), **607**
asthma
acute, 127
chronic
control difficulties, 128
management, 126
definition, 126
diagnosis, 126
features, **127**
history taking, 125–126
approach, 125
pathophysiology, 126
patient discharge criteria, **128**
precipitating factors, 125
pregnancy, 127
red flag seeking, 125–126
referral indications, **127**
symptoms, 125
treatment, 127, **127**
asymmetrical septal hypertrophy (ASH), *376*
ataxia
cerebellar disease, *443*
Friedreich's, 447–449, **448**
atherosclerosis, 152–153
infection, 153
inflammation, 152, 153
lesions
evolution, 152–153
types, 153
plaque rupture, 153
posterior circulation strokes, **437**
statin therapy, 180
atopic eczema, **606**
treatment, 605
atopy, 126
atorvastatin, 148
atrial fibrillation (AF), **171**
classification, **172**
complications, **171**
history taking, 170–175
approach, 170–171
management, 172–175
mechanism, 171–172
multiple sources hypothesis, 172
single focus hypothesis, 171–172
non-pharmacological therapies, 175
rate control, 173, **173**
recurrence, 172
rhythm control, **173**
stroke, 425
sustained, 172
symptoms, **171**
tachycardia, 172
ventricular ectopic beats *vs.*, 171
ventricular rate, 173
see also specific types
atrial flutter, 175
atrial septal defect (ASD), 373–375
atrioventricular node (AVN), Wolff–
Parkinson–White syndrome, 168
atrioventricular re-entrant tachycardias
(AVRTs), 168

atrophy, **600**
audiograms, sensorineural hearing loss, 418
Auer rods, 97
aura, **302**
Auspitz sign, 602, 603
autoantibodies
systemic lupus erythematosus, 657
tests, **637**
type 1 diabetes mellitus, 217
autografts, 367
autoimmune cytopenias, 264
autoimmune haemolytic anaemia (AIHA), 263
treatment, 263–264
types, 263
autoimmune hepatitis (AIH), 79–81
classification, **80**
decompensation, 80
diagnostic criteria, **79**
spider naevi, *79*
symptoms, 80
treatment, 80–81
autoimmune polyglandular syndromes, 710
autoimmune skin disease, 617–618, **618**
autoimmune tests
joints examination, 635, **637**
thyrotoxicosis, 696
autoimmunity, 324–325
anergy, 325
T-cell receptors, 325
autopsy requests, 569–571
'a' wave, **346**
abnormalities, **348**
axillary freckling, *625*
axillary nerve lesions, 459
azathioprine, renal transplants, **109**

background diabetic retinopathy (BDR), 675, **675**
back pain
history taking, 205–210
approach, 205–206
'red flags', 205
spondyloarthropathies, **652**
bacteraemia
infective endocarditis, 371
Staphylococcus, 331
bacterial endocarditis, 372
bacterial meningitis, 191
bad news, breaking *see* breaking bad news
balance tests, falls, 294
'barrel chest', COPD, *16*
Barrett's oesophagus, 130
Bartter's syndrome, 259
basement membrane nephropathy, 244
battery
advanced directives, 562
definition, 532
risks, 532
BCG immunisation, 36
behaviour, threatening, **508**
Behçet's disease, 247–248

Bell's palsy, 419
  treatment, 419–420
  viral causes, 419
beneficence, **487**
benign paroxysmal positional vertigo, **293**
beta blockers
  acute coronary syndrome, **161**
  aortic root dilation, 669
  atrial fibrillation, 173
  heart failure, **164**, 165, 378
  hypertension, **186**
  hyperthyroidism, 696–697
  older people, 493
beta cell failure, type 2 diabetes mellitus,
  222
bias, 586
bilateral hilar lymphadenopathy (BHL),
  44, 46, **47**
bile acid sequestrants, **181**
bileaflet valves, 367
biliary sepsis, 139
bilirubin
  metabolism, 71–72
  net absorption, 191
  in urine, 72
Binet classification, chronic lymphocytic
  leukaemia, 102
biopsy
  myositis, 477
  nerve, 467
bisphosphonates, **209**
biventricular pacing, heart failure, 166
bladder
  capacity, 316
  control, incontinence, **315**
  neurological inputs, 316
Blalock–Taussig shunting, 375
Blatchford score, **134**
blindsight, 433
blind spot, **675**
blistering disorders, 608–612
  differential diagnoses, **611**
  see also specific disorders
blood pressure
  ambulatory monitoring, 185
  definitions, **185**
  lowering
    acute coronary syndrome, **161**
    cardiovascular disease reduction, **149**
    type 2 diabetes mellitus, 225
  palpation, 347
  targets
    cardiovascular disease, 148, **148**
    type 2 diabetes mellitus, 225–226
blood transfusion, vitamin B12 deficiency,
  263
B lymphocytes, 321
body mass index (BMI), **145**
bone
  formation, 207
    stimulation, osteoporosis, 209
  Paget's disease, 667
  resorption, 206–207
  types, 206

bone densitometry, **206**
bone marrow
  anaemia, **262**
  chronic myeloid leukaemia, 95
  examination, 96–97
  failure, 101
bone marrow transplants (BMT), 98, 282
bone mineral density (BMD)
  measurement, 208
  osteoporosis, 207
bone remodelling, 206–207
  abnormalities, **207**
  formation, 207
  fractures, 208
  regulation, 207
Boutonnière deformity, 646, *646*
bowel habit, altered, 139–143
  history taking, 139–140
    approach, 140
    large bowel causes, 140
    presentation, 140
    symptom exploration, 140
  see also diarrhoea
bradycardia, 169
  acute haemorrhage, 133
bradykinesia, **438**
brain
  middle temporal area, 433
  plasticity, 430
  V4 area, 433, 434
  visual external world perception, 433
  see also specific regions
brain death, 567, **567**
brain imaging, transient ischaemic attack,
  194
brainstem
  function assessment, 566
  lesions, 381, **382**, 408
  multiple sclerosis, **199**
brainstem death, 565–567
  persistent vegetative state *vs.*, 565
brainstem strokes, 419
brainstem syndromes, *436*, **567**
branch occlusion, 685
breaking bad news, 514–523
  cancer
    incurable, 516–518
    patient not fit for active treatment,
      518–520
    potentially curable, 514–516
  chronic disease, 520–522
  mistakes, **516**
  to relatives, 522–523
breathlessness, 121–125
  exertional, 356
  functional scale, **16**
  history taking, 121–125
    approach, 121–122
    symptoms, 121
    trigger factors, 121
breath sounds, 13–14
British Hypertension Society (BHS)
  hypertension definition, 184
  intervention thresholds, **185**

  treatment guidelines, 187
  treatment targets, 185
Broca's area, 389
bronchial breath sounds, **13**
bronchial obstruction, 30
bronchiectasis, 30–32
bronchiolitis obliterans organising
    pneumonia (BOOP), **40**
bronchiolitis obliterans syndrome, 61
bronchitis
  acute, 22
  chronic, 17
bronchoalveolar lavage, 39
bronchodilators, COPD, **18**
Brown–Séquard syndrome, 443–446, *444*
Brugada syndrome, 169
bruising see purpura
buccal mucosa, lichen planus, *608*
Budd–Chiari syndrome (hepatic vein
    thrombosis), 69
bulbar function, 385–386
bulbar palsy, 420–421, **421**
  investigations, 421
  management, 421
  pseudobulbar palsy *vs.*, **390**
bulla, **600**
bullous pemphigoid, 608–609

C1 (esterase) inhibitor deficiency, 324
C8 root lesions, 459
cachexia, COPD, *16*
café-au-lait spots, *625*, 626–627
caged-ball valves, 367
CAGE questions, **583**
calcific aortic stenosis, 360, 361
calcitonin, 209
calcium
  hyperkalaemia, 233
  hypomagnesaemia, 251
  serum regulation, 250
  supplementation, osteoporosis, 210
calcium channel blockers
  atrial fibrillation, 173
  hypertension, **186**
California scores, 196
caloric intake, cardiovascular disease,
    147
cancer
  AIDS-related, 289
  breaking bad news see breaking bad
    news
  C-reactive protein, 334
  patient support
    active treatment impossibilities, 520
    incurable disease, 517
    potentially curable disease, 515–516
  see also malignancy; *individual cancers*
candidiasis, oesophageal, 288
cannon wave, **348**
capacity, 520, 533–542, **534**
  consent and, 533–537
  legal necessity, 534–535
  resuscitation-status, **545**
  self-harm, 541

withholding/withdrawing treatment, **552**, 554
Capgrass syndrome, 433
Caplan's syndrome, 44
caput medusa, 62, *63*
carbimazole, 696–697
carbon monoxide (CO), 124–125
carbon monoxide transfer factor (TLCO), 124–125
carcinoid syndrome, 93–94
  complications, 93
  decompensation, 93
  diagnosis, 93
  liver metastases, 93
  management, 94
carcinoid tumours, 93
cardiac catheterisation, mitral stenosis, 357
cardiac resynchronisation therapy (CRT), 370
cardiac tamponade, constrictive pericarditis *vs.*, **379**
cardiac troponin levels, 159
cardiac valves *see* heart valves
cardiomyopathy
  definition, 377
  dilated, 369, 378
  hypertrophic *see* hypertrophic (obstructive) cardiomyopathy
  implantable cardioverter–defibrillators, 369, **369**
  restrictive, 378
cardiopulmonary resuscitation (CPR), 544–546
  patient discussion, 544
  see also resuscitation-status
cardiorenal failure, 231
cardiovascular disease (CVD)
  cholesterol, 179
  chronic kidney disease and, 238
  dementia, 313
  history taking, 144–151
    approach, 144–145
  lifestyle interventions, 147–148
  lipid-lowering therapy, 179–180
  premature, 145–146
  prevention, 144–151
    drug strategies, **149**
    folate, 278
    high-risk patients, **146**
    Joint British Societies' guidelines, 145, **147**
  risk assessment, 145–149
    on-treatment, 146
    risk factors, **146**
    stroke endpoint, 146
    total risk *vs.* single risk factors, 146–147
  unaccustomed exercise, 148
cardiovascular system, 346–379
  anaesthesia effects, 594–595
  auscultation, 349–355
    sites, 349–350, *350*
    valve abnormality prediction, 349, **349**

inspection, 346–347
palpation, 347–349
percussion, 349
see also specific conditions
cardioversion, atrial fibrillation, 172
  acute onset, 175
  recurrence predictors, 172
  sinus rhythm maintenance, 172–173
carotid artery dissection, 196, 437–438
carotid atherosclerosis, stroke, 425
carotid dopplers, transient ischaemic attack, **194**
carotid endarterectomy, stroke, 430
carotid pulse, **346**
carotid sinus hypersensitivity (CSH), 299
carotid stenosis
  endarterectomy, 195
  transient ischaemic attack, 193
  warfarin, 195
carpal tunnel syndrome, 454–455
  causes, **455**
  clinical tests, 454
  thenar wasting, 454, *454*
  treatment, 455
carvedilol, 165
case–control (retrospective) studies, 586
casts, renal disease, 241
cataracts, 690–691
  age-related macular degeneration and, 688
cauda equina, 452
  lesions, **453**
cauda equina syndrome, 452–454
  lumbar disc disease *vs.*, 452–454
cavernous sinus lesions, 408
CD4 lymphocytes, HIV infection, 286
CD8 lymphocytes, HIV infection, 286
cellulitis, *632*
central cyanosis, 15
central herniation, **567**
central pontine myelinosis (CPM), 254
central retinal artery occlusion, *684*, 684–685
  branch occlusion *vs.*, 685
central retinal vein occlusion, *683*, 683–684
central scotoma, 406
cerebellar ataxia, *443*
cerebellar disease, *392*, 442–443
  causes, 442
  conditions associated, 443
  signs, **392**
cerebellar gait, **405**
cerebellar lesions, 411
cerebellar tremor, **203**
cerebellopontine angle (CPA), 416, *417*
cerebellopontine angle syndrome, 416–418
cerebellum, multiple sclerosis, **199**
cerebral artery
  anterior, *423*
  middle, *423*
cerebral salt wasting, 254
cerebral toxoplasmosis, 288

cerebral venous sinus thrombosis (CVST), 192
cerebrospinal fluid (CSF), 191
  normal pressure hydrocephalus, 312
  oligoclonal bands, multiple sclerosis, 201
cervical myeloradiculopathy, 451–452
cervical spondylosis, 452
CETP gene, 180
CHADS$_2$ scoring system, 174
Charcot–Marie–Tooth disease, 468–469
  type 1, 468
  type 2, 469
Charles Bonnet syndrome, 312
chemokines, 321
  atherosclerosis, 153
  disease associations, **322–323**
  roles, **322–323**
chemotherapy
  lung cancer, 27
  myeloma, 282
chest
  chronic obstructive pulmonary disease, 15
  expansion assessment, *11*
  inspection, 10
  palpation, 10–11
  size, **10**
chest pain, **152**
  acute coronary syndrome, 156
  differential diagnoses, 152
  dyspepsia *vs.*, 495
  history taking, 151–155
    approach, 151–152
  risk factors, 152
  symptoms, 151–152
  see also angina
chest wall, cardiovascular system inspection, 346–347
chest X-ray
  aortic regurgitation, 363
  Fallot's tetralogy, 375
  HIV-associated tuberculosis, 286
  mitral regurgitation, 359
  mitral stenosis, 357
  pericardial disease, 379
  silicosis, 122
Childs–Pugh score, 66, **66**
cholestatic jaundice, 72–73
cholesteatoma, facial nerve palsy, 419
cholesterol
  cardiovascular disease, 179
  synthesis, 179
cholesterol absorption inhibitors, **181**
chorea, **393**
chorioretinitis, 682, *682*
choroidal haemorrhage, *687*
chronic disease
  breaking bad news, 520–522
  definition, 501
  management negotiation, 500–502
chronic fatigue syndrome, 336
chronic inflammatory demyelinating polyradiculopathy (CIDP), 467, 469

chronic kidney disease (CKD), 233–239
  acute renal failure *vs.*, 236
  anaemia, 237
  cardiovascular disease and, 238
  classification, 234, **235**
  early detection, 234
  glomerulonephritis, 241
  history taking, 234
    approach, 234
  hypertension management, 236
  lipid-lowering therapy, 238
  management, 234, **235**
  mineral disturbance correction, 238
  progression slowing strategies, **236**
chronic liver disease (CLD), 66–71
  bleeding, **69**
  differential diagnoses, 67
  hepatic failure, 67–68
  portal hypertension, 69
  severity, 66
  signs, 67
  transplantation, 70, **70**
chronic lymphocytic leukaemia (CLL),
    101–103
  staging, 102
  treatment, **103**
chronic myeloid leukaemia (CML),
    95–98
  bone marrow failure, 95
  decompensation, 95
  diagnosis, 96
  genetic abnormalities, 95
  monitoring, 96
  signs/symptoms, 95, 95
  splenomegaly, 95
  treatment, **96**
chronic obstructive pulmonary disease
    (COPD), 15–19
  acid–base disturbance, 257
  acute respiratory failure management,
    19
  α1-antitrypsin deficiency, 17
  arterial blood gases, **19**
  breathlessness, functional scale, **16**
  causes, 17
  cor pulmonale, 19, 49
  decompensation, 16
  definition, 16–17
  exacerbations, 17–19, **18**, 22
  invasive ventilation, 549
  long-term oxygen therapy, 17, **17**
  non-invasive positive pressure
    ventilation, 19, **20**
  oxygen therapy, 19
  pathogenesis, 17
  pneumothorax *vs.*, 57
  pulmonary hypertension, 17
  staging, **18**
  treatment, **18**
chronic plaque psoriasis, 600, 602
chronic renal failure *see* chronic kidney
    disease (CKD)
Churg–Strauss syndrome (CSS), **41**, 245
chylomicrons, 178

ciclosporin
  psoriasis, **603**
  renal transplants, **109**
Circle of Willis, *423*
cirrhosis, 68–69
  bleeding risk, 69
clarification, facilitating skills, 117
'claw hand', 457, *457*
clinical errors, 580
clinical governance (CG), 572–588
  critical incidents, 572–575
  definition, 573
  fitness to practise, 578–584
  randomised controlled trials,
    recruitment, 584–588
clinical investigations
  cognitive impairment, 491–492
  consent, 530–533
  older patients, 491–492
  patient explanations, 489–492, **490**
    approach, 490
    with dementia, 490–491
  see also individual tests
clinical management discussions
  complications, 494–495
  diagnosis *see* diagnosis explanations
  investigations *see* clinical investigations
  management, 494–495, **495**
  prognosis, 494–495, 523
  risk, 497–500, **500**
  treatment *see* treatment
clinical reasoning, 114
clinical stations, 6–7
  abdominal system *see* abdominal system
  cardiovascular system *see*
    cardiovascular system
  communication skills *see*
    communication skills
  criteria, **3**
  discussion, 7
  endocrine system *see* endocrine system
  eyes *see* eye(s)
  history-taking skills *see* history-taking
    skills
  instruction, 6
  interpretation, 6–7
  locomotor system *see* locomotor system
  nervous system *see* nervous system
  recognition, 6
  respiratory system *see* respiratory system
  skin *see* skin
clinical trials, 586
clopidogrel
  acute coronary syndrome, 158
  stroke, secondary prevention, 430
  transient ischaemic attack, 195
closed questions, 117
Clostridium difficile, 141
Clostridium difficile-associated diarrhoea
    (CDAD), 141–142
  control, 142
  haematobiochemical disturbances, 141
  treatment, 141–142
clubbing (fingers) *see* finger clubbing

cluster headaches, 190
coagulation, 271
  disorders, **271**
coagulation 'jigsaw', *269*, 271
coal worker's pneumoconiosis (CWP), 44,
    44
coeliac disease, **142**, 263
cognitive enhancer drugs, dementia, 313
cognitive impairment, mild, 307–314
  approach to case, 308–310
  reversible causes, 309
cogwheel rigidity, 395
cohort (prospective) study design, 586
colchicine, 664
cold agglutinins, 324
collapsing pulse, **349**
collecting duct, 259
colobomata, 681
colon, arterial supply, 138
colonoscopy, 143
colorectal cancer (CRC), 142–143
  family history, 143
  management, 143
  risks, 142, 143
  screening, 143
  symptoms, 143
coma
  measurement, 565
  persistent vegetative state *vs.*, 565
comfort feeding, 555
communicating artery, anterior, *423*
communication, 585–598
  angry patients/relatives, 506–508
  appropriate language, 118
  breaking bad news *see* breaking bad news
  capacity *see* capacity
  clinical governance *see* clinical
    governance
  clinical management *see* clinical
    management discussions
  complaints management, 575–578
  concordance, 502–504
  confidentiality *see* confidentiality
  consent *see* consent
  criteria, **4**
  cross-cultural, 505–506
  delayed discharge, 511–513
  doctor-centred, 486–487
  effective, 486
  eliciting skills, 117–118
  end-of-life issues *see* end-of-life issues
  facilitating skills, 117–118
  history taking, 116–119
  listening, 116–117
  negligence, 575–578
  in PACES, 718–719
  patient-centred, 486–487
  patient explanations *see* clinical
    management discussions
  self-discharge, 509–511
  smoking cessation, 504
  special circumstances, 505–513
  station *see* communication skills and
    ethics station

summarising, 118–119
upset/distressed relatives, 508–509
communication skills and ethics station
(Station 4), 2, **4**, 719
candidate information, 5
case settings, 5–6
documents, 5–6
examiner information, 6
patient/subject information, 5–6
community-acquired pneumonia (CAP), 23
community geriatricians, 502
complaints
formal, 507
levels, **577**
management, 575–578
procedures, 576
complement proteins, 324
compliance, 124
complications, discussion with patient,
494–495
computed tomography (CT)
colorectal cancer, 143
intestinal ischaemia, 139
normal pressure hydrocephalus, 312
parenchymal infarction, acute, 427
Parkinson's disease, 441
pleural effusion, 55
stroke, 427
sub-arachnoid haemorrhage, 190–191
computed tomography (CT) angiography,
vascular occlusion, 427
computed tomography pulmonary
angiography (CTPA), 51
concordance, 502–504
confidence interval (CI), 587
confidentiality, 524–530
breaches, **525**, 526–529
driving, 528–529, **529**
implied consent and, 530
legal points, 524–525
relatives/third parties, 529–530
confusion, acute
causes, **306**
history taking, 304–307
approach, 305, 307
risk factors, **306**
treatment, 307, **308**
problems, 307
Confusion Assessment Method (CAM), 305
delirium diagnosis, **306**
congenital acyanotic heart disease, **373**,
373–375
complications, **374**
diagnosis, **374**
congenital adrenal hyperplasia (CAH), 712
congenital erythropoietic porphyria
(CEP), **613**
conjecture, 118
Conn's syndrome, 184
consent, 530–542
capacity and, 533–537
clinical investigations, 530–533
Coroner's autopsy, 571
definition, 532

express, 530, **532**
implied, 530, **532**
informed, **532**
organ donation, 569
refusal, 537–540, **540**
third party disclosure, 530
to treatment, 530–533
valid, 532, **532**
verbal, 530
consolidation, *15*, 19–20
constipation, 142
constrictive pericarditis, 379, **379**
contact dermatitis, 605
continuing care, 513
continuous murmurs, **353**
contraceptive pill, systemic lupus
erythematosus and, 658–659
conus medullaris, 452
coordination examination, 390–392
dominance, 391
lower limbs, 402
corneal melt, 692
corneal reflex, 382
coronary angiography, **154**
high-risk lesions, 154
coronary artery bypass grafting (CABG),
154
heart failure, 166
coronary artery disease (CAD)
development predictions, 151
microvascular, 169
coronary heart disease (CHD)
risk assessment, 146
sudden cardiac death syndrome, 169
Coroner's autopsy, consent, 571
cor pulmonale, 49
COPD, 19, 49
heart failure *vs.*, 166
Kartagener's syndrome, 34
obstructive sleep apnoea–hypopnoea
syndrome, 60
cortical blindness, 407
cortical bone, 206
cortical lesions, **382**
cortical representation (body), 422, *424*
cortical vision, 434
corticobasal degeneration (CBD), 440
corticospinal tracts, 381, *381*, 393
absent ankle jerks, **448**
extensor plantars, **448**
corticosteroids
autoimmune hepatitis, 80
chronic obstructive pulmonary disease,
18
giant cell arteritis, 327, **327**
iatrogenic hypoadrenalism, 710–711
potency, **607**
pulmonary sarcoidosis, 47
renal transplants, **109**
rheumatoid arthritis, 651
cough, 121
Court Appointed Deputies, 537
Court of Protection, 537
crackles, **13**

cranial diabetes insipidus (CDI), **256**
cranial nerves, 380–381
anatomy, *381*
coordination, swallowing, 386
examination, 380–387
lesions, 381, 382
supranuclear control, **425**
see also specific nerves
cranial nerve syndromes, **382**
C-reactive protein (CRP), 320
cancer, 334
measurement, **321**
creams, ointments *vs.*, 605
creatine phosphokinase monitoring, statin
therapy, 180
creatinine, glomerular filtration rate *vs.*,
234–236
crescendo transient ischaemic attacks, 194
Creutzfeld–Jakob disease (CJD), 311–312
new variant, 312
sporadic, 312
critical appraisal guidelines, 586
critical incidents, 572–575
definition, 573–574
criticism, 507, 512
Crohn's disease (CD), 87–90
clinical subtypes, **89**
epidemiology, 88–89
extra-intestinal associations, 88
immunological basis, 89
perioral aphthous ulceration, **88**
surgery, 90
therapy, 90
cross-cultural communication, 505–506
cross-sectional (descriptive) study design,
586
cryoglobulins, 324
cryptococcal meningitis, 288
Cryptococcus neoformans, meningitis, 288
cryptogenic organising pneumonia (COP),
40
Cryptosporidium parvum, 288
crystal arthropathy, 662–664, **664**
CT scanning *see* computed tomography
(CT)
cue recognition, 118
Cushing's syndrome, 705–707
causes, 705, **707**
diagnosis, **708**
investigations, **708**
signs, *475*, 705, **705**, *706*
treatment, 705–707
cutaneous porphyria, 610
cyanosis, **15**
cyanotic heart disease, 375
cyclooxygenase-2 (COX-2) inhibitors, 155
cyclophosphamide, 282
cystic fibrosis (CF), 32–34
diagnosis, 33
gene therapy, 33–34
pathophysiology, 33
severity/complications, 32–33
symptoms, **32**
treatments, **33**

cystic fibrosis transmembrane regulator (CFTR) gene, 33
cystinuria, 258
cysts, renal, 106
cytokines, 319

dactylitis, **655**
DaT scan, Parkinson's disease, 204, 441
DDD dual chamber pacing, 368
D-dimer testing
    pulmonary embolism, 51, **52**
    venous thromboembolism, 275, **275**
death, legal definition, 567
decision making
    ethical, 487
    incapacitated patients, **535**
deep vein thrombosis (DVT)
    history taking, 273–276
        approach, 274
    ideas, concerns and expectations, 115
    symptoms, 274
    treatment, 429
    Wells scoring system, **274**
dehydration, 298
    osmolality and, 253
delayed discharge, 511–513
delayed transfer of care (DTOC), 513
deliberate self-harm, 540–542
    capacity, 541
delirium
    diagnosis, 305, **306**
    pathophysiology, 307
demargination, 97
dementia, 309
    AIDS-related, 288
    behavioural problems, **311**
    cardiovascular disease, 313
    cognitive enhancer drugs, 313
    definition, **309**
    driving, 313
    history taking, 307–314
        approach, 308–310
    investigation explanations, 490–491
    neuroimaging, 311
    prevention, 312–313
    see also individual types
dementia with Lewy bodies (DLB), 309, **309**, 311
    Parkinsonian features, **309**
demyelinating optic neuritis, 681
De Quervain's tenosynovitis, 635
dermatitis, 605–607
    types, **606**
    see also individual types
dermatomes, 395
dermatomyositis, 615, 615, **618**
    malignancy screening, 477
descriptive (cross-sectional) study design, 586
desquamative interstitial pneumonia (DIP), 40
dexamethasone suppression tests, Cushing's syndrome, **708**
dextrose, hyperkalaemia, 233

diabetes insipidus, **256**
diabetes mellitus
    acute coronary syndrome risks, 159
    definition, 148
    diagnosis, **148**
    eye complication, 678
    glycaemic monitoring, 217
    peripheral neuropathy, 462
    skin manifestations, 623
    type 1 see type 1 diabetes mellitus
    type 2 see type 2 diabetes mellitus
    types, **216**
diabetic amyotrophy, 461
diabetic cheiropathy, 457
diabetic ketoacidosis (DKA), 217, **217**
diabetic maculopathy, 676
diabetic nephropathy, 226–227, **242**
    proteinuria quantification, **226**
diabetic neuropathy, 227, **227**, 462
    treatment, 467
diabetic retinopathy (DR), 675–678
    management, 678
    non-proliferative, 675, **676**
    preproliferative, **675**
    proliferative, 675
    screening, 677–678
diagnosis explanations, 488–489
    uncertainty, 496–497
dialysis, 238–239
    fluid, 239
diarrhoea
    acute bloody, 141
    acute watery, 140–141
    antimicrobial treatment, 141
    chronic bloody, 141
    chronic watery, 141
    Clostridium difficile see Clostridium difficile-associated diarrhoea (CDAD)
    HIV-associated, 288
    inflammatory bowel disease, 140
    norovirus, 141
    Shiga-toxin-producing E. coli, 141
    small bowel causes, **141**
    type determination, 140
diastolic heart failure, 166, **166**
diastolic murmurs, **353**
diffuse cutaneous systemic sclerosis (DcSSc), 660–661
diffuse parenchymal lung disease (DPLD), 37–41
    causes, 41
    classification, **38**
    diagnosis, 39
    differential diagnosis, **39**
    symptoms, **37**
dignity, 487
digoxin
    atrial fibrillation, 173
    heart failure, **164**
    Wolff–Parkinson–White syndrome, 168
1,25-dihydroxyvitamin D (1,25(OH)$_2$D), 250

diplopia
    false images, 409
    ophthalmoplegia, 409
dipyridamole, stroke, 429
direct thrombin inhibitors (DTIs), 53, 276
disability, 596
discharge
    delayed, 511–513
    early supported, 512
    planning, 512
    self, 509–511
discharge assessment teams (DATs), 512–513
discoid lesions, **600**
discoid lupus erythematosus (DLE), 614, 614
discoid/nummular dermatitis, **606**
disc prolapse, 452
disease-modifying antirheumatic drugs (DMARDs), 651
dissection
    stroke, 193
    transient ischaemic attack, 193
disseminated intravascular coagulation (DIC), 270
distal interphalangeal (DIP) joints, **456**
distal symmetrical polyneuropathy, 465
DMPK gene, 481
doctor-centred communication, 486–487
doctrine of double effect, palliative care, 560
domiciliary visits, 502
'do not attempt resuscitation' (DNAR), **546**
    challenges, 545
    guidelines, 544
    Human Rights Act, 544
    incapacitated adults, **548**
    policies, 544
dopamine agonists, restless leg syndrome, 204
dorsal columns, 381, 382
    absent ankle jerks, **448**
    extensor plantars, **448**
dorsal interosseus muscle wasting, **459**
double lumen catheters, 239
Driver and Vehicle Licensing Agency (DVLA)
    confidentiality, 528–529, **529**
    informing, **596**
driving
    dementia, 313
    diabetes mellitus, 595–596
    epilepsy, 528
    patient fitness, 595–596
    post-seizures, 596
    syncope, 300
    visual requirements, 596
drug-eluting stents (DES), 158–159
drug-induced conditions
    large pupils, 414
    movement disorders, **393**
    rash, 605
drusen, 686–688, 687
dual antiplatelet therapy (DAPT), 159

dual energy X-ray absorption (DEXA)
  bone mineral density measurement, 208
  osteoporosis prevention, 210
Dubin–Johnson syndrome, 72
Duchenne muscular dystrophy, 477
Duke criteria, infective endocarditis, **372**
duodenal ulcers, 131, **132**
Dupuytren's contractions, *75*
dynamic volumes, pulmonary function
        testing, 122–123
dysaesthesia, diabetic neuropathy and, 467
dysarthria, 390, *391*, 431
  bulbar palsy, 420
  examination, 390
  types, 390
dyskinesia, **393**
dyslipidaemia
  classification, **177**
  diabetic, 226
  history taking, 175–182
    approach, 176
  mixed, 180
dyspepsia, 129
  cardiac chest pain *vs.*, 495
  causes, **129**
  differential diagnosis, 129
  endoscopy, 132
  functional, **129**
  Helicobacter pylori, 131
  history taking, 129–133
    approach, 129–130
dysphagia, 133–136
  alarm features, 134
  aspiration risks, 136
  causes, **135**
  history taking, 133–136
    approach, 134–135
  management, **136**
  oesophageal, **135**, *136*
  pharyngeal, **135**, *136*
  swallowing assessment, 135
dysphasia, 431
  examination, 389–390
  expressive, **389**
  receptive, **389**
  types, 389
dysphonia, 390
dysplastic naevus syndrome, 629
dyspnoea *see* breathlessness
dystonia, 391–392
  acute, **393**
  types, **393**

early supported discharge, 512
Ebstein's anomaly, 364
echocardiography
  aortic stenosis, 361
  hypertrophic cardiomyopathy, 377
  mitral stenosis, 357
  pericarditis, 379
  transient ischaemic attack, **194**
  transoesophageal, 172
'economy class syndrome', 50–51
eczema, 605

eczema craquelé (asteatotic dermatitis),
        607
Ehlers–Danlos syndrome, 670–671, *671*
  genetics, 671
Eisenmenger's syndrome, 375
ejection click/sound, **351**
elastic recoil, 124
elbow movement examination, *399*, 638,
        640
elderly *see* older people
electrocardiogram (ECG)
  aortic regurgitation, 363
  aortic stenosis, 361
  Fallot's tetralogy, 375
  hypertrophic cardiomyopathy, 377
  mitral regurgitation, 359
  mitral stenosis, 357
  myocardial infarction, 159
  pericarditis, 379
  pulmonary embolism, 52–53
  syncope, 298
  transient ischaemic attack, **194**
electrodiagnostic studies, peripheral
        neuropathy, 462–463, **463**
electroencephalogram (EEG), epilepsy, 303
electromyography (EMG)
  myasthenia gravis, 474
  myositis, 477
electrophysiological study, 169–170
eliciting skills, 117–118
emphysema, 17
  elastic recoil, 124
empty sella syndrome, 702
empyema, 56
  parapneumonic effusion *vs.*, **56**
encephalopathies, **307**
  hepatic, 69
  HIV-associated, 288
  transmissible spongiform, 311–312
encouragement, 117
endarterectomy, carotid stenosis, 195
endocarditis
  bacterial, 372
  infective *see* infective endocarditis
  prosthetic valve, 371
endocrine system, 693–714
  stimulation tests, 706
  suppression tests, 706
end-of-life issues, 543–571
  advance directives, 561–563, **562**
  autopsy requests, 569–571
  intensive therapy unit transfer, 548–550
  options, **560**
  organ donation *see* organ donation
  percutaneous endoscopic gastronomy
        feeding, 556–558
  resuscitation-status, decision-making,
        543–548
  treatment withholding/withdrawal,
        550–555
  see also palliative care
endoscopy
  dyspepsia, 132
  gastro-oesophageal reflux disease, 130

endothelial cells, glomerulonephritides,
        243
energy intake–expenditure balance, CVD
        prevention, 147
English Mental Capacity Act (2005), 535
enhanced external counterpulsation,
        angina, 155
Entamoeba histolytica, 85
enteric stomas, 92–93
enthesitis, **655**
enzymopathies, anaemia, 266
eosinophilic lung disease, **41**
eosinophilic lung diseases, 41
eosinophilic pneumonia, **41**
epilepsy, 302–303
  diagnosis, 303
  driving, 528
  juvenile myoclonic, 303
  treatment, 303–304
episcleritis, 692
epithelial cells, glomerulonephritides, **242**
Epstein–Barr virus (EBV), 110
erosion, **600**
erythema multiforme, *633*
erythema nodosum, *89*, 621, *622*, **624**
erythrocyte abnormalities, 265–266
erythrocyte sedimentation rate (ESR), 320
  influencing factors, **321**
erythrocytosis, 98
erythrodermic psoriasis, **602**
erythropoeitic protoporphyria (EPP), **613**
erythropoietin (EPO), 237
essential thrombocythaemia (ET), 100
essential tremor, **203**, 441
etanercept, **651**
ethics, 5–6, 8, 487
  criteria, **4**
  decision-making, 487
  mark-sheet, 3–4
  principles, 487, **487**
ethnicity, 505–506
ethylene glycol poisoning, 258
euthanasia, 560
euvolaemic patients, 298
evidence-based medicine (EBM), 585
examiners, 2–3, 716
  feedback from, 718
  personalities, 717
exam technique, 716–719
  answering questions, 719
  communication skills, 718–719
  on the day, 716–719
  equipment required, 716
  ethics station, 719
  if things go wrong, 719
  patients, examination, 717
  patients, importance of, 716–717
  post PACES, 719
  practice, 716
  presenting, 717–718
  prior to exam, 716
  rapport, 717
  running commentary avoidance, 717
  unclear diagnosis, 718

excoriation, **600**
exercise
  murmurs, **354**
  unaccustomed, cardiovascular disease,
    148
exercise tolerance test (ETT)
  chest pain, 154, **154**
  metabolic equivalents, 594, **594**
exertional dyspnoea, 356
exophthalmos, 694
expiratory flow rates, lung disease,
  123–124
expiratory splitting, **352**
express consent, 530, **532**
extensor plantars, 447–449
extracellular fluid, 253, **253**
extradural haematoma, **426**
extrinsic allergic alveolitis (EEA), *42*,
  42–43
  acute *vs.* chronic, **43**
exudates, diabetic retinopathy, **675**, *677*
eye(s), 673–692
  anatomy, 673, *673*
  cranial nerve testing, 382–384
  examination, 673–675
  movement
    abducens nerve testing, 383–384
    abnormal, 411–412
    muscles associated, 408–409, *409*
    oculomotor nerve testing, 383–384
    trochlear nerve testing, 383–384
  resting position, brainstem assessment,
    566
eye disease
  advanced, 676, **677**
  thyroid, *694*
  see also specific conditions

face
  abdominal system examination, 62
  acromegaly, 703
  cardiovascular system examination, 346
  myotonic dystrophy, 479
  respiratory system examination, 10
  scleroderma, 617, 659
'face blindness', 432–433
facial nerve (VII), 385
  bilateral weakness, 419
  examination, *385*
  lesions, 418, *419*
  palsy, 418–420, *419*
  supranuclear control, *425*, **425**
facial rash, 612–617
  features, **616**
  see also specific rashes
facial sensation, *384*
facilitating skills, communication, 117–118
  cue recognition, 118
  encouragement, 117
  interpretation, 117
  legitimising, 118
  questioning, 117–118
factor replacement, haemophilia, 273
factor Va, 271

factor VIIa, 271
factor Xa, 271
faecal occult blood testing, colorectal
  cancer, 143
Fallot's tetralogy, 375
falls
  causes, **291**
  disequilibrium, **292**
  environmental factors, 292
  history taking, 291–295
    approach, 291–293
  interventions, 294
  patient discharge, 294
  risk assessment, 292, **292**, 294
    balance tests, 294
    strength, 294
  vitamin D deficiency, 294
false images, diplopia, 409
familial adenomatous polyposis (FAP),
  142
familial combined hyperlipidaemia (FHC),
  177
familial hypercholesterolaemia (FH), **177**
familial hypocalciuric hypercalcaemia
  (FHH), 249
family members *see* relatives
fascioscapulohumeral muscular dystrophy,
  477
fasting plasma glucose (FPG), 148, **148**
  targets, **149**
fat intake, CVD prevention, 147
Felty's syndrome, 87, **649**
femoral nerve lesion, 461
fever, 191
fibrates, **181**
finger clubbing
  cardiovascular disease, 346
  lung cancer, *25*
  nail lesions, **621**
  phases, **620**
finger deformities, rheumatoid arthritis,
  645, *646*, *647*
finger movement examination, *400*
finger–nose test, *392*
Finkelstein's test, *639*
first dorsal interosseus wasting, **459**
first (S1) heart sound, 350–351
  abnormalities, **350**
Fischer syndrome, 470
fish oils, **181**
fissures, **600**
fitness to drive, 595–596
fitness to practise
  colleague health problems, 582–584
  misconduct, 580–582
  poor colleague performance, 578–580
flashes, 685, **686**
flexible sigmoidoscopy, colorectal cancer,
  143
flexor digitorum profundus (FDP), **456**
flexural psoriasis, **602**
floaters, 685, **686**
flow rates, restrictive lung disease,
  123–124

flow volume loops, 124, *124*
fludrocortisone, 710
fluid distribution, 253
focal and segmental glomerulosclerosis
  (FSGS), **242**
folate, 278
folate deficiency, **263**
folate supplementation, 263, 278
follicle-stimulating hormone (FSH)
  deficiency, **700**
foot drop, *460*, **461**
foot examination, **645**
forced expiratory volume over one second
  (FEV$_1$), 122–123, *123*
forced vital capacity (FVC), 122–123, *123*
formal complaints, 507
Foster–Kennedy syndrome, 680
fourth (S4) heart sound, **351**
fractures
  bone remodelling, 208
  osteoporosis, 205
Framingham data, cardiovascular disease
  risk, 147
Friedreich's ataxia, 447–449, **448**
Froment's sign, 456, *457*
frontal lobe, 387–388
  disease effects, **387**
  functions, **387**
fundoscopy, 673–674, *674*
fungal infection, HIV-associated, 286
funnel vision, 683

gait
  abnormalities, 403, **405**, 406
  examination, 403–406
gait, arms, legs, spine (GALS) screen, 635,
  635, *636*
galactorrhoea, 713
gastric cancer, 131
gastric ulcers, **132**
gastrin, 131
gastroenteritis, type 2 diabetes mellitus,
  223
gastrointestinal pathology, skin signs, **62**
gastronomy feeding, 557–558
gastro-oesophageal reflux disease
  (GORD), 130
  anti-secretory treatment relationship,
    132
  complications, **130**
  endoscopy, 130
  hiatus hernias, 130
  symptoms, **129**
  treatment, **131**
Gegenhalten, 395–396
generalisation, 588
generalised seizures, **303**
gene therapy, cystic fibrosis, 33–34
genetic testing, 589–590
  long-term QT syndrome, 169
  neurofibromatoses, 627
geographic atrophy, 687–688
geriatricians, community, 502
germline mutation, 95–96

Gerstmann's syndrome, **435**
ghrelin, 705
giant cell arteritis (GCA), 325–327
   diagnosis, 326
   differential diagnoses, **326**
   raised inflammatory markers, 326
   symptoms, **326**
   temporal artery biopsy, 326–327
   treatment, 327, **327**
Gilbert's syndrome, 71–72
Gitelman's syndrome, 259
Glasgow Coma Score, **565**
glaucoma, 689–690
   acute, 692
   aqueous flow obstruction, 689–690
glenohumeral disease, **642**
Global Initiative for Chronic Obstructive
   Lung Disease (GOLD), **18**
glomerular disease, acute renal failure,
   230
glomerular filtration rate (GFR), 231–232
   ACE inhibitors effects, 237
   angiotensin II receptor blockers effects,
      237
   calculation, 234
   serum creatinine vs., 234–236
glomerulonephritis, 239–244
   classification, 240, **241**
   history taking, 239–240
      approach, 240
   infection-associated, **243**
   mesangiocapillary, **243**
   pathology, **242–243**
   prevalence, 241
   progression, 241
   treatment, **242–243**
   types, 241
glossopharyngeal nerve (IX) examination,
   385–386
glucagon-like peptide (GLP-1), 223
glucocorticoid-induced osteoporosis, 210
glucocorticoid-remediable aldosteronism
   (GRA), **184**
glucose-dependent insulinotropic
   polypeptide (GIP), 223
glutamic acid decarboxylase (GAD), 217
glycaemic control
   type 1 diabetes mellitus, 219
   type 2 diabetes mellitus, 222
   vascular complications, 222–223
glycogen storage, myalgia, 477
glycosuria, 258
goitre, 699–700
good medical practice, **580**
Goodpasture's disease, 244, 247
gout
   acute, 662
   chronic tophaceous, 663, *663*
   diagnosis, 664
   risk factors, **663**
   treatment, 664
GPIIbIIIa inhibitors, 158
graft versus host disease, 98
granular casts, 241

Graves' disease, 693–697
   ophthalmopathy, *694*, **694**, 696
      treatment, 697
   pregnancy and, 697
Graves' thyrotoxicosis, 539, **694**
growth hormone
   deficiency, **700**, **705**
   therapy, 705
Guillain–Barré syndrome, 469–472
   diagnosis, 470
   differential diagnosis, 469
   investigations, **472**
   pathophysiology, 470
   progression, 469
   subtypes, 469, **471**
   treatment, 470, 472
guttate psoriasis, **602**
gynaecomastia, *712*, 712–713
   causes, **712**

HACEK microorganisms, infective
   endocarditis, 371
haematemesis, 133
haematological problems, 260–283
   bone marrow examination, 96–97
haematuria, 240
   detection, 241
haemochromatosis, 82–84
   clinical manifestations, 83
   decompensation, 83
   diagnosis, 83
   genetic basis, 83
   screening, 83–84
   treatment, 83
haemodialysis
   acute, **231**
   complications, 239
   principles, 239
haemoglobin A_{1c} (HbA_{1c}), 217
haemoglobinopathies, 266
haemolysis, **265**
haemolytic anaemia, 263, **264**
   laboratory findings, 263
haemolytic uraemic syndrome, 270
haemophagocytic lymphohistiocytosis
   (HLH), 321–322
haemophagocytic syndrome, 321–322
haemophilia, 271–273
   activated partial thromboplastin time, 272
   bleeding management, 273
   forms, 272
   history taking, 271–272
      approach, 272
haemopoietic stem cells (HSCs), 96
haemopoietic stem cell transplantation
   (HSCT), 98
   indications, 98
   myeloma, 282
   non-Hodgkin's lymphoma, 105
haemoptysis, 121
haemorrhage
   acute, bradycardia in, 133
   choroidal, *687*
   diabetic retinopathy, **675**, *676*, *677*

intracerebral, 175, **426**, 430
intracranial, **426**
sub-arachnoid see sub-arachnoid
   haemorrhage (SAH)
vitreous, 685–686, **686**
haemorrhagic stroke, 425
haemostasis regulation, 268, *269*
   endothelium role, 268–269, *269*
   platelet adhesion, *269*
haemothorax, 56
hallucinations, recurrent, **309**
haloperidol, **308**
Hamman–Rich syndrome, **40**
hand(s)
   acromegaly, 704
   examination, 635, **638**, 638–640
      abdominal system inspection, 62
      cardiovascular system inspection, 346
      respiratory system inspection, 10
   Felty's syndrome, 87
   scleroderma, 617, 659
   small muscles
      examination, 398, *401*
      wasting, **459**, 459–460, *460*
Hashimoto's thyroiditis, 698
headache, 188–192
   causes, **189**
   history taking
      approach, 188–190
      past medical history, 189–190
   patterns, 188–189
   primary, **189**
   scans, **191**
   secondary, **189**
   symptoms, **189**
   see also specific types
hearing tests, 385
heart failure, 161–166
   biventricular pacing, 166
   causes, **163**
   cor pulmonale vs., 166
   definition, 163
   diastolic, 166, **166**
   differential diagnosis, 162
   history taking, 161–163
      approach, 162–163
   New York Heart Association
      classification, **162**
   orthostatic hypotension management,
      298
   pathophysiology, 163
   symptoms, 162
   systolic, **166**
   treatment, 165–166, 378
heart murmurs see murmurs
heart sounds
   auscultation, 350–351
   extra, **351**
   palpable, 348–349
heart valves
   abnormalities
      prediction, 349, **349**
      right-sided, 364
      see also specific abnormalities

prosthetic *see* prosthetic valves
replacement, 367, 368
  complications, **367**
trauma, infective endocarditis, 371
see also prosthetic valves
Heberden's nodes, *664*
heel–shin test, *392*
Helicobacter pylori, 131–132
  diagnosis, 132
  eradication, 132
  gastric cancer, 131
  location–clinical outcome relationship, 131
  proton pump inhibitors, 131–132
  serology, 132
hemianopia
  bitemporal, 406
  homonymous, 406, 434
Henoch–Schönlein purpura, 247
heparin, 275
  low-molecular-weight heparin *vs.*, 158
  mechanism of action, 275
hepatic decompensation, 67–68, **68**
hepatic encephalopathy, 69
hepatic failure, 67–68
hepatic vein thrombosis (Budd–Chiari syndrome), 69
hepatitis, autoimmune *see* autoimmune hepatitis (AIH)
hepatitis B virus infection, 76–78
  carriers, 76
  markers, 76
  phases, **77**
  pre-core mutant disease, 76
  treatment, 76, 78
hepatitis C virus infection, 78–79
hepatocellular carcinoma (HCC), 70–71
hepatomegaly, 85–86
  infective causes, 85
hepatorenal syndrome (HRS), 69–70
hepatosplenomegaly, 86
hepcidin, 267
hereditary coporphyria (HC), **613**
hereditary haemorrhagic telangiectasia (HHT), 619
hereditary non-polyposis colon cancer (HNPCC), 142
hereditary sensory and motor neuropathy (HSMN), 469, *469*
hereditary spherocytosis, 266
herpes zoster, chronic myeloid leukaemia, *95*
hiatus hernia, gastro-oesophageal reflux disease, 130
hibernation, 153–154
high-density lipoproteins (HDL), 180
higher cortical function, 387
  examination, 387–389
highly active antiretroviral therapy (HAART), 289
high stepping gait, *405*
hip examination, 640–641, **643**
  movement, *403*, *643*

hirsutism, *711*, 711–712
histology, *Helicobacter pylori*, 132
history taking, 7–8, 114–343
  abdominal problems, 129–143
  assumptions, 115
  cardiovascular problems, 144–187
  clinical reasoning, 114
  common faults, **119**
  communication skills, 116–119
  criteria, **3**
  elderly care problems, 291–300, 325–327, 333–336
  endocrine problems, 215–227
  eye problems, 213–214
  haematological problems, 260–283
  HIV infection, 284–290
  locomotor problems, 205–215
  metabolic problems, 228–259
  neurological problems, 188–204
  patient-centred, 116
  patient's perspective, 114–116
    preconceptions, 115
  questioning *see* questioning (of patients)
  renal problems, 228–259
  respiratory problems, 121–128
  traditional medical history model, 114
    content plus process, 119, **120**
    content *vs.* process, 119
  see also specific conditions
history-taking station (Station 2), 2
  candidate information, 4–5
  case settings, 4–5
  documents, 4–5
  examiner information, 5
  patient/subject information, 5
HIV-associated respiratory disease, 284, 286–287
HIV encephalopathy, 288
HIV infection, 284–290
  antiretroviral treatment, 289
    failure, 289
  confidentiality, 527
  diarrhoea, 288
  emerging treatments, 289
  epidemiology, 285
  history taking, 284–285
    approach, 284–285
  immune response, 285–286
    antibodies, 286
    CD4 lymphocytes, 286
    CD8 lymphocytes, 286
  lipodystrophy, 289
  'long-term non-progressors', 286
  malignancy, 290
  neurological manifestations, 288
  opportunistic infections, 286, 290
  pathogenesis, 285
  screening, 289
  stages, **287**
  transmission risks, 592–593
  tuberculosis, 286–287
  types, 285
  vaccination, 290
  virion structure, 285

virus replication, 285
wasting, 288
HIV lipodystrophy, 289
HIV testing, 590–591
  needlestick injuries, 591–593
  pregnancy, 592
Hodgkin's lymphoma, **105**
Hoffmann's sign, *402*
Holmes–Adie pupil, 413–414
homeopathic treatment, 539–540
homeostasis, 151
homografts, 367
horizontal voluntary conjugate gaze, **410**, *410*, 410–411
hormone replacement therapy (HRT)
  osteoporosis, 209
  pituitary hormones, **702**
  systemic lupus erythematosus and, 658–659
hormones
  deficiencies *see* specific deficiencies
  types, 707
  see also specific hormones
Horner's syndrome, *415*, 415–416
  features, 415
  lesions, 415–416
  Pancoast's syndrome, 28
  small pupils, 414
hospital management, 574
Howell–Jolly bodies, 264
human herpes virus 8, 288
human immunodeficiency virus (HIV) infection *see* HIV infection
human leucocyte antigen (HLA) *see* major histocompatibility complex (MHC)
Human Rights Act (1998), 544
Human Tissue Act (1969), 569, 571
Human Tissue Authority, 571
human tissue retention, 570
Huntington's disease, 589–590
hyaline casts, 241
hydatid disease, 85–86
hydrocortisone, 710
hyperaldosteronism, **184**
hyperapobetalipoproteinaemia, **177**, 182
hypercalcaemia, 248–252
  causes, 249, **249**
  history taking, 248–249
    approach, 248–249
  patient surveillance, 249
  surgical treatment, 249–250
    complications, 250
  symptoms, 248
hypergonadotrophic hypogonadism, 712
hyperhomocysteinaemia, 277–278
hyperinflation, **15**
hyperkalaemia, **232**, 232–233
  treatment, 233
hyperlipidaemia
  secondary, **177**
  treatment, 494
hyperlipoproteinaemia, type III, **177**
hypernatraemia, 254

hyperosmolar non-ketotic coma (HONC), 220
hyperparathyroidism, 250
  renal osteodystrophy, 238
hyperpigmentation, Addison's disease, 707, *709*
hyperprolactinaemia, 702, **702**
hypersensitivity, **324**
hypertension, 182–187
  cardiovascular disease risks, 183
  chronic kidney disease, 236
  definition, 184
  history taking, 182–183
    approach to, 182–183
  idiopathic intracranial, 191–192
  lifestyle measures, 185
  refractory, 187
  renin–angiotensin–aldosterone system, 184, **184**
  secondary care referral, 182–183
  secondary causes, **183**
  supine, 299
  target organ damage, **183**
  therapy, 185–187, **186**
    indications/contraindications, 187
hypertensive retinopathy, *678*, 678–679
hyperthyroidism, 693–697
  biochemical abnormalities, 696
  subclinical, 697
  thyrotoxicosis *vs.*, 695
  treatment, 696–697
hypertrichosis, 711
hypertriglyceridaemia, **177**
hypertrigyceridaemic phenotype, 151
hypertrophic (obstructive) cardiomyopathy, 375–378
  aortic stenosis *vs.*, **376**
  diagnosis, 377
  dynamic manoeuvre effects, **376**
  ECG features, 377
  lifestyle consequences, 378
  risk stratification, **377**
  screening, 378
  severity, 377
  symptoms, **376**
  treatment, 377–378
hypertrophic pulmonary osteoarthropathy, 25
hypoadrenalism, 707–711
  complications, 709–710
  decompensation, 709–710
  hypopituitarism *vs.*, 710
  severity, 709–710
  symptoms, **709**
  treatment, 710–711
hypoaldosteronism, primary, **184**
hypocalcaemia
  causes, **250**
  clinical features, **251**
  treatment, 251
hypoglossal nerve (XII) examination, 386
hypoglycaemia, 219–220
  causes, 336
  detection, 219

nocturnal, 220
normal responses, 219, **219**
prevention, 220
treatment, 220
hypoglycaemia-associated autonomic failure (HAAF), 219–220
hypoglycaemic agents, oral, **224**
hypoglycaemic unawareness, 219–220
hypogonadism, 712–713
hypogonadotrophic hypogonadism, 712
hypokalaemia, **232**, 232–233
  treatment, 233
hypolipidaemia, 180, 182
hypomagnesaemia, 251
hyponatraemia, 252–256
  consequences, 254
  history taking, 252–253
    approach, 252–253
  stages, **255**
  treatment, 254
hypoparathyroidism, 251, 713
hypophosphataemia, 252
hypopituitarism, 700–702, *701*
  causes, **701**
  hypoadrenalism *vs.*, 710
  signs/symptoms, **700**
hypotension, orthostatic *see* orthostatic hypotension
hypothesis testing, 115
hypothetico-deductive reasoning, 114
hypothyroidism, *697*, 697–698
  causes, **698**
  complications, 698
  subclinical, 698
  symptoms, **698**
  treatment, 698
hypoxia, pulmonary embolism, 51

ideas, concerns and expectations (ICE), 114–116
  patient's thoughts, 114–115
idiopathic myelofibrosis (IMF), 100
idiopathic pulmonary artery hypertension (IPAH), 48–49
idiopathic pulmonary fibrosis (IPF), 37–41
  treatment, 39
idiopathic sensorineural hearing loss (ISNHL), 417–418
idiopathic thrombocytopenic purpura (ITP), 270
idraparinux, 174
ileal disease, active, **89**
ileocaecal disease, active, **89**
  management, 90
immune-mediated inflammatory disorders, 320
  see also specific disorders
immune system, 318
  acute-phase response, 319–320
  antigen response, 318, *318*
  autoimmunity, 324–325
  tolerance, 324–325
immunodeficiency disorders, **290**
immunoglobulin(s), 323

immunoglobulin A (IgA) nephropathy, **242**
immunoglobulin A (IgA) vasculitis, 631
immunoglobulin M (IgM), 324
immunomodulators, dermatitis, 605
immunosuppression, myasthenia gravis, **474**
impaired fasting glucose (IFG), 148, **148**
impaired glucose tolerance (IGT), 148, **148**
implantable cardioverter-defibrillator (ICD), 369
  acute coronary syndrome, **161**
  ischaemic cardiomyopathy, **369**
implied consent, 530, **532**
incapacitated patients
  decision making, **535**
  'do not attempt resuscitation', **548**
  legal representation, 535
  withholding/withdrawing treatment, **552**, 554–555
incidence, 499
incontinence, 314–316
  history taking, 314–316
    approach, 314–316
  types, **315**
'incurable conditions', diagnosis explanation, 489
indomethacin, 664
industrial injury benefits, 596–597
infection
  atherosclerosis, 153
  pyrexia, **329**
  skin, 632–634
  see also individual infections
infective endocarditis, 370–372
  assessment, 370
  bacteraemia, 371
  complications, **371**
  diagnosis, **372**
  emergence, 371
  mitral valve prolapse, 371
  peripheral signs, **346**, 370
  rheumatic valves, 371
  surgical indications, 372
  vasculitic rash, *370*
inferior mesenteric artery (IMA), 138
inflammation
  atherosclerosis, 152
  pyrexia, **330**
  raised inflammatory markers, 317–325
  sepsis, 330–331
inflammatory bowel disease (IBD), 89, 91
  diarrhoea, 140
  differential diagnoses, 90
  extra-intestinal associations, **89**
  see also Crohn's disease (CD); ulcerative colitis
inflammatory markers, raised, 317–325
  'biological therapies', 320
  giant cell arteritis, 326
  history taking, 317
    approach, 317
  tests, 320
inflammatory response syndrome
  fluid management, 254, 256
  sodium management, 254, 256

infliximab, **651**
informed consent, **532**
inquests, 577–578
inspiratory splitting, **352**
insulin
 hyperkalaemia, 233
 lipid transport, 178
insulin regimens
 type 1 diabetes mellitus, **218**
 type 2 diabetes mellitus, **225**
insulin resistance, type 2 diabetes mellitus, 222
integrated care pathway (ICP), 512
intensive therapy unit (ITU) transfer
 advance directives, 563
 age affecting outcome, 549
 appropriateness, 548–550
intention to treat (ITT) analysis, 588
intercostal drain, pneumothorax, 58
interferon-β, multiple sclerosis, 202
interferon-γ (IFN-γ), allergy, 324
interleukin-2 (IL-2), renal transplants, **109**
intermediate care, 513
international normalised ratio (INR), stroke, 174–175
internuclear ophthalmoplegia, 409–411, *410*
 horizontal voluntary gaze, 410, *410*, **410**
interpretation, facilitating skills, 117
interpreters, 506, **506**
interstitial nephritis, **230**
interstitial pneumonia, 38
 acute, **40**
 classification, **40**
intestinal ischaemia, 139
intracellular fluid, 253, **253**
intracerebral haemorrhage (ICH), 175, **426**, 430
intracranial haemorrhage, **426**
intracranial hypertension, idiopathic, 191–192, 680
intracranial pressure, raised, **189**
invasive ventilation, COPD, 549
investigations *see* clinical investigations
iodine, radioactive, 697
iritis, 692
 old, *691*
iron
 anaemia, **262**
 overload, 267
 restless leg syndrome, 204
 storage, 261
 transport, 261
 uptake, 261
iron deficiency anaemia, **262**
irritant contact dermatitis (ICD), **606**
ischaemia
 intestinal, 139
 reversible, 427
ischaemic cardiomyopathy, **369**
ischaemic colitis, 139
ischaemic heart disease, 155

ischaemic stroke, **426**
 treatment, 429
islet cell antibodies, 217
isotretinoin, 617
itching, 605

Janeway lesions, infective endocarditis, **346**, 370
jaundice, 71–73
 bilirubin metabolism, 71–72
 causes, **71**
 cholestatic, 72–73
 chronic liver disease, 71
Joint British Societies' guidelines (JBS 2), cardiovascular disease prevention, 145
joint examination, 635
 approaches, **648**
 autoimmune tests, 635
 symptoms, 635
joint pain, 211–212
 differential diagnoses, 211, *212*
 history taking, 211–212
 approach, 211–212
 patient perspective, 211
 symptoms, 211
jugular foramen syndrome, 418
jugular venous pulse (JVP), 346
 carotid pulse *vs.*, **346**
 measurement, *347*
 waveforms, **346**, *347*
 abnormal, **348**
justice, **487**
juvenile myoclonic epilepsy, 303
juvenile plantar dermatosis, **607**

Kaposi's sarcoma, 288–289
Kartagener's syndrome, 34
Kawasaki disease, 246
Kayser–Fleischer rings, 84, *84*
Kennedy's disease, 451
keratitis, 692
 marginal, 692
kidney
 amyloidosis, 283
 palpation, 64, **65**
 see also entries beginning renal
knee movement examination, *403*, **644**
Köbner's phenomenon, 602
Korotkoff sounds, 347
Kussmaul's sign, **348**

labyrinthitis, acute (vestibular neuronitis), **293**
lacunar stroke (LACS), 422, **422**, 424–425
Lambert–Eaton myasthenic syndrome (LEMS), 474
language, appropriate use, 118
language examination, 389–390
language therapy, dysphagia, 136
lateral cutaneous nerve lesion, 461
lateral herniation, **567**
lateral medullary syndrome, *436*
lead-pipe rigidity, 395

lead poisoning, 612
left parasternal heave, 348, *350*
left ventricular failure (LVF), 162
left ventricular outflow obstruction, 360
left ventricular systolic dysfunction (LVSD), 162
 non-pharmacological treatment, 165–166
 pharmacological treatment, **164**
leg examination, 640–642
leg ulceration, 624
leprosy, 457
 bilateral ulnar nerve palsy, *458*
leptin, 150
leucocytoplastic vasculitis, 631
leucoerythroblastic change, 97
leukaemia
 acute *vs.* chronic, 97
 see also individual leukaemias
Lewy bodies, 441
Lewy body dementia, 309, **309**
 withholding/withdrawing treatment, 555
lichenification, **600**
lichen planus, 607–608
 buccal mucosa, *608*
 nail lesions, 620
Liddle's syndrome (pseudohyperaldosteronism), **184**
life-prolonging treatment, withholding/ withdrawing, 550–555
 antibiotics, 550–552
 artificial hydration and nutrition, 550–555
 capacity, **552**, 554–555
 drugs, 550–552
 guidelines, 552, **555**
lifestyle interventions, **147**
 cardiovascular disease, 147–148
light flashes, 685, **686**
light reflex, **383**, *384*
limb examination, 394–397
 lower limbs *see* lower limb examination
 power, 394–395, **395**
 reflexes, 396–397, **397**
 tone, 395–396
 upper limbs *see* upper limb examination
 weakness patterns, 395, **396**
limb girdle muscular dystrophies (LGMDs), 477
limbic system, 389
limited cutaneous systemic sclerosis (LcSSc), 660–661
linoleic acid, 147
lipid-lowering therapy, 149, 180, **181**
 acute coronary syndrome, **161**
 cardiovascular disease, 179–180, 182
 chronic kidney disease, 238
 diabetes mellitus, 226
lipid targets
 cardiovascular disease, 148, **148**
 diabetes mellitus, 226
lipid transport, **178**, 178–179
 dietary, 178–179
 endogenous, 179

lipodystrophy, HIV, 289
lipoprotein lipase (LPL), 178–179
lipoproteins, 176
listening, 116–117
  active, 117
liver
  infective disorders, 86
  infiltrative disorders, 86
  palpation, 63, **64**
  regeneration, 68
  see also entries beginning hepatic/hepato-
liver disease
  alcoholic, 74–75
  chronic *see* chronic liver disease (CLD)
liver metastases, carcinoid syndrome, 93
Liverpool Care Pathway, 560
'liver screen' blood tests, **72**
liver transplantation, chronic liver disease, 70, **70**
'living wills', 561–563, **562**
lobar collapse, *15*, 30
lobectomy, 30
lobe syndromes, 387
'locked-in' syndrome, 565
locomotor system, 635–672
  joint examination, 635
  see also individual parts and conditions
Loeffler syndrome, **41**
Löfgren's triad, **47**
long-term care, assessment, 513
long-term conditions (LTC), 501
  management negotiation, 500–502
'long-term non-progressors' (LTNPs), HIV, 286
long-term oxygen therapy (LTOT), COPD, 17, **17**
long-term QT syndrome (LQTS), 169
long tracts, spinal cord, 381–382, 393, *394*
loop diuretics, 258–259
  heart failure, **164**
loop of Henle, 258–259
lorazepam, **308**
low-density lipoprotein (LDL), 179
  atherosclerosis, 152–153
low-density lipoprotein, small dense, **177**
lower limb examination, 402–403
  coordination, 402
  power, 402
  reflexes, *404*
  tone, 402, *403*
lower motor neuron weakness, **396**
lower oesophageal sphincter (LOS), transient, 130
low-molecular-weight heparin (LMWH), 275
  heparin *vs.*, 158
  non-ST elevation myocardial infarction, 158
  pulmonary embolism, 53
lumbar disc disease, 452
  cauda equina syndrome *vs.*, 452, 454
lumbar puncture, sub-arachnoid haemorrhage, 190–191

lung(s)
  lobes, 11, *11*
  volumes, 122, *122*
  see also entries beginning pulmonary
lung abscess, 23–24
lung base, dullness, 21
lung biopsy, diffuse parenchymal lung disease, 39
lung cancer, 24–28
  classification, 26–27
  clinical signs, 24–25
  diagnosis, *26*
  differential diagnoses, 25
  palliative care, **28**
  paraneoplastic syndromes, **25**
  prognosis, 27
  WHO/Zubrod performance status scale, **25**
  see also individual types
lung disease
  asbestos-related, 43–44, **597**
  eosinophilic, 41, *41*
  flow rates, 123–124
  interstitial, 124–125
  obstructive, **123**
  restrictive, **123**
  scleroderma, 617, 661
  see also specific conditions
lung transplant, 60–61
  indications, **61**
lupus erythematosus, 616
lupus pernio, *46*, *615*
lupus vulgaris, 615
luteinising hormone (LH) deficiency, **700**
lymphadenopathy, 103–105
  differential diagnosis, **103**
lymphocytes, 96
lymphocytic interstitial pneumonia, **40**
lymphoid neoplasms
  WHO classification, **105**
  see also specific neoplasms
lymphoma, 103–105
  central nervous system prophylaxis, 105
  non-Hodgkin's *see* non-Hodgkin's lymphoma (NHL)

macrocytosis, 261–262
macrophages, atherosclerosis, 153
macula, **675**
  fundoscopy, 674
macule, **600**
maculopathy, **677**
magnetic resonance angiography
  intestinal ischaemia, 139
  posterior circulation strokes, 438
magnetic resonance imaging (MRI)
  acute parenchymal infarction, 427
  diabetic neuropathy, 467
  hypertrophic cardiomyopathy, 377
  multiple sclerosis, 201
  myeloma, 281
  normal pressure hydrocephalus, 312
  Parkinson's disease, 441

spinal cord syndromes, 446
stroke, 427
major histocompatibility complex (MHC), 318
  class I-peptide complex distress signal, 318
  class II-peptide complex distress signal, 318–319
malabsorption, **140**
malar flush, 346
malar rash, *614*
malignancy
  alarm symptoms, 121
  dermatomyositis, 477
  endocrine manifestations, 250, **250**
  nervous system effects, **198**
  occult, 51
  pleural effusion, 55
  polymyositis, 477
  see also cancer
malignant melanoma, 629
  assessment, **630**
  risk factors, 629
  types, **630**
management plans, 486
  chronic disease/long-term condition, 500–502
mandibular nerve, 417
marche à petit pas, **405**
Marfan's syndrome, 668–670
  complications, 670
  decompensation, 670
  diagnostic criteria, **669**
  management, 670
  pregnancy, 670
  severity, 670
  signs, *668*
marginal keratitis, 692
margination, 96
mark-sheets, 3–4, **4**
maturity onset diabetes of the young (MODY), 222
maxillary nerve, 417
maximal expiratory flow rates (MEFR), lung disease, 123–124
McArdle's disease, 477
McDonald diagnostic criteria, multiple sclerosis, 200, **201**
medial longitudinal fasciculus, **410**, *410*
median nerve, **455**
  lesion *see* carpal tunnel syndrome
mediastinal mass, anterior, 30
megaloblastic anaemia, 261
melanoma, malignant *see* malignant melanoma
melphalan, 282
membranous nephropathy, **242**
Ménière's disease, **293**
meningitis
  bacterial, 191
  cryptococcal, 288
  symptoms, **189**
meningococcal disease, warning signs, **191**

Mental Capacity Act
  innovations, **536**
  patient restraint, 537
  principles, **535**
Mental Health Act, 542
  sections, **542**
meralgia paraesthetica, 461
mesangial cells, glomerulonephritides, **242**
mesenteric ischaemia
  acute, 138, **139**
  chronic, 138
mesothelioma, **45**
meta-analyses, 586
metabolic acidosis, 258, **258**
  anion gap, 258
metabolic alkalosis, 258
metabolic disturbance, 256–259
metabolic syndrome, **151**
metered dose inhalers (MDIs), 127
metformin, **224**
methanol poisoning, 258
methicillin-resistant *Staphylococcus aureus*
      (MRSA), 331
  treatment, **332**
methotrexate, **603**
methylprednisolone, 202
metoprolol, 165
microaneurysms, diabetic retinopathy,
      675, *676*
microcytic anaemia, 261
  altered iron status *vs.*, **262**
microscopic colitis, 92
microscopic polyarteritis (MPA), **245**, 246
microvascular coronary artery disease, 169
mid-systolic (non-ejection) click, **351**
migraine, 190
Milwaukee shoulder, 664
mini-mental state examination (MMSE),
      308, *388*
  dementia, 313
miosis, 415
  age-related, 414
'mirror agnosia', 434
misconduct, 580–582
  types, 581–582
mitochondrial cytopathies, 477, 479
mitral regurgitation, 357–359
  differential diagnosis, 358
  mitral stenosis *vs.*, **365**
  pathophysiology, 359
  severity, **358**
  signs, 358, *358*
  treatments, 359
mitral stenosis, 355–357
  first heart sound, **350**
  mitral regurgitation *vs.*, **365**
  severity, 355, **355**
  signs, *356*
  symptoms, 356
  treatment, 357
  valve pathology, 356
mitral valve prolapse, 365–367
  complications, 366
  dynamic manoeuvre effects, **366**

infective endocarditis, 371
  pathophysiology, 367
  signs, *366*
mitral valve replacement, 368
mixed valve disease, 365
mobilisation, acute coronary syndrome,
      161
model of end-stage liver disease (MELD)
      score, 66, **66**
modified Schober's test, *652*
monoclonal gammopathies of
      undetermined significance
      (MGUS), 282–283
mononeuropathy
  causes, **463**
  definition, 463–464
  diagnosis, 464
mononeuropathy multiplex, 464, **465**
morphea, 661
motor cortex, 390–391
motor neurone disease, 449–451
  complications, 449
  decompensation, 449
  definition, 450
  diagnosis, 450
  differential diagnosis, 449
  long-term survival indicators, **450**
  palsy, *450*
  severity, 449
  symptom control, 451
  treatment, 450–451
  wasting, *450*
motor neuron weakness
  lower, **396**
  upper, **396**
motor tracts, 393
mouth ulcers, **619**
movement disorders, 391–392
  drug-induced, **393**
  types, **393**
MRSA *see* methicillin-resistant
      Staphylococcus aureus (MRSA)
multi-drug resistant (MDR) tuberculosis,
      287
multiple endocrine neoplasia (MEN)
      syndromes, 94, **94**
multiple sclerosis, 198–202
  definition, 200
  demyelination sites, **199**
  diagnostic criteria, 200, **201**
  differential diagnosis, **200**
  disabling paraparesis, 202
  disease course, 202
  history taking, 198–200
    approach, 199–200
  pathogenesis, 200
  prognosis, 202
  symptoms, 199, **199**
  treatment, **201**
    acute relapse, 202
    disease modifying, 202
  types, 199
multiple sources hypothesis, atrial
      fibrillation, 172

multiple system atrophy (MSA), 440
murmurs, 351–355
  character, **353**
  continuous, **353**
  diastolic, **353**
  dynamic auscultation effects, **354**,
      354–355
  exercise effects, **354**
  intensity, **353**
  location, **353**
  palpable, 348–349
  physiological manoeuvres and, 354–355
  radiation, **353**
  respiration and, 354
  right-sided, 364–365
    decompensation, 364
    differential diagnosis, 364
  systolic, **353**
  timing, **353**
muscle imbalance, rehabilitation, 295
muscle wasting, hands, **459**, 459–460, *460*
muscle weakness, **396**
muscular dystrophies, 477
  see also specific muscular dystrophies
myalgia, 477
myasthenia gravis, 472–474, *473*
  differential diagnosis, **472**
  investigations, 473–474
  pupils, 413
  remission, **474**
  respiratory muscles, 472
  subtypes, **473**
  treatment, **474**
  weakness, 472, *473*
mycobacterial infection, HIV-associated,
      286–287
Mycobacterium avium–intracellulare
      complex, 287
Mycobacterium tuberculosis, 35–36
mycophenolate mofetil, **109**
mydriatic drugs, 414
myelinated nerve fibres, 688–689
myelodysplastic syndromes (MDSs),
      98–101
  splenomegaly, 98
  treatment, **101**
  WHO classification, **101**
myeloma, 279–283
  clinical features, **280**
  definition, 281
  diagnosis, 281, **282**
  history taking, 279–281
    approach, 279–281
  incidence, 281
  paraprotein levels, 282
  prognosis, 282, **282**
  radiology, 281
  treatments, 282
myelopathy
  acute transverse, **445**
  HIV infection, 445
  treatment, **446**
myeloproliferative disorders (MPDs),
      98–101, **100**

myocardial damage markers, 159
myocardial infarction
    angiotensin-converting enzyme
        inhibitors, 150
    complications, 161
    see also individual types
myocardial ischaemia
    investigation, **154**
    protection mechanisms, 153
myocardial perfusion scan, 154
myocarditis, 378
myoclonus, **393**
myopathy, 474–479, **475**
    differential diagnoses, **475**
myositis, 474–479, **477**
    biopsy, 477
    definition, 476
    polymyalgia *vs.*, 479
    types, **478–479**
myotomes, **394**
myotonia, 480
myotonia congenita, 481
myotonic dystrophy, 413, 479–481
    complications, 479
    decompensation, 479
    genetics, 480–481
    severity, 479
    signs, *480, 481*
    wasting, *481*
myxoedema coma, 698

nail(s)
    discoloration, **621**
    lesions, 620–621
    lines, 620
nasogastric tubes (NGT), insertion
        complications, 557
National Institute for Health Severity
        Score (NIH-SS), stroke, 428
National Patient Safety Agency (NPSA),
        574, **574**
native valve endocarditis, 371
neck
    cardiovascular system inspection, 346
    lumps, 699–700
    palpation, 10
    respiratory system inspection, 10
necrobiosis lipoidica diabeticorum, 623
    clinical features, 622, *623*
    ulcerated, *624*
necrotising fasciitis, 632–633, *633*
    treatment, 634
needlestick injuries, HIV
    action, **592**
    testing, 591–593
    transmission risks, 592–593
negative predictive value (PPV), 491
negligence, 577–578
    conditions for, 577, **577**
    suing, 577
neoplasm, pyrexia, **329**
neoplastic skin lesions, 628–630
neovascularization, **676**, *676*
nephritic syndrome, **241**

nephrogenic diabetes insipidus (NDI), **256**
nephropathy
    basement membrane, 244
    diabetic *see* diabetic nephropathy
    membranous, **242**
    non-diabetic, 236–237
nephrotic syndrome, 107, **241**
nerve biopsy, peripheral neuropathy, 467
nerve conduction studies, peripheral
        neuropathy, 463
nerve fibres, myelinated, 688–689
nerve lesions *see specific lesions*
nerve stretch tests, 642
nervous system
    anatomy, *381*
        cranial nerves, *381*
        long tracts, 381–382
    examination, 380–406
        anatomical interpretation, 380
        pathological interpretation, 380
    history taking, 380
    levels, 380, **380**
net bilirubin absorption (NBA), 191
neurally mediated syncope (NMS), *297*
neurodegenerative disease, 311
neurodermatitis, **607**
neurofibromatosis, 625–627
    complications, 625
    decompensation, 625
    definition, 625
    genetics, 626
    genetic testing, 627
    severity, 625
neurofibromatosis 1 (NF1)
    clinical features, **626**
    complications, 625, **626**
    diagnostic criteria, **625**
neurofibromatosis 2 (NF2)
    clinical features, 627, **627**
    diagnostic criteria, **627**
neuroimaging
    dementia, 311
    Parkinson's disease, 441
    see also specific techniques
neurological diseases, HIV-associated, 288
neuromuscular junction weakness, **396**
neuropathy
    diabetic *see* diabetic neuropathy
    hereditary, 469
    peripheral *see* peripheral neuropathy
    trigeminal, 417
neuropsychiatric porphyria, 610
neutropenia, 97
neutrophilia, 97
neutrophils, 96
new variant Creutzfeld–Jakob disease
        (nvCJD), 312
NHS Litigation Authority, 577
nicotinic acids, **181**
nocturnal hypoglycaemia, 220
nodule, **600**
non-alcoholic fatty liver disease
        (NAFLD), 75
non-ejection (mid-systolic) click, **351**

non-Hodgkin's lymphoma (NHL), 103–
        105, *104*
    management, 104–105
    prognosis, 103–104
    staging, 104
    treatment concordance, 503–504
non-invasive positive pressure ventilation
        (NIV), COPD, **20**
non-limb girdle muscular dystrophies
        (LGMDs), 477
non-maleficence, **487**
non-proliferative diabetic retinopathy
        (NPDR), 675, **676**
non-small-cell lung cancer (NSCLC),
        26–27
    prognosis, 27
    staging, **27**, *28*
    treatment, 27
non-specific interstitial pneumonia (NSIP),
        40
non-ST elevation myocardial infarction
        (NSTEMI)
    cerebral infarction, warfarin
        administration, 195
    management, 157–158
non-steroidal anti-inflammatory drugs
        (NSAIDs)
    ischaemic heart disease, 155
    rheumatoid arthritis, 651
non-verbal cues, 118
normal pressure hydrocephalus (NPH),
        312
normochromic normocytic anaemia, 261
noroviral diarrhoea, 141
nuclear medicine, thyrotoxicosis, 696
null hypothesis, 587
number needed to harm (NNH), 500
number needed to treat (NNT), 500
nutrient absorption, 142
nystagmus, 411–412, *412*
    peripherally *vs.* centrally provoked, **411**,
        411–412

obesity, 144, 150
    abdominal, 151
    body mass index, **145**
    patient perspective, 145
    risks, **145**
    secondary causes, **144**
oblique muscles, eye, 409
obstructive cardiomyopathy *see*
        hypertrophic (obstructive)
        cardiomyopathy
obstructive lung disease (OLD), **123**
    compliance, 124
obstructive sleep apnoea–hypopnoea
        syndrome (OSAHS), 59–60
    cor pulmonale, 60
    symptoms, **60**
obturator nerve lesion, 461
occipital lobe, 389
occlusive stroke, 424–425
occult malignancy, 51
ocular myasthenia, **474**

ocular nerves
lesions, 407–409, *408*
basal area, 408
muscles innervated, 409
see also individual nerves
oculocephalic response, 567
oculomotor nerve (III)
eye movement, 383–384
lesions, 407–408
palsy
large pupil, 413
ptosis, 413
pupil examination, 383
oculopharyngeal muscular dystrophy, 477
oculovestibular response, 567
odds, 499
odds ratio, 499
oedema, 253
oesophageal candidiasis, HIV infection, 288
oesophageal diseases, HIV infection, 288
oesophageal pain, 130
oesophageal ulceration, HIV infection, 288
oesophagitis, 129, 130
see also dyspepsia
oesophagogastroduodenoscopy (OGD), 497
ointments, creams *vs.*, 605
older people
coronary syndrome, 493
diagnostic uncertainty, 497
explaining treatment, 493, **493**
hyperlipidaemia, 494
investigations, 491
management, 495, **495**
prescription, 493, **493**
stress tests, 497
warfarin, 494
oliguric acute renal failure, 230, **231**
onchyomycosis, *620*, 621
opening snap (OS) heart sound, 351
open questions, 116
ophthalmic nerve, 417
ophthalmopathy, Graves' disease *see*
Graves' disease
ophthalmoplegia, 409
diplopia and, 409
internuclear *see* internuclear
ophthalmoplegia
optic atrophy, **675**, *680*, 680–681, **681**
optic disc, **675**
appearance, *674*
examination, 674
fundoscopy, 674
glaucoma, 690
swelling, **675**, 679–680, *680*, *683*
optic nerve (II)
damage, **406**, **681**
multiple sclerosis, **199**
pupils, 383
visual acuity, 382
visual fields, 382–383
optic neuritis, **681**
demyelinating, 681

optokinetic nystagmus, 411
oral glucose tolerance test (OGTT), **148**
oral hairy leucoplakia, 287–288
oral hypoglycaemic agents, **224**
oral lesions, 619
organ donation, 568–569
consent, 569
live, 568–569
organ retention, 570
orthostatic hypotension
management, 298–299
in heart failure, 298
supine hypertension and, 299
syncope and, *297*
orthostatic tremor, **203**
Ortner's phenomenon, 355
Osler's nodes, infective endocarditis, **346**, 370
osmolality, 253
dehydration and, 253
osteoarthritis, 664–666
adhesive capsulitis *vs.*, **642**
differential diagnoses, **665**
natural history, 665
prevalence, 665
risk factors, **665**
spondyloarthropathies *vs.*, **653**
symptoms, 665
treatment, 665–666, **666**
osteoblast maturation, 207
osteogenesis imperfecta, *671*, 671–672
cause, 672
management, 672
types, **672**
osteomalacia, 210, 238
osteoporosis, 205–210
bone loss, 207–208
definition, 208
glucocorticoid-induced, 210
incidence, 206
pathophysiology, 207–208
bone mineral density, 207
peak bone mass acquisition, 207
physiology, 209
prevention, 209–210
secondary investigations, **208**
symptoms, **205**
testosterone deficiency, 210
treatment, 208–209, **209**
ostium primum atrial septal defect (OP
ASD), 373
ostium secundum atrial septal defect (OS
ASD), 373
surgery, 375
overdose, 257, 540–542
overdrive pacing, tachyarrhythmia, 369
oxygen therapy, COPD, 19

pacemakers, permanent, *368*, 368–370
indications, 368
PACES, 2–5
aims, 2
examiners *see* examiners
marking system, 3

stations, 2, *2*, **4**
structure, 2, *2*
technique *see* exam technique
timing, 716
pacing, types, 368
Paget's disease, 666–668
bone changes, 667
skull, *666*
tibia, *667*
treatment, 668
pain *see specific types*
pain perception, 434
palliative care, 558–561
doctrine of double effect, 560
lung cancer, **28**
Parkinson's disease, 441
palmar erythema, *68*
palpation *see specific systems/organs*
palpitations, 166–170
electrophysiological study indications, 169–170
history taking, 166–168
approach, 167–168
risk factors, 167
Pancoast's syndrome, 28–29
pancytopenia, 264
Panton–Valentine leucocidin *(PVL)* gene, 332
papilloedema, 679–680
pathophysiology, 680
papule, **600**
paraneoplastic syndromes, **198**
characteristics, 198
lung cancer, **25**
parapneumonic effusion, **56**
paraprotein, myeloma, 282
parathyroid hormone (PTH), 250
parathyroid hormone (PTH)-related
peptide (PTH-rp), tumour
produced, **250**
paratonia, 395–396
parenchymal infarction, acute, 427
parietal lobe, 388–389
disease manifestations, **389**
dominance, 388–389
lesions, 388–389
Parkinsonian gait, **405**
Parkinsonian-plus syndromes, 440
Parkinsonian tremor, **203**, 438
Parkinson's disease, 438–442, *439*
clinical features, **440**
complex, 441
diagnosis, 438, **439**, 441
dysphagia, 136
neuroimaging, 441
non-motor symptoms, 441
palliative care, 441
pathology, 441
posture, *438*
'red flags', **440**
risk factors, 441
severity, 439
staging, 440–441
treatment, 441, **442**

Parkinson's disease dementia (PDD), 311
parotid enlargement/swelling, 74–75
　facial nerve palsy, 419
paroxysmal atrial fibrillation (PAF), 173
　anticoagulation, 175
paroxysmal nocturnal haemoglobinuria, 264
partial anterior circulation stroke (PACS), 422, **422**
partial seizures, **303**
patch, **600**
patent ductus arteriosus (PDA), 373
patent foramen ovale, 193
patient(s)
　angry, 506–508
　denial, 521–522
　　confidentiality, 524
　perspective, history taking, 114–116
　reactions, need for treatment, 492
　vulnerable, 537
patient-centred communication, 486–487
patient-centred history taking, 116
patient restraint, Mental Capacity Act, 537
pattern recognition, clinical reasoning, 114
peak expiratory flow rates (PEFR), 123
pemphigoid, 608–609, 609
　pemphigus vs., **612**
pemphigus, 609, 610
　complications, 610
　pemphigoid vs., **612**
　severity, 610
pendular nystagmus, 411
penetrating artery disease, **437**
Penfield's homunculus, 'phantom limb syndrome', 424, 430
peptic ulcer disease, **129**
　bleeding management, 133
　development, 131
　pathophysiology, 131
　persistent symptom management, 132–133
percussion
　abdominal system, 65
　cardiovascular system, 349
　respiratory system, 11, 12
percutaneous coronary intervention (PCI), **154**
　acute coronary syndrome, 158
　older patients, 159
percutaneous endoscopic gastrostomy (PEG) feeding, 556–558
percutaneous endoscopic gastrostomy (PEG) tube
　displacement, 558
　management, 558
　stomas, 92–93
percutaneous interventional electrophysiology, 170
performance tremor, **203**
pericardial disease, 378–379
pericardial effusion, 379
pericardial knock, **351**
pericardial rub, **351**, 378–379

pericarditis, 378–379
　constrictive, 379, **379**
　electrocardiogram, 379
　management, 379
perindopril, 186
peripheral blood films, anaemia, 262, **262**
peripheral cyanosis, **15**
peripheral neuropathy, 461–468
　clinical evaluation, 462–463, **463**, 464
　definition, 462
　lesion types, 463–464
　nerve biopsy, 467
　stocking distribution, 462
　symptoms, **462**
　tests, **468**
　treatment, 467
permanent pacemakers see pacemakers, permanent
'pernicious' anaemia, 262
peroneal nerve lesions, 460–461, **461**
persistent vegetative state (PVS), 563–565
　brainstem death vs., 565
　coma vs., 565
　definition, 564
　future care considerations, **565**
　life-sustaining treatment, 564–565
petechial rash, chronic myeloid leukaemia, 95
Peutz–Jeghers syndrome, 619
phaeochromocytoma, 184
Phalen's sign, 454
'phantom limb syndrome', 430
photocoagulation scars, 676
photosensitive dermatitis, **606**
phototherapy, psoriasis, **603**
physical activity, CVD prevention, 147
physiological splitting, accentuated, **352**
pigmented lesions, 628–629
'pill rolling', 438
pimecrolimus, 605
pinprick tests, 397
pituitary adenoma, 701
pityriasis rosea, 608
pityriasis versicolor, 608
plaque, **600**
plaque psoriasis, chronic, 600, 602
plasma cell(s), 96
plasma cell disorders, **281**
plasmacytoma, 283
plasma viscosity (PV), 320, **321**
platelets
　aspirin, 270
　thrombus formation, 269, 270
pleural disease, benign, **45**
pleural effusion, **54**, 54–56
　fluid analyses, **55**
　Light's criteria, **55**
　malignancy, 55, 56
　patterns, 15
　sampling, 55
pleural rub, **13**, 56–57
pleurodesis, pneumothorax, 58–59

pneumoconiosis, 43–44
　coal worker's, 44, **44**
　silicosis, 44, 122
Pneumocystis jirovecii, 284, **284**
pneumonectomy, 30
pneumonia, 21–24
　atypical, 23, **24**
　clinical instability, **23**
　collapse, 30
　community acquired, 23
　complications, **22**
　CURB score, 22
　decompensation, 22
　differential diagnoses, 23
　eosinophilic, **41**
　interstitial see interstitial pneumonia
　symptoms, **22**
　see also individual types
pneumothorax, **15**, **57**, 57–59
　chronic obstructive pulmonary disease vs., 57
　management
　　primary spontaneous, 58
　　secondary spontaneous, 58
　pleurodesis, 58–59
　predisposition, 58
　size, **57**
poisoning, 256–259
　ethylene glycol, 258
　history taking, 256–257
　　approach, 257
　lead, 612
　methanol, 258
polyarteritis nodosa, 247
polycystic kidney disease (PKD), 106–107
　extra-renal manifestations, **106**
　genetics, 106
　renal manifestations, 106
polycystic ovarian syndrome (PCOS), 711–712
　treatment, 712
polycythaemia, 39
polycythaemia vera, 98–101, 99
　complications, 99
　decompensation, 99
　diagnostic criteria, **100**
　management, 99
　splenomegaly, 98
　symptoms, **98**
　transformation, 99–100
polygenic hypercholesterolaemia, **177**
polymyalgia, myositis vs., 479
polymyalgia rheumatica (PMR), 327, **327**
　corticosteroid-reducing regimen, **327**
　history taking, 325–326
　　approach, 325–326
polymyositis
　autoantibody tests, **637**
　malignancy screening, 477
polyneuropathy
　causes, **466–467**
　classification, 465, 467
　　acute, 465
　　chronic, 465

chronic axonal, 465, 467
    chronic demyelinating, 465
clinical types, 465
symptom progression, **465**
Polypill, 150
polyps, malignant transformation, 142
polyuria, 256
pompholyx, **607**
poor performance, fitness to practise,
    578–580
porphyria(s), 610, **613**
    acquired, 610
    acute, 610
    cutaneous, 610
    diagnosis, 611
    malignant potential, 612
    neuropsychiatric, 610
    treatment, 612
porphyria cutanea tarda (PCT), 611, **613**
portal hypertension, 69
portal vein, 69
portosystemic shunting, 69
Poser diagnostic criteria, multiple
    sclerosis, 200
positive predictive value (PPV), 491
positron-emission tomography (PET),
    lung cancer, 26
posterior circulation stroke (POCS), 422,
    424, *424*
    embolic, **437**
    presentation patterns, **437**
posterior circulation stroke (POCS)
    syndromes, **435**, 435–438
posterior fossae, blood supply, *423*
posterior vitreous detachment, 685
    symptoms, 686
post mortem requests, 569–571
post-test probability, 491
post-transplantation lymphoproliferative
    disease (PTLD), 110
postural disequilibrium, **292**
postural equilibrium, **292**
posture
    Parkinson's disease, *438*
    rehabilitation, 295
potassium
    regulation, 232–233
        aldosterone, **232**
        depletion, **232**
        redistribution, **232**
    serum concentration, 233
power
    examination, 392–397
        limbs, 394–395
    grading, 395, **395**
power of attorney (PA), 535–536
Practical Assessment of Clinical
    Examination Skills (PACES) *see*
    PACES
prandial glucose regulators, **224**
predictive values, 491, **491**
prednisolone
    gout, 664
    polymyalgia rheumatica, 327

pregnancy
    anti-epileptic drugs, **304**
    asthma, 127
    Graves' disease, 697
    HIV testing, 592
    hormone changes, 707
    Marfan's syndrome, 670
    pulmonary embolism, 53–54
    systemic lupus erythematosus, 658–659
    venous thromboembolism, 275
premalignant sun-related lesions, 629
preproliferative diabetic retinopathy
    (PPDR), **675**
pre-renal acute renal failure, 230, **231**
prescribed disability, 596
pressure ulcers, 634, **634**
pre-test probability, 491
pretibial myxedema, 622, *624*, 694
    histology, 623
    prevalence, 499
Prevost's sign, 422
primary biliary cirrhosis (PBC), 81–82
    diagnosis, **82**
    symptoms, 81
    treatment, 81
primary hyperparathyroidism (PHPT)
    hypercalcaemia, 248
        end-organ damage, 248
    surgical indications, **249**
primary open-angle glaucoma (POAG),
    689–690
primary percutaneous coronary
    intervention (PPCI), 159
primary sclerosing cholangitis (PSC), 82
primary torsion dystonia, 392
primitive reflexes, **387**
prions, 311–312
Procurator Fiscal, 571
proerythroblasts, 96
prognosis, patient explanation, 494–495,
    523
progressive multifocal
    leucoencephalopathy, 288
progressive supranuclear palsy (PSP), 440
pro-inflammatory response, sepsis, 331
proliferative diabetic retinopathy (PDR),
    675
proprioception, 397, *397*
prosopagnosia, 432–433
prospective disability, 596
prospective (cohort) study design, 586
prostate cancer, 316
prostate-specific antigen (PSA) testing,
    316
prosthetic valve endocarditis, 371
prosthetic valves, 367–368
    aortic, 367
    bio-prosthetic, 367
    mechanical, 367
    mitral, 367
    sounds, 351
protease inhibitors, HIV, 289
protein C deficiency, **277**
protein S deficiency, **277**

proteinuria
    diabetic nephropathy, **226**
    types, 241
prothrombinase complex, 271
prothrombotic tendency,
    hyperhomocysteinaemia, 277–278
proton pump inhibitors (PPIs),
    Helicobacter pylori, 131–132
proximal tubule, 258
    disorders, 258
pseudobulbar palsy, *431*, 431–432, **432**
    bulbar palsy *vs.*, **390**
'pseudogout', 664
pseudohyperaldosteronism (Liddle's
    syndrome), **184**
pseudohypoaldosteronism, **184**
pseudohyponatraemia, 254
pseudohypoparathyroidism, 251, 713
pseudopapilloedema, 680
pseudopseudohypoparathyroidism, 251, 713
pseudoseizure, 303
psoriasis, 600–604
    chronic plaque, 600, 602
    distribution, *601*, 654
    facial, **602**
    immunopathology, 603
    nail lesions, **602**, 620, 621
    treatments, **603**
        immunomodulatory therapies, 603,
        604, *604*
    variants, 602, **602**
psoriatic arthritis, 653–654
    rheumatoid arthritis *vs.*, 646
psoriatic arthropathy, **603**, *654*
psychogenic polydipsia, **255**
ptosis, 384, 412–413, **413**, *413*
pulmonary artery hypertension (PAH), 48
    scleroderma, 661
pulmonary artery pressure (PAP), 47–48
pulmonary embolism (PE), 49–54
    acute, **50**
    clinical probability, **52**
    hypoxia, 51
    investigations, 51–52
    pregnancy, 53–54
    risk factors, **50**
        'economy class syndrome', 50–51
    syncope, 53
pulmonary function testing, dynamic
    volumes, 122–123
pulmonary hypertension, 47–49, 356–357
    chronic obstructive pulmonary disease,
    17
    classification, **48**
    decompensation, 47
    investigation, 48
    treatment, 49
pulmonary infiltration, **47**
pulmonary regurgitation, *364*
pulmonary rehabilitation, COPD, **18**
pulmonary sarcoidosis, 44–47
    differential diagnoses, 46
    extrapulmonary features, **46**
    management, **47**

pathogenesis, 46
skin manifestations, 46
treatment, 47
pulsus alternans, **349**
pulsus paradoxus, **349**
pupil(s)
brainstem function assessment, 566
large, 413–414
drug-induced, 414
myasthenia gravis, 413
optic nerve, 383
small, 414–415
purpura, 267–271
history taking, 267–268
approach, 268
platelet problems *vs.* coagulopathy, **268**
vascular disorders, **269**
pustular psoriasis, **602**
pustule, **600**
pyoderma gangrenosum, 621, *622*, **624**
treatment, 624
ulcerative colitis, *91*
variants, 621
pyogenic abscess, 85
pyramidal tracts *see* corticospinal tracts
pyrexia, 327–333
history taking, 327–330
approach, 328–330
pyrexia of unknown origin (PUO), 328,
329–330

quadrantanopia, 407
qualitative research, 585
quantitative research, 585
questioning (of patients)
facilitating skills, 117–118
history taking, 115, 116
closed questions, 117
open questions, 116, 117

radial nerve, **459**
lesions, 457–459, *458*
radiculopathies, 394, **394**
radioactive iodine, thyrotoxicosis, 697
radiotherapy, lung cancer, 27
Rai classification, chronic lymphocytic
leukaemia, **102**
raised inflammatory markers *see*
inflammatory markers, raised
raised intracranial pressure, **189**
raloxifene, 208–209
ramipril, 236–237
Ramsay–Hunt syndrome, 419
randomised controlled trials (RCT)
bias, 586–587
generalisation, 588
intention to treat analysis, 588
null hypothesis, 587
'*P*' value, 587
recruitment, 584–588
sample size, 587
study design, 585–586
rapport, 717
rate, 499

rate ratio, 499
Raynaud's phenomenon, **618**, 660
reactive arthritis, 654
receptor activator of nuclear factor κB
(RANK), 206–207
receptor activator of nuclear factor κB
ligand (RANKL), 206–207
Recognition–Interpretation–Discussion
(RID) sequence, 717, 718
rectus muscles, 408–409, *409*
red blood cell abnormalities, 265–266
red eye, 691–692
red reflex, 673
refeeding syndrome, 558
reflexes
examination, 396–397
grading, **397**
inverted, **452**
lower limbs, *404*
primitive, **387**
upper limbs, *402*
see also specific reflexes
refractory hypertension, 187
rehabilitation, 295
stroke, 430
Reiter's syndrome, 654
relative risk (RR), 499–500
relative risk reduction (RRR), 500
relatives
angry, 506–508
breaking bad news, 522–523
confidentiality, 529–530
resuscitation-status, **545**
upset/distressed, 508–509
relevant disability, 596
renal artery stenosis (RAS), 165, 237, *237*
renal cell carcinoma, 332
symptoms, 332
treatment, 332–333
renal cysts, 106
renal disease, genetic, 107
renal failure, amyloidosis, 283
renal osteodystrophy, 238
mixed, 238
osteomalacia, 238
renal replacement therapy, 233–239
renal transplant, 107–110, *108*, 290
anti-rejection therapy, 109, **109**
complications, **109**
immunosuppression-related, *108*
recurrent diseases, **110**
renal tubules, 232
renal tubular acidosis (RTA), 259
type 1 (distal), 259
type 2 (proximal), 259
type 4 (associated aldosterone
deficiency), 259
renin, 184
renin–angiotensin–aldosterone system
(RAAS)
abnormalities, **184**
hypertension, 184
research, types, 585
residual volume, 122

respect, **487**
respiration, heart murmurs, 354
respiratory acidosis, primary, 257, 258
respiratory alkalosis, 257
respiratory-bronchiolitis-associated
interstitial lung disease (RBAILD),
40
respiratory failure
acute, management, 19
definition, 125
respiratory pattern, brainstem function
assessment, 566–567
respiratory system, 10–61
auscultation, 11–12
breath sounds, **13–14**
vocal resonance, 12
focal abnormalities, *15*
history taking, 121–128
HIV-associated disease, 284
inspection, 10
integration, *15*
occult malignancy, 51
palpation, 10–11
chest, 10–11
neck, 10
paraneoplastic syndromes, **25**
percussion, 11, *12*
pre-auscultation sounds, **10**
see also specific conditions
response efficacy, treatment, 499
restless leg syndrome (RLS), 204
restrictive lung disease (RLD), **123**
resuscitation-status discussions
with patients, 543–546
with relatives, 547–548
reticular skin lesions, **600**
reticulocytes, 96
reticulocytosis, 263
retina, 673, **675**
retinal detachment, *685*, 685–686
risk factors, **686**
symptoms, 686
retinal tear, 686
retinitis pigmentosa, *682*, 682–683
retinopathy
diabetic *see* diabetic retinopathy (DR)
hypertensive, *678*, 678–679
retrospective (case–control) study, 586
reverse cholesterol transport impairment,
180
reversed splitting, **352**
reverse transcriptase inhibitors (RTIs),
HIV, 289
rheumatic fever, **357**
rheumatic heart disease, 355
rheumatic valves, infective endocarditis,
371
rheumatoid arthritis, 643–651
anaemia, 650
biological agents, **651**
cause, 648
diagnostic criteria, **648**
differential diagnosis, 646
extra-articular features, **649**

finger deformities, *646, 647*
joints affected, 648
onset patterns, 648
prognosis, **647**
radiological features, 648
skin signs, **618**
spondyloarthropathies *vs.*, **653**
swelling, 645
treatment, 651
rheumatoid factor (RF), 648–650
rheumatoid hands, *639*, 643, 645–651
rheumatoid lung, 42, **649**
rheumatoid nodules, *648*, **649**
rheumatological symptoms, **637**
right coronary artery (RCA) occlusion, 161
right ventricular failure (RVF), 162
right ventricular heave, 348, *350*
right ventricular infarction (RVI), 159–160
right ventricular parasternal lift, 348, *350*
rigidity, Parkinson's disease, 438
riluzole, 450–451
Rinne's test, hearing, 385, *386*
risk, 499
risk communication, 497–500, **498**
risk management teams, 574
risk ratio, 499
rituximab, **651**, 657–658
Rockall score, upper gastrointestinal
   bleeding, 133, **134**
rosacea, *614*, 614–615
   cause, 616
   treatment, 616
rosuvastatin, 148
rotator cuff disease, 640
Roth's spots, **346**
rubral tremor, **203**
running commentary, 717

sacroiliitis, **655**
salbutamol, 233
sarcoidosis *see* pulmonary sarcoidosis
scars/scarring
   abdominal system, *63*
   photocoagulation, *676*
   thoracotomy, *31*
scheme-inductive reasoning, 114
Schiavo, Terri, 564–565
schistocytosis, 264
Schober's test, modified, *652*
sciatic nerve, 460
   stretch test, 642
scleritis, 692
scleroderma, *39*, 617–618, *618, 659*, 659–662
   antibodies associated, 661
   classification, **660**
   complications, 660, 661
      skin, 661
   face, 617, 659
   hands, 617, 659
   lung disease, 617
   management, **662**
   pathogenesis, **660**
scleroderma renal crisis (SRC), 662
scotoma, central, **675**

screening
   colorectal cancer, 143
   criteria, 491
   diabetic retinopathy, 677–678
   thrombophilia, 278–279
seborrhoeic dermatitis, **606**, *607*
second (S2) heart sound, 351
   abnormalities, **351**
   splitting, **352**
sedation, emergency, **308**
seizures, 300–304, **302**
   classification, **302**
   definition, 301
   driving and, 596
   generalised, **303**
   history taking, 300–301
      approach, 301
   monotherapy resistant, 304
   partial, **303**
   pseudoseizure *vs.*, 303
   syncope *vs.*, **296**
   treatment, 304
self-discharge, 509–511
self efficacy, treatment, **499**
sensation examination, 397
sensitivity, communication, 491, **491**
sensorineural hearing loss (SNHL), 417–418
   audiogram features, 418
   vertigo, 418
sensory ataxic gait, **405**
sensory inattention, 434
sensory loss patterns, **398**
sensory neglect, 434
sensory tracts, 393
sepsis
   bacterial role, 330
   cause, 330
   history taking, 327–333
   markers, 330–331
   pro-inflammatory response, 331
septic arthritis, 212
septic shock, 330
sequestration crises, **265**
severe combined immunodeficiency
   (SCID), X-linked, 319
Shamroth's sign, **620**
Sheehan's syndrome, 701
Shiga-toxin-producing *E. coli* (STEC),
   diarrhoea, 141
shin lesions, 621–624
short stature, **713**
shoulder
   anatomy, *639*
   examination, *399*, 638–640, **641**
   glenohumeral disease, **642**
   subacromial disease, 640
shunting assessment, 312
sick euthyroid syndrome, 696
sickle cell disease (SCD), 264–267
   clinical consequences, **265**
   history taking, 264–265
      approach, 265
   sickling spectrum, **266**
   underlying abnormality, 266

sideroblastic anaemia, 261, **262**
silicon dioxide, **44**
silicosis, 44, **44**, 122
single focus hypothesis, atrial fibrillation,
   171–172
single photon emission tomography
   (SPECT), Parkinson's disease, 441
sinus rhythm maintenance, atrial
   fibrillation, 173
Sjögren's syndrome, 650
   autoantibody tests, **637**
   clinical manifestations, **650**
skin, 600–634
   autoimmune disease, 617–618, **618**
   examination, 600
   gastrointestinal pathology signs, **62**
   infection, 632–634
   inspection, 62
   lesions
      distribution, 600
      neoplastic, 628–630
      terminology, **600**
      see also specific conditions
   rheumatoid arthritis, 645
skin vasculitis, 630–631, **631**, *631*
skull, Paget's disease, *666*
small-cell lung cancer (SCLC), 26–27
   staging, **28**
   treatment, **28**
small dense low-density lipoprotein, **177**
small intestine
   arterial supply, 138
   nutrient absorption, 142
SMN gene, 444–445
smoking cessation, 504
Snellen wall chart, 382
sodium
   daily requirements, 254
   regulation, 253
somatic mutation, 95–96
spastic gait, **405**
spasticity, 395
spastic paraparesis, 443–446, *444*
   hereditary, 445
speech, 385–386
   examination, 389–390
speech therapy, dysphagia, 136
spider naevi
   autoimmune hepatitis, *79*
   chronic liver disease, *68*
spinal arteriovenous malformations
   (AVMs), 444
spinal cord, 392–394
   blood supply, 444
   compressive disorders, 444
   infarction, 444
   lesions, 394, **394**
   multiple sclerosis, **199**
   non-compressive disorders, **445**
   subacute combined degeneration,
      447–449
   syndrome investigations, 445
spinal examination, 642–643, **646**
spinal muscular atrophy, 444–445, 451

spinocerebellar tracts, 449
spinothalamic tracts, 382–383
  absent ankle jerks, **448**
  extensor plantars, **448**
spironolactone, 165
spleen
  infective disorders, 86
  infiltrative disorders, 86
  palpation, 63–64, **65**
splenomegaly, 86
  chronic myeloid leukaemia, 95
  Felty's syndrome, 87
  myelodysplasia, 98
  polycythaemia vera, 98
splinter haemorrhages, **346**
splitting, second heart sounds, **352**
spondyloarthropathies, 652–655, **653**
  back pain, **652**
  clinical investigations, 654
  musculoskeletal features, **655**
  osteoarthritis vs., **653**
  rheumatoid arthritis vs., **653**
  treatment, 655
  see also ankylosing spondylitis
squint, 409
Staphylococcus
  bacteraemia, 331
  infective endocarditis, 371
  Panton–Valentine leucocidin gene, 332
Staphylococcus aureus, 331–332
  infective endocarditis, 371
statins, **181**
  acute coronary syndrome, **161**
  atherosclerosis, 180
  cardiovascular disease prevention, 148,
    149–150
  creatine phosphokinase monitoring, 180
  heart failure, **164**
  hypertension, 187
  stroke, 180
  transaminase monitoring, 180
  transient ischaemic attack, 195
stations, 2, *2*, **4**
  clinical *see* clinical stations
  communication skills and ethics *see*
    communication skills and ethics
    station (Station 4)
  history taking *see* history-taking station
    (Station 2)
status epilepticus, 304
  see also epilepsy
ST elevation in myocardial infarction
    (STEMI), **159**
  management, 159, *160*
stem cells, haemopoietic, 96
stenosing tenosynovitis (trigger finger),
    635
steroids, 707
Still's disease, 323
stomach
  anatomy, 131
  normal secretions, 131
strabismus, 409
strength testing, falls, 294

streptococci, infective endocarditis, 371
Streptococcus pneumoniae, 21
stress tests, older patients, 497
stroke
  atrial fibrillation, 173–174, **174**, 425
  brain imaging, 427, **428**
  brainstem, 419
  care advances, 427
  carotid atherosclerosis, 425
  CHADS₂ scoring system, 174
  definition, 425
  dissection, 193
  mimics, 427
  outcome predictors, 430–431
  patent foramen ovale, 193
  prevention
    ACC/AHA/ESC guidelines, 174
    antithrombotic therapy, 173–174,
      174
    international normalised ratio,
      174–175
    secondary, 429–430
  statin therapy, 180
  thrombolysis, 428, **429**
  total anterior circulation stroke, 422
  treatment, 428–430
stroke units, 428
strontium ranelate, 209
structural cardiac cardiopulmonary disease,
    297
stunning, 153–154
subacromial disease, 640
subacute bacterial endocarditis (SBE),
    372
subacute combined degeneration of the
    cord, 447–449, **448**
subarachnoid haemorrhage (SAH), **426**
  diagnosis, 190–191
  symptoms, **189**
subdural haematoma, **426**
sudden arrhythmic death syndrome
    (SADS), 169
sudden cardiac death (SCD), 169
  family members, 169
  prevention, 378
  at-risk patients, 170
suicide attempts
  capacity, 542
  patient assessment, **541**
suing, 577
sulphonylureas, **224**
sun-related lesions, premalignant, 629
superior colliculus, 433
superior mesenteric artery (SMA), 138
superior vena cava obstruction (SVCO),
    29, 29–30
supine hypertension, orthostatic
    hypotension and, 299
supranuclear fibres, 381, 382
supraspinatus tendonitis, 640
supraventricular tachycardia (SVT)
  treatment, 168
  types, 168
  Wolff–Parkinson–White syndrome, 168

swallowing, 385–386
  assessment
    dysphagia, 135
    speech/language therapists role, 136
  brainstem function assessment, 566
  phases, 135–136
    oesophageal, 136
    oral, 135
    pharyngeal, 135–136
swan neck deformities, 645, *646*
swinging light test, **384**
synaesthesia, 434–435
syncope, 295–300, *297*
  definition, **296**
  driving, 300
  ECG abnormalities, 298
  history taking, 295–298
    approach, 296
  neurally mediated, *297*, 299, **300**
  prognosis, 299
  pulmonary embolism, 53
  seizures vs., **296**
  tilt table testing, 299–300
syndrome of inappropriate ADH excess
    (SIADH), **255**
synovial fluid, rheumatoid arthritis, 648
synovitis, *639*
syphilis, 449
syringobulbia, 446, *447*
syringomyelia, 446, *447*
systematic reviews, 586
system error, 574
systemic lupus erythematosus (SLE),
    655–659
  antiphospholipid syndrome and, 658
  autoantibody tests, **637**
  complications, 656
  contraceptive pill and, 658–659
  definition, 656
  diagnosis, **656**
    patient explanations, 488
  diagnostic criteria, **656**
  drug-induced, 656
  hormone replacement therapy,
    658–659
  pathogenesis, 656
  pregnancy, 658–659
  serological tests, 656–657
  severity, 656
  skin signs, 612–614, **618**
  system reviews, **657**
  treatment, 657–658, **658**
systemic sclerosis (SSc), 660–661
  autoantibody tests, **637**
systemic sclerosis (SSc) *sine* scleroderma,
    661
systolic heart failure, **166**
systolic murmurs, **353**

T1 root lesions, 459
tabes, **448**
tachyarrhythmia
  pacing, 369
  types, 168

tachycardia
   atrial fibrillation, 172
   mitral stenosis, 356
tacrolimus
   dermatitis, 605
   renal transplants, **109**
tardive dyskinesia, **393**
tar staining, fingers, *16*
task-specific tremor, **203**
T-cell activation, atherosclerosis, 153
T-cell activation inhibitors, psoriasis, **604**
T cell receptors, 325
telangiectasia, **600**, *619*
telomere shortening, 313
temperature sensation examination, 397
temporal artery biopsy, giant cell arteritis,
   326–327
temporal lobe, 389
temporary pacing, acute coronary
   syndrome, 161
Tensilon test, 474
tension headache, 190
teriparatide, 209
terminal distal tubule, 259
   aldosterone effects, 259
testosterone deficiency, 712–713
   osteoporosis, 210
tetraparesis, 443
thalassaemia, 264–267
   management, 267
α-thalassaemia, 266, **267**
β-thalassaemia, 266, **267**
thalassaemia trait, **262**
thalidomide, myeloma, 282
T helper cell(s), 319
   activation, 319
T helper 1 (Th1) cells, 319
   pathway, 319, *320*
   response, 319, 321
T helper 2 (Th2) cells, 319, *320*, 321
thenar wasting, carpal tunnel syndrome,
   454
thiazide diuretics, 259
   hypertension, **186**
thienopyridines, 158
third (S3) heart sound, **351**
Thomas's test, 641
thoracic outlet syndrome, 416
thoracotomy scar, *31*
threatening behaviour, **508**
'thrifty gene' hypothesis, weight gain, 144
thrills, 348–349
thrombin, 271
thrombocytopenia, 271
thromboembolic disease
   prevention, 53
   symptoms, 50
thrombolysis
   primary angioplasty *vs.*, 159
   pulmonary embolism, 53
   stroke, 428, **429**
Thrombolysis in Myocardial Infarction
   (TIMI) score, 158, **158**
thrombolytic agents, 493

thrombophilia, 277
   inherited, 51, **277**
   screening, 278–279
thrombophilic tendency, 276–279
   history taking, 276–277
      approach, 276–277
thrombosis, polycythaemia vera, 99
thrombotic thrombocytopenic purpura
   (TTP), 270
thrombus formation, 270
thumbs, Z-shaped, 646, *646*
thymus, myasthenia gravis, 473
thyroid
   examination, 693, *693*
   malignancy, **699**
thyroid lumps, **699**, 699–700
thyroid stimulating hormone (TSH)
   deficiency, **700**
   suppression, 696
thyrotoxicosis
   anticoagulants, 174
   autoimmune tests, 696
   causes, **695**
   hyperthyroidism *vs.*, 695
   nuclear medicine assessments, 696
   radioactive iodine, 697
   symptoms, **694**
thyrotoxic storms, 697
tibia, Paget's disease, *667*
tic, **393**
tilting disc valves, 367
tilt table testing (TTT), syncope,
   299–300
Tinea pedis, 605
Tinel's sign, 454, *454*
tinnitus, 418
tiredness, 334–336
   cause, **335**
   history taking, 334–336
      approach, 335–336
tissue factor (TF)
   acute coronary syndromes, 153
   coagulation, 271
toe movement examination, *404*
tolerance, immunity, 324–325
tone examination, 395–396
   lower limbs, 402, *403*
   upper limbs, 397
tongue
   hypoglossal nerve, 386
   pseudobulbar palsy, 431
tonsillar herniation, **567**
torsion dystonia, primary, 392
total anterior circulation stroke (TACS),
   422, **422**, *424*
total lung capacity (TLC), 122
toxoplasmosis, cerebral, 288
trabecular bone, 206
trachea, position determination, *10*
traditional medical history model, 114
transaminases, 180
transfer coefficient (KCO), 124–125
transfer factor (TLCO), 124–125
transient global amnesia, 303

transient ischaemic attack (TIA), 192–196
   carotid stenosis, 193
   crescendo, 194
   differential diagnoses, 193
   dissection, 193
   history taking, 192–193
      approach, 192–193
   investigations, **194**
   recurrent, 193
      anticoagulation, 195
   secondary prevention, **195**
   stroke risk, 196
   symptoms, **192**
transmissible spongiform encephalopathy
   (TSE), 311–312
transoesophageal echocardiography, 172
transplantation
   bone marrow, 98, 282
   haemopoietic stem cell *see* haemopoietic
      stem cell transplantation (HSCT)
   kidney *see* renal transplant
   liver, 70, **70**
   see also organ donation
treatment
   consent, 530–533
   discussions, 492–494
   end-of-life issues *see* end-of-life issues
   goals, 545
   homeopathic, 539–540
   life-prolonging *see* life-prolonging
      treatment,
         withholding/withdrawing
   patient explanations, 492–494
      benefits, 493
      cancer, 518
      effects, 497–500
      older patients, 493
      side-effects, 493
   provision, 552
tremor, 202–204, **393**
   history taking, 202–204
      approach, 203–204
   types, **203**
   see also individual types
Trendelenberg's test, 641
triceps reflex, radial nerve lesions, 458
tricuspid regurgitation, 363–364
   differential diagnosis, 363
   severity, 364
   signs, *363*
trigeminal autonomic cephalalgias
   (TACs), 190
trigeminal nerve (V)
   examination, 384–385
   functions, 416–417
trigeminal neuralgia, 417
trigeminal neuropathies, 417
trigger finger (stenosing tenosynovitis),
   635
triptans, 190
trochlear nerve (IV)
   eye movement, 383–384
   lesions, 408
trunk inspection, 62

T scores, osteoporosis, **208**
tuberculin sensitivity, 36
tuberculosis (TB), 34–37
  atypical, HIV-associated, 286
  BCG immunisation, 36
  complications, 35
  diagnosis, 36
  differential diagnosis, 46
  extrapulmonary manifestations, **35**
    HIV-associated, 286
  HIV-associated, 286–287
  multi-drug resistant, 287
  post-primary, 36, *37*
  primary, 35–36
    outcomes, **36**
tuberose sclerosis, 627–628, **628**
tubular injury, acute renal failure, **230**
tumour necrosis factor-α (TNF-α)
    inhibitors, psoriasis, **604**
tunnel vision, 683
Turner's syndrome, 713
type 1 diabetes mellitus, 215–220
  admission indications, **215**
  autoantibodies, 217
  classification, 217
  definition, 217
  glycaemic monitoring, 217
  glycaemic targets, 217–218
  history taking, 215–216
    approach, 215–216
  hyperosmolar non-ketotic coma, 220
  insulin regimens, **218**
  nutrition principles, 219
  presentation, 215, **215**
  prevention, 151
type 2 diabetes mellitus, 220–227
  blood pressure targets, 225–226
  causes, 221–222
    beta cell failure, 222
    insulin resistance, 222
  complications, 221
  history taking, 220–221
    approach, 221
  insulin dose management, 223, **225**
  management, **222**
  pathogenesis, 223
  prevalence, 221
  prevention, 150
  symptoms, 221, **221**

UK Prospective Diabetes Study
    (UKPDS), 223
ulcerative colitis (UC), 90–92
  clinical subtypes, **91**
  colorectal cancer risks, 142
  epidemiology, 88
  extra-intestinal associations, 88, 91
  maintenance therapy, **92**
  severity, 92
  surgery, 92
  treatment, **91**
ulcer/ulceration
  definition, **600**
  duodenal, 131, **132**

gastric, **132**
leg, 624
mouth, **619**
oesophageal, 288
pressure, 634, **634**
treatment, **634**
ulnar nerve, **457**
  lesions, 455–457, *456*
    low *vs.* high, *456*
    sensory loss, *456*
    wasting, *455*
ultrasound, intestinal ischaemia, 139
underdrive pacing, tachyarrhythmia, 369
unstable angina, 154
upper gastrointestinal bleeding, **133**
  risk assessment, 133, **134**
upper gastrointestinal malignancy, **129**
upper limb examination, 397–402
  coordination, 398
  power, 398
  reflexes, *402*
  tone, 397
upper motor neuron weakness, **396**
uraemic emergency, 231, **231**
urea breath test, *Helicobacter pylori*,
    132–133
urinary stomas, 92–93
urobilinogen, 72
urodynamic studies, 316
urticaria, 605, 607
usual interstitial pneumonia (UIP), **40**
uveal tract, 692
uveitis, 691–692

vagus nerve (X) examination, 386
valid consent, 532, **532**
Valsalva release phase, heart murmurs,
    354
Valsalva strain phase, heart murmurs, **354**
valsartan, 150
valves, cardiac *see* heart valves
varices, 69
  management, 69, **70**
variegate porphyria (VC), **613**
vascular access, 239
vascular dementia (VaD), 309, **310**
  Alzheimer's dementia *vs.*, 311
vascular occlusion imaging, 427
vasculitic rash, infective endocarditis, *370*
vasculitis, **649**
  autoantibody tests, **637**
  classification, 246, **246**
  systemic, 244–248
    symptoms, 244–245
vaso-occlusive crises, **265**
vegetation, 371
venous dermatitis, **606**
venous thromboembolism (VTE)
  clinical model, 274
  D-dimer testing, 275, **275**
  occult cancer, 51
  pregnancy and, 275
  prevention, 53
  risk factors, 274

ventilation/perfusion (V/Q) scan,
    pulmonary embolism, 52
ventricular arrhythmias, 369
ventricular ectopic beats, 171
ventricular septal defect (VSD), 373–375
  treatment, 375
  types, 374
ventricular tachycardia (VT)
  clinical features, 168–169
  ECG features, 168–169
  management, 169, 170
verapamil, 168
verbal consent, 530
verbal cues, 118
vertebral artery, bilateral, *423*
vertebral artery dissection (VAD),
    436–438
  posterior circulation strokes, **437**
vertigo, **293**
  sensorineural hearing loss, 418
vesicle, **600**
vestibular neuronitis (acute labyrinthitis),
    293
vestibulo-ocular reflex (VOR) pathway,
    567
vibration, sensation examination, 397,
    397
vicarious liabilities, 577
'victim mode', 716
viral hepatitis, 75–79
  hepatitis B *see* hepatitis B virus
    infection
  hepatitis C, 78–79
viridans streptococci, infective
    endocarditis, 371
virilisation, 711
visual acuity (VA), 382, 673
visual centres, 433
visual cortex, 433
visual fields (VF), 382–383
  defects, *406*, 406–407, *407*
  testing, *383*, *406*
visual hallucinations, recurrent, **309**
visual loss, 213, 213–214
  history taking, 213–214
    approach, 213–214
vital capacity (VC), 122
vitamin B12 deficiency
  blood transfusions, 263
  causes, **263**
  complications, 262
  subacute combined degeneration of the
    cord, 449
  treatment, 263
vitamin D deficiency
  clinical manifestations, 251
  falls, 294
  hypocalcaemia, **250**
  'simple', 251
  treatment, 251–252
vitamin D supplementation
  chronic kidney disease, 238
  osteoporosis, 210
vitiligo, 617–618, **618**, *618*

vitreous haemorrhage, 685–686, **686**
vocal resonance, 12
Volkmann's ischaemic contracture, 457
von Willebrand disease (VWD), 273
vulnerable patients, 537
VVI pacing, 368

waddling, **405**
wall–occiput test, *652*
warfarin
  atrial fibrillation, 174, 195
  carotid stenosis, 195
  mechanism of action, 275
  non-ST elevation myocardial infarction
     and cerebral infarction, 195
  older people, 494
  pulmonary embolism, 53
wasting, 196–198
  hand muscles, **459**, 459–460, *460*
  HIV infection, 288
  motor neurone disease, *450*
  myotonic dystrophy, *481*
  rheumatoid arthritis, 646
  ulnar nerve lesions, *455*

water deprivation test, 256
weakness, 196–198, **197**
  myasthenia gravis, 472
  patterns, 395, **396**
Weber's syndrome, *436*
Weber's test, hearing, 385, *386*
Wegener's granulomatosis (WG), **245**, 246
weight gain
  'abdominal phenotype', 144
  prevention, 144–151
  'thrifty gene' hypothesis, 144
weight loss, **197**, **333**, 333–334
  history taking, 333–334
    approach, 333–334
Wells scoring system, deep vein
    thrombosis, **274**
Wernicke's area, 389
wheals, 605
wheeze, **13**
  breathlessness, 121
whispering pectoriloquy, 12, 20
WHO/Zubrod performance status scale,
    lung cancer, **25**

wide and fixed splitting, **352**
Wilson's disease, 84–85
  cause, 84
  extrahepatic features, **84**
  hepatic features, 84
  Kayser–Fleischer rings, 84, *84*
  treatment, 85
Wolff–Parkinson–White (WPW)
    syndrome, 168
  supraventricular tachycardia, 168
wrist drop, *458*
wrist movement examination, *400*, **638**

xanthelasmata, 631–632, *632*
xanthochromia, 191
xanthomata, 631–632
xenografts, 367
ximelagatran, 174
X-rays
  chest *see* chest X-ray
  intestinal ischaemia, 139
  osteogenesis imperfecta, 672

Zollinger–Ellison syndrome, 132